PTEXAM: The Complete Study Guide

Scott M. Giles PT, DPT, MBA

President, Scorebuilders

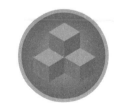

SCOREBUILDERS

Your Source for Examination Preparation

Scorebuilders

P.O. Box 7242
Scarborough, Maine 04070-7242

Toll Free: (866) PTEXAMS
Phone: (207) 885-0304
Fax: (207) 883-8377
Web Site: **www.scorebuilders.com**

Acknowledgments

The 2010 edition of **PTEXAM: The Complete Study Guide** was possible in large part due to the significant contributions of a talented group of individuals.

Dedication

This edition and every future edition of **PTEXAM: The Complete Study Guide** is dedicated to Gwenn Hoyt. Thanks for your years of support, love, and expertise. You are greatly missed for so many reasons.

Contributors

Therese Giles PT, MS

I would like to thank my wife, Traci, for her substantial contributions to all areas of the project. You are a great teammate and, of course, my best friend.

Michael Fillyaw PT, MS

I would like to thank Mike for his many contributions to this project, most notably, item writing and explanation of answers.

Paula Hould PT, MEd

I would like to thank Paula for her contributions to the explanation of answers.

Jon Stuart

I would like to thank Jon for his technical expertise and willingness to create and adapt the CD to the many nuances associated with the current National Physical Therapy Examination.

David Timm

I would like to thank David for his support and assistance with a wide variety of activities throughout the duration of the project.

Ryan Bailey DPT
Rachel Sargeant DPT
Amanda Pothier SPT
Suzanne Joyal SPT

I would like to thank Ryan, Rachel, Amanda, and Suzanne for their assistance and attention to detail throughout the editing process.

Erin Giles
Grace Farnkoff

I would like to thank Erin and Grace for sharing a portion of their summer with Scorebuilders.

Book and Cover Design

Lucian Burg, LuDesign, Portland, Maine

I would like to thank Lucian for his technical and artistic expertise throughout the creation of the new edition.

Special Thanks

To my children Meghan, Erin, and Alex. Thanks for your continued support and assistance. You are a talented group who continue to make valuable contributions to the business. Love always.

To the hundreds of students from academic programs throughout the country that served as reviewers throughout the project.

What's In The New Edition

The new edition of our best selling review book *PTEXAM: The Complete Study Guide* has been updated with a variety of enhancements that will be of great benefit to candidates preparing for the National Physical Therapy Examination. The changes in the book represent the most meaningful new edition release in our 20 year history.

New Edition Features

☆ The explanation of answers for the sample questions includes a thorough description of why each correct answer is correct and why each incorrect answer is incorrect. This new feature allows candidates to improve academic content knowledge and decision making when answering challenging multiple-choice questions.

☆ A complete index has been added for the academic review. The index allows candidates to quickly access the page numbers associated with specific subject matter. This feature significantly increases the efficiency of the academic review process and allows candidates to quickly access necessary academic content during remedial activities.

☆ The sample examinations better reflect the relative difficulty and structure of the National Physical Therapy Examination. This was accomplished by reducing the number of sample examinations from four to three and by adding new questions in many of the areas emphasized on the Federation of State Boards Physical Therapist Content Outline. The detail associated with the explanation of answers provides candidates with another valuable source of academic review material.

☆ A complete index has been added for the sample examinations. Candidates can use the index to locate specific subject matter within the sample examinations. For example, questions related to breathing exercises are located in Examination Two: Questions 146,152; Examination Three: Question 8. This feature makes it possible for candidates to quickly review questions related to specific subject matter after taking the various sample examinations.

☆ The entire layout of the book has been redesigned to make the look and feel of the resource more visually pleasing and user friendly for candidates. The addition of a second color and consistent use of formatting throughout the academic review makes it even easier for candidates to extract relevant information.

Scorebuilders strives to ensure that our review products provide candidates with the most current information available for the National Physical Therapy Examination. We look forward to assisting you with your preparation for this important examination.

Introduction

PTEXAM: The Complete Study Guide

Preparing for a comprehensive examination that potentially encompasses all elements of a physical therapy academic program can be an overwhelming task. Students are often exhausted after completing a rigorous academic program and suddenly are faced with the daunting task of taking a comprehensive examination. Anxiety, economics, and a strong desire to practice as a physical therapist only increase a candidate's sense of urgency. Often when faced with such an overwhelming task the reaction is to either procrastinate or to wander aimlessly through study sessions without direction or focus.

Our text **PTEXAM: The Complete Study Guide** provides candidates with a number of powerful study tools each designed to prepare candidates for the breadth and depth associated with the current National Physical Therapy Examination. A brief description of each unit in the study guide is listed below.

Unit One: National Physical Therapy Examination

The section provides candidates with information on the purpose, development, scoring, and administration of the National Physical Therapy Examination. Candidates are introduced to a systematic approach to answering multiple-choice questions and are exposed to recent developments in item construction.

Unit Two: Academic Review

The section provides candidates with an efficient method to review didactic information from a physical therapy curriculum. The academic review avoids attempting to cover every aspect of a physical therapist's academic training and instead focuses on the most essential information necessary to maximize examination performance. Since the examination is designed to assess entry-level practice it is likely that candidates will encounter the information presented in the academic review frequently on the actual examination. Mastery of the information can significantly increase candidates' scores on the National Physical Therapy Examination.

Unit Three: Clinical Application Templates

The section includes a description of the physical therapy management of 60 commonly encountered medical diagnoses on the National Physical Therapy Examination. By utilizing the clinical application templates candidates can expand their applied clinical knowledge while at the same time reinforce existing knowledge. Since the majority of examination questions are presented in an applied manner it is essential that candidates possess requisite knowledge related to these medical diagnoses. As candidates become increasingly familiar with the information they will be better able to make informed decisions when answering challenging multiple-choice questions. An executive summary section assists candidates to recall essential information from each of the presented clinical application templates.

Unit Four: Study Concepts

The section consists of ten Study Concepts dealing with a wide range of topics including learning style, time management, golden rules, truths and myths, assessment, automaticity, levels of knowledge and understanding, blood pressure, emergent conditions, and lines, tubes, and equipment. Inclusion of specific Study Concepts serves to remind candidates that preparing for the National Physical Therapy Examination requires more than simply reviewing academic content and answering sample examinations. Candidates who are able to effectively integrate this type of information into an existing study plan increase their probability of being successful on the National Physical Therapy Examination.

Unit Five: National Physical Therapy Examination Blueprint

The section provides a detailed analysis of each of the content outline and system specific areas of the National Physical Therapy Examination. By exploring the categories and subcategories of each of the content outline and system specific areas candidates gain a better understanding of the breadth and depth of the current examination and as a result spend less time covering topics that are not clinically relevant.

Unit Six: Computer-Based Examinations

The section consists of three, 200 question sample examinations located on a CD. The examinations were developed based on selected specifications from the current content outline and are designed to expose candidates to the nuances of computer-based testing. Candidates are able to generate a detailed performance analysis summary that identifies current strengths and weaknesses according to content outline and system specific areas. The examinations provide candidates with the opportunity to refine their test taking skills and to assess their current preparedness for the examination. An answer key includes an explanation specifying why the correct answer is correct and an explanation specifying why each incorrect answer is incorrect. The answer key also includes a cited resource with page number, and the assigned content outline and system specific area.

*Additional resources to assist candidates with their preparation for the National Physical Therapy Examination are located at the conclusion of the text.

Author's Note

Congratulations on your decision to purchase **PTEXAM: The Complete Study Guide**. Leave no stone unturned in your preparation for this important examination and strive to make your examination score reflect your academic knowledge. Candidates that have a firm grasp of didactic information combined with a meaningful study plan emphasizing applied knowledge are often richly rewarded on this challenging examination. We are confident that our text will be a valuable component of your comprehensive study program. Although undoubtedly there will be many magical moments in your life, you will never forget the moment when you become licensed as a physical therapist. Best of luck on the examination and in your future career endeavors!

Table of Contents

Unit Three: Clinical Application Templates · 247

National Physical Therapy Examination

The National Physical Therapy Examination is a 250 question (200 scored, 50 pre-test), multiple-choice examination designed to determine if candidates possess the minimal competency necessary to practice as physical therapists.

The examination is created under the auspices of the Federation of State Boards of Physical Therapy (FSBPT). According to the *National Physical Therapy Examination Candidate Handbook*, the examination program serves three important purposes:

1. Provide examination services to regulatory authorities charged with the regulation of physical therapists and physical therapist assistants.

2. Provide a common element in the evaluation of candidates so that standards will be comparable from jurisdiction to jurisdiction.

3. Protect the public interest in having only those persons who have the requisite knowledge of physical therapy be licensed to practice physical therapy.

There are two primary methods to obtain a license to practice as a physical therapist in the United States. They are termed examination and endorsement. Licensure by examination is obtained after a candidate meets or exceeds the minimum scoring requirement on the National Physical Therapy Examination and has satisfied all other state requirements. This form of obtaining licensure is the traditional method for candidates seeking initial licensure.

Licensure by endorsement makes it possible for candidates who have already been licensed in a state by virtue of an examination to potentially gain licensure in another state without retaking the examination. Examination scores can be transferred to any physical therapy state licensing agency via the Federation of State Boards of Physical Therapy Score Transfer Service. The web site address for the Federation of State Boards of Physical Therapy is available in the Appendix.

Although the National Physical Therapy Examination is 250 questions, 50 of the questions serve only as pre-test items and are not officially scored. The pre-test items allow new examination questions to be evaluated throughout the year and eliminate lengthy delays in score reporting when new examinations are introduced. Candidates are unable to differentiate between pre-test and scored items on the examination.

The 250 questions are administered to candidates in five sections consisting of 50 questions each. Each section contains scored items and pre-test items, although the number of pre-test and scored items in each section may vary slightly. Candidates have five hours to complete the five sections at their own pace. Since the sections are not timed individually it is important for candidates to effectively manage their allotted time as they progress through each of the five sections. Candidates have the opportunity to take one scheduled break at the conclusion of section two, immediately prior to beginning section three. Additional unscheduled breaks can be taken at the conclusion of a given section, however, the elapsed time will not stop. If a candidate does not want to take the break or prefers a shorter break they can end the break by following the directions displayed on the computer screen. Candidates can leave the examination only when either a scheduled or unscheduled break message is displayed on the computer. Leaving the testing room while not on a designated break will result in an examination irregularity being reported to the FSBPT.

Candidates are unable to return to previously completed sections once a new section is initiated. The academic content is randomized within each section and scoring is based only on the number of questions a candidate answers correctly out of the 200 scored items. As a result, each of the examinations in *PTEXAM: The Complete Study Guide* consists of only 200 questions (four sections, each consisting of 50 questions). Candidates will have four hours to complete each of the 200 question sample examinations.

The FSBPT publishes a content outline which describes the specific categories and subcategories of the examination. The categories and subcategories are based on the tasks and roles that comprise the practice of physical therapy. Once established, the content outline remains active for a period of approximately five years. The most recent version was implemented in March of 2008. The six main categories of the examination are listed here, although the entire content outline will be discussed in detail in Unit Five.

Examination Content Outline

Clinical Application of Foundational Sciences

Examination

Foundations for Evaluation, Differential Diagnosis, & Prognosis

Interventions

Equipment & Devices; Therapeutic Modalities

Safety & Professional Roles; Teaching/Learning; Research

According to the FSBPT, the involvement of a large representative group of practicing physical therapists and other professionals at each stage of examination development ensures that the examinations are relevant to the practice of physical therapy. Individual physical therapists are responsible for writing examination questions. The physical therapists involved are required to attend item-writing workshops that are taught by experienced testing professionals. Questions, once completed, are analyzed independently to make sure they are reflective of the current examination content outline. Examination questions tend to focus on decision making and not purely rote memorization of fact. Successful candidates on the examination must demonstrate the ability to apply knowledge in a safe and effective manner.

Examination Scoring

The questions on the examination are multiple-choice with four possible answers to each question. Each option is listed as 1, 2, 3, 4. Options such as "none of the above", "all of the above", and "1 and 2 only" are not included on the examination. Candidates are asked to identify the best answer to each of the questions. Each question has only one best answer while the other possible answers serve as distracters. A candidate's score is determined based on the number of scored questions answered correctly. Since there is no penalty for questions answered incorrectly it is imperative that candidates answer all of the available questions. A candidate's cumulative score is termed the total raw score. The maximum total raw score for the National Physical Therapy Examination is 200.

Criterion-referenced scoring is used to determine passing scores on the National Physical Therapy Examination. Passing scores are based on the judgment of selected experts on the minimum number of questions that should be answered correctly by a minimally qualified candidate. Criterion-referenced passing scores are determined independently of candidate performance and are designed to reflect the difficulty level of each examination. For example, if a given examination was judged to be particularly difficult, the criterion-referenced passing score would be lower than the criterion-referenced passing score for another examination that was judged to be less difficult. All state licensing agencies have adopted the FSBPT criterion-referenced passing score and therefore do not individually determine passing scores at the state level. As a result, a passing score for a given examination will always be the same in all jurisdictions.

Since the minimum passing score varies based on the difficulty level of each examination it is impossible to determine an automatic passing score. Criterion-referenced passing scores often range from 135 - 145. If the criterion-referenced passing score was established as 142 for a given examination, a total raw score of greater than or equal to 142 would be considered a passing score, while a total raw score of less than 142 would be considered a failing score. Within a given examination cycle, criterion-referenced passing scores usually fluctuate in a relatively small range, perhaps by as few as five questions.

An individual examination score is often reported to candidates in the form of a scaled score. Scaled scores range from 200 - 800 with the minimum passing score always being equal to a scaled score of 600. Scaled scores are necessary as a method of equating examinations with different criterion-referenced passing scores. A few state licensing agencies use a slightly different scaled score system where the minimum passing score is equivalent to a scaled score of 75.

Applying for the Examination

Candidates planning to take the examination should request an application from the state licensing agency in the jurisdiction where they intend to practice as a physical therapist. Candidates are not permitted to apply for the examination in more than one jurisdiction at a time. The address of each agency, phone number, and web site are provided in the Appendix. All state licensing agencies offer online registration for the examination through the FSBPT.

Each state licensing agency can establish its own criteria to be eligible to sit for the National Physical Therapy Examination. A variety of items may be required as part of the application process. These items often include a photograph, a notarized birth certificate, an official transcript from an accredited school, professional reference letters, and a check or money order for the required application, examination, and licensing fees. Candidates should recognize that even a small departure from the established eligibility criteria can lead to a significant delay in processing a candidate's application. To avoid such delays, it is prudent to read the application carefully and to inquire as to the status of the application approximately two weeks after the completed application has been submitted.

Foreign trained therapists are often subjected to a myriad of requirements before they are eligible to become licensed in the United States. Since the requirements vary significantly by state, it is recommended that candidates contact the state licensing agency within the state they intend to practice. The state licensing agency can provide detailed information on their individual requirements.

There are two general requirements for foreign trained therapists that seem to be consistent in all states:

- Applicants are required to submit their educational credentials for evaluation of their equivalence to the United States trained applicant.
- Applicants must meet or exceed the minimum scoring requirement on the National Physical Therapy Examination.

Other state requirements can include, but are not limited to, the following:

- Demonstrate proficiency in written and spoken English
- Submit letters of reference
- Obtain a valid visa and resident alien card
- Complete an internship or period of supervised practice
- Appear for an interview
- Attain the United States equivalent of a grade of "C" or higher in all professional coursework

Some states offer candidates with verifiable employment the opportunity to practice prior to being licensed by issuing a temporary license. Typically, candidates are required to have a completed application on file and have met all other qualifications for licensure before being considered for the temporary license. In most states temporary licenses are revoked if a candidate receives notification they were unsuccessful on the National Physical Therapy Examination.

In addition to the National Physical Therapy Examination, a significant number of states require candidates to successfully complete a jurisprudence examination. This type of examination is based on the state rules and regulations governing physical therapy practice. The examination can include multiple-choice items, short-answer questions or fill in the blanks. States can administer the examination using computer-based testing or even as a take-home examination.

After the necessary application forms have been completed, the information is returned along with any necessary fees to the state licensing agency or an identified intermediary. The FSBPT then issues candidates an "authorization to test" letter that includes instructions on how to schedule an appointment to take the examination. Candidates must sit for the examination within 60 days of the date on their letter. It is important to schedule an appointment relatively early in the 60 day window in order to ensure availability at a local Prometric Testing Center. Once an examination appointment is scheduled candidates retain the right to reschedule or cancel the appointment as long as it is done at least three days in advance of the scheduled testing date. Rescheduling between 3-29 days prior to the scheduled appointment will result in a $25 fee paid to Prometric (there is no charge to reschedule 30 days or more prior to the exam date). Failure to take the examination within the designated 60 day period will require a candidate to go through a modified application process.

Candidates should schedule their examination at a time consistent with their optimal level of functioning. For example, if a candidate tends to be a "morning person" it would be prudent to schedule the examination early in the morning. Candidates with significant anxiety may also want an early appointment in order to avoid worrying about the examination throughout the day. If candidates are not familiar with the exact location of the examination site, it may be desirable to travel to the site before the actual examination date. The trip will provide candidates with an accurate idea of the time necessary to travel to the site and avoid the possibility of getting lost and subsequently being late for the examination.

Examination Administration

The examination is offered on computer at over 300 Prometric Testing Centers within the United States. A list of participating Prometric Testing Centers by state is located in the Appendix. Testing is typically offered Monday through Saturday from 9:00 AM - 6:00 PM. Within each Prometric Testing Center candidates can concentrate on the examination without environmental distracters. Private, modular booths provide adequate work space with proper lighting and ventilation. All Prometric Testing Centers are fully accessible and in compliance with the Americans with Disabilities Act. Candidates requesting accommodation for a documented disability must do so through the state licensing agency. Candidates are not limited to the testing centers within the state they are applying for licensure. For example, a candidate that has recently graduated from a physical therapy program in Maine could apply for licensure in California and take the required examination while still residing in Maine.

Candidates must arrive 30 minutes prior to their scheduled appointment with two forms of acceptable identification which include a government issued photo ID and another piece of identification preprinted with a name and a signature. The first and last names on both forms of ID must match the name on the Authorization to Test letter issued by the FSBPT. Candidates are photographed and a digital image of their fingerprint is taken prior to beginning the examination. Candidates cannot bring any electronic devices (e.g., watches, cell phones) or food and drink into the testing area. A locker will be provided to store personal items. Candidates can request headphones if they want to minimize background noise.

It is important to note that computer skills are not necessary with computer-based testing. Prior to beginning the examination, candidates utilize a tutorial that explains topics such as selecting answers and navigating within the examination. Time spent on the computer tutorial does not count toward the allotted time for the actual examination. The tutorial typically takes candidates less than ten minutes and if necessary candidates can go through the tutorial a second time.

Candidates have the option of entering their answers using a computer keyboard or mouse. Candidates can go back to previously answered or unanswered questions and make any desired changes within a given section of 50 questions. Once a candidate submits a given section they are unable to return to the questions within the section. Paper and pencil are not permitted in the Prometric Testing Centers, however, candidates are given an erasable note board or an electronic writing board to utilize during the examination.

The FSBPT is responsible for scoring the examination and reporting results to the individual state licensing agencies. The state licensing agencies then notify candidates as to their performance on the examination. Formal notification typically occurs through the mail, however, many state licensing agencies have web sites that allow candidates to determine their licensing status online. Some states permit candidates to access their examination status online within two days through the FSBPT. In most instances, candidates' scores are available within 2-10 business days.

If a candidate successfully completes the examination, in most cases they have fulfilled the final requirement for licensure. Conversely, if a candidate is unsuccessful on the examination, they are required to reapply to the state licensing agency. With computer-based testing there is no mandatory waiting period before retaking the examination, however, some states limit the number of times a candidate can take the examination as well as mandate remedial coursework. In all states, candidates are prohibited from taking the examination more than three times in a 12 month period.

Candidates that were unsuccessful on the National Physical Therapy Examination can receive role feedback from the FSBPT. The role feedback report compares individual examination performance using the content outline and system specific categories with the performance of other candidates exposed to the same examination. Additional information on role feedback is available through the FSBPT.

Test Taking Skills

Test taking skills are specific skills that allow individuals to utilize the characteristics and format of a selected examination in order to maximize their performance. These skills can be valuable when taking an examination such as the National Physical Therapy Examination. Despite the importance of this topic, very little, if any, academic time is set aside to address test taking skills. The good news is that test taking skills can be learned and that through dedication, desire, and determination, these skills can serve to improve examination performance.

The National Physical Therapy Examination consists of multiple-choice questions with four potentially correct answers to each question. Candidates are instructed to select the "best answer" to complete each question. Before exploring selected test taking strategies, we need to identify the various components of a multiple-choice question. Multiple-choice questions can be dissected into specific identifiable components:

Item   An item refers to an individual multiple-choice question and the corresponding potential answers. The National Physical Therapy Examination contains 200 scored items and 50 pre-test items. Each item consists of a stem and four options. Items may vary in content and length, but should utilize a consistent format.

Stem   The stem refers to the statement that asks the question. Typically, the stem conveys to the reader the necessary information needed to respond correctly to the question. In addition to the necessary information, extraneous information may be included in the stem. This information, when not recognized by the candidate as unnecessary, often can serve as a significant distracter.

The stem commonly takes on the form of a complete sentence or an incomplete sentence. The stem can be expressed in a positive or negative form. A positive form requires a candidate to identify correct information, while a negative form requires a candidate to identify incorrect information. It is important to scrutinize each stem, since a single key word such as "NOT," "EXCEPT" or "LEAST" can turn a positive stem into a negative stem. Failure to identify this can lead to the identification of an incorrect answer.

Options   The options refer to the potential answers to the question asked. One option in each item will be the "best answer," while the others are considered distracters. Options can take on a variety of forms, including a single word, a group of words, an incomplete sentence, a complete sentence or a group of sentences. The method for analyzing each option does not change, regardless of form.

Approach for Answering Multiple-Choice Questions

On the National Physical Therapy Examination there are 250 items (200 scored, 50 pre-test) that candidates must answer within a five hour time period. Due to the length of the examination and the time constraints associated with it, candidates need to approach the examination in a systematic and organized fashion. Loss of control during the examination will yield poor results that are not reflective of a candidate's actual knowledge. To assist candidates to minimize the impact of this potential pitfall, we will introduce a systematic approach to utilize when answering sample examination items.

The following six-step approach is recommended as a method for answering examination items:

1. Read the stem carefully to become familiar with the item and to determine the command words that indicate the desired action

2. Read the stem again and identify relevant words or groups of words based on the identified command words

3. Attempt to generate an answer to the stem

4. Examine each option completely before moving to the next option

5. Attempt to identify the best option

6. Utilize deductive reasoning strategies

The six-step approach begins with a candidate reading the stem. Candidates should read the stem initially to determine the command words and the associated desired action. Once this has been determined candidates can reread the stem and attempt to extract the necessary components including relevant words or groups of words.

Perhaps the most important step in the six-step approach is to have candidates attempt to generate an answer to each question based on the identified command words. This is the only opportunity a candidate will have to objectively evaluate the question prior to exposing each of the options. Once a candidate exposes the options they are no longer able to examine the question in a fully objective manner and instead become more likely to have their interpretation of the question influenced by a presented option. If for some reason a candidate is unable to generate a specific answer, they should attempt to think about the general topic and recall related information. Once a possible answer is generated, candidates should then begin to examine each option one at a time. It is important to read the entire option, since one word can often make a potentially correct answer incorrect. If the generated answer is consistent with one of the available options, the candidate should give the option strong consideration, however, since more than one option can be correct it is imperative to analyze each presented option.

If candidates finish analyzing an item and are still unable to select one of the available options they should consider using a deductive reasoning strategy. Deductive reasoning strategies allow candidates to improve examination scores without direct knowledge of subject matter. This type of strategy should be applied only when candidates are unable to identify the correct response using academic knowledge. Deductive reasoning strategies often allow candidates to eliminate one or more of the potential answers. Elimination of any option significantly increases the probability of identifying the correct answer. On the National Physical Therapy Examination, eliminating one option increases the chance of selecting a correct answer from 25% to 33%. Eliminating two options increases the chance of selecting a correct answer to 50%. On the surface this may not seem terribly significant, however, on an examination such as the National Physical Therapy Examination this can often be the difference between a passing and a failing score. Selected deductive reasoning strategies that can be used effectively on the National Physical Therapy Examination are presented.

Absurd options

Many times a multiple-choice item will include an option that is not consistent with what the stem is asking or with the other options. In many cases, this option can be eliminated. Rapid elimination of specific options will allow candidates to spend additional time analyzing other more viable options.

Similar options

When two or more options have a similar meaning or express the same fact, they often imply each other's incorrectness. For this reason, candidates can often eliminate both options.

Obtainable information

There is a great deal of factual material that candidates must sift through when taking the National Physical Therapy Examination. In some instances, the material can provide candidates with valuable information that can assist them when answering other examination questions.

Degree of qualification

Particularly in the sciences, there seems to be many exceptions to general rules. Therefore, specific wording such as "always" or "never" often overqualify an option.

Activity One

In this activity, three sample questions are presented. Candidates should attempt to identify the best answer to each question by utilizing the six-step approach.

An analysis section immediately follows each of the three sample questions. The analysis section begins by showing the sample question with key terms underlined and command words in bold type. A brief narrative follows, which describes how the six-step approach can be applied to the sample question.

An answer key located at the conclusion of the exercise indicates the best answer and an explanation for each question.

Sample Question One

A physical therapist instructs a patient with a Foley catheter in ambulation activities. During ambulation the therapist should position the collection bag:

1. above the level of the patient's bladder
2. below the level of the patient's bladder
3. above the level of the patient's heart
4. below the level of the patient's heart

Analysis:

A physical therapist instructs a patient with a <u>Foley catheter in ambulation activities</u>. During ambulation the therapist should **position** <u>the collection bag</u>:

1. above the level of the patient's bladder
2. below the level of the patient's bladder
3. above the level of the patient's heart
4. below the level of the patient's heart

A candidate should attempt to generate an answer to the question after reading the stem and identifying the pertinent information and command words. The candidate should then begin to reveal each of the available options one at a time. If a generated answer is consistent with one of the available options, there is a high probability that the answer is correct.

If a candidate was not able to generate an answer, they should expose the first option and give it careful consideration before moving on to the next option. They should progress through the remaining options in a similar manner. Candidates should remember it is possible to have more than one option that satisfactorily answers the question. It is then the candidate's responsibility to select the best answer from the viable options.

Sample Question Two

A group of physical therapists attempts to determine the relationship between two variables on an examination form. Which of the following correlation coefficients would indicate the strongest relationship?

1. +.86
2. +.45
3. -.34
4. -.89

Analysis:

A group of physical therapists attempts to determine <u>the relationship between two variables</u> on an examination form. Which of the following <u>correlation coefficients</u> would indicate the **strongest relationship**?

1. +.86
2. +.45
3. -.34
4. -.89

After reading the stem and identifying the pertinent information and command words, a candidate should recognize that it is virtually impossible to generate an answer prior to viewing the available options. A candidate should, however, begin to think about correlation coefficients and determining the strength of the relationship between variables. The candidate should then expose each of the available options and attempt to identify the correct response.

Although the six-step approach does not directly supply a candidate with the correct response, by carefully reading the stem, a candidate can avoid an unnecessary mistake. In this item, the stem asks the candidate to identify the correlation coefficient that indicates the strongest relationship between the two variables. If a candidate does not read the question carefully, they may make an assumption that the stem is asking for the strongest positive relationship and subsequently answer the question incorrectly.

It is important that a candidate answer each item based only on the given information. By making even small assumptions or by not reading each item carefully, a candidate can make careless mistakes.

Sample Question Three:

A physical therapist completes an isokinetic examination on an 18-year-old male rehabilitating from a medial meniscectomy. The therapist notes that the patient generates 140 ft/lbs of force using the uninvolved quadriceps at 60 degrees per second. Assuming a normal ratio of hamstrings to quadriceps strength, which of the following would be an acceptable hamstrings value at 60 degrees per second?

1. 64 ft/lbs
2. 84 ft/lbs
3. 114 ft/lbs
4. 116 ft/lbs

Analysis:

A physical therapist completes an isokinetic examination on an 18-year-old male rehabilitating from a medial meniscectomy. The therapist notes that the patient generates 140 ft/lbs of force using the uninvolved quadriceps at 60 degrees per second. Assuming a normal ratio of hamstrings to quadriceps strength, which of the following would be **an acceptable hamstrings value at 60 degrees per second?**

3:2

1. 64 ft/lbs
2. 84 ft/lbs
3. 114 ft/lbs
4. 116 ft/lbs

For the purpose of discussion, let's assume a candidate has no idea of the normal ratio of quadriceps/hamstrings strength at 60 degrees per second. Lack of specific academic knowledge will result in a candidate not being able to identify the correct answer using the first five steps of the six-step approach. However, by utilizing deductive reasoning strategies, a candidate can significantly increase their chances of identifying the best answer without applying direct academic knowledge.

In this item, the stem asks a candidate to identify a value that would be representative of a normal quadriceps/hamstrings ratio at 60 degrees per second. As with many measurements in physical therapy, precise normal values are difficult to ascertain, and therefore often are expressed in ranges. Since options 3 and 4 are so close in value they likely imply each other's incorrectness and can therefore be eliminated. Although in this example deductive reasoning strategies were not able to identify the correct answer, they were able to eliminate two of the four possible options. By eliminating two options, a candidate now has a 50% chance of identifying the best answer, even without utilizing any direct academic or clinical knowledge.

Activity One – Answer Key

1. **Correct Answer: 2**

   The effect of gravity necessitates the collection bag being below the level of the patient's bladder. (Pierson p. 290)

2. **Correct Answer: 4**

   Correlation coefficients range from +1.00 to -1.00. Since the question does not ask for a positive or negative correlation, the strongest relationship is indicated by -.89. (Portney p. 533)

3. **Correct Answer: 2**

   A gross estimate of quadriceps:hamstrings ratio is 3:2. Option 2, 84 ft/lbs is therefore the most consistent with the expressed ratio. (Hamill p. 236)

Recent Developments in Item Construction

There have been a number of changes in item construction on the National Physical Therapy Examination within the past few years, most notably the introduction of graphically enhanced items. Although representing a relatively small percentage of the total examination, candidates need to be comfortable answering this type of item. Graphically enhanced items will be incorporated into each of the sample examinations.

Graphically Enhanced Items

Graphically enhanced items consist of figures, diagrams, pictures or other static images that are combined with traditional text in an examination item.

Activity Two

Two graphically enhanced items are presented. Candidates should attempt to identify the best answer to each question. An answer key located at the conclusion of the exercise indicates the best answer and an explanation for each question.

The following image should be used to answer question 1:

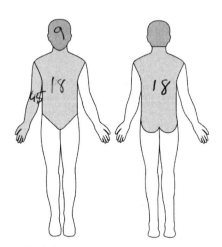

1. A 32-year-old male sustained extensive burns in a house fire. The shaded portion of the body diagrams represents the areas affected by the burns. Using the rule of nines, what percentage of the patient's body was involved?

   1. 40.5%
   2. 44.0%
   3. 49.5%
   4. 54.5%

The following image should be used to answer question 2:

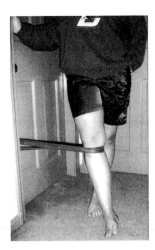

2. A physical therapist instructs a patient to complete an exercise activity using a piece of elastic band as pictured. The patient is a 14-year-old female rehabilitating from a lower extremity injury sustained in a soccer contest. The therapist's primary objective for the activity is to:

    1. strengthen the right hip abductor muscles
    2. strengthen the right hip adductor muscles
    3. stretch the right hip abductor muscles
    4. stretch the right hip adductor muscles

Activity Two – Answer Key

1. Correct Answer: 3

The percentage of the body surface burned in an adult can be calculated using the rule of nines: anterior thorax (18%) + posterior thorax (18%) + head (9%) + anterior arm (4.5%) = 49.5%. (Rothstein p. 963)

2. Correct Answer: 2

Successful completion of the activity requires the adductor muscles to exert a force greater than the tension supplied by the elastic band while moving into hip adduction. Muscles acting to adduct the hip include the adductor longus, adductor brevis, adductor magnus, and gracilis. (Magee p. 672)

Time Constraints

Like many objective examinations, candidates have a specific allotted time to complete the National Physical Therapy Examination. For physical therapists, the available time is five hours. Since the examination consists of 250 questions, candidates will have 72 seconds available to answer each question. This number, although correct when viewing the examination as a whole, can be misleading. There will be many questions that a candidate will be able to answer in much less than 72 seconds, whereas other questions will take somewhat longer. The key to success lies in progressing through the examination in a consistent and predictable manner.

Although 72 seconds per question does not seem like a great deal of time, the majority of candidates will have ample time to complete the examination. Despite this fact, it is important to pay attention to the elapsed time during the examination. It also is important to know your test taking history. Are you typically one of the first, one of the last, or somewhere in the middle of individuals completing an examination? This information is important as you plan your test taking strategy. In order to make sure your pace is appropriate during practice sessions and during the actual examination, it is important to formally check on the elapsed time, at a very minimum, when completing each section of 50 questions. This action will allow candidates to assess their progress and modify their pace, if necessary.

Preparing for the Examination

The simple thought of preparing for a comprehensive examination such as the National Physical Therapy Examination can be overwhelming. Many candidates ask themselves how it is possible to prepare adequately for an examination that encompasses up to three years of professional coursework. To further complicate matters the majority of candidates take the National Physical Therapy Examination shortly after graduation. This can be a very anxious and unsettled time. Candidates often are actively seeking employment or are attempting to adjust to a new job. As a result, it is critical that candidates outline a well conceived and deliberate study plan for the examination.

One of the largest advantages of taking an examination such as the National Physical Therapy Examination is that it does not require candidates to demonstrate mastery of new material. On the surface this may not seem like a significant advantage, but since candidates are, in effect, only reviewing or relearning previously presented information, their level of attainment should be significantly greater. Many candidates fail to utilize this advantage. Candidates who attempt to learn large quantities of new information, instead of focusing on understanding and applying basic concepts, often do themselves a tremendous disservice. It is true that there undoubtedly will be questions that contain information that was not part of a selected curriculum, but to attempt to study this new information in any significant detail would be a large mistake for most candidates. Instead, candidates should focus on reviewing or relearning basic concepts that are an integral component of all accredited physical therapy programs. It is this type of information that will make up the vast majority of the examination. Individuals who take this common sense approach optimize their chances of success.

In physical therapy academic programs, candidates constantly are learning new information on a variety of topics. Although students typically exhibit mastery of selected material during a scheduled examination, they do not always retain the information for later use. Often times, simply reviewing information is enough for candidates to relearn the material, however, in some cases, a more in-depth approach is necessary.

It is recommended that candidates pay particular attention to their practice-oriented professional coursework. Practice-oriented professional coursework includes, but is not limited to, study of the musculoskeletal, neuromuscular, cardiopulmonary, and integumentary systems. The recent content outline from the FSBPT clearly demonstrates the need for candidates to also review "other systems" (i.e., metabolic and endocrine, gastrointestinal, genitourinary, multi-system). In addition, candidates usually have coursework in patient care skills, physical agents, administration, ethics, research, and education. Each of these topics are important components of the content outline for the National Physical Therapy Examination, although the weighting of each item differs significantly. Unit Five will offer specific information on the relative weighting of each area according to systems and non-systems categories.

Special attention must be taken not to become bogged down in one specific area for any significant amount of time. General concepts that are understood should be scanned quickly, while other concepts that are more difficult for a candidate should be read carefully. Concepts that remain unclear after being reviewed should be written down for future study sessions.

Other foundational coursework encountered earlier in the professional curriculum can be consulted as needed during various study sessions. This type of coursework often includes, but is not limited to anatomy and physiology, neuroanatomy, exercise physiology, and kinesiology. It is important to limit the amount of time spent reviewing this type of foundational coursework. Candidates often can make better use of their allotted time by reviewing coursework encountered later in the curriculum that may be more practice-oriented. By reviewing practice-oriented information, candidates not only keep their studying consistent with the format of the examination, but also at the same time indirectly review much of the information presented in the foundational coursework.

Before beginning to study, develop specific goals for each study session. Ideally, these goals should be established on a weekly basis. Establishing goals will ensure that candidates cover the desired material and will serve as a mechanism to keep them on schedule with their study plan. Candidates should be realistic with the goals they establish and should not attempt to cover more material than is possible in a particular study session.

Unit 2

Academic Review

The National Physical Therapy Examination is a generalist examination that attempts to determine if candidates possess the minimal qualifications necessary to practice as an entry-level physical therapist. The examination requires candidates to exhibit familiarity with the management of commonly encountered medical diagnoses and then apply the information to challenging clinically-oriented multiple-choice questions. In order to accomplish this objective it is essential that candidates have a firm understanding of the basic didactic information included in a physical therapy academic program.

The academic review unit of **PTEXAM: The Complete Study Guide** is designed to provide candidates with an efficient method to review didactic information. The academic review avoids attempting to cover every aspect of a physical therapy curriculum and instead focuses on the most essential information necessary to maximize examination performance. The unit presents information arranged in seven distinct chapters. A detailed listing of the content of each chapter is located in the table of contents. A complete index of the various topics included in the academic review section is available at the conclusion of the review book. The majority of information presented in the academic review should be familiar to candidates, however, due to the sheer volume of information included in a physical therapy academic program there will be many didactic areas that will need to be reviewed prior to the examination.

Candidates should remember that the examination is designed to reflect current clinical practice and as a result topics that are commonly encountered in clinical practice will represent a vast majority of the actual questions on any version of the examination. Candidates should make sure that they are thoroughly familiar with basic content prior to expanding the breadth and depth of their academic review. This pragmatic approach allows candidates to significantly increase the utility of their study sessions and increase their examination score.

A prime example of this basic premise is as follows. Assume that a candidate is reviewing orthopedic special tests by utilizing the textbook *Orthopedic Assessment* by David Magee. The textbook offers a complete description of hundreds of special tests organized by area of the body. Although the textbook is a wonderful resource for students and faculty the sheer volume of special tests makes it impractical to attempt to review all of the presented information related to special tests. In contrast, the academic review section of **PTEXAM: The Complete Study Guide** offers a summary of the most commonly encountered special tests organized by body part and by specific condition that the test is designed to identify.

Candidates have numerous resources that they can rely on for additional information such as the textbook by Magee, however, as this example illustrates candidates must have a firm grasp on the basics before expanding the scope of their academic review.

Chapter 1

Musculoskeletal System

Foundational Science: Anatomy and Physiology

Joint Classification

Fibrous Joints (Synarthroses)

Fibrous joints are composed of bones that are united by fibrous tissue and are nonsynovial. Movement is minimal to none with the amount of movement permitted at the joint dependent on the length of the fibers uniting the bones.

Suture – (e.g., sagittal suture of the skull)
- Union of two bones by a ligament or membrane
- Immovable joint
- Eventual fusion is termed a synostosis

Syndesmosis – (e.g., the tibia and fibula with interosseous membrane)
- Bone connected to bone by a dense fibrous membrane or cord
- Very little motion

Gomphosis – (e.g., a tooth in its socket)
- Two bony surfaces connect as a peg in a hole
- The teeth and corresponding sockets in the mandible/maxilla are the only gomphosis joints in the body
- The periodontal membrane is the fibrous component of the joint

Cartilaginous Joints (Amphiarthroses)

Cartilaginous joints have a hyaline cartilage or fibrocartilage that connects one bone to another. These are slightly moveable joints.

Synchondrosis – (e.g., sternum and true rib articulation)
- Hyaline cartilage
- Cartilage adjoins two ossifying centers of bone
- Provides stability during growth
- May ossify to a synostosis once growth is completed
- Slight motion

Symphysis – (e.g., pubic symphysis)
- Generally located at the midline of the body
- Two bones covered with hyaline cartilage
- Two bones connected by fibrocartilage
- Slight motion

Synovial Joints (Diarthroses)

Synovial joints provide free movement between the bones they join. They have five distinguishing characteristics: joint cavity, articular cartilage, synovial membrane, synovial fluid, and fibrous capsule. The joints are the most complex and vulnerable to injury and are further classified by the type of movement and by the shape of articulating bones.

Uniaxial joint – one motion around a single axis in one plane of the body
- Hinge (ginglymus) – elbow joint
- Pivot (trochoid) – atlantoaxial joint

Biaxial joint – movement occurs in two planes and around two axes through the convex/concave surfaces
- Condyloid – metacarpophalangeal joint of a finger
- Saddle – carpometacarpal joint of the thumb

Multi-axial joint – movement occurs in three planes and around three axes
- Plane (gliding) – carpal joints
- Ball and socket – hip joint

Specific Joints

Shoulder

The shoulder complex consists of four separate articulations.

Sternoclavicular joint: Composed of the clavicle articulating with the manubrium of the sternum.

Acromioclavicular joint: Composed of the lateral end of the clavicle articulating with the acromion of the scapula.

Glenohumeral joint: Classified as a ball and socket joint, in which the round head of the humerus articulates with the shallow glenoid cavity of the scapula. The capsule of the glenohumeral joint is reinforced by the superior glenohumeral ligament, middle glenohumeral ligament, inferior glenohumeral ligament, and the coracohumeral ligament.

Scapulothoracic articulation: Composed of the articulation between the scapula and the posterior rib cage. The articulation is not considered to be a joint since it lacks connection by fibrous, cartilaginous or synovial tissue.

Elbow

The elbow is classified as a hinge joint. It is composed of the humerus, ulna, and radius. Flexion and extension occur at the articulation of the trochlea with the semilunar notch of the ulna. The joint capsule is reinforced by the ulnar collateral ligament and the radial collateral ligament.

Wrist and Hand

The wrist complex consists of the radiocarpal and midcarpal joints. Motions at the wrist include flexion, extension, radial and ulnar deviation. The hand consists of the metacarpophalangeal joints, the proximal and distal interphalangeal joints, and the carpometacarpal joints.

Hip

The hip is classified as a ball and socket joint. It is formed by the articulation of the femur with the innominate bone. The head of the femur inserts into a deep socket called the acetabulum.

Stability is provided to the hip joint by the following:

- Acetabulum
- Iliofemoral ligament
- Pubofemoral ligament
- Ischiofemoral ligament

Knee

The knee is classified as a hinge joint. It is formed by the articulation of the tibia with the femur. The knee is extremely weak in terms of its bony arrangement.

Stability is provided to the knee joint by the following ligaments:

- Anterior cruciate ligament
- Posterior cruciate ligament
- Medial collateral ligament
- Lateral collateral ligament
- Deep medial capsular ligament

Ankle

The ankle is classified as a hinge joint which is formed by the articulation of the tibia and fibula with the talus. The distal ends of the tibia and fibula form a mortise that borders the talus. The bony arrangement provides the ankle with good lateral stability.

The ankle is structurally strong secondary to the bony and ligamentous arrangement.

Medial Ligaments: Deltoid

Lateral Ligaments:
Anterior tibiofibular
Anterior talofibular
Calcaneofibular
Lateral talocalcaneal
Posterior talofibular

Joint Receptors

Free Nerve Endings

Location	Joint capsule, ligaments, synovium, fat pads
Sensitivity	One type sensitive to non-noxious mechanical stress; other type sensitive to noxious mechanical or biochemical stimuli
Primary Distribution	All joints

Golgi Ligament Endings

Location	Ligaments, adjacent to ligaments' bony attachment
Sensitivity	Tension or stretch on ligaments
Primary Distribution	Majority of joints

Golgi-Mazzoni Corpuscles

Location	Joint capsule
Sensitivity	Compression of joint capsule
Primary Distribution	Knee joint, joint capsule

Pacinian Corpuscles

Location	Fibrous layer of joint capsule
Sensitivity	High frequency vibration, acceleration, and high velocity changes in joint position
Primary Distribution	All joints

Ruffini Endings

Location	Fibrous layer of joint capsule
Sensitivity	Stretching of joint capsule, amplitude, and velocity of joint position
Primary Distribution	Greater density in proximal joints particularly in capsular regions

Muscle Action

Head

Temporomandibular Joint

Depress:
- Lateral pterygoid
- Suprahyoid
- Infrahyoid

Elevate:
- Temporalis
- Masseter
- Medial pterygoid

Protrusion:
- Masseter
- Lateral pterygoid
- Medial pterygoid

Retrusion:
- Temporalis
- Masseter
- Digastric

Side to Side:
- Medial pterygoid
- Lateral pterygoid
- Masseter
- Temporalis

Spine

Cervical Intervertebral Joints

Flexion:
- Sternocleidomastoid
- Longus coli
- Scalenus muscles

Extension:
- Splenius cervicis
- Semispinalis cervicis
- Iliocostalis cervicis
- Longissimus cervicis
- Multifidus
- Trapezius

Rotation and Lateral Bending:
- Sternocleidomastoid
- Scalenus muscles
- Splenius cervicis
- Longissimus cervicis
- Iliocostalis cervicis
- Levator scapulae
- Multifidus

Thoracic and Lumbar Intervertebral Joints

Flexion:
- Rectus abdominis
- Internal oblique
- External oblique

Extension:
- Erector spinae
- Quadratus lumborum
- Multifidus

Rotation and Lateral Bending:
- Psoas major
- Quadratus lumborum
- External oblique
- Internal oblique
- Multifidus
- Longissimus thoracis
- Iliocostalis thoracis
- Rotatores

Upper Extremity

Scapula

Elevation:
- Upper trapezius
- Levator scapulae

Depression:
- Latissimus dorsi
- Pectoralis major
- Pectoralis minor
- Lower trapezius

Protraction:
- Serratus anterior
- Pectoralis major
- Pectoralis minor

Retraction:
- Trapezius
- Rhomboids

Upward Rotation:
- Upper trapezius
- Serratus anterior
- Lower trapezius

Downward Rotation:
- Rhomboids
- Levator scapulae
- Pectoralis minor

Shoulder Joint

Flexion:
- Anterior deltoid
- Coracobrachialis
- Pectoralis major
- Biceps brachii
- Supraspinatus

Extension:
- Latissimus dorsi
- Subscapularis
- Posterior deltoid
- Teres major

Abduction:
- Middle deltoid
- Supraspinatus

Adduction:
- Pectoralis major
- Latissimus dorsi
- Teres major

Lateral Rotation:
- Teres minor
- Infraspinatus
- Posterior deltoid

Medial Rotation:
- Subscapularis
- Teres major
- Pectoralis major
- Latissimus dorsi
- Anterior deltoid

Upper Extremity (continued)

Elbow Joint

Flexion:
- Biceps brachii
- Brachialis
- Brachioradialis

Extension:
- Triceps brachii
- Anconeus

Radioulnar Joint

Supination:
- Biceps brachii
- Supinator

Pronation:
- Pronator teres
- Pronator quadratus

Wrist Joint

Flexion:
- Flexor carpi radialis
- Flexor carpi ulnaris
- Palmaris longus

Extension:
- Extensor carpi radialis longus
- Extensor carpi radialis brevis
- Extensor carpi ulnaris

Radial Deviation:
- Extensor carpi radialis
- Flexor carpi radialis
- Extensor pollicis longus and brevis

Ulnar Deviation:
- Extensor carpi ulnaris
- Flexor carpi ulnaris

Lower Extremity

Hip Joint

Flexion:
- Iliopsoas
- Sartorius
- Rectus femoris
- Pectineus

Extension:
- Gluteus maximus and medius
- Semitendinosus
- Semimembranosus
- Biceps femoris

Abduction:
- Gluteus medius
- Gluteus minimus
- Piriformis
- Obturator internus

Adduction:
- Adductor magnus
- Adductor longus
- Adductor brevis
- Gracilis

Medial Rotation:
- Tensor fasciae latae
- Gluteus medius
- Gluteus minimus
- Pectineus
- Adductor longus

Lateral Rotation:
- Gluteus maximus
- Obturator externus
- Obturator internus
- Piriformis
- Gemelli
- Sartorius

Knee Joint

Flexion:
- Biceps femoris
- Semitendinosus
- Semimembranosus
- Sartorius

Extension:
- Rectus femoris
- Vastus lateralis
- Vastus intermedius
- Vastus medialis

Medial Rotation of Flexed Leg:
- Sartorius
- Popliteus
- Semitendinosus
- Semimembranosus

Lateral Rotation of Flexed Leg:
- Biceps femoris

Ankle Joint

Plantar Flexion:
- Tibialis posterior
- Gastrocnemius
- Soleus
- Peroneus longus
- Peroneus brevis
- Plantaris
- Flexor hallucis

Dorsiflexion:
- Tibialis anterior
- Extensor hallucis longus
- Extensor digitorum longus
- Peroneus tertius

Inversion:
- Tibialis posterior
- Tibialis anterior
- Flexor digitorum longus

Eversion:
- Peroneus longus
- Peroneus brevis
- Peroneus tertius

Kinesiology

Planes of the Body

Motions are described as occurring around three cardinal planes of the body (frontal, sagittal, transverse). Movement in the cardinal planes occurs around three corresponding axes (anterior-posterior, medial-lateral, vertical).

Frontal plane (coronal)

The frontal (or coronal) plane divides the body into anterior and posterior sections. Motions in the frontal plane such as abduction and adduction occur around an anterior-posterior axis.

Sagittal plane

The sagittal plane divides the body into right and left sections. Motions in the sagittal plane such as flexion and extension occur around a medial-lateral axis.

Transverse plane

The transverse plane divides the body into upper and lower sections. Motions in the transverse plane such as medial and lateral rotation occur around a vertical axis.

Classes of Levers

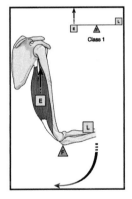

Class 1 Lever

A class 1 lever has the axis of rotation (fulcrum) between the effort (force) and resistance (load). There are very few class 1 levers in the body. A class 1 lever is illustrated with the triceps brachii force on the olecranon with an external counter force pushing on the forearm. Another example of a class 1 lever is a seesaw.

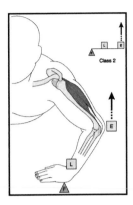

Class 2 Lever

A class 2 lever has the resistance (load) between the axis of rotation (fulcrum) and the effort (force). The length of the effort arm is always longer than the resistance arm. In most instances, gravity is the effort and muscle activity is the resistance, however, there are class 2 levers that the muscle is the effort when the distal attachment is on a weight bearing segment. An example of a class 2 lever is a wheelbarrow.

Class 3 Lever

A class 3 lever has the effort (force) between the axis of rotation (fulcrum) and the resistance (load). The length of the effort arm is always shorter than the length of the resistance arm. Shoulder abduction with weight at the wrist is a class 3 lever. Class 3 levers usually permit large movements at rapid speeds and are the most common type of lever in the body. An example of a class 3 lever is elbow flexion.

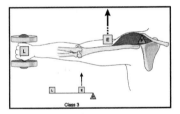

Exercise Physiology

Energy Systems

ATP-PC or Phosphagen System
Anaerobic Glycolysis or Lactic Acid System
Aerobic or Oxygen System

Anaerobic Metabolism

ATP-PC System

This energy system is used for ATP production during high intensity, short duration exercise such as sprinting 100 meters. Phosphocreatine decomposes and releases a large amount of energy that is used to construct ATP. There is two to three times more phosphocreatine in cells of muscles than ATP. This process occurs almost instantaneously allowing for ready and available energy needed by the muscles. The system provides energy for muscle contraction for up to 15 seconds.

The phosphagen system represents the most rapidly available source of ATP for use by the muscle. Reasons for this rapid availability are as follows:

- It does not depend on a long series of chemical reactions.
- It does not depend on transporting the oxygen we breathe to the working muscles.
- Both ATP and PC are stored directly within the contractile mechanisms of the muscle.

Anaerobic Glycolysis

This energy system is a major supplier of ATP during high intensity, short duration activities such as sprinting 400 or 800 meters. Stored glycogen is split into glucose, and through glycolysis, split again into pyruvic acid. The energy released during this process forms ATP. The process does not require oxygen. This system is nearly 50% slower than the phosphocreatine system and can provide a person with 30 to 40 seconds of muscle contraction.

Anaerobic glycolysis results in the formation of lactic acid, which causes muscular fatigue.
- It does not require the presence of oxygen.
- It uses only carbohydrates (glycogen and glucose).
- It releases enough energy for the resynthesis of only small amounts of ATP.

Aerobic Metabolism

The aerobic system is used predominantly during low intensity, long duration exercise such as running a marathon. The oxygen system yields by far the most ATP, but it requires several series of complex chemical reactions. This system provides energy through the oxidation of food. The combination of fatty acids, amino acids, and glucose with oxygen releases energy that forms ATP. This system will provide energy as long as there are nutrients to utilize.

Muscle Physiology

Classification of Muscle Fibers

Type I	Type II
Aerobic	Anaerobic
Red	White
Tonic	Phasic
Slow twitch	Fast twitch
Slow-oxidative	Fast-glycolytic

Functional Characteristics of Muscle Fibers

Type I	Type II
Low fatigability	High fatigability
High capillary density	Low capillary density
High myoglobin content	Low myoglobin content
Smaller fibers	Larger fibers
Extensive blood supply	Less blood supply
Large amount of mitochondria	Fewer mitochondria
Example: marathon, swimming	Example: high jump, sprinting

Muscle Receptors

Muscle Spindle

Muscle spindles are distributed throughout the belly of the muscle. They function to send information to the nervous system about muscle length and/or the rate of change of its length. The muscle spindle is important in the control of posture and with the help of the gamma system, involuntary movements.

Golgi Tendon Organ

Golgi tendon organs are encapsulated sensory receptors through which the muscle tendons pass immediately beyond their attachment to the muscle fibers. They are very sensitive to tension especially when produced from an active muscle contraction. They function to transmit information about tension or the rate of change of tension within the muscle.

An average of 10-15 muscle fibers are usually connected in series with each Golgi tendon organ. The Golgi tendon organ is stimulated through the tension produced by muscle fibers. Golgi tendon organs provide the nervous system with instantaneous information on the degree of tension in each small muscle segment.

Types of Muscular Contraction

Concentric: A concentric contraction occurs when the muscle shortens while developing tension.

Eccentric: An eccentric contraction occurs when the muscle lengthens while developing tension.

Isometric: An isometric contraction occurs when tension develops but there is no change in the length of the muscle.

Isotonic: An isotonic contraction occurs when the muscle shortens or lengthens while resisting a constant load.

Isokinetic: An isokinetic contraction occurs when the tension developed by the muscle, while shortening or lengthening at a constant speed, is maximal over the full range of motion.

Open-Chain versus Closed-Chain Activities

Open-Chain: Open-chain activities involve the distal segment, usually the hand or foot, moving freely in space. An example of an open-chain activity is kicking a ball with the lower extremity.

Closed-Chain: Closed-chain activities involve the body moving over a fixed distal segment. An example of a closed-chain activity is a squat lift.

Resistive and Overload Training

Isometric Exercise: Muscular force is generated without a change in muscle length. Isometric exercises are often performed against an immovable object. Submaximal isometric exercises are traditionally used in rehabilitation programs.

Isotonic Exercise: Muscular contraction in which the muscle exerts a constant tension. This can also be thought of as muscle movement with a constant load. Isotonic exercises are performed against resistance often employing equipment such as handheld weights.

Isokinetic Exercise: Exercise with a constant maximal speed and variable load. In isokinetic exercise the reaction force is identical to the force applied to the equipment. Cybex, Biodex, and Lido are a few of the companies making isokinetic exercise equipment.

Exercise Programs

DeLorme	Protocol
First Set	10 repetitions x 50% of 10 repetition maximum
Second Set	10 repetitions x 75% of 10 repetition maximum
Third Set	10 repetitions x 100% of 10 repetition maximum

Oxford Technique	Protocol
First Set	10 repetitions x 100% of 10 repetition maximum
Second Set	10 repetitions x 75% of 10 repetition maximum
Third Set	10 repetitions x 50% of 10 repetition maximum

Musculoskeletal System Examination

Upper Quarter Screening

The upper quarter screen provides a rapid assessment of mobility and neurologic function of the cervical spine and upper extremities. The screen is traditionally performed with the patient in sitting.

The following are components of an upper extremity screening:

Posture

- Postural assessment

Range of Motion

- Active range of motion of the cervical spine
- Active range of motion of the upper extremities
- Passive overpressure of the cervical spine and upper extremities, if the patient does not exhibit signs and symptoms of pathology

Resistive Testing (C1 – T1)

Resistive Test	Innervation Level
Cervical rotation	C1
Shoulder elevation	C2 – C4
Shoulder abduction	C5
Elbow flexion	C5 – C6
Wrist extension	C6
Elbow extension	C7
Wrist flexion	C7
Thumb extension	C8
Finger adduction	T1

Reflex Testing (C5 – C7)

Reflex	Innervation Level
Biceps	C5
Brachioradialis	C6
Triceps	C7

Dermatome Testing (C2 – T1)

Area of Skin	Innervation Level
Posterior head	C2
Posterior-lateral neck	C3
Acromioclavicular joint	C4
Lateral Arm	C5
Lateral forearm and thumb	C6
Palmar distal phalanx – middle finger	C7
Little finger and ulnar border of the hand	C8
Medial forearm	T1

Lower Quarter Screening

The lower quarter screen provides a rapid assessment of mobility and neurologic function of the lumbosacral spine and lower extremities. The screen is traditionally performed with the patient in standing or sitting.

The following are components of a lower extremity screening:

Posture

- Postural assessment

Range of Motion

- Active range of motion of the lumbosacral spine
- Active range of motion of the lower extremities
- Passive overpressure of the lumbosacral spine and lower extremities, if the patient does not exhibit signs and symptoms of pathology

Functional Testing (L4 – S1)

Functional Test	Innervation Level
Heel walking	L4 – L5
Toe walking	S1
Straight leg raise	L4 – S1

Resistive Testing (L1 – S1)

Resistive Test	Innervation Level
Hip flexion	L1 – L2
Knee extension	L3 – L4
Ankle dorsiflexion	L4 – L5
Great toe extension	L5
Ankle plantar flexion	S1

Reflex Testing (L4 – S1)

Reflex	Innervation Level
Patella	L4
Achilles	S1

Dermatome Testing (L2 – S5)

Area of Skin	Innervation Level
Anterior thigh	L2
Middle third of anterior thigh	L3
Patella and medial malleolus	L4
Fibular head and dorsum of foot	L5
Lateral and plantar aspect of foot	S1
Medial aspect of posterior thigh	S2
Perianal area	S3 – S5

Scanning Examination to Rule Out Referral of Symptoms from Other Tissues

History

↓

Observation

↓

Scanning Examination

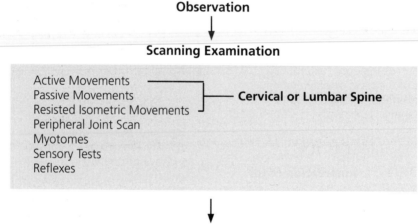

Active Movements ⎤
Passive Movements ⎥— **Cervical or Lumbar Spine**
Resisted Isometric Movements ⎦
Peripheral Joint Scan
Myotomes
Sensory Tests
Reflexes

↓

Decision: Spinal Joints or Peripheral Joints?
(Educated Guess)

Spine
(cervical or lumbar)

Peripheral Joint

Special Tests
 – (Sensory Tests)
 – (Reflexes)
Joint Play
Palpation
Imaging Techniques

Active Movements ⎤
Passive Movements ⎥ **Peripheral**
Resisted Isometric ⎥— **Joint**
 Movements ⎦ **Movement**
Special Tests
 – (Sensory Tests)
 – (Reflexes)
Joint Play
Palpation
Imaging Techniques

From Magee, DJ: Orthopedic Physical Assessment. W.B. Saunders Company, Philadelphia 2002, p.15, with permission.

Body Composition

Body composition is defined as the relative percentage of body weight that is comprised of fat and fat-free tissue. There are multiple methods for testing the percentage of body fat including hydrostatic weighing, skinfold, measurements, plethysmography, body mass index, and bioelectrical impedance analysis. A healthy range of body fat is 12-18% for males and 18-23% for females.

Densitometry

Hydrostatic Weighing: This method calculates the density of the body by immersing a person in water and measuring the amount of water that becomes displaced. The percentage of body fat is then determined by calculating the measured amount of water displaced in an equation based on Archimedes' principle. This method is the most widely used laboratory procedure to determine body density. Limitations of this method include the need to account for residual lung volume during submersion and evaluating patients that must tolerate water submersion during the testing. The standard error for this method is estimated at 2 to 2.5%.

Plethysmography: This method calculates the density of the body utilizing the amount of air displacement during testing within a specialized closed chamber. The change in pressure within the chamber is measured and converted to the percentage of body fat using a standardized equation.

Anthropometry

Skinfold Measurement: This method determines the overall percentage of body fat through the measurement of nine standardized sites. The correlation relies on the theory that the amount of subcutaneous fat is proportional to the total fat in the body. Limitations of this method include the requisite of an experienced examiner as well as variance from the standards based on gender, age, and ethnicity. Accuracy of measurement is within +/-3% with appropriate technique and equipment.

Skinfold Measurement Procedure

- All measurements should be taken on the right side of the body
- Take multiple measurements at each site to ensure accuracy and retest if the difference is greater than one to two millimeters
- Skinfold calipers should be positioned one centimeter away from the examiner's fingers when pinching the side, positioned perpendicular to the skinfold, and centered between the base and top of the fold
- Wait one to two seconds before reading the caliper
- Maintain pinching of the site during the reading of the caliper

Standard Skinfold Sites

Abdominal	Midaxillary
Triceps *	Subscapular *
Biceps	Suprailiac
Chest/pectoral	Thigh
Medial calf	

There are seven-site and three-site formulas to calculate the percentage of body fat using particular sites. There are also specific formulas for gender, sport, ethnicity, and age.
* Indicates the most commonly utilized sites

Other Techniques

Body Mass Index (BMI)

This formula is designed to assess risk potential for obesity-related health issues by calculating an estimated percentage of body fat. The formula divides body weight in kilograms by height in meters squared (kg/m^2). There is evidence that an increase in BMI is associated with an increase in mortality rate secondary to heart disease, diabetes, and cancer. Limitation of this formula is that it does not measure proportional composition of the body or percentage of fat. The standard error with estimating percent fat using BMI is approximately 5%.

BMI Classification System

< 18.5 kg/m^2 underweight
$20 - 24.9$ kg/m^2 desirable
$25 - 29.9$ kg/m^2 overweight
$30 - 34.9$ kg/m^2 class 1 obesity
$35 - 39.9$ kg/m^2 class 2 obesity
> 40 kg/m^2 class 3 obesity

Bioelectrical Impedance Analysis (BIA)

This method of assessing body composition uses a small electrical current and measures the resistance or opposition to the current flow. This technique is based on the principle that resistance to electrical current is inversely related to the composition of water within the body. The formula of $height^2/resistance$ is used for the general population while population-specific equations are also available. The standard error compares to the accuracy of skinfold measurements at approximately +/- 3%. Limitations include the requisite for the subjects to be properly hydrated as well as following all guidelines for the testing protocol.

BIA Protocol

- Abstain from eating or drinking within four hours prior to testing
- Abstain from vigorous physical activity within 12 hours prior to testing
- Urinate within 30 minutes prior to testing
- Avoid alcohol consumption for 48 hours prior to testing
- Avoid excessive water intake prior to testing

Posture

GOOD AND FAULTY POSTURE: SUMMARY CHART

Good Posture	Part	Faulty Posture
In standing, the longitudinal arch has the shape of a half dome. Barefoot or in shoes without heels, the feet toe-out slightly. In shoes with heels the feet are parallel. In walking with or without shoes, the feet are parallel and the weight is transferred from the heel along the outer border to the ball of the foot. In sprinting the feet are parallel or toe-in slightly. The weight is on the balls of the feet and toes because the heels do not come in contact with the ground.	**Foot**	Low longitudinal arch or flat foot. Low metatarsal arch, usually indicated by calluses under the ball of the foot. Weight borne on the inner side of the foot (pronation). "Ankle rolls in." Weight borne on the outer border of the foot (supination). "Ankle rolls out." Toeing-out while walking, or while standing in shoes with heels ("slue-footed"). Toeing-in while walking or standing ("pigeon-toed").
Toes should be straight, that is, neither curled downward nor bent upward. They should extend forward in line with the foot and not be squeezed together or overlap.	**Toes**	Toes bend up at the first joint and down at middle joints so that the weight rests on the tips of the toes (hammer toes). This fault is often associated with wearing shoes that are too short. Big toe slants inward toward the midline of the foot (hallux valgus). "Bunion." This fault is often associated with wearing shoes that are too narrow and pointed at the toes.
Legs are straight up and down. Kneecaps face straight ahead when feet are in good position. Looking at the knees from the side, the knees are straight, i.e., neither bent forward nor locked backward.	**Knees and Legs**	Knees touch when feet are apart (knock-knees). Knees are apart when feet touch (bowlegs). Knee curves slightly backward (hyperextended knee). "Back-knee." Knee bends slightly forward, that is, it is not as straight as it should be (flexed knee). Kneecaps face slightly toward each other (medially rotated femurs). Kneecaps face slightly outward (laterally rotated femurs).
Ideally, the body weight is borne evenly on both feet, and the hips are level. One side is not more prominent than the other as seen from front or back, nor is one hip more forward or backward than the other as seen from the side. The spine does not curve to the left or the right side. (A slight deviation to the left in right-handed individuals and to the right in left-handed individuals is not uncommon. Also, a tendency toward a slightly low right shoulder and slightly high right hip is frequently found in right-handed people, and vice versa for left-handed people).	**Hips, Pelvis, and Spine Back View**	One hip is higher than the other (lateral pelvic tilt). Sometimes it is not really much higher but appears so because a sideways sway of the body has made it more prominent. (Tailors and dressmakers often notice a lateral tilt because the hemline of skirts or length of trousers must be adjusted to the difference.) The hips are rotated so that one is farther forward than the other (clockwise or counter clockwise rotation).

GOOD AND FAULTY POSTURE: SUMMARY CHART

Good Posture	Part	Faulty Posture
The front of the pelvis and the thighs are in a straight line. The buttocks are not prominent in back but slope slightly downward. The spine has four natural curves. In the neck and lower back the curve is forward, in the upper back and lowest part of the spine (sacral region) it is backward. The sacral curve is a fixed curve while the other three are flexible.	**Spine and Pelvis Side View**	The low back arches forward too much (lordosis). The pelvis tilts forward too much. The front of the thigh forms an angle with the pelvis when this tilt is present. The normal forward curve in the low back has straightened. The pelvis tips backward as in swayback and flat-back postures. Increased backward curve in the upper back (kyphosis or round upper back). Increased forward curve in the neck. Almost always accompanied by round upper back and seen as a forward head. Lateral curve of the spine (scoliosis); toward one side (C-curve), toward both sides (S-curve).
In young children up to about the age of 10, the abdomen normally protrudes somewhat. In older children and adults it should be flat.	**Abdomen**	Entire abdomen protrudes. Lower part of the abdomen protrudes while the upper part is pulled in.
A good position of the chest is one in which it is slightly up and slightly forward (while the back remains in good alignment). The chest appears to be in a position about halfway between that of a full inspiration and a forced expiration.	**Chest**	Depressed, or "hollow-chest" position. Lifted and held up too high, brought about by arching the back. Ribs more prominent on one side than on the other. Lower ribs flaring out or protruding.
Arms hang relaxed at the sides with palms of the hands facing toward the body. Elbows are slightly bent, so forearms hang slightly forward. Shoulders are level and neither one is more forward or backward than the other when seen from the side. Shoulder blades lie flat against the rib cage. They are neither too close together or too wide apart. In adults, a separation of about 4 inches is average.	**Arms and Shoulders**	Arms held stiffly in any position forward, backward, or out from the body. Arms turned so that palms of hands face backward. One shoulder higher than the other. Both shoulders hiked-up. One or both shoulders drooping forward or sloping. Shoulders rotated either clockwise or counterclockwise. Shoulder blades pulled back too hard. Shoulder blades too far apart. Shoulder blades too prominent, standing out from the rib cage (winged scapulae).
Head is held erect in a position of good balance.	**Head**	Chin up too high. Head protruding forward. Head tilted or rotated to one side.

From Kendall F, McCreary E, Provance P: Muscle Testing and Function. Lippencott, William & Wilkins, Baltimore 1993, p.115-116, with permission.

Positioning of a Joint

Loose Packed Position of Joints

Joint:	Position:
Facet (spine)	Midway between flexion and extension
Temporomandibular	Mouth slightly open (freeway space)
Glenohumeral	55° abduction, 30° horizontal adduction
Acromioclavicular	Arm resting by side in normal physiological position
Ulnohumeral (elbow)	70° flexion, 10° supination
Radiohumeral	Full extension, full supination
Proximal radioulnar	70° flexion, 35° supination
Distal radioulnar	10° supination
Radiocarpal (wrist)	Neutral with slight ulnar deviation
Carpometacarpal	Midway between abduction - adduction and flexion - extension
Metacarpophalangeal	Slight flexion
Interphalangeal	Slight flexion
Hip	30° flexion, 30° abduction, slight lateral rotation
Knee	25° flexion
Talocrural (ankle)	10° plantar flexion, midway between maximum inversion and eversion
Subtalar	Midway between extremes of range of movement
Midtarsal	Midway between extremes of range of movement
Tarsometatarsal	Midway between extremes of range of movement
Metatarsophalangeal	Neutral
Interphalangeal	Slight flexion

From Magee, DJ: Orthopedic Physical Assessment. W.B. Saunders Company, Philadelphia 2002, p.50, with permission.

Close Packed Position of Joints

Joint:	Position:
Facet (spine)	Extension
Temporomandibular	Clenched teeth
Glenohumeral	Abduction and lateral rotation
Acromioclavicular	Arm abducted to 90°
Sternoclavicular	Maximum shoulder elevation
Ulnohumeral (elbow)	Extension
Radiohumeral	Elbow flexed 90°, forearm supinated 5°
Proximal radioulnar	5° supination
Distal radioulnar	5° supination
Radiocarpal (wrist)	Extension with radial deviation
Metacarpophalangeal (fingers)	Full flexion
Metacarpophalangeal (thumb)	Full opposition
Interphalangeal	Full extension
Hip	Full extension, medial rotation
Knee	Full extension, lateral rotation of tibia
Talocrural (ankle)	Maximum dorsiflexion
Subtalar	Supination
Midtarsal	Supination
Tarsometatarsal	Supination
Metatarsophalangeal	Full extension
Interphalangeal	Full extension

From Magee, DJ: Orthopedic Physical Assessment. W.B. Saunders Company, Philadelphia 2002, p.50, with permission.

Descriptions of Specific Positions

	Loose Packed	Close Packed
Stress on joint	Minimal	Maximal
Congruency of joint	Minimal	Full
Ligament position	Great laxity	Full tightness
Joint surface	No volitional separation	Compressed

Common Capsular Patterns of Joints

Joint:	Restriction:*
Temporomandibular	Limitation of mouth opening
Atlanto-occipital	Extension, side flexion equally limited
Cervical spine	Side flexion and rotation equally limited, extension
Glenohumeral	Lateral rotation, abduction, medial rotation
Sternoclavicular	Pain at extreme of range of movement
Acromioclavicular	Pain at extreme of range of movement
Ulnohumeral	Flexion, extension
Radiohumeral	Flexion, extension, supination, pronation
Proximal radioulnar	Supination, pronation
Distal radioulnar	Full range of movement, pain at extremes of rotation
Wrist	Flexion and extension equally limited
Trapeziometacarpal	Abduction, extension
Metacarpophalangeal and interphalangeal	Flexion, extension
Thoracic spine	Side flexion and rotation equally limited, extension
Lumbar spine	Side flexion and rotation equally limited, extension
Sacroiliac, symphysis pubis, and sacrococcygeal	Pain when joints are stressed
Hip**	Flexion, abduction, medial rotation (sometimes medial rotation is most limited)
Knee	Flexion, extension
Tibiofibular	Pain when joint stressed
Talocrural	Plantar flexion, dorsiflexion
Talocalcaneal (subtalar)	Limitation of varus range of movement
Midtarsal	Dorsiflexion, plantar flexion, adduction, medial rotation
First metatarsophalangeal	Extension, flexion
Second to fifth metatarsophalangeal	Variable
Interphalangeal	Flexion, extension

* Movements are listed in order of restriction.**For the hip, flexion, abduction, and medial rotation are always the movements most limited in a capsular pattern. —From Magee, DJ: Orthopedic Physical Assessment. W.B. Saunders Company, Philadelphia 2002, p.28, with permission.

End-Feel

Normal End-feel

End-feel is the type of resistance that is felt when passively moving a joint through the end range of motion. Certain tissues and joints have a consistent end-feel and are described as firm, hard or soft. Pathology can be identified through noting the type of abnormal end-feel within a particular joint.

Firm (stretch)

Examples: Ankle dorsiflexion
Finger extension
Hip medial rotation
Forearm supination

Hard (bone to bone)

Example: Elbow extension

Soft (soft tissue approximation)

Examples: Elbow flexion
Knee flexion

Abnormal End-feel

Abnormal end-feel would consist of any end-feel that is felt at an abnormal or inconsistent point in the range of motion or in a joint that normally presents with a different end-feel.

Empty (cannot reach end-feel, usually due to pain)

Examples: Joint inflammation
Fracture
Bursitis

Firm

Examples: Increased tone
Tightening of the capsule
Ligament shortening

Hard

Examples: Fracture
Osteoarthritis
Osteophyte formation

Soft

Examples: Edema
Synovitis
Ligament instability/tear

Muscle Testing

Manual Muscle Testing Grades

Zero
(0/5)
The subject demonstrates no palpable muscle contraction.

Trace
(1/5)
The subject's muscle contraction can be palpated, but there is no joint movement.

Poor Minus
(2-/5)
The subject does not complete range of motion in a gravity-eliminated position.

Poor
(2/5)
The subject completes range of motion with gravity-eliminated.

Poor Plus
(2+/5)
The subject is able to initiate movement against gravity.

Fair Minus
(3-/5)
The subject does not complete the range of motion against gravity, but does complete more than half of the range.

Fair
(3/5)
The subject completes range of motion against gravity without manual resistance.

Fair Plus
(3+/5)
The subject completes range of motion against gravity with only minimal resistance.

Good Minus
(4-/5)
The subject completes range of motion against gravity with minimal-moderate resistance.

Good
(4/5)
The subject completes range of motion against gravity with moderate resistance.

Good Plus
(4+/5)
The subject completes range of motion against gravity with moderate-maximal resistance.

Normal
(5/5)
The subject completes range of motion against gravity with maximal resistance.

Positioning for Muscle Testing

Supine

Abdominals	Anterior deltoid*
Biceps	Brachioradialis
Finger flexors	Finger extensors
Iliopsoas	Infraspinatus
Lateral rotators of shoulder*	Medial rotators of shoulder*
Neck flexors	Pectoralis major
Pectoralis minor	Peroneals
Pronators	Sartorius
Serratus anterior	Supinators
Tensor fasciae latae	Teres minor
Thumb muscles	Tibialis anterior
Tibialis posterior	Toe extensors
Toe flexors	Triceps*
Wrist extensors	Wrist flexors

Sidelying

Gluteus medius	Gluteus minimus
Hip adductors	Lateral abdominals

Prone

Back extensors	Gastrocnemius
Gluteus maximus	Hamstrings*
Lateral rotators of the shoulder*	Latissimus dorsi
Lower trapezius	Medial rotators of the shoulder*
Middle trapezius	Neck extensors
Posterior deltoid*	Quadratus lumborum
Rhomboids	Soleus
Teres major	Triceps*

Sitting

Coracobrachialis	Deltoid*
Hip flexors*	Lateral rotators of hip
Medial rotators of hip	Quadriceps
Upper trapezius	Serratus anterior*

Standing

Ankle plantar flexors	Serratus anterior*

*Indicates multiple acceptable positions for muscle testing

Gait

Standard versus Rancho Los Amigos Terminology

	Standard Terminology	Rancho Los Amigos Terminology
Stance Phase (60% of gait cycle)	Heel strike Foot flat Midstance Heel off Toe off	Initial contact Loading response Midstance Terminal stance Pre-swing
Swing Phase (40% of gait cycle)	Acceleration Midswing Deceleration	Initial swing Midswing Terminal swing

Standard Terminology

Stance Phase

Heel strike: Heel strike is the instant that the heel touches the ground to begin stance phase.

Foot flat: Foot flat is the point in which the entire foot makes contact with the ground and should occur directly after heel strike.

Midstance: Midstance is the point during the stance phase when the entire body weight is directly over the stance limb.

Heel off: Heel off is the point in which the heel of the stance limb leaves the ground.

Toe off: Toe off is the point in which only the toe of the stance limb remains on the ground.

Swing Phase

Acceleration: Acceleration begins when toe off is complete and the reference limb swings until positioned directly under the body.

Midswing: Midswing is the point when the swing limb is directly under the body.

Deceleration: Deceleration begins directly after midswing as the swing limb begins to extend and ends just prior to heel strike.

Rancho Los Amigos Terminology

Stance Phase

Initial contact: Initial contact is the beginning of the stance phase that occurs when the foot touches the ground.

Loading response: Loading response corresponds to the amount of time between initial contact and the beginning of the swing phase for the other leg.

Midstance: Midstance corresponds to the point in stance phase when the other foot is off the floor until the body is directly over the stance limb.

Terminal stance: Terminal stance begins when the stance limb's heel rises and ends when the other foot touches the ground.

Pre-swing: Pre-swing phase begins when the other foot touches the ground and ends when the stance foot reaches toe off.

Swing Phase

Initial swing: Initial swing phase begins when the stance foot lifts from the floor and ends with maximal knee flexion during swing.

Midswing: Midswing phase begins with maximal knee flexion during swing and ends when the tibia is perpendicular with the ground.

Terminal swing: Terminal swing phase begins when the tibia is perpendicular to the floor and ends when the foot touches the ground.

Normal Gait

	SWING 40 %			STANCE 60 %				
	Initial Swing	Midswing	Terminal Swing	Initial Contact	Loading Response	Midstance	Terminal Stance	Pre-Swing
Trunk	Erect Neutral	Erect Neutral	Erect Neutral	Erect Neutral	Erect Neutral	Erect Neutral	Erect Neutral	Erect Neutral
Pelvis	Level: Backward Rotation 4-5°	Level: Neutral Rotation	Level: Forward Rotation 4-5°	Level: Maintains Forward Rotation	Level: Less Forward Rotation	Level: Neutral Rotation	Level: Backward Rotation 4-5°	Level: Backward Rotation 4-5°
Hip	Flexion 20°	Flexion 20° - 30°	Flexion 30°	Flexion 30°	Flexion 30°	Extending to Neutral	Apparent Hyperextension 10°	Neutral Extension
	Neutral: Rotation Abduction Adduction	Neutral: Rotation Abduction Adduction	Neutral: Rotation Abduction Adduction	Neutral: Rotation Abduction Adduction	Neutral: Rotation Abduction Adduction	Neutral: Rotation Abduction Adduction	Neutral: Rotation Abduction Adduction	Neutral: Rotation Abduction Adduction
Knee	Flexion 60°	From 60° to 30° Flexion	Extension to 0°	Full Extension	Flexion 15°	Extending to Neutral	Full Extension	Flexion 35°
Ankle	Plantar Flexion 10°	Neutral	Neutral	Neutral Heel First	Plantar Flexion 15°	From Plantar Flexion to 10° Dorsiflexion	Neutral with Tibia Stable and Heel Off Prior to Initial Contact Opposite Foot	Plantar Flexion 20°
Toes	Neutral	Neutral	Neutral	Neutral	Neutral	Neutral	Neutral IP Extended MP	Neutral IP Extended MP

From Rancho Los Amigos National Rehabilitation Center: Normal and Pathological Gait Syllabus, p. 11, Downey, California, with permission.

Peak Muscle Activity During the Gait Cycle

Tibialis anterior: Peak activity is just after heel strike. Responsible for eccentric lowering of the foot into plantar flexion.

Gastroc-soleus group: Peak activity is during late stance phase. Responsible for concentric raising of the heel during toe off.

Quadriceps group: Two periods of peak activity. In periods of single support during early stance phase and just before toe off to initiate swing phase.

Hamstrings group: Peak activity is during late swing phase. Responsible for decelerating the unsupported limb.

Range of Motion Requirements for Normal Gait

Hip flexion:	**0 – 30 degrees**
Hip extension:	**0 – 10 degrees**
Knee flexion:	**0 – 60 degrees**
Knee extension:	**0 degrees**
Ankle dorsiflexion:	**0 – 10 degrees**
Ankle plantar flexion:	**0 – 20 degrees**

Gait Terminology

Base of support: The distance measured between the left and right foot during progression of gait. The distance decreases as cadence increases. The average base of support for an adult is two to four inches.

Cadence: The number of steps an individual will walk over a period of time. The average value for an adult is 110–120 steps per minute.

Degree of toe-out: The angle formed by each foot's line of progression and a line intersecting the center of the heel and second toe. The average degree of toe-out for an adult is seven degrees.

Double support phase: The double support phase refers to the two times during a gait cycle where both feet are on the ground. The time of double support increases as the speed of gait decreases. This phase does not exist with running.

Gait cycle: The gait cycle refers to the sequence of motions that occur from one initial contact of the heel to the next consecutive initial contact of the same heel.

Pelvic rotation: Rotation of the pelvis opposite the thorax in order to maintain balance and regulate speed. The pelvic rotation during gait for an adult is a total of 8 degrees (4 degrees forward with the swing leg and 4 degrees backward with the stance leg).

Single support phase: The single support phase occurs when only one foot is on the ground and occurs twice during a single gait cycle.

Step length: The distance measured between right heel strike and left heel strike. The average step length for an adult is 13 to 16 inches.

Stride: The distance measured between right heel strike and the following right heel strike. The average stride length for an adult is 26 to 32 inches.

Abnormal Gait Patterns

Antalgic: A protective gait pattern where the involved step length is decreased in order to avoid weight bearing on the involved side usually secondary to pain.

Ataxic: A gait pattern characterized by staggering and unsteadiness. There is usually a wide base of support and movements are exaggerated.

Cerebellar: A staggering gait pattern seen in cerebellar disease.

Circumduction: A gait pattern characterized by a circular motion to advance the leg during swing phase; this may be used to compensate for insufficient hip or knee flexion or dorsiflexion.

Double step: A gait pattern in which alternate steps are of a different length or at a different rate.

Equine: A gait pattern characterized by high steps; usually involves excessive activity of the gastrocnemius.

Festinating: A gait pattern where a patient walks on toes as though pushed. It starts slowly, increases, and may continue until the patient grasps an object in order to stop.

Hemiplegic: A gait pattern in which patients abduct the paralyzed limb, swing it around, and bring it forward so the foot comes to the ground in front of them.

Parkinsonian: A gait pattern marked by increased forward flexion of the trunk and knees; gait is shuffling with quick and small steps; festinating may occur.

Scissor: A gait pattern in which the legs cross midline upon advancement.

Spastic: A gait pattern with stiff movement, toes seeming to catch and drag, legs held together, hip and knee joints slightly flexed. Commonly seen in spastic paraplegia.

Steppage: A gait pattern in which the feet and toes are lifted through hip and knee flexion to excessive heights; usually secondary to dorsiflexor weakness. The foot will slap at initial contact with the ground secondary to the decreased control.

Tabetic: A high stepping ataxic gait pattern in which the feet slap the ground.

Trendelenburg: A gait pattern that denotes gluteus medius weakness; excessive lateral trunk flexion and weight shifting over the stance leg.

Vaulting: A gait pattern where the swing leg advances by compensating through the combination of elevation of the pelvis and plantar flexion of the stance leg.

Gait Deviations

	Foot slap	Toe down instead of heel strike	Clawing of toes	Heel lift during midstance	No toe off
Ankle and Foot	• Weak dorsiflexors • Dorsiflexor paralysis	• Plantar flexor spasticity • Plantar flexor contracture • Weak dorsiflexors • Dorsiflexor paralysis • Leg length discrepancy • Hindfoot pain	• Toe flexor spasticity • Positive support reflex	• Insufficient dorsiflexion range • Plantar flexor spasticity	• Forefoot/toe pain • Weak plantar flexors • Weak toe flexors • Insufficient plantar flexion range of motion
	Exaggerated knee flexion at contact	**Hyperextension in stance**	**Exaggerated knee flexion at terminal stance**	**Insufficient flexion with swing**	**Excessive flexion with swing**
Knee	• Weak quadriceps • Quadriceps paralysis • Hamstrings spasticity • Insufficient extension range of motion	• Compensation for weak quadriceps • Plantar flexor contracture	• Knee flexion contracture • Hip flexion contracture	• Knee effusion • Quadriceps extension spasticity • Plantar flexor spasticity • Insufficient flexion range of motion	• Flexor withdrawal reflex • Lower extremity flexor synergy
	Insufficient hip flexion at initial contact	**Insufficient hip extension at stance**	**Circumduction during swing**	**Hip hiking during swing**	**Exaggerated hip flexion during swing**
Hip	• Weak hip flexors • Hip flexor paralysis • Hip extensor spasticity • Insufficient hip flexion range of motion	• Insufficient hip extension range of motion • Hip flexion contracture • Lower extremity flexor synergy	• Compensation for weak hip flexors • Compensation for weak dorsiflexors • Compensation for weak hamstrings	• Compensation for weak dorsiflexors • Compensation for weak knee flexors • Compensation for extensor synergy pattern	• Lower extremity flexor synergy • Compensation for insufficient hip flexion or dorsiflexion

Range of Motion

Process for Conducting Goniometric Measurements

1. Place the subject in the recommended testing position.
2. Stabilize the proximal joint segment.
3. Move the distal joint segment through the available range of motion. Make sure that the passive range of motion is performed slowly, the end of the range is attained, and the end-feel determined.
4. Make a clinical estimate of the range of motion.
5. Return the distal joint segment to the starting position.
6. Palpate bony anatomical landmarks.
7. Align the goniometer.
8. Read and record the starting position. Remove the goniometer.
9. Stabilize the proximal joint segment.
10. Move the distal segment through the full range of motion.
11. Replace and realign the goniometer. Palpate the anatomical landmarks again if necessary.
12. Read and record the range of motion.

Adapted from Norkin and White: Measurement of Joint Motion: A Guide to Goniometry. F.A. Davis Company, Philadelphia, 2003, p.35, with permission.

Average Adult Range of Motion for the Upper and Lower Extremities

Upper Extremity

Shoulder

Flexion	0-180
Extension	0-60
Abduction	0-180
Medial rotation	0-70
Lateral rotation	0-90

Elbow

Extension	0
Flexion	0-150

Forearm

Pronation	0-80
Supination	0-80

Wrist

Flexion	0-80
Extension	0-70
Radial deviation	0-20
Ulnar deviation	0-30

Thumb

Carpometacarpal

Abduction	0-70
Flexion	0-15
Extension	0-20
Opposition	Tip of thumb to base of fifth digit

Metacarpophalangeal

Flexion	0-50

Interphalangeal

Flexion	0-80

Digits – Second to Fifth

Metacarpophalangeal

Flexion	0-90
Hyperextension	0-45

Proximal interphalangeal

Flexion	0-100

Distal interphalangeal

Flexion	0-90
Hyperextension	0-10

Lower Extremity

Hip

Flexion	0-120
Extension	0-30
Abduction	0-45
Adduction	0-30
Medial rotation	0-45
Lateral rotation	0-45

Knee

Flexion	0-135

Ankle

Dorsiflexion	0-20
Plantar flexion	0-50
Inversion	0-35
Eversion	0-15

Subtalar

Inversion	0-5
Eversion	0-5

Goniometric Technique

Upper Extremity

Shoulder

Flexion

Axis: acromial process
Stationary arm: midaxillary line of the thorax
Moveable arm: lateral midline of the humerus using the lateral epicondyle of the humerus for reference

Extension

Axis: acromial process
Stationary arm: midaxillary line of the thorax
Moveable arm: lateral midline of the humerus using the lateral epicondyle of the humerus for reference

Abduction

Axis: anterior aspect of the acromial process
Stationary arm: parallel to the midline of the anterior aspect of the sternum
Moveable arm: medial midline of the humerus

Adduction

Axis: anterior aspect of the acromial process
Stationary arm: parallel to the midline of the anterior aspect of the sternum
Moveable arm: medial midline of the humerus

Medial rotation

Axis: olecranon process
Stationary arm: parallel or perpendicular to the floor
Moveable arm: ulna using the olecranon process and ulnar styloid for reference

Lateral rotation

Axis: olecranon process
Stationary arm: parallel or perpendicular to the floor
Moveable arm: ulna using the olecranon process and ulnar styloid process for reference

Elbow

Flexion

Axis: lateral epicondyle of the humerus
Stationary arm: lateral midline of the humerus using the center of the acromial process for reference
Moveable arm: lateral midline of the radius using the radial head and radial styloid process for reference

Extension

Axis: lateral epicondyle of the humerus
Stationary arm: lateral midline of the humerus using the center of the acromial process for reference
Moveable arm: lateral midline of the radius using the radial head and radial styloid process for reference

Forearm

Pronation

Axis: lateral to the ulnar styloid process
Stationary arm: parallel to the anterior midline of the humerus
Moveable arm: dorsal aspect of the forearm, just proximal to the styloid process of the radius and ulna

Supination

Axis: medial to the ulnar styloid process
Stationary arm: parallel to the anterior midline of the humerus
Moveable arm: ventral aspect of the forearm, just proximal to the styloid process of the radius and ulna

Wrist

Flexion

Axis: lateral aspect of the wrist over the triquetrum
Stationary arm: lateral midline of the ulna using the olecranon and ulnar styloid process for reference
Moveable arm: lateral midline of the fifth metacarpal

Extension

Axis: lateral aspect of the wrist over the triquetrum
Stationary arm: lateral midline of the ulna using the olecranon and ulnar styloid process for reference
Moveable arm: lateral midline of the fifth metacarpal

Radial deviation

Axis: over the middle of the dorsal aspect of the wrist over the capitate
Stationary arm: dorsal midline of the forearm using the lateral epicondyle of the humerus for reference
Moveable arm: dorsal midline of the third metacarpal

Ulnar deviation

Axis: over the middle of the dorsal aspect of the wrist over the capitate
Stationary arm: dorsal midline of the forearm using the lateral epicondyle of the humerus for reference
Moveable arm: dorsal midline of the third metacarpal

Thumb

Carpometacarpal flexion

Axis: over the palmar aspect of the first carpometacarpal joint
Stationary arm: ventral midline of the radius using the ventral surface of the radial head and radial styloid process for reference
Moveable arm: ventral midline of the first metacarpal

Carpometacarpal extension

Axis: over the palmar aspect of the first carpometacarpal joint
Stationary arm: ventral midline of the radius using the ventral surface of the radial head and radial styloid process for reference
Moveable arm: ventral midline of the first metacarpal

Carpometacarpal abduction

Axis: over the lateral aspect of the radial styloid process
Stationary arm: lateral midline of the second metacarpal using the center of the second metacarpophalangeal joint for reference
Moveable arm: lateral midline of the first metacarpal using the center of the first metacarpophalangeal joint for reference

Carpometacarpal adduction

Axis: over the lateral aspect of the radial styloid process
Stationary arm: lateral midline of the second metacarpal using the center of the second metacarpophalangeal joint for reference
Moveable arm: lateral midline of the first metacarpal using the center of the first metacarpophalangeal joint for reference

Fingers

Metacarpophalangeal flexion

Axis: over the dorsal aspect of the metacarpophalangeal joint
Stationary arm: over the dorsal midline of the metacarpal
Moveable arm: over the dorsal midline of the proximal phalanx

Metacarpophalangeal extension

Axis: over the dorsal aspect of the metacarpophalangeal joint
Stationary arm: over the dorsal midline of the metacarpal
Moveable arm: over the dorsal midline of the proximal phalanx

Metacarpophalangeal abduction

Axis: over the dorsal aspect of the metacarpophalangeal joint
Stationary arm: over the dorsal midline of the metacarpal
Moveable arm: dorsal midline of the proximal phalanx

Metacarpophalangeal adduction

Axis: over the dorsal aspect of the metacarpophalangeal joint
Stationary arm: over the dorsal midline of the metacarpal
Moveable arm: dorsal midline of the proximal phalanx

Proximal interphalangeal flexion

Axis: over the dorsal aspect of the proximal interphalangeal joint
Stationary arm: over the dorsal midline of the proximal phalanx
Moveable arm: over the dorsal midline of the middle phalanx

Proximal interphalangeal extension

Axis: over the dorsal aspect of the proximal interphalangeal joint
Stationary arm: over the dorsal midline of the proximal phalanx
Moveable arm: over the dorsal midline of the middle phalanx

Distal interphalangeal flexion

Axis: over the dorsal aspect of the distal interphalangeal joint
Stationary arm: over the dorsal midline of the middle phalanx
Moveable arm: over the dorsal midline of the distal phalanx

Distal interphalangeal extension

Axis: over the dorsal aspect of the distal interphalangeal joint
Stationary arm: over the dorsal midline of the middle phalanx
Moveable arm: over the dorsal midline of the distal phalanx

Lower Extremity

Hip

Flexion

Axis: over the lateral aspect of the hip joint using the greater trochanter of the femur for reference
Stationary arm: lateral midline of the pelvis
Moveable arm: lateral midline of the femur using the lateral epicondyle for reference

Extension

Axis: over the lateral aspect of the hip joint using the greater trochanter of the femur for reference
Stationary arm: lateral midline of the pelvis
Moveable arm: lateral midline of the femur using the lateral epicondyle for reference

Abduction

Axis: over the anterior superior iliac spine (ASIS) of the extremity being measured
Stationary arm: align with imaginary horizontal line extending from one ASIS to the other ASIS
Moveable arm: anterior midline of the femur using the midline of the patella for reference

Adduction

Axis: over the anterior superior iliac spine (ASIS) of the extremity being measured
Stationary arm: align with imaginary horizontal line extending from one ASIS to the other ASIS
Moveable arm: anterior midline of the femur using the midline of the patella for reference

Medial rotation

Axis: anterior aspect of the patella
Stationary arm: perpendicular to the floor or parallel to the supporting surface
Moveable arm: anterior midline of the lower leg using the crest of the tibia and a point midway between the two malleoli for reference

Lateral rotation

Axis: anterior aspect of the patella
Stationary arm: perpendicular to the floor or parallel to the supporting surface
Moveable arm: anterior midline of the lower leg using the crest of the tibia and a point midway between the two malleoli for reference

Knee

Flexion

Axis: lateral epicondyle of the femur
Stationary arm: lateral midline of the femur using the greater trochanter for reference
Moveable arm: lateral midline of the fibula using the lateral malleolus and fibular head for reference

Extension

Axis: lateral epicondyle of the femur
Stationary arm: lateral midline of the femur using the greater trochanter for reference
Moveable arm: lateral midline of the fibula using the lateral malleolus and fibular head for reference

Ankle

Dorsiflexion

Axis: lateral aspect of the lateral malleolus
Stationary arm: lateral midline of the fibula using the head of the fibula for reference
Moveable arm: parallel to the lateral aspect of the fifth metatarsal

Plantar flexion

Axis: lateral aspect of the lateral malleolus
Stationary arm: lateral midline of the fibula using the head of the fibula for reference
Moveable arm: parallel to the lateral aspect of the fifth metatarsal

Inversion

Axis: anterior aspect of the ankle midway between the malleoli
Stationary arm: anterior midline of the lower leg using the tibial tuberosity for reference
Moveable arm: anterior midline of the second metatarsal

Eversion

Axis: anterior aspect of the ankle midway between the malleoli
Stationary arm: anterior midline of the lower leg using the tibial tuberosity for reference
Moveable arm: anterior midline of the second metatarsal

Subtalar

Inversion

Axis: posterior aspect of the ankle midway between the malleoli
Stationary arm: posterior midline of the lower leg
Moveable arm: posterior midline of the calcaneus

Eversion

Axis: posterior aspect of the ankle midway between the malleoli
Stationary arm: posterior midline of the lower leg
Moveable arm: posterior midline of the calcaneus

Muscle Insufficiency

A muscle contraction that is less than optimal due to an extremely lengthened or shortened position of the muscle. There are two types of insufficiency:

Active: when a two-joint muscle contracts across both joints simultaneously

Passive: when a two-joint muscle is lengthened over both joints simultaneously

Dynamometry

Dynamometry is the process of measuring forces that are doing work. A dynamometer is a device that measures strength through the use of a load cell or spring loaded gauge. There are various kinds of dynamometers that are used based on treatment objectives. Three types of dynamometry that will be discussed here include the handheld dynamometer that measures grip strength, the handheld dynamometer used to measure strength of the extremities through isometric contraction, and the dynamometer used to measure strength through isokinetic contraction. Handheld dynamometry demonstrates intrarater reliability of > .94. The same dynamometer should be used each session and the same tester should consistently measure the patient.

- **A handheld dynamometer** can be used to assess the grip strength of a patient. Normally, a patient's dominant grip strength is five to ten pounds greater than the non-dominant grip strength. Handheld dynamometry is also used to measure muscle group strength by having the patient exert maximal force against the dynamometer. Portable, non-electric units include a hydraulic or spring-load system and display the force on a gauge. Electrical units use load cells or strain gauges and display force digitally.

- **Isometric dynamometry** measures the static strength of a muscle group without any movement. The extremity is restrained by stabilization straps or stabilized with only verbal instruction.
  Benefits include attaining peak and average force data, reaction time data, rate of motor recruitment, and maximal exertion data. This method is relatively safe, simple to use, easy to interpret data, and incurs a relative low cost.
  Disadvantages include the inability to convert data to functional activities, as well as the need for caution with patients with acute orthopedic injury, osteoporosis or hernia. This method is contraindicated for patients with fractures and significant hypertension.

- **Isokinetic dynamometry** measures the strength of a muscle group during a movement with constant, predetermined speed. This device will alter the resistance to accommodate for the change in the length-tension ratio and lever arm throughout the entire arc of motion. The muscle group will therefore maximally contract throughout the motion. Common speeds of motion include 60, 120, and 180 degrees per second.

Benefits include the ability to test the muscle strength at various speeds, the ability to measure the patient's power, and that the patient will never have more resistance than they can handle during the isokinetic testing.

Disadvantages include the high cost of operation for the device, limitations in patterns of movement, a higher level of understanding required by the patient, and that this method doesn't truly correlate to function since people do not perform at a constant velocity during daily activities.

Make Test:

A make test is an evaluation procedure where a patient is asked to apply a force against the dynamometer.

Break Test:

A break test is an evaluation procedure where a patient is asked to hold a contraction against pressure that is applied in the opposite direction to the contraction.

Special Tests

Special Tests Outline

Upper Extremity

Shoulder

Dislocation

Apprehension test for anterior shoulder dislocation
Apprehension test for posterior shoulder dislocation

Biceps Tendon Pathology

Ludington's test
Speed's test
Yergason's test

Rotator Cuff Pathology/Impingement

Drop arm test
Hawkins-Kennedy impingement test
Neer impingement test
Supraspinatus test

Thoracic Outlet Syndrome

Adson maneuver
Allen test
Costoclavicular syndrome test
Roos test
Wright test (hyperabduction test)

Miscellaneous

Glenoid labrum tear test

Elbow

Ligamentous Instability

Varus stress test
Valgus stress test

Epicondylitis

Cozen's test
Lateral epicondylitis test
Medial epicondylitis test
Mill's test

Neurological Dysfunction

Tinel's sign

Wrist/Hand

Ligamentous Instability

Ulnar collateral ligament instability test

Vascular Insufficiency

Allen test
Capillary refill test

Contracture/Tightness

Bunnel-Littler test
Tight retinacular ligament test

Neurological Dysfunction

Froment's sign
Phalen's test
Tinel's sign

Miscellaneous

Finkelstein test
Grind test
Murphy sign

Lower Extremity

Hip

Contracture/Tightness

Ely's test
Ober's test
Piriformis test
Thomas test
Tripod sign
90-90 straight leg raise test

Pediatric Tests

Barlow's test
Ortolani's test

Hawkins-Kennedy impingement test

The patient is positioned in sitting or standing. The therapist flexes the patient's shoulder to 90 degrees and then medially rotates the arm. A positive test is indicated by pain and may be indicative of shoulder impingement involving the supraspinatus tendon.

Neer impingement test

The patient is positioned in sitting or standing. The therapist positions one hand on the posterior aspect of the patient's scapula and the other hand stabilizing the elbow. The therapist elevates the patient's arm through flexion. A positive test is indicated by a facial grimace or pain and may be indicative of shoulder impingement involving the supraspinatus tendon.

Supraspinatus test

The patient is positioned with the arm in 90 degrees of abduction followed by 30 degrees of horizontal adduction with the thumb pointing downward. The therapist resists the patient's attempt to abduct the arm. A positive test is indicated by weakness or pain and may be indicative of a tear of the supraspinatus tendon, impingement or suprascapular nerve involvement.

Thoracic Outlet Syndrome

Adson maneuver

The patient is positioned in sitting or standing. The therapist monitors the radial pulse and asks the patient to rotate his/her head to face the test shoulder. The patient is then asked to extend his/her head while the therapist laterally rotates and extends the patient's shoulder. A positive test is indicated by an absent or diminished radial pulse and may be indicative of thoracic outlet syndrome.

Allen test

The patient is positioned in sitting or standing with the test arm in 90 degrees of abduction, lateral rotation, and elbow flexion. The patient is asked to rotate the head away from the test shoulder while the therapist monitors the radial pulse. A positive test is indicated by an absent or diminished pulse when the head is rotated away from the test shoulder. A positive test may be indicative of thoracic outlet syndrome.

Costoclavicular syndrome test

The patient is positioned in sitting. The therapist monitors the patient's radial pulse and assists the patient to assume a military posture. A positive test is indicated by an absent or diminished radial pulse and may be indicative of thoracic outlet syndrome caused by compression of the subclavian artery between the first rib and the clavicle.

Roos test

The patient is positioned in sitting or standing with the arms positioned in 90 degrees of abduction, lateral rotation, and elbow flexion. The patient is asked to open and close their hands for three minutes. A positive test is indicated by an inability to maintain the test position, weakness of the arms, sensory loss or ischemic pain. A positive test may be indicative of thoracic outlet syndrome.

Wright test (hyperabduction test)

The patient is positioned in sitting or supine. The therapist moves the patient's arm overhead in the frontal plane while monitoring the patient's radial pulse. A positive test is indicted by an absent or diminished radial pulse and may be indicative of compression in the costoclavicular space.

Miscellaneous

Glenoid labrum tear test

The patient is positioned in supine. The therapist places one hand on the posterior aspect of the patient's humeral head while the other hand stabilizes the humerus proximal to the elbow. The therapist passively abducts and laterally rotates the arm over the patient's head and then proceeds to apply an anterior directed force to the humerus. A positive test is indicated by a clunk or grinding sound and may be indicative of a glenoid labrum tear.

Elbow

Ligamentous Instability

Varus stress test

The patient is positioned in sitting with the elbow in 20 to 30 degrees of flexion. The therapist places one hand on the elbow and the other hand proximal to the patient's wrist. The therapist applies a varus force to test the lateral collateral ligament while palpating the lateral joint line. A positive test is indicated by increased laxity in the lateral collateral ligament when compared to the contralateral limb, apprehension or pain. A positive test may be indicative of a lateral collateral ligament sprain.

Valgus stress test

The patient is positioned in sitting with the elbow in 20 to 30 degrees of flexion. The therapist places one hand on the elbow and the other hand proximal to the patient's wrist. The therapist applies a valgus force to test the medial collateral ligament while palpating the medial joint line. A positive test is indicated by increased laxity in the medial collateral ligament when compared to the contralateral limb, apprehension or pain. A positive test may be indicative of a medial collateral ligament sprain.

Epicondylitis

Cozen's test

The patient is positioned in sitting with the elbow in slight flexion. The therapist places his/her thumb on the patient's lateral epicondyle while stabilizing the elbow joint. The patient is asked to make a fist, pronate the forearm, radially deviate, and extend the wrist against resistance. A positive test is indicated by pain in the lateral epicondyle region or muscle weakness and may be indicative of lateral epicondylitis.

Lateral epicondylitis test

The patient is positioned in sitting. The therapist stabilizes the elbow with one hand and places the other hand on the dorsal aspect of the patient's hand distal to the proximal interphalangeal joint. The patient is asked to extend the third digit against resistance. A positive test is indicated by pain in the lateral epicondyle region or muscle weakness and may be indicative of lateral epicondylitis.

Medial epicondylitis test

The patient is positioned in sitting. The therapist palpates the medial epicondyle and supinates the patient's forearm, extends the wrist, and extends the elbow. A positive test is indicated by pain in the medial epicondyle region and may be indicative of medial epicondylitis.

Mill's test

The patient is positioned in sitting. The therapist palpates the lateral epicondyle and pronates the patient's forearm, flexes the wrist, and extends the elbow. A positive test is indicated by pain in the lateral epicondyle region and may be indicative of lateral epicondylitis.

Neurological Dysfunction

Tinel's sign

The patient is positioned in sitting with the elbow in slight flexion. The therapist taps with the index finger between the olecranon process and the medial epicondyle. A positive test is indicated by a tingling sensation in the ulnar nerve distribution of the forearm, hand, and fingers. A positive test may be indicative of ulnar nerve compression or compromise.

Wrist/Hand

Ligamentous Instability

Ulnar collateral ligament instability test

The patient is positioned in sitting. The therapist holds the patient's thumb in extension and applies a valgus force to the metacarpophalangeal joint of the thumb. A positive test is indicated by excessive valgus movement and may be indicative of a tear of the ulnar collateral and accessory collateral ligaments. This type of injury is referred to as gamekeeper's or skier's thumb.

Vascular Insufficiency

Allen test

The patient is positioned in sitting or standing. The patient is asked to open and close the hand several times in succession and then maintain the hand in a closed position. The therapist compresses the radial and ulnar arteries. The patient is then asked to relax the hand and the therapist releases the pressure on one of the arteries while observing the color of the hand and fingers. A positive test is indicated by delayed or absent flushing of the radial or ulnar half of the hand and may be indicative of an occlusion in the radial or ulnar artery.

Capillary refill test

The patient is positioned in sitting or standing. The therapist compresses the patient's nailbed and after releasing the pressure notes the amount of time taken for the color to return to the nail. A positive test is indicated by a delayed or muted response (greater than two seconds) and may be indicative of arterial insufficiency.

Contracture/Tightness

Bunnel-Littler test

The patient is positioned in sitting with the metacarpophalangeal joint held in slight extension. The therapist attempts to move the proximal interphalangeal joint into flexion. If the proximal interphalangeal joint does not flex with the metacarpophalangeal joint extended, there may be a tight intrinsic muscle or capsular tightness. If the proximal interphalangeal joint fully flexes with the metacarpophalangeal joint in slight flexion, there may be intrinsic muscle tightness without capsular tightness.

Tight retinacular ligament test

The patient is positioned in sitting with the proximal interphalangeal joint in neutral and the distal interphalangeal joint flexed. If the therapist is unable to flex the distal interphalangeal joint the retinacular ligaments or capsule may be tight. If the therapist is able to flex the distal interphalangeal joint with the proximal interphalangeal joint in flexion, the retinacular ligaments may be tight and the capsule may be normal.

Neurological Dysfunction

Froment's sign

The patient is positioned in sitting or standing and is asked to hold a piece of paper between the thumb and index finger. The therapist attempts to pull the paper away from the patient. A positive test is indicated by the patient flexing the distal phalanx of the thumb due to adductor pollicis muscle paralysis. If at the same time the patient hyperextends the metacarpophalangeal joint of the thumb it is termed Jeanne's sign. Both objective findings may be indicative of ulnar nerve compromise or paralysis.

Phalen's test

The patient is positioned in sitting or standing. The therapist flexes the patient's wrists maximally and asks the patient to hold the position for 60 seconds. A positive test is indicated by tingling in the thumb, index finger, middle finger, and lateral half of the ring finger and may be indicative of carpal tunnel syndrome due to median nerve compression.

Tinel's sign

The patient is positioned in sitting or standing. The therapist taps over the volar aspect of the patient's wrist. A positive test is indicated by tingling in the thumb, index finger, middle finger, and lateral half of the ring finger distal to the contact site at the wrist. A positive test may be indicative of carpal tunnel syndrome due to median nerve compression.

Miscellaneous

Finkelstein test

The patient is positioned in sitting or standing and is asked to make a fist with the thumb tucked inside the fingers. The therapist stabilizes the patient's forearm and ulnarly deviates the wrist. A positive test is indicated by pain over the abductor pollicis longus and extensor pollicis brevis tendons at the wrist and may be indicative of tenosynovitis in the thumb (de Quervain's disease).

Grind test

The patient is positioned in sitting or standing. The therapist stabilizes the patient's hand and grasps the patient's thumb on the metacarpal. The therapist applies compression and rotation through the metacarpal. A positive test is indicated by pain and may be indicative of degenerative joint disease in the carpometacarpal joint.

Murphy sign

The patient is positioned in sitting or standing and is asked to make a fist. A positive test is indicated by the patient's third metacarpal remaining level with the second and fourth metacarpals. A positive test may be indicative of a dislocated lunate.

Hip

Contracture/Tightness

Ely's test

The patient is positioned in prone while the therapist passively flexes the patient's knee. A positive test is indicated by spontaneous hip flexion occurring simultaneously with knee flexion and may be indicative of a rectus femoris contracture.

Ober's test

The patient is positioned in sidelying with the lower leg flexed at the hip and the knee. The therapist moves the test leg into hip extension and abduction and then attempts to slowly lower the test leg. A positive test is indicated by an inability of the test leg to adduct and touch the table and may be indicative of a tensor fasciae latae contracture.

Piriformis test

The patient is positioned in sidelying with the test leg positioned toward the ceiling and the hip flexed to 60 degrees. The therapist places one hand on the patient's pelvis and the other hand on the patient's knee. While stabilizing the pelvis, the therapist applies a downward (adduction) force on the knee. A positive test is indicated by pain or tightness, and may be indicative of piriformis tightness or compression on the sciatic nerve caused by the piriformis.

Thomas test

The patient is positioned in supine with the legs fully extended. The patient is asked to bring one of his/her knees to the chest in order to flatten the lumbar spine.

The therapist observes the position of the contralateral hip while the patient holds the flexed hip. A positive test is indicated by the straight leg rising from the table and may be indicative of a hip flexion contracture.

Tripod sign

The patient is positioned in sitting with the knees flexed to 90 degrees over the edge of a table. The therapist passively extends one knee. A positive test is indicated by tightness in the hamstrings or extension of the trunk in order to limit the effect of the tight hamstrings.

90-90 straight leg raise test

The patient is positioned in supine and is asked to stabilize the hips in 90 degrees of flexion with the knees relaxed. The therapist instructs the patient to alternately extend each knee as much as possible while maintaining the hips in 90 degrees of flexion. A positive test is indicated by the knee remaining in 20 degrees or more of flexion and is indicative of hamstrings tightness.

Pediatric Tests

Barlow's test

The patient is positioned in supine with the hips flexed to 90 degrees and the knees flexed. The therapist tests each hip individually by stabilizing the femur and pelvis with one hand while the other hand moves the test leg into abduction while applying forward pressure posterior to the greater trochanter. A positive test is indicated by a click or a clunk and may be indicative of a hip dislocation being reduced. The test is considered to be a variation of Ortolani's test.

Ortolani's test

The patient is positioned in supine with the hips flexed to 90 degrees and the knees flexed. The therapist grasps the legs so that their thumbs are placed along the patient's medial thighs and the fingers are placed on the lateral thighs toward the buttocks. The therapist abducts the infant's hips and gentle pressure is applied to the greater trochanters until resistance is felt at approximately 30 degrees. A positive test is indicated by a click or a clunk and may be indicative of a dislocation being reduced.

Miscellaneous

Craig's test

The patient is positioned in prone with the test knee flexed to 90 degrees. The therapist palpates the posterior aspect of the greater trochanter and medially and laterally rotates the hip until the greater trochanter is parallel with the table. The degree of anteversion corresponds to the angle formed by the lower leg with the perpendicular axis of the table. Normal anteversion for an adult is 8-15 degrees.

Patrick's test (Faber test)

The patient is positioned in supine with the test leg flexed, abducted, and laterally rotated on the opposite leg. The therapist slowly lowers the test leg in abduction toward the

table. A positive test is indicated by a failure of the test leg to abduct below the level of the opposite leg and may be indicative of iliopsoas, sacroiliac or hip joint abnormalities.

Quadrant scouring test

The patient is positioned in supine. The therapist passively flexes and adducts the hip with the knee in maximal flexion. The therapist applies a compressive force through the shaft of the femur while continuing to passively move the patient's hip. A positive test is indicated by grinding, catching or crepitation in the hip and may be indicative of pathologies such as arthritis, avascular necrosis or an osteochondral defect.

Trendelenburg test

The patient is positioned in standing and is asked to stand on one leg for approximately ten seconds. A positive test is indicated by a drop of the pelvis on the unsupported side and may be indicative of weakness of the gluteus medius muscle on the supported side.

Knee

Ligamentous Instability

Anterior drawer test

The patient is positioned in supine with the knee flexed to 90 degrees and the hip flexed to 45 degrees. The therapist stabilizes the lower leg by sitting on the forefoot. The therapist grasps the patient's proximal tibia with two hands and places their thumbs on the tibial plateau and administers an anterior directed force to the tibia on the femur. A positive test is indicated by excessive anterior translation of the tibia on the femur with a diminished or absent end-point and may be indicative of an anterior cruciate ligament injury.

Lachman test

The patient is positioned in supine with the knee flexed to 20-30 degrees. The therapist stabilizes the distal femur with one hand and places the other hand on the proximal tibia. The therapist applies an anterior directed force to the tibia on the femur. A positive test is indicated by excessive anterior translation of the tibia on the femur with a diminished or absent end-point and may be indicative of an anterior cruciate ligament injury.

Lateral pivot shift test

The patient is positioned in supine with the hip flexed and abducted to 30 degrees with slight medial rotation. The therapist grasps the leg with one hand and places the other hand over the lateral surface of the proximal tibia. The therapist medially rotates the tibia and applies a valgus force to the knee while the knee is slowly flexed. A positive test is indicated by a palpable shift or clunk occurring between 20 and 40 degrees of flexion and is indicative of anterolateral rotary instability. The shift or clunk results from the reduction of the tibia on the femur.

Posterior drawer test

The patient is positioned in supine with the knee flexed to

90 degrees and the hip flexed to 45 degrees. The therapist stabilizes the lower leg by sitting on the forefoot. The therapist grasps the patient's proximal tibia with two hands and places their thumbs on the tibial plateau and administers a posterior directed force to the tibia on the femur. A positive test is indicated by excessive posterior translation of the tibia on the femur with a diminished or absent end-point and may be indicative of a posterior cruciate ligament injury.

Posterior sag sign

The patient is positioned in supine with the knee flexed to 90 degrees and the hip flexed to 45 degrees. A positive test is indicated by the tibia sagging back on the femur and may be indicative of a posterior cruciate ligament injury.

Slocum test

The patient is positioned in supine with the knee flexed to 90 degrees and the hip flexed to 45 degrees. The therapist rotates the patient's foot 30 degrees medially to test anterolateral instability or 15 degrees laterally to test anteromedial instability. The therapist stabilizes the lower leg by sitting on the forefoot. The therapist grasps the patient's proximal tibia with two hands and places their thumbs on the tibial plateau and administers an anterior directed force to the tibia on the femur. A positive test is indicated by movement of the tibia occurring primarily on the lateral side and may be indicative of anterolateral instability.

Valgus stress test

The patient is positioned in supine with the knee flexed to 20-30 degrees. The therapist positions one hand on the medial surface of the patient's ankle and the other hand on the lateral surface of the knee. The therapist applies a valgus force to the knee with the distal hand. A positive test is indicated by excessive valgus movement and may be indicative of a medial collateral ligament sprain. A positive test with the knee in full extension may be indicative of damage to the medial collateral ligament, posterior cruciate ligament, posterior oblique ligament, and posteromedial capsule.

Varus stress test

The patient is positioned in supine with the knee flexed to 20-30 degrees. The therapist positions one hand on the lateral surface of the patient's ankle and the other hand on the medial surface of the knee. The therapist applies a varus force to the knee with the distal hand. A positive test is indicated by excessive varus movement and may be indicative of a lateral collateral ligament sprain. A positive test with the knee in full extension may be indicative of damage to the lateral collateral ligament, posterior cruciate ligament, arcuate complex, and posterolateral capsule.

Meniscal Pathology

Apley's compression test

The patient is positioned in prone with the knee flexed to 90 degrees. The therapist stabilizes the patient's femur using one hand and places the other hand on the patient's heel. The therapist medially and laterally rotates the tibia while applying a compressive force through the tibia. A positive test is indicated

by pain or clicking and may be indicative of a meniscal lesion.

Bounce home test

The patient is positioned in supine. The therapist grasps the patient's heel and maximally flexes the knee. The patient's knee is extended passively. A positive test is indicated by incomplete extension or a rubbery end-feel and may be indicative of a meniscal lesion.

McMurray test

The patient is positioned in supine. The therapist grasps the distal leg with one hand and palpates the knee joint line with the other. With the knee fully flexed the therapist medially rotates the tibia and extends the knee. The therapist repeats the same procedure while laterally rotating the tibia. A positive test is indicated by a click or pronounced crepitation felt over the joint line and may be indicative of a posterior meniscal lesion.

Swelling

Brush test

The patient is positioned in supine. The therapist places one hand below the joint line on the medial surface of the patella and strokes proximally with the palm and fingers as far as the suprapatellar pouch. The other hand then strokes down the lateral surface of the patella. A positive test is indicated by a wave of fluid just below the medial distal border of the patella and is indicative of effusion in the knee.

Patellar tap test

The patient is positioned in supine with the knee flexed or extended to a point of discomfort. The therapist applies a slight tap over the patella. A positive test is indicated if the patella appears to be floating and may be indicative of joint effusion.

Miscellaneous

Clarke's sign

The patient is positioned in supine with the knees extended. The therapist applies slight pressure with the web space of their hand over the superior pole of the patella. The therapist then asks the patient to contract the quadriceps muscle while maintaining pressure on the patella. A positive test is indicated by failure to complete the contraction without pain and may be indicative of patellofemoral dysfunction.

Hughston's plica test

The patient is positioned in supine. The therapist flexes the knee and medially rotates the tibia with one hand while the other hand attempts to move the patella medially and palpate the medial femoral condyle. A positive test is indicated by a popping sound over the medial plica while the knee is passively flexed and extended.

Noble compression test

The patient is positioned in supine with the hip slightly flexed and the knee in 90 degrees of flexion. The therapist places the thumb of one hand over the lateral epicondyle of the

femur and the other hand around the patient's ankle. The therapist maintains pressure over the lateral epicondyle while the patient is asked to slowly extend the knee. A positive test is indicated by pain over the lateral femoral epicondyle at approximately 30 degrees of knee flexion and may be indicative of iliotibial band friction syndrome.

Patellar apprehension test

The patient is positioned in supine with the knees extended. The therapist places both thumbs on the medial border of the patella and applies a laterally directed force. A positive test is indicated by a look of apprehension or an attempt to contract the quadriceps in an effort to avoid subluxation and may be indicative of patella subluxation or dislocation.

Ankle

Ligamentous Instability

Anterior drawer test

The patient is positioned in supine. The therapist stabilizes the distal tibia and fibula with one hand, while the other hand holds the foot in 20 degrees of plantar flexion and draws the talus forward in the ankle mortise. A positive test is indicated by excessive anterior translation of the talus away from the ankle mortise and may be indicative of an anterior talofibular ligament sprain.

Talar tilt

The patient is positioned in sidelying with the knee flexed to 90 degrees. The therapist stabilizes the distal tibia with one hand while grasping the talus with the other hand. The foot is maintained in a neutral position. The therapist tilts the talus into abduction and adduction. A positive test is indicated by excessive adduction and may be indicative of a calcaneofibular ligament sprain.

Miscellaneous

Homans' sign

The patient is positioned in supine. The therapist maintains the leg in extension and passively dorsiflexes the patient's foot. A positive test is indicated by pain in the calf and may be indicative of deep vein thrombophlebitis.

Thompson test

The patient is positioned in prone with the feet extended over the edge of a table. The therapist asks the patient to relax and proceeds to squeeze the muscle belly of the gastrocnemius and soleus muscles. A positive test is indicated by the absence of plantar flexion and may be indicative of a ruptured Achilles tendon.

Tibial torsion test

The patient is positioned in sitting with the knees over the edge of a table. The therapist places the thumb and index finger of one hand over the medial and lateral malleolus. The therapist then measures the acute angle formed by the axes

of the knee and ankle. Normal lateral rotation of the tibia is considered to be 12-18 degrees in an adult.

True leg length discrepancy test

The patient is positioned in supine with the hips and knees extended and the legs 15 to 20 cm apart with the pelvis in balance with the legs. Using a tape measure the therapist measures from the distal point of the anterior superior iliac spines to the distal point of the medial malleoli. A positive test is indicated by a bilateral variation of greater than one centimeter and may by indicative of a true leg length discrepancy.

Spine

Cervical Region

Foraminal compression test

The patient is positioned in sitting with the head laterally flexed. The therapist places both hands on top of the subject's head and exerts a downward force. A positive test is indicated by pain radiating into the arm toward the flexed side and may be indicative of nerve root compression.

Vertebral artery test

The patient is positioned in supine. The therapist places the patient's head in extension, lateral flexion, and rotation to the ipsilateral side. A positive test is indicated by dizziness, nystagmus, slurred speech or loss of consciousness and may be indicative of compression of the vertebral artery.

Lumbar/Sacroiliac Region

Sacroiliac joint stress test

The patient is positioned in supine. The therapist crosses their arms placing the palms of the hands on the patient's anterior superior iliac spines. The therapist applies a downward and lateral force to the pelvis. A positive test is indicated by unilateral pain in the sacroiliac joint or gluteal area and may be indicative of sacroiliac joint dysfunction.

Sitting flexion test

The patient is positioned in sitting with the knees flexed to 90 degrees and the feet on the floor. The patient's hips should be abducted to allow the patient to bend forward. The therapist places his/her thumbs on the inferior margin of the posterior superior iliac spines and monitors the movement of the bony structures as the patient bends forward and reaches toward the floor. A positive test is indicated by one posterior superior iliac spine moving further in a cranial direction and may be indicative of an articular restriction.

Standing flexion test

The patient is positioned in standing with the feet 12 inches apart. The therapist places his/her thumbs on the inferior margin of the posterior superior iliac spines and monitors the movement of the bony structures as the patient bends forward with the knees extended. A positive test is indicated by one posterior superior iliac spine moving further in a cranial direction and may be indicative of an articular restriction.

Osteokinematic and Arthrokinematic Motions

Upper Extremity Joints - Osteokinematic and Arthrokinematic Motion

Joint	Resting Position	Convex/Concave	Osteokinematic/ Arthrokinematic Motion
Sternoclavicular	Anatomical position	*Elevation/depression* Convex: clavicle Concave: sternum *Protraction/retraction* Convex: sternum Concave: clavicle	Opposite direction Same direction
Acromioclavicular	Anatomical position	Convex: clavicle Concave: acromion	Opposite direction
Glenohumeral	55 degrees abduction, 30 degrees horizontal adduction	Convex: humerus Concave: glenoid	Opposite direction
Ulnohumeral	70 degrees flexion, 10 degrees supination	Convex: humerus Concave: ulna	Same direction
Radiohumeral	Full extension, full supination	Convex: humerus Concave: radius	Same direction
Proximal radioulnar	70 degrees flexion, 35 degrees supination	Convex: radius Concave: ulna	Opposite direction

Upper Extremity Joints - Osteokinematic and Arthrokinematic Motion (continued)

Joint	Resting Position	Convex/Concave	Osteokinematic/ Arthrokinematic Motion
Distal radioulnar	10 degrees supination	Convex: ulna Concave: radius	Same direction
Radiocarpal	Neutral with slight ulnar deviation	Convex: carpals Concave: radius	Opposite direction
Metacarpophalangeal joints of digits 2-5	Slight flexion	Convex: metacarpals Concave: phalanges	Same direction
Proximal and distal interphalangeal joints of the hands 2-5	Slight flexion	Convex: proximal phalanges Concave: distal phalanges	Same direction

Lower Extremity Joints - Osteokinematic and Arthrokinematic Motion

Joint	Resting Position	Convex/Concave	Osteokinematic/ Arthrokinematic Motion
Hip	30 degrees flexion, 30 degrees abduction, slight lateral rotation	Convex: femur Concave: acetabulum	Opposite direction
Tibiofemoral	25 degrees flexion	Convex: femur Concave: tibia	Same direction
Patellofemoral	25 degrees flexion	Convex: patella Concave: femur	Opposite direction
Proximal tibiofibular	0 degrees plantar flexion	Convex: tibia Concave: fibula	Same direction
Distal tibiofibular	0 degrees plantar flexion	Convex: fibula Concave: tibia	Opposite direction
Talocrural	10 degrees plantar flexion, midway between maximum inversion and eversion	Convex: talus Concave: tibia and fibula	Opposite direction
Subtalar	Midway between extremes of range of movement	Convex: anterior and middle talus Concave: anterior and middle calcaneus Convex: posterior calcaneus Concave: posterior talus	Same direction Opposite direction
Midtarsal	Midway between extremes of range of movement	Convex: more medial metatarsals Concave: more lateral metatarsals	Same direction
Metatarsophalangeal	Neutral	Convex: metatarsals Concave: phalanges	Same direction
Interphalangeal joints of the toes	Slight flexion	Convex: proximal phalanges Concave: distal phalanges	Same direction

Miscellaneous Joints - Osteokinematic and Arthrokinematic Motion

Joint	Resting Position	Convex/Concave	Osteokinematic/ Arthrokinematic Motion
Temporomandibular	Mouth slightly open (freeway space)	Convex: mandible Concave: temporalis	Opposite direction

Mobilization

Mobilization is a passive movement technique designed to improve joint function.

Indications: restricted joint mobility, restricted accessory motion, desired neurophysiological effects

Contraindications: active disease, infection, advanced osteoporosis, articular hypermobility, fracture, acute inflammation, muscle guarding, joint replacement

Grades of Movement

Grade I	Small amplitude movement performed at the beginning of range.
Grade II	Large amplitude movement performed within the range, but not reaching the limit of the range and not returning to the beginning of range.
Grade III	Large amplitude movement performed to the limit of range.
Grade IV	Small amplitude movement performed at the limit of range.
Grade V	Small amplitude, high velocity thrust technique performed to snap adhesions at the limit of range.

Convex-Concave Rule

Determines the direction of decreased joint gliding and the appropriate direction for the mobilizing force.

Convex surface moving on a concave surface:
- Roll and slide occur in the opposite direction
- Mobilizing force should be applied in the opposite direction of the bone movement

Concave surface moving on a convex surface:
- Roll and slide occur in the same direction
- Mobilizing force should be applied in the same direction as the bone movement

Mobilization Technique

- The patient should have a general understanding of the purpose of mobilization.
- The patient should be completely relaxed during treatment.
- The therapist should be in a comfortable position while performing mobilization activities.
- The therapist's position should allow for optimal control of movement. Explain specific mobilization techniques to the patient prior to beginning treatment. Complete a general examination of each patient prior to beginning mobilization activities.
- Use gravity to assist with mobilization whenever possible.
- Mobilization activities are usually performed initially with the joint in a loose packed position.
- Maintain contact with the mobilizing hand as close to the joint space as possible.
- Allow one digit to palpate the joint line when possible.
- Mobilize one joint in one direction at a time.
- Use a mobilization belt or wedge to assist with stabilization when necessary.
- Constantly modify mobilization techniques based on individual patient response.
- Compare the quality and quantity of joint play bilaterally.
- Reassess each patient prior to each treatment session.

Musculoskeletal System Profile

Examination

- Past medical history
- History of current condition
  - Surgical procedures
  - Precautions/contraindications
- Social history
- Medications
- Living environment
- Systems review
  - Vital signs
- Observation/inspection
- Postural assessment
- Reflex assessment
- Special tests
- Pain
- Range of motion
- Gait
- Mobility skills
- Strength

Intervention

- Exercise training
- Edema control
- Pain management
- Electrotherapeutic modalities
- Physical agents
- Joint mobilization
- Mobility training
- Patient/caregiver teaching:
  - Precautions/contraindications
  - Exercise program
  - Positioning
  - Competence with an assistive device
  - Proper body mechanics

Goals

- Maximize functional mobility skills
- Reduce edema to the affected areas
- Maximize strength and endurance
- Maximize range of motion
- Minimize pain
- Maximize proper posture
- Maximize tissue healing
- Maximize patient/caregiver competence with:
  - Safe use of assistive device
  - Body mechanics
  - Home exercise program
- Safe positioning for mobility

Musculoskeletal System Surgical Procedures

Total Hip Arthroplasty

Surgical Indications:

- Osteoarthritis
- Rheumatoid arthritis
- Failed internal fixation of a fracture
- Developmental dysplasia
- Osteomyelitis
- Avascular necrosis

Surgical Contraindications:

- Poor periarticular support
- Sepsis
- Active infection

Types of Total Hip Arthroplasty:

- **Cemented**
  - Immediate weight bearing as tolerated
  - May require more bone tissue removal
  - May experience loosening of the prosthesis
- **Noncemented**
  - Toe touch weight bearing for up to six weeks
  - Longer life expectancy than cemented
  - Allows a larger amount of bone tissue to remain intact
  - Allows for continued tissue growth

Potential Post-surgical Complications:

- Deep vein thrombosis
- Infection
- Heterotopic ossification
- Sciatic nerve injury
- Periprosthetic fracture
- Dislocation/subluxation of the femoral head
- Pulmonary embolus

General Post-operative Precautions (Posterolateral approach):

- Use an abduction pillow
- Maintain appropriate weight bearing status
- Avoid hip adduction
- Avoid hip medial rotation
- Avoid hip flexion > 90 degrees
- Do not sit on low surfaces
- Do not bend over towards the ground
- Do not lean over to get up from a chair
- Do not bend over to tie shoes
- Do not pivot towards the surgical side
- Do not cross the legs when sitting or lying down
- Use a pillow between the legs when sidelying

Physical Therapy Intervention:

- ✓ Maintain appropriate weight bearing status
- ✓ Mobility training using hip precautions
- ✓ Early ambulation training
- ✓ Initiate strengthening with isometric exercises and progress as tolerated
- ✓ Implement gentle stretching using hip precautions

Total Knee Arthroplasty

Surgical Indications:

- Disabling pain
- Failed conservative treatment
- Impaired mobility due to advanced arthritis

Surgical Contraindications:

- Active infection
- Advanced osteoporosis
- Severe peripheral vascular disease
- Sepsis
- Morbid obesity

Types of Total Knee Arthroplasty:

- **Cemented**
  - Immediate weight bearing as tolerated
  - Used with older and sedentary patients
- **Hybrid**
  - Toe touch weight bearing for up to six weeks
  - Cemented tibial component and noncemented femoral and patellar components
- **Noncemented**
  - Toe touch weight bearing for up to six weeks
  - Femoral, tibial, and patellar components are all noncemented
  - Longer life expectancy than cemented

Potential Post-surgical Complications:

- Deep vein thrombosis
- Infection
- Chronic joint effusion
- Periprosthetic fracture
- Restricted range of motion
- Pulmonary embolus
- Peroneal nerve palsy

General Post-operative Precautions:

- Maintain appropriate weight bearing status
- Post-surgical use of knee immobilizer for stability

Physical Therapy Intervention:

- ✓ Maintain appropriate weight bearing status
- ✓ Mobility training
- ✓ Early ambulation training with knee immobilizer
- ✓ Use of a continuous passive motion machine (CPM)
- ✓ Initiate strengthening with isometric exercises

- ✓ Initiate passive range of motion to attain 90 degrees of knee flexion and 0 degrees of knee extension
- ✓ Use compression stockings for excess edema
- ✓ Wean from the knee immobilizer once the patient gains quadriceps control

Continuous Passive Motion Machine

The continuous passive motion machine (CPM) is a mechanical device designed to provide continuous motion for a particular joint using a predetermined range and speed. Robert Salter first developed this device based on research that continuous passive motion had beneficial healing effects for joints and surrounding soft tissues. Subsequent studies looking at the beneficial effects using a CPM machine versus not using a CPM machine vary in conclusion. Some studies show no significant difference in short-term outcome for CPM use versus an alternate form of early motion. Others show benefits from using the CPM to include earlier motion resulting in shorter hospitalizations. The primary indication for CPM use is to improve range of motion that may have been impaired secondary to a surgical procedure. Any joint may be indicated for CPM use, however, the knee is the most common joint treated with a CPM machine.

Therapeutic Effects:

- May lessen the debilitating effects from immobilization
- May improve the rate of recovery
- May provide a stimulating effect on tissue healing

- May provide a quicker increase in range of motion
- May decrease post-operative pain
- May reduce edema by assisting venous and lymphatic return

Contraindications:

- If the CPM increases a patient's pain
- If the CPM causes unwanted translation of opposing bones
- Particular anticoagulant therapy that may place the patient at risk for an intracompartment hematoma

Treatment Parameters:

- ✓ CPM can be applied immediately after surgery.
- ✓ Specific protocols apply for each individual joint regarding time of use and degrees of motion.
- ✓ The patient must be instructed in the use of the CPM and all associated safety information (including how to stop the machine in case of emergency).
- ✓ The patient's joint must be positioned to correctly align with the fulcrum of the CPM in order to receive effective and safe treatment.
- ✓ The patient will usually begin with a small arc of motion and progress approximately 10 degrees per day or as tolerated.
- ✓ CPMs may be utilized at home after discharge from the hospital, if necessary. A patient or caregiver must be independent with the CPM protocol for home use.

Musculoskeletal System Pathology

Rheumatism

A condition found in a number of disorders characterized by inflammation, degeneration or metabolic derangement of the connective tissue, soreness, joint pain, and stiffness of muscles. Some conditions that present with rheumatism include: osteoarthritis, rheumatoid arthritis, juvenile rheumatoid arthritis, gout, systemic lupus erythematosus, and ankylosing spondylitis.

Physical Therapy Examination:

- Measurement of independence with functional activities
- Measurement of joint inflammation
- Measurement of joint range of motion
- Determination of limiting factors including pain, weakness, and fatigue

Physical Therapy Goals:

Short-Term Goals (Acute or Exacerbation)
- Alleviate pain
- Decrease inflammation
- Maintain strength and endurance to activity
- Provide splinting and/or assistive devices to increase safety

Long-Term Goals
- Patient independence and competence with:
  – Proper body mechanics
  – Reduction of biomechanical stressors
  – Exercise program

- Maximize functional mobility
- Maximize endurance to tolerate activities of daily living
- Demonstrate safety with ambulation and all mobility
- Management of pain

Osteoarthritis

A chronic disease that primarily involves the weight bearing joints. Osteoarthritis causes a degeneration of articular cartilage. Subsequent deformity and thickening of subchondral bone occurs with an outcome of impaired functional status. Any joint may be involved, however, the most commonly affected sites include cervical spine (C5-C6),

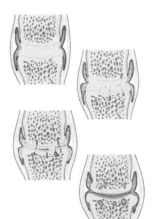

lumbar spine, hips, and knees. It is common to be diagnosed with osteoarthritis after age 40. The disease affects men more than women. Risk factors include trauma, repetitive microtrauma, and obesity.

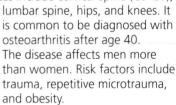

Pathogenesis:

- Cartilage becomes soft and damaged
- Osteophytes form
- Subchondral bone thickens
- Synovitis is mild to moderate

Clinical Presentation:

- Pain present at the affected joint
- Usually localized to a few joints
- Increased pain after exercise
- Increased pain with weather changes
- Joints may become enlarged
- Joint motion limitation
- Heberden's nodes
- Gradual onset
- Joint crepitus
- Joint stiffness < 15 minutes
- Bouchard's nodes

Physical Therapy Intervention:

- ✓ Rest required for the affected joints
- ✓ Patient education on disease process, energy conservation, body mechanics, and joint protection techniques
- ✓ Splinting
- ✓ Use of cold and/or heat
- ✓ Ultrasound, hydrotherapy, paraffin
- ✓ Use of assistive devices to reduce weight bearing on affected joints
- ✓ Weight loss
- ✓ Isometric exercise followed by gradual progression to isotonic exercise
- ✓ Transcutaneous electrical nerve stimulation
- ✓ NSAIDs
- ✓ Orthopedic surgical intervention

Rheumatoid Arthritis

Rheumatoid arthritis is a systemic autoimmune disorder of unknown etiology. The disease presents with a chronic inflammatory reaction in the synovial tissues of a joint that results in erosion of cartilage and supporting structures within the capsule. One to two percent of the American population is affected. Women are affected three times more than men and the most common age of onset falls between thirty and fifty years of age. Onset of rheumatoid arthritis may occur first at any joint, but it is common to find it in the small joints of the hand, foot, wrist, and ankle. This disease has periods of exacerbation and remission.

 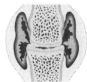 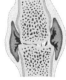

Pathogenesis:

- Thickening of synovial membrane in affected joints
- Colonization of lymphocytes which synthesize the rheumatoid factor
- Subsequent erosion of cartilage and supporting structures

Clinical Presentation:

- Onset may be gradual or immediate
- Symmetrical polyarthritis
- Pain and tenderness of affected joints
- Morning stiffness > one hour
- Warm joints
- Decrease in appetite
- Boutonniere deformity – DIP extension, PIP flexion
- Malaise and increased fatigue
- Redness at joints
- Swan neck deformity – DIP flexion, PIP hyperextension

Physical Therapy Intervention:

- ✓ Complete bed rest or regular rest periods may be indicated
- ✓ NSAIDs or other medications
- ✓ Patient education on disease process, energy conservation, body mechanics, and joint protection techniques
- ✓ Modalities such as hydrotherapy, hot pack, paraffin, or use of cold - avoid deep heat
- ✓ Splinting
- ✓ Use of assistive devices
- ✓ Passive range of motion during acute stage
- ✓ Active range of motion once in the subacute stages
- ✓ Hydrotherapy and isometrics once in the subacute stages

Types of Fractures

Avulsion fracture: A portion of a bone becomes fragmented at the site of tendon attachment from a traumatic and sudden stretch of the tendon.

Closed fracture: A break in a bone where the skin over the site remains intact.

Comminuted fracture: A bone that breaks into fragments at the site of injury.

Compound fracture: A break in a bone that protrudes through the skin.

Greenstick fracture: A break on one side of a bone that does not damage the periosteum on the opposite side. This type of fracture is often seen in children.

Nonunion fracture: A break in a bone that has failed to unite and heal after nine to twelve months.

Stress fracture: A break in a bone due to repeated forces to a particular portion of the bone.

Spiral fracture: A break in a bone shaped as an "S" due to torsion and twisting.

Musculoskeletal System Terminology

Bursitis: A condition caused by acute or chronic inflammation of the bursae. Symptoms may include a limitation in active range of motion secondary to pain and swelling.

Contusion: A sudden blow to a part of the body that can result in mild to severe damage to superficial and deep structures. Treatment includes active range of motion, ice, and compression.

Edema: An increased volume of fluid in the soft tissue outside of a joint capsule.

Effusion: An increased volume of fluid within a joint capsule.

Genu valgum: A condition where the knees touch while standing with the feet separated. Genu valgum will increase compression of the lateral tibial condyle and increase stress to the medial structures. Genu valgum is also termed knock-knee.

Genu varum: A condition where there is bowing of the legs with added space between the knees while standing with the feet together. Genu varum will increase compression of the medial tibial condyle and increase stress to the lateral structures. Genu varum is also termed bowleg.

Kyphosis: An excessive curvature of the spine in a posterior direction usually identified in the thoracic spine. Common causes include osteoporosis, compression fractures, and poor posture secondary to paralysis.

Lordosis: An excessive curvature of the spine in an anterior direction usually identified in the cervical or lumbar spine. Common causes include weak abdominal muscles, pregnancy, excessive weight in the abdominal area, and hip flexion contractures.

Myositis ossificans: A condition of heterotopic bone formation that occurs three to four weeks after a contusion or trauma within the soft tissue.

Osteoporosis: The thinning of bone matrix with eventual bone loss and an increased risk for fracture. Osteoporosis is usually found in postmenopausal women.

Causative factors for osteoporosis include decreased weight bearing, inactivity, family history, smoking, and drinking. Diagnosis of osteoporosis is made through bone density screening. Medications used to slow the process of osteoporosis include estrogen, calcium, vitamin D, calcitonin, and fluoride.

Q angle: The degree of angulation present when measuring from the midpatella to the anterosuperior iliac spine and to the tibial tubercle. A normal Q angle measured in supine with the knee straight is 13 degrees for a male and is 18 degrees for a female. An excessive Q angle can lead to pathology and abnormal tracking.

Scoliosis: A lateral curvature of the spine. Scoliosis can occur in the cervical, thoracic or lumbar curves. Classifications of scoliosis include idiopathic, non-structural, and structural.

Shoulder dislocation: A true separation of the humerus from the glenoid fossa.

Shoulder separation: A disruption in the stability of the acromioclavicular joint.

Sprain: An acute injury involving a ligament.

- **Grade I** – mild pain and swelling, little to no tear of the ligament
- **Grade II** – moderate pain and swelling, minimal instability of the joint, minimal to moderate tearing of the ligament, decreased range of motion
- **Grade III** – severe pain and swelling, substantial joint instability, total tear of the ligament, substantial decrease in range of motion

Strain: An injury involving the musculotendinous unit that involves a muscle, tendon or their attachments to bone.

- **Grade I** – localized pain, minimal swelling, and tenderness
- **Grade II** – localized pain, moderate swelling, tenderness, and impaired motor function
- **Grade III** – a palpable defect of the muscle, severe pain, and poor motor function

Tendonitis: A condition caused by acute or chronic inflammation of a tendon. Symptoms may include gradual onset, tenderness, swelling, and pain.

Musculoskeletal System Pediatric Pathology

Congenital Hip Dysplasia

Congenital hip dysplasia is a condition also known as developmental dysplasia. Presentation includes a malalignment of the femoral head with the acetabulum. The condition develops during the last trimester in utero.
- **Causative factors** may include cultural predisposition, malposition, and environmental and genetic influences.
- **Characteristics** include asymmetrical hip abduction with tightness and apparent femoral shortening of the involved side. Testing for this condition includes the Ortolani test, Barlow maneuver, and ultrasound.
- **Treatment** is dependent on age, severity, and initial attempts to reposition the femoral head within the acetabulum through the constant use of a harness, bracing, splinting or traction. Open reduction with subsequent application of a hip spica cast may be required if conservative treatment fails. Physical therapy may be indicated after cast removal for stretching, strengthening, and caregiver education.

Congenital Limb Deficiencies

A congenital limb deficiency is a malformation that occurs in utero secondary to an impaired developmental course. Congenital limb deficiencies are classified as longitudinal or transverse.
- The **causative factor** of a longitudinal limb deficiency

is an abnormality present at conception where a bone lacks potential to form. The **causative factors** of a transverse limb deficiency can include environmental factors, teratogen (thalidomide), trauma or infection.

- The primary **characteristic** of a longitudinal limb deficiency is a missing long bone such as the radius. A transverse limb deficiency is a limb that does not develop beyond a particular point.
- **Treatment** may focus on symmetrical movements, strengthening, range of motion, weight bearing activities, and prosthetic training.

Congenital Torticollis

Congenital torticollis is characterized by a unilateral contracture of the sternocleidomastoid musculature.

- Etiology is unknown, however, **causative factors** include malposition in utero, breech position in utero, and birth trauma. An infant is usually diagnosed within the first three weeks after birth.
- **Characteristics** include lateral flexion to the same side as the contracture, rotation toward the opposite side, and facial asymmetries.
- **Treatment** is usually conservative for the first year with emphasis on stretching, active range of motion, positioning, and caregiver education. Surgical management is indicated when conservative options have failed and the child is over one year of age. A surgical release followed by physical therapy may be indicated for range of motion and proper alignment.

Legg-Calve-Perthes Disease

Legg-Calve-Perthes disease is characterized by degeneration of the femoral head due to a disturbance in the blood supply (avascular necrosis). The disease is self-limiting and has four distinct stages: condensation, fragmentation, re-ossification, and remodeling.

- **Causative factors** include trauma, genetic predisposition, synovitis, vascular abnormalities, and infection.
- **Characteristics** include pain, decreased range of motion, antalgic gait, and a positive Trendelenburg sign.
- **Treatment** methods may vary but the primary focus is to relieve pain, maintain the femoral head in the proper position, and improve range of motion. Physical therapy may be required intermittently for stretching, splinting, crutch training, aquatic therapy, traction, and exercise. Orthotic devices and surgical intervention may be indicated depending on classification and severity of the condition.

Osgood-Schlatter Disease

Osgood-Schlatter disease is a condition also known as traction apophysis that results from repetitive traction on the tibial tuberosity apophysis.

- The **causative factor** is the repeated tension to the patella tendon over the tibial tuberosity in young athletes, which results in a small avulsion of the tuberosity and swelling.
- **Characteristics** of this self-limiting condition include point tenderness over the patella tendon at the insertion on the tibial tubercle, antalgic gait, and pain with increasing activity.
- **Treatment** is usually conservative with focus on education, icing, flexibility exercises, and eliminating activities that place strain on the patella tendon such as squatting, running or jumping.

Osteogenesis Imperfecta

Osteogenesis imperfecta is a connective tissue disorder that affects the formation of collagen during bone development. There are four classifications of osteogenesis imperfecta that vary in levels of severity.

- The **causative factor** is genetic inheritance with type I and IV considered autosomal dominant traits, and types II and III considered autosomal recessive traits.
- **Characteristics** of this condition include pathological fractures, osteoporosis ("brittle bones"), hypermobile joints, bowing of the long bones, weakness, scoliosis, and impaired respiratory function.
- **Treatment** begins at birth with caregiver education on proper handling and facilitation of movement. Use of orthotics, active and symmetrical movements, positioning, functional mobility, and fracture management are essential areas of treatment. In severe cases where ambulation is not realistic, wheelchair prescription and training is indicated.

Scoliosis

Scoliosis is a lateral curvature of the spine that can be classified as infantile, juvenile, adolescent or adult.

- **Causative factors** include unknown etiology, altered development of the spine in utero, association with cerebral palsy, muscular dystrophy, other neuromuscular conditions and leg length discrepancy.
- **Characteristics** indicate whether a scoliosis is a structural or non-structural curve. A structural curve cannot be corrected with active or passive movement and there is rotation of the vertebrae towards the convexity of the curve. This results in a rib hump over the thoracic region on the convex side of the curve. Asymmetries will be visually noted at the shoulders, scapulae, pelvis, and skinfolds. A non-structural curve will correct with lateral bending towards the apex of the curve. This type of curve is typically non-progressive with minimal rotation. The primary **causative factor** for a non-structural curve is a leg length discrepancy.
- **Treatment** is based on the type and severity of the curve, age, and previous management. Generally, curves that are less than 25 degrees require monitoring; curves between 25 and 40 degrees are treated with orthotic management and physical therapy intervention for posture, flexibility, respiratory function, and body mechanics. Curves that progress beyond 40 degrees require surgical intervention to improve spinal stability.

Talipes Equinovarus

Talipes equinovarus is a deformity of the ankle and foot also known as "clubfoot."

- **Causative factors** are unclear, however, theories postulate familial tendency, positioning in utero or defect in the ovum. This condition accompanies other neuromuscular abnormalities including spina bifida and arthrogryposis, and may result from the lack of movement that assists with repositioning in utero.
- **Characteristics** of this deformity involve adduction of the forefoot, various positioning of the hindfoot, and equinus at the ankle. Severe cases can include deformity of the lower leg.
- **Treatment** begins soon after birth and includes splinting and serial casting. The goal of intervention is to restore proper positioning of the foot and ankle. Failed management or severe involvement will require surgical intervention and subsequent casting.

Juvenile Rheumatoid Arthritis

Juvenile rheumatoid arthritis (JRA) is the most common chronic rheumatic disease in children and presents with inflammation of the joints and connective tissues.

- The exact etiology is unknown, however, it is theorized that **causative factors** include an external source such as a virus, infection or trauma that may trigger an autoimmune response producing JRA in a child with a genetic predisposition.
- **Characteristics** depend on the classification of JRA. *Systemic juvenile rheumatoid arthritis* occurs in 10% to 20% of children with JRA and presents with acute onset, high fevers, rash, enlargement of the spleen and liver, and inflammation of the lungs and heart. *Polyarticular juvenile rheumatoid arthritis* accounts for 30-40% of children with JRA and presents with high female incidence, RF+ majority, and arthritis in more than five joints with symmetrical joint involvement. *Oligoarticular (Pauciarticular) juvenile rheumatoid arthritis* accounts for 40-60% of children with JRA and affects less than five joints with asymmetrical joint involvement. General **characteristics** include inflammation, malaise, pain with palpation and movement, stiffness, iritis, fever, and rash.
- **Treatment** includes pharmacological management to relieve inflammation and pain through NSAIDs, corticosteroids, and antirheumatic and immunosuppressive agents. Physical therapy management includes passive and active range of motion, positioning, splinting and orthotic prescription, strengthening, endurance, weight bearing activities, postural training, and functional mobility. Pain management includes use of modalities such as paraffin, ultrasound, warm water, and cryotherapy. A realistic home program must be a constant priority. Surgical intervention may be indicated secondary to pain, contractures or irreversible joint destruction.

Pharmacology

Pharmacological Intervention for Pain/Musculoskeletal System Management

Nonopioid Agents

	Acetylsalicylic Acid
Provide analgesia and pain relief, produce anti-inflammatory effects, anti-pyretic (reduces fever) properties	Aspirin (Bayer, Ascriptin)
	Acetaminophen (Tylenol, Panadol)
	Nonsteroidal Anti-inflammatories
	Diclofenac (Voltaren)
May produce gastrointestinal distress with long-term use	Ibuprofen (Motrin, Advil)
	Indomethacin (Indocin)
	Ketorolac (Toradil)
	Naproxen sodium (Aleve)
	Celecoxib (Celebrex)

Opioid Agents (narcotics)

Provide analgesia for acute severe pain management	Morphine (MS Contin)
	Hydromorphone (Dilaudid)
	Meperidine (Demerol)
	Codeine (Codeine)
May produce mood swings, sedation, confusion, and physical dependence	Oxycodone (Oxycontin)
	Naloxone (Narcan)
	Propoxyphene (Darvon)
	Fentanyl (Sublimaze)

Glucocorticoid Agents (corticosteroids)

Produce hormonal, anti-inflammatory, and metabolic effects	Cortisol (Hydrocortone)
	Prednisone (Deltasone, Prednisone)
Suppression of articular and systemic disease processes	Dexamethasone (Decadron)
	Prednisolone (Prelone, Pediapred)
May produce muscle atrophy, gastrointestinal distress, and glaucoma	Methylprednisolone (Medrol)

*selected pharmaceutical drugs and their respective trade names in parentheses, not intended to be a complete listing

Miscellaneous

Craig's test
Patrick's test (Faber test)
Quadrant scouring test
Trendelenburg test

Knee

Ligamentous Instability

Anterior drawer test
Lachman test
Lateral pivot shift test
Posterior drawer test
Posterior sag sign
Slocum test
Valgus stress test
Varus stress test

Meniscal Pathology

Apley's compression test
Bounce home test
McMurray test

Swelling

Brush test
Patellar tap test

Miscellaneous

Clarke's sign
Hughston's plica test
Noble compression test
Patellar apprehension test

Ankle

Ligamentous Instability

Anterior drawer test
Talar tilt

Miscellaneous

Homans' sign
Thompson test
Tibial torsion test
True leg length discrepancy test

Spine

Cervical Region

Foraminal compression test
Vertebral artery test

Lumbar/Sacroiliac Region

Sacroiliac joint stress test
Sitting flexion test
Standing flexion test

Descriptions of Special Tests

Shoulder

Dislocation

Apprehension test for anterior shoulder dislocation

The patient is positioned in supine with the arm in 90 degrees of abduction. The therapist laterally rotates the patient's shoulder. A positive test is indicated by a look of apprehension or a facial grimace prior to reaching an end point.

Apprehension test for posterior shoulder dislocation

The patient is positioned in supine with the arm in 90 degrees of flexion and medial rotation. The therapist applies a posterior force through the long axis of the humerus. A positive test is indicated by a look of apprehension or a facial grimace prior to reaching an end point.

Biceps Tendon Pathology

Ludington's test

The patient is positioned in sitting and is asked to clasp both hands behind the head with the fingers interlocked. The patient is then asked to alternately contract and relax the biceps muscles. A positive test is indicated by absence of movement in the biceps tendon and may be indicative of a rupture of the long head of the biceps.

Speed's test

The patient is positioned in sitting or standing with the elbow extended and the forearm supinated. The therapist places one hand over the bicipital groove and the other hand on the volar surface of the forearm. The therapist resists active shoulder flexion. A positive test is indicated by pain or tenderness in the bicipital groove region and may be indicative of bicipital tendonitis.

Yergason's test

The patient is positioned in sitting with 90 degrees of elbow flexion and the forearm pronated. The humerus is stabilized against the patient's thorax. The therapist places one hand on the patient's forearm and the other hand over the bicipital groove. The patient is directed to actively supinate and laterally rotate against resistance. A positive test is indicated by pain or tenderness in the bicipital groove and may be indicative of bicipital tendonitis.

Rotator Cuff Pathology/Impingement

Drop arm test

The patient is positioned in sitting or standing with the arm in 90 degrees of abduction. The patient is asked to slowly lower the arm to their side. A positive test is indicated by the patient failing to slowly lower the arm to their side or by the presence of severe pain and may be indicative of a tear in the rotator cuff.

Orthotics

Types of Orthoses

Lower Extremity

Foot Orthotics

A semirigid or rigid insert worn inside a shoe that corrects foot alignment and improves function. May also be used to relieve pain. Foot orthotics are custom molded and are often designed for a specific level of functioning.

Ankle-foot Orthosis (AFOs)

A metal ankle-foot orthosis consists of two metal uprights connected proximally to a calf band and distally to a mechanical ankle joint and shoe. The ankle joint may have the ability to be locked and not allow any motion, or set to have limited anterior/posterior capability depending on the patient's need. A plastic ankle-foot orthosis is fabricated by a cast mold of the patient's lower extremity. The use of plastic is more cosmetic, lighter, and requires that if a patient presents with edema it does not significantly fluctuate. Proper fit of a plastic ankle-foot orthosis requires that a patient be casted in a subtalar neutral position. A footplate can be incorporated into the ankle-foot orthosis to assist with tone reduction. Solid ankle-foot orthoses control dorsiflexion/plantar flexion and also inversion/eversion with a trim line anterior to the malleoli. They can be fabricated to keep an ankle positioned at 90 degrees or can be fabricated with an articulating ankle joint. This articulation allows the tibia to advance over the foot during the mid to late stance phase of gait. A posterior leaf spring is a plastic AFO with a trim line posterior to the malleoli. Its primary purpose is to assist with dorsiflexion and prevent foot drop. It requires adequate medial/lateral control by the patient. Ankle-foot orthoses can also influence knee control. A floor reaction AFO assists with knee extension during stance through positioning of a calf band and/or positioning at the ankle. Ankle-foot orthoses are commonly prescribed for patients with peripheral neuropathy, nerve lesions or hemiplegia.

Knee-ankle-foot Orthosis (KAFOs)

Knee-ankle-foot orthoses provide support and stability to the knee and ankle. The orthoses can be fabricated using two metal uprights extending from the foot/shoe to the thigh with calf and thigh bands. Plastic knee-ankle-foot orthoses are fabricated by a cast mold of the patient's lower extremity. A plastic thigh shell is connected to a plastic ankle-foot orthosis through metal uprights lateral and medial to the knee joint. Both types allow for a lock mechanism at the knee that provides stability. The ankle is also held in proper alignment.

Craig-Scott knee-ankle-foot Orthosis

A knee-ankle-foot orthosis designed specifically for persons with paraplegia. This design allows a person to stand with a posterior lean of the trunk.

Hip-knee-ankle-foot Orthosis (HKAFOs)

A hip-knee-ankle-foot orthosis is indicated for patients with hip, foot, knee, and ankle weakness. It consists of bilateral knee-ankle-foot orthoses with an extension to the hip joints with use of a pelvic band. The orthosis can control rotation at the hip and abduction/adduction. The orthosis is heavy and restricts patients to a swing-to or swing-through gait pattern.

Reciprocating Gait Orthosis (RGOs)

Reciprocating gait orthoses are a derivative of the HKAFO and incorporate a cable system to assist with advancement of the lower extremities during gait. When the patient shifts weight onto a selected lower extremity, the cable system advances the opposite lower extremity. The orthoses are used primarily for patients with paraplegia.

Parapodiums

A standing frame designed to allow a patient to sit when necessary. It is a prefabricated frame and ambulation is achieved by shifting weight and rocking the base across the floor. It is primarily used by the pediatric population.

Spine

Corset

A corset is constructed of fabric and may have metal uprights within the material to provide abdominal compression and support. Corsets are utilized to provide pressure and relieve pain associated with mid and low back pathologies.

Halo Vest Orthosis

The halo vest is an invasive cervical thoracic orthosis that provides full restriction of all cervical motion. A metal ring with four posts that attach to a vest is placed on a patient and secured by inserting four pins through the ring into the skull. This orthosis is commonly used with cervical spinal cord injuries to prevent further damage or dislocation during the recovery period. A patient will wear a halo vest until the spine becomes stable.

Milwaukee Orthosis

The Milwaukee orthosis is designed to promote realignment of the spine due to scoliotic curvature. The orthosis is custom made and extends from the pelvis to the upper chest. Corrective padding is applied to the areas of severity of the curve.

Taylor Brace

The Taylor brace is a thoracolumbosacral orthosis that limits trunk flexion and extension through a three-point control design.

Thoracolumbosacral Orthosis (TLSO)

A custom molded TLSO is utilized to prevent all trunk motions and is commonly utilized as a means of post-surgical stabilization. The rigid shell is fabricated from plastics in a bivalve style using straps/Velcro to secure the orthosis.

Orthotic Basics

Functions of Orthotics

- Prevent deformity
- Assist function of a weak limb
- Maintain proper alignment of joints
- Inhibit tone
- Protect against injury of a weak joint
- Allow for maximal functional independence
- Facilitate motion

Orthotic Considerations

- Cost
- Energy efficiency
- Cosmesis
- Temporary versus permanent
- Dynamic versus static
- Encourage normal movement

Orthotic Profile

Examination

- Past medical history
- History of current condition
- Social history (caregiver support)
- Medications
- Living environment
- Systems review
- Skin assessment
- Edema/girth measurements
- Postural tone assessment
- Pathological reflex assessment
- Sensation, proprioception, and kinesthesia
- Range of motion
- Motor assessment/strength
- Mobility skills

Intervention

- Ensure continued proper fit
- Donning/doffing orthosis
- Implement progressive wearing schedule
- Patient/caregiver teaching:
  - Skin inspection
  - Care of orthosis
- Mobility training with orthosis

Goals

- Maximize functional mobility skills with orthosis
- Maximize independence with donning/doffing
- Maximize independence with wearing schedule
- Maximize independence with skin inspection
- Maximize competence with care of orthosis

Amputations and Prosthetics

Factors that Influence Vascular Disease

- Hypertension
- Aging
- Diabetes mellitus
- Infection
- Poor nutrition
- Cigarette smoking

Risk Factors for Amputation

- Vascular disease
  - Atherosclerosis/arteriosclerosis
  - Venous insufficiency
  - Buerger's disease
  - Diabetes mellitus
- Malignancy/tumor
  - Osteosarcoma
- Congenital deformities
- Infection
- Trauma

Types of Lower Extremity Amputations

Hemicorporectomy: Surgical removal of the pelvis and both lower extremities

Hemipelvectomy: Surgical removal of one half of the pelvis and the lower extremity

Hip Disarticulation: Surgical removal of the lower extremity from the pelvis

Transfemoral: Surgical removal of the lower extremity above the knee joint

Knee Disarticulation: Surgical removal through the knee joint

Transtibial: Surgical removal of the lower extremity below the knee joint

Syme's: Surgical removal of the foot at the ankle joint with removal of the malleoli

Chopart's: Disarticulation at the midtarsal joint

Transmetatarsal: Surgical removal of the midsection of the metatarsals

Considerations for Prosthetic Training

Hemipelvectomy and Hip Disarticulation

- All functions of the hip, knee, ankle, and foot are absent
- Most common cause is malignancy
- Does not allow for activation of the prosthesis through a residual limb
- Prosthetic motion must be initiated through weight bearing

Transfemoral Amputation

- Length of the residual limb with regard to leverage and energy expenditure
- No ability to weight bear through the end of the residual limb
- Susceptible to hip flexion contracture
- Adaptation required for balance, weight of prosthesis, and energy expenditure

Knee Disarticulation

- Loss of all knee, ankle, and foot function
- The residual limb can weight bear through its end
- Susceptible to hip flexion contracture
- Knee axis of the prosthesis is below the natural axis of the knee
- Gait deviations can occur secondary to the malalignment of the knee axis

Transtibial Amputation

- Loss of ankle and foot functions
- Residual limb does not allow for weight bearing at its end
- Weight bearing in the prosthesis should be distributed over the total residual limb
- Patella tendon should be the area of primary weight bearing
- Adaptations required for balance
- Susceptible to knee flexion contracture

Syme's Amputation

- Loss of all foot functions
- Residual limb can weight bear through its end
- Residual limb is bulbous with a non-cosmetic appearance
- Dog ears must be reduced for proper prosthetic fit
- Adaptation required for the increased weight of the prosthesis
- Adaptation required due to diminished toe off during gait

Transmetatarsal and Chopart's Amputation

- Loss of forefoot leverage
- Loss of balance
- Loss of weight bearing surface
- Loss of proprioception
- Tendency to develop equinus deformity

Potential Complications

Neuroma
A neuroma is a bundle of nerve endings that group together and can produce pain due to scar tissue, pressure from the prosthesis or tension on the residual limb.

Phantom Limb
Phantom limb refers to a painless sensation where the patient feels that the limb is still present. This is seen soon after the amputation and will usually subside with desensitization and prosthetic use, however, may continue for extended periods of time for some patients.

Phantom Pain
Phantom pain refers to the patient's perception of some form of painful stimuli. The pain can be continuous or intermittent, local or general, and short-term or permanent. This type of pain can disable the patient and interfere with successful rehabilitation. Treatment options include TENS, ultrasound, icing, relaxation techniques, desensitization techniques, and prosthetic use.

Wrapping Guidelines

- ✓ Elastic wrap should not have any wrinkles
- ✓ Diagonal and angular patterns should be used
- ✓ Do not wrap in circular patterns
- ✓ Provide pressure distally to enhance shaping
- ✓ Anchor wrap above the knee for transtibial amputations
- ✓ Anchor wrap around pelvis for transfemoral amputations
- ✓ Promote full knee extension for transtibial amputations
- ✓ Promote full hip extension for transfemoral amputations
- ✓ Secure the wrap with tape; do not use clips
- ✓ Use 3-4 inch wrap for transtibial amputations
- ✓ Use 6 inch wrap for transfemoral amputations
- ✓ Rewrap frequently to maintain adequate pressure

Types of Post-Operative Dressings

Rigid (Plaster of Paris)

Advantages	Disadvantages
Allows early ambulation with pylon	Immediate wound inspection is not possible
Promotes circulation and healing	Does not allow for daily dressing change
Stimulates proprioception	Requires professional application
Provides protection	
Provides soft tissue support	
Limits edema	

Semi-rigid (Una paste, air splint)

Advantages	Disadvantages
Reduces post-operative edema	Does not protect as well as the rigid dressing
Provides soft tissue support	Requires more changing than rigid dressing
Allows for earlier ambulation	May loosen and allow for development of edema
Provides protection	
Easily changed	

Soft (Ace wrap, shrinker)

Advantages	Disadvantages
Reduces post-operative edema	Tissue healing is interrupted by frequent dressing changes
Provides some protection	Joint range of motion may delay the healing of the incision
Relatively inexpensive	Increased risk of joint contractures
Easily removed for wound inspection	Less control of residual limb pain
Allows for active joint range of motion	Cannot control the amount of tension in the bandage
	Risk of a tourniquet effect

Components of a Prosthesis

	Transfemoral	Transtibial
Socket	• Quadrilateral socket • Ischial containment socket	• Patella tendon bearing socket (PTB) • Supracondylar patella tendon socket (PTS) • Supracondylar – suprapatellar socket (SC-SP)

Suspension	• Complete suction
	• Partial suction
	  – Silesian bandage
	  – Pelvic belt/band
		• Supracondylar cuff
		• Thigh corset
		• Supracondylar brim
		• Rubber sleeve suspension
		• Waist belt with fork strap

Knee	• Single axis knee
	• Polycentric knee
	
	Friction mechanisms:
	  – Constant friction
	  – Variable friction
	  – Sliding friction
	  – Hydraulic friction
	  – Pneumatic friction
		• Not needed

Shank	• Exoskeleton – rigid exterior • Endoskeleton – pylon covered with foam	• Same as transfemoral shank
Foot	• Solid ankle cushion heel (SACH) • Stationary attachment flexible endoskeleton (SAFE) • Single axis foot • Multi-axis foot	• Same as transfemoral foot

Gait Deviations

Prosthetic Causes	Amputee Causes

Lateral Bending

Prosthetic Causes	Amputee Causes
Prosthesis may be too short Improperly shaped lateral wall High medial wall Prosthesis aligned in abduction	Poor balance Abduction contracture Improper training Short residual limb Weak hip abductors on prosthetic side Hypersensitive and painful residual limb

Abducted Gait

Prosthetic Causes	Amputee Causes
Prosthesis may be too long High medial wall Poorly shaped lateral wall Prosthesis positioned in abduction Inadequate suspension Excessive knee friction	Abduction contracture Improper training Adductor roll Weak hip flexors and adductors Pain over lateral residual limb

Circumducted Gait

Prosthetic Causes	Amputee Causes
Prosthesis may be too long Too much friction in the knee Socket is too small Excessive plantar flexion of prosthetic foot	Abduction contracture Improper training Weak hip flexors Lacks confidence to flex the knee Painful anterior distal stump Inability to initiate prosthetic knee flexion

Excessive Knee Flexion During Stance

Prosthetic Causes	Amputee Causes
Socket set forward in relation to foot Foot set in excessive dorsiflexion Stiff heel Prosthesis too long	Knee flexion contracture Hip flexion contracture Pain anteriorly in residual limb Decrease in quadriceps strength Poor balance

Vaulting

Prosthetic Causes	Amputee Causes
Prosthesis may be too long Inadequate socket suspension Excessive alignment stability Foot in excess plantar flexion	Residual limb discomfort Improper training Fear of stubbing toe Short residual limb Painful hip/residual limb

Rotation of Forefoot at Heel Strike

Prosthetic Causes	Amputee Causes
Excessive toe-out built in Loose fitting socket Inadequate suspension Rigid SACH heel cushion	Poor muscle control Improper training Weak medial rotators Short residual limb

Forward Trunk Flexion

Prosthetic Causes	Amputee Causes
Socket too big Poor suspension Knee instability	Hip flexion contracture Weak hip extensors Pain with ischial weight bearing Inability to initiate prosthetic knee flexion

Medial or Lateral Whip

Prosthetic Causes	Amputee Causes
Excessive rotation of the knee Tight socket fit Valgus in the prosthetic knee Improper alignment of toe break	Improper training Weak hip rotators Knee instability

Amputation and Prosthetic Profile

Examination

- Past medical history
- History of current condition
- Social history (caregiver support)
- Medications
- Living environment
- Systems review
- Residual limb assessment
  - Level of healing
  - Color
  - Shape
  - Pulses
  - Edema
  - Girth and length
- Sensation
- Skin assessment
- Range of motion
- Balance
- Endurance
- Pain
  - Phantom limb sensation
  - Phantom pain
  - Neuroma
- Mobility skills

Preprosthetic Intervention

- Positioning
  - Prone lying
- Residual limb care
- Patient/caregiver teaching:
  - Nutrition
  - Desensitization
  - Positioning
  - Wrapping technique
  - Skin inspection and care
- Range of motion
- Strengthening
- Edema control
- Physical agents
- Electrotherapeutic modalities
- Pain management
- Endurance activities
- Balance activities
- Mobility training
- Gait training
- Wheelchair prescription
- Assistive device training

Prosthetic Intervention

- Proper adjustment/alignment of prosthesis
- Development of wearing schedule
- Skin inspection with prosthetic use
- Donning/doffing prosthesis
- Mobility training with prosthesis

Preprosthetic Goals

- Maximize functional mobility
- Maximize range of motion
- Maximize strength and endurance
- Reduce edema and promote proper shaping
- Maximize independence with wheelchair management and assistive devices
- Maximize balance
- Maximize patient/caregiver competence with:
  - Skin care and inspection
  - Wrapping
  - Desensitization techniques
  - Positioning

Prosthetic Goals

- Maximize functional mobility using prosthesis
- Maximize independence with donning/doffing prosthesis
- Maximize wearing tolerance of prosthesis
- Maximize competence with prosthetic care and use

Chapter 2 · Neuromuscular & Nervous Systems

Foundational Science: Neuroanatomy

Central Nervous System (CNS)

- Brain
- Spinal cord

Peripheral Nervous System (PNS)

- Cranial nerves and their ganglia
- Spinal nerves, their ganglia and plexuses
- Efferent and afferent somatic nerves outside the CNS
- Autonomic nervous system (ANS)
  - Sympathetic (fight or flight)
  - Parasympathetic (activated during time of rest)

Brain (Encephalon)

- **Brainstem** (midbrain or mesencephalon, pons, medulla oblongata)
- **Cerebellum**
- **Diencephalon** (hypothalamus, infundibulum, optic chiasm)
- **Cerebral hemispheres** (cortex, white matter, basal nuclei)
  - Two hemispheres, deep white matter, basal ganglia, lateral ventricles

Fissures

- **interhemispheric fissure:** separates the two cerebral hemispheres
- **Sylvian or lateral fissure:** (anterior portion) separates the temporal from frontal lobes; (posterior portion) separates temporal from parietal lobes

Sulci

- **central sulcus:** separates frontal and parietal lobes laterally
- **parieto-occipital sulcus:** separates the parietal and occipital lobes medially
- **calcarine sulcus:** separates the occipital lobe into superior and inferior halves

Meninges

Meninges is the term to describe the three layers of connective tissue covering the brain and spinal cord.

- **dura mater:** outer most meninge, has four folds, lines the periosteum of the skull
- **arachnoid:** the middle meninge, surrounds the brain in a loose manner
- **pia mater:** inner most meninge, covers the contours of the brain, forms choroid plexus in the ventricular system

Ventricular System

The ventricular system is designed to protect and nourish the brain; comprised of four ventricles and multiple foramen that allow the passage of cerebrospinal fluid (CSF). CSF acts as a cushion around the brain and spinal cord and is produced by the choroid plexus of each ventricle.

Dural Spaces

- **epidural space:** space occupied between the skull and outer dura mater
- **subdural space:** space occupied between the dura and arachnoid meninges
- **subarachnoid space:** space occupied between the arachnoid and pia mater that contains CSF and the circulatory system for the cortex

Ascending and Descending Tracts

Corticospinal tract (anterior): pyramidal motor tract responsible for ipsilateral voluntary movement

Corticospinal tract (lateral): pyramidal motor tract responsible for contralateral voluntary fine movement

Fasciculus gracilis: sensory tract for trunk and lower extremity proprioception, two-point discrimination, vibration, and graphesthesia

Fasciculus cuneatus: sensory tract for trunk, neck and upper extremity proprioception, vibration, two-point discrimination, and graphesthesia

Rubrospinal tract: extrapyramidal motor tract responsible for motor input of gross postural tone

Spinocerebellar tract (dorsal): sensory tract for ipsilateral and contralateral subconscious proprioception

Spinocerebellar tract (ventral): sensory tract for ipsilateral subconscious proprioception

Spinothalamic tract (lateral): sensory tract for pain, light touch, and temperature

Tectospinal tract: extrapyramidal motor tract responsible for contralateral posture muscle tone associated with auditory/visual stimuli

Vestibulospinal tract: extrapyramidal motor tract responsible for ipsilateral gross postural adjustments subsequent to head movements

Nerve Root Dermatomes, Myotomes, Reflexes, and Paresthetic Areas

Nerve Root	Dermatome*	Muscle Weakness (Myotome)	Reflexes Affected	Paresthesias
C1	Vertex of skull	None	None	None
C2	Temple, forehead, occiput	Longus colli, sternocleidomastoid, rectus capitis	None	None
C3	Entire neck, posterior cheek, temporal area, prolongation forward under mandible	Trapezius, splenius capitis	None	Cheek, side of neck
C4	Shoulder area, clavicular area, upper scapular area	Trapezius, levator scapulae	None	Horizontal band along clavicle and upper scapula
C5	Deltoid area, anterior aspect of entire arm to base of thumb	Supraspinatus, infraspinatus, deltoid, biceps	Biceps, brachioradialis	None
C6	Anterior arm, radial side of hand to thumb and index finger	Biceps, supinator, wrist extensors	Biceps, brachioradialis	Thumb and index finger
C7	Lateral arm and forearm to index, long, and ring fingers	Triceps, wrist flexors (rarely, wrist extensors)	Triceps	Index, long, and ring fingers
C8	Medial arm and forearm to long, ring, and little fingers	Ulnar deviators, thumb extensors, thumb adductors (rarely, triceps)	Triceps	Little finger alone or with two adjacent fingers; not ring or long fingers, alone or together (C7)
T1	Medial side of forearm to base of little finger	Disk lesions at upper two thoracic levels do not appear to give rise to root weakness. Weakness of intrinsic muscles of the hand is due to other pathology (e.g., thoracic outlet pressure, neoplasm of lung, and ulnar nerve lesion). Dural and nerve root stress has T1 elbow flexion with arm horizontal. T1 and T2 scapulae forward and backward on chest wall. Neck flexion at any thoracic level.		
T2	Medial side of upper arm to medial elbow, pectoral and midscapular areas			
T3 – T12	T3-T6, upper thorax; T5-T7, costal margin; T8-T12, abdomen and lumbar region	Articular and dural signs and root pain are common. Root signs (cutaneous analgesia) are rare and have such indefinite area that they have little localizing value. Weakness is not detectable.		
L1	Back, over trochanter and groin	None	None	Groin; after holding posture, which causes pain
L2	Back, front of thigh to knee	Psoas, hip adductors	None	Occasionally anterior thigh
L3	Back, upper buttock, anterior thigh and knee, medial lower leg	Psoas, quadriceps, thigh atrophy	Knee jerk sluggish, PKB positive, pain on full SLR	Medial knee, anterior lower leg
L4	Medial buttock, lateral thigh, medial leg, dorsum of foot, big toe	Tibialis anterior, extensor hallucis	SLR limited, neck flexion pain, weak or absent knee jerk, side flexion limited	Medial aspect of calf and ankle

Nerve Root Dermatomes, Myotomes, Reflexes, and Paresthetic Areas (continued)

Nerve Root	Dermatome*	Muscle Weakness (Myotome)	Reflexes Affected	Paresthesias
L5	Buttock, posterior and lateral thigh, lateral aspect of leg, dorsum of foot, medial half of sole, first, second, and third toes	Extensor hallucis, peroneals, gluteus medius, dorsiflexors, hamstring and calf atrophy	SLR limited one side, neck flexion painful, ankle decreased, crossed-leg raising pain	Lateral aspect of leg, medial three toes
S1	Buttock, thigh, and leg posterior	Calf and hamstrings, wasting of gluteals, peroneals, plantar flexors	SLR limited, Achilles reflex weak or absent	Lateral two toes, lateral foot, lateral leg to knee, plantar aspect of foot
S2	Same as S1	Same as S1 except peroneals	Same as S1	Lateral leg, knee, and heel
S3	Groin, medial thigh to knee	None	None	None
S4	Perineum, genitals, lower sacrum	Bladder, rectum	None	Saddle area, genitals, anus, impotence, massive posterior herniation

*In any part of which pain may be felt. PKB = prone knee bending; SLR = straight leg raising.

From Magee, DJ: Orthopedic Physical Assessment. W.B. Saunders Company, Philadelphia 2002, p.16, with permission.

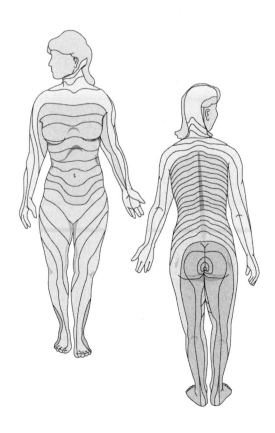

Nerves of the Brachial Plexus

Origin	Nerves	Muscles
From the rami of the plexus	Dorsal scapular	Rhomboids Levator scapulae
	Long thoracic	Serratus anterior
From the trunks of the plexus	Nerve to subclavius	Subclavius
	Suprascapular	Infraspinatus Supraspinatus
From the lateral cord of the plexus	Lateral pectoral	Pectoralis major Pectoralis minor
	Musculocutaneous	Coracobrachialis Biceps brachii Brachialis
	Lateral root of the median	Flexor muscles in the forearm, except flexor carpi ulnaris, and five muscles in the hand
From the medial cord of the plexus	Medial pectoral	Pectoralis major Pectoralis minor
	Ulnar	1 ½ muscles of the forearm and most small muscles of the hand
	Medial root of the median	Flexor muscles in the forearm, except flexor carpi ulnaris, and five muscles of the hand
From the posterior cord of the plexus	Upper subscapular	Subscapularis
	Thoracodorsal	Latissimus dorsi
	Lower subscapular	Subscapularis Teres major
	Axillary	Deltoid Teres minor
	Radial	Brachioradialis and the extensor muscles of the forearm

Lower Extremity Innervation

Lumbar Plexus:

Psoas major
Psoas minor

Sciatic Nerve-Tibial Division:

Semitendinosus
Soleus
Popliteus
Semimembranosus
Plantaris
Tibialis posterior
Gastrocnemius
Biceps femoris (long head)
Flexor hallucis longus
Flexor digitorum longus

Sacral Plexus:

Piriformis
Superior gemelli
Obturator internus
Inferior gemelli
Quadratus femoris

Sciatic Nerve-Common Peroneal Division:

Biceps femoris (short head)

Inferior Gluteal Nerve:

Gluteus maximus

Deep Peroneal Nerve:

Extensor digitorum longus
Tibialis anterior

Superior Gluteal Nerve:

Gluteus medius
Tensor fasciae latae
Gluteus minimus

Superficial Peroneal Nerve:

Peroneus longus
Peroneus brevis

Femoral Nerve:

Iliacus
Vastus lateralis
Rectus femoris
Vastus medialis
Sartorius
Vastus intermedius
Pectineus

Obturator Nerve:

Adductor longus
Gracilis
Adductor brevis
Obturator externus
Adductor magnus

Medial Plantar Nerve:

Abductor hallucis
Lumbricale I
Flexor digitorum brevis
Flexor hallucis longus

Lateral Plantar Nerve:

Abductor digiti minimi
Dorsal interossei
Quadratus plantae
Adductor hallucis
Lumbricale II, III, IV
Plantar interossei
Flexor digiti minimi brevis

Cranial Nerves and Methods of Testing

Nerve	Afferent (Sensory)	Efferent (Motor)	Test
Olfactory	Smell: Nose		Identify familiar odors (e.g., chocolate, coffee)
Optic	Sight: Eye		Test visual fields
Oculomotor		Voluntary motor: Levator of eyelid; superior, medial, and inferior recti; inferior oblique muscle of eyeball Autonomic: Smooth muscle of eyeball	Upward, downward, and medial gaze Reaction to light
Trochlear		Voluntary motor: Superior oblique muscle of eyeball	Downward and lateral gaze
Trigeminal	Touch, pain: Skin of face, mucous membranes of nose, sinuses, mouth, anterior tongue	Voluntary motor: Muscles of mastication	Corneal reflex Face sensation Clench teeth; push down on chin to separate jaws
Abducens		Voluntary motor: Lateral rectus muscle of eyeball	Lateral gaze
Facial	Taste: Anterior tongue	Voluntary motor: Facial muscles Autonomic: Lacrimal, submandibular, and sublingual glands	Close eyes tight Smile and show teeth Whistle and puff cheeks Identify familiar tastes (e.g., sweet, sour)
Vestibulocochlear (acoustic nerve)	Hearing: Ear Balance: Ear		Hear watch ticking Hearing tests Balance and coordination test
Glossopharyngeal	Touch, pain: Posterior tongue, pharynx Taste: Posterior tongue	Voluntary motor: Unimportant muscle of pharynx Autonomic: Parotid gland	Gag reflex Ability to swallow
Vagus	Touch, pain: Pharynx, larynx, bronchi Taste: Tongue, epiglottis	Voluntary motor: Muscles of palate, pharynx, and larynx Autonomic: Thoracic and abdominal viscera	Gag reflex Ability to swallow Say "Ahhh"
Accessory		Voluntary motor: Sternocleidomastoid and trapezius muscle	Resisted shoulder shrug
Hypoglossal		Voluntary motor: Muscles of tongue	Tongue protrusion (if injured, tongue deviates toward injured side)

From Magee, DJ: Orthopedic Physical Assessment. W.B. Saunders Company, Philadelphia 2002, p.69, with permission.

Sensory Testing

Light touch	Cotton ball; light pressure with finger	**Kinesthesia**	Identify direction and extent of movement of a joint or body part
Deep pain	Squeeze the forearm or calf muscle	**Temperature**	Hot and cold test tubes
Superficial pain	Pen cap, paper clip end, pin	**Stereognosis**	Identify an object without sight
Vibration	Tuning fork	**Graphesthesia**	Draw a number or letter on the skin with your finger; then identify without sight
Proprioception	Identify a static position of an extremity/part	**Two-point discrimination**	Two-point caliper on skin; identify one or two points without sight

Cranial Nerve Testing

The cranial nerves refer to twelve pairs of nerves that have their origin in the brain. The majority of cranial nerves contain both sensory and motor fibers, however, there are several exceptions. Since lesions affecting the cranial nerves produce specific and predictable alterations, it is often prudent to perform cranial nerve testing as part of a neurological examination. The following information is a summary of some of the more common methods of testing selected cranial nerves.

Cranial Nerve I - Olfactory

The patient is positioned in sitting with the eyes closed or blindfolded. The therapist places an item with a familiar odor under the patient's nostril and the patient is asked to identify the odor. A positive test may be indicated by an inability to identify familiar odors.

Cranial Nerve II - Optic

The patient is positioned in standing a selected distance from a chart or diagram. The therapist asks the patient to identify objects or read selected items from the chart or diagram. A positive test may be indicated by an inability to identify objects at a reasonable distance.

Cranial Nerve III - Oculomotor

The patient is positioned in sitting and is asked to follow an object such as a writing utensil with their eyes as it is moved vertically, horizontally, and diagonally. The therapist should make sure the patient does not rotate their head during the testing and should inspect the patient's eyes for asymmetry or ptosis. A positive test is indicated by an identified tracking deficit, asymmetry or ptosis.

Cranial Nerve IV - Trochlear

The patient is positioned in sitting and asked to follow an object such as a writing utensil with their eyes as it is moved in an inferior direction. The therapist should make sure the patient does not move his head downward. A positive test results by an inability to depress the eyes and/or complaints of diplopia.

Cranial Nerve V - Trigeminal

The patient is positioned in sitting and is asked to close their eyes. The therapist uses a piece of cotton and a safety pin to alternately touch the patient's face. The patient is asked to classify each contact with the face as "sharp" or "dull." A positive test for the sensory component may be identified by impaired or absent sensation or the inability to differentiate between "sharp" or "dull." The motor component is tested by asking the patient to perform mandibular protrusion, retrusion, and lateral deviation. A positive test may be indicated by an impaired ability to move the mandible through the specified motions.

Cranial Nerve VI - Abducens

The patient is positioned in sitting. The therapist asks the patient to abduct their eyes without rotating the head. A positive test is indicated by an inability to abduct the eyes.

Cranial Nerve VII - Facial

The patient is positioned in sitting and is asked to distinguish between sweet and salty substances placed on the anterior portion of the tongue. A positive test for the sensory component may be identified by an inability to accurately identify sweet and salty substances. The motor component is tested by performing a manual muscle test of selected muscles involved in facial expression. A positive test for the motor component may be indicated by an inability to mimic selected facial expressions due to muscle impairment.

Cranial Nerve VIII - Vestibulocochlear

The patient is positioned in sitting in a quiet location. The therapist, positioned behind the patient and to one side, slowly brings a ticking watch toward the patient's ear. The therapist records the distance from the ear when the patient is able to identify the ticking sound. The therapist repeats the procedure on the contralateral ear and compares the measurements. A positive test is indicated by an inability to hear the ticking sound at 18-24 inches or a significant bilateral difference. Alternate tests include the Weber and Rinne tests which require a 512 Hz tuning fork.

Cranial Nerve IX - Glossopharyngeal

The patient is positioned in sitting. The therapist touches the pharynx with a tongue depressor. A positive test may be indicated by lack of gagging or an inability to feel the tongue depressor touch the back of the throat. The sensory component is tested by assessing the patient's ability to distinguish objects by taste after they are placed on the posterior portion of the tongue. A positive test for the sensory component may be identified by an inability to accurately identify tasted substances, especially sour and bitter substances, placed on the posterior third of the tongue.

Cranial Nerve X - Vagus

The patient is positioned in sitting. The therapist touches the pharynx with a tongue depressor. A positive test may be indicated by a lack of gagging or an inability to feel the tongue depressor touch the back of the throat. (Same description for Cranial Nerve IX - Glossopharyngeal). If the gag reflex is absent the therapist should carefully assess the movement of the soft palate and uvula.

Cranial Nerve XI - Accessory

The patient is positioned in sitting with the arms at the side. The therapist asks the patient to shrug their shoulders and maintain the position while the therapist applies resistance through the shoulders in the direction of shoulder depression. A positive test may be indicated by an inability to maintain the test position against resistance.

Cranial Nerve XII - Hypoglossal

The patient is positioned in sitting. The therapist asks the patient to protrude the tongue. A positive test may be indicated by an inability to fully protrude the tongue or the tongue deviating to one side during protrusion.

Deep Tendon Reflexes (DTR)

A reflex is a motor response to a sensory stimulation that is used in an assessment to observe the integrity of the nervous system. Deep tendon reflexes (DTR) elicit a muscle contraction when the muscle's tendon is stimulated.

Procedure Guidelines

✓ The patient should be relaxed.
✓ The muscle should be placed on a slight stretch.
✓ A reflex hammer taps the tendon with an anticipated immediate response.
✓ Both sides of the body should be assessed.
✓ Reflexes can be graded as normal, exaggerated (hyper) or depressed (hypo) or on a scale of 0-4.

Grading

0 = no response
1+ = diminished/depressed response
2+ = active normal response
3+ = brisk/exaggerated response
4+ = very brisk/hyperactive; abnormal response

Common DTR Sites

Biceps tendon	C5-C6 spinal level
Brachioradialis tendon	C5-C6 spinal level
Triceps tendon	C7-C8 spinal level
Patellar tendon	L3-L4 spinal level
Tibialis posterior tendon	L4-L5 spinal level
Achilles tendon	S1-S2 spinal level

DTR Normal Response

Biceps tendon	Contraction of the biceps muscle
Brachioradialis tendon	Elbow flexion and/or forearm pronation
Triceps tendon	Elbow extension or contraction of the triceps muscle
Patellar tendon	Knee Extension
Tibialis posterior tendon	Plantar flexion/inversion of the foot
Achilles tendon	Plantar flexion of the foot

Peripheral Nerves

The peripheral nervous system is the nervous system that lies outside of the brain and spinal cord. The peripheral nervous system (PNS) consists of motor, sensory, and autonomic neurons. These neurons are located in cranial, spinal, and peripheral nerves. The PNS consists of 12 pairs of cranial nerves, 31 pairs of spinal nerves, and all associated ganglia and sensory receptors. Most peripheral nerves contain motor (efferent) and sensory (afferent) components.

A Fibers

- Large fibers
- Myelinated
- High conduction rate
- Contained in the alpha and gamma motor systems
- Sensory components include:
  - Muscle spindle (primary afferent ending): primary for low-threshold stretch
  - Muscle spindle (secondary afferent endings): receptors that respond to change in length
  - Golgi tendon organ: responds to tension/stretch of a tendon
  - Bare nerve endings: joint receptors, mechanoreceptors of soft tissues, exteroceptors of pain, cold, and touch.

B Fibers

- Medium fibers
- Myelinated
- Reasonably fast conduction rate
- Pre-ganglionic fibers of the autonomic system

C Fibers

- Small nerve fibers
- Poorly myelinated or unmyelinated
- Slowed conduction rate
- Post-ganglionic fibers of sympathetic system
- Exteroceptors for pain, temperature, and touch

Types of Nerve Injury

Nerve injury can occur through many mechanisms of injury. Possible etiologies include: mechanical (compression injury), crush and percussion (fracture, compartment syndrome), laceration, penetrating trauma (stab wound), stretch (traction injury), high velocity trauma (MVA), and cold (frostbite).

Neurapraxia

- Mildest form of injury
- Conduction block usually due to myelin dysfunction
- Axonal continuity conserved
- Nerve conduction is preserved proximal and distal to the lesion
- Nerve fibers are not damaged
- Recovery will occur within 4-6 weeks

Axonotmesis

- A more severe grade of injury to a peripheral nerve
- Reversible injury to damaged fibers
- Damage occurs to the axons with preservation of the endoneurium (neural connective tissue sheath), epineurium, Schwann cells, and supporting structures
- Distal Wallerian degeneration can occur
- The nerve can regenerate distal to the site of lesion at a rate of one millimeter per day

Neurotmesis

- The most severe grade of injury to a peripheral nerve
- Axon, myelin, connective tissue components are all damaged or transected
- Irreversible injury; no possibility of regeneration
- All motor and sensory loss distal to lesion becomes permanently impaired.

Peripheral Nervous System Pathology

Anterior Horn Cell	Peripheral Polyneuropathy
• Sensory component intact • Motor weakness and atrophy • Fasciculation • Decreased DTR • Example: ALS, polio	• Sensory impairments; "stocking glove" distribution • Motor weakness and atrophy; weaker distally than proximally; may have fasciculations • Decreased DTR • Example: diabetic peripheral neuropathy

Spinal Roots and Nerves	Neuromuscular Junction
• Sensory component will have corresponding dermatomal deficits • Motor weakness in an innervated pattern; may have fasciculations • Decreased DTR • Example: herniated disc	• Sensory component intact • Motor fatigue noted • Normal DTR • Example: myasthenia gravis

Peripheral Nerve (mononeuropathy)	Muscle
• Sensory loss along the nerve route • Motor weakness and atrophy in a peripheral distribution; may have fasciculations • Example: trauma	• Sensory component intact • Motor weakness; fasciculations are rare • Normal or decreased DTR • Example: muscular dystrophy

Upper versus Lower Motor Neuron Disease

	UMND	LMND
Reflexes	Hyperactive	Diminished or absent
Atrophy	Mild from disuse	Present
Fasciculations	Absent	Present
Tone	Hypertonic	Hypotonic to flaccid

Upper Motor Neuron Disease

An upper motor neuron disease is characterized by a lesion found in descending motor tracts within the cerebral motor cortex, internal capsule, brainstem or spinal cord. Symptoms include weakness of involved muscles, hypertonicity, hyperreflexia, mild disuse atrophy, and abnormal reflexes. Damaged tracts are in the lateral white column of the spinal cord.

Examples of upper motor neuron lesions include cerebral palsy, hydrocephalus, CVA, birth injuries, multiple sclerosis, and brain tumors.

Lower Motor Neuron Disease

A lower motor neuron disease is characterized by a lesion that affects nerves or their axons at or below the level of the brainstem, usually within the "final common pathway." The ventral gray column of the spinal cord may also be affected. Symptoms include flaccidity or weakness of the involved muscles, decreased tone, fasciculations, muscle atrophy, and decreased or absent reflexes.

Examples of lower motor neuron lesions include poliomyelitis, tumors involving the spinal cord, trauma, infection, and muscular dystrophy.

Blood Supply to the Brain

Posterior cerebral artery (PCA)

- Portion of midbrain
- Subthalamic nucleus
- Basal nucleus
- Thalamus
- Inferior temporal lobe
- Occipital and occipitoparietal cortices

Middle cerebral artery (MCA)

- Most of outer cerebrum

- Basal ganglia
- Posterior and anterior internal capsule
- Putamen
- Pallidum
- Lentiform nucleus

Vertebrobasilar artery

- Medulla
- Cerebellum
- Pons
- Middle occipital cortex

Cerebral Hemisphere Function

Frontal Lobe	Parietal Lobe	Temporal Lobes	Occipital Lobe
precentral gyrus, supplementary motor area, prefrontal pole, paracentral lobule, Broca's area	postcentral gyrus, parietal pole, optic radiation, Wernicke's area, Gustatory cortex	superior temporal gyrus-auditory cortex, middle/inferior temporal gyri, limbic lobe and olfactory cortex, Wernicke's area	optic radiation, striate and parastriate cortices
Responsibilities	**Responsibilities**	**Responsibilities**	**Responsibilities**
– Voluntary motor function – Advanced motor planning – Initiation of action – Cranial nerves III, IV, VI, IX, X, XII – Interpretation of emotion – Personality center – Judgment, conscience – Planning, motivation – Bladder & bowel inhibition – Broca's motor speech center (dominant); – Appreciation of intonation, understanding gestures (nondominant)	– Process perceptual and sensory information – Body schema – Contralateral pain, posture, touch, and proprioception (to arm, trunk, and leg) – Perform calculations – Spatial awareness – Sensory: speech comprehension center (dominant) – Appreciation of tone of voice and other emotional language (nondominant) – Visual tract – Taste perception	– Auditory and limbic processing – Appreciation of language (dominant) – Appreciation of music and sound (nondominant) – Memory – Learning – Affective mood centers (primitive behaviors, visceral emotions) – Short-term memory – Same responsibilities for Wernicke's area (as parietal lobe)	– Primary processing area of visual information – Visual tract – Perception of vision
Impairments	**Impairments**	**Impairments**	**Impairments**
– Contralateral weakness – Contralateral head and eye paralysis – Personality changes, antisocial behavior – Ataxia, primitive reflexes – Broca's aphasia (language deficits) – Delayed or poor initiation	– Agraphia, finger agnosia (dominant) – Constructional apraxia, dressing apraxia, anosognosia (nondominant) – Wernicke's aphasia (receptive) – Homonymous visual deficits – Impaired language comprehension – Impairment in taste	– Auditory impairment – Hearing impairment (dominant) – Impaired appreciation of music (nondominant) – Memory deficits – Learning deficits – Wernicke's aphasia – Antisocial behaviors	– Homonymous hemianopsia – Impaired extraocular muscle movement

Cerebellum

anterior, posterior, flocculonodular lobes	
Responsibilities	**Impairments**
– Coordination of motor skills – Postural tone – Sensory/motor input for trunk and extremities – Coordination of gait – Sensory/motor input from eyes and head for coordination of eye/head movement and balance	– Ataxia – Discoordination of trunk and extremities – Intention tremor – Balance deficits – Ipsilateral facial sensory loss – Dysdiadochokinesia

Cerebral Hemisphere Function (continued)

Diencephalon	Brainstem
Thalamus (specific and association nuclei)	**Midbrain** (superior cerebellar peduncles, superior/inferior colliculi, reticular formation, cerebral aqueduct, medial/lateral lemniscus, III, IV nuclei)
Responsibilities	**Responsibilities**
– Cortical arousal – Memory – Communicates information to and from the cerebral cortex	– Communication pathways between higher and lower brain centers – Auditory and visual reflexes
Hypothalamus (mamillary bodies, optic chiasm, infundibulum)	**Pons** (middle cerebellar peduncles, anterior wall of 4th ventricle, respiratory center, V, VI, VII, VIII nuclei)
Responsibilities	**Responsibilities**
– Controls basic life functions (body temperature, thirst, hunger, sleep/wake cycles) – Centers for sympathetic and parasympathetic responses – Regulates anterior pituitary gland	– Communication pathways between higher and lower brain centers
Epithalamus (pineal body, posterior commissure)	**Medulla** (inferior cerebellar peduncles, decussation of pyramidal tracts, inferior olivary nuclei, nucleus cuneatus and gracilis, IX, X, XI, XII nuclei}
Responsibilities	**Responsibilities**
– Limbic system association	– Center for respiratory, cardiac, and vasomotor homeostasis

Subthalamus
(substantia nigra, red nuclei)

Responsibilities

– Association for motor control

Pituitary
(anterior and posterior lobes)

Responsibilities

– Reproductive hormones
– Secretion of ADH/oxytocin

Internal Capsule
(tracts connecting thalamus to cortex)

Responsibilities

– Communication between cortex and spinal cord

Diencephalon	Brainstem
Impairments	**Impairments**
– Altered consciousness – Contralateral hemiparesis, hemiplegia – Dyskinesia – Visual deficits – Headache – Autonomic function	– Altered consciousness – Contralateral hemiparesis, hemiplegia – Cranial nerve injury (palsy) – Altered respiratory pattern – Attention deficits

Hemisphere Specialization/Dominance

Left	Right
• Language • Sequence and perform movements • Understand language • Produce written and spoken language • Analytical • Controlled • Logical • Rational • Mathematical calculations • Express positive emotions such as love and happiness • Process verbally coded information in an organized, logical, and sequential manner	• Nonverbal processing • Process information in a holistic manner • Artistic abilities • General concept comprehension • Hand-eye coordination • Spatial relationships • Kinesthetic awareness • Understand music • Understand nonverbal communication • Mathematical reasoning • Express negative emotions • Body image awareness

Cerebellum

• Balance • Higher level muscular movements • Integration and coordination of multi-joint movements	• Creative • Pictorial • Intuitive • Initiation, timing, and sequencing of muscle contraction

Balance

Balance can be defined as "a state of physical equilibrium," "maintenance and control of the center of gravity," and "achieving and maintaining an upright posture." All definitions assume integrated somatosensory, visual, and vestibular information within the central nervous system.

Somatosensory input

Somatosensory receptors are located in the joints, muscles, ligaments, and skin to provide proprioceptive information regarding length, tension, pressure, pain, and joint position. Proprioceptive and tactile input from the ankles, knees, hips, neck, and eye musculature provide balance information to the brain.

Visual input

Visual receptors allow for perceptual acuity regarding verticality, motion of objects and self, environmental orientation, postural sway, and movements of the head/neck. Children rely heavily on this system for maintenance of balance.

Vestibular input

The vestibular system provides the central nervous system with feedback regarding the position and movement of the head with relation to gravity. The labyrinth (which lies within the otic capsule of the temporal bone) consists of three semicircular canals filled with endolymph and two otolith organs. Semicircular canals respond to the movement of fluid with head motion. Otoliths measure the effects of gravity and movement with regard to acceleration/deceleration.

Balance Reflexes

Vestibuloocular reflex (VOR): VOR allows for head/eye movement coordination. This reflex supports gaze stabilization where the eyes can move while the head is fixed; visual tracking can also occur when both the eyes and head are moving.

Vestibulospinal reflex (VSR): VSR attempts to stabilize the body and control movement. The reflex assists with stability while the head is moving as well as coordination of the trunk during upright postures.

Automatic postural strategies: Automatic postural strategies are automatic motor responses that are used to maintain the center of gravity over the base of support. These responses always react or respond to a particular stimulus.

Ankle strategy: The ankle strategy is the first strategy to be elicited by a small range and slow velocity perturbation when the feet are on the ground. Muscle groups contract in a distal to proximal fashion to control postural sway from the ankle joint.

Hip strategy: The hip strategy is elicited by a greater force, challenge or perturbation through the pelvis and hips. The hips will move (in the opposite direction from the head) in order to maintain balance. Muscle groups contract in a proximal to distal fashion in order to counteract the loss of balance.

Suspensory strategy: The suspensory strategy is used to lower the center of gravity during standing or ambulation in order to better control the center of gravity. Examples of this strategy include knee flexion, crouching or squatting. This strategy is often used when both mobility and stability are required during a task (such as surfing).

Stepping strategy: The stepping strategy is elicited through unexpected challenges or perturbations during static standing or when the perturbation produces such a movement that the center of gravity is beyond the base of support. The lower extremities step and/or upper extremities reach to regain a new base of support.

Vertigo

Vertigo is used to describe a sense of movement and rotation of oneself or the surrounding environment. True vertigo is caused by inner ear disease.

Common causes of peripheral vertigo include benign paroxysmal positional vertigo, vestibular neuronitis, Meniere disease, and immune-mediated inner ear disease.

Common causes of central dizziness include migraine headaches and associated syndromes. Other causes include cerebellar lesions, acoustic tumors or demyelination.

Nystagmus

Nystagmus is abnormal eye movement that entails nonvolitional, rhythmic oscillation of the eyes. The speed of movement is faster in one direction than the other direction. A patient with nystagmus will also commonly complain of vertigo.

Spontaneous nystagmus: an imbalance of vestibular signals to the oculomotor neuron that causes a constant drift in one direction that is countered by a quick movement in the opposite direction.

Peripheral nystagmus: occurs with a peripheral vestibular lesion and is inhibited when the patient fixates their vision on an object.

Central nystagmus: occurs with a central lesion of the brain stem/cerebellum and is not inhibited by visual fixation on an object.

Vestibular Rehabilitation

Vestibular rehabilitation is a therapeutic intervention that can be highly successful for patients with vestibular or central balance system disorders. Exercise protocols for vestibular retraining utilize compensation, adaptation, and plasticity to increase the brain's sensitivity, restore symmetry, improve vestibuloocular control, and subsequently increase motor control and movement.

Goals for Vestibular Rehabilitation

✓ Improve balance
✓ Improve trunk stability
✓ Increase strength and range of motion in order to improve musculoskeletal balance responses and strategies
✓ Decrease the rate and risk of falls
✓ Minimize dizziness

Balance Testing

Static Standing Tests	Outcome Measurement Tools	Vertigo
• Romberg test • One-legged stance test • Timed standing test • Nudge/push test • Postural Stress test • Motor control test • The Clinical Test for Sensory Interaction on Balance	• Tinetti Performance Oriented Mobility Assessment • Berg Balance Scale • Get up and Go test • Timed Get up and Go test • Gait Assessment Rating Scale	• Hallpike-Dix test • VOR test • Oculomotor tests • Fukuda stepping test • Semicircular canal function • Hamid vestibular stress test

Nystagmus	Active Standing Tests	Other
• Head-shaking test • Head thrust test • Positional testing • Hallpike-Dix test • Electrooculo-graphy • Saccadic test • Gaze test	• The Functional Reach test • The Multi-Directional Reach test • The Sensory Organization test • Gait observation	• The Fregley-Graybiel Ataxia Test Battery • Fugl-Meyer Sensorimotor Assessment of Balance Performance Battery

Pharmacological Intervention for Vestibular Management

Antihistamine Agents Treats vertigo	Meclizine (Antivert) Dimenhydrinate (Dramamine)
Anticholinergic Agents Decreases conduction in vestibular-cerebellar pathways	Scopolamine (Isopto) Glycopyrrolate (Robinul)
Benzodiazepine Agents Treats vertigo and emesis	Diazepam (Valium)
Phenothiazine Agents Treats emesis	Promethazine (Phenergan) Prochlorperazine (Compazine)
Monoaminergic Agents Treats vertigo	Ephedrine (Pretz-D)

*Selected pharmaceutical and trade names in parentheses, not intended to be a complete listing

Vestibulooccular Retraining Therapeutic Guidelines

✓ Vestibuloocular reflex (VOR) stimulation exercises

✓ Ocular motor exercises

✓ Balance exercises

✓ Gait exercises

✓ Combination exercises (obstacle courses, functioning at the mall)

✓ Habituation training exercises (use only with appropriate patients)

✓ Individualize each program based on the patient's specific impairments (rehabilitation vs. compensation training)

✓ Use of practice, feedback, and repetition are vital for skill refinement

✓ Use of gravity, varying surface conditions, visual conditions, and environmental cues should be included in therapeutic planning

✓ The center of gravity must be controlled at each stage of treatment

✓ Strategy (hip, ankle, stepping, suspense) training that should be implemented during treatment so strategies become automatic responses

✓ Forceplate systems, electromyographic biofeedback, optokinetic visual stimulation, and videography are all technical systems that can provide feedback to motor learning during vestibular rehabilitation

✓ Foam, mirrors, rocker boards, BAPS boards, Swiss balls, foam roller, trampolines, and wedges are lower "tech" treatment tools that are successfully used for vestibular rehabilitation

Communication Disorders

Aphasia (Dysphasia)

Aphasia is an acquired neurological impairment of processing for receptive and/or expressive language. Aphasia is the result of brain injury, head trauma, CVA, tumor or infection. There are multiple forms of aphasia; diagnosis is based on the site of lesion in the brain and the blood vessels involved. Patients with aphasia are classified based on observation of:

- Fluent versus non-fluent
- Good versus poor comprehension
- Good versus poor repetition

Fluent Aphasia

- Lesion often in temporoparietal lobe of dominant hemisphere
- Word output is functional
- Speech production is functional
- Prosody is acceptable
- "Empty speech" or jargon
- Speech lacks any substance
- Use of paraphasias (substitution of incorrect words)

Wernicke's Aphasia

- Lesion found at the posterior region of the superior temporal gyrus
- Major fluent aphasia
- Also known as receptive aphasia
- Comprehension (reading/auditory) impaired
- Use of paraphasias
- Good articulation
- Use of neologism (fabricated words)
- Impaired writing
- Poor naming ability

Conduction Aphasia

- Lesion of the supramarginal gyrus and arcuate fasciculus
- Major fluent aphasia
- Severe impairment with repetition
- Intact fluency
- Good comprehension
- Speech interrupted by word-finding difficulties
- Reading intact
- Writing impaired

Anomic Aphasia

- Lesion of angular gyrus
- Minor fluent aphasia
- Word finding difficulties with writing and speech
- Functional comprehension
- Good repetition skills
- Speech can seem empty; words regarding content are dropped

Non-fluent Aphasia

- Lesion often in frontal region of the dominant hemisphere
- Poor word output
- Increased effort for producing speech
- Poor articulation
- Dysprosodic speech
- Content of speech is present, but syntactical words are impaired

Broca's Aphasia

- Major non-fluent aphasia
- Also known as "expressive aphasia"
- Most common form of aphasia
- Lesions of the 3rd convolution of the frontal lobe
- Intact auditory and reading comprehension
- Impaired repetition and naming skills
- Frequent frustration regarding language skill errors

Global Aphasia

- Major non-fluent aphasia
- Lesion of frontal, temporal, and parietal lobes
- Comprehension (reading and auditory) is severely impaired
- Impaired naming and writing skills
- Impaired repetition skills
- May involuntarily verbalize; usually without correct context
- May use nonverbal (gestures) skills for communication

Prognosis is dependent on the individual patient, location, and extent of lesion. The following characteristics associated with aphasia are often associated with a poor prognosis: perseveration of speech, severe auditory comprehension impairments, unreliable yes/no answers, and the use of empty speech without recognition of impairments.

Verbal Apraxia

Apraxia is a non-dysarthric and non-aphasic impairment of prosody and articulation of speech. Verbal expression is impaired secondary to deficits in motor planning. A patient is unable to initiate learned movement (articulation of speech) even though they understand the task. Lesions are usually found in the left frontal lobe adjacent to Broca's area.

Dysarthria

Dysarthria is a motor disorder of speech that is caused by an upper motor neuron lesion that affects the muscles that are used to articulate words and sounds. Speech is often noted as "slurred" and there may also be an effect on respiratory or phonatory systems due to the weakness.

Cerebrovascular Accident (CVA)

Types of Cerebrovascular Accidents

Completed Stroke

A CVA that presents with total neurological deficits at the onset.

Stroke in Evolution

A CVA, usually caused by a thrombus that gradually progresses. Total neurological deficits are not seen for one to two days after onset.

Ischemic Stroke

Once there is a loss of perfusion to a portion of the brain (within just seconds) there is a central area of irreversible infarction surrounded by an area of potential ischemia.

– Embolus (20% of ischemic CVAs)

Associated with cardiovascular disease, an embolus may be a solid, liquid or gas, and can originate in any part of the body. The embolus travels through the bloodstream to the cerebral arteries causing occlusion of a blood vessel and a resultant infarct. The middle cerebral artery is most commonly affected by an embolus from the internal carotid arteries. Due to the sudden onset of occlusion, tissues distal to the infarct can sustain higher permanent damage than those of thrombotic infarcts. An embolic CVA occurs rapidly with no warning, and often presents with a headache. Common cardiac disorders that can lead to embolism include valvular disease (i.e., rheumatic mitral stenosis), ischemic heart disease, acute myocardial infarction, arrhythmias (i.e., atrial fibrillation), patent foramen ovale, cardiac tumors, and post cardiac catheterization.

– Thrombus

An atherosclerotic plaque develops in an artery and eventually occludes the artery or a branching artery causing an infarct. This type of CVA is extremely variable in onset where symptoms can appear in minutes or over several days. A thrombotic CVA usually occurs during sleep or upon awakening, after a myocardial infarction or post-surgical procedure.

Hemorrhage (10 - 15% of CVAs)

An abnormal bleeding in the brain due to a rupture in blood supply. The infarct is due to disruption of oxygen to an area of the brain and compression from the accumulation of blood. Hypertension is usually a precipitating factor causing rupture of an aneurysm or arteriovenous malformation. Trauma can also precipitate hemorrhage and subsequent CVA. Characteristics include severe headache, vomiting, high blood pressure, and abrupt onset of symptoms. Hemorrhage usually occurs during the day with symptoms evolving in relation to the speed of the bleed. Approximately 50% of deaths from hemorrhagic stroke occur within the first 48 hours.

Transient Ischemic Attack (TIA)

A transient ischemic attack is usually linked to an atherosclerotic thrombosis. There is a temporary interruption of blood supply to an area. The effects may be similar to a CVA, but symptoms resolve quickly. A TIA most often occurs in the carotid and vertebrobasilar arteries and may indicate future CVA.

Risk Factors for Cerebrovascular Accident

Primary	Secondary
• Hypertension • Heart disease • Diabetes mellitus • Cigarette smoking • Transient ischemic attacks	• Obesity • High cholesterol • Behaviors related to hypertension • Physical inactivity • Increased alcohol consumption

Expected Impairment Based on Vascular Involvement

Anterior Cerebral Artery	Posterior Cerebral Artery	Middle Cerebral Artery	Lacunar Infarct

• Lower extremity involvement
• Loss of bowel and bladder control
• Loss of behavioral inhibition
• Significant mental changes
• May see neglect
• May see aphasia
• May see apraxia and agraphia
• Perseveration
	• Pain and temperature sensory loss
	• Contralateral hemiplegia (central area)
	• Ataxia, athetosis or choreiform movement
	• Quality of movement is impaired
	• Thalamic pain syndrome
	• Anomia
	• Prosopagnosia with occipital infarct
	• Hemiballismus
	• Visual agnosia
	• Homonymous hemianopsia
	• Mild hemiparesis
	• Memory impairment
	• Dyschromatopsia
	• Palinopsia, micropsia, macropsia
	• Alexia, dyslexia
	• Achromatopsia
		• Most common site of a CVA
		• Wernicke's aphasia in dominant hemisphere
		• Homonymous hemianopsia
		• Apraxia
		• Flat affect in right hemisphere
		• Superficial MCA - greater face and arm involvement
		• Deep MCA - pure motor hemiplegia without sensory impairment
		• Impaired spatial relations
		• Anosognosia in non-dominant hemisphere
		• Impaired body schema
			• Cystic cavity after infarct
			• Contralateral weakness
			• Sensory loss
			• Ataxia
			• Dysarthria
			• Deep regions of the brain:
			  – internal capsule
			  – thalamus
			  – basal ganglia
			  – pons

Vertebral-Basilar Artery

- Loss of consciousness
- Hemiplegia or tetraplegia
- Comatose or vegetative state
- Inability to speak
- Locked-in syndrome
- Vertigo
- Nystagmus
- Dysphagia
- Dysarthria
- Syncope
- Ataxia

Characteristics of a Cerebrovascular Accident

Right Hemisphere

- Weakness, paralysis of the left side
- Decreased attention span
- Left hemianopsia
- Decreased awareness and judgment
- Memory deficits
- Left inattention
- Decreased abstract reasoning
- Emotional lability
- Impulsive behaviors
- Decreased spatial orientation

Left Hemisphere

- Weakness, paralysis of the right side
- Increased frustration
- Decreased processing
- Possible aphasia (expressive, receptive, global)
- Possible dysphagia

- Possible motor apraxia (ideomotor and ideational)
- Decreased discrimination between left and right
- Right hemianopsia

Brainstem

- Unstable vital signs
- Decreased consciousness
- Decreased ability to swallow
- Weakness on both sides of the body
- Paralysis on both sides of the body

Cerebellum

- Decreased balance
- Ataxia
- Decreased coordination
- Nausea
- Decreased ability for postural adjustment
- Nystagmus

Synergy Patterns

When the central nervous system is damaged as with a CVA, the higher centers of the brain are also damaged. The higher centers are responsible for both complex motor patterns and the inhibition of massive gross motor patterns. Synergy patterns result when the higher centers of the brain lose control and the uncontrolled or partially controlled stereotyped patterns of the middle and lower centers emerge.

Upper Limb

	Flexor Synergy	Extensor Synergy
Scapula	Elevation and retraction	Depression and protraction
Shoulder	Abduction and lateral rotation	Medial rotation and adduction
Elbow	Flexion	Extension
Forearm	Supination	Pronation
Wrist	Flexion	Extension
Fingers	Flexion with adduction	Flexion with adduction
Thumb	Flexion and adduction	Adduction and flexion

- **The flexor synergy is seen when the patient attempts to lift up their arm or reach for an object.**

Lower Limb

	Flexor Synergy	Extensor Synergy
Hip	Abduction and lateral rotation	Extension, medial rotation and adduction
Knee	Flexion	Extension
Ankle	Dorsiflexion with supination	Plantar flexion with inversion
Toes	Extension	Flexion and adduction

- **The flexor synergy is characterized by great toe extension and flexion of the remaining toes secondary to spasticity.**

Theories of Neurological Rehabilitation

Bobath: Neuromuscular Developmental Treatment

Neuromuscular Developmental Treatment (NDT)

An approach developed by Karl and Berta Bobath based on the hierarchical model of neurophysiologic function. Abnormal postural reflex activity and abnormal muscle tone is caused by the loss of central nervous system control at the brainstem and spinal cord levels. The concept recognizes that interference of normal function of the brain caused by central nervous system dysfunction leads to a slowing down or cessation of motor development and the inhibition of righting reactions, equilibrium reactions, and automatic movements. The patient should learn to control movement through activities that promote normal movement patterns that integrate function.

Key Terminology

Facilitation: A technique utilized to elicit voluntary muscular contraction.

Inhibition: A technique utilized to decrease excessive tone or movement.

Key points of control: Specific handling of designated areas of the body (shoulder, pelvis, hand, and foot) will influence and facilitate posture, alignment, and control.

Placing: The act of moving an extremity into a position that the patient must hold against gravity.

Reflex inhibiting posture: Designated static positions that Bobath found to inhibit abnormal tonal influences and reflexes.

Intervention

- ✓ Inhibition of abnormal patterns with facilitation of normal patterns
- ✓ Alteration of abnormal tone and influencing isolated active movement
- ✓ Avoid utilization of abnormal reflexes
- ✓ Manual contact and handling through key points of control for facilitation and inhibition
- ✓ Achieve a balance between muscle groups
- ✓ Use of developmental sequence
- ✓ Provide the patient with the sensation of normal movement by inhibiting abnormal postural reflex activity
- ✓ Use of dynamic reflex inhibiting patterns
- ✓ Use of functional activities with varying levels of difficulty
- ✓ Treatment should be active and dynamic
- ✓ Avoid associated reactions
- ✓ Emphasize the component of rotation during treatment activities
- ✓ Orientation to midline control by moving in and out of midline with dynamic activity
- ✓ Compensation techniques are avoided and perceived as unnecessary

Brunnstrom: Movement Therapy in Hemiplegia

Movement Therapy in Hemiplegia

Movement therapy in hemiplegia developed by Signe Brunnstrom is based on the hierarchical model by Hughlings Jackson. This approach created and defined the term synergy and initially encouraged the use of synergy patterns during rehabilitation. The belief was to immediately practice synergy patterns and subsequently develop combinations of movement patterns outside of the synergy. Synergies are considered primitive patterns that occur at the spinal cord level as a result of the hierarchical organization of the central nervous system. Reinforcing synergy patterns is rarely utilized now as research has indicated that reinforced synergy patterns are very difficult to change. Brunnstrom developed the *seven stages of recovery*, which are used for evaluation and documentation of patient progress.

Key Terminology

Associated reactions: An involuntary and automatic movement of a body part as a result of an intentional active or resistive movement in another body part.

Homolateral synkinesis: A flexion pattern of the involved upper extremity facilitates flexion of the involved lower extremity.

Limb synergies: A group of muscles that produce a predictable pattern of movement in flexion or extension patterns.

Raimiste's phenomenon: The involved lower extremity will abduct/adduct with applied resistance to the uninvolved lower extremity in the same direction.

Souque's phenomenon: Raising the involved upper extremity above 100 degrees with elbow extension will produce extension and abduction of the fingers.

Stages of recovery: Brunnstrom separates neurological recovery into seven separate stages based on progression through abnormal tone and spasticity. These seven stages of recovery describe tone, reflex activity, and volitional movement.

Seven Stages of Recovery

Stage 1: No volitional movement initiated.

Stage 2: The appearance of basic limb synergies. The beginning of spasticity.

Stage 3: The synergies are performed voluntarily; spasticity increases.

Stage 4: Spasticity begins to decrease. Movement patterns are not dictated solely by limb synergies.

Stage 5: A further decrease in spasticity is noted with independence from limb synergy patterns.

Stage 6: Isolated joint movements are performed with coordination.

Stage 7: Normal motor function is restored.

Brunnstrom: Movement Therapy in Hemiplegia (continued)

Intervention

- ✓ Evaluation of strength focuses on patterns of movement rather than straight plane motion at a joint
- ✓ Sensory examination is required to assist with treating motor deficits
- ✓ Initially limb synergies are encouraged as a necessary milestone for recovery

- ✓ Encourage overflow to recruit active movement of the weak side
- ✓ Use of repetition of task and positive reinforcement
- ✓ A patient will follow the stages of recovery, but may experience a plateau at any point so that full recovery is not achieved
- ✓ Movement combinations that deviate from the basic limb synergies should be introduced in stage 4 of recovery

Kabat, Knott, and Voss: Proprioceptive Neuromuscular Facilitation (PNF)

Proprioceptive Neuromuscular Facilitation (PNF)

PNF was introduced in the early 1950's using the hierarchical model as its framework. The original goal of treatment was to lay down gross motor patterns within the central nervous system. This approach is based on the premise that stronger parts of the body are utilized to stimulate and strengthen the weaker parts. Normal movement and posture is based on a balance between control of antagonist and agonist muscle groups. Development will follow the normal sequence through a component of motor learning. This theory places great emphasis on manual contacts and correct handling. Short and concise verbal commands are used along with resistance throughout the full movement pattern. The PNF approach utilizes methods that promote or hasten the response of the neuromuscular mechanism through stimulation of the proprioceptors. Movement patterns follow diagonals or spirals that each possess a flexion, extension, and rotatory component and are directed toward or away from midline.

Key Terminology

Chopping: A combination of bilateral upper extremity asymmetrical extensor patterns performed as a closed-chain activity.

Developmental sequence: A progression of motor skill acquisition. The stages of motor control include mobility, stability, controlled mobility, and skill.

Mass movement patterns: The hip, knee, and ankle move into flexion or extension simultaneously.

Overflow: Muscle activation of an involved extremity due to intense action of an uninvolved muscle or group of muscles.

Intervention

- ✓ A patient learns diagonal patterns of movement
- ✓ Techniques must have accurate timing, specific commands, and correct hand placement
- ✓ Verbal commands must be short and concise
- ✓ Repetition is important in motor learning
- ✓ Resistance given during the movement pattern is greater if the objective is stability, less if the objective is mobility
- ✓ Techniques utilize isometric and isotonic muscle contractions
- ✓ Treatment objectives will dictate the use of techniques through either full movement or at points within the range
- ✓ Developmental sequence is used in conjunction with PNF techniques in order to increase the balance between agonists and antagonists
- ✓ PNF techniques are implemented to progress a patient through the stages of motor control
- ✓ Functional patterns of movement are used to increase control
- ✓ Techniques should be utilized that increase strength or improve relaxation by enhancing irradiation from the stronger to the weaker muscles

PNF Diagonal Patterns – Upper Extremity Responses

	D1 Flexion Pattern	D1 Extension Pattern	D2 Flexion Pattern	D2 Extension Pattern
Scapula	Elevation Abduction Upward rotation	Depression Adduction Downward rotation	Elevation Adduction Upward rotation	Depression Abduction Downward rotation
Shoulder	Flexion Adduction Lateral rotation	Extension Abduction Medial rotation	Flexion Abduction Lateral rotation	Extension Adduction Medial rotation
Elbow	Flexion or extension	Flexion or extension	Flexion or extension	Flexion or extension
Radioulnar	Supination	Pronation	Supination	Pronation
Wrist	Flexion Radial deviation	Extension Ulnar deviation	Extension Radial deviation	Flexion Ulnar deviation
Thumb	Adduction	Abduction	Extension	Opposition

PNF Diagonal Patterns – Lower Extremity Responses

	D1 Flexion Pattern	D1 Extension Pattern	D2 Flexion Pattern	D2 Extension Pattern
Pelvis	Protraction	Retraction	Elevation	Depression
Hip	Flexion Adduction Lateral rotation	Extension Abduction Medial rotation	Flexion Abduction Medial rotation	Extension Adduction Lateral rotation
Knee	Flexion or extension	Flexion or extension	Flexion or extension	Flexion or extension
Ankle and Toes	Dorsiflexion Inversion	Plantar flexion Eversion	Dorsiflexion Eversion	Plantar flexion Inversion

Levels of Motor Control

Mobility

The ability to initiate movement through a functional range of motion.

Stability

The ability to maintain a position or posture through cocontraction and tonic holding around a joint. Unsupported sitting with midline control is an example of stability.

Controlled Mobility

The ability to move within a weight bearing position or rotate around a long axis. Activities in prone on elbows or weight shifting in quadruped are examples of controlled mobility.

Skill

The ability to consistently perform functional tasks and manipulate the environment with normal postural reflex mechanisms and balance reactions. Skill activities include ADLs and community locomotion.

PNF Therapeutic Exercises

Technique	Mobility		Stability	Controlled Mobility	Skill		Strength
	Increased ROM	Initiate Movement			Distal Functional Movement	Proximal Dynamic Stability	
Agonistic Reversals				X		X	
Alternating Isometrics			X				X
Contract-Relax	X						
Hold-Relax	X						
Hold-Relax Active Movement		X					
Joint Distraction	X	X					
Normal Timing					X		
Repeated Contractions		X					X
Resisted Progression						X	X
Rhythmic Initiation		X					
Rhythmical Rotation	X	X					
Rhythmic Stabilization	X		X				
Slow Reversal			X	X	X		
Slow Reversal Hold			X	X	X		
Timing for Emphasis							X

PNF Therapeutic Exercise Descriptions

*Italicized terms indicate level of developmental sequence.

Agonistic Reversals (AR)

Controlled mobility, skill: An isotonic concentric contraction performed against resistance followed by alternating concentric and eccentric contractions with resistance. AR requires use in a slow and sequential manner, and may be used in increments throughout the range to attain maximum control.

Alternating Isometrics (AI)

Stability: Isometric contractions are performed alternating from muscles on one side of the joint to the other side without rest. AI emphasizes endurance or strengthening.

Contract-Relax (CR)

Mobility: A technique used to increase range of motion. As the extremity reaches the point of limitation the patient performs a maximal contraction of the antagonistic muscle group. The therapist resists movement for eight to ten seconds with relaxation to follow. The technique is repeated until no further gains in range of motion are noted during the session.

Hold-Relax (HR)

Mobility: An isometric contraction used to increase range of motion. The contraction is facilitated for all muscle groups at the limiting point in the range of motion. Relaxation occurs and the extremity moves through the newly acquired range to the next point of limitation until no further increases in range of motion occur. The technique is often used for patients that present with pain.

Hold-Relax Active Movement (HRAM)

Mobility: A technique to improve initiation of movement to muscle groups tested at 1/5 or less. An isometric contraction is performed once the extremity is passively placed into a shortened range within the pattern. Overflow and facilitation may be used to assist with the contraction. Upon relaxation the extremity is immediately moved into a lengthened position of the pattern with a quick stretch. The patient is asked to return the extremity to the shortened position through an isotonic contraction.

Joint Distraction

Mobility: A proprioceptive component used to increase range of motion around a joint. Consistent manual traction is provided slowly and usually in combination with mobilization techniques. It can also be used in combination with quick stretch to initiate movement.

Normal Timing (NT)

Skill: A technique used to improve coordination of all components of a task. NT is performed in a distal to proximal sequence. Proximal components are restricted until the distal components are activated and initiate movement. Repetition of the pattern produces a coordinated movement of all components.

Repeated Contractions (RC)

Mobility: A technique used to initiate movement and sustain a contraction through the range of motion. Repeated contractions is used to initiate a movement pattern, throughout a weak movement pattern or at a point of weakness within a movement pattern. The therapist provides a quick stretch followed by isometric or isotonic contractions.

Resisted Progression (RP)

Skill: A technique used to emphasize coordination of proximal components during gait. Resistance is applied to an area such as the pelvis, hips, or extremity during the gait cycle in order to enhance coordination, strength or endurance.

Rhythmic Initiation (RI)

Mobility: A technique used to assist initiating movement when hypertonia exists. Movement progresses from passive ("let me move you"), to active assistive ("help me move you"), to slightly resistive ("move against the resistance"). Movements must be slow and rhythmical to reduce the hypertonia and allow for full range of motion.

Rhythmical Rotation (RR)

Mobility: A passive technique used to decrease hypertonia by slowly rotating an extremity around the longitudinal axis. Relaxation of the extremity will increase range of motion.

Rhythmic Stabilization (RS)

Mobility, stability: A technique used to increase range of motion and coordinate isometric contractions. The technique requires isometric contractions of all muscles around a joint against progressive resistance. The patient should relax and move into the newly acquired range and repeat the technique. If stability is the goal, RS should be applied as a progression from AI in order to stabilize all muscle groups simultaneously around the specific body part.

Slow Reversal (SR)

Stability, controlled mobility, skill: A technique of slow and resisted concentric contractions of agonists and antagonists around a joint without rest between reversals. This technique is used to improve control of movement and posture.

Slow Reversal Hold (SRH)

Stability, controlled mobility, skill: Using slow reversal with the addition of an isometric contraction that is performed at the end of each movement in order to gain stability.

Timing for Emphasis (TE)

Skill: Used to strengthen the weak component of a motor pattern. Isotonic and isometric contractions produce overflow to weak muscles.

Motor Control: A Task-Oriented Approach

Theories of motor control have been documented since the late nineteenth century when Sir Charles Sherrington postulated the reflex theory of motor control. Motor control refers to the ability to produce, regulate, and alter mechanisms that produce movement and control posture. The various theories are based on a specific interpretation of how the brain functions and interacts with other body systems. A task-oriented approach to motor control utilizes a systems theory of motor control that views the entire body as a mechanical system with many interacting subsystems that all work cooperatively in managing internal and environmental influences. The task-oriented approach utilizes an examination that consists of observation of functional performance, analysis of strategies used to accomplish tasks, and assessment of impairments. Treatment attempts to resolve impairments, design and implement effective recovery and compensatory strategies, and retrain using functional activities.

Key Terminology

Compensation: The ability to utilize alternate motor and sensory strategies due to an impairment that limits the normal completion of a task.

Motor learning: The ability to perform a movement as a result of internal processes that interact with the environment and produce a consistent strategy to generate the correct movement.

Plasticity: The ability to modify or change at the synapse level either temporarily or permanently in order to perform a particular function.

Postural control: The ability of the motor and sensory systems to stabilize position and control movement.

Recovery: The ability to utilize previous strategies to return to the same level of functioning.

Strategy: A plan used to produce a specific result or outcome that will influence the structure or system.

Intervention

- ✓ Models of motor control vary based on the interpretation of brain function
- ✓ Evaluation determines the degree of impairment
- ✓ Intervention is designed at the level of impairment
- ✓ Sensory, motor, and cognitive strategies are used to acquire postural control
- ✓ Focus is both on recovery and compensatory techniques
- ✓ Tasks are broken down into components of the task for practice
- ✓ Sensory, motor, and perceptual input contribute to motor control
- ✓ Movement is based around a behavioral goal
- ✓ Variable practice allows for training in a different and changing environment
- ✓ Type and amount of feedback (visual, verbal) should be evaluated for each individual patient
- ✓ Emphasis on postural control, alignment, and sequencing of movements is essential
- ✓ Intervention should create multiple ways to solve a movement disorder
- ✓ Environmental factors must be considered with intervention, planning, and implementation

Rood

This theory is based on Sherrington and the reflex stimulus model. Rood believed that all motor output was the result of both past and present sensory input. Treatment is based on sensorimotor learning. It takes into account the autonomic nervous system and emotional factors as well as motor ability. Rood used a developmental sequence, which was seen as "key patterns" in the enhancement of motor control. A goal of this approach is to obtain homeostasis in motor output and to activate muscles and perform a task independently of a stimulus. Exercise is seen as a treatment technique only if the response is correct and if it provides sensory feedback that enhances the motor learning of that response. Once a response is obtained during treatment the stimulus should be withdrawn. Rood introduced the use of sensory stimulation to facilitate or inhibit responses such as icing and brushing in order to elicit desired reflex motor responses.

Sensory Stimulation Techniques

Facilitation	Inhibition
• Approximation • Joint compression • Icing • Light tough • Quick stretch • Resistance • Tapping • Traction	• Deep pressure • Prolonged stretch • Warmth • Prolonged cold • Carotid reflex

Key Terminology

Heavy work: A method used to develop stability by performing an activity (work) against gravity or resistance. Heavy work focuses on the strengthening of postural muscles.

Light work: A method used to develop controlled movement and skilled function by performing an activity (work) without resistance. Light work focuses on the extremities.

Key patterns: A developmental sequence designed by Rood that directs patients' mobility recovery from synergy patterns through controlled motion.

Intervention

- ✓ Use of sensory stimulation to achieve motor output
- ✓ Movement is considered autonomic and noncognitive
- ✓ Homeostasis of all systems is essential
- ✓ Use of techniques such as neutral warmth, maintained pressure, and slow rhythmical stroking to calm a patient
- ✓ Tactile stimulation is used to facilitate normal movement
- ✓ Exercise must provide proper sensory feedback in order to be therapeutic

Pharmacological Intervention for CVA Management

Thrombolytic Agents – Produces anticoagulation effects, destroys thrombus/emboli	Heparin Ximelagatran Alteplase (Activase) Warfarin (Coumadin) Tissue-type plasminogen activator (tPA)
Antiplatelet Agents – Reduce atherosclerotic events and decrease the risk for CVA	Aspirin (Bayer, Ascriptin) Ticlopidine (Ticlid) Clopidogrel (Plavix) Dipyridamole (Persantine)
Cholesterol-lowering Agents – Decrease the triglycerides and low-density lipoproteins in the bloodstream	Atorvastatin (Lipitor) Lovastatin (Mevacor) Pravastatin (Pravachol) Simvastatin (Zocor) Gemfibrozil (Lopid)
Neuroprotective Agents – Administered only within the acute stage of CVA	N-methyl-D-aspartate (NMDA)
Antiarrhythmic Agents – Prevention of arrhythmias, ischemia and hypertension – Sodium channel blockers – Beta-blockers (cardiac medications p. 113) – Refractory period alterations – Calcium channel blockers (cardiac medications p. 113)	**Sodium channel blockers** Encainide (Enkaid) Lidocaine (Xylocaine) Procainamide (Pronestyl) Quinidine (Biquin) Disopyramide (Norpace) **Refractory period alterations** Amlodarone (Cordarone) Ibutilide fumarate

Antihypertensive Agents
– Assist to lower blood pressure; decrease tension within the circulation system
	Diuretics
	  Thiazide
	  Furosemide (Lasix)
	  Chlorothiazide (Divril)
	  Bumetanide (Bumex)
	  Amiloride (Midamor)
	Beta-blockers
	  Acebutolol (Sectral)
	  Pindolol (Visken)
	  Ateolol (Tenormin)
	  Propanolol (Inderal)
	  Metoprolol (Lopressor)
	Calcium channel blockers
	  Amlodipine (Norvasc)
	  Diltiazem (Cardizem)
	  Nicardipine (Cardene)
	  Verapamil (Calan)
	Alpha-blockers
	  Phenoxybenzamine (Dibenzyline)
	  Prazosin (Minipress)
	  Terazosin (Hytrin)
	  Doxazosin (Cardura)

*selected pharmaceutical drugs and their respective trade names in parentheses, not intended to be a complete listing

Neuromuscular and Nervous Systems Profile

Examination

- Past medical history
- History of current condition
- Social history (caregiver support)
- Medications
- Living environment
- Systems review
- Cognitive and language assessment
- Respiratory assessment
- Postural tone assessment
- Righting and equilibrium reaction assessment
- Pathological reflex assessment
- Pain
- Sensation, proprioception, and kinesthesia
- Range of motion
- Motor assessment
- Mobility skills

Intervention

- Postural control
- Positioning
- Therapeutic exercise
- Developmental activities training
- Facilitation/inhibition techniques
- Motor function retraining
- Sensory integration
- Wheelchair and orthotic prescription
- Mobility training

Goals

- Maximize functional mobility
- Normalize tonal abnormalities
- Maximize active isolated movement and strength
- Maximize range of motion and joint integrity
- Maximize independence with adaptive equipment
- Maximize static and dynamic balance
- Maximize patient/caregiver competence with:
  - Positioning
  - Use of adaptive equipment and orthotic devices
  - Home exercise programs

Neuromuscular and Nervous Systems Terminology

Agnosia: The inability to interpret information.

Agraphesthesia: The inability to recognize symbols, letters or numbers traced on the skin.

Agraphia: The inability to write due to a lesion within the brain.

Akinesia: The inability to initiate movement; commonly seen in patients with Parkinson's disease.

Aphasia: The inability to communicate or comprehend due to damage to specific areas of the brain.

Apraxia: The inability to perform purposeful learned movements, although there is no sensory or motor impairment.

Astereognosis: The inability to recognize objects by sense of touch.

Ataxia: The inability to perform coordinated movements.

Athetosis: A condition that presents with involuntary movements combined with instability of posture. Peripheral movements occur without central stability.

Bradykinesia: Movement that is very slow.

Chorea: Movements that are sudden, random, and involuntary.

Clonus: A characteristic of an upper motor neuron lesion; involuntary alternating spasmodic contraction of a muscle precipitated by a quick stretch reflex.

Constructional apraxia: The inability to reproduce geometric figures and designs. This person is visually unable to analyze how to perform a task.

Decerebrate rigidity: A characteristic of a corticospinal lesion at the level of the brainstem that results in extension of the trunk and all extremities.

Decorticate rigidity: A characteristic of a corticospinal lesion at the level of the diencephalon where the trunk and lower extremities are positioned in extension and the upper extremities are positioned in flexion.

Diplopia: Double vision

Dysarthria: Slurred and impaired speech due to a motor deficit of the tongue or other muscles essential for speech.

Dysdiadochokinesia: The inability to perform rapidly alternating movements.

Dysmetria: The inability to control the range of a movement and the force of muscular activity.

Dysphagia: The inability to properly swallow.

Dystonia: Closely related to athetosis, however, there is larger axial muscle involvement rather than appendicular muscles.

Emotional lability: A characteristic of a right hemisphere infarct where there is an inability to control emotions and outbursts of laughing or crying that are inconsistent with the situation.

Hemiballism: An involuntary and violent movement of a large body part.

Hemiparesis: A condition of weakness on one side of the body.

Hemiplegia: A condition of paralysis on one side of the body.

Homonymous hemianopsia: The loss of the right or left half of the field of vision in both eyes.

Ideational apraxia: The inability to formulate an initial motor plan and sequence tasks where the proprioceptive input necessary for movement is impaired.

Ideomotor apraxia: A condition where a person plans a movement or task, but cannot volitionally perform it. Automatic movement may occur, however, a person cannot impose additional movement on command.

Kinesthesia: The ability to perceive the direction and extent of movement of a joint or body part.

Neglect: The inability to interpret stimuli on the left side of the body due to a lesion of the right frontal lobe of the brain.

Perseveration: The state of repeatedly performing the same segment of a task or repeatedly saying the same word/phrase without purpose.

Proprioception: The ability to perceive the static position of a joint or body part.

Rigidity: A state of severe hypertonicity where a sustained muscle contraction does not allow for any movement at a specified joint.

Synergy: A result of brain damage that presents with mass movement patterns that are primitive in nature and coupled with spasticity.

Spinal Cord Injury

Types of Spinal Cord Injury

Complete lesion: A lesion to the spinal cord where there is no preserved motor or sensory function below the level of lesion.

Incomplete lesion: A lesion to the spinal cord with incomplete damage to the cord. There may be scattered motor function, sensory function or both below the level of lesion.

Specific Incomplete Lesions

Anterior Cord Syndrome

An incomplete lesion that results from compression and damage to the anterior part of the spinal cord or anterior spinal artery. The mechanism of injury is usually cervical flexion. There is loss of motor function and pain and temperature sense below the lesion due to damage of the corticospinal and spinothalamic tracts.

Brown-Sequard's Syndrome

An incomplete lesion usually caused by a stab wound, which produces hemisection of the spinal cord. There is paralysis and loss of vibratory and position sense on the same side as the lesion due to the damage to the corticospinal tract and dorsal columns. There is a loss of pain and temperature sense on the opposite side of the lesion from damage to the lateral spinothalamic tract. Pure Brown-Sequard's syndrome is rare since most spinal cord lesions are atypical.

Cauda Equina Injuries

An injury that occurs below the L1 spinal level where the long nerve roots transcend. Cauda equina injuries can be complete, however, they are frequently incomplete due to the large number of nerve roots in the area. A cauda equina injury is considered a peripheral nerve injury. Characteristics include flaccidity, areflexia, and impairment of bowel and bladder function. Full recovery is not typical due to the distance needed for axonal regeneration.

Central Cord Syndrome

An incomplete lesion that results from compression and damage to the central portion of the spinal cord. The mechanism of injury is usually cervical hyperextension that damages the spinothalamic tract, corticospinal tract, and dorsal columns. The upper extremities present with greater involvement than the lower extremities and greater motor deficits exist as compared to sensory deficits.

Posterior Cord Syndrome

A relatively rare syndrome that is caused by compression of the posterior spinal artery and is characterized by loss of pain perception, proprioception, two-point discrimination, and stereognosis. Motor function is preserved.

Potential Complications of Spinal Cord Injury

Autonomic Dysreflexia

Autonomic dysreflexia is perhaps the most dangerous complication of spinal cord injury and can occur in patients with lesions above T6. A noxious stimulus below the level of the lesion triggers the autonomic nervous system causing a sudden elevation in blood pressure. Common causes include distended or full bladder, kink or blockage in the catheter, bladder infections, pressure ulcers, extreme temperature changes, tight clothing, or even an ingrown toenail. If not treated, this condition can lead to convulsions, hemorrhage, and death.

Symptoms: High blood pressure, severe headache, blurred vision, stuffy nose, profuse sweating, goose bumps below the level of the lesion, and vasodilation (flushing) above the level of injury.

Treatment: The first reaction to this medical crisis is to check the catheter for blockage. The bowel should also be checked for impaction. A patient should remain in a sitting position. Lying a patient down is contraindicated and will only assist to further elevate blood pressure. The patient should be examined for any other irritating stimuli. If the cause remains unknown, the patient should receive immediate medical intervention.

Deep Vein Thrombosis (DVT)

Deep vein thrombosis results from the formation of a blood clot that becomes dislodged and is termed an embolus. This is considered a serious medical condition since the embolus may obstruct a selected artery. A patient with a spinal cord injury has a greater risk of developing a DVT due to the absence or decrease in the normal pumping action by active contractions of muscles in the lower extremities. Homans' sign is a special test designed to confirm the presence of a DVT. Prevention of a DVT should include prophylactic anticoagulant therapy, maintaining a positioning schedule, range of motion, proper positioning to avoid excessive venous stasis, and use of elastic stockings.

Symptoms: Swelling of the lower extremity, pain, sensitivity over the area of the clot, and warmth in the area.

Treatment: Once a DVT is suspected there should be no active or passive movement performed to the involved lower extremity. Bed rest and anticoagulant drug therapy are usually indicated. Surgical procedures can be performed if necessary.

Ectopic Bone

Ectopic bone or heterotopic ossification refers to the spontaneous formation of bone in the soft tissue. It typically occurs adjacent to larger joints such as the knees or the hips. Theories regarding etiology range from tissue hypoxia to abnormal calcium metabolism.

Symptoms: Early symptoms include edema, decreased range of motion, and increased temperature of the involved joint.

Treatment: Drug intervention usually involves diphosphates that inhibit ectopic bone formation. Physical therapy and surgery are often incorporated into treatment. Physical therapy must focus on maintaining functional range of motion and allowing the patient the most independent functional outcome possible.

Orthostatic Hypotension

Orthostatic hypotension or postural hypotension occurs due to a loss of sympathetic control of vasoconstriction in combination with absent or severely reduced muscle tone. Venous pooling is fairly common during the early stages of rehabilitation. A decrease in systolic blood pressure greater than 20 mm Hg after moving from a supine position to a sitting position is typically indicative of orthostatic hypotension.

Symptoms: Complaints of dizziness, light-headedness, nausea, and "blacking out" when going from a horizontal to a vertical position.

Treatment: Monitoring vital signs assists with minimizing the effects of orthostatic hypotension. The use of elastic stockings, ace wraps to the lower extremities, and abdominal binders are common. Gradual progression to a vertical position using a tilt table is often indicated. Drug intervention may be indicated in order to increase blood pressure.

Pressure Ulcers

A pressure ulcer is caused by sustained pressure, friction, and/or shearing to a surface. The most common areas susceptible to pressure ulcers are the coccyx, sacrum, ischium, trochanters, elbows, buttocks, malleoli, scapulae, and prominent vertebrae. Pressure ulcers require immediate medical intervention and often can significantly delay the rehabilitation process.

Symptoms: A reddened area that persists; an open area.

Treatment: Prevention is of greatest importance. A patient should change position frequently, maintain proper skin care, sit on an appropriate cushion, consistently weight shift, and maintain proper nutrition and hydration. Surgical intervention is often necessary with advanced pressure ulcers.

Spasticity

Spasticity can occasionally be useful to a patient with a spinal cord injury, however, more often serves to interfere with functional activities. Spasticity can be enhanced by both internal and external sources such as stress, decubiti, urinary tract infections, bowel or bladder obstruction, temperature changes or touch.

Symptoms: Increased involuntary contraction of muscle groups, increased tonic stretch reflexes, excessive deep tendon reflexes.

Treatment: Medications are usually administered in an attempt to reduce the degree of spasticity (Dantrium, Baclofen, Lioresal). Aggressive treatment includes phenol blocks, rhizotomies, myelotomies, and other surgical intervention. Physical therapy intervention includes positioning, aquatic therapy, weight bearing, functional electrical stimulation, range of motion, resting splints, and inhibitive casting.

Functional Outcomes for Complete Lesions				
Functional Skills	**Level of Assistance Required (by SCI level groups)**			
	High Tetraplegia (C1-C5)	**Mid-Level Tetraplegia (C6)**	**Low Tetraplegia (C7-C8)**	**Paraplegia**
Bed Mobility • Rolling side to side • Rolling supine/prone • Supine/sitting • Scooting all directions	– Dependent (C1-C4) – Moderate to maximal assistance (C5) – Verbally direct	– Minimal assistance to modified independent with equipment – Verbally direct	– Independent with all	– Independent
Transfers • Bed • Car • Toilet • Bath equipment • Floor • Upright wheelchair	– Dependent (C1-C4) – Maximal assistance with level sliding board transfers (C5) – Verbally direct	– Minimal assistance to modified independent for sliding board transfers – Dependent with wheelchair loading in car – Dependent with floor transfers and uprighting wheelchair – Verbally direct	– Modified independent to independent with level surface transfer (sliding board) – Moderate assistance to modified independent with car transfer – Maximal to moderate assistance with floor transfers and uprighting wheelchair – Verbally direct	– Independent with level surface and car transfers (depression) – Minimal assistance to independent with floor transfers and uprighting wheelchair – Verbally direct

Functional Outcomes for Complete Lesions

Functional Skills	Level of Assistance Required (by SCI level groups)			
	High Tetraplegia (C1-C5)	Mid-Level Tetraplegia (C6)	Low Tetraplegia (C7-C8)	Paraplegia
Weight Shifts • Pressure relief • Repositioning in wheelchair	– Setup to modified independent with power recline/tilt weight shift – Dependent with manual recline/tilt/lean weight shift – Verbally direct	– Modified independent with power recline/tilt weight shift – Minimal assistance to modified independent with side to side/forward lean weight shift – Verbally direct	– Modified independent with side to side/forward lean, or depression weight shift	– Modified independent with depression weight shift
Wheelchair Management • Wheel locks • Armrests • Footrests/legrests • Safety strap(s) • Cushion adjustment • Anti-tip levers • Wheelchair maintenance	– Dependent with all – Able to verbally direct	– Some assistance required – Able to verbally direct	– May require assistance with cushion adjustment, anti-tip levers, and wheelchair maintenance – Able to verbally direct	– Independent with all
Wheelchair Mobility • Smooth surfaces • Up/down ramps • Up/down curbs • Rough terrain • Up/down steps (manual wheelchair only)	– Supervision/setup to modified independent on smooth, ramp, and rough terrain with power wheelchair – Modified independent with manual wheelchair on smooth surface in forward direction (C5) – Maximal assistance to dependent with manual wheelchair in all other situations (C5) – Able to verbally direct	– Modified independent in smooth, ramp, and rough terrain with power wheelchair – Dependent to maximal assistance up/down curb with power wheelchair – Modified independent on smooth surfaces with manual wheelchair – Moderate to minimal assistance on ramps and rough terrain with manual wheelchair – Maximal to moderate assistance up/down curbs with manual wheelchair – Able to verbally direct	– Modified independent on smooth, ramp, and rough terrain with power wheelchair – Dependent to maximal assistance up/down curb with power wheelchair – Modified independent on smooth surfaces and up/down ramps with manual wheelchair – Minimal assistance to modified independent on rough terrain – Moderate to minimal assistance up/down curbs with manual wheelchair – Dependent to maximal assistance up/down steps with manual wheelchair – Can verbally direct	– Minimal assistance to modified independent up/down 6″ curbs with manual wheelchair – Modified independent with descending steps with manual wheelchair – Maximal to minimal assistance to ascend steps with manual wheelchair – Able to verbally direct
Gait • Don/doff orthoses • Sit/stand • Smooth surfaces • Up/down ramps • Up/down curbs • Up/down steps • Rough terrain • Safe falling	– Not applicable	– Not applicable	– Not applicable	– Abilities range from: – exercise only with KAFOs* – household gait with KAFOs – limited community gait with KAFOs or AFOs* – functional community ambulation with or without orthoses

Functional Outcomes for Complete Lesions

Functional Skills	Level of Assistance Required (by SCI level groups)			
	High Tetraplegia (C1-C5)	Mid-Level Tetraplegia (C6)	Low Tetraplegia (C7-C8)	Paraplegia
ROM/Positioning • PROM to trunk, legs, and arms • Pad/position in bed	– Dependent – Able to verbally direct	– Moderate assistance to modified independent with all – Able to verbally direct	– Minimal assistance to modified independent with all – Able to verbally direct	– Independent
Feeding • Drinking • Finger feeding • Utensil feeding	– Dependent (C1-C4) – Minimal assistance with adaptive equipment (C5) – Able to verbally direct	– Modified independent with adaptive equipment	– Modified independent with adaptive equipment (C7)	– Independent
Grooming • Face • Teeth • Hair • Makeup • Shaving face	– Dependent (C1-C4) – Minimal assistance with adaptive equipment for face, teeth, makeup/shaving (C5) – Maximal/moderate assistance for hair grooming (C5) – Able to verbally direct	– Modified independent with adaptive equipment	– Modified independent	– Independent
Dressing • Dressing and undressing (in bed or wheelchair) • Upper body/lower body (in bed or wheelchair)	– Dependent – Able to verbally direct	– Modified independent for upper body in bed or wheelchair – Minimal assistance with lower body dressing in bed – Moderate assistance with lower body undressing in bed – Able to verbally direct	– Modified independent for upper/lower body dressing in bed – Minimal assistance with lower body dressing/undressing in wheelchair (C7) – Modified independent for upper/lower body dressing/undressing in wheelchair (C8) – Able to verbally direct	– Modified independent
Bathing • Bathing and drying off • Upper body and lower body	– Dependent – Able to verbally direct	– Minimal assistance for upper body bathing and drying – Moderate assistance for lower body bathing and drying – Use of shower or tub chair – Able to verbally direct	– Modified independent with all using shower or tub chair	– Modified independent with all on tub bench or tub bottom cushion
Bowel/Bladder Problems • Intermittent catheterization • Leg bag care • Condom application • Clean up • In bed/wheelchair (bladder) • Feminine hygiene • Bowel program	– Dependent – Able to verbally direct	**Bladder:** – Minimal assistance for male in bed or wheelchair – Moderate assistance for female in bed **Bowel:** – Moderate assistance with use of equipment – Able to verbally direct	**Bladder:** – Modified independent for male in bed or wheelchair – Modified independent for female in bed; moderate assistance for female in wheelchair **Bowel:** – Minimal assistance to modified independent with use of equipment – Able to direct	**Bladder:** – Modified independent for male and female **Bowel:** – Modified independent for male and female

*KAFO = knee-ankle-foot orthosis; AFO = ankle-foot orthosis

From Umphred DA: Neurological Rehabilitation. Mosby-Year Book, Inc. 1995, p. 502-505, with permission.

Pharmacological Intervention for SCI Management

Corticosteroid Agents Administered within eight hours after injury to prevent overall decline in white matter within the cord. Allows for enhanced blood flow and reduces post-traumatic ischemia	Methylprednisolone (Adlone, DepoMedrol, Medrol) Dexamethasone (AK-Dex, Baldex, Decadron) GM-1 (GM-1 is a complex acidic glycolipid administered with methylprednisolone to enhance recovery)	**Biphosphonate Agents** Prevent demineralization and SCI-induced osteoporosis	Pamidronate (Aredia) Cyclical Etidronate (Didronel) Clodronate (Bonetos) Ibandronate (Boniva)
Antispasticity Agents reduces tension in the muscles	Baclofen (Lioresal) Tizanidine Clonidine (Catapres) Diazepam (Valium) Gabapentin Dantrolene (Dantrium)	**Agents for Bladder Program**	Minipress Probanthine Ditropan Urecholine
Anticonvulsant Agents Treatment of neurogenic pain	Gabapentin	**Agents for Bowel Program**	Dulcolax Glycerine Docusate sodium Mylicon Pericolace
Tricyclic Antidepressants Treatment of neurogenic pain	Amitriptyline (Elavil) Doxepin (Sinequan) Desipramine (Norpramin) Clomipramine (Anafranil) Nortriptiline (Pamelor)	**Antibone Resorption Agents** Treats heterotopic ossification through inhibiting bone resorption and formation and prevents ossification	Etidronate (Didronel) Alendronate (Fosamax)
Parathyroid Hormone Promotes new bone formation and an increase in bone mineral density	Teriparatide (Forteo)	**Anticoagulation Agents** Prevents deep vein thrombus	Warfarin (Coumadin) Heparin (unfractionated heparin) Enoxaparin (Lovenox)

*selected pharmaceutical drugs and their respective trade names in parentheses, not intended to be a complete listing

Spinal Cord Injury Profile

Examination

- Past medical history
- History of current condition
- Social history (caregiver support)
- Medications
- Living environment
- Systems review
- Cognitive assessment
- Skin assessment
- American Spinal Cord Injury Association (ASIA) Standard Neurological Classification
  - Sensory examination
  - Motor examination
- American Spinal Cord Injury Association (ASIA) impairment scale
- Respiratory assessment
  - Cough
  - Chest expansion
  - Accessory muscle use
  - Vital capacity
- Range of motion
- Pain
- Mobility skills

Intervention

- Positioning
- Family/caregiver teaching
- Respiratory training
  - Assisted cough and secretion clearance
  - Breathing exercises
- Wheelchair, cushion, and orthotic prescription
- Pressure relief
- Range of motion
- Motor function retraining
- Mobility training
- Gait training (T9 or lower)

Goals

- Maximize functional mobility based on level of injury (please refer to "functional outcome" chart)
- Maximize respiratory function
- Attain functional range of motion for all joints
- Maximize strength of available muscle groups
- Maximize patient/caregiver competence with:
  - Pressure relief
  - Positioning
  - Range of motion
  - Strengthening
  - Wheelchair management

Spinal Cord Injury Terminology

Cauda equina injury: A term used to describe injuries that occur below the L1 level of the spine. A cauda equina injury is considered to be a lower motor neuron lesion.

Dermatome: Designated sensory areas based on spinal segment innervation.

Myelotomy: A surgical procedure that severs certain tracts within the spinal cord in order to decrease spasticity and improve function.

Myotome: Designated motor areas based on spinal segment innervation.

Neurectomy: A surgical removal of a segment of a nerve in order to decrease spasticity and improve function.

Neurogenic bladder: The bladder empties reflexively for a patient with an injury above the level of S2. The sacral reflex arc remains intact.

Neurologic level: The lowest segment (most caudal) of the spinal cord with intact strength and sensation. Muscle groups at this level must receive a grade of fair.

Nonreflexive bladder: The bladder is flaccid as a result of a cauda equina or conus medullaris lesion. The sacral reflex arc is damaged.

Paraplegia: A term used to describe injuries that occur at the level of the thoracic, lumbar or sacral spine.

Rhizotomy: A surgical resection of the sensory component of a spinal nerve in order to decrease spasticity and improve function.

Sacral sparing: An incomplete lesion where some of the innermost tracts remain innervated. Characteristics include sensation of the saddle area, movement of the toe flexors, and rectal sphincter contraction.

Spinal shock: A physiologic response that occurs between 30 and 60 minutes after trauma to the spinal cord and can last up to several weeks. Spinal shock presents with total flaccid paralysis and loss of all reflexes below the level of injury.

Tenotomy: A surgical release of a tendon in order to decrease spasticity and improve function.

Tetraplegia (quadriplegia): A term adopted by the American Spinal Cord Injury Association to describe injuries that occur at the level of the cervical spine.

Zone of preservation: A term used to describe poor or trace motor or sensory function for up to three levels below the neurologic level of injury.

Traumatic Brain Injury

Types of Injury

Open Injury

An injury of direct penetration through the skull to the brain. Location, depth of penetration, and pathway determine the extent of brain damage. Examples include gunshot wound, knife or sharp object penetration, skull fragments, and direct trauma.

Closed Injury

An injury to the brain without penetration through the skull. Examples include concussion, contusion, hematoma, injury to extracranial blood vessels, hypoxia, drug overdose, near drowning, and acceleration or deceleration injuries.

Primary Injury

Initial injury to the brain sustained by impact. Examples include skull penetration, skull fractures, and contusions to gray and white matter.

Coup lesion: A direct lesion of the brain under the point of impact. Local brain damage is sustained.

Contrecoup lesion: An injury that results on the opposite side of the brain. The lesion is due to the rebound effect of the brain after impact.

Secondary Injury

Brain damage that occurs as a response to the initial injury. Examples include hematoma, hypoxia, ischemia, increased intracranial pressure, and post-traumatic epilepsy.

Epidural hematoma: A hemorrhage that forms between the skull and dura mater.

Subdural hematoma: A hemorrhage that forms due to venous rupture between the dura and arachnoid.

Acute Diagnostic Management

- **Glasgow Coma Scale:** level of arousal and cerebral cortex function
- **CAT Scan:** observe intracranial structures
- **X-Ray:** fractures
- **MRI:** observe intracranial structures
- **Cerebral angiography:** observe blood vessels and internal anatomy of the brain
- **Evoked potential/electroencephalogram:** localizing structural damage
- **Positron emission tomography:** cerebral metabolic abnormalities
- **Ventriculography:** radiography used to observe cerebral

ventricles following cerebrospinal fluid removal

- **Radioisotope imaging:** allows for a two dimensional concentrated view of the brain

Levels of Consciousness

Coma: A state of unconsciousness and a level of unresponsiveness to all internal and external stimuli.

Stupor: A state of general unresponsiveness with arousal occurring from repeated stimuli.

Obtundity: A state of consciousness that is characterized by a state of sleep, reduced alertness to arousal, and delayed responses to stimuli.

Delirium: A state of consciousness that is characterized by disorientation, confusion, agitation, and loudness.

Clouding of consciousness: A state of consciousness that is characterized by quiet behavior, confusion, poor attention, and delayed responses.

Consciousness: A state of alertness, awareness, orientation, and memory.

Glasgow Coma Scale

A neurological assessment tool used initially after injury to determine arousal and cerebral cortex function. A total score of eight or less correlates to coma in 90% of patients. Scores of 9 to 12 indicate moderate brain injuries and scores from 13 to 15 indicate mild brain injuries.

Glasgow Coma Scale

Eye Opening	E
Spontaneous	4
To speech	3
To pain	2
Nil	1
Best Motor Response	**M**
Obeys commands	6
Localizes pain	5
Withdraws	4
Abnormal flexion	3
Extensor response	2
Nil	1
Verbal Response	**V**
Oriented	5
Confused conversation	4
Inappropriate words	3
Incomprehensible sounds	2
Nil	1

Coma Score (E+M+V) = 3 to 15

From Management of Head Injuries by Bryan Jennett and Graham Teasdale, Copyright-1981 by Oxford University Press, Inc. Used by permission of Oxford University Press, Inc.

Rancho Los Amigos Levels of Cognitive Functioning

I.   NO RESPONSE

Patient appears to be in a deep sleep and is completely unresponsive to any stimuli.

II.   GENERALIZED RESPONSE

Patient reacts inconsistently and non-purposefully to stimuli in a nonspecific manner. Responses are limited and often the same regardless of stimulus presented. Responses may be physiological changes, gross body movements, and/or vocalization.

III.   LOCALIZED RESPONSE

Patient reacts specifically but inconsistently to stimuli. Responses are directly related to the type of stimulus presented. May follow simple commands such as closing the eyes or squeezing the hand in an inconsistent, delayed manner.

IV.   CONFUSED-AGITATED

Patient is in a heightened state of activity. Behavior is bizarre and non-purposeful relative to the immediate environment. Does not discriminate among persons or objects; is unable to cooperate directly with treatment efforts. Verbalizations frequently are incoherent and/or inappropriate to the environment; confabulation may be present. Gross attention to environment is very brief; selective attention is often nonexistent. Patient lacks short and long-term recall.

V.   CONFUSED-INAPPROPRIATE

Patient is able to respond to simple commands fairly consistently. However, with increased complexity of commands or lack of any external structure, responses are non-purposeful, random, or fragmented. Demonstrates gross attention to the environment but is highly distractible and lacks the ability to focus attention on a specific task. With structure, may be able to converse on a social automatic level for short periods of time. Verbalization is often inappropriate and confabulatory. Memory is severely impaired; often shows inappropriate use of objects; may perform previously learned tasks with structure, but is unable to learn new information.

VI.   CONFUSED-APPROPRIATE

Patient shows goal-directed behavior, but is dependent on external input or direction. Follows simple directions consistently and shows carryover for relearned tasks such as self-care. Responses may be incorrect due to memory problems, but they are appropriate to the situation. Past memories show more depth and detail than recent memory.

VII.   AUTOMATIC-APPROPRIATE

Patient appears appropriate and oriented within the hospital and home settings; goes through daily routine automatically, but frequently robot-like. Patient shows minimal to no confusion and has shallow recall of activities. Shows carryover for new learning, but at a decreased rate. With structure is able to initiate social or recreational activities; judgment remains impaired.

VIII. PURPOSEFUL-APPROPRIATE

Patient is able to recall and integrate past and recent events and is aware of and responsive to environment. Shows carryover for new learning and needs no supervision once activities are learned. May continue to show a decreased ability relative to premorbid abilities, abstract reasoning, tolerance for stress, and judgment in emergencies or unusual circumstances.

From Professional Staff Association, Rancho Los Amigos Hospital, p.87-88, with permission.

Memory Impairments

Anterograde memory: The inability to create new memory. Anterograde memory is usually the last to recover after a comatose state. Contributing factors include poor attention, distractibility, and impaired perception of stimuli.

Post-traumatic amnesia: The time between the injury and when the patient is able to recall recent events. The patient does not recall the injury or events up until this point of recovery. Post-traumatic amnesia is used as an indicator of the extent of damage.

Retrograde amnesia: An inability to remember events prior to the injury. Retrograde amnesia may progressively decrease with recovery.

Treatment Guidelines for Brain Injury

- ✓ Emphasis on motivation
- ✓ Promote independence
- ✓ Therapy should be goal-directed, functional, and recreational
- ✓ Focus on orientation
- ✓ Focus on behavior modification activities
- ✓ The use of repetition may be helpful
- ✓ Educate patient in compensatory strategies for success
- ✓ Structure is essential depending on the level of the patient
- ✓ Avoid overstimulation during therapy
- ✓ Use of calm voice and simple commands
- ✓ Perform activities that are both familiar and enjoyable for the patient
- ✓ Family education and support can enhance and assist in the rehabilitation process
- ✓ Allow patient to choose activities on occasion
- ✓ Flexibility in treatment is needed based on patient's immediate needs and state of mind

Pharmacological Intervention for TBI Management

Diuretic Agents – Decreases the volume of fluid in the brain and the intracranial pressure	Mannitol Furosemide Glycerol Urea Osmitrol Resectisol
Antidepressant Agents – Reduce disruptive or aggressive behavior	Elavil Marplan Nardil Pemelor Ritalin Paroxetine (Paxil) Fluoxetine (Prozac) Sertraline (Zoloft)
Anticonvulsant Agents – Prevention of early seizures in head injury	Phenytoin (Dilantin) Carbamazepine (Tegretol) Clonazepam (Klonopin) Phenobarbital Valproic acid (Depakane)
Electrolytes – Adequate stores are needed during the acute phase of head injury	Magnesium sulfate
Calcium Channel Blocker Agents – May improve outcome for traumatic subarachnoid hemorrhage	Nimodipine (Nimotop)
Psychostimulant Agents – Improve alertness and cognition	Methylphenidate (Ritalin) Pemoline (Cylert)
Dopamine Agonist Agents – May improve alertness or with post-traumatic Parkinsonism	Levodopa (Dopar, Larodopa)
Selective Serotonin Reuptake Inhibitor Agents – May benefit patients with head injury and emotional inhibition/impairment	Sertraline (Zoloft) Fluoxetine (Prozac) Paroxetine (Paxil)
Antispasticity Agents – May assist with relaxing increased muscle tone and/or cramping	Tizanidine hydrochloride (Zanaflex) Baclofen (Lioresal) Dantrolene (Dantrium) Diazepam (Valium)

*selected pharmaceutical drugs and their respective trade names in parentheses, not intended to be a complete list

Traumatic Brain Injury Profile

Examination

- Past medical history
- History of current condition
- Social history (caregiver support)
- Medications
- Living environment
- Systems review
- Cognitive and language assessment
- Behavioral assessment
- Safety assessment
- Skin assessment
- Postural tone assessment
- Sensation, proprioception, and kinesthesia
- Range of motion
- Motor assessment
- Endurance assessment
- Mobility skills

Intervention

- Cognitive and orientation training
- Therapeutic exercise
- Positioning
- Sensory integration
- Balance and vestibular training
- Range of motion
- Motor function training
- Wheelchair and adaptive equipment prescription
- Splinting and serial casting
- Mobility training

Goals

- Maximize functional mobility
- Maximize community independence
- Maximize strength
- Maximize range of motion and prevent heterotopic ossification
- Maximize static and dynamic balance
- Maximize endurance
- Maximize patient/caregiver competence with:
  - Positioning
  - Use of adaptive equipment and orthotic/splinting devices
  - Home exercise program

Pediatrics

Developmental Gross and Fine Motor Skills

Gross Motor Skills	Fine Motor Skills
Newborn to 1 Month:	
Prone Physiological flexion Lifts head briefly Head to side **Supine** Physiological flexion Rolls partly to side **Sitting** Head lag in pull to sit **Standing** Reflex standing and walking	Regards objects in direct line of sight Follows moving object to midline Hands fisted Arm movements jerky Movements may be purposeful or random

Gross Motor Skills	Fine Motor Skills
2 to 3 Months:	
Prone Lifts head 90 degrees briefly Chest up in prone position with some weight through forearms Rolls prone to supine **Supine** Asymmetrical tonic neck reflex (ATNR) influence strong Legs kick reciprocally Prefers head to side **Sitting** Head upright but bobbing Variable head lag in pull to sitting position Needs full support to sit **Standing** Poor weight bearing Hips in flexion, behind shoulders	Can see further distances Hands open more Visually follows through 180 degrees Grasp is reflexive Uses palmar grasp

Developmental Gross and Fine Motor Skills

Gross Motor Skills	Fine Motor Skills
4 to 5 Months:	
Prone Bears weight on extended arms Pivots in prone to reach toys **Supine** Rolls from supine to side position Plays with feet to mouth **Sitting** Head steady in supported sitting position Turns head in sitting position Sits alone for brief periods **Standing** Bears all weight through legs in supported stand	Grasps and releases toys Uses ulnar-palmar group
6 to 7 Months:	
Prone Rolls from supine to prone position Holds weight on one hand to reach for toy **Supine** Lifts head **Sitting** Lifts head and helps when pulled to sitting position Gets to sitting position without assistance Sits independently **Mobility** May crawl backward	Approaches objects with one hand Arm in neutral when approaching toy Radial-palmar grasp "Rakes" with fingers to pick up small objects Voluntary release to transfer objects between hands

Gross Motor Skills	Fine Motor Skills
8 to 9 Months:	
Prone Gets into hands-knees position **Supine** Does not tolerate supine position **Sitting** Moves from sitting to prone position Sits without hand support for longer periods Pivots in sitting position **Standing** Stands at furniture Pulls to stand at furniture Lowers to sitting position from supported stand **Mobility** Crawls forward Walks along furniture (cruising)	Develops active supination Radial-digital grasp develops Uses inferior pincer grasp Extends wrist actively Points with index finger Pokes with index finger Release of objects is more refined Takes objects out of container
10 to 11 Months:	
Standing Stands without support briefly Pulls to stand using half-kneel intermediate position Picks up object from floor from standing with support **Mobility** Walks with both hands held Walks with one hand held Creeps on hands and feet (bear walk)	Fine pincer grasp developed Puts objects into container Grasps crayon adaptively
12 to 15 Months:	
Mobility Walks without support Fast walking Walks backward Walks sideways Bends over to look between legs Creeps or hitches upstairs Throws ball in sitting	Marks paper with crayon Builds tower using two cubes Turns over small container to obtain contents

Developmental Gross and Fine Motor Skills

Gross Motor Skills	Fine Motor Skills
16 to 24 Months:	
Squats in play Walks upstairs and downstairs with one hand held-both feet on step Propels ride-on toys Kicks ball Throws ball Throws ball forward Picks up toy from floor without falling	Folds paper Strings beads Stacks six cubes Imitates vertical and horizontal strokes with crayon on paper Holds crayon with thumb and fingers
2 Years:	
Rides tricycle Walks backward Walks on tiptoe Runs on toes Walks downstairs alternating feet Catches large ball Hops on one foot	Turns knob Opens and closes jar Able to button large buttons Uses child-size scissors with help Does 12 to 15 piece puzzles Folds paper or clothes
Preschool Age (3 to 4 Years):	
Throws ball 10 feet Walks on a line 10 feet Hops 2-10 times on one foot Jumps distances of up to two feet Jumps over obstacles up to 12 inches Throws and catches small ball Runs fast and avoids obstacles	Controls crayons more effectively Copies a circle or cross Matches colors Cuts with scissors Draws recognizable human figure with head and two extremities Draws squares May demonstrate hand preference

Gross Motor Skills	Fine Motor Skills
Early School Age (5 to 8 Years):	
Skips on alternate feet Gallops Can play hopscotch, balance on one foot, controlled hopping, and squatting on one leg Jumps with rhythm, control (jump rope) Bounces large ball Kicks ball with greater control Limbs growing faster than trunk allowing greater speed, leverage	Hand preference is evident Prints well, starting to learn cursive writing Able to button small buttons
Later School Age (9 to 12 Years):	
Mature patterns of movement in throwing, jumping, running Competition increases, enjoys competitive games Improved balance, coordination, endurance, attention span Boys may develop preadolescent fat spurt Girls may develop prepubescent and pubescent changes in body shape (hips, breasts)	Develops greater control in hand usage Learns to draw Handwriting is developed
Adolescence (13 Years+):	
Rapid growth in size and strength, boys more than girls Puberty leads to changes in body proportions: center of gravity rises toward shoulders for boys, lower to hips for girls Balance and coordination skills, eye-hand coordination, endurance may plateau during growth spurt	Develops greater dexterity in fingers for fine tasks (knitting, sewing, art, crafts)

From Ratliffe KT: Clinical Pediatric Physical Therapy: A Guide for the Physical therapy Team. Mosby Company Inc., Philadelphia 1998, p.45-47, with permission.

Concepts of Development

Cephalic to Caudal: A person develops head and upper extremity control prior to trunk and lower extremity control. There is a general skill acquisition from the direction of head to toe.

Gross to Fine: A general trend for large muscle movement acquisition with progression to small muscle skill acquisition.

Mass to Specific: A general trend for a person to acquire simple movements and progress towards complex movements.

Proximal to Distal: A concept that uses the midline of the body as the reference point. Trunk control (midline stability) is acquired first with subsequent gain in distal control (extremities).

Pediatric Therapeutic Positioning

Proper positioning is essential to obtain maximum function for the pediatric population. Positioning is used for many purposes including facilitation of desired patterns of movement, inhibition of abnormal reflexes, normalization of tone, midline orientation, enhancement of respiratory capacity, pulmonary hygiene, maintaining skin integrity, and prevention of contractures.

Federal Legislation Affecting Health and Education for Children with Disabilities

Perkins Vocational and Applied Technology Act (enacted 1990)
Reauthorization and modification of the Education for all Handicapped Children (EHA). Provides free appropriate education in the least restrictive environment for individuals with disabilities from age 3 – 21.

IDEA Amendments (enacted 1991)
Reauthorized early intervention; established Federal Interagency Coordination Council.

Rehabilitation Act Amendments (enacted 1992)
Transition planning at high school graduation includes coordination of assistive technology services and rehabilitation system.

IDEA Amendments (enacted 1997)
Restructuring of IDEA into four distinct and individual parts.

Ideal Positioning

	Supine	Prone	Sidelying	Sitting
Pelvis and Hips	Pelvis in line with trunk. Hips in 30 to 90 degrees of flexion. Neutral rotation of pelvis. Hips symmetrically abducted 10 to 20 degrees.	Pelvis in line with trunk. Hips in extension. Neutral rotation of pelvis. Hips symmetrically abducted 10-20 degrees.	Pelvis in line with trunk. Hips in flexion. Neutral rotation. Hips in 10 to 20 degrees abduction.	Pelvis in line with trunk. Hips at 90 degrees flexion. Neutral rotation of pelvis. Hips symmetrically abducted 10 to 20 degrees.
Trunk	Straight. Shoulders in line with hips. Neutral rotation of trunk.	Straight. Shoulders in line with hips. Neutral rotation.	Straight. Shoulders in line with hips. Slight sidebending okay.	Straight. Shoulders over hips. Not rotated.
Head and Neck	Head in neutral position. Facing forward. Slight cervical flexion.	Head in neutral position. Facing to one side. Slight cervical flexion.	Head in neutral position. Facing forward. Slight cervical flexion.	Head in neutral position. Facing forward. Head evenly on shoulders.
Shoulders and Arms	Arms fully supported. Arms forward of trunk. Forearms rest on trunk or pillow.	Arms fully supported. Arms forward of trunk. Flexion at shoulders. Flexion at elbows.	Both arms supported. Lower arm forward, not lying on point of shoulders. Lower arm neutral rotation. Upper arm may have 0 to 40 degrees medial rotation.	Arms fully supported. Elbows in flexion. 0 to 45 degrees internally rotated shoulders.
Legs and Feet	Knees supported in flexion. Feet held at 90 degrees.	Knees extended. Feet supported at 90 degrees.	Knees in flexion. Feet positioned at 90 degrees. Pillow between knees.	Knees at 90 degrees. Ankles at 90 degrees. Feet fully supported. Thighs fully supported.

From Ratliffe KT: Clinical Pediatric Physical Therapy: A Guide for the Physical Therapy Team. Mosby Inc., Philadelphia 1998, p.266, with permission.

Infant Reflexes and Possible Effects if Reflex Persists Abnormally

Primitive Reflex	Possible Negative Effect on Movement with Abnormal Persistence of Reflex

Asymmetrical Tonic Neck Reflex (ATNR)

Stimulus: Head position, turned to one side
Response: Arm and leg on face side are extended, arm and leg on scalp side are flexed, spine curved with convexity toward face side
Normal age of response: Birth to 6 months

Interferes with:
- Feeding
- Visual Tracking
- Midline use of hands
- Bilateral hand use
- Rolling
- Development of crawling
- Can lead to skeletal deformities (e.g., scoliosis, hip subluxation, hip dislocation)

Symmetrical Tonic Neck Reflex (STNR)

Stimulus: Head position, flexion or extension
Response: When head is in flexion, arms are flexed, legs extended. When head is in extension, arms are extended, legs are flexed
Normal age of response: 6 to 8 months

Interferes with:
- Ability to prop on arms in prone position
- Attaining and maintaining hands-and-knees position
- Crawling reciprocally
- Sitting balance when looking around
- Use of hands when looking at object in hands in sitting position

Tonic Labyrinthine Reflex (TLR)

Stimulus: Position of labyrinth in inner ear - reflected in head position
Response: In the supine position, body and extremities are held in extension; in the prone position, body and extremities are held in flexion
Normal age of response: Birth to 6 months

Interferes with:
- Ability to initiate rolling
- Ability to prop on elbows with extended hips when prone
- Ability to flex trunk and hips to come to sitting position from supine position
- Often causes full body extension, which interferes with balance in sitting or standing

Galant Reflex

Stimulus: Touch to skin along spine from shoulder to hip
Response: Lateral flexion of trunk to side of stimulus
Normal age of response: 30 weeks of gestation to 2 months

Interferes with:
- Development of sitting balance
- Can lead to scoliosis

Palmar Grasp Reflex

Stimulus: Pressure in palm on ulnar side of hand
Response: Flexion of fingers causing strong grip
Normal age of response: Birth to 4 months

Interferes with:
- Ability to grasp and release objects voluntarily
- Weight bearing on open hand for propping, crawling, protective responses

Plantar Grasp Reflex

Stimulus: Pressure to base of toes
Response: Toe flexion
Normal age of response: 28 weeks of gestation to 9 months

Interferes with:
- Ability to stand with feet flat on surface
- Balance reactions and weight shifting in standing

Rooting Reflex

Stimulus: Touch on cheek
Response: Turning head to same side with mouth open
Normal age of response: 28 weeks of gestation to 3 months

Interferes with:
- Oral-motor development
- Development of midline control of head
- Optical righting, visual tracking, and social interaction

Infant Reflexes and Possible Effects if Reflex Persists Abnormally (continued)

Primitive Reflex	Possible Negative Effect on Movement with Abnormal Persistence of Reflex

Moro Reflex

Stimulus: Head dropping into extension suddenly for a few inches
Response: Arms abduct with fingers open, then cross trunk into adduction; cry
Normal age of response: 28 weeks of gestation to 5 months

Interferes with:
- Balance reactions in sitting
- Protective responses in sitting
- Eye-hand coordination, visual tracking

Startle Reflex

Stimulus: Loud, sudden noise
Response: Similar to Moro response but elbows remain flexed and hands closed
Normal age of response: 28 weeks of gestation to 5 months

Interferes with:
- Sitting balance
- Protective responses in sitting
- Eye-hand coordination, visual tracking
- Social interaction, attention

Positive Support Reflex

Stimulus: Weight placed on balls of feet when upright
Response: Stiffening of legs and trunk into extension
Normal age of response: 35 weeks of gestation to 2 months

Interferes with:
- Standing and walking
- Balance reactions and weight shift in standing
- Can lead to contractures of ankles into plantar flexion

Walking (Stepping) Reflex

Stimulus: Supported upright position with soles of feet on firm surface
Response: Reciprocal flexion/extension of legs
Normal age of response: 38 weeks of gestation to 2 months

Interferes with:
- Standing and walking
- Balance reactions and weight shifting in standing
- Development of smooth, coordinated reciprocal movements of lower extremities

From Ratliffe KT: Clinical Pediatric Physical Therapy: A Guide for the Physical Therapy Team. Mosby Inc., Philadelphia 1998, p.266, with permission.

Neuromuscular and Nervous Systems Pediatric Pathology

Arthrogryposis Multiplex Congenita

Arthrogryposis multiplex congenita is a non-progressive neuromuscular disorder that is estimated to occur during the first trimester in utero. The restriction in utero allows for fibrosis of muscles and structures within the joints.

- An exact etiology is unknown, but **causative factors** include poor movement during early development due to myopathic, neuropathic or joint abnormalities. The causative factor for a small percentage of children with this condition is genetic inheritance as an autosomal dominant trait.

- **Characteristics** include cylinder-like extremities with minimal definition, significant and multiple contractures, dislocation of joints, and muscle atrophy.

- The goal of **treatment** is to attain the maximum level of developmental skills through positioning, stretching, strengthening, splinting, and use of adaptive equipment.

Significant family involvement is required for the home program. Surgical intervention may be indicated.

Cerebral Palsy

Cerebral palsy is an umbrella term used to describe movement disorders due to brain damage that are non-progressive and are acquired in utero, during birth or infancy. The brain damage decreases the brain's ability to monitor and control nerve and voluntary muscle activity.

- **Causative factors** before or during birth include a lack of oxygen, maternal infections, drug and alcohol abuse, placental abnormalities, toxemia, prolonged labor, prematurity, and Rh incompatibility. Causative factors that are seen in acquired cerebral palsy include meningitis, CVA, seizures, and head injury.

Characteristics vary from mild and undetectable to severe loss of control accompanied by profound mental retardation. All types of cerebral palsy demonstrate abnormal muscle tone, impaired modulation of movement, presence of abnormal reflexes, and impaired mobility.

- **Cerebral Palsy Primary Motor Patterns (mixed motor patterns exist)**

    Spastic - indicating a lesion in the motor cortex of the cerebrum; upper motor neuron damage
    Athetoid - indicating a lesion involving the basal ganglia; cerebellum and cerebellar pathways

- **Distribution of Involvement**

    Monoplegia - one extremity

    Diplegia - primarily bilateral lower extremity involvement, however, upper extremities may be affected

    Hemiplegia - unilateral involvement of the upper and lower extremities

    Quadriplegia - involvement of the entire body

- **Treatment** of cerebral palsy is a lifelong process. Intervention includes ongoing family and caregiver education, normalization of tone, stretching, strengthening, motor learning and developmental milestones, positioning, weight bearing activities, and mobility skills. Splinting, assistive devices, and specialized seating may be indicated. Surgical intervention may be required for orthopedic management or reduction of spasticity.

Down Syndrome

Down syndrome is a genetic abnormality consisting of an extra twenty-first chromosome, termed trisomy 21.

- **Causative factors** include incomplete cell division of the 21st pair of chromosomes due to nondisjunction, translocation or mosaic classification. Advanced maternal age increases the risk of genetic imbalance.

- **Characteristics** of this syndrome include mental retardation, hypotonia, joint hypermobility, flattened nasal bridge, narrow eyelids with epicanthal folds, small mouth, feeding impairments, flat feet, scoliosis, congenital heart disease, and visual and hearing loss.

- **Treatment** should emphasize exercise and fitness, stability, maximizing respiratory function, and education for caregivers. Surgical intervention may be indicated for cardiac abnormalities.

Duchenne Muscular Dystrophy

Duchenne muscular dystrophy is a progressive disorder caused by the absence of the gene required to produce the muscle proteins dystrophin and nebulin. Without dystrophin and nebulin, cell membranes weaken, myofibrils are destroyed, and muscle contractility is lost. Fat and connective tissue eventually replace muscle, and death usually occurs from cardiopulmonary failure prior to age 25, usually in the teenage years.

- The **causative factor** is inheritance as an X-linked recessive trait. The child's mother is a silent carrier and only male offspring will manifest the disease.

- **Characteristics** usually manifest between two and five years of age. Progressive weakness, disinterest in running, falling, toe walking, excessive lordosis, and pseudohypertrophy of muscle groups are common symptoms. Progressive impairment with ADLs and mobility begins around age five and the inability to ambulate follows.

- **Treatment** focuses on family and caregiver education, respiratory function, submaximal exercise, mobility skills, splinting, orthotics, and adaptive equipment. Medical management includes the use of immunosuppressants, steroids, and surgical intervention for orthopedic impairments.

Prader-Willi Syndrome

Prader-Willi syndrome is a genetic condition that is diagnosed by physical attributes and patterns of behavior rather than genetic testing.

- The **causative factor** is a partial deletion of chromosome 15.

- **Characteristics** include physical and behavioral attributes such as small hands, feet, and sex organs, hypotonia, almond shaped eyes, obesity, and a constant desire for food. This child will present with coordination impairments and mental retardation.

- **Treatment** includes postural control, exercise and fitness, and gross and fine motor skills training.

Spina Bifida

Spina bifida is a developmental abnormality due to insufficient closure of the neural tube by the 28th day of gestation. This defect usually occurs in the low thoracic, lumbar or sacral regions and affects the central nervous, musculoskeletal, and urinary systems.

- A single etiology has not been identified, however, **causative factors** include genetic predisposition, environmental influence, low levels of maternal folic acid, maternal hyperthermia, and certain classifications of drugs.

- **Types of Spina Bifida**

    Spina Bifida Occulta - An impairment and non-fusion of the spinous processes of a vertebrae, however, the spinal cord and meninges remain intact. There is usually no associated disability.

    Spina Bifida Cystica - Presents with a cyst-like protrusion through the non-fused vertebrae, which results in impairment.

- **Forms of Spina Bifida Cystica**

    Meningocele - Herniation of meninges and cerebrospinal fluid into a sac that protrudes through the vertebral defect. The spinal cord remains within the canal.

Myelomeningocele - A severe form characterized by herniation of meninges, cerebrospinal fluid, and the spinal cord extending through the defect in the vertebrae. The cyst may or may not be covered by skin.

- **Characteristics** and associated impairments of myelomeningocele include motor loss below the level of defect in the spinal cord, sensory deficits, hydrocephalus, Arnold-Chiari Type II malformation, osteoporosis, clubfoot, scoliosis, tethered cord syndrome, latex allergy, bowel and bladder dysfunction, and learning disabilities.

- Initial **treatment** for this population prioritizes significant family teaching regarding positioning, handling, range of motion, and therapeutic exercise. Ongoing treatment in physical therapy includes range of motion, facilitation of developmental milestones, skin care, strengthening, balance and mobility training, adaptive equipment, splinting, orthotic prescription, and wheelchair prescription. Physical therapy is ongoing through adolescence and is based on the severity of impairments and needs of the child.

Spinal Muscular Atrophy (SMA)

Spinal muscular atrophy is a condition of progressive degeneration of the anterior horn cell.

- Categories of Spinal Muscular Atrophy

    Acute Infantile SMA (Werdnig-Hoffmann disease) - Occurs between birth and two months of age. Motor degeneration progresses quickly and life expectancy is less than one year.

    Chronic Childhood SMA (type II muscular atrophy, chronic Werdnig-Hoffmann disease) - Presents after six months to one year and has slower progression than infantile SMA. Impairment is steady, however, a child can survive into adulthood.

    Juvenile SMA (Kugelberg-Welander SMA) - Occurs later in childhood from 4-17 years of age. This population can also survive into adulthood.

- The **causative factor** of spinal muscular atrophy is an autosomal recessive genetic inheritance. Certain types of this disease involve a mutation on chromosome 5. Characteristics for all categories of the disease are the same, and vary in onset and speed of progression.

- **Characteristics** include progressive muscle weakness and atrophy, diminished or absent deep tendon reflexes, normal intelligence, intact sensation, and end stage respiratory compromise.

- **Treatment** includes positioning, vestibular and visual stimulation, and access to play. Treatment for the slower progressing categories is primarily supportive including educating caregivers, mobility training, and use of assistive devices and adaptive equipment.

Pediatric Profile

Examination

- Past medical history
- History of current condition
- Social history (caregiver support)
- Medications
- Living environment
- Systems review
- Pediatric assessment tools
- Gross and fine motor skill acquisition
- Pathological reflexes
- Neurological assessment
- Strength
- Range of motion
- Respiratory assessment
- Postural tone assessment
- Reassessment of existing adaptive equipment, orthotics and splinting

Intervention

- Progression through pediatric milestones
- Therapeutic exercise
- Sensory integration
- Postural control
- Therapeutic positioning
- Therapeutic play
- Wheelchair and orthotic prescription
- Chest physical therapy
- Family/caregiver teaching
- Mobility training

Goals

- Maximize functional mobility
- Maximize range of motion
- Maximize strength and postural control
- Maximize patient/caregiver competence with:
    - Home program
    - Disease process and its progression
    - Therapeutic positioning and handling
- Maximize independence with use of equipment

Chapter 3

Cardiac, Vascular, and Pulmonary Systems

Foundational Science: Cardiac and Vascular Systems

Anatomy of the Heart

Apex: Located at the fifth intercostal space at the midclavicular line; this represents the tip of the left ventricle.

Base: Located at the second intercostal space behind the sternum on the posterior aspect of the heart; it lies adjacent to the vertebral bodies of T6 through T9.

Endocardium: A thin layer of tissue that lines the inside surface of the heart and valves.

Epicardium: The outer layer of the cardiac wall that covers the surface to protect against trauma or infection.

Myocardium: The thick layer of muscle of the heart that provides the pumping force for the ventricles.

Pericardium: A double-walled connective tissue sac (fibrous layer and serous layer) that surrounds the heart and protects it from trauma or infection.

Right atrium: Receives venous blood from the superior and inferior vena cava.

Right ventricle: Receives venous blood from the right atrium through the tricuspid valve. Pushes blood into the pulmonary artery and pulmonary circulation.

Left atrium: Receives arterial blood from the pulmonary veins.

Left ventricle: Receives blood from the left atrium. Pushes blood into the aorta and the systemic circulation.

Tricuspid valve: Prevents right ventricular blood from going back into the right atrium.

Pulmonic valve: Prevents blood from returning to the right ventricle.

Mitral valve: Prevents left ventricular blood from returning to the left atrium.

Aortic valve: Prevents the systemic blood from returning to the left ventricle.

Atrioventricular valves: Blood from each atria flows to each ventricle through these valves. The valves close upon ventricular contraction to avoid backflow.

Semilunar valves: Blood from each ventricle flows out of the heart through these valves. The valves close upon the subsequent diastole to avoid backflow of the blood into the heart.

Aorta: Largest artery which carries the total cardiac output. Divisions include the carotids, subclavians, and descending aorta.

- **Ascending aorta:** provides blood to the head, neck, and arms

- **Descending aorta:** provides blood to the lower body and visceral tissues

Superior vena cava: The primary vein that drains venous blood from the head, neck, and upper body into the right atrium.

Inferior vena cava: The primary vein that drains venous blood from the lower body and viscera into the right atrium.

Pulmonary artery: The primary artery that carries blood to the lungs from the right ventricle.

Coronary Arteries

Left coronary artery supplies:

- Left atrium
- Left ventricle (majority)
- Right ventricle (a portion of)
- Interventricular septum (majority)
- AV bundle
- SA node (40-45% of population)

Left coronary artery bifurcates into:

- Left anterior descending artery
- Left circumflex artery

Right coronary artery supplies:

- Right atrium
- Right ventricle (majority)
- Left ventricle (small portion)
- Interventricular septum (small portion)
- AV node and bundle of His (80% population)
- SA node (55-60% population)

Right coronary artery gives branches to:

- Right marginal artery
- Atrioventricular nodal artery (70% population)

Right coronary artery turns into:

- Posterior interventricular artery

Cardiac Conduction System

Sinoatrial node (SA): The sinoatrial node is located in the right atrium near the superior vena cava and is the primary pacemaker of the heart.

Atrioventricular node (AV): The atrioventricular node or junctional node is located in the inferior wall of the right atrium close to the tricuspid valve.

Bundle of His: The Bundle of His is a group of fibers that initiates at the atrioventricular node, enters the interventricular system, and splits into the left and right ventricles. The fibers branch into small Purkinje fibers.

Purkinje fibers: Purkinje fibers compose the last part of the electrical conduction system of the heart. The fibers relay the electrical impulses to the muscle cells of the heart.

Cardiac Reflexes

There are several quick-acting nervous system mechanisms that influence heart rate when triggered. The reflexes are divided into the baroreceptor reflex, Bainbridge reflex, and chemoreceptor reflex.

Baroreceptor Reflex
The baroreceptor reflex is produced by a group of mechanoreceptors that are found within the walls of the heart, intrathoracic vessels, the large arteries (especially the aorta), the carotid arteries, and carotid sinuses. This reflex is activated when pressure rises within the large arteries above 60 mm Hg. The mechanoreceptors that are sensitive to stretch and pressure peak in activity at approximately 180 mm Hg. Activation results in vasodilation secondary to inhibition of the vasomotor centers within the medulla as well as a decrease in heart rate and strength of contraction secondary to vagal stimulation.

Bainbridge Reflex
The Bainbridge reflex occurs when mechanoreceptors embedded within the right atrial myocardium respond to an increase in pressure and stretch (distention of the right atrium). This reflex stimulates the vasomotor centers of the medulla and results in increased sympathetic input and heart rate. This reflex can also influence a decrease in heart rate when the heart is beating too fast.

Chemoreceptor Reflex
The chemoreceptor reflex responds to the need for increased depth and rate of ventilation. Chemoreceptors are located on the carotid and aortic bodies and detect lack of oxygen, thus responding to an increase in arterial CO_2 levels.

Cardiac Facts

Cardiac Output
Cardiac output is the amount of blood pumped out of the heart through the aorta each minute. Normal cardiac output for an adult male at rest is 5.6 L/min with women producing 10 to 20% less. A person can increase the cardiac output to upwards of 25 L/min during extensive exercise. Cardiac output = stroke volume (x) heart rate.

Venous Return
Venous return is the amount of blood that comes from the veins to the right atrium each minute. This is similar in volume to the cardiac output.

Stroke Volume
Stroke volume is the amount of blood ejected from the ventricles with each contraction. Factors that can influence stroke volume include "preload" (influenced by end-diastolic volume), "afterload," and contractility.

Cardiac Index
The cardiac index is the amount of blood pumped out of the heart per minute per square meter of body mass. Normal cardiac index ranges between 2.5 to 4.2 liters/min/meter^2.

Blood Volume
Blood volume in an adult is usually 7-8% of their body weight. The blood is pumped through the body at 30 cm/sec with a total circulation time of 20 seconds.

Heart Sounds

S1	"lub" mitral and tricuspid valves closing at the onset of systole
S2	"dub" aortic and pulmonic valves closing at the onset of diastole
S3	(ventricular gallop) abnormal in older adults; noncompliant left ventricle; may be associated with congestive heart failure
S4	Pathological sound of vibration of the ventricular wall with ventricular filling and atrial contraction; may be associated with hypertension, stenosis, hypertensive heart disease or myocardial infarction

Common Circulatory Pulse Locations

Artery	Location
Carotid	Anterior to sternocleidomastoid
Brachial	Medial aspect of arm midway between shoulder and elbow
Radial	At wrist, lateral to flexor carpi radialis tendon
Ulnar	At wrist, between flexor digitorum superficialis and flexor carpi ulnaris tendons
Femoral	In femoral triangle (sartorius, adductor longus, and inguinal ligament)
Popliteal	Posterior aspect of knee (deep and hard to palpate)
Posterior tibial	Posterior aspect of medial malleolus
Dorsalis pedis	Between first and second metatarsal bones on superior aspect of the foot

From Magee, DJ: Orthopedic Physical Assessment. W.B. Saunders Company, Philadelphia 2002, p.52, with permission.

Laboratory/Diagnostic Testing

Laboratory Testing

Hematocrit

Hematocrit is the percentage of packed red blood cells in total blood volume. Hematocrit is commonly used in the identification of abnormal states of hydration, polycythemia, and anemia. A low hematocrit may result in a feeling of weakness, chills or dyspnea. A high hematocrit may result in an increased risk of thrombus.

Hemoglobin

Hemoglobin is the iron containing pigment of the red blood cells. Hemoglobin's function is to carry oxygen from the lungs to the tissues. This test is used to assess blood loss, anemia, and bone marrow suppression. Low hemoglobin may indicate anemia or recent hemorrhage, while elevated hemoglobin suggests hemoconcentration caused by polycythemia or dehydration.

Partial thromboplastin time

Partial thromboplastin time is most commonly used to monitor oral anticoagulant therapy or to screen for selected bleeding disorders. The test examines all of the clotting factors of the intrinsic pathway with the exception of platelets. Partial thromboplastin time is more sensitive than prothrombin time in detecting minor deficiencies.

Platelet count

Platelet count refers to the number of platelets per milliliter of blood. Platelets play an important role in blood coagulation, homeostasis, and blood thrombus formation. Low platelet counts increase the risk of bruising and bleeding. High platelet counts increase the risk of thrombosis.

Prothrombin time

Prothrombin time is most commonly used to monitor oral anticoagulant therapy or to screen for selected bleeding disorders. The test examines extrinsic coagulation factors V, VII, X, prothrombin, and fibrinogen.

White blood cell count

White blood cell count refers to the number of white blood cells per milliliter of blood. White blood cell count is commonly used to identify the presence of infection, allergens, bone marrow integrity or the degree of immunosuppression. An increase in white blood cell count can occur after hemorrhage, surgery, coronary occlusion or malignant growth.

Reference Values for Clinical Chemistry - (Blood, Serum, Plasma)

		Conventional Units	SI Units
Cholesterol, serum or EDTA plasma	Desirable range	< 200 mg/dL	< 5.18 mmol/L
	LDL cholesterol	60 - 120 mg/dL	600 - 1200 mg/L
	HDL cholesterol	40 - 80 mg/dL	400 - 800 mg/L
Oxygen, blood, arterial, room air	Partial pressure (PaO$_2$)	80 - 100 mm Hg	80 - 100 mm Hg
	Saturation (SaO$_2$)	95 - 98%	95 - 98%
pH, arterial blood		7.35 - 7.45	7.35 - 7.45

From Miller-Keane: Encyclopedia and Dictionary of Medicine, Nursing, and Allied Health. W.B. Saunders Company, Philadelphia 1997, p.1844, with permission.

Reference Values in Hematology

Cell Counts		Conventional Units	SI Units
Erythrocytes			
Males		4.6 - 6.2 million/mm³	4.6 - 6.2 X 10^{12}/L
Females		4.2 - 5.4 million/mm³	4.2 - 5.4 X 10^{12}/L
Children (varies with age)		4.5 - 5.1 million/mm³	4.5 - 5.1 X 10^{12}/L
Leukocytes			
Total		4,500 - 11,000/mm³	4.5 - 11.0 X 10^{9}/L

Differential	**Percentage**	**Absolute**	**Absolute**
Myelocytes	0	0/mm³	0/L
Band neutrophils	3 - 5	150 - 400/mm³	150 - 400 X 10^{6}/L
Segmented neutrophils	54 - 62	3000 - 5800/mm³	3000 - 5800 X 10^{6}/L
Lymphocytes	25 - 33	1500 - 3000/mm³	1500 - 3000 X 10^{6}/L
Monocytes	3 - 7	300 - 500/mm³	300 - 500 X 10^{6}/L
Eosinophils	1 - 3	50 - 250/mm³	50 - 250 X 10^{6}/L
Basophils	0 - 1	15 - 50/mm³	15 - 50 X 10^{6}/L

	Conventional Units	SI Units
Platelets	150,000 - 400,000/mm³	150 - 400 X 10^{9}/L
Reticulocytes	25,000 - 75,000/mm³ (0.5 - 1.5% of erythrocytes)	25 - 75 X10^{9}/L
	20 - 165 mg/dL	0.20 - 1.65 g/L

Hematocrit

	Conventional Units	SI Units
Males	40 - 54 mL/dL	0.40 - 0.54 volume fraction
Females	37 - 47 mL/dL	0.37 - 0.47 volume fraction
Newborns	49 - 54 mL/dL	0.49 - 0.54 volume fraction
Children (varies with age)	35 - 49 mL/dL	0.35 - 0.49 volume fraction

Hemoglobin

	Conventional Units	SI Units
Males	14.0 - 18.0 gm/dL	2.17 - 2.79 mmol/L
Females	12.0 - 16.0 gm/dL	1.86 - 2.48 mmol/L
Newborns	16.5 - 19.5 gm/dL	2.56 - 3.02 mmol/L
Children (varies with age)	11.2 - 16.5 gm/dL	1.74 - 2.56 mmol/L

From Miller-Keane: Encyclopedia and Dictionary of Medicine, Nursing, and Allied Health. W.B. Saunders Company, Philadelphia 1997, p. 1843, with permission.

Diagnostic Tests for Cardiac Dysfunction

Procedure	Description
Cardiac catheterization (for angiography)	The coronary arteries are injected with a contrast dye, and the arterial system can be seen with cinefluoroscopy: narrowing or occlusion of arteries can be evaluated.
Cardiac catheterization	Catheterization is used to measure intracardiac, transvalve, and pulmonary artery pressures and measure blood gas pressures to determine cardiac output and evaluate shunting.
Continuous hemodynamic monitoring	Pulmonary artery catheterization (Swan-Ganz) provides immediate cardiopulmonary pressure measurements. An invasive bedside (ICU) procedure that evaluates left ventricular function. A balloon-tipped, flow-directed catheter, connected to a transducer and a monitor, is used to allow measurements of pulmonary artery pressure; pulmonary capillary wedge pressure; cardiac output; and mixed venous saturation, which evaluates pulmonary vascular resistance and tissue oxygenation.
Echocardiography a. Transthoracic (TTE)	The reflections of ultrasound waves from cardiac surfaces are analyzed. It is used to evaluate left ventricular systolic function and the structure and function of cardiac walls, valves, and chambers; it can identify abnormal conditions such as tumors or pericardial effusion.
b. Transesophageal (TEE)	Transesophageal echocardiography is performed through the esophagus and stomach by a modified gastroscopy probe with one or two ultrasound transducers at its tip. TEE provides better image resolution and superior images of posterior cardiac structures. Continuous imaging is possible during operations or invasive procedures.

Procedure	Description
Electrocardiogram (ECG)	Surface electrodes record the electrical activity of the heart. A 12-lead ECG provides 12 views of the heart; it is used to assess cardiac rhythm, to diagnose the location, extent, and acuteness of myocardial ischemia and infarction; and to evaluate changes with activity.
Hemodynamic monitoring	See Continuous hemodynamic monitoring
Exercise stress tests	Numerous protocols for exercise tests have been used to assess responses to increased workloads with steps, treadmills, or bicycle ergometers. In conjunction with ECG and blood pressure recordings, patients are evaluated for exercise capacity, cardiac dysrhythmias, and diagnosis, prognosis, and management of coronary artery disease.
Holter monitoring	Continuous ambulatory ECG monitoring done by tape recording the cardiac rhythm for up to 24 hours. It is used to evaluate cardiac rhythm, efficacy of medications, transient symptoms that may indicate cardiac disease, and pacemaker function; and to correlate symptoms with activity.
Pharmacologic stress tests	A non-invasive assessment for patients with coronary artery disease who are unable to achieve adequate cardiac stress with exercise.
a. Dipyridamole thallium	This potent vasodilator markedly enhances blood flow to normally perfused myocardium, whereas myocardium fed by stenotic coronary arteries demonstrates relative hypoperfusion and diminished thallium activity.
b. Dobutamine echocardiography	An incremental infusion is given causing an increase in the myocardial oxygen demand. Simultaneous evaluation of wall motion abnormalities, ECG, and BP are performed.

Diagnostic Tests for Cardiac Dysfunction (continued)

Procedure	Description
Phonocardiography	This test records cardiac sounds. It is used to time the events of the cardiac cycle and to confirm auscultatory findings.
Radionuclide angiography	Red blood cells tagged (marked) with a radionuclide are injected into blood. Ventricular wall motion can be evaluated and the ejection fraction determined; abnormal blood flow with valve and congenital defects can be detected. Techniques include gated-pool equilibrium studies and first-pass techniques.
Technetium-99m scanning (hot spot imaging)	Technetium-99m injected into blood is taken up by damaged myocardial tissue; this identifies and localizes acute myocardial infarctions.
Thallium-201 myocardial perfusion imaging (cold spot imaging)	Thallium-201 injected into blood at peak exercise; scanning identifies ischemic and infarcted myocardium, which does not take up thallium-201. It is used to diagnose coronary artery disease and perfusion, particularly when ECG is equivocal.

From Rothstein J, Roy S, Wolf S: The Rehabilitation Specialist's Handbook. F. A. Davis Company Inc, Philadelphia 1998, p.624-626, with permission.

Electrocardiogram

ECG: Measures the electrical activity of the heart

12-lead Electrocardiogram

- Six limb leads (I, II, III, aVR, aVL, aVF)
- Six precordial leads (V1, V2, V3, V4, V5, V6)
- Provides 12 different views of the heart
- Leads I, II, III are bipolar limb leads that form a triangle connecting the right arm, left arm, and left foot; the heart should be at the center of the triangle
- Leads aVR, aVL, aVF are unipolar augmented leads

Precordial Lead Placement

V1 – right of sternum, 4th intercostal space
V2 – left of sternum, 4th intercostal space
V3 – half way between V2 and V4
V4 – midclavicular line in the 5th intercostal space
V5 – halfway between V4 and V6
V6 – Midaxillary line in the 5th intercostal space

P wave: Atrial depolarization

PR interval: Time required for conduction from the SA node to AV node. The time between atrial and ventricular depolarization. This is normally .12 to .2 seconds.

QRS complex: Ventricular depolarization and atrial repolarization.

QT interval: Electrical systole that is measured by the time elapsed from the start of the Q wave to the end of the T wave. This is normally .32 to .40 seconds.

ST segment: Delay before repolarization of the ventricles; useful in assessing myocardial ischemia.

T wave: Ventricular repolarization

Pathological Changes in an ECG

Depressed QRS: Heart failure, ischemia, pericardial effusion, obesity, chronic obstructive pulmonary disease

Ectopic foci: A location where abnormal myocardial depolarization originates. This can occur if the rhythmicity of the ectopic pacemaker increases; the rhythmicity of normal pacemakers is inhibited or if the conduction path from the normal pacemakers to the ectopic foci is blocked. These beats should be monitored.

Elevated QRS: Hypertrophy of the myocardium

Q Wave: Previous myocardial infarction

ST Segment Elevation: Acute myocardial infarction

Atrial fibrillation (A. fib)

- Irregular atrial rhythm
- No rate
- No P waves
- "F" waves absent
- Quivers noted
- Ventricular rhythm varies

Common causes include: hypertension, congestive heart failure, coronary artery disease, rheumatic heart disease, cor pulmonale, pericarditis, and illegal drug use.

Supraventricular tachycardia

- Rate varies between 160 to 250 bpm
- Regular rhythm
- Originates from a location above the AV node
- Will start and stop without cause

Common causes include: mitral valve prolapse, cor pulmonale, digitalis toxicity, and rheumatic heart disease.

Premature atrial contractions (PAC)

- Occur when an ectopic focus in the atrium fires and supersedes the SA node
- The P wave is premature with abnormal configuration
- Rate normal between 60-100 bpm
- Irregular rhythm that can be regularly irregular such as consistently skipping every third beat
- Can be indicative of ischemia or valve pathology

Common causes include: intake of caffeine, emotional stress, smoking, and pathologies such as coronary artery disease, electrolyte imbalance, infection, and congestive heart failure.

Ventricular tachycardia (VT)

- Rate usually > 100 bpm
- Rhythm usually regular
- No P wave or it appears after QRS complex with retrograde conduction
- Requires immediate medical attention

Common causes include: post myocardial infarction, rheumatic heart disease, coronary artery disease, and cardiomyopathy.

Ventricular fibrillation (V. fib)

- No regular rate or rhythm
- Emergency
- Requires immediate medical intervention

Common causes include: long-term or severe heart disease, post myocardial infarction, hypercalcemia, hypokalemia, and hyperkalemia.

Multifocal ventricular tachycardia

- Rate > 150 bpm
- Irregular rhythm
- No P waves
- QRS complex is wide
- Requires immediate medical intervention

Common causes include: hypokalemia, hypomagnesemia, hypothermia, and drug-induced through antiarrhythmic medications.

Premature ventricular contractions (PVC)

- Occur when an ectopic focus in the ventricles or Purkinje fibers fires and supersedes normal conduction
- Focal PVCs occur from one ectopic foci and have the same waveform
- Multifocal PVCs have multiple ectopic foci that result in different waveforms
- Rate is normal between 60-100 bpm
- The P wave is absent, the ST segment is distorted, and the QRS complex occurs early
- Irregular rhythm that can be regularly irregular such as consistently skipping every third beat
- A couplet is known as two skips in a row; bigeminy is a skip every other beat; trigeminy is a skip every third beat

Common causes include: intake of caffeine, emotional stress, smoking, pathologies such as coronary artery disease, digitalis toxicity, cardiomyopathy, and myocardial infarction.

Complete heart block (third-degree AV block)

- Regular rhythm
- Atrial rate > ventricular rate
- Requires immediate medical intervention (pacemaker)

Common causes include: infection, electrolyte imbalance, coronary artery disease, anteroseptal myocardial infarction, and impairment with the AV conduction system.

Asystole

- No rhythm
- Absence of P wave, QRS, and T waves
- Can have abrupt onset
- Requires immediate medical attention

Common causes include: failure of all pacemakers to initiate, conduction system failure, acute myocardial infarction and ventricular rupture.

Vital Signs

Blood Pressure

Normal blood pressure values are accepted as:

Infants:	60-90 / 30-55 mm Hg
Child:	90-110 / 50-70 mm Hg
Adult:	100-140 / 60-90 mm Hg

Systole: A period of contraction of the cardiac muscle.

Diastole: A period of relaxation of the cardiac muscle.

Atrial systole: A period that is initially comprised of atrial emptying of blood into the ventricles through the pressure gradient between the chambers as well as contraction of the cardiac muscle.

Atrial diastole: A period of atrial filling secondary to pressure from the venous circulation.

Ventricular systole: A period of a ventricular contraction that causes a rapid ejection of blood.

Ventricular diastole: A period of ventricular filling secondary to the pressure gradient from the atria in combination with atrial contraction.

Blood Pressure Classification

Hypertension

The American Heart Association defines hypertension as an adult blood pressure greater than or equal to 140 mm Hg systolic pressure or greater than or equal to 90 mm Hg diastolic pressure. Factors that can influence the onset of hypertension include age, level of physical fitness, genetic predisposition, smoking, sedentary life, obesity, and diabetes mellitus.

Hypertension exists if:

Children: Based on percentile within normative data for age and height

Adult Prehypertension: 120-139 mm Hg systolic or 80-89 mm Hg diastolic

Adult Stage 1: 140-159 mm Hg systolic or 90-99 mm Hg diastolic

Adult Stage 2: ≥ 160 mm Hg systolic or 100 mm Hg diastolic

Hypotension exists if:

Systolic pressure < 100 mm Hg

- This condition is not dangerous, however, a patient may experience periods of dizziness especially when changing position.

Korotkoff's Sounds

Phase I: the first clear sound detected that indicates systolic pressure

Phase II: the sounds now have a muffle or swishing sound

Phase III: the sounds are louder and clear compared to the initial sounds

Phase IV: the sounds abruptly become muffled, as if a whisper; this is the indication of diastolic pressure

Phase V: the sounds disappear, there is nothing heard through auscultation

Preparation and Procedure

- ✓ Requires sphygmomanometer and stethoscope
- ✓ Ensure proper size cuff for children, adults, and obese patients
- ✓ Width of bladder should equal 40% of the circumference of the midpoint of the extremity (adult: 3-6 inches wide)
- ✓ Values are usually slightly higher when measured in the left upper extremity versus the right upper extremity; be consistent with which side the blood pressure is taken
- ✓ Expose the antecubital space and palpate the pulse
- ✓ Place arrow on cuff over brachial artery
- ✓ Wrap the cuff above the antecubital space with a snug fit (false readings will occur if too loose)
- ✓ Palpate the brachial pulse, inflate the cuff and note the reading when the pulse disappears
- ✓ Release the cuff and wait 30-60 seconds
- ✓ Inflate the cuff to 20 mm Hg above this reading (where the brachial pulse disappears)
- ✓ Slowly deflate the cuff observing the needle gauge
- ✓ The first Korotkoff's sound indicates the systolic pressure,

the last audible sound indicates the diastolic pressure
- ✓ The thigh is an alternate site to obtain a blood pressure reading

Ankle-Brachial Index (ABI)

The ankle-brachial index is a test that measures arterial perfusion using a Doppler unit. Blood pressures are measured in both upper extremities (using the brachial arteries) and lower extremities (using the dorsalis pedis or tibialis posterior artery). The patient is tested in the supine position for all measurements. The highest lower extremity systolic pressure is divided by the brachial systolic pressure. The ratio for normal blood flow is 1.0. A ratio of .9 at rest or .85 after exercise indicates peripheral artery disease.

ABI Scale

1.0	Normal
.5 – .9	Arterial occlusion
	Impairment with wound healing
	Therapeutic exercise beneficial
< .5	Severe arterial occlusion
	Exercise is unrealistic
	Poor to no wound healing

Heart Rate/Pulse

Heart rate indirectly measures the rate of contraction of the left ventricle through a peripheral pulse site.

Normal heart rate values are accepted as:

Infant:	100 to 130 bpm
Child:	80 to 100 bpm
Adult:	60 to 100 bpm

Pulse sites for measurement include: brachial, carotid, dorsal pedal, femoral, popliteal, posterior tibial, radial, and temporal pulses. The carotid and radial pulse sites are the most common sites for measuring a patient's pulse rate.

Bradycardia: a condition of a heart rate consistently below 60 bpm

Tachycardia: a condition of a heart rate consistently above 100 bpm

Strong/regular: adequate force and consistent beats

Weak: poor force with contraction

Irregular: inconsistency during heart rate measurement with regard to strength and beat of the heart

Preparation and Procedure

- ✓ A regular and strong heart beat may be taken for 15 seconds and multiplied by four to total the per minute heart rate
- ✓ If there is any form of irregularity the pulse should be

taken for a full 60 seconds
- ✓ Find the appropriate pulse site and use a timepiece with a seconds hand (stop watch)
- ✓ Use the index and middle fingers to measure the heart rate, never the thumb
- ✓ Assess and document the rhythm as regular or irregular
- ✓ Assess and document the strength or amplitude of the pulse as strong, medium or weak
- ✓ An alternate method to obtain heart rate is to auscultate over the apical pulse for one minute

Peripheral Pulse Assessment Grading Systems

0-3 scale

0	absent
1+	weak/thready pulse
2+	normal
3+	full, firm pulse

Pulse Amplitude Classification

0	absent
1+	diminished
2+	normal
3+	moderately increased
4+	markedly increased

Respiratory Rate

Inspiration: to breathe air into the lungs

Expiration: to breathe air out of the lungs

Normal respiration rates are:

Infants:	30 to 50 respirations per minute
Adults:	12 to 18 respirations per minute

Values above 20 respirations or lower than 10 respirations per minute for an adult are considered abnormal.

Preparation and Procedures

- ✓ Observe the patient at rest breathing for 60 seconds
- ✓ Use a timepiece with a seconds hand (stop watch)
- ✓ Assess and document any accessory muscle use
- ✓ Assess and document the patient's respiration rate, rhythm of respiration, depth of respiration, and any deviation away from quiet respiration
- ✓ An alternate method to measure respiration rate is to place your hand over the patient's upper thorax and observe and feel movement with each respiration

Metabolic Equivalents (METS)

A MET is the amount of oxygen consumed per kilogram of body weight per minute to perform a given activity. At rest a person consumes 3.5 ml/kg/minute. The following list identifies METS associated with common activities of daily living.

MET Chart

Eating	1
Toileting	1 – 2
Driving a car	1 – 2
Dressing	2
Walking (2 mph)	2 – 2.5
Bathing	2 – 3
Cooking	2 – 3
Light housework	2 – 4
Light gardening	3 – 4
Showering	3.5 – 4
Sexual intercourse	4 – 5
Dancing	4 – 5
Walking (4 mph)	4.5 – 5.5
Swimming	4 – 8
Shoveling snow	6 – 7
Mowing the lawn	6 – 7

Borg's Rating of Perceived Exertion Scale and the Revised 10-Grade Scale

RPE:		10-Grade Rating Scale:	
6		0	Nothing at all
7	Very, very light	0.5	Very, very weak (just noticeable)
8		1.0	Very weak
9	Very light	2.0	Weak (light)
10		3.0	Moderate
11	Fairly light	4.0	Somewhat strong
12		5.0	Strong (heavy)
13	Somewhat hard	6.0	
14		7.0	Very strong
15	Hard	8.0	
16		9.0	
17	Very hard	10.0	Very, very strong (almost maximum)
18			Maximal
19	Very, very hard		

From Borg GAV: Psychophysical Bases of Perceived Exertion. Med Sci Sports Exerc 14:377, 1982, American College of Sports Medicine, with permission.

Methods to Determine Exercise Intensity

Target Heart Rate Formula
Target heart rate formula is a method for obtaining an appropriate demand on the heart during exercise. The age-adjusted maximum heart rate is determined by subtracting the patient's age from 220. The training heart rate is determined by multiplying the age-adjusted maximum heart rate by the appropriate percentage of intensity that the patient should maintain during exercise. Normal training intensity ranges from 60-90% of the age-adjusted maximum heart rate. A patient with cardiac pathology must have exercise intensity determined from the results of a stress test.

Karvonen's Formula: Heart Rate Reserve Method
The Karvonen formula is a method to obtain an appropriate range for training heart rate. The maximum heart rate is obtained by an exercise stress test (or the age-adjusted maximum heart rate) and the resting heart rate is subtracted from it. This number is termed the heart rate reserve. The heart rate reserve is multiplied by both ends of the prescribed range (e.g., HR reserve x 60% and HR reserve x 80%). The resting heart rate is then added to each of the two numbers to identify the upper and lower limits of the prescribed target heart rate.

Cardiac Pathology

Comparisons of Right and Left-Sided Heart Failure

Right	Left
Elevated end-diastolic right ventricular pressure	Elevated end-diastolic left ventricular pressure
Systemic congestion: – Enlarged liver – Ascites – Jugular venous distention – Dependent (pitting) edema	Pulmonary congestion: – Pulmonary edema – Dyspnea, orthopnea – Paroxysmal nocturnal dyspnea – Cough – Bronchospasm
Fatigue	Fatigue
Oliguria, nocturia	Oliguria
Cyanosis (capillary stasis)	Cyanosis (central)
Pleural effusion (R>L)	Tachycardia
Anorexia and bleeding Unexplained weight gain	

Etiology	Etiology
– Mitral stenosis – Pulmonary parenchymal or vascular disease – Pulmonic or tricuspid valvular disease – Infective endocarditis	– Hypertension – Coronary artery disease – Aortic valve disease – Cardiomyopathies – Congenital heart defects – Infective endocarditis – High output conditions – Various connective tissue disorders

From Rothstein J, Roy S, Wolf S: The Rehabilitation Specialist's Handbook. F. A. Davis Company, Philadelphia 1998, p.654-655, with permission.

Risk Factors for Cardiac Pathology

Modifiable Factors
- Cholesterol – greater than 200 mg/dL
- Hypertension
- Smoking
- Atherogenic diet
- Culture
- Physical inactivity
- Stress

Non-Modifiable Factors
- Age – risk increases with age
- Sex – male > female (after menopause female equal to male)
- Family history
- Culture

Secondary Factors
- Alcohol consumption
- Obesity
- Coping with stress
- Diabetes mellitus
- Peripheral vascular disease

Symptoms of Cardiac Pathology
- Chest pain
- Shortness of breath
- Cardiac arrhythmia (palpitation)
- Fainting
- Claudication
- Cyanosis of lips and nailbeds
- Fatigue
- Edema

Symptoms of Myocardial Infarction
- Severe chest pain
- Chest heaviness
- Radiating pain down one or both arms
- Weakness
- Nausea
- Vomiting
- Diaphoresis
- Shortness of breath

Diagnosis of Myocardial Infarction
- Abnormal ECG
- Elevation in enzyme level
  - Creatine phosphokinase (CPK)
  - Aspartate aminotransferase (AST)
  - Lactate dehydrogenase

Cardiac Rehabilitation

Indications for Cardiac Rehabilitation

- Myocardial infarction
- Angina (stable)
- Coronary artery bypass surgery
- Compensated heart failure
- Cardiac surgery
- High risk for coronary artery disease
- High risk for high blood pressure
- End-stage renal disease
- Status post pacemaker insertion
- Cardiomyopathy
- Peripheral vascular disease
- Heart transplant
- High risk for diabetes

Relative Contraindications to Stop Exercising during Cardiac Rehabilitation

- Abnormal heart rate that increases > 50 bpm with low-level activity
- Blood pressure that increases > 210 mm Hg systolic during exercise
- Blood pressure that increases > 110 mm Hg diastolic during exercise
- Decrease in systolic pressure > 10 mm Hg during low-level exercise
- Any ST segment changes
- Severe lower extremity claudication
- Angina
- Confusion
- Extreme fatigue
- Ventricular gallop

Contraindications for Cardiac Rehabilitation

- Uncontrolled atrial/ventricular arrhythmias
- Recent diagnosis of embolism
- Resting diastolic pressure > 110 mm Hg
- Thrombophlebitis
- Orthostatic blood pressure (> 20 mm Hg drop)
- Acute infection
- Resting ST segment displacement of > 2 mm
- Unstable angina
- Resting systolic pressure > 200 mm Hg
- Uncompensated congestive heart failure

Absolute Contraindications for Treatment of an Unstable Cardiac Patient

- Third-degree heart block
- Uncompensated congestive heart failure
- PVCs of ventricular tachycardia at rest
- Multifocal PVCs
- Chest pain with ST segment changes
- ECG changes that indicate ischemia
- Dissecting aortic aneurysm

Absolute Contraindications to Exercise Testing

- ECG changes that denote cardiac ischemia
- Recent myocardial infarction < 48 hrs
- Multifocal PVCs
- Uncontrolled heart failure
- Unstable angina
- Uncontrolled cardiac arrhythmias
- Untreated heart block (2nd or 3rd degree)
- Pulmonary embolism
- Acute infection

Benefits of Routine Exercise

- Decrease myocardial oxygen cost
- Decrease heart rate and blood pressure
- Increase maximal oxygen uptake
- Decrease minute ventilation
- Decrease in depression and/or anxiety
- Decrease serum triglycerides
- Decrease risk of heart disease
- Decrease percent body fat
- Improve glucose tolerance
- Increase HDL cholesterol

Description of a Cardiac Rehabilitation Program

Phase I

A Phase I program begins with the physician referral to the cardiac rehabilitation program. Patients are referred to the inpatient program when they are medically stable. Phase I consists of patient and family education, self-care evaluation, continuous monitoring of vital signs, group discussions, and low-level exercise. Exercise activities include active range of motion, ambulation, and self-care. Exercise intensity is often prescribed according to heart rate and by rating on a perceived exertion scale. A Phase I program typically concludes with a low-level exercise test, although this activity may not be appropriate for high-risk clients. The trend toward early hospital discharge following a cardiac event has resulted in Phase I programs averaging 3-5 days.

Phase II

A Phase II program begins immediately after hospitalization and lasts from 2-12 weeks depending on the patient's ability to tolerate the exercise training. Patients are monitored closely during the Phase II program and are supervised during all activities. Goals for a Phase II program include increasing functional capacity through exercise, educating the patient on risk factor modification, and developing independence in self-monitoring. Frequency of visits in a Phase II program averages 2-3 times a week. Patients typically progress to a Phase III program when they are clinically stable, independent with self-monitoring techniques, and do not require ECG monitoring.

Phase III

A Phase III program is often viewed as a continuation of a Phase II program and lasts approximately 6-8 weeks. Exercise training, physical fitness, level of endurance, and risk factor modification are the primary emphasis of the program. Phase III programs often include exercise, education, and counseling. A maximal symptom-limited exercise test is required to assess fitness level and appropriately plan for exercise intensity. The average frequency of the program is once per week.

Phase IV

A Phase IV program lasts throughout the patient's lifetime and is designed to promote optimal health. Requirements for participation in a Phase IV program include independence with self-monitoring of exercise, stable cardiac status, no contraindications to exercise, and at least a 5 MET capacity for activities.

Therapist Role During Inpatient Cardiac Rehabilitation

- ✓ Provide constant monitoring of heart rate, blood pressure, and ECG interpretation before, during, and after each session
- ✓ Develop program within the guidelines of the patient's prescribed training heart rate
- ✓ Use of exertion scales to identify subjective intensity of exercise
- ✓ Promote proper technique and breathing patterns during exercise
- ✓ Progress activities based on METs tolerated

Therapist Role During Outpatient Cardiac Rehabilitation

- ✓ Initially close monitoring of ECG, heart rate, and blood pressure throughout session is required
- ✓ Constant measurement of vital signs should decrease and self-monitoring of heart rate and perceived exertion by the patient should guide exercise sessions
- ✓ Development of an exercise program should be based on a symptom-limited treadmill test and determined target heart rate
- ✓ Exercise should be gradual in progression; the session should generally include warm-up for 5-10 minutes, aerobic activity for 20-60 minutes, and a cool down for 5-10 minutes
- ✓ Warm-up should include stretching as well as low-

intensity activity which will slowly increase heart rate
- ✓ Exercise may include walking, stationary bicycling, as well as isotonic strengthening (low resistance)
- ✓ Isometrics are contraindicated

Cardiopulmonary Resuscitation

CPR Adult Flow Chart

No Movement or response

↓

Phone 911; emergency response

↓

Open airway; check breathing

↓

If NO breathing-administer 2 breaths that make chest rise

↓

If NO response-check pulse

↓

If pulse-rescue breathing only at 10-12 breaths/minute

↓

If NO pulse-begin CPR with 30 compressions and 2 breaths. Push hard and fast (100/min) and release completely. Minimize interruptions during compressions.

↓

Continue to perform CPR until medical assistance arrives, breathing, coughing or other signs of circulation return, the patient begins to move or you cannot physically continue due to exhaustion.

Cardiopulmonary ABC's

Airway – maintain an open airway
Breathing (rescue breathing) – "Look, listen, and feel"
Circulation (compressions) – check pulse

CPR – Adult (eight years +)

Breathing with CPR	2 initial breaths; CPR 8-10 breaths/minute
Rescue breathing only	10-12 breaths/minute
Compressions	100/minute
Depth of compressions	1 ½ to 2 inches
Placement for chest compressions	Lower half of sternum, between nipples
One-rescuer ratio of compressions:ventilations	30:2
Two-rescuer ratio of compressions:ventilations	30:2

CPR – Child (one to eight years old)

Breathing with CPR	2 initial effective breaths; CPR 8-10 breaths/minute
Rescue breathing only	12-20 breaths/minute
Compressions	100/minute
Depth of compressions	1/3-1/2 the depth of chest
Placement for chest compressions	Lower half of sternum, between nipples
One-rescuer ratio of compressions:ventilations	30:2
Two-rescuer ratio of compressions:ventilations	15:2

CPR – Infant (less than one year old)

Breathing with CPR	2 initial effective breaths; CPR 8-10 breaths/minute
Rescue breathing only	12-20 breaths/minute
Compressions	100/minute
Depth of compressions	1/3-1/2 the depth of chest
Placement for chest compressions	Just below nipple line; lower half of sternum
One-rescuer ratio of compressions:ventilations	30:2
Two-rescuer ratio of compressions:ventilations	15:2

From American Heart Association, 2005.

Cardiac System Profile

Examination

- Past medical history
- History of current condition
  - Cardiac testing
- Social history (caregiver support)
- Medications
- Living environment
- Risk factors profile
- Systems review
  - Vital signs
  - Auscultation of heart and lung sounds
- Skin assessment
  - Cyanosis
  - Edema
  - Pallor
  - Diaphoresis
- Cognitive assessment
- Pain
- Strength as tolerated
- Endurance
- Mobility skills as tolerated

Intervention

- Patient/caregiver teaching:
  - Risk factor modification
  - Signs and symptoms of pathology
  - Measurement of vital signs
  - Nutrition
- Breathing exercises
- Endurance/exercise training
- Mobility training
- Relaxation techniques

Inpatient Goals

- Maximize self-care skills
- Maximize functional mobility skills
- Maximize endurance
- Maximize patient/caregiver competence with:
  - Safe activity guidelines
  - Modification of risk factors
  - Monitoring of vital signs
  - Breathing exercises
  - Stress management
- Perform low-level exercise test (4-6 METS)
- Maximize energy conservation techniques

Outpatient Goals

- Maximize functional mobility skills
- Maximize endurance
- Maximize aerobic capacity
- Maximize patient/caregiver competence with:
  - Nutritional education
  - Monitoring of vital signs
  - Energy conservation techniques
  - Warning signs of cardiac pathology
  - Home exercise program

Cardiac System Pathology

Aneurysm

An aneurysm is a weakening in the wall of a vessel that produces a sac-like area. By definition there is a 50% increase in the normal vessel diameter with weakening of all layers of the arterial (or venous) wall. Etiology can include genetic disposition, trauma or infection. The most common sites include aorta, abdominal aorta, femoral, and popliteal arteries. Surgical repair prior to rupture has a good prognosis; a ruptured aneurysm is a medical emergency with high mortality rates.

Symptoms

– Dependent on site of aneurysm
– Intermittent or constant pain
– Abnormal heart beat
– Serious complications can occur including MI, stroke, renal failure, and embolization

Angina Pectoris

A transient process that occurs when the coronary arteries are unable to supply the heart with adequate oxygen. Sudden onset is common once the myocardial oxygen demand is higher than the supply. Coronary artery disease accounts for 90% of all angina. The four most common types of angina pectoris are as follows:

- **Nocturnal:** Angina that will wake someone up from his or her sleep with the same characteristics as angina from exertion. This may be related to congestive heart failure.
- **Prinzmetal's:** Angina that occurs while at rest secondary to coronary artery disease or spasm. This can be severe and not readily relieved by nitroglycerin.
- **Stable:** Angina that usually occurs at a predictable level of exertion, exercise or stress and responds to rest or nitroglycerin.
- **Unstable:** Angina that can occur at rest or with exertion and has changed intensity, frequency, and/or duration.

Symptoms

– Temporary pain
– Sudden onset
– Pain may radiate
– Usually lasts one to five minutes
– Usually relieved with rest or nitroglycerin

Atherosclerosis

Atherosclerosis is a condition of progressive accumulation of fatty plaques on the inner walls of vessels that ultimately produces stenosis.

This process begins in childhood and usually effects medium sized arteries. Over time the plaque that produces stenosis inside the vessel can also block blood flow. Heart attack or stroke can result from atherosclerosis.

Cardiomyopathy

Cardiomyopathy refers to a group of conditions that affect the myocardium muscle itself, impairing the ability for the heart to contract and relax. Three types of cardiomyopathy are dilated, hypertrophic, and restrictive.

Symptoms

– Dependent on the type of cardiomyopathy
– Symptoms are the same as heart failure
– Neck vein distension
– Fatigue, weakness
– Possible chest pain
– Sudden death (hypertrophic)
– Exercise intolerance

Congestive Heart Failure (CHF)

Congestive heart failure is a condition that usually results from coronary artery disease when the heart is unable to maintain an adequate cardiac output. CHF is characterized by abnormal retention of fluid and results in diminished blood flow to the tissue and congestion of the pulmonary and/or systemic circulation. This is not a disease, but rather a symptom of pathology within the heart muscle itself or the cardiac valves.

Symptoms

– Dependent on type of CHF
– Pulmonary edema
– Dyspnea when lying down (orthopnea)
– Cough (nonproductive)
– S3 gallop
– Exertional hypotension
– Weight gain within hours
– Increased resting heart rate
– See chart on page 106 for symptoms

Coronary Artery Disease (CAD)

Coronary artery disease is the narrowing or blockage of the coronary arteries that may produce ischemia and necrosis of the myocardium. There is an inability for vasodilation and as a result the arteries cannot meet the metabolic demands. This will produce ischemia and ultimately necrosis. CAD includes thrombus, vasospasms, and atherosclerosis. CAD results from inheritance, environment, culture, nutrition, and smoking.

Symptoms

– Appear after significant blockage is present > 75%
– Pain in the occluded artery's region
– If untreated, MI or sudden death

Heart Failure

Heart failure is a condition where there is an inability of the heart to maintain a proper cardiac output of four liters per minute while at rest. The most common etiology associated with heart failure is chronic hypertension.

Infective Endocarditis

Endocarditis causes inflammation of the endothelium that lines the heart and cardiac valves. This condition most commonly damages the mitral valve, then the aortic and tricuspid valves. Endocarditis is commonly caused by bacteria that are normally present in the body. It can also occur after an invasive medical or dental procedure. At risk individuals can easily prevent endocarditis with antibiotic prophylaxis, however, once infected it is not easily diagnosed or treated.

Symptoms

- May have sudden onset or be asymptomatic for months
- Valvular dysfunction
- May affect organ systems
- Chest pain, CHF, clubbing
- Arthralgia, arthritis, acidosis
- Myalgia, low back pain
- Meningitis, stroke, confusion

Myocardial Infarction (MI)

A myocardial infarction causes irreversible damage to a segment of heart muscle due to prolonged ischemia. The causative factors include narrowing of coronary arteries due to atherosclerotic occlusion, poor coronary perfusion secondary to hemorrhage or occlusion of one of the major coronary arteries.

Symptoms

- Sudden constant pain and/or pressure
- May radiate up neck, down arm
- Shortness of breath
- Profuse perspiration
- Unexplained fatigue

Area of Infarct	Expected Damage
Anterior heart	– Left anterior descending artery – High risk of large infarction – Heart failure – Sudden death
Inferior heart	– Right coronary artery – Right ventricle damage – AV block – Medium infarct possible
Lateral heart and/or Superior heart	– Least area of muscle affected – Usually the least overall damage – Minor impairment or complications

Myocarditis

Myocarditis refers to an uncommon condition of inflammation to the myocardium muscle itself, usually due to infection. This condition can be treated with antimicrobial therapy, however, left untreated can quickly progress to a dilated cardiomyopathy with heart failure.

Symptoms

- Mild, low-level chest pain
- Soreness in the epigastric region
- Fatigue
- Palpitations

Pericarditis

Pericarditis refers to an inflammation of the pericardium (the outer membrane) of the heart. This condition may be acute or chronic (constrictive pericarditis) and can be painful or asymptomatic. Etiology is often unknown; however, causes such as infection, myocardial infarction, radiation therapy, post cardiac surgery, metabolic disorders, and aortic dissection have been linked to this diagnosis. Prognosis is usually good, however, if left untreated a patient can experience shock or death.

Symptoms

- Symptoms are varied and based on the underlying etiology
- Auscultation reveals pericardial friction rub
- Pleuretic chest pain
- Diffuse ST segment elevation
- Retrosternal chest pain
- Cough and hoarseness
- Fever, fatigue, and weakness
- Joint pain

Rheumatic Heart Disease

Rheumatic heart disease is the result of damage to the heart secondary to inflammation from rheumatic fever. Rheumatic fever can occur from streptococcal group A bacteria (i.e., strep throat) and is classified as an autoimmune disease. It can affect all connective tissues of the heart, joints, and central nervous system and frequently damages the cardiac valves. Acute rheumatic fever has a low mortality rate; however, recurrent or chronic rheumatic disease has significant influence on long-term outcome and level of disability.

Symptoms

- Carditis with chest pain
- Acute onset of polyarthritis
- Chorea
- Arthralgias and weakness
- Fever
- Palpitations

Cardiac and Pulmonary Systems Pediatric Pathology

Asthma

Asthma is a reversible condition of airway hypersensitivity and bronchoconstriction within the lungs.

- **Causative factors** are extrinsic or intrinsic by nature. Extrinsic factors include allergens such as foods, animals, dust, smoke, and pollen. Intrinsic factors include exercise, stress, viral infections, and overall fatigue.

- **Characteristics** can range from mild to severe depending on the level of airway restriction. A mild asthma attack presents with wheezing, chest tightness, and slight shortness of breath. A severe asthma attack presents with dyspnea, flaring nostrils, diminished wheezing, anxiety, cyanosis, and the inability to speak. A severe attack left untreated will result in respiratory failure.

- **Treatment** includes pharmacological intervention using bronchodilators. Physical therapy management includes caregiver education, bronchial drainage and hygiene, breathing exercises, relaxation, endurance, and strength training.

Cystic Fibrosis

Cystic fibrosis is a disease of the exocrine glands that primarily affects the respiratory and gastrointestinal systems.

- The **causative factor** is a mutation of chromosome seven to include the cystic fibrosistransmembrane conductance regulator (CFTR). Cystic fibrosis is an autosomal recessive genetic disorder and a terminal disease.

- **Characteristics** change with the progression of the disease and include increased secretion of thick mucus, gastrointestinal distress, abnormal bowels, recurrent pulmonary infection, salty tasting skin, wheezing, productive cough, barrel chest, dyspnea, and progressive use of accessory muscles with respiration.

- **Treatment** has improved survival rates from seven years in the late 1960's to a mean age of 32 years today. Pharmacological interventions include antibiotics used to control pulmonary infections, nutritional supplements, pancreatic enzyme replacements, mucus thinning medications, and bronchodilators. Physical therapy treatment is essential and includes bronchial drainage, percussion, vibration, suctioning, breathing techniques, assisted cough, and ventilatory muscle training for optimal pulmonary function. General exercise is indicated to improve overall strength and endurance except with severe lung disease. Family involvement with a home program is vital for the child's ongoing pulmonary needs.

Patent Ductus Arteriosus

Patent ductus arteriosus is a disorder where the ductus arteriosus, which normally shunts blood in utero from the pulmonary artery directly to the descending aorta, fails to close shortly after birth.

- **Causative factors** for this condition include premature birth, respiratory distress syndrome, fetal alcohol syndrome, Trisomy 13 (Patau's syndrome), and Trisomy 18 (Edwards' syndrome).

- **Characteristics** of this condition depend on the size of the ductus. A small ductus may be asymptomatic where as a large ductus may present with tachycardia, respiratory distress, poor nutrition, weight loss, and congestive heart failure.

- Initial **treatment** attempts to non-surgically reduce the size of the ductus with use of diuretics and indomethacin when indicated. Surgical repair may be necessary for a large ductus or when initial management fails.

Respiratory Distress Syndrome (RDS)

Respiratory distress syndrome is a pulmonary condition seen in neonates born before 37 weeks of gestation. RDS is also known as hyaline membrane disease and is the leading cause of death in the neonate.

- **Causative factors** are due to the immaturity of the lungs and the inability to produce necessary levels of surfactant. This deficit results in increased alveolar tension, alveolar collapse, atelectasis, and difficulty breathing. Associated factors with RDS include being the second born twin, cesarean delivery, hypoxia, and acidosis.

- **Characteristics** are observed immediately as the infant works hard to breathe and re-inflate the collapsed lung. Tachypnea, flaring of the nostrils, use of accessory muscles, and respiratory distress are observed within one to two hours. Untreated, the infant lacks oxygen and presents with metabolic acidosis and acute respiratory failure.

- **Treatment** will vary and can include mechanical ventilation, supplemental oxygen, administration of artificial surfactant, nutritional support, bronchial drainage, and chest physical therapy. As a child recovers from RDS there is an increase in secretions from oxygen therapy and mechanical ventilation that requires short-term chest physical therapy.

Tetralogy of Fallot

Tetralogy of Fallot is the most common cyanotic heart defect where the following four abnormalities exist:
- Ventricular septal defect
- Right ventricular hypertrophy
- Aortic override of the interventricular septum
- Pulmonary stenosis

- The **causative factors** are congenital defect, association with Down syndrome and fetal alcohol syndrome.

- **Characteristics** vary depending on the extent of the defects and include dyspnea, hypoxia, failure to gain weight, cyanosis, and poor development.

- **Treatment** usually includes pharmacological intervention, reopening of the ductus arteriosus or surgical reconstruction of the defects.

Pharmacology

There are multiple medications that are administered for various cardiac conditions. General classifications of drugs with example medications are listed. The list is designed to serve as a general overview of major cardiac medications.

Pharmacological Intervention for Cardiac Management

Diuretic Agents

Increase sodium and water excretion to manage hypertension, congestive heart failure Types: Thiazide, Loop, Potassium sparing	Furosemide (Lasix) Hydrochlorothiazide (Esidrix, Microzide, Hydrodiuril) Chlorthalidone (Thalitone, Hygroton) Spirondactone (Aldactone) Amiloride (Midamor)

Nitrates

Decrease ischemia through smooth muscle relaxation of preload and afterload	Nitroglycerin (Nitrostat) Isosorbide dinitrate (Isordil) Erythrityl tetranitrate (Tetranitrol)

Beta-adrenergic Blocking Agents (Beta-blockers)

Decrease the heart's oxygen demand through decreasing heart rate and contractility. Treat angina, arrhythmias, and hypertension	Bisoprolol (Zebeta) Atenolol (Tenormin) Metoprolol (Lopressor) Propanolol (Inderal)

Alpha-adrenergic Blocking Agents

Block post-synaptic alpha 1-adrenergic receptors which dilates arterioles and veins; decreases blood pressure	Prazosin (Minipress) Terazosin (Hytrin) Doxazosin (Cardura)

Angiotensin-converting Enzyme Inhibitor (ACE) Agents

Decrease blood pressure, and afterload in patients with congestive heart failure and hypertension	Captorpril (Capoten) Enalapril (Vasotec) Lisinopril (Prinivil) Fosinopril (Monopril) Benazepril (Lotensin) Ramipril (Altace)

Angiotensin II Receptor Antagonist Agents

Used when patients cannot tolerate ACE inhibitors	Losartan (Cozaar) Diltiazem (Cardizem) Verapamil (Calan)

Antiarrhythmic Agents

Alter conductivity in order to correct ectopic stimuli or other electrical abnormality	Lidocaine (Xylocaine) Amiodarone (Cordarone) Bretylium tosylate Procainamide (Procanbid)

Calcium Channel Blocker Agents

Decreases the heart's oxygen demand by reducing the flow of calcium. Allows for peripheral vasodilation that further reduces demand on the heart	Amlodipine (Norvasc) Nifedipine (Procardia XL) Verapamil (Calan) Diltiazem (Cardizem)

*selected pharmaceutical drugs and their respective trade names in parentheses, not intended to be a complete listing

Foundational Science: Pulmonary System

Breath Sounds

Normal tracheal and bronchial sounds

These are loud and tubular sounds with a high-pitch noted during inspiration and expiration, pausing between the two components.

Vesicular breath sounds

These are normal, soft, and low-pitched sounds heard over the more distal airways primarily during inspiration. During expiration the soft sound is diminished and only heard during the beginning of expiration.

Abnormal breath sounds

These are sounds that are heard outside of their normal location or phase of respiration.

Adventitous breath sounds

These are abnormal breath sounds heard using a stethoscope with inspiration and/or expiration. These sounds can be continuous or discontinuous sounds.

Wheeze

These are continuous adventitious breath sounds that are high-pitched and varying in duration. These are usually heard during expiration but may also be present on inspiration. Wheezes are typically a sign of airway obstruction from retained secretions or due to bronchoconstriction or bronchospasm with quality similar to whistling. Wheezes found with inspiration occur with movement of air through secretions.

Rhonchi

These are continuous adventitious breath sounds that are

low-pitched and occur with both inspiration and expiration. Rhonchi are associated with an obstructive process of the larger or more central airways with quality similar to snoring.

Stridor

A continuous adventitious sound comprised of a very high-pitched wheeze that can be heard with inspiration and expiration and also indicates upper airway obstruction. A stridor that is heard without a stethoscope can indicate an emergency.

Crackle (formerly rales)

A discontinuous adventitious sound heard with a stethoscope that "bubbles" or "pops." Crackles typically represent the movement of fluid or secretions during inspiration (wet crackles) or occur from the sudden opening of closed airways (dry crackles). Crackles that occur during the latter half of inspiration typically represent atelectasis, fibrosis, pulmonary edema or pleural effusion. Crackles secondary to the movement of secretions are usually low-pitched and can be heard during inspiration and/or expiration.

Bronchial breath sounds

These sounds are abnormal breath sounds when heard in locations that vesicular sounds are normally present. Pneumonia may produce these sounds.

Decreased or diminished sounds

A less audible sound may indicate severe congestion, emphysema or hypoventilation.

Absent breath sounds

Absent lung sounds may indicate pneumothorax or lung collapse.

Voice Sounds

Egophony, bronchophony, and whispering pectoriloquy are techniques to further assess lung pathology. If there is an abnormal transmission of sound it can further substantiate particular lung abnormalities.

- **Egophony:** While auscultating lung segments the patient repeatedly says the letter "e." If when auscultating the distal segments it sounds like "a," fluid is expected in the air spaces or lung parenchyma.

- **Bronchophony:** While auscultating lung segments throughout the chest the patient repeatedly says "99." If the word is clearly audible in distal lung fields the test is positive for consolidation. If the word is less audible, softer or weaker sounding, the test is positive for hyperinflation.

- **Whispering pectoriloquy:** While auscultating lung segments the patient repeatedly whispers words. The clearly audible and less audible words indicate the same findings as bronchophony testing.

Pulmonary Function Testing

Anatomic dead space volume (VD): The volume of air that occupies the non-respiratory conducting airways.

Expiratory reserve volume (ERV): Maximal volume expired after normal expiration.

Forced expiratory volume (FEV): The amount of air exhaled in the 1st, 2nd, and 3rd second of a forced vital capacity test.

Forced vital capacity (FVC): The amount of air forcefully expired after a maximal inspiration.

Functional residual capacity (FRC): Volume in the lungs after normal exhalation.

Inspiratory capacity (IC): The amount of air that can be inspired after a normal exhalation.

Inspiratory reserve volume (IRV): Maximal volume inspired after normal inspiration.

Minute volume ventilation (VE): The amount of air expired in one minute. This is equal to the product of the tidal volume and the respiratory rate.

Peak expiratory flow (PEF): The maximum flow of air during the beginning of a forced expiratory breath.

Residual volume (RV): Lung volume remaining in the lungs at the end of a maximal expiration.

Tidal volume (TV): Total volume inspired and expired per breath.

Total lung capacity (TLC): Lung volume measured at the end of a maximal inspiration.

Vital capacity (VC): Maximal volume forcefully expired after a maximal inspiration.

Pulmonary Function Reference Values

Values are calculated for an individual patient based on variables such as height, weight, sex, and age. A value is usually considered abnormal if it is less than 80% of the reference value.

Determining Lung Capacities

Total Lung Capacity (TLC) =	Inspiratory Reserve Volume (IRV) + Tidal Volume (TV) + Expiratory Reserve Volume (ERV) + Residual Capacity (RC)
Vital Capacity (VC) =	Inspiratory Reserve Volume (IRV) + Tidal Volume (TV) + Expiratory Reserve Volume (ERV)
Inspiratory Capacity (IC) =	Tidal Volume (TV) + Inspiratory Reserve Volume (IRV)
Functional Residual Capacity (FRC) =	Expiratory Reserve Volume (ERV) + Residual Volume (RV)

Typical Lung Volumes and Capacities

Tidal Volume =	500 mL
Expiratory Reserve Volume =	1000 mL
Vital Capacity =	4000-5000 mL
Inspiratory Capacity =	3000-4000 mL 75-80% of vital capacity 55-60% of total lung capacity

Forced Expiratory Volumes

Forced Expiratory Volume in one second (FEV1):	83% of VC
Forced Expiratory Volume in two seconds (FEV2):	94% of VC
Forced Expiratory Volume in three seconds (FEV3):	97% of VC

Gas Pressure (mm Hg)

Gas	Dry Air	Moist Tracheal Air	Alveolar Gas	Arterial Blood	Mixed Venous Blood
PO_2	159.1	149.2	104.0	100.0	40.0
PCO_2	0.3	0.3	40.0	40.0	46.0
PH_2O	0.0	47.0	47.0	47.0	47.0
PN_2	600.6	563.5	569.0	573.0	573.0
PTOTAL	760.0	760.0	760.0	760.0	760.0

From Rothstein, JM: Rehabilitation Specialist's Handbook. F.A. Davis Company, Philadelphia 1998, p.528, with permission.

Arterial Blood Gases (ABG)

The study of blood gases is used as a tool to determine the effectiveness of alveolar ventilation. Values are expressed as the partial pressure of the gas. PaO_2, the partial pressure of oxygen within the arterial system, is normally 95-100 mm Hg. Supplemental oxygen is usually required for oxygen saturation rates less than 90%. The body cannot carry out vital functions with oxygen saturation less than 70%. $PaCO_2$, the partial pressure of carbon dioxide within the arterial system, is normally 35-45 mm Hg. The range for the acid-base balance or pH is 7.35-7.45. Changes in the $PaCO_2$ directly affect the balance of pH in the body. Prolonged imbalance of the pH in either direction can affect the nervous system and in some cases cause convulsions or coma.

Hypercapnia: an increased amount of CO_2 in the blood.

Hyperkalemia: an increased amount of potassium in the blood.

Hypocapnia: a decreased amount of CO_2 in the blood.

Hypoxemia: when the PaO_2 is less than 80 mm Hg.

Physical Signs Observed in Various Disorders

Condition	Breath Sounds	Adventitious Sounds	Voice	Inspection	Tactile Fremitus	Percussion
Normal	Nl	None	Muffled, distant, indistinct	Trachea midline, symmetric chest expansion	Nl	Nl
Asthma, acute moderately severe attack	↓ Bronchial, prolonged expiration	Inspiratory plus expiratory wheezes	↓	↑ Use of accessory muscles, tachypnea	↓	Nl - ↑
Atelectasis	↓ or 0	Crackles	↓ or 0	Trachea deviated to affected side	↓	↓ - ↓↓
Bronchiectasis	Nl	Crackles	Nl	↓ Expansion AS, tachypnea, clubbing	↑ Rhonchal fremitus	Nl
Bronchitis	Nl, possible prolonged expiration	Crackles, wheezes	Nl	Possible↓ motion, occasional use of accessory muscles	↓ Bilaterally	↑ Bilaterally
COPD	↓ - ↓↓ Prolonged expiration	None versus Crackles and wheezes	↓ or 0 bilaterally	Barrel-shaped chest, moves as a unit, ↑ use of accessory muscles	↓ Bilaterally	↑ Bilaterally
Consolidation	Bronchial	Crackles	Whispered pectoriloquy	↓ Motion AS	↑	↓
Fibrosis						
• Localized	↓	Crackles	↓	↓ Motion over area	↓ or 0	↓
• Generalized	↓	Crackles	↓	↓ Motion bilaterally	↓ or 0	↓
Heart failure	Nl	Dependent crackles	Nl	Nl chest expansion, tachypnea	Nl	Nl
Pleural effusion (moderate to large)	↓ or 0,* Bronchial**	Possible pleural rub	↓ * ↑**	↓ Motion AS, ↑ RR, trachea deviated to OS	↓ or 0	↓ - ↓↓
Pneumothorax (>15%)	↓ or 0	None	↓ or 0	↓ Motion AS Trachea deviated to unaffected side	↓ or 0	

Nl = normal, ↓ = decreased, ↓↓ = very decreased, ↑ = increased, 0 = absent, AS = on affected side, COPD = chronic obstructive pulmonary disease, RR = respiratory rate, OS = opposite side; *Over the effusion; **Above the fluid.

From Watchie, J: Cardiopulmonary Physical Therapy: A Clinical Manual. W.B. Saunders Company, Philadelphia 1995, p.193, with permission.

Interpretation of Abnormal Acid-Base Balance

Type	pH	PaCO$_2$	HCO$_3$	Causes	Signs and Symptoms
Respiratory alkalosis	↑	↓	WNL	Alveolar hyperventilation	Dizziness, syncope, tingling, numbness, early tetany
Respiratory acidosis	↓	↑	WNL	Alveolar hypoventilation	Early: anxiety, restlessness, dyspnea, headache; late: confusion, somnolence, coma
Metabolic alkalosis	↑	WNL	↑	Bicarbonate ingestion, vomiting, diuretics, steroids, adrenal disease	Vague symptoms: weakness, mental dullness, possibly early tetany
Metabolic acidosis	↓	WNL	↓	Diabetic, lactic, or uremic acidosis, prolonged diarrhea	Secondary hyperventilation (Kussmaul's breathing), nausea and vomiting, cardiac dysrhythmias, lethargy, and coma

From Rothstein, JM: Rehabilitation Specialist's Handbook. F.A. Davis Company, Philadelphia 1998, p.529, with permission.

Normal Values

pH	7.4
PCO$_2$	40 mm Hg
PO$_2$	97 mm Hg
HCO$_3$	24 mEq/L
%Sat	95 - 98%

Metabolic alkalosis   pH > 7.45
Metabolic acidosis   pH < 7.35
Acute alveolar hyperventilation   pH > 7.5
Acute ventilatory failure   pH < 7.3
Respiratory alkalosis   PCO$_2$ < 40 mm Hg   *hypocapnia   *hyperventilation
Respiratory acidosis   PCO$_2$ > 40 mm Hg   *hypercapnia   *hypoventilation

Chest Physical Therapy

Indications for Chest Physical Therapy

- Patients who have acute or chronic respiratory problems
- The inability to expel pulmonary secretions
- An ineffective cough
- Patients with increased secretions
- Patients with pneumonia
- Patients with atelectasis
- Patients with neurological impairments that cause swallowing difficulties

Contraindications for Postural Drainage

- Congestive heart failure
- Significant pulmonary edema
- Significant pleural effusion
- Pneumothorax
- Cardiac arrhythmia
- History of recent myocardial infarction
- Unstable angina
- Pulmonary embolism

Contraindications for Percussion

- Over a fracture
- Over a spinal fusion site
- Over osteoporotic bone
- Unstable angina
- Low platelet count
- Anticoagulation therapy
- Pulmonary embolism

Guidelines for Chest Physical Therapy

- ✓ Treatment should be administered prior to eating or at least one hour after meals.
- ✓ Percuss and vibrate over each segment to be treated for at least 3-5 minutes.
- ✓ Cough after each segment is treated.
- ✓ Allow for a rest period after each segment is treated.
- ✓ Review breathing exercises in each drainage position.
- ✓ Treatment should not exceed 45-60 minutes secondary to patient fatigue.

Goals for Chest Physical Therapy

✓ Mobilize secretions
✓ Expel secretions
✓ Improve breathing patterns
✓ Improve ventilation throughout all lobes
✓ Improve overall function

Technique

Percussion

Percussion is a technique using cupped hands that strike over a particular lung segment in alternating fashion during inspiration and expiration in order to mobilize secretions. This rhythmic sequence should last for several minutes and should not be painful.

Vibration

Vibration is a technique using both hands (one on top of another) directly over the chest wall to provide pressure and manual vibration during exhalation. Vibration should be used in conjunction with percussion and only during expiration. Pressure should be applied in the same direction as chest wall movement during expiration.

Positioning

Trendelenburg position

The Trendelenburg position places the person in a "head down" position in supine with the bottom of the bed inclined to approximately 45°. This position is ideal to assist with secretion drainage from the lower lobes of the lungs. It can also assist with increasing blood pressure in the case of hypotension. Patients with congestive heart failure, pulmonary edema, hypertension, shortness of breath or other circulatory problems will not tolerate this position.

Reverse Trendelenburg position

The reverse Trendelenburg position places a person in supine with their head raised above their trunk and lower extremities. This position is opposite of the Trendelenburg position, resulting in its name. This position may be used with patients diagnosed with hypertension or other cardiac conditions. This position also decreases the weight of the abdominal contents on the diaphragm providing it with less resistance to movement during breathing.

Semi-Fowler's position

The semi-Fowler's position places a patient in supine with the head of the bed elevated to 45° and pillows under the patient's knees for support and maintenance of a proper lumbar curve. This position is used quite often for patients with congestive heart failure or other cardiac conditions.

Bronchial Drainage

Upper Lobes

- **Apical Segment: Left and Right Anterior**
  Sitting: Lean back against a pillow; clap above the clavicles between the neck and shoulder.

- **Apical Segment: Left and Right Posterior**
  Sitting: Lean forward onto a pillow; clap on both sides of the back above the scapula. Fingers should be positioned slightly over the shoulder.

- **Anterior Segment: Left and Right**
  Supine: Lie flat on back with pillow under knees for comfort; clap on both sides just below the clavicles and above the nipple line.

- **Left Posterior Segment**
  Side: Lie on right side with head and shoulders elevated on pillows. Make 1/4 turn forward; clap over the left scapula.

- **Right Posterior Segment**
  Side: Lie on left side. Place a pillow in front from the shoulders to the hips and roll slightly forward onto it; clap over the right scapula.

- **Left Lingula**
  Side: Elevate bottom of bed 14-16 inches. Lie on right side. Place pillow behind from the shoulders to the hips and roll slightly back onto it; clap over left nipple.

Middle Lobe

- **Right Middle Lobe**
  Side: Elevate bottom of bed 14-16 inches. Lie on left side. Place pillow behind from the shoulders to the hips and roll slightly back onto it; clap over selected lobe.

Lower Lobes

- **Superior Segments: Left and Right**
  Prone: Lie flat on stomach; place pillow under the stomach area for added comfort and clap over the middle back at the tip of the scapula.

- **Lateral Basal Segment: Left and Right**
  Side: Elevate bottom of bed 20 inches. Lie on opposing side; clap at lower ribs. A pillow under the waist may help to keep the spine straight.

- **Anterior Basal Segment: Left and Right**
  Supine: Elevate bottom of bed 18-20 inches. Lie on back and place a pillow under the knees; clap at the lower ribs on both sides.

- **Posterior Basal Segment: Left and Right**
  Prone: Elevate bottom of bed 18-20 inches. Lie on stomach and place pillow under the hips; clap at the lower ribs on both sides.

Breathing Exercises

Inspiratory Muscle Training

Inspiratory muscle training attempts to increase ventilating capacity and decrease dyspnea through the strengthening of the diaphragm and intercostal muscles. This is commonly used with patients that exhibit decreased chest expansion, shortness of breath, bradypnea, and decreased breath sounds.

Treatment Protocol

✓ Teach the patient proper use of inspiratory muscles
✓ Two to four sessions of 30 to 60 minutes of deep breathing with proper diaphragmatic breathing
✓ Use "sniffing" to increase awareness regarding the proper use of the diaphragm when breathing
✓ Strength training through resisted inhalation (for patients that have tidal volumes > 500 ml)
✓ Strength training through active breathing exercises (for patients that have tidal volumes < 500 ml)

Goals for Breathing Retraining

✓ Improve overall ventilation and respiration
✓ Decrease accumulation of secretions and prevent complications
✓ Decrease the work of breathing
✓ Improve the efficiency of coughing
✓ Strengthening respiratory muscles
✓ Improve chest wall mobility

Diaphragmatic Breathing

Diaphragmatic breathing attempts to enhance movement of the diaphragm upon inspiration and expiration and diminish accessory muscle use.

- Position the patient in bed with head and trunk elevated 45 degrees.
- Place dominant hand over the rectus abdominis muscles.
- Place non-dominant hand over the sternum.
- Direct the patient to inspire slowly and feel the dominant hand rise.
- Instruct the patient to control both inspiration and expiration.
- The non-dominant hand should have only minimal movement.

Low-frequency Breathing

Low-frequency breathing is slow deep breathing designed to improve alveolar ventilation and oxygenation.

- Instruct the patient to breathe slowly, taking long and deep breaths.
- Ensure the patient is not at risk for hyperventilation.

Incentive Spirometry

Incentive spirometry is used to increase inspiration using a device that provides immediate feedback to the patient regarding performance. This type of intervention is commonly utilized to treat patients status post surgery in order to strengthen weak inspiratory muscles and to prevent alveolar collapse.

- Position the patient in a comfortable setting.
- Instruct the patient to breathe into the spirometer.
- Instruct the patient to perform a maximal inhalation into the spirometer.
- Repeat 7 to 10 times per session and repeat the session 3-4 times per day.
- Increase volume expectations on regular intervals until the patient is within normal range.

Pursed-lip Breathing

Pursed-lip breathing attempts to improve ventilation by decreasing the respiratory rate and increasing the tidal volume. This technique assists with shortness of breath that is commonly encountered in patients with COPD.

- Position the patient in a comfortable setting.
- Instruct the patient to avoid using the abdominals.
- Instruct the patient to place a hand over the abdominal muscles while breathing.
- Slowly inhale.
- Relax and loosely purse lips during exhalation.
- Expiration should be twice as long as inspiration.

Segmental Breathing

Segmental breathing is used to prevent accumulation of fluid and to increase chest mobility by directing inspired air to predetermined areas.

- Position the patient in a comfortable setting based on the targeted lung segment.
- Place hands on target area and apply pressure downward and inward during exhalation.
- Apply a quick stretch immediately before inspiration.
- Instruct the patient to slowly inspire air into the target lung area under your hands. Give mild resistance during inspiration.
- Observe accessory muscles during exercise in order to limit their use.

Pulmonary System Profile

Examination

- Past medical history
- History of current condition
  - Pulmonary function testing
  - Arterial blood gases
- Social history (caregiver support)
- Medications
- Living environment
- Systems review
  - Pulse oximetry
  - Auscultation of the lungs
  - Vital signs
  - Cough
- Observation of breathing/use of accessory muscles
- Postural assessment
- Cognitive assessment
- Pain
- Strength
- Endurance
- Mobility skills

Intervention

- Breathing exercises
- Coughing techniques
- Postural drainage, chest physical therapy
- Endurance/exercise training
- Relaxation techniques
- Patient/caregiver teaching:
  - Energy conservation
  - Breathing and coughing techniques
  - Stress management
  - Measurement of vital signs
- Mobility training

Goals

- Maximize independence in secretion clearance
- Maximize self-care skills
- Maximize functional mobility skills
- Maximize aerobic capacity
- Maximize independence with performing and monitoring home exercise program
- Maximize patient/caregiver competence with:
  - Energy conservation techniques
  - Breathing techniques
  - Stress management techniques

Pulmonary System Pathology

Asthma

Asthma is a reversible, obstructive lung condition characterized by increased responsiveness of the trachea and bronchi to stimuli, inflammation, and overproduction of mucous glands with widespread narrowing of the airways. Asthma attacks may be mild or life threatening. Clinical symptoms include increased respiration rate, prolonged expiration time with wheezing, increased use of accessory muscles, episodes of dyspnea, and a non-productive cough. Immediate medical intervention and the use of bronchodilators may be warranted.

Bronchiectasis

Bronchiectasis is a progressive obstructive lung disease that produces abnormal dilation of a bronchus. This is an irreversible condition that is usually associated with chronic infections, aspiration, cystic fibrosis or immune system impairment. The bronchial walls weaken over time secondary to infection and allow for permanent dilation of bronchi and bronchioles. Symptoms include a consistent productive cough, hemoptysis, weight loss, anemia, crackles, wheezes, and loud breath sounds.

Chronic Bronchitis

Chronic bronchitis is characterized by increased mucus secretions from the bronchioles as well as structural changes to the bronchi. A productive cough is usually present for three months during two consecutive years. The major impairments include hypertrophy of the mucus secreting glands and insufficient oxygenation of the alveoli due to mucus blockage. Clinical symptoms include increased pulmonary artery pressure, thick sputum, increased use of accessory muscles, persistent cough, wheezing, dyspnea, and cyanosis. Patients with chronic bronchitis are often called "blue bloaters."

Chronic Obstructive Pulmonary Disease (COPD)

Chronic obstructive pulmonary disease is characterized by increased resistance to the passage of air in and out of the lungs due to narrowing of the bronchial tree. COPD symptoms include dyspnea, chronic productive cough, and excessive mucus production. Progression of the disease includes alveolar destruction and subsequent increases in the amount of air that remains in the lungs. Patients with COPD have an overall increased total lung capacity with a significant increase in residual volume. The disease is diagnosed by determining the amount of air forcibly expired from the lungs in one second. Chronic obstructive pulmonary disease includes bronchitis, emphysema, asthma, and bronchiectasis.

Cor Pulmonale

Cor pulmonale is considered to be a medical emergency. There is a sudden dilatation of the right ventricle of the heart secondary to a pulmonary embolus. Right-sided heart failure will occur if the condition is not treated. As the condition progresses symptoms resemble congestive heart failure. Clinical symptoms include chronic cough, chest pain, distal swelling (bilateral), dyspnea, fatigue, and weakness.

Emphysema

Emphysema is a condition that develops from a long history of chronic bronchitis. The alveolar walls present with significant pathology and the air spaces are permanently over inflated. Expiration is difficult and dead space increases within the lungs. Emphysema is categorized as centrilobular, panlobular or paraseptal. Clinical symptoms include dyspnea, chronic cough, orthopnea, barrel chest, increased use of accessory muscles, and increased respiration rate.

Restrictive Pulmonary Disease

Restrictive pulmonary disease is characterized by the lungs' failure to fully expand due to a weakened diaphragm, structural inability of the chest wall to expand, and a decrease in the elasticity of lung tissue. Clinical symptoms include shortness of breath, a persistent non-productive cough, and increased respiratory rate. There may be chronic inflammation of the alveoli or plaques that develop and result in progressive fibrosis and a decreased lung capacity. Restrictive pulmonary disease results in a decrease in all lung volumes. Restrictive pulmonary diseases include scoliosis, atelectasis, pneumonia, and adult respiratory distress syndrome.

Tuberculosis (TB)

Tuberculosis is a bacterial infection that is transmitted in an airborne fashion (coughing, sneezing, and speaking). The lungs are primarily involved, however, TB can occur in kidneys, lymph nodes, and meninges. Lesions in the lungs can be seen with x-ray. Clinical symptoms include fatigue, weight loss, loss of appetite, low-grade fever, productive cough, chest discomfort, and dyspnea. Treatment includes anti-tuberculosis drug therapy. Prevention of TB through immunization is recommended for children.

Pharmacology

Pharmacological Intervention for Pulmonary Management

Bronchodilator Agents

Relieve bronchospasm, increase size of the airway, and reduce resistance and subsequent obstruction. Three subsets: anticholinergic, beta-adrenergic, methylxanthine	Albuterol (Proventil) Epinephrine (Primatene Mist) Pirbuterol acetate (Maxair) Salmeterol (Serevent) Aminophylline (Phyllocontin) Theophylline (Slo-bid)

Inhaled Corticosteroid Agents

Control inflammation of the airways; decrease bronchospasm and stabilize inflammatory response in the respiratory tract	Beclomethasone (Vanceril) Budesonide (Pulmicort) Fluticasone propionate (Flovent) Dexamethasone (Decadron)

Mucolytic Agents

Thin mucous secretions by altering the composition and consistency of mucus	Acetylcysteine (Mucosil) Dornase alpha (Pulmozyme)

Expectorant Agents

Increase removal of mucus through transport from the lungs	Guaifenesin (Anti-Tuss) Iodinated glycerol (Iophen) Terpin hydrate

Antiasthmatic Agents

Stabilize mast cells; inhibit the release of inflammatory medications	Cromolyn sodium (Intal) Nedocromil sodium (Tilade)

*selected pharmaceutical drugs and their respective trade names in parentheses, not intended to be a complete list

Chapter 4 — Integumentary System

Integumentary System

The integumentary system (or skin) is the largest organ within the body and consists of the dermal and epidermal layers, hair follicles, nails, sebaceous glands, and sweat glands. Each layer is stratified into several layers. The dermis is known as the true skin, is well vascularized, and is characterized as elastic, flexible, and tough. The epidermis is avascular and consists of the outermost layer of skin.

Key Functions of the Integumentary System

- Excretion of sweat
- Protection
- Sensation
- Thermoregulation
- Vitamin D synthesis

Ulcers

Type of Ulcers

Arterial insufficiency ulcers

Wounds resulting from arterial insufficiency occur secondary to ischemia from inadequate circulation of oxygenated blood often due to complicating factors such as atherosclerosis. (See Table)

Venous insufficiency ulcers

Wounds resulting from venous insufficiency occur secondary to inadequate functioning of the venous system resulting in inadequate circulation and eventual tissue damage and ulceration. (See Table)

Pressure ulcers

Pressure ulcers, often called decubitus ulcers, result from sustained or prolonged pressure at levels greater than the level of capillary pressure on the tissue. Pressure against the skin over a bony prominence results in localized ischemia and/or tissue necrosis. Factors contributing to pressure ulcers include shear, moisture, heat, friction, medication, muscle atrophy, malnutrition, and debilitating medical conditions.

Neuropathic ulcers

Neuropathic ulcers are a secondary complication usually associated with a combination of ischemia and neuropathy. Most often neuropathic ulcers are associated with diabetes. Neuropathic ulcers are frequently found on the plantar surface of the foot, often beneath the metatarsal heads. The wound is typically well defined by a prominent callus rim. The wound has good granulation tissue and little or no drainage. Patients rarely report pain with neuropathic ulcers in part due to altered sensation. Pedal pulses are most often diminished or absent. The distal limb may appear to be shiny and appear somewhat cool to touch. The periwound skin often appears to be dry or cracked.

Characteristics of Arterial and Venous Insufficiency Ulcers

	Arterial Ulcers	Venous Ulcers
Location	Lower one-third of leg, toes, web spaces (distal toes, dorsal foot, lateral malleolus)	Proximal to the medial malleolus
Appearance	Smooth edges, well defined; lack granulation tissue; tend to be deep	Irregular shape; shallow
Pain	Severe	Mild to moderate
Pedal Pulses	Diminished or absent	Normal
Edema	Normal	Increased
Skin Temperature	Decreased	Normal
Tissue Changes	Thin and shiny; hair loss; yellow nails	Flaking, dry skin; brownish discoloration
Miscellaneous	Leg elevation increases pain	Leg elevation lessens pain

Intervention and Treatment Recommendations

Intervention for arterial insufficiency ulcers focuses on:

- Cleansing the ulcer
- Rest
- Reducing risk factors
- Limb protection

General Recommendations

- ✓ Wash and dry feet thoroughly
- ✓ Avoid unnecessary leg elevation
- ✓ Inspect legs and feet daily
- ✓ Wear appropriately sized shoes with clean, seamless socks
- ✓ Use bandages as necessary and avoid any unnecessary pressure
- ✓ Avoid using heating pads or soaking feet in hot water

Intervention for venous insufficiency ulcers focuses on:

- Cleansing the ulcer
- Compression to control edema

General Recommendations

- ✓ Elevate legs above heart when resting or sleeping
- ✓ Attempt active exercise including frequent range of motion
- ✓ Inspect legs and feet daily
- ✓ Wear appropriately sized shoes with clean, seamless socks
- ✓ Use bandages as necessary and avoid scratching or other forms of direct contact

Types of Dressings

Hydrocolloids

Hydrocolloid dressings consist of gel-forming polymers such as gelatin, pectin, and carboxymethylcellulose with a strong film or foam adhesive backing. The dressings vary in permeability, thickness, and transparency. Hydrocolloids absorb exudate by swelling into a gel-like mass and vary from being occlusive to semipermeable. The dressing does not attach to the actual wound itself and is instead anchored to intact skin surrounding the wound.

Indications: Hydrocolloids are useful for partial and full-thickness wounds. The dressings can be used effectively with granular or necrotic wounds.

Advantages

- Provides a moist environment for wound healing
- Enables autolytic debridement
- Offers protection from microbial contamination
- Provides moderate absorption
- Does not require a secondary dressing
- Provides a waterproof surface

Disadvantages

- May traumatize surrounding intact skin upon removal
- May tend to roll in areas of excessive friction
- Cannot be used on infected wounds

Hydrogels

Hydrogels consist of varying amounts of water and varying amounts of gel-forming materials such as glycerin. The dressings are available in sheet form or amorphous form.

Indications: Hydrogels are commonly used on superficial and partial-thickness wounds (e.g., abrasions, blisters, pressure ulcers) that have minimal drainage. Rather than absorb drainage, hydrogels are moisture retentive.

Advantages

- Provides a moist environment for wound healing
- Enables autolytic debridement
- May reduce pressure and diminish pain
- Can be used as a coupling agent for ultrasound
- Minimally adheres to wound

Disadvantages

- Potential for dressings to dehydrate
- Cannot be used on wounds with significant drainage
- Typically requires a secondary dressing

Foam Dressings

Foam dressings are composed from a hydrophilic polyurethane base. The dressings are hydrophilic at the wound contact surface and are hydrophobic on the outer surface. The dressings allow exudates to be absorbed into the foam through the hydrophilic layer. The dressings are most commonly available in sheets or pads with varying degrees of thickness. Semipermeable foam dressings are produced in adhesive and non-adhesive forms. Non-adhesive forms require a secondary dressing.

Indications: Foam dressings are used to provide protection over partial and full-thickness wounds with varying levels of exudate. They can also be used as secondary dressings over amorphous hydrogels.

Advantages

- Provides a moist environment for wound healing
- Available in adhesive and non-adhesive forms
- Provides prophylactic protection and cushioning
- Encourages autolytic debridement
- Provides moderate absorption

Disadvantages

- May tend to roll in areas of excessive friction
- Adhesive form may traumatize periwound area upon removal
- Lack of transparency makes inspection of wound difficult

Transparent Film

Film dressings are thin membranes made from transparent polyurethane with water resistant adhesives. The dressings are permeable to vapor and oxygen, but are mostly impermeable to bacteria and water. They are highly elastic, conform to a variety of body contours, and allow easy visual inspection of the wound since they are transparent.

Indications: Film dressings are useful for superficial wounds (scalds, abrasions, lacerations) or partial-thickness wounds with minimal drainage.

Advantages

- Provides a moist environment for wound healing
- Enables autolytic debridement
- Allows visualization of the wound
- Resistant to shearing and frictional forces
- Cost effective over time

Disadvantages

- Excessive accumulation of exudates can result in periwound maceration
- Adhesive may traumatize periwound area upon removal
- Cannot be used on infected wounds

Gauze

Gauze dressings are manufactured from yarn or thread and are the most readily available dressing used in an inpatient environment. Gauze dressings come in many shapes and sizes (e.g., sheets, squares, rolls, packing strips). Impregnated gauze is a variation of woven gauze in which various materials such as petrolatum, zinc or antimicrobials have been added.

Indications: Gauze dressings are commonly used on infected or non-infected wounds of any size. The dressings can be used for wet-to-wet, wet-to-moist or wet-to-dry debridement.

Advantages

- Readily available, cost effective dressings
- Can be used alone or in combination with other dressings or topical agents
- Can modify number of layers to accommodate for changing wound status
- Can be used on infected or uninfected wounds

Disadvantages

- Has a tendency to adhere to wound bed
- Highly permeable and therefore requires frequent dressing changes (prolonged use decreases cost effectiveness)
- Increased infection rate compared to occlusive dressings

Alginates

Alginate dressings consist of calcium salt of alganic acid that is extracted from seaweed. Alginates are highly permeable and non-occlusive. As a result, they require a secondary dressing. Alginate dressings are based on the interaction of calcium ions in the dressing and the sodium ions in the wound exudate.

Indications: Alginates are typically used on partial and full-thickness draining wounds such as pressure wounds or venous insufficiency ulcers. Alginates are often used on infected wounds due to the likelihood of excessive drainage.

Advantages

- High absorptive capacity
- Enables autolytic debridement
- Offers protection from microbial contamination
- Can be used on infected or uninfected wounds
- Non-adhering to wound

Disadvantages

- May require frequent dressing changes based on level of exudate
- Requires a secondary dressing
- Cannot be used on wounds with an exposed tendon, joint capsule or bone

Occlusion and Moisture

Occlusion refers to the ability of a dressing to transmit moisture, vapor or gases from the wound bed to the atmosphere. A truly occlusive substance would be completely impermeable, while a truly non-occlusive substance would be completely permeable. Dressings are classified according to this continuum.

The following list of dressings is arranged from most occlusive to non-occlusive:

- Hydrocolloids, hydrogels, semipermeable foam, semipermeable film, impregnated gauze, alginates, and traditional gauze

Dressings can also be classified by their ability to retain moisture. The following list of dressings is arranged from most moisture retentive to least moisture retentive:

- Alginates, semipermeable foam, hydrocolloids, hydrogels, semipermeable films

Primary Versus Secondary Dressings

A **primary dressing** comes into direct contact with the wound.

A **secondary dressing** is placed directly over the primary dressing to provide protection, absorption, and/or occlusion.

Red-Yellow-Black System

Color	Wound Description	Goals
Red	Pink granulation tissue	Protect wound; maintain moist environment
Yellow	Moist yellow slough	Debride necrotic tissue; Absorb drainage
Black	Black, thick eschar firmly adhered	Debride necrotic tissue

Selective Debridement

Selective debridement involves removing only nonviable tissues from a wound. Selective debridement is most often performed by sharp debridement, enzymatic debridement, and autolytic debridement.

Sharp Debridement

Sharp debridement requires the use of scalpel, scissors, and/or forceps to selectively remove devitalized tissues, foreign materials or debris from a wound. Sharp debridement is most often used for wounds with large amounts of thick, adherent, necrotic tissue; however, it is also used in the presence of cellulitis or sepsis. Sharp debridement is the most expedient form of removing necrotic tissue. Physical therapists are permitted to perform sharp debridement in the majority of states.

Enzymatic Debridement

Enzymatic debridement refers to the topical application of enzymes to the surface of necrotic tissue. Enzymatic debridement can be used on infected and non-infected wounds with necrotic tissue. This type of debridement may be used in wounds that have not responded to autolytic debridement or in conjunction with other debridement techniques. Enzymatic debridement can be slow to establish a clean wound bed and should be discontinued after removal of devitalized tissues in order to avoid damage.

Autolytic Debridement

Autolytic debridement refers to using the body's own mechanisms to remove nonviable tissue. Common methods of autolytic debridement include transparent films, hydrocolloids, hydrogels, and alginates. Autolytic debridement results in a moist wound environment that permits rehydration of the necrotic tissue and eschar and allows enzymes to digest the nonviable tissue. Autolytic debridement can be used with any amount of necrotic tissue and is non-invasive and pain free. Patients and caregivers can be instructed to perform autolytic debridement with relative ease; however, this type of debridement requires a longer period of time for overall wound healing to occur. Autolytic debridement should not be performed on infected wounds.

Non-selective Debridement

Non-selective debridement involves removing both viable and nonviable tissues from a wound. Non-selective debridement is often termed "mechanical" and is most commonly performed by wet-to-dry dressings, wound irrigation, and hydrotherapy (whirlpool).

Wet-to-dry Dressings

Wet-to-dry dressings refer to the application of a moistened gauze dressing placed in an area of necrotic tissue. The dressing is then allowed to dry completely and is later removed along with the necrotic tissue that has adhered to the gauze. Wet-to-dry dressings are most often used to debride wounds with moderate amounts of exudate and necrotic tissue. This type of debridement should be used sparingly on wounds with both necrotic tissue and viable tissue since granulation tissue will be traumatized in the process. Removal of dry dressings from granulation tissue may cause bleeding and be extremely painful.

Wound Irrigation

Wound irrigation removes necrotic tissue from the wound bed using pressurized fluid. Pulsatile lavage is an example of wound irrigation that uses a pressured stream of irrigation solution. This type of debridement is most desirable for wounds that are infected or have loose debris. Most devices permit varying pressure settings and provide suction for removal of the exudate and debris.

Hydrotherapy

Hydrotherapy is most commonly employed using a whirlpool tank with agitation directed toward a wound that requires debridement. This process results in the softening and loosening of adherent necrotic tissue. Physical therapists must be aware of the side effects of hydrotherapy such as dependent positioning of the lower extremities, systemic effects such as a drop in blood pressure, and maceration of surrounding skin.

Wound Terminology

Abrasion: An abrasion is a wound that occurs from the scraping away of the surface layers of the skin, often as a result of trauma.

Contusion: A contusion is an injury in which the skin is not broken. The injury is characterized by pain, swelling, and discoloration.

Hematoma: A hematoma is a swelling or mass of blood localized in an organ, space or tissue, usually caused by a break in a blood vessel.

Laceration: A laceration is a wound or irregular tear of tissues that is often associated with trauma.

Penetrating wound: A penetrating wound is a wound that enters into the interior of an organ or cavity.

Puncture: A puncture is a wound that is made by a sharp pointed instrument or object by penetrating through the skin into underlying tissues.

Ulcer: An ulcer is a lesion on the surface of the skin or the surface of a mucous membrane, produced by the sloughing of inflammatory, necrotic tissue.

Factors Influencing Wound Healing

There are a variety of factors that are not inherent to the actual wound that can significantly impact the rate and degree of wound healing.

Age: A decreased metabolism in older adults tends to decrease the overall rate of wound healing.

Illness: Compromised medical status such as cardiovascular disease may significantly delay healing. This often results secondary to diminished oxygen and nutrients at the cellular level.

Infection: An infected wound will impact essential activity associated with wound healing including fibroblast activity, collagen synthesis, and phagocytosis.

Lifestyle: Regular physical activity results in increased circulation that enhances wound healing. Lifestyle choices such as smoking negatively impacts wound healing by limiting the blood's oxygen carrying capacity.

Medication: There are a variety of pharmacological agents that can negatively impact wound healing. Medications falling into this category include steroids, anti-inflammatory drugs, heparin, antineoplastic agents, and oral contraceptives. Undesirable physiologic effects include delayed collagen synthesis, reduced blood supply, and decreased tensile strength of connective tissues.

Scar Management

Immediately after an injury, homeostasis attempts to occur and the acute inflammatory response is triggered. The proliferative or fibroplastic phase of wound repair includes granulation tissue formation and reepithelialization. The maturation or remodeling phase includes the remodeling of the tissue and scar formation. Scars can form in an organized manner termed normotrophic scarring or in a disorganized manner such as seen with hypertrophic or keloid scars.

General Treatment Guidelines

✓ Massage using cream twice per day (once the wound is completely healed)

✓ Use of sun block and vitamin E over the scar

✓ Use of silicone gel (softens scar)

✓ Pressure garments

✓ Consider ultrasound treatment

✓ Consider electrical stimulation treatment

Exudate Classifications

Serous: Presents as clear, light color with a thin, watery consistency. Serous exudate is considered to be normal in a healthy healing wound.

Sanguineous: Presents as red with a thin, watery consistency. Sanguineous exudate appears to be red due to the presence of blood or may be brown if allowed to dehydrate. This type of exudate may be indicative of new blood vessel growth or the disruption of blood vessels.

Serosanguineous: Presents as light red or pink color with a thin, watery consistency. Serosanguineous exudate can be normal in a healthy healing wound.

Seropurulent: Presents as opaque, yellow or tan color with a thin, watery consistency. Seropurulent exudate may be an early warning sign of an impending infection.

Purulent: Presents as yellow or green color with a thick, viscous consistency. Purulent exudate is generally an indicator of wound infection.

Pressure Ulcer Staging*

Stage I

An observable pressure related alteration of intact skin whose indicators as compared to an adjacent or opposite area on the body may include changes in skin color, skin temperature, skin stiffness or sensation.

Stage II

A partial-thickness skin loss that involves the epidermis and/or dermis. The ulcer is superficial and presents clinically as an abrasion, a blister or a shallow crater.

Stage III

A full-thickness skin loss that involves damage or necrosis of subcutaneous tissue that may extend down to, but not through, underlying fascia. The ulcer presents clinically as a deep crater with or without undermining adjacent tissue.

Stage IV

A full-thickness skin loss with extensive destruction, tissue necrosis or damage to muscle, bone or supporting structures (e.g., tendon, joint capsule).

*Resource: NPAUP The Pressure Ulcer Staging System

The Wagner Ulcer Grade Classification Scale

The Wagner Ulcer Grade Classification Scale is commonly used as an assessment instrument for the evaluation of diabetic foot ulcers.

Grade

0	No open lesion but may possess pre-ulcerative lesions; healed ulcers; presence of bony deformity
1	Superficial ulcer not involving subcutaneous tissue
2	Deep ulcer with penetration through the subcutaneous tissue; potentially exposing bone, tendon, ligament or joint capsule
3	Deep ulcer with osteitis, abscess or osteomyelitis
4	Gangrene of digit
5	Gangrene of foot requiring disarticulation

Bony Prominences Associated with Pressure Injuries

Supine	Prone	Sidelying	Sitting (Chair)
Occiput	Forehead	Ears	Spine of the scapula
Spine of scapula	Anterior portion of acromion process	Lateral portion of acromion process	Vertebral spinous processes
Inferior angle of scapula	Anterior head of humerus	Lateral head of humerus	Ischial tuberosities
Vertebral spinous processes	Sternum	Lateral epicondyle of humerus	
Medial epicondyle of humerus	Anterior superior iliac spine	Greater trochanter	
Posterior iliac crest	Patella	Head of fibula	
Sacrum	Dorsum of foot	Lateral malleolus	
Coccyx		Medial malleolus	
Heel			

Burns

Types of Burns

Thermal burn: Caused by conduction or convection. Examples include hot liquid, fire or steam.

Electrical burn: Caused by the passage of electrical current through the body. Typically there is an entrance and an exit wound. Complications can include cardiac arrhythmias, respiratory arrest, renal failure, neurological damage, and fractures. Lightning is an example of an electrical burn.

Chemical burn: Occurs when certain chemical compounds come in contact with the body. The reaction will continue until the chemical compound is diluted from the site. Compounds that cause chemical burns include sulfuric acid, lye, hydrochloric acid, and gasoline.

Burn Classification

The extent and severity of a burn is dependent on gender, age, duration of burn, type of burn, and affected area. Burns are most appropriately classified according to the depth of tissue destruction.

Superficial Burn: A superficial burn involves only the outer epidermis. The involved area may be red with slight edema. Healing occurs without evidence of scarring.

Superficial Partial-Thickness Burn: A superficial partial-thickness burn involves the epidermis and the upper portion of the dermis. The involved area may be extremely painful and exhibit blisters. Healing occurs with minimal to no scarring.

Deep Partial-Thickness Burn: A deep partial-thickness burn involves complete destruction of the epidermis and the majority of the dermis. The involved area may appear to be discolored with broken blisters and edema. Damage to nerve endings may result in only moderate levels of pain. Healing occurs with hypertrophic scars and keloids.

Full-Thickness Burn: A full-thickness burn involves complete destruction of the epidermis and dermis along with partial damage of the subcutaneous fat layer. The involved area often presents with eschar formation and minimal pain. Patients with full-thickness burns require grafts and may be susceptible to infection.

Subdermal Burn: A subdermal burn involves the complete destruction of the epidermis, dermis, and subcutaneous tissue. Subdermal burns may involve muscle and bone and as a result often require surgical intervention.

Zones of Injury

Zone of coagulation: The area of the burn that received the most severe injury along with irreversible cell damage.

Zone of stasis: The area of less severe injury that possesses reversible damage and surrounds the zone of coagulation.

Zone of hyperemia: The area surrounding the zone of stasis that presents with inflammation, but will fully recover without any intervention or permanent damage.

Positioning and Splinting

Effective management of burns includes proper positioning and splinting. A patient that sustains a burn is prone to develop contractures due to hypertrophic scarring and overall lack of motion. A general rule is to position the affected joint in the opposite direction from which it will contract. The identified position should, if at all possible, be a position of function. Splints are usually left on overnight, worn intermittently during the day, and require frequent observation to ensure proper fit. Ideal positioning includes placing the neck in extension, upper extremities abducted to 90 degrees, shoulder lateral rotation, and supination of the forearm. The lower extremities should align in neutral hip extension, 20 degrees abduction, full extension of the knee, and ankle dorsiflexion.

Rule of Nines

Allows for a gross approximation of the percentage of the body affected by a burn.

Adult Values

Head and neck	9%
Anterior trunk	18%
Posterior trunk	18%
Bilateral anterior arm, forearm, and hand	9%
Bilateral posterior arm, forearm, and hand	9%
Genital region	1%
Bilateral anterior leg and foot	18%
Bilateral posterior leg and foot	18%
Total	**100%**

Children Values

A child under one year has 9% taken from the lower extremities and added to the head region. Each year of life, 1% is distributed back to the lower extremities until age nine when the head region is considered to be the same as an adult.

Topical Agents Used in Burn Care

Topical Agent	Advantages	Disadvantages
Silver Sulfadiazine	Can be used with or without dressings Is painless Can be applied to wound directly Broad-spectrum Effective against yeast	Does not penetrate into eschar
Silver Nitrate	Broad-spectrum Non-allergenic Dressing application is painless	Poor penetration Discolors, making assessment difficult Can cause severe electrolyte imbalances Removal of dressings is painful
Povidone-iodine	Broad-spectrum Antifungal Easily removed with water	Not effective against Pseudomonas May impair thyroid function Painful application
Mafenide Acetate	Broad-spectrum Penetrates burn eschar May be used with or without occlusive dressings	May cause metabolic acidosis May compromise respiratory function May inhibit epithelialization Painful application
Gentamicin	Broad-spectrum May be covered or left open to air	Has caused resistant strains Ototoxic Nephrotoxic
Nitrofurazone	Bacteriocidal Broad-spectrum	May lead to overgrowth of fungus and Pseudomonas Painful application

From Trofino, RB: Nursing Care of the Burn-Injured Patient. F.A. Davis Company, Philadelphia 1991, p.46, with permission.

Skin Graft Procedures

Allograft (homograft): A temporary skin graft taken from another human, usually a cadaver, in order to cover a large burned area.

Autograft: A permanent skin graft taken from a donor site on the patient's own body.

Heterograft (xenograft): A temporary skin graft taken from another species.

Mesh graft: A skin graft that is altered to create a mesh-like pattern in order to cover a larger surface area.

Sheet graft: A skin graft that is transferred directly from the donor site to the recipient site.

Split-thickness skin graft: A skin graft that contains only a superficial layer of the dermis in addition to the epidermis.

Full-thickness skin graft: A skin graft that contains the dermis and the epidermis.

Anticipated Deformities Based on Burn Location

Area	Anticipated deformity	Splinting type	Area	Anticipated deformity	Splinting type
Anterior neck	Flexion with possible lateral flexion	Soft collar, molded collar, Philadelphia collar	Hip	Flexion and adduction	Anterior hip spica, abduction splint
Anterior chest and axilla	Shoulder adduction, extension, and medial rotation	Axillary or airplane splint, shoulder abduction brace	Knee	Flexion	Conforming splint, three-point splint, air splint
Elbow	Flexion and pronation	Gutter splint, conforming splint, three-point splint, air splint	Ankle	Plantar flexion	Posterior foot drop splint, posterior ankle conforming splint, anterior ankle conforming splint
Hand and wrist	Extension or hyperextension of the MCP joints; flexion of the IP joints; adduction and flexion of the thumb; flexion of the wrist	Wrist splint, thumb spica splint, palmar or dorsal extension splint			

Burn Profile

Examination

- Past medical history
- History of current condition
- Social history (caregiver support)
- Medications
- Living environment
- Systems review
- Respiratory assessment
- Neurological assessment
- Edema/girth measurements
- Sensation
- Range of motion
- Flexibility
- Strength
- Pain
- Mobility skills

Intervention

- Positioning
- Splinting
- Edema control
- Scar management
- Passive range of motion
- Massage
- Conditioning exercises
- Endurance training
- Joint mobilization
- Electrotherapeutic modalities
- Compression devices
- Hydrotherapy
- Physical agents
- Mobility training

Goals

- Maximize functional mobility
- Maintain range of motion to all affected joints
- Maximize strength and endurance
- Reduce edema to the affected areas
- Maximize proper positioning and reduce scar contracture
- Maximize patient/caregiver competence with:
  - Positioning of joints
  - Use of splinting
  - Pressure garments
  - Stretching and strengthening programs

Burn Terminology

Dermis: The vascular layer of skin below the epidermis that contains hair follicles, sebaceous glands, and sweat glands.

Donor site: A site where healthy skin is taken and used as a graft.

Epidermis: The superficial avascular layer of skin that contains the hair follicles, sebaceous glands, and sweat glands.

Eschar: The necrotic and nonviable tissue resulting from a deep burn. This skin is hard, dry, and does not possess qualities of normal skin.

Escharotomy: A surgical procedure that removes eschar from a burn site and subsequently enhances circulation.

Hypertrophic scarring: An abnormal and disorganized scar formation characterized by a raised, firm scar with collagen fibers that do not follow any pattern.

Normotrophic scarring: A scar with organized formation of collagen fibers that align in a parallel fashion.

Pressure garments: A custom-made garment that applies sustained pressure in order to improve the structure of a scar. Pressure garments are worn 22-23 hours per day and may be required for up to two years.

Recipient site: A site that has been burned and requires a graft.

Z-plasty: A surgical procedure to eliminate a scar contracture. An incision in the shape of a "z" allows the contracture to change configuration and lengthen the scar.

Chapter 5

Other Systems

Metabolic System

The metabolic system governs the chemical and physical changes that take place within the body that enable it to continue to grow and function. Metabolism involves the breakdown of complex organic compounds within the body in order to generate energy for all bodily processes. It also generates energy for the synthesis of complex substances that form the tissues and organs. During metabolism, organic compounds are broken down to provide heat and energy in the process called **catabolism**. Simple molecules are also used to build more complex compounds like proteins for growth and repair of tissues as part of **anabolism**. Many metabolic processes are facilitated by enzymes. The overall speed at which an organism carries out its metabolic processes is termed its metabolic rate (or when the organism is at rest, its basal metabolic rate).

Metabolic System Terminology

Metabolism: The physical and chemical processes of cells burning food to produce and use energy. Examples include digestion, elimination of waste, breathing, thermoregulation, muscular contraction, brain function, and circulation.

Mitochondria: The part of the cell that is responsible for energy production. The mitochondria are also responsible for converting nutrients into energy and other specialized tasks.

Osteomalacia: softening of the bones

Osteopenia: low bone mass; deprivation of bone

Osteopetrosis: increased bone density

Osteoporosis: decreased bone density

DNA (deoxyribonucleic acid): A double helix molecule that contains the genes that provide the blueprint for all of the structures and functions of a living being.

pH: A measure of the hydrogen ion concentration in body fluid.

Gene: a fundamental unit of heredity

Metabolic System Pathology

Inherited Metabolic Disorders

Metabolic disorders that are present at birth occur due to genetic mutations in genes that code for enzymes. The enzyme deficiency leads to accumulation of the substrate and a subsequent deficiency in the intended enzyme's product. There are many different disorders that can occur genetically and these are grouped according to the substrate that has been affected (i.e., carbohydrates, amino acids). **Symptoms** tend to be nonspecific and can include neurologic symptoms, autonomic symptoms, developmental delay, urine changes, atypical odors in body fluids, growth delay, altered ammonia levels, altered liver function, and organomegaly. If symptoms are evident immediately at and after birth, the disorder is more dangerous and symptoms may include lethargy, vomiting, difficulty feeding, seizures, and weakness. Disorders that do not present immediately tend to affect growth and development. **Treatment** varies and is based on degree and area of deficiency.

Phenylketonuria (amino acid/organic acid metabolic disorder)

Phenylketonuria (PKU) is a syndrome that consists of mental retardation as well as behavioral and cognitive issues secondary to an elevation of serum phenylalanine. There is a deficiency in the enzyme phenylalanine hydroxylase. This is an autosomal recessive inherited trait and is most common in white populations. Normally, excessive phenylalanine is converted to tyrosine by phenylalanine hydroxylase. When this process does not occur and there is an excess of phenylalanine, the brain is the primary organ that becomes affected. Children in the United States are tested at birth for PKU and levels greater than 6 mg/dl of phenylalanine require some form of treatment. **Symptoms** present within a few months of birth as the phenylalanine accumulates. If left untreated, severe mental retardation will occur. These children may also experience gait disturbances, hyperactivity, psychoses, abnormal body odor, and display features that are lighter in coloring when compared to other family members. **Treatment** is through dietary restriction of phenylalanine throughout the person's lifetime. Adequate prevention will avoid all manifestations of the disease.

Tay-Sachs Disease (lysosomal storage disorder)

Tay-Sachs disease is the absence or deficiency of hexosaminidase A. This produces an accumulation of gangliosides (GM_2) within the brain. This disease is an autosomal recessive inherited trait and carried primarily in the Eastern European (Ashkenazi) Jewish population. At approximately six months of age the child will start to miss developmental milestones and will continue to deteriorate in motor and cognitive skills. As **symptoms** progress, the patient develops significant mental retardation, paralysis, and will usually die by the age of five. There is currently no effective **treatment** for this condition; genetic testing in high risk populations to identify the carriers prior to pregnancy is important in order to avoid this disorder.

Mitochondrial Disorders

Mitochondrial disorders result from genetically inherited or spontaneous mutations in the DNA that lead to impaired function of proteins found within the mitochondria. There are over one hundred different forms of mitochondrial disease and each produces a different spectrum of disability and clinical manifestations. These diagnoses are relatively new and **treatment** is as varied as the symptomology and presentation of the disease. Treatment is aimed at alleviating the current symptoms and slowing the progression of the disease process.

Wilson's Disease (hepatolenticular degeneration)

Wilson's disease is an autosomal recessive inherited trait that produces a defect in the body's ability to metabolize copper. The copper accumulates over time within the brain, liver, cornea, kidneys, and other tissues. **Symptoms** usually begin to appear after the age of six and include Kayser-Fleischer rings surrounding the iris of the eye secondary to copper deposits, degenerative changes in the brain especially within the basal ganglia, hepatitis, cirrhosis of the liver, athetoid

movements, and ataxic gait patterns. There may also be emotional and behavioral changes as the copper continues to accumulate. Over time and with severe disease there will be deformities of the musculoskeletal system, pathologic fractures, osteomalacia, muscle atrophy, and contractures. **Treatment** consists of continual pharmacological intervention using vitamin B6 and D-penicillamine; both promote the excretion of excess copper from the body. Treatment will also focus on prevention of hepatic disease since a patient will die from hepatic failure if the condition is left untreated.

Rehabilitation Considerations for Patients with Inherited Metabolic Disease

- **Must be familiar** with all signs and symptoms of the particular inherited metabolic disease in order to refer patients to a physician if a change in their status occurs
- **Must have an awareness** of dietary restrictions
- **Patient and family training** to prevent deleterious effects from the metabolic disease
- **Adapt treatment** to facilitate developmental milestones within patient tolerance
- **Symptoms** of excessive or inadequate pharmacological treatment
- **Side effects** from commonly used pharmacological agents
- **Avoidance of treatments** that exacerbate the condition

Acid-Base Metabolic Disorders

The process of metabolism is regulated by the endocrine and nervous systems. The rate of metabolism can be influenced by:
- Body temperature
- Exercise
- Hormone activity
- Digestion activity

If proper fluid and acid-base balance is compromised, it can alter metabolic function and cause many signs and symptoms of the dysfunction.

Metabolic Alkalosis

Metabolic alkalosis is a condition that occurs when there is an increase in bicarbonate accumulation or an abnormal loss of acids. This commonly occurs when there has been continuous vomiting, ingestion of antacids or other basic substances, diuretic therapy or may be associated with hypokalemia or nasogastric suctioning. As a result, the pH rises above 7.45. **Symptoms** include nausea, diarrhea, prolonged vomiting, confusion, muscle fasciculations, muscle cramping, neuromuscular hyperexcitability, convulsions, paresthesias, and hypoventilation. If left untreated the patient can become comatose, experience seizures, and respiratory paralysis. **Treatment** includes managing the underlying cause, correcting coexisting electrolyte imbalances, and administering potassium chloride to the patient.

Metabolic Acidosis

Metabolic acidosis is a condition that occurs when there is an accumulation of acids due to an acid gain or bicarbonate loss.

This commonly occurs with conditions such as renal failure, lactic acidosis, starvation, diabetic or alcoholic ketoacidosis, severe diarrhea or poisoning by certain toxins. As a result, the pH drops below 7.35. **Symptoms** include compensatory hyperventilation, vomiting, diarrhea, headache, weakness and malaise, hyperkalemia, and cardiac arrhythmias. If left untreated the continued increase in acid can induce coma and eventual death. **Treatment** includes managing the underlying cause, correcting any coexisting electrolyte imbalances, and administering $NaCO_3$.

Rehabilitation Considerations for Patients with Acid-Base Imbalances

- **Must have awareness** of patients at higher risk for imbalances:
  - Renal, cardiovascular, pulmonary disease
  - Burns, fever, sepsis
  - Patients on mechanical ventilation
  - Insulin dependent diabetes mellitus
  - Patients currently vomiting with diarrhea or enteric drainage
- **Patient and family training** to prevent episodes of acid-base imbalances
- **Signs of dehydration** in a diabetic patient
- **Injury prevention** and safety measures during involuntary muscular contractions
- **Patients using diuretic therapy** may be at risk for potassium depletion
- **Awareness of the Trousseau's sign** during blood pressure measurements may indicate calcium deficiency and the early stages of tetany

Metabolic Bone Disease

Metabolic bone disease is a classification for particular diagnoses where there has been a disruption in normal metabolism within the skeletal system. The skeletal system houses calcium and phosphorus and also continuously balances the remodeling of the cortical and trabecular bone in order to optimize the structure of the skeleton. Disruption in the homeostasis of skeletal metabolic processes will result in deformity, bone loss, fracture, softening of the bone, arthritis, and pain.

Osteomalacia

Osteomalacia is a metabolic condition where bones become soft secondary to a calcium or phosphorus deficiency. There is adequate bone matrix, however, there is insufficient calcification of the matrix due to the deficiency. The calcium is usually lost secondary to inadequate intestinal absorption and the phosphorus is lost secondary to an increase in renal excretion. A deficiency in vitamin D will also cause osteomalacia. **Symptoms** can include a vague presentation of aching, fatigue, and weight loss. Myopathy and sensory polyneuropathy may also occur along with periarticular tenderness and pain, thoracic kyphosis deformity, and bowing of the lower extremities. The patient may also struggle to perform transfers and assuming a standing position. **Treatment** will focus on the underlying etiology. Increased nutrition is recommended and pharmacological intervention may include vitamin D or phosphate supplements.

Osteoporosis

Osteoporosis is a metabolic condition that presents with a decrease in bone mass that subsequently increases the risk of fracture. Primary osteoporosis can include idiopathic, postmenopausal or involutional (senile) osteoporosis. Secondary osteoporosis can occur as a result of another primary condition or with use of certain medications. Osteoporosis affects primarily trabecular and cortical bone where the rate of bone resorption accelerates while the rate of bone formation declines. Declining osteoblast function coupled with the loss of calcium and phosphate salts will cause the bones to become brittle. **Symptoms** include compression and other bone fractures, low thoracic or lumbar pain, loss of lumbar lordosis, deformities such as kyphosis, decrease in height, dowager's hump, and postural changes. **Treatment** of primary osteoporosis includes vitamin and pharmacological intervention, proper nutrition, assistive and adaptive device prescription, and patient education. Surgical intervention may be required for fracture stabilization.

Paget's Disease

Paget's disease is a metabolic condition characterized by heightened osteoclast activity. This process of excessive bone formation lacks true structural integrity. The bone appears enlarged, but lacks strength due to the high turnover of bone secondary to abnormal osteoclastic proliferation. This disease has a genetic component as well as geographical incidence, and most commonly affects patients over 50 years of age. **Symptoms** include musculoskeletal pain accompanied by bony deformities (kyphosis, coxa varus, bowing of the long bones, vertebral compression). The skull, pelvis, femur, spine and tibia are common sites that will exhibit bony changes. Symptoms of advanced progression of the disease include continued pain, vertigo, hearing loss, mental deterioration, fatigue, increased cardiac output and heart failure (secondary to an increased cardiac output). **Treatment** relies heavily on pharmacological intervention using biphosphonates in order to inhibit bone resorption and improve the quality of the involved bone. Exercise, weight control, and cardiac fitness are all key components in a program to maintain strength and motion.

Rehabilitation Considerations for Patients with Metabolic Bone Disease

- **Must be familiar** with all signs and symptoms of metabolic bone diseases in order to refer patients to a physician if a change in their status occurs
- **Must have awareness** of signs of compression fracture and of patients at higher risk for all forms of fracture
- **Patient and family training** to prevent exacerbation of metabolic bone disease
- **Focus on both resistance training and endurance training** to build bone density and increase strength
- **Symptoms** of excessive or inadequate pharmacological treatment
- **Side effects** from commonly used pharmacological agents (cramping, dizziness)
- **Avoidance of treatments** that exacerbate the condition or put patients at risk for fracture

Endocrine System

The endocrine system consists of endocrine glands (specialized ductless glands) that secrete hormones that travel through the bloodstream to signal specific target cells throughout the body. The hormones travel throughout the body to the target organs upon which they act. They will bind selectively to receptor sites on the surface of the receptor cells. The endocrine system and nervous system both function to achieve and maintain stability of the internal environment (homeostasis). The systems are capable of working alone or in concert with each other. The endocrine and nervous systems work together to regulate metabolism, response to stress, sexual reproduction, blood pressure, and water and salt balances.

Endocrine System
- Secreting cells send hormones through the bloodstream to signal specific target cells
- Hormones diffuse into the blood and travel long distances to virtually every area of the body
- Endocrine effectors consist of virtually all tissues
- Regulatory effects are slow and tend to last for long periods

Nervous System
- Neurons secrete neurotransmitters to signal nearby cells that have an appropriate receptor site
- Neurotransmitters are sent very short distances across a synapse
- Nervous effectors are limited to muscle and glandular tissue
- Regulatory effects appear rapidly and are often short lived

Glands of the Endocrine System

Hypothalamus

The hypothalamus is part of the diencephalon located below the thalamus and cerebral hemisphere. The hypothalamus connects to the pituitary gland through the infundibular or pituitary stalk. It is responsible for regulation of the autonomic nervous system (body temperature, appetite, sweating, thirst, sexual behavior, rage, fear, blood pressure, sleep) and other endocrine glands through its impact on the pituitary gland.

Pituitary Gland

The pituitary gland is normally the size of a pea and is located at the base of the brain just beneath the hypothalamus. The pituitary gland consists of two separate glands; the adenohypophysis (anterior) and the neurohypophysis (posterior). The pituitary gland is considered the most important part of the endocrine system since it releases hormones that regulate several other endocrine glands. This "master gland" is influenced by factors such as seasonal changes or emotional stress. The pituitary gland secretes endorphins that act on the nervous system and reduce a person's sensitivity to pain. It also controls ovulation and works as a catalyst for the testes and ovaries to create sex hormones.

Thyroid Gland

The thyroid gland is located on the anterior and lateral surfaces of the trachea immediately below the larynx and is shaped like a "bow tie" or "butterfly" with two halves (lobes); a right lobe and a left lobe joined by an isthmus. The thyroid produces thyroxine and triiodothyronine that act to control the rate at which cells burn the fuel from food. An increase in thyroid hormones will increase the rate of the chemical reactions within the body.

Parathyroid Glands

There are four parathyroid glands found on the posterior surface of the thyroid's lateral lobes. These glands produce parathyroid hormone which functions as an antagonist to calcitonin and is important for the maintenance of normal blood levels of calcium and phosphate. Parathyroid hormone increases the reabsorption of calcium and phosphate from bones to the blood. Secretion of parathyroid hormone is stimulated by hypocalcemia and inhibited by hypercalcemia. Normal clotting, neuromuscular excitability, and cell membrane permeability are dependent on normal calcium levels.

Adrenal Glands

The two adrenal glands are located on top of each kidney; the outer portion is called the adrenal cortex and the inner portion is called the adrenal medulla. The adrenal cortex and the adrenal medulla secrete different hormones. The adrenal cortex produces corticosteroids that will regulate water and sodium balance, the body's response to stress, the immune system, sexual development and function, and metabolism. The adrenal medulla produces epinephrine that increases heart rate and blood pressure when there is an increase in stress.

Pancreas

The pancreas is located in the upper left quadrant of the abdominal cavity extending from the duodenum to the spleen. The pancreas includes both endocrine and exocrine tissues. The islets of Langerhans are the hormone-producing cells of the pancreas. Alpha cells produce glucagon and beta cells produce insulin. These hormones work in combination to ensure a consistent level of glucose within the bloodstream and properly maintain stores of energy within the body.

Ovaries

The ovaries are located in the pelvic cavity on each side of the uterus. The ovaries provide estrogen and progesterone that contribute to regulation of the menstrual cycle and pregnancy. Estrogen is secreted by the ovarian follicles which are responsible for the development and maintenance of female sex characteristics such as breast development and the cycles of the female reproductive system. Progesterone is produced by the corpus luteum and functions to maintain the lining of the uterus at a level necessary for pregnancy.

Testes

The testes are located in the scrotum between the upper thighs. The testes secrete androgens (most importantly testosterone) that regulate body changes associated with sexual development and support the production of sperm.

Classes of Hormones

Prostaglandins (Steroid hormone)

All cells create prostaglandins from the phospholipids of the cell membranes. They are unique from other hormones since they do not circulate in the blood and instead exert their effects only where they are produced. Prostaglandins are capable of producing a wide variety of effects; some effects as it pertains to rehabilitation are related to inflammation, pain mechanisms, vasodilation, vasoconstriction, nutrient metabolism, and blood clotting.

Epinephrine (Amino acid derivative)

Catecholamines (epinephrine, norepinephrine, and dopamine) are synthesized from chromaffin cells within the adrenal medulla. Sympathetic nervous system stimulation releases the catecholamines into the bloodstream. Epinephrine has one of the largest effects on the sympathetic nervous system and creates the "fight or flight" response. The target areas for epinephrine are receptor sites in the cardiovascular and metabolic systems. Other functions of catecholamines include increasing cardiac contraction, constriction of blood vessels, activation of glycogen breakdown, blocking of insulin secretion, increasing metabolic rate, and dilation of the airways within the lungs.

Insulin (Peptide hormone)

Insulin is a hormone secreted by the beta cells of the islets of Langerhans within the pancreas. Insulin is released when there is an elevation in the level of blood glucose. The insulin produces an increase in cellular uptake of glucose for metabolism. Insulin also stimulates the skeletal muscle and liver to store the glucose and increases amino acid transport across hepatic, muscle, and adipose tissues. Insulin release affects all systems of the body with its primary goal of reducing blood glucose levels.

Endocrine System: Hormone, Function, and Regulation of Secretion

Hormone	Function	Regulation of Secretion
Hypothalamus		
Growth hormone-releasing hormone Target: pituitary gland	Increases the release of growth hormone	Central nervous system feedback; circulating levels of hormones
Growth hormone-inhibiting hormone Target: pituitary gland	Decreases the release of growth hormone	Central nervous system feedback; circulating levels of hormones
Gonadatropin-releasing hormone Target: pituitary gland	Increases the release of luteinizing hormone and follicle-stimulating hormone	Central nervous system feedback; circulating levels of hormones
Thyrotropin-releasing hormone Target: pituitary gland	Increases the release of thyroid stimulating hormone	Central nervous system feedback; circulating levels of hormones
Corticotropin-releasing hormone Target: pituitary gland	Increases the release of adrenocorticotropic hormone	Central nervous system feedback; circulating levels of hormones
Prolactin-releasing hormone Target: pituitary gland	Stimulates the release of prolactin	Central nervous system feedback; circulating levels of hormones
Prolactin-inhibitory factor; dopamine Target: pituitary gland	Decreases the release of prolactin	Central nervous system feedback; circulating levels of hormones
Pituitary		
Growth hormone Target: bone and muscle	Promotes growth and development; increases the rate of protein synthesis	Hypothalamus
Follicle-stimulating hormone Target: ovaries and testes	Promotes follicular development and the creation of estrogen in females; promotes spermatogenesis in males	Hypothalamus
Luteinizing hormone Target: ovaries and testes	Promotes ovulation along with estrogen/progesterone synthesis from the corpus luteum in females; promotes testosterone synthesis in males	Hypothalamus
Thyroid-stimulating hormone Target: thyroid gland	Increases the synthesis of thyroid hormones T3 and T4	Hypothalamus
Adrenocorticotropic hormone Target: adrenal cortex	Increases cortisol synthesis (adrenal steroids)	Hypothalamus
Prolactin Target: mammary glands	Allows for the process of lactation	Hypothalamus
Oxytocin Target: uterus and mammary glands	Increases contraction of uterine muscles; promotes release of milk from mammary glands	Nerve impulses from the hypothalamus; stretching of cervix; nipple stimulation
Antidiuretic hormone Target: kidneys	Increases water reabsorption; conserves water; increases blood pressure through stimulating contraction of muscles in small arteries	Decreased water content

Endocrine System: Hormone, Function, and Regulation of Secretion (Continued)

Hormone	Function	Regulation of Secretion
Adrenal Cortex		
Androgen Target: ovaries and testes	Increases masculinization; promotes growth of pubic hair in males and females	Influenced by the hypothalamic production and release of GnRH and LH
Aldosterone (mineralocorticoid) Target: kidneys	Increases reabsorption of sodium ions by the kidneys to the blood; increases excretion of potassium ions by the kidney into the urine	Low blood sodium level; high blood potassium level
Cortisol (glucocorticoid) Target: gastrointestinal system	Influences metabolism of food molecules; anti-inflammatory effect in large amounts	Adrenocorticotropic hormone
Adrenal Medulla		
Epinephrine Target: cardiovascular and metabolic systems	Increases heart rate and force of contraction; increases energy production; vasodilation in skeletal muscle	Sympathetic impulses from the hypothalamus in stress situations
Norepinephrine Target: cardiovascular and metabolic systems	Vasoconstriction in skin, viscera, and skeletal muscles	
Ovaries		
Estrogen, progesterone Target: uterus and mammary glands	Involved in regulation of the female reproductive system and female sexual characteristics	Cyclical rise and fall of hormone levels
Pancreas		
Glucagon Target: liver	Glucagon increases blood glucose by stimulating the conversion of glycogen to glucose	Hypoglycemia
Insulin Target: all body systems	Insulin decreases blood glucose and increases the storage of fat, protein, and carbohydrates	Hyperglycemia
Parathyroids		
Parathormone Target: bone, kidney, intestinal mucosa	Increases blood calcium	Hypocalcemia
Testes		
Testosterone Target: pituitary gland	Involved in the process of spermatogenesis and male sexual characteristics	Influenced by pituitary release of LH
Thyroid		
Thyroxine (T4), Triiodothyronine (T3) Target: all tissues	Involved with normal development; increases cellular level metabolism	Thyroid-stimulating hormone
Calcitonin Target: plasma	Increases calcium storage in bone; decreases blood calcium levels	Hypercalcemia

Endocrine System Dysfunction: General Signs and Symptoms

Neuromuscular

- Muscle weakness
- Periarthritis
- Myalgia
- Arthralgia
- Stiffness
- Osteoarthritis
- Muscle atrophy
- Adhesive capsulitis

Systemic

- Polydipsia
- Growth dysfunction
- Skin pigmentation dysfunction
- Polyuria
- Increased vital signs
- Hair dysfunction
- Nervousness or anxiety

Endocrine System Pathology

The endocrine system is multifaceted and can develop pathology in one or more areas due to hyperfunction or hypofunction of one or more glands. In many instances, it is the hypothalamus or the pituitary gland that effects the function of other endocrine glands when they experience direct or indirect dysfunction.

Hyperfunction of an endocrine gland: usually secondary to overstimulation of the pituitary gland or in many cases, hyperplasia or neoplasia of the gland itself.

Hypofunction of an endocrine gland: usually secondary to understimulation of the pituitary gland. This can also occur from congenital or acquired disorders.

There are other instances where direct damage to the hypothalamus or pituitary gland creates dysfunction:

Hypothalamus dysfunction

- Hypothalamus tumors (i.e., ependymomas)
- Inflammatory processes (i.e., sarcoidosis)
- Surgical transection
- Trauma (i.e., skull fracture)

Pituitary dysfunction

- Pituitary tumors (i.e., adenomas)
- Ischemic necrosis or infarction of the pituitary gland
- Infiltrative disorders (i.e., hemochromatosis)
- Inflammatory processes (i.e., meningitis)
- Iatrogenic (i.e., irradiation)

Hypopituitarism: This condition occurs when there is a decrease or absent hormonal secretion from the anterior pituitary gland. This is a rare disorder and **symptoms** are dependent on the age of the affected person and deficit hormones. Typical disorders may include short stature (dwarfism), delayed growth and puberty, sexual and reproductive disorders, and diabetes insipidus. **Treatment** is also based on the deficit hormones and usually includes pharmacological replacement therapy.

Hyperpituitarism: This condition occurs when there is an excessive secretion of one or multiple hormones under the pituitary gland's control (frequently growth hormone that produces acromegaly in adults). Disorders and **symptoms** are dependent on the hormone(s) that are affected. Some disorders include gigantism or acromegaly, galactorrhea (abnormal lactation in males or females), amenorrhea, infertility, and impotence. **Treatment** is hormone and

site dependent and can include tumor resection, surgery, radiation therapy, and hormone suppression or replacement (if gland becomes dysfunctional after treatment).

Rehabilitation Considerations for Patients with Pituitary Dysfunction

- **Must be familiar** with symptoms of disproportionate pharmacological treatment
- **Avoidance of treatments** that exacerbate the condition
- **Ambulation/exercise** encouraged within 24 hours of surgery (post tumor/gland removal)
- **Increased awareness** for signs of hypoglycemia
- **Bilateral carpal tunnel syndrome** is often common with hyperpituitarism
- **Arthritis, osteophyte formation**
- **Orthostatic hypotension** may be present with hypopituitarism
- **Bilateral hemianopsia** requires special consideration during treatment (hypopituitarism)

Adrenal dysfunction: (Addison's disease, Cushing's syndrome)

Addison's disease: This form of adrenal dysfunction occurs when there is progressive hypofunctioning of the adrenal cortex. Subsequently there is decreased production of both cortisol (glucocorticoid) and aldosterone (mineralocorticoid). **Symptoms** include a widespread metabolic dysfunction secondary to cortisol deficiency as well as fluid and electrolyte imbalances secondary to aldosterone dysfunction. The person may experience weakness, anorexia, weight loss, altered pigmentation, and if left untreated this condition will result in shock and death. **Treatment** primarily consists of long-term pharmacological intervention using synthetic corticosteroids and mineralocorticoids.

Cushing's syndrome: This form of adrenal dysfunction occurs when excessive amounts of cortisol (glucocorticoid) are produced. If the pituitary gland produces excessive ACTH with subsequent hypercortisolism it is termed Cushing's disease. **Symptoms** evolve over years and can include persistent hyperglycemia, growth failure, truncal obesity, "moon shaped face," weakness, acne, and hypertension. Mental changes can include depression, poor concentration, and memory loss. **Treatment** may include pharmacological

intervention to block the production of the hormones, radiation therapy, chemotherapy or surgery.

Rehabilitation Considerations for Patients with Adrenal Dysfunction

- **Must be familiar** with symptoms of excessive pharmacological treatment
- **Avoidance of treatments** that exacerbate the condition
- **Signs of stress** and exhaustion
- **Physician notification** with any signs of illness; medications may need to be altered
- **Orthostatic hypotension** secondary to long-term cortisol therapy
- **Report sleep disturbances** to physician
- **Degenerative myopathy**, tendon ruptures
- **Increased incidence of osteoporosis** and bone fractures
- **Delayed wound healing**

Thyroid dysfunction: (hypothyroidism, hyperthyroidism, Graves' disease)

Hypothyroidism: This condition occurs when there are decreased levels of thyroid hormones in the bloodstream. This deficiency slows the processes within the body and **symptoms** may include fatigue, weakness, decreased heart rate, weight gain, constipation, delayed puberty, and retarded growth and development. Common causes of hypothyroidism are Hashimoto's thyroiditis or an underdeveloped thyroid gland. **Treatment** includes oral thyroid hormone replacement therapy.

Hyperthyroidism: This condition occurs when there are excessive levels of thyroid hormones in the bloodstream. **Symptoms** can include an increase in nervousness, excessive sweating, weight loss, increase in blood pressure, bulging

eyes, myopathy, chronic periarthritis, and an enlarged thyroid gland. **Treatment** may include pharmacological intervention, radioactive iodine, and surgery.

Graves' disease: This condition is a form of hyperthyroidism that is specifically caused by an autoimmune disease in which specific antibodies produced by the immune system stimulate the thyroid gland to become overactive. **Symptoms** are similar to hyperthyroid presentation. The classic signs of Graves' disease include mild enlargement of the thyroid gland (goiter), heat intolerance, nervousness, weight loss, tremor, and palpitations. **Treatment** includes pharmacological intervention and/or removal of the thyroid gland using radiation or surgical intervention.

Hypothyroidism

- Depression and/or anxiety, increased lethargy, fatigue, headache, slowed speech, slowed mental function, impaired short-term memory

- Proximal muscle weakness, carpal tunnel syndrome, trigger points, myalgia, increased bone density, cold intolerance, paresthesias

- Dyspnea, bradycardia, CHF, respiratory muscle weakness, decreased peripheral circulation, angina, increase in blood pressure and cholesterol

- Anorexia, constipation, weight gain, decreased absorption of food and glucose

- Infertility, irregular menstrual cycle, increased menstrual bleeding

Hyperthyroidism

- Tremors, hyperkinesis, nervousness, increased DTRs, emotional lability, insomnia, weakness, atrophy, fatigue

- Chronic periarthritis, heat intolerance, flushed skin hyperpigmentation, increased hair loss

- Tachycardia, palpitations, increased respiratory rate, decrease in blood pressure, arrhythmias

- Hypermetabolism, increased appetite, increased peristalsis, nausea, vomiting, diarrhea, dysphagia

- Polyuria, infertility, increased first trimester miscarriage, amenorrhea

Rehabilitation Considerations for Patients with Thyroid Dysfunction

- **Must be familiar** with symptoms of excessive pharmacological treatment
- **Avoidance of treatments** that exacerbate the condition
- **Avoid cardiovascular stress** to eliminate secondary complications from hypotension, goiter, Graves' disease
- **Avoid exercise** in a hot aquatic or gym setting due to heat intolerance (Graves' disease)
- **Close monitoring** of vital signs
- **Effects of radioiodine therapy**
- **Recognize reduced exercise capacity** and fatigue
- **Risk of rhabdomyolysis** (hypothyroidism)

Parathyroid dysfunction: (hypoparathyroidism, hyperparathyroidism)

Hypoparathyroidism: This condition occurs due to hyposecretion or low-level production of parathyroid hormone by the parathyroid gland. **Symptoms** may include hypocalcemia, neurological symptoms such as seizures, cognitive defects, short stature, tetany (life-threatening) muscle spasms, muscle pain, and cramps. **Treatment** of acute hypoparathyroidism requires rapid elevation in serum calcium levels through intravenous calcium. Long-term treatment includes pharmacological management and dietary modifications.

Hyperparathyroidism: This condition occurs due to excessive levels of hormone production by the parathyroid gland that leads to disruption of calcium, phosphate, and bone metabolism. **Symptoms** may include renal stones and kidney damage, depression, memory loss, muscle wasting, bone deformity, and myopathy. Acute **treatment** may include pharmacological intervention that produces an immediate lowering of serum calcium using diuretics or antiresorption medications. Surgical intervention is usually required to remove the diseased parathyroid gland. Pharmacological intervention may be used prior to surgery or for long-term management.

Hypoparathyroidism

- Decreased bone resorption
- Hypocalcemia
- Elevated serum phosphate levels
- Shortened 4th and 5th metacarpals (pseudohypoparathyroidism)
- Compromised breathing due to intercostal muscle and diaphragm spasms
- Cardiac arrhythmias and potential heart failure
- Increased neuromuscular activity that can result in tetany

Hyperparathyroidism

- Increased bone resorption
- Hypercalcemia
- Decreased serum phosphate levels
- Osteitis fibrosa, subperiosteal resorption, arthritis, bone deformity
- Nephrocalcinosis, renal hypertension, and significant renal damage
- Gout
- Decreased neuromuscular irritability

Rehabilitation Considerations for Patients with Parathyroid Dysfunction

- **Must be familiar** with symptoms of excessive pharmacological treatment
- **Avoidance of treatments** that exacerbate the condition
- **Effects of hypercalcemia** (hyperparathyroidism)
- **Effects of hypocalcemia** (hypoparathyroidism)
- **Increased risk for fractures**
- **Effects from osteogenic synovitis** (Achilles, triceps, and obturator tendons most affected)

Pancreas dysfunction: Type 1 diabetes mellitus (DM), Type 2 diabetes mellitus (DM)

Type 1 diabetes mellitus (DM): This form of diabetes occurs when the pancreas fails to produce enough or any insulin. **Symptoms** include a rapid onset of symptoms, polyphagia, weight loss, polyuria, polydipsia, blurred vision, dehydration, and fatigue. **Treatment** includes exogenous insulin injections that are required to maintain proper glucose blood levels and avoid complications. Proper nutritional management is also required for blood glucose control. Insulin pumps may be indicated for continuous administration of insulin. Since there is no cure for type 1 DM at this time the goal is to control the regulation of blood glucose levels. This form of diabetes is normally diagnosed in childhood.

Type 2 diabetes mellitus (DM): This form of diabetes occurs when the body cannot properly respond to insulin. Obesity is found to contribute to this condition by increasing insulin resistance. **Symptoms** are relatively the same as with type 1, however, ketoacidosis does not occur since insulin is still produced. **Treatment** of type 2 diabetes includes blood glucose control through diet, exercise, oral medications or insulin injections when necessary. There has been an increase in children diagnosed with type 2 diabetes secondary to a rise in childhood obesity.

Type 1 Diabetes Mellitus (insulin-dependent, juvenile diabetes)	**Type 2 Diabetes Mellitus** (non-insulin dependent, adult onset diabetes)
<ul><li>Onset: usually less than 25 years of age</li><li>Abrupt onset</li><li>5-10 % of all cases</li><li>Etiology: destruction of islet of Langerhans cells secondary to possible autoimmune or viral causative factor</li><li>Insulin production: very little or none</li><li>Ketoacidosis can occur</li><li>Treatment includes insulin injection, exercise and diet</li></ul>	<ul><li>Onset: usually older than 40 years of age</li><li>Gradual onset</li><li>90-95% of all cases</li><li>Etiology: resistance at insulin receptor sites usually secondary to obesity; ethnic prevalence</li><li>Insulin production: variable</li><li>Ketoacidosis will rarely occur</li><li>Treatment includes weight loss, oral insulin, exercise, and diet</li></ul>

Rehabilitation Considerations for Patients with Diabetes Mellitus

- **Must be familiar** with symptoms of excessive pharmacological treatment
- **Avoid treatments** that exacerbate the condition
- **Peripheral neuropathies**
- **Small vessel angiopathy**
- **Tissue ischemia** and ulceration
- **Impaired** wound healing
- **Tissue necrosis** and amputation
- **Acute metabolic changes**
- **Sudden hypoglycemia**
- **Inconsistent management** of insulin intake
- **Diet and physical activity**
- **Proper skin care** and shoe evaluation

Testes and ovaries dysfunction: (poor development/underdevelopment of sex organs)

In males, the hypothalamus produces GnRH and the pituitary responds by producing LH and FSH. The Leydig cells of the testes respond to these hormones with the production of testosterone. This cycle normally occurs on a daily basis.

Male hypogonadism: Primary hypogonadism is defined as a deficiency of testosterone secondary to failure of the testes to respond to the FSH and LH (produced by the pituitary and hypothalamus). The most common cause of primary hypogonadism is Klinefelter's syndrome. Secondary hypogonadism occurs when there is a failure of the hypothalamus or pituitary to produce the hormones that will subsequently stimulate the production of testosterone.

If a male experiences this prior to puberty **symptoms** will include sparse body hair, underdevelopment of skeletal muscles, and long arms and legs secondary to a delay in the closure of the epiphyseal growth plates. Adult-onset testosterone deficiency will present with a decreased libido, erectile dysfunction, infertility, decrease in cognitive skills, mood changes, and sleep disturbances. **Treatment** includes hormone replacement pharmacological intervention.

In females, the hypothalamus produces GnRH and the pituitary responds by producing LH and FSH. In the ovaries, LH acts on theca and interstitial cells to produce progestins and androgens, and FSH acts on granulosa cells to stimulate the precursor steroids to estrogen.

Female hypogonadism: Primary hypogonadism results if the gonad does not produce the amount of sex steroid sufficient to suppress secretion of LH and FSH at normal levels. The most common cause of primary hypogonadism is Turner syndrome. Secondary hypogonadism occurs when there is a failure of the hypothalamus or pituitary to produce the hormones that subsequently stimulate the production of estrogen. If a female experiences this prior to puberty **symptoms** will include gonadal dysgenesis, a short stature, failure to progress through puberty or primary amenorrhea, and premature gonadal failure. When hypogonadism occurs in postpubertal females, secondary amenorrhea is the primary symptom. **Treatment** includes hormone replacement pharmacological intervention.

Pharmacological Intervention for Endocrine System Management

Endocrine pharmacological intervention will either consist of replacement therapy that will provide the deficient hormones or hyperfunction therapy which inhibits the oversecretion of the target hormones. The chart below is an overview that lists only the general process for treatment.

Replacement Therapy Administer extract or synthetic hormone replacement when hypofunction exists within the endocrine system	Deficient hormone replacement agents
Hyperfunction Therapy Inhibition of hormone function when an endocrine gland is secreting excessive amounts of hormone	Hormone antagonist agents

Endocrine System Profile

Key Points of Examination for Endocrine Dysfunction

(Endocrine system pathology will normally affect multiple systems within the body; the parentheses contain an example for the symptoms or characteristics provided)

Pituitary Dysfunction

- Multiple endocrinopathies may result from pituitary dysfunction

Adrenal Dysfunction

- May present with ataxic gait
- May present with cognitive defects
- Papilledema and other signs of increased intracranial pressure

Thyroid Dysfunction

- Reduced motor velocity with delayed relaxation of muscle stretch reflexes
- Median neuropathy usually presents at wrists
- Inspect for goiter

Parathyroid Dysfunction

- Tetany is common
- Cataracts may be present
- Occasional increased intracranial pressure

Pancreatic Dysfunction

- Glucose tolerance test
- Monitor blood glucose levels, especially with exercise

Gonad Dysfunction

- Hirsutism
- Amenorrhea
- May present with weakness and underdeveloped skeletal muscles

Past Medical History

History of Current Condition

Medications

Laboratory Studies

- Blood work analyzing hormone levels will assist to distinguish area of dysfunction
- Creatine kinase levels may be increased (hypothyroidism)

Other Testing

- EMG
- Ultrasound
- Needle biopsy
- CT scan
- Radioisotope scan
- Muscle biopsy
- Testing for bilateral carpal tunnel syndrome
- Pulse (rate, strength, rhythm)
- Blood pressure for hypertension (Cushing's), hypotension (Addison's), Trousseau's sign (hypocalcemia)
- Muscle weakness (hypothyroid, Cushing's)
- Peripheral neuropathy (DM)

Visual Examination

- Syndrome's signs and appearance
- Stature
- Weight
- Nails
- Hands
  Oversized hands (acromegaly)
  Heat (hyperthyroid)
  Tremor (hyperthyroid)
  Palmar erythema (hyperthyroid)
  Pigmentation of palmar crease (Addison's)
  4th, 5th metacarpals shortened
    (pseudohypoparathyroid)
- Acanthosis nigricans (acromegaly)
- Axillary hair loss (hypopituitary)
- Skin tags (acromegaly)

Key Points of Examination for Endocrine Dysfunction (continued)

(Endocrine system pathology will normally affect multiple systems within the body;
the parentheses contain an example for the symptoms or characteristics provided)

- Face
  Syndrome symptoms
  Acne, oily skin (Cushing's)
  Hirsutism (panhypopituitary)
  Chin enlargement (acromegaly)
- Eyes-Exophthalmos (hyperthyroid)
- Mouth
  Buccal pigmentation (Addison's)
  Tongue enlargement (acromegaly)

- Neck
  Inspect buffalo hump (Cushing's)
  Palpate supraclavicular fat pads (Cushing's)
  Inspect webbed neck (Turner's)
- Chest
  Pigmented nipple (Addison's)
  Loss, gain of chest hair
  Male gynecomastia (Cushing's)
  Reduced female breast size (panhypopituitary)
- Abdomen
  Purple striae (Cushing's)
  Disproportionate abdominal fat (Cushing's)

Gastrointestinal System

Gastrointestinal Anatomy and Function

Upper GI

Mouth	Initiation of mechanical and chemical digestion
Esophagus	Transports food from mouth to stomach
Stomach	Grinding of food, secretion of hydrochloric acid and other exocrine functions, secretion of hormones that release digestive enzymes from the liver, pancreas, and gallbladder to assist with digestion

Lower GI – Small Intestine

Duodenum	Neutralizes acid in food from stomach and mixes pancreatic and biliary secretions with food
Jejunum	Absorbs water, electrolytes, and nutrients
Ileum	Absorbs bile and intrinsic factors to be recycled

Lower GI – Large Intestine
(including cecum and appendix)

Ascending colon	
Transverse colon	Continues to absorb water and electrolytes; stores and eliminates undigested food as feces
Descending colon	
Sigmoid	
Rectum	
Anus	

Gland Organs

Gall bladder	Stores and releases bile into the duodenum to assist with digestion
Liver	Bile is produced and is necessary for absorption of lipid soluble substances, assists with red blood cell and vitamin K production, regulates serum level of carbohydrates, proteins and fats
Pancreas	Exocrine-secretes bicarbonate and digestive enzymes into duodenum; endocrine-secretes insulin, glucagon, and other hormones into the blood to regulate serum glucose level

Gastrointestinal System Pathology

GI Components	Common Pathologies
Esophagus	Hiatal hernia, gastroesophageal reflux disease, esophageal cancer, dysphagia, esophageal varices, Barrett's esophagus
Stomach	Gastritis, peptic ulcer disease, gastric cancer, gastrointestinal hemorrhage, motility and emptying disorders
Intestines	Malabsorption syndrome, appendicitis, irritable bowel syndrome, Crohn's disease, ulcerative colitis, colon cancer, intestinal hernia, diverticular diseases
Rectum and anus	Rectal or anal cancer, hemorrhoids, anorectal fistula, rectal fissure
Gall bladder	Gallstones (cholelithiasis), cholecystitis, gallbladder cancer
Liver	Cirrhosis, jaundice, hepatitis A, B, C, D, E, ascites, hepatic encephalopathy, liver cancer, hepatomegaly
Pancreas	Pancreatitis (acute and chronic), diabetes mellitus, pancreatic cancer

Esophagus

Gastroesophageal Reflux Disease (GERD)

GERD is diagnosed when there is an incompetence of the lower esophageal sphincter (LES) that results in reflux of gastric contents. This backwards movement of stomach acids and contents can cause tissue injury within the esophagus over time as well as other pathology. GERD is estimated to occur in 20-30% of adults and can be found in some newborns or infants. Etiology includes weakness of the LES, intermittent relaxation of the LES, direct damage of the LES through NSAIDs, alcohol, infectious agents, smoking, and certain prescription medications. Clinical **symptoms** include heartburn, regurgitation of gastric contents, belching, chest pain, hoarseness and coughing, esophagitis, and hematemesis. If GERD is left untreated the patient may develop esophageal strictures, esophagitis, aspiration pneumonia, asthma, Barrett's esophagitis, and esophageal adenocarcinoma. **Treatment** is primarily through pharmacological intervention.

Rehabilitation Considerations for Patients with GERD

- **Avoidance of certain exercise** secondary to an increase in symptoms with activity
- **Neck and head discomfort** secondary to a feeling of a lump in the throat and subsequent compensation
- **Recumbency** will induce symptoms
- **Left sidelying** preferred since right sidelying may promote acid flowing into the esophagus
- **Chronic bronchitis, asthma, pulmonary fibrosis** may all present with GERD
- **Tight clothing, exercise, constipation** may all precipitate GERD
- **Positioning during postural drainage** may encourage acid to move into the esophagus

Stomach

Gastritis

Gastritis is the inflammation of the gastric mucosa or inner layer of the stomach. **Symptoms** are similar to GERD, however, they tend to have a higher intensity. Gastritis is classified as erosive or non-erosive based on the level and zone of injury.

Erosive gastritis (acute gastritis): Etiology includes bleeding from the gastric mucosa secondary to stress, NSAIDs, alcohol utilization, viral infection or direct trauma. **Symptoms** include dyspepsia, nausea, vomiting, and hematemesis. At times, the patient is asymptomatic. **Treatment** is supportive with removal of stimulus of the disease process and pharmacological intervention. Surgical procedures may be required if the bleeding continues.

Non-erosive gastritis (chronic type B gastritis): Etiology is usually a result of the helicobacter pylori infection (H. pylori). The patient is usually asymptomatic but will show **symptoms** if the gastritis progresses. H. pylori is a carcinogen and must be **treated** aggressively, usually with a proton pump inhibitor and antibiotics.

Rehabilitation Considerations for Patients with Gastritis

- **Patient may be asymptomatic** but may have gastritis based on chronic NSAID use
- **Blood in stool** should result in physician referral
- **Educate** the patient to take medications with food and avoid certain types of food and drink

Peptic Ulcer Disease

Peptic ulcer disease is a condition where there is a disruption or erosion in the gastrointestinal mucosa. There is an imbalance between the protective mechanisms of the stomach and the secretion of acids within the stomach. Many ulcers are caused by the H. pylori infection and chronic NSAID use. Irritants that increase risk of ulcer include stress, alcohol, particular medications, foods, and smoking. **Symptoms** are dependent on location and severity of ulceration (gastric or duodenal) and can include epigastric pain, burning or heartburn, nausea, vomiting, bleeding, bloody stools, pain that comes in waves, and is relieved by eating. Symptoms specific to the etiology of H. pylori can also include halitosis, rosacea (facial red acne), and flushing. Complications can include hemorrhage, perforation, obstruction (secondary to scarring), and malignancy. **Treatment** is primarily through pharmacological intervention, however, in more severe cases surgical intervention may be required.

Rehabilitation Considerations for Patients with Peptic Ulcer Disease

- **Asymptomatic patient** with history of ulcer should be monitored for signs of bleeding
- **Fatigue level, pallor, and exercise tolerance** must be monitored for signs of bleeding
- **Heart rate increase or blood pressure decrease** may be signs of bleeding
- **Back pain** is a sign of a perforated ulcer located on the posterior wall of the stomach and duodenum
- **Pain that radiates** from the midthoracic back to the right upper quadrant and shoulder may signify blood and acid within the peritoneal cavity secondary to a perforated and bleeding ulcer

Diarrhea/Constipation

Diarrhea is defined as an abnormal frequency or volume of stool and can appear as a symptom of certain gastrointestinal pathologies. Constipation is defined as the infrequent or difficult passage of stool secondary to an increase in the hardness of the stool and can also appear as a symptom of certain gastrointestinal pathologies.

Pathologies Associated with Diarrhea and Constipation

Diarrhea	Constipation
• Irritable bowel syndrome • Hypothyroidism • Electrolyte imbalance • Endocrine disorder • Incomplete obstruction of the bowel • Diverticulitis • Certain medications • Caffeine • Diet • Malabsorption • Pelvic inflammatory disease	• Multiple sclerosis • Spinal cord tumors • Irritable bowel syndrome • Duchenne muscular dystrophy • Endocrine disorder • CVA • Inactivity • Bowel obstruction or fecal impaction • Pregnancy • Diet • Certain medications • Hemorrhoids (or other rectal lesions)

Intestines

Malabsorption Syndrome

Malabsorption syndrome is a condition characterized by a group of pathologies where there is reduced intestinal absorption and inadequate nutrition secondary to defects in digestion and/or the inability of the intestinal mucosa to absorb the nutrients from digested food. Celiac disease, cystic fibrosis, pancreatic carcinoma, pernicious anemia, AIDS, Crohn's disease, and Addison's disease are a few pathologies that may present with malnutrition syndrome. Although each patient's **symptoms** are based on the root pathology and co-morbidities that may exist; the primary symptoms are weight loss, chronic diarrhea, and anemia. Other symptoms can include fatigue, abdominal bloating, steatorrhea (oil covered stools), abdominal cramps, indigestion, bone pain, and excessive gas. Once diagnosed, **treatment** includes avoidance of the underlying cause for the malabsorption, probiotics, antibiotics, dietary modification, and nutritional support including vitamins, minerals, and electrolytes.

Rehabilitation Considerations for Patients with Malabsorption Syndrome

- **Osteoporosis** may occur and place patient at an increased risk for pathologic fracture
- **Fatigue level, pallor, and exercise tolerance** must be monitored
- **Weight loss and abdominal bloating**
- **Bone pain** must be considered during treatment
- **Muscle spasms** present secondary to electrolyte imbalances
- **Generalized swelling** present secondary to protein depletion

Irritable Bowel Syndrome (IBS)

Irritable bowel syndrome consists of recurrent symptoms of the upper and lower gastrointestinal system that interfere with the normal functioning of the colon. The etiology is unknown, but one theory believes that the colon or large intestine may be sensitive to certain foods or stress. Other theories hypothesize that the immune system, serotonin, and bacterial infections may all be causative factors. IBS typically occurs in as many as 20% of adults, more commonly in females, and begins prior to the age of 30 in 50% of patients. Females tend to have a slightly higher rate of instance which may be triggered by food sensitivities, stress, anxiety, caffeine, smoking, alcohol or high fat intake. **Symptoms** can include abdominal pain, bloating or distention of the abdomen, nausea, vomiting, anorexia, changes in form and frequency of stool, and passing of mucus in the stool. IBS is normally a diagnosis of exclusion from other GI diagnoses and **treatment** is usually multifactorial. Change in lifestyle and nutrition, decrease in stress, pharmacological intervention, adequate sleep, exercise, and psychotherapy may all assist in alleviating symptoms. Patients with IBS should avoid large meals, milk, wheat, rye, barley, alcohol, and caffeine. Although the symptoms can be severe, it does not lead to serious disease. Symptoms can typically be controlled by diet, pharmacological intervention, and stress management.

Rehabilitation Considerations for Patients with Irritable Bowel Syndrome

- **Physical activity** assists the bowel function and can relieve stress
- **Breathing techniques** will assist in stress reduction and with breath-holding patterns
- **Biofeedback training** may be beneficial
- **No link between IBS and bowel malignancy**

Diverticulitis

Diverticulitis is the condition of having inflamed or infected diverticula. This occurs in approximately 20-25% of the population that has diverticulosis.

Diverticulosis is the condition of having diverticula. These are pouch-like protrusions occurring in the colon. Approximately 10% of the population over 40 years of age develops diverticulosis. **Symptoms** may include bloating, mild cramping, and constipation but is asymptomatic in 80%. **Treatment** includes an increased amount of fiber (20-35 grams per day recommended) in a patient's diet to avoid diverticulitis.

The exact etiology of diverticulitis is unknown; however, a dominant theory is that the disease results from a low fiber diet. Abdominal pain is the primary symptom of diverticulitis. Tenderness over the left side of the lower abdomen, cramping, constipation, nausea, fever, chills, and vomiting

can also occur. **Treatment** includes diet modification, controlling the underlying infection, and lowering internal colonic pressure through increased fiber intake. In more severe cases, a nasogastric tube may be required to give the intestines a rest. Surgical intervention is indicated for severe obstruction, perforation or necrosis. Complications can include bleeding infections, intestinal blockage, abscess, perforations or tears in the colon, fistulas or peritonitis.

Rehabilitation Considerations for Patients with Diverticular Disease

- **Physical activity** assists the bowel function and is extremely important during periods of remission
- **Breathing techniques** will assist in stress reduction and with breath-holding patterns
- **Avoid** any increase in intra-abdominal pressure with exercise or activity
- **Back pain and/or referred hip pain** must be examined for possible medical diseases

Colorectal Cancer

Colorectal cancer accounts for approximately 15% of deaths from cancer annually. Adenocarcinoma and primary lymphoma account for the majority of intestinal cancers. Risk factors include increasing age, history of polyps, ulcerative colitis, Crohn's disease, diet high in fat and low in fiber, and family history. Colon cancer does not provide early signs of disease and the most prominent **symptom** is a continuous change in bowel habits. Bright red blood from the rectum is another prominent sign of colon cancer. The patient may experience symptoms of fatigue, weight loss, anemia, and overt rectal bleeding. **Treatment** is based on the type and staging of the cancer and may include surgical resection of the tumor and potentially a portion of the bowel, with subsequent radiation therapy and/or chemotherapy.

Rehabilitation Considerations for Patients with Colorectal Cancer

- **Physical activity** must be modified based on the treatment regimen of the patient
- **Urinary or bowel incontinence** may occur
- **Incontinence** provides an increased risk for skin breakdown
- **Chest, shoulder, and arm pain** may be present secondary to metastases (through the hemorrhoidal plexus)

Liver

Hepatitis is an inflammatory process within the liver. Viral hepatitis is most common and is classified as hepatitis A, B, C, D, E or G. Hepatitis A, B, and C are the most common and discussed briefly below. Other etiologies of hepatitis include a chemical reaction, drug reaction or alcohol abuse. Other virus' that can cause hepatitis include Epstein-Barr virus, herpes virus I and II, varicella-zoster virus, and measles. Acute viral hepatitis usually resolves with medical treatment but can become chronic in some cases. Chronic hepatitis may result in the need for liver transplant. **Symptoms** of hepatitis include fever, flu-like symptoms, abrupt onset of fatigue, anorexia, headache, jaundice, darkened urine, lighter stool, enlarged spleen and liver, and intermittent pruritus.

Hepatitis A (HAV)

Hepatitis A is a virus that affects the liver and its function. Transmission occurs by close personal contact with someone that has the infection or through the fecal-oral route (i.e., contaminated water and food sources). The flu-like symptoms are an acute infection only and this form does not progress to chronic disease or cirrhosis of the liver. Patients usually recover in six to ten weeks. **Treatment** is supportive and the virus is self-limiting.

Hepatitis B (HBV)

Hepatitis B is a virus that affects the liver and its function. Transmission of this virus occurs through the sharing of needles, intercourse with an infected person, exposure to an infected person's blood, semen or maternal-fetal exposure. Approximately 10% of cases progress to chronic hepatitis since the body cannot always rid itself of HBV. **Treatment** includes hepatitis B immunoglobulin (HBIG) for the unvaccinated patient within 24 hours of exposure. The patient should then receive the vaccination series at one and six months. If the patient is already vaccinated they may require another dose of the HBV vaccine. Chronic hepatitis is now being treated with interferon alfa-2b providing remission for some.

Hepatitis C (HCV)

Hepatitis C is a virus that affects the liver and its function. It's one of the primary etiologies for chronic liver disease and eventual liver failure. Transmission of this virus occurs through the sharing of needles, intercourse with an infected person, exposure to an infected person's blood, semen, body fluids or maternal-fetal exposure. The virus accounts for 90% of cases of hepatitis post transfusion. Like hepatitis B, this virus is often asymptomatic and the acute infection can be mild. Hepatitis C has an increased frequency of manifestations such as Hashimoto's thyroid disease, diabetes mellitus, and corneal ulceration. **Treatment** may include the use of interferon alfa-2b to reduce the inflammation and liver damage but only a small percentage of patients with hepatitis C benefit from the medication. There is no vaccine to prevent this virus and no immunoglobulin fully effective in treating the infection. Chronic hepatitis occurs in 50% of cases and 20% of those cases progress to cirrhosis of the liver.

Rehabilitation Considerations for Patients with Hepatitis

- **Health care workers** that are at risk for contact with hepatitis should receive all immunizations for HBV
- **Health care workers** that are exposed to blood or body fluids of an infected person must receive immunoglobulin therapy immediately
- **Standard precautions** should be followed at all times for protection
- **Enteric precautions** are required for patients with hepatitis A and E
- **Arthralgias** may be noted, especially in older patients
- **Arthralgias** secondary to hepatitis will not respond to traditional therapy and therefore may require consultation with the primary physician
- **Energy conservation techniques and pacing skills** should be incorporated into therapy
- **Balance activity and periods of rest**; avoid prolonged bed rest
- **Patient education** regarding signs and symptoms of relapse or chronic hepatitis

Cirrhosis of the Liver

Cirrhosis of the liver is a condition where the healthy tissue of the liver is replaced with scar tissue that blocks the flow of blood through the organ and prevents the liver from properly functioning. The etiology is usually alcoholism or hepatitis C. Alcohol tends to block the normal metabolism of protein, fats, and carbohydrates. This condition will normally occur after a patient has been heavily drinking for more than a decade. Inflammation of the liver secondary to hepatitis C is also a large causative factor for cirrhosis. Persistent inflammation and slow damage to the liver will result in cirrhosis of the liver after several decades of infection. Other causes include hepatitis B and D, certain drugs, infections, and toxins, specific hereditary diseases, nonalcoholic steatohepatitis, and blocked bile ducts. **Symptoms** include fatigue, decreased appetite, nausea, weakness, abdominal pain, spider angiomas, and weight loss. Common complications from cirrhosis include ascites (water accumulation in the abdomen secondary to decreased production of albumin by the liver), edema in the lower extremities, jaundice, gallstones, increased itching, ecchymosis, bleeding, an increase in sensitivity to medications, accumulation of toxins in the brain, portal vein hypertension, development of varices (enlarged blood vessels in the stomach and esophagus), immune system dysfunction, encephalopathy, and liver cancer. **Treatment** cannot reverse the process or damage, but can slow the process. Treatment is based on the causative factors and is implemented until symptoms cannot be controlled. A liver transplant may be necessary to sustain life.

Rehabilitation Considerations for Patients with Cirrhosis of the Liver

- **Ascites** may develop as well as fluid accumulation in the ankles and feet
- **Report any blood loss** through nose bleeds, gum bleeds, tarry stools or excessive bruising
- **Avoid** all activities that produce the Valsalva maneuver (increase in intra-abdominal pressure)
- **Adequate rest** is required to lower the demands on the liver and improve circulation
- **Avoid unnecessary fatigue** during therapy or daily activities

Pancreas

Diabetes Mellitus

Please refer to the clinical application template on diabetes mellitus for full details on page 292.

Pancreatic Cancer

Pancreatic cancer is a prominent type of cancer with an extremely high mortality rate. Most pancreatic cancers develop from the exocrine cells in the ducts and are called ductal adenocarcinomas. Symptoms are very vague during the initial stages of the disease which often results in delayed diagnosis. Common **symptoms** include epigastric pain that can radiate to the thoracic region, weight loss, and jaundice. An advanced cancer may present with severe pain that may indicate that the cancer has metastasized. **Treatment** is usually directed to assist in the relief of symptoms. Pancreatic cancer has a very poor survival rate with a mortality rate of almost 100%. Surgical resection along with chemotherapy and radiation assist to relieve symptoms and minimally prolong life.

Rehabilitation Considerations for Patients with Pancreatic Cancer

- **Vague back pain** can be the first symptom of pancreatic cancer
- **Cervical lymphadenopath**y (Virchow's node) may be the first symptom of metastases, (palpate a large supraclavicular lymph node)
- **Paraneoplastic syndrome** can be associated with pancreatic cancer and is an abnormality in blood coagulation (thrombophlebitis, dermatomyositis)
- **Chronic pain clinic** may be appropriate for patients with severe back pain
- **Pain management** is the primary focus of rehabilitation
- **The use of TENS, biofeedback, and relaxation techniques** is often warranted

Gallbladder

Cholecystitis and Cholelithiasis

Cholecystitis refers to inflammation of the gallbladder that may be acute or chronic. The most common etiology is that gallstones become impacted within the cystic duct. Gallstones (cholelithiasis) develop from hypomobility of the gallbladder, supersaturation of the bile with cholesterol or crystal formation from bilirubin salts. These stones can also cause infection which exacerbate the condition. Many times gallstones are asymptomatic, however, the most common **symptom** is right upper quadrant pain. If the gallstone becomes lodged within the cystic duct, then the patient can experience many problems including severe right upper quadrant pain with muscle guarding, tenderness, and rebound pain. These symptoms can radiate to the interscapular region. Other symptoms include jaundice, fever, nausea, vomiting, anorexia, and abdominal rigidity. **Treatment** is not recommended for the patient with asymptomatic gallstones, but a diet low in fat intake can decrease the stimulation of the gallbladder if mild symptoms are present. If patients are symptomatic a lithotripsy procedure can be used in an attempt to break up and dissolve the stones. Primary treatment is a laparoscopic cholecystectomy to remove the gallbladder and the lodged stones from the ducts. Acute cholecystitis should resolve itself within a week with analgesics, antibiotics, and intravenous alimentary feedings.

Rehabilitation Considerations for Patients with Cholecystitis and Cholelithiasis

- **Awareness** of signs and symptoms of disease
- **Post-surgical exercises** would apply if the person has had a laparoscopic cholecystectomy (breathing exercises, splinting while coughing, mobility training)
- **Ambulation** should be implemented as soon as advised for the post-surgical patient

Pharmacology

Pharmacological intervention is normally related to gastrointestinal disorders that are caused by gastric acid secretion and abnormal food movement through the gastrointestinal tract.

Pharmacological Intervention for Gastrointestinal System Management

Antacids

– Used to chemically neutralize gastric acid; increases the intragastric pH; used for minor or transient discomfort	Aluminum-containing agents (Basaljel) Magnesium-containing agents (Milk of Magnesia) Calcium carbonate-containing agents (Tums) Sodium bicarbonate-containing agents (Bromo Seltzer)

H^2 Receptor Blockers

– Binds specifically to histamine receptors to prevent the histamine-activated release of gastric acid during the stimulation by food; used for dyspepsia and GERD	Cimetidine (Tagamet) Famotidine (Pepcid) Nizatidine (Axid) Ranitidine (Zantac)

Proton Pump Inhibitors (PPI)

– Inhibit the H+, K+, ATPase enzyme that is responsible for secretion of acid from gastric cells into the stomach; may possess antibacterial effects against H. pylori infection; used for gastric, duodenal ulcers, and GERD	Lansoprazole (Prevacid) Esomeprazole (Nexium) Omeprazole (Prilosec) Pantoprazole (Protonix) Rabeprazole (AcipHex)

Anticholinergics

– Blocks the effects of acetylcholine on parietal cells in the stomach and decreases the release of gastric acid; selective for muscarinic receptors	Muscarinic cholinergic antagonist Pirenzepine (Gastrozepin)

Antibiotics

– Used for the treatment of H. pylori when its present with a gastric ulcer	Metronidazole Tetracycline Clarithromycin Amoxicillin

Antidiarrheal Agents

– Used to retard serious debilitating effects from dehydration found with prolonged diarrhea; there are multiple classes of Antidiarrheal agents	Attapulgite (Donnagel) Kaolin (Kapectolin) (Pepto-Bismol) Difenoxine (Motofen) Loperamide (Imodium)

Laxative Agents

– Used for evacuation of the bowel; promote defecation; should be used sparingly	Methylcellulose (Citrucel) Psyllium (Metamucil) Docusate (Colace) Glycerin (Fleet Glycerin suppository) Magnesium hydroxide (Phillips' Milk of Magnesia) Bisacodyl (Correctol) Senna (Senokot)

Emetic Agents

– Used to induce vomiting; usually after ingestion of a toxic substance	Apomorphine Ipecac

Antiemetic Agents

– Used to decrease nausea and vomiting; usually post surgical procedure, in conjunction with oncology treatments or for motion sickness	Anticholinergic agents (Scopolamine) Antihistamine agents (Meclizine) 5-HT3 receptor antagonist agents (Dolasetron)

*selected pharmaceutical names and their respective trade names in parentheses, not intended to be a complete listing

Gastrointestinal System Profile

Abdominal Pain Quadrant and Potential Etiologies

Left upper quadrant	Right upper quadrant	Left lower quadrant	Right lower quadrant
Gastric ulcer	Hepatomegaly	Perforated colon	Kidney stone
Perforated colon	Duodenal ulcer	Ileitis	Ureteral stone
Pneumonia	Cholecystitis	Sigmoid diverticulitis	Meckel diverticulum
Spleen injury	Pneumonia	Kidney stone	Appendicitis
Spleen rupture	Hepatitis	Ureteral stone	Cholecystitis
Aortic aneurysm	Biliary stones	Intestinal obstruction	Intestinal obstruction

Key Points of Examination for Gastrointestinal Dysfunction

Past Medical History

- Abdominal or other pain (duration and location) Type: burning, dull, knife-like, cramping
- Vomiting, nausea
- Urine and stool characteristics

History of Current Condition

Medications

Laboratory Studies

- Blood work may include bilirubin, amylase/lipase, ALT/AST, albumin, thrombin/prothrombin time, platelet count, hepatitis antigens
- CBC

Other Testing

- Ultrasound
- CT scan, MRI
- Pulse (rate, strength, rhythm)
- Blood pressure
- Endoscopy
- Barium swallow fluoroscopy
- Colonoscopy, sigmoidoscopy

Visual Examination

- General appearance, contour, symmetry
- Scars, rash, lesion, ascites, presence of mass

Palpation

- Tenderness, guarding, rebound, rigidity

Percussion and Auscultation of Abdomen

- Perform in all four quadrants

Rehabilitation Considerations for Patients with Gastrointestinal Disease

- **Electrolyte imbalance** from diarrhea, vomiting, weight loss
- **Orthostatic hypotension** secondary to electrolyte imbalance
- **Muscle cramping** secondary to alteration in the sodium-potassium pump
- **Difficulty swallowing** secondary to disk protrusion or esophageal pathology
- **Thoracolumbar junction pain (back pain and/or shoulder pain)** secondary to an acute ulcer or GI bleeding
- **Kehr's sign** present indicating free air or blood within the abdominal cavity

Genitourinary System

The genitourinary system consists of all the reproductive organs and the urinary system. These are often considered together due to their common embryological origin.

Renal system	Male genital system	Female genital system
• Kidneys • Ureters • Urinary bladder • Urethra	• Testes/scrotum • Penis • Epididymis • Vas deferens • Seminal vesicles • Prostate gland • Cowper's gland	• Ovaries • Fallopian tubes • Uterus • Vagina • External genitalia • Bartholin's glands • Skene's gland

Genital System

The genital system is a complex system comprised of the male and female gonads and associated ducts, external genitalia, and associated hormones that all function to reproduce the species.

Urinary System

The urinary system consists of two kidneys, two ureters, the urinary bladder, and the urethra. The kidneys function to form urine while the remainder of the urinary system is responsible for eliminating the urine.

Genitourinary System Anatomy

Male Reproductive Anatomy

The male reproductive anatomy consists of the testes (housed within the temperature controlled scrotum) which creates the immature sperm. The sperm travel to the epididymis for storage and to further develop. Glands that create ejaculation fluids include the prostate gland, vas deferens, and the seminal vesicles. The penis, vas deferens, urethra, and Cowper's gland are all used during intercourse to deposit the sperm into the female for reproduction.

Female Reproductive Anatomy

The female reproductive anatomy is a complex system comprised of organs and glands. The ovaries are attached to the uterus by the fallopian tubes and they are responsible for the release of an ovum at intervals of approximately 28 days. The ovum will pass into the uterus and will either become fertilized by a male sperm or remain unfertilized and pass with the endometrium through menstruation on a 28-day cycle. The vagina is attached to the uterus and is a receptacle for the male sperm as well as a birth canal for a baby.

Kidney Anatomy

Kidneys are bean shaped organs that are located around the mid-back just below the rib cage. A kidney processes approximately 200 quarts of blood each 24 hours and extracts waste products that are excreted as urine. The waste must be removed from the blood so damage to the body does not occur. Filtering of the blood occurs within the nephrons that are located inside the kidneys. There are approximately one million nephrons found within each kidney.

The kidneys also release three important hormones:

- Erythropoietin (stimulates the bone marrow to create red blood cells)
- Renin (regulates blood pressure)
- Calcitriol (active form of vitamin d that maintains calcium for bones and promotes chemical balance)

The kidneys serve several critical roles:

Homeostasis

The kidney is an important contributor to homeostasis. These essential functions include acid-base balance, regulation of electrolyte concentrations, control of blood volume, and regulation of blood pressure. The kidneys accomplish these functions independently and in conjunction with other organs through the control of hormones that are secreted into the bloodstream.

Acid-base balance

The kidneys regulate the acid-base balance of the blood (pH) by excretion or conservation of ions such as H^+ ions or HCO_3^- ions.

Blood pressure

Regulation of blood pressure is maintained by the kidneys' ability to excrete enough sodium chloride to maintain normal sodium balance, extracellular fluid volume, and blood volume. Kidney disease is the most common cause of secondary hypertension. Kidney disease allows for chronic increases in extracellular fluid and blood volumes, which results in increased blood pressure.

Plasma volume

A drop in plasma osmolality will be detected by the hypothalamus and cause the pituitary gland to secrete antidiuretic hormone. This will result in water reabsorption by the kidney and an increase in urine concentration.

Hormone secretion

The kidneys secrete a variety of hormones including erythropoietin, urodilatin, rennin, and calcitriol.

Urination

An adult will excrete approximately one to two liters of urine per 24 hours. The exact amount depends on factors such as medications, fluid intake, and amount of fluid lost through breathing and exercise.

Genitourinary System Terminology

Anuria: Inadequate urine output in a 24-hour period; less than 100 ml (severe dehydration, shock, end stage renal disease).

Benign prostatic hypertrophy: A non-cancerous enlargement of the prostate gland that is progressive. Common in males over 60 and can interfere with normal voiding.

Cystocele: Bulging of the bladder into the vagina.

Ectopic: Implantation of a fertilized ovum outside of the uterus (fallopian tube is the most common site of an ectopic pregnancy).

Endometrium: The inner lining of the uterus that is shed monthly in response to hormonal influence.

Glomerular filtration rate: An estimate of the filtering capacity of the kidneys; volume of filtrate produced per minute by the kidneys.

Glomerulonephritis: Inflammation of the glomerular portion of the kidney.

Glomerulus: The specialized tuft of capillaries that are needed for the filtration of fluid as blood passes through the arterioles of the kidneys.

Hematuria: Presence of blood in urine (cancer, faulty catheterization, serious disease).

Impotence: Impairment with ejaculation, orgasm, erection, and/or libido.

Intermittent hemodialysis: The patient's arterial blood is circulated mechanically through semipermeable tubing to clean the blood and return it to the body.

Myometrium: The muscular outer layer of the uterus.

Nephrolithiasis: Urinary stones that develop in the kidneys.

Nocturia: Urinary frequency at night (diabetes mellitus, congestive heart failure).

Oliguria: Inadequate urine output in a 24-hour period; less than 400 ml (acute renal failure, diabetes mellitus).

Overflow incontinence: A loss of urine secondary to bladder distention; associated with urinary retention (spinal cord injury, diabetes mellitus).

Peritoneal dialysis: A form of renal replacement therapy that uses the peritoneal cavity as a semipermeable membrane to exchange between the dialysate fluid and blood vessels of the abdominal cavity.

Polyuria: Large volume of urine excreted at one time (diabetes mellitus, chronic renal failure).

Perimetrium: The serous peritoneal coat of the uterus.

Radical mastectomy: A surgical procedure in which the entire breast, pectoral muscles, axillary lymph nodes, and some skin are removed usually secondary to breast cancer.

Rectocele: The bulging of the anterior wall of the rectum into the vagina secondary to weakening of the pelvic supporting structures.

Seminiferous tubules: Coiled tubes found within each lobe of the testes where spermatogenesis takes place.

Stress incontinence: Intermittent loss of urine due to an increase in abdominal pressure (coughing, straining, and sneezing in combination with weakness in pelvic musculature).

Urea: Major nitrogen-containing end product of protein metabolism normally cleared from the blood by the kidney into the urine.

Urge incontinence: Having the feeling that there is a need to urinate with a sudden involuntary loss of urine (neurologic disease of bladder).

Urgency: Strong desire to urinate.

Obstetrics

Exercise and Pregnancy

Recommended exercise activities

- Swimming
- Walking
- Stretching
- Low impact aerobics
- Golfing
- Stationary cycling

Exercise activities to avoid

- High-level balance activities
- Skiing
- Water skiing
- Scuba diving
- Horseback riding

- Contact sports
- Skating
- Strenuous lifting

Pregnant women are encouraged to continue with exercise activity at a moderate rate during a low risk pregnancy. Guidelines permit women to remain at 50-60% of their maximal heart rate for approximately thirty minutes per session. Women must monitor their heart rate intermittently to ensure that they are maintaining their target heart rate. Non-weight bearing activities are preferred due to the continuous change in the center of gravity and balance. Loose clothing is advised to allow for adequate heat loss, and adequate fluids are required during exercise. Women should avoid becoming overtired and should not exercise in the supine position after the first trimester.

American College of Obstetricians and Gynecologists (ACOG) Recommendations for Exercise in Pregnancy and Postpartum

1. During pregnancy, women can continue to exercise and derive health benefits even from mild to moderate exercise routines. Regular exercise (at least three times per week) is preferable to intermittent activity.

2. Women should avoid exercise in the supine position after the first trimester. Such a position is associated with decreased cardiac output in most pregnant women. Since the remaining cardiac output will be preferentially distributed away from splanchnic beds (including the uterus) during vigorous exercise, such regimens are best avoided during pregnancy. Prolonged periods of motionless standing should also be avoided.

3. Women should be aware of the decreased oxygen available for aerobic exercise during pregnancy. They should be encouraged to modify the intensity of their exercise according to maternal symptoms. Pregnant women should stop exercising when fatigued and not exercise to exhaustion. Weight bearing exercises may, under some circumstances, be continued at intensities similar to those prior to pregnancy throughout pregnancy. Non-weight bearing exercises, such as cycling or swimming, will minimize the risk of injury and facilitate the continuation of exercise during pregnancy.

4. Morphologic changes in pregnancy should serve as a relative contraindication to types of exercise in which loss of balance could be detrimental to maternal or fetal well-being, especially in the third trimester. Further, any type of exercise involving the potential for even mild abdominal trauma should be avoided.

5. Pregnancy requires an additional 300 kcal/day in order to maintain metabolic homeostasis. Thus, women who exercise during pregnancy should be particularly careful to ensure an adequate diet.

6. Pregnant women who exercise in the first trimester should augment heat dissipation by ensuring adequate hydration, appropriate clothing, and optimal environmental surroundings during exercise.

7. Many of the physiological and morphological changes of pregnancy persist four to six weeks postpartum. Thus, pre-pregnancy exercise routines should be resumed gradually based upon a woman's physical capability.

From American College of Obstetricians and Gynecologists. Exercise During Pregnancy and the Postpartum Period. (Technical Bulletin No. 189). Washington, DC, copyrights ACOG, February 1994, with permission.

Physiological Changes during Pregnancy

- Weight gain between 25 and 35 pounds
- Increased depth of respiration
- Increased tidal volume
- Increased minute ventilation
- Increased oxygen consumption per minute (15-20%)
- Abdominals become overstretched

- Ligaments become lax secondary to hormonal changes
- Joints may become hypermobile
- Increased blood volume (40-50%)
- Anemia may occur
- Hypotension in supine position during late pregnancy from pressure on the inferior vena cava
- Increased cardiac output (30-60%)

Postural Changes

- Change in the center of gravity
- Forward head posture
- Increased cervical lordosis
- Increased base of support in standing

Diastasis Recti

Diastasis recti is a separation of the rectus abdominis muscle along the linea alba that can occur during pregnancy. The exact cause is unknown, however, theories indicate biomechanical and hormonal changes in women may cause the separation. Testing should be performed on all pregnant women for diastasis recti prior to prescribing exercises that require the use of the abdominals. A therapist should place a hand horizontally over the umbilicus as the pregnant woman lies in a hooklying position. A patient is considered to have diastasis recti if the therapist detects a separation greater than the width of two fingers when the woman lifts her head and shoulders off the plinth. The therapist must note how many fingers fit into the separation and modify treatment accordingly. Diastasis recti requires stabilization and support with abdominal strengthening exercises. A newborn can also have diastasis recti secondary to incomplete development, however, in infants this condition usually resolves itself without intervention.

Pelvic Floor Weakness

The pelvic floor is comprised of a group of muscles that stretch between the pubis and coccyx and create the inferior stability of the pelvic cavity. The pubococcygeal muscles can become lax and overstretched during delivery or can become disrupted by an episiotomy. Weakness of the vaginal canal and stress incontinence are two problems that can result from childbirth and may require physical therapy intervention. Pubococcygeal or Kegel exercises should begin during pregnancy for prevention of pubococcygeal muscle weakness. The exercises require a patient to contract or squeeze as if she was stopping the flow of urine. The isometric contraction should be held five to ten seconds with complete relaxation after each contraction. Five to ten contractions should be performed in a series and three to four series should be performed each day.

Contraindications for Exercise During Pregnancy

- Pregnancy induced hypertension
- Preterm rupture of membrane
- Preterm labor during the prior or current pregnancy
- Incompetent cervix
- Persistent second to third trimester bleeding
- Intrauterine growth retardation

From American College of Obstetricians and Gynecologists. Exercise During Pregnancy and the Postpartum Period. Technical Bulletin No. 189). Washington, DC, copyrights ACOG, February 1994, with permission.

Genitourinary System Pathology

Kidneys and Bladder

Renal failure

Renal pathology usually occurs secondary to diabetes mellitus or hypertension, but can also occur from poison, trauma, and genetics. The nephrons are usually damaged and they lose their ability to filter the blood.

Renal failure can be classified as:

- Acute (damage occurs quickly)
- Chronic (damage occurs slowly)
- End-stage (nearly total or total renal failure, dialysis required)

Acute Renal Failure (ARF): (sudden decline in renal function)

- Increase in BUN and creatinine
- Oliguria
- Hyperkalemia
- Sodium retention
- **Prerenal etiology (secondary to a decrease in blood flow)**
  Shock, hemorrhage, burn, pulmonary embolism
- **Postrenal etiology (obstruction distal to the kidney)**
  Neoplasm, kidney stone, prostate hypertrophy
- **Intrarenal (primary damage of renal tissue)**
  Toxins, intrarenal ischemia, vascular disorders

Chronic Renal Failure (CRF): (progressive deterioration in renal function)

- Diabetes mellitus
- Severe hypertension
- Glomerulopathies
- Obstructive uropathy
- Interstitial nephritis
- Polycystic kidney disease

Stages of Kidney Disease According to the National Kidney Foundation

Stage 1	kidney damage with normal GFR (90 or greater)
Stage 2	mild decrease in GFR (60-89)
Stage 3	moderate decrease in GFR (30-59)
Stage 4	severe reduction in GFR (15-29)
Stage 5	kidney failure (GFR less than 15)

Symptoms of renal failure vary based on severity of the condition and can include nausea, vomiting, lethargy, weakness, hiccups, anorexia, ulceration within the GI tract, sleep disorders, headache, peripheral neuropathy, anemia, pruritus, osteomalacia, ecchymosis, pulmonary edema, seizures, and coma. **Treatment** of ARF includes management of primary etiology, pharmacological intervention, diuretics, nutritional support, hydration, dialysis and/or transfusions if applicable. **Treatment** of CRF includes conservative management and renal replacement therapy. Conservative management assists with slowing the process and assisting the body in its compensation. Nutritional support, hydration, avoidance of protein, and pharmacological intervention are usually the primary basis of intervention. Renal replacement therapy includes some form of dialysis and/or organ transplant.

Hemodialysis

Hemodialysis is a treatment process for patients with advanced and permanent kidney failure. Kidney failure creates excess toxic waste, increased blood pressure, retention of excess body fluids, and a decrease in red blood cell production. Hemodialysis removes the blood from the body along with waste, excess sodium, and fluids. The process cleanses the blood and returns it to the body. A patient requires this process on average three times per week and each visit requires three to five hours to complete the treatment. Side effects that may be associated with dialysis include anemia, renal osteodystrophy, pruritus (itching), sleep disorders ("restless legs"), and dialysis-related amyloidosis.

Rehabilitation Considerations for Patients with Renal Failure/Dialysis

- **Modify** treatment plan based on fluid and electrolyte status
- **Standard precautions** should be followed at all times for protection
- **Understand patient's abilities** post dialysis and potential for dehydration and hypotension
- **Monitor vital signs** closely
- **Mobilization activities** are contraindicated during dialysis
- **Energy conservation techniques and pacing skills** should be incorporated into therapy
- **Avoid placement of the blood pressure cuff over the fistula**
- **Patient education** regarding signs and symptoms of relapse or chronic hepatitis

Neurogenic Bladder

Neurogenic bladder is a dysfunction where there is damage to the cerebral control that allows for controlled micturation resulting in urinary dysfunction. If the urine cannot be properly released there may be an increase in urinary tract infections and kidney damage. The etiology of neurogenic bladder can include diabetes, diminished bladder capacity, hyperactive detrusor muscle, CVA, other disease processes, infection, and nerve damage. **Symptoms** include frequent urinary tract infections, leakage of urine, inability to empty the bladder or loss of the urge to urinate when the bladder is full. Diagnosis should include an evaluation by a physician, X-rays, and urodynamics to assist with diagnosis. **Treatment** is dependent on the actual etiology with a goal of preventing bladder overdistention, UTIs, and renal damage. Patient education, bladder techniques, lower abdominal massage, temporary catheterization, pharmacological intervention, and a timed urination program may be indicated.

Urinary Tract Infection (UTI)

Urinary tract infections (UTI) occur when bacteria infiltrates the urethra (termed urethritis) or further into the bladder itself (cystitis). Untreated, this type of infection can spread and cause a kidney infection (pyelonephritis). **Symptoms** of a UTI include increased frequency of urination, pain and/or burning with urination, cloudy urine, pressure above the pubic bone in women, shakiness, fever, back pain, and fatigue. Diagnosis is confirmed with urinalysis. Frequent UTIs may require ultrasound, intravenous pyelogram, and cystoscopy to further assess the function of the bladder. Early **treatment** has the best results; delay in treatment may allow for serious infection to occur. Pharmacological treatment includes bacteria-specific antibiotics based on the bacteria found in the bladder. Patients are also encouraged to drink an excess of fluids to assist with treatment of the infection.

Urinary Incontinence

Please refer to clinical application template on page 378.

Gonads

Erectile dysfunction (ED)

Erectile dysfunction, also known as impotence, is estimated to range from 25-85% in men with diabetes, which makes this population three times more likely than the general population. Onset of ED in individuals with diabetes usually occurs 10-15 years earlier than in men without diabetes. Other risk factors include coronary heart disease, hypertension, hypothyroidism, hypopituitarism, multiple sclerosis, psychiatric disorders, excessive alcohol consumption or alcoholism, smoking, vessel disease, kidney disease, pharmacological side effects, and hormonal imbalances. This condition is diagnosed with the primary **symptom** as the consistent inability to maintain an erection adequate for sexual intercourse. **Treatment** varies and includes pharmacological intervention, surgical intervention, and injections directly to the penis.

Prostate Cancer

Adenocarcinoma of the prostate is the most common form of prostate cancer. Risk factors include family history, geographic location, increasing age (over 50), African American race, high fat diet, and occupations related to the use of cadmium. **Symptoms** are varied and in many instances prostate cancer is found accidentally. The initial signs that may be noted include difficulty with urination, pain, weight loss, and fatigue. Areas of pain vary depending on the site and size of the tumor or lesion, as well as if there is metastasis of the cancer. Areas of pain can include the rectum, sacrum, thoracic and lumbar spine, and scapular area. **Treatment** is dictated by the diagnosis of prostate cancer and the staging at the time of diagnosis. Treatment can include surgical intervention, radiation therapy, and hormonal therapy.

Rehabilitation Considerations for Patients with Prostate Cancer

- **Modify** treatment plan based on patient endurance status
- **Monitor** for signs of infection post surgery
- **Monitor pain** and watch for signs of metabolic spread
- **Monitor for complications** from radiation therapy
- **Understand the side effects** associated with hormonal manipulation
- **Educate** the patient to use pacing and other skills with functional daily activities

Cystocele

Cystocele or a "fallen bladder" occurs due to weakness in the wall between the vagina and bladder. This weakness allows the bladder to fall into the vagina and produces impairment with emptying the bladder. There are three grades of cystocele with progressive **symptoms**; grade 1 is classified as mild and is characterized by the bladder drooping only a small amount into the vagina; grade 2 is classified as a more significant cystocele and is characterized by drooping far enough into the vagina to reach the opening; and stage 3 is the most severe classification demonstrating a bladder that protrudes through the opening of the vagina. Other symptoms include urinary frequency and urgency, cystitis, and pain with a "bearing down" sensation in the perineal area. Etiology may include strain from the birth process, hormonal changes that occur after menopause, diabetic neuropathy, straining repetitively during activities or bowel movements. Diagnosis can be made by observation and examination as well as by participating in a voiding cystourethrogram. **Treatment** may range from no treatment to surgical intervention depending on the degree of cystocele. Physical therapy may be indicated to educate the patient regarding lifting and avoidance of straining during activities. Pelvic floor strengthening should be incorporated into all post-surgical rehabilitation programs. The physician may need to prescribe a pessary which is a device that is placed into the vagina to hold the bladder in place. A severe cystocele will require surgical treatment in order to place the bladder back into the correct position.

Breast Cancer

Breast cancer is the most common form of cancer in women with the majority of the cases involving adenocarcinomas. Risk factors currently include family history and genetics, gender, race, age, menstrual history, geographical location, and history of pregnancy. The most common initial **symptom** for many women is a hard, irregular, painless, palpable mass. Other symptoms can include a change in breast shape, discharge from the nipple, and erythema. **Treatment** depends on the staging of the disease and may include surgical intervention, radiation therapy, chemotherapy or hormone therapy. The current 5-year survival rate for localized tumors is 92%; this drops to 72% if there is nodal involvement. If the patient is stage III or IV the treatment becomes palliative.

Rehabilitation Considerations for Patients with Breast Cancer

- **Examination of the shoulder girdle** should include inspection of the outer and upper quadrant of the breast and axilla where most tumors (and metastases) are detected
- **Mass in the muscle** should change during contraction of the muscle
- **Monitor** for signs of infection post surgery
- **Awareness** of the signs associated with breast cancer (i.e., may develop cancer in the other breast)
- **Monitor side effects** from adjunctive therapy post surgery
- **Monitor for complications** from radiation therapy, chemotherapy
- **Scheduling** of therapy around times of fatigue
- **Educate** the patient to use pacing and other skills with functional daily activities; post-mastectomy intervention focuses on breathing and coughing techniques, edema prevention, phantom pain

Pharmacological Intervention for Genitourinary System Management

CHEMOTHERAPEUTIC AGENTS for Genitourinary Oncology

Alkylating Agents

– Used as part of chemotherapy to exert cytotoxic effects by preventing DNA function and replication	Altretamine (Hexalen) ovarian Cyclophosphamide (Cytoxan) breast, ovary Ifosfamide (IFEX) testicular Melphalan (Alkeran) ovarian Thiotepa (thioplex) breast, ovary, bladder

Anti-metabolites

– Cancer drugs similar to endogenous metabolites, the drugs compete with certain compounds during DNA synthesis. They interfere with normal metabolites	Capecitabine (Xeloda) breast

Anti-neoplastic Antibiotics

– Used primarily in neoplastic diseases secondary to their high toxicity; exert anti-neoplastic effects	Bleomycin (Blenoxane) penis, testicle, vulva, cervical Dactinomycin (Cosmegen) testicle, endometrium Doxorubicin (Adriamycin) bladder, breast, ovary Mitoxantrone (Novantrone) prostate Plicamycin (Mithracin) testicular

Plant Alkaloids

– Used to directly impair cell division; disrupt mitotic apparatus	Docetaxel (taxotere) breast Etoposide (Etopophos) testes Paclitaxel (Taxol) breast, ovary Topotecan (Hycamtin)

CHEMOTHERAPEUTIC AGENTS for Genitourinary Oncology (continued)

Anti-neoplastic Hormones

– Used in certain hormone-sensitive types of cancer to either mimic or block the effects	*Androgens*-breast *Anti-androgens*-prostate *Aromatase inhibitors*-breast *Estrogens*-breast, prostate *Anti-estrogens*-breast *Progestins*-breast, endometrium, prostate, renal *Gonadatropin-releasing hormone*-prostate, breast

OTHER AGENTS used with Genitourinary Treatment

Heavy Metal Compounds

	Carboplatin (Paraplatin) ovary Cisplatin (Platinol) bladder, ovary, testicles

Diuretic Agents

– Increase sodium and water excretion to manage hypertension Types: Thiazide, Loop, Potassium sparing	Furosemide (Lasix) Hydrochlorothiazide (Esidrix, Microzide, Hydrodiuril) Chlorthalidone (Thalitone, Hygroton) Spirondactone (Aldactone) Amiloride (Midamor)

Urinary Anti-infective Agents

– Antibiotics that are specifically used in the treatment of kidney and urine infections	Cinoxacin (Cinobac) Fosfomycin (Monurol) Nitrofurantoin (Macrobid)

Overactive Bladder

	Oxybutynin (Ditropan) Tolterodine tartrate (Detrol)

Genitourinary System Profile

Key Points of Examination for Genitourinary Dysfunction

Past Medical History

- Abdominal or other pain (duration and location)
  Type of pain, burning, dull, knife-like, cramping
- Vomiting, nausea
- Urine and stool characteristics
- Hernia
- Incontinence
- History of previous cancer

History of Current Condition

Medications

Laboratory Studies

- Glomerular filtration rate (GFR)
- Blood creatinine
- Blood urea nitrogen (BUN)
- Urinalysis
- CBC
- Microalbuminuria and proteinuria

Other Testing

- CT scan, MRI
- IV urography (pyelography)
- Percutaneous anterograde urography
- Retrograde urography
- Angiography
- Ultrasound
- Radionuclide scanning
- Bladder catheterization
- Biopsy
- Cystoscopy
- Uroflowmetry
- Renography or renal scan

Visual Examination

- Abdominal/genital
  Rash, lesion, hernia, mass
- Edema within the extremities

Palpation

- Tenderness, guarding, rebound, rigidity

Multi-System

Diagnostic Tests

Arteriography

Arteriography refers to a radiograph that visualizes injected radiopaque dye in an artery. The test can be used to identify arteriosclerosis, tumors or blockages.

Arthrography

Arthrography is an invasive test utilizing a contrast medium to provide visualization of joint structures through radiographs. Soft tissue disruption can be identified by leakage from the joint cavity and capsule. The test is commonly used at peripheral joints such as the hip, knee, ankle, elbow, and wrist.

Bone Scan

A bone scan is an invasive test that utilizes isotopes to identify stress fractures, infection, and tumors. Bone scans can identify bone disease or stress fractures with as little as 4-7% bone loss.

Computed Tomography

Computed tomography produces cross-sectional images based on x-ray attenuation. A computerized analysis of the changes in absorption produces a detailed reconstructed image. The test is commonly used to diagnose spinal lesions and in diagnostic studies of the brain.

Doppler Ultrasonography

Doppler ultrasonography is a non-invasive test that evaluates blood flow in the major veins, arteries, and cerebrovascular system. The test relies on the transmission and reflection of high frequency sound waves to produce cross-sectional images in a variety of planes. Doppler ultrasonography is safer, less expensive, and requires a shorter time period than more invasive tests such as arteriography and venography.

Electrocardiography

Electrocardiography is the recording of the electrical activity of the heart. The test identifies three distinct waveforms: P wave (atrial depolarization), QRS complex (ventricular depolarization), and the T wave (ventricular repolarization). Electrocardiography is used to help identify conduction abnormalities, cardiac arrhythmias, and myocardial ischemia.

Electroencephalography

Electroencephalography is the recording of the electrical activity of the brain. The electrical activity is collected by examining the difference between the electrical potential of two electrodes placed at different locations on the scalp. Electroencephalography is used to assess seizure activity, metabolic disorders, and cerebellar lesions.

Diagnostic Tests (continued)

Electromyography

Electromyography is the recording of the electrical activity of a selected muscle or muscle groups at rest and during voluntary contraction. Electromyography is performed by inserting a needle electrode percutaneously into a muscle or through the use of surface electrodes. The test is commonly used to assess peripheral nerve injuries and to differentiate between various neuromuscular disorders.

Fluoroscopy

Fluoroscopy is designed to show motion in joints through x-ray imaging. The technique permits objects placed between a fluorescent screen and a roentgen tube to become visible. Fluoroscopy is not used commonly due to excessive radiation exposure.

Magnetic Resonance Imaging

Magnetic resonance imaging is a non-invasive technique that utilizes magnetic fields to produce an image of bone and soft tissue. The test is valuable in providing images of soft tissue structures such as muscles, menisci, ligaments, tumors, and internal organs. Magnetic resonance imaging requires the patient to remain still for prolonged periods of time and is extremely expensive.

Myelography

Myelography is an invasive test that combines fluoroscopy and radiography to evaluate the spinal subarachnoid space. The test utilizes a contrast medium that is injected into the epidural space by spinal puncture. Myelography is used to identify bone displacement, disk herniation, spinal cord compression or tumors.

Venography

Venography refers to a radiograph that visualizes injected radiopaque dye in a vein. The test can be used to identify tumors or blockages in the venous network.

X-ray

X-ray is a radiographic photograph commonly used to assist with the diagnosis of musculoskeletal problems such as fractures, dislocations, and bone loss. X-ray produces planar images and as a result often requires images to be taken in multiple planes in order to visualize a lesion's location and size.

Oncology

Oncology Terminology

Benign neoplasm: An abnormal cell growth that is usually slow growing and harmless; it closely resembles the adjacent tissue composition.

Cancer (malignancy, tumor, carcinoma): Cancer can be defined as groups of diseases characterized by uncontrolled cell proliferation with mutation and spreading of the abnormal cells. The etiology is based on the type and location of the cancer. The most common causes include cigarette smoking, diet and nutrition, chemical agents, physical agents, environmental causes, viral causes, and genetics.

Dysplasia: The process of normal change in shape, size, and type of normal cells.

Hyperplasia: An increase in cell number that may be normal or abnormal.

Malignant neoplasm: An abnormal cell growth that grows uncontrollably, invades and destroys adjacent tissues, and may metastasize to other sites and systems of the body.

Metaplasia: A change in a cell from one type to another that may be normal or abnormal.

Tumor (neoplasm): A tumor is an abnormal new growth of tissue that increases the overall tissue mass. Tumors are benign (non-cancerous) or malignant (cancerous) as well as primary or secondary. Primary tumors form from cells that belong to the area of the tumor. Secondary tumors grow from cells that have metastasized (spread) from another affected area within the body.

Tumor classification is defined by cell type, tissue of origin, amount of differentiation, benign versus malignant, and anatomic site.

Tissue and Tumor Classification

Tissue Classification	Examples	Tumor Classification
Epithelium Protect, absorb, and excrete	– Skin – Lines internal cavities – Mucous membrane – Lining of bladder	Carcinoma Glandular tissue-adenocarcinoma
Pigmented Cells	– Moles	Malignant Melanoma
Connective Tissues Elastic, collagen, fibrous	– Striated muscle – Blood vessels – Bone – Cartilage – Fat – Smooth muscle	Sarcoma Fibrosarcoma Liposarcoma Chondrosarcoma Osteosarcoma Hemangiosarcoma Leiomyosarcoma Rhabdomyosarcoma
Nerve Tissues Neurons, nerve fibers, dendrites, glial cells	– Brain – Nerves – Spinal cord – Retina	Astrocytoma Glioma Neurilemic sarcoma Neuroblastoma Retinoblastoma
Lymphoid Tissues	– Where ever lymph tissue is present throughout the body – Lymph nodes – Spleen – Can appear in stomach, intestines, skin, CNS, bone and tonsils	Lymphoma
Hematopietic Tissues	– Bone marrow – Plasma cells	Leukemia Myelodysplasia Myeloproliferative syndromes Multiple myeloma

General Signs and Symptoms of Cancer

C – Change in bowel/bladder routine

A – A sore that will not heal

U – Unusual bleeding/discharge

T – Thickening/lump develops

I – Indigestion or difficulty swallowing

O – Obvious change in wart/mole

N – Nagging cough/hoarseness

**Unexplained weight loss, fatigue, anorexia, anemia, pain, and/or weakness are other general symptoms that may indicate cancer.

Staging

Staging of a malignancy is diagnosed through determining the extent of the disease, the lymph node involvement, and determining if metastases exist in other areas. Staging allows for appropriate treatment and course of intervention and can assist with predicting outcome and prognosis.

Leading Cause of Deaths

Male		Female	
Lung	30%	Lung	26%
Prostate	9%	Breast	15%
Colon	9%	Colon	9%
Pancreas	6%	Pancreas	6%
Leukemia	4%	Ovary	5%
Esophagus	4%	Non-Hodgkin's Lymphoma	4%
Liver	4%	Leukemia	3%
Bladder	3%	Uterine	3%
Kidney	3%	Brain	2%
Non-Hodgkin's Lymphoma	3%	Liver	2%
Other	25%	Other	25%

* Cancer is the leading cause of death in the United States
* Data taken from the American Cancer Society, www.cancer.org

Diagnostic Tools

• Family history	• Pap smear
• Physical examination	• Blood tests
• Radiography	• Biopsy
• CT scan	• Mammography
• Bone scan	• Endoscopy
• Stool guaiac	• Isotope scan

Risk Factors

• Increasing age	• Poor diet
• Tobacco use	• Stress
• Alcohol use	• Occupational hazards
• Gender	• Ethnic background
• Virus exposure	• Genetic influence
• Environmental influence	• Sexual/reproductive behavior

Common Sites of Metastasis

• Lymph nodes	• Brain
• Liver	• Bone
• Lung	

Cancer Prevention

Primary Prevention	• Screening for high risk population • Elimination of modifiable risk factors • Use of natural agents (i.e., teas, vitamins) to prevent cancer • Cancer vaccine
Secondary Prevention	• Early detection • Selective preventative pharmacological agents (e.g., Tamoxifen) • Multifactorial risk reduction
Tertiary Prevention	• Prevent disability that can occur secondary to cancer and its treatment • Manage symptoms • Limit complications

Oncology Pathology

Skin Cancer

Basal Cell Carcinoma

- Slow growing
- Originates from epidermis
- Rarely metastasizes
- Sun exposure is a common cause
- Prognosis is good; can be cured

Squamous Cell Carcinoma

- Usually develops in sun-damaged skin
- Usually found in fair-skinned people
- Peak incidence at 60 years
- Can be difficult to diagnose
- Can metastasize
- Prognosis with treatment is excellent

Malignant Melanoma

- Originates from melanocytes
- Cutaneous melanoma can be classified as: superficial spreading, nodular, lentigo, maligna or acral lentiginous melanomas
- Peak incidence is between 40-60 years
- Risk factors include blonde/red hair, fair skin, blue eyes, sunburn easily
- Associated with intensity of sun exposure (as opposed to duration of exposure)
- Treatment requires surgical excision and radiation/chemotherapy
- Early diagnosis is vital to prognosis
- Can spread and metastasize quickly
- Metastases to the brain, lungs, liver, bone, skin, and CNS are fatal within 12 months
- 100% curable with early diagnosis

Breast Cancer

- Most common female malignancy, but can also occur in men
- Second leading cause of female death from cancer
- 70% of breast cancer occurs to patients over 50 years of age
- Risk factors include genetics, gender, age, menstrual history, and geography
- Presents as a lump; usually found by the woman
- Mass is typically firm, irregular, and non-painful
- Common metastases to the lymph nodes, lungs, bones, skin, and brain

- Treatment may include surgery, radiation, chemotherapy or hormonal manipulation
- Curable if diagnosed prior to metastases
- Survival rate decreases as the stage of the cancer increases
- If the cancer recurs, it is usually within two years of the initial diagnosis

Lung Cancer

- Cancer of the epithelium within the respiratory tract
- Most frequent cause of death from all cancers
- Incidence of death increases from age 45 and levels off at approximately 74 years of age
- Risk factors include cigarette smoking, environmental exposure, geographic location, occupational hazards, age, and family history
- Early symptoms include cough, sputum, and dyspnea
- Rapid metastasis can occur through the pulmonary vascular system, adrenal gland, brain, bone, and liver
- Poor prognosis in most cases secondary to expedited metastasis (less than 14% for a five-year survival rate)

Pancreatic Cancer

- Fourth leading cause of death by cancer
- Cancer of the exocrine cells within the ducts (ductal adenocarcinoma) is the most common form of pancreatic cancer
- Peak incidence occurs during a person's 7th and 8th decades
- Most common in African American men
- Risk factors include tobacco use, gender, increasing age, and cholecystectomy
- Early symptoms are nondescript and include decreased appetite, abdominal pain, and weight loss
- Later symptoms include jaundice, obstruction, and back pain
- Metastasizes to the liver, lungs, pleura, colon, stomach, and spleen; poor prognosis

Brain Cancer

- Most primary cancers metastasize to the brain
- Primary CNS cancers rarely metastasize outside the CNS
- Signs and symptoms are based on location of the tumor within the brain
- Signs and symptoms include headache, seizures, increased intracranial pressure, cognitive and emotional impairment, and decreased motor and sensory function
- Symptoms progress rapidly
- Usually a poor prognosis with both primary brain cancer and brain metastases

Leukemia

- Malignant neoplasm of the white blood cells
- Replaces normal cells with lymphocytic or myelogenous cells
- Two acute forms, two chronic forms
- Main symptoms include anemia, infection, bruising/bleeding tendencies
- The five-year survival rate has increased for acute

leukemias to 75% for children and 44% for adults
- Chronic myelogenous leukemia has a less favorable prognosis due to limitations in treatment
- Chronic lymphocytic leukemia is fatal with no curative treatment
- Treatment can include chemotherapy, radiation, bone marrow transplant, stem cell transplant, and hormone therapy

Lymphoma

- Cancers that develop in the lymphatic system and occupy lymph tissues
- A painless lump is usually the first sign
- Lymphomas are categorized as Hodgkin's disease or non-Hodgkin's lymphoma
- Hodgkin's disease is distinguished by the presence of the Reed-Sternberg cells that are part of the tissue macrophage system
- Hodgkin's disease can metastasize to extralymphatic sites including the liver, bone marrow, spleen, and lungs
- Risk factors for Hodgkin's disease include association with Epstein-Barre virus, immunosuppressant use, drug abuse, obesity, chronic or autoimmune diseases
- Hodgkin's disease is one of the most curable cancers depending on age, disease stage, overall health, and responsiveness to treatment at diagnosis
- Non-Hodgkin's lymphomas are solid tumors found within the lymphatic system
- Lymphomas are classified according to size, B-cell and T-cell markers, grading, and pattern of growth
- Risk factors for non-Hodgkin's lymphoma include exposure to benzene (i.e., cigarette smoke), auto emissions, pollution, and food containing high levels of polychlonnated biphenyls (i.e., meats, dairy, fish)
- Treatment options are based on the patient's age and staging classification and include chemotherapy, chemotherapy with radiation, stem cell transplant, and highly active antiretroviral therapy
- Prognosis of non-Hodgkin's lymphoma varies based on classification, co-morbidities, and response to treatment

Multiple Myeloma

- A primary malignant neoplasm of plasma cells
- Most often found in bone marrow
- Initially found in bone marrow of flat bones will infiltrate other bone marrow and then other organs
- Slow progression with initial signs of bone pain, altered red blood cell, leukocyte, and platelet production
- Peak age of incidence is between 50 and 70 years
- Anemia, bleeding tendencies, and increased susceptibility to infection result
- The pre-symptomatic period of the disease can last from 5 to 20 years
- Treatment can include chemotherapy with high potency biphosphonates, stem cell therapy, bone marrow transplant
- Median duration of remission is three years
- Median length of survival is six years
- Currently, there is no curative treatment

Sarcoma (Bone Tumor)

- Most common bone tumors are osteosarcoma, chondrosarcoma, Ewing's sarcoma, and angiosarcoma
- Bone tumors are classified as osteoblastic or osteolytic
- Pain is the predominant sign; other signs include weight loss, failure to relieve pain, night pain, age, history of cancer, swelling, and fever
- Sarcomas usually metastasize to the lungs, liver, and other bones
- Diagnosis is made through biopsy; testing that assists diagnosis includes X-ray, MRI, and bone scan
- Treatment is based on staging of the cancer and ranges from radiation or chemotherapy to surgical excision or amputation
- Prognosis varies based on grade of malignancy and stage of tumor

Colon Cancer

- Adenocarcinoma is the primary cancer that affects the bowel
- Third leading cause of death from cancer for men and women
- Risk factors include genetic syndromes, increasing age, male gender, Crohn's disease, polyps, colitis, sedentary life style, cigarette smoking, and high fat diet
- Signs are not often seen in early stages; primary symptoms include a change in bowel habits, bright red blood noted during a bowel movement, and stomach pain
- Will metastasize to the liver, lungs, bone, and brain
- Treatment requires surgical removal of the tumor with adjunct chemotherapy or radiation
- Colostomy may be required
- Prognosis is good with early diagnosis when the cancer is contained
- Prognosis is poor if it has metastasized

Liver Cancer

- Hepatocellular carcinoma is the most common liver cancer
- Risk increases with age, especially after 60 years
- There is a link between HBV, hepatitis C, and hepatocellular cancer
- Risk factors include male gender, alcohol abuse, anabolic steroids, and oral contraceptives
- Symptoms are usually nondescript initially but can

include gastrointestinal pain, abdominal distention, anorexia and/or weight loss, change in bowel habits, and jaundice
- Definitive diagnosis requires a liver biopsy
- Prognosis is currently at a five year survival rate of 35% with treatment; if treatment is unsuccessful, 4 to 6 months

Prostate Cancer

- Adenocarcinoma is the most common prostate cancer
- Second highest cause of death from cancer in men
- The majority of prostate cancer affects men over 50 years of age
- Risk factors include increased age, high fat diet, genetic predisposition, African American descent, and exposure to cadmium
- Can metastasize to the bladder, musculoskeletal system, lungs, and lymph nodes
- Most times this is asymptomatic until the cancer reaches the advanced stages
- Symptoms include urinary obstruction, pain, urgency, and decreased stream/flow of urine
- Diagnosis is found through prostate biopsy
- Treatment varies and can include surgical incision of the prostate gland, radiation, and hormonal therapy
- Prognosis is good with appropriate treatment, approximately 10% fatality rate from this diagnosis

Cervical Cancer

- Cervical cancer is slow growing
- The human papilloma virus is the primary cause of cervical cancer
- Other risk factors include smoking, maternal use of diethylstilbestrol (DES), African American ethnicity, oral contraceptive use, and certain sexually transmitted diseases
- Symptoms are not common during the early stages
- Symptoms can include abnormal bleeding, pelvic and low back pain, impairment with bladder and bowel function
- Annual cervical screening is recommended
- Diagnosis is made through a Pap test (smear)
- Treatment varies with the stage of the disease process and can include laser therapy, excision, cryotherapy, or hysterectomy with adjunct chemotherapy or radiation
- Prognosis is good with appropriate intervention

Oncology Pediatric Pathology

Astrocytoma

An astrocytoma is a classification that accounts for approximately fifty percent of pediatric brain tumors. The etiology of pediatric cancers is usually unknown.

- **Causative factors** include genetic predisposition, environmental influence, radiation and toxin exposure, and association with certain childhood disorders.

- There are two types of astrocytoma with **characteristics** as follows:

  Cerebellar - clumsiness, ataxic gait, headache, change in personality, and vomiting

  Supratentorial - headache, seizures, change in personality, visual impairments, and vomiting

- **Treatment** for cerebellar tumors consists of surgical resection with an 80-90% cure rate. **Treatment** for supratentorial tumors requires surgery to resect the tumor with radiation and/or chemotherapy.

Leukemia

Leukemia is a cancer of the blood that occurs when leukocytes change into malignant cells. These immature cells proliferate, accumulate in bone marrow, and ultimately cease the production of normal cells. This process will spread to lymph nodes, liver, spleen, and other areas of the body.

- The exact etiology is unknown, however, **causative factors** include environmental, chemical or toxin exposure, genetic predisposition, and viral association. There are many types of leukemia with acute lymphoblastic leukemia (ALL), and acute myelogenous leukemia (AML) occurring most frequently in children.
- **Characteristics** of these types include an abrupt onset with high fever, bleeding, enlarged lymph nodes and spleen, progressive weakness, fatigue, and painful joints. Blood work will indicate anemia, leukocyte count greater than 500,000 mm^3 and thrombocytopenia.
- **Treatment** will vary based on the type and degree of leukemia. Options include immunotherapy, cytotoxic agents, chemotherapy or radiation, and bone marrow transplant. Over 90% of patients with ALL achieve complete remission with treatment, while patients with AML achieve complete remission at a rate of 70-80%.

Neuroblastoma

A neuroblastoma is a tumor that initiates from primitive ectodermal cells of the neural plate and is found within the sympathetic nervous system, primarily seen in the adrenal glands or paraspinal ganglions. This is the most common malignant tumor seen in children.

- The etiology remains unknown, but **causative factors** include genetic predisposition, familial incidence, environmental influence, radiation and toxin exposure or viral association.
- **Characteristics** vary with the site and include an abdominal mass, change in personality, anemia, sweating, pain, and diarrhea.
- **Treatment** includes surgical resection, chemotherapy, and radiation. Prognosis is best for children diagnosed in the first year of life. A neuroblastoma will spontaneously regress in rare cases.

Non-Hodgkin's Lymphoma

Non-Hodgkin's lymphoma is a cancer of the lymphatic system with peak incidence between 7 - 10 years of age.

- The etiology is unknown, however, a likely **causative factor** is viral infection.
- **Characteristics** can differ from adults and include abdominal pain, swallowing issues, anemia, and swelling. Nodular histologies are rare in children.
- **Treatment** is based on the site/extent of the cancer and includes surgery, chemotherapy, and radiation.

Osteogenic Sarcoma

An osteogenic sarcoma is a cancer that occurs at the epiphyses of long bones. Osteogenic sarcoma is the most common form of bone cancer in children with a peak incidence between the ages of 10 to 20.

- **Causative factors** are unknown, however, there is a correlation between immunoincompetence and rate of tumor progression. Osteogenic sarcoma can metastasize quickly.
- **Characteristics** include presence of a mass, rapid metastases, and associated pain. Diagnosis can be made with a biopsy.
- **Treatment** includes amputation with proximal resection to ensure proper removal of affected tissue or surgical procedures that attempt to resect the tumor and salvage the limb. Chemotherapy is beneficial, however, radiation is not effective with this type of tumor.

Wilms' Tumor

Wilms' tumor is an embryonal adenomyosarcoma found in the kidney. Most cases are diagnosed between one and four years of age.

- **Causative factors** include genetic inheritance as an autosomal dominant disease or a non-inherited form with an unknown etiology.
- **Characteristics** include an abdominal mass, pain, hematuria, fever, nausea, and vomiting.
- **Treatment** includes resection of the kidney and the associated lymphatic tissue followed by chemotherapy and/or radiation. Dactinomycin is also administered due to the drug's antitumor properties. The five-year cure rate is approximately 75%.

Oncology Treatment Options

Surgery

Surgery is used to resect and excise a neoplasm. Surgery is indicated only after consideration of the size, type, and location of the malignancy as well as the patient's age and overall health status. Surgery may be curative or palliative and usually requires a combination of other treatment modalities secondary to potential metastases. These adjunct therapies assist to alleviate all residual cancer cells. Common side effects include fatigue, pain, deformity, scar tissue formation, and infection.

Radiation

Radiation is administered as either ionizing radiation or particle radiation and can be delivered by teletherapy (external beam), brachytherapy (a sealed source) or system therapy (unsealed source). Radiation destroys the hydrogen bonds between the DNA strands within the cancer cells. Radiation may be used prior to surgical intervention to shrink a tumor and/or post-surgical intervention to ensure destruction of residual cancer cells. Radiation is most useful with localized cancer. Common side effects include headache, bone marrow suppression, skin reactions, neuropathy, visual disturbances, nausea, vomiting, urinary frequency, diarrhea, delayed wound healing, and infection.

Chemotherapy

Chemotherapy consists of a group of drugs that are administered to destroy cancer cells. Chemotherapeutic agents include alkylating agents, antimetabolite agents, steroid hormones, plant alkaloid agents, interferons, and anti-tumor antibiotics. Each class of chemotherapeutic agents has a different mechanism of action to destroy cancer cells. Chemotherapy is most useful with widespread cancer and metastatic cancer, but is also used to induce remission, cure and/or eradicate residual cancer cells. The drugs can be administered orally, subcutaneously, intramuscularly, intravenously or intracavitarily. Common side effects include nausea, vomiting, electrolyte imbalance, sexual dysfunction, hair loss, pain, and a decrease in platelet, red, and white blood cell counts.

Biotherapy (Immunotherapy)

Biotherapy utilizes various agents and/or techniques to change the relationship between the cancer and its host. Biologic response modifiers strengthen the person's

biological response to the cancer cells. Common agents or procedures used with this treatment include interferons, interleukin-2, bone marrow transplant, stem cell transplant, monoclonal antibodies, hormonal therapy, and colony-stimulating factors. These forms of biotherapy are used in conjunction with other forms of curative cancer treatment (i.e., chemotherapy) in order to decrease unnecessary damage to the patient and support the overall therapeutic goals. Common side effects include fever, chills, nausea, vomiting, anorexia, central nervous system impairment, inflammatory reactions, leukopenia, and fatigue.

Antiangiogenic Therapy

Antiangiogenic therapy focuses on the use of thalidomide and its suppression of blood supply formation. It has had initial success in the treatment of multiple myeloma. There is research to support inhibition in the growth of primary tumors through blocking the process of tumor growth as opposed to destruction of an already formed mass.

Palliative Treatment (provide relief)

Palliative treatment for the management of cancer can include radiation, chemotherapy, physical therapy, chiropractics, acupuncture, alternative and homeopathic medicines, relaxation, biofeedback, pharmacological intervention, and hospice.

Oncology Profile

Examination

- Past medical history
- Risk factor profile
- History of current condition
- Medical management
- Precautions/contraindications
- Social history
- Medications
- Living environment
- Systems review
- Safety assessment
- Skin assessment
- Range of motion
- Motor assessment
- Endurance assessment
- Mobility skills
- Cancer pain assessment

Intervention

- Mobility training
- Positioning
- Therapeutic exercise (to tolerance)
- Energy conservation techniques
- Relaxation training
- Therapeutic modalities
- Assistive device/adaptive equipment training
- Wheelchair and orthotic prescription
- Pain management

Goals

- Maximize functional mobility
- Maximize strength
- Maximize endurance
- Maximize pain management techniques
- Maximize independence with adaptive equipment
- Maximize static and dynamic balance
- Maximize patient/caregiver competence with:
  - Pain management/relaxation
  - Use of adaptive equipment and orthotic devices
  - Home exercise programs

Modality Contraindications in the Treatment of Cancer

Modality	Contraindications

Superficial heat

Hot pack Paraffin Infrared Hydrotherapy	• Over irradiated areas • Over bleeding areas • Over inflammation • Over a tumor

Deep Heat

Diathermy Ultrasound	• Over acute hemorrhage • Over growing epiphyses • Over inflammation • Over irradiated or insensitive skin • Over a tumor • Over implants

Electrotherapy

Neuromuscular electrical nerve stimulation TENS	• Potential pathological fracture • Cardiopulmonary insufficiency • Deep bone pain

Modality	Contraindications

Cryotherapy

Cold pack Ice massage Cold hydrotherapy Vapocoolant spray Cold compression	• Over dysvascular tissue/ irradiated tissue • Impaired sensation to the treatment area • Delayed wound healing • Radiation or chemotherapy-induced nerve injury • When chemotherapy exacerbates-Raynaud's disease or peripheral vascular disease

Mechanical Agents

Traction	• Presence of tumor • Presence of infection • Previous radiation therapy

Treatment Guidelines

✓ A patient post-surgical skin grafting may require bed rest and bedside therapy per physician protocol

✓ Physical therapy is contraindicated while a patient is receiving radiation with implanted radioactive seeds

✓ Massage and heat are contraindicated over a radiated area for a minimum of 12 months

✓ Special care is required for a person undergoing radiation therapy in the areas marked as sites for treatment (where the beam radiation is delivered)

✓ It is important to notify the nurse/physician if a patient vomits during therapy, especially when the patient is taking antiemetic medication to control nausea and vomiting

✓ Always check the status of a patient undergoing chemotherapy regarding their level of toxicity and risk levels for contact with the other patients and staff

✓ Always modify treatment as necessary secondary to the side effects of medical treatment

✓ Always check physician orders prior to treatment of a patient with bone metastases for proper weight bearing status and clearance to perform mobility

✓ A physical therapist should minimize excessive shear force during mobility, especially over treatment areas

✓ Always check a patient's blood values daily, especially the platelet and hematocrit counts to determine if it is safe for the patient to be mobile and exercise

✓ Understanding the staging and grading of a patient's cancer and how the measure impacts the goals and anticipated outcomes

✓ Always encourage patient and family education in all aspects of care and mobility

✓ Exercise should be conducted at a range of 40-65% of the peak heart rate, heart rate reserve, VO_2 max or below the anaerobic threshold

✓ Perceived exertion should never exceed a 12 during exercise using the Borg's Rating of Perceived Exertion Scale

✓ Schedule therapeutic exercise during the day at the time of the patient's peak level of energy

Psychological Disorders

Affective Disorders

Affective disorders are classified by disturbances in mood or emotion. States of extreme happiness or sadness occur and mood can alternate without cause. These extreme emotions can become intense and unrealistic.

Depression

- Slower mental and physical activity
- Poor self-esteem
- Immobilized from everyday activities
- Sadness, hopelessness, and helplessness
- Desire to withdraw
- Delusions in severe cases

Mania

- Constantly active
- Impulses immediately expressed
- Unrealistic activity
- Elation and self-confidence
- Disagreement with a patient may produce patient aggression
- Disorganized thoughts and speech
- Very few patients are diagnosed with only a manic disorder

Bipolar

- Alternating periods of depression and mania
- Females are at greater risk
- Usually begins in a patient's twenties

Neuroses Disorders

Neuroses refer to a group of disorders that are characterized by individuals exhibiting fear and maladaptive strategies in dealing with stressful or everyday stimuli. Patients with neuroses are not dealing with psychosis, do not have delusions, and usually realize that they have a problem.

Obsessive-compulsive Disorder

- Obsessions – persistent thoughts that will not leave
- Compulsions – repetitive ritual behaviors the patient cannot stop performing
- Thoughts or ritual behaviors that interfere with daily living
- Unable to control irrational behavior
- Most commonly begins in young adulthood

Anxiety Disorder

- Constant high tension
- Overreacts in certain instances
- Presents with apprehension

- Chronic worry
- Acute anxiety attacks
  - Lasts a few minutes in duration
  - Excitation of the sympathetic autonomic nervous system
  - Fear of impending doom or death
  - Shortness of breath, heart palpitations, dizziness, nausea
  - Initiated by unconscious and internal mechanisms

Phobia Disorder

- Excessive fear of objects, occurrences or situations
- Fear is considerably out of proportion and irrational
- Fear creates difficulty in everyday life
- Subclassifications include agoraphobia, social phobia, and simple phobia
- May develop from traumatic experiences, observation, classical conditioning
- Simple phobias are the easiest to treat
  - **Acrophobia:** fear of heights
  - **Agoraphobia:** fear of open spaces
  - **Astraphobia:** fear of thunderstorms
  - **Belonephobia:** fear of needles
  - **Claustrophobia:** fear of being in closed-in places
  - **Pathophobia:** fear of disease
  - **Pyrophobia:** fear of fire
  - **Zoophobia:** fear of animal(s)

Dissociative Disorders

Dissociative disorders develop when a person unconsciously dissociates (separates) one part of the mind from the rest.

Psychogenic Amnesia

- Produced by the mind
- No physical cause
- Forgets all aspects of the past

Multiple Personality

- A rare dissociative disorder
- Two or more independent personalities
- Each personality may or may not know about the other
- Causative factors are not understood
- Believed to allow a person to engage in behaviors that are against the patient's morality and normally produce guilt

Somatoform Disorders

Somatoform disorders are classified based on the physical symptoms present in each disorder.

Somatization Disorder

- Primarily in women
- Often chronic and long lasting
- Complaints of symptoms with no physiological basis
- Symptoms usually lead to medications and medical visits
- Symptoms alter the patient's life
- Resembles hypochondriasis disorder
- Has familial association

Conversion Disorders

- Physical complaints of neurological basis with no underlying cause
- Paralysis is the most common finding
- Other findings include deafness, blindness, paresthesia
- Freud believes this is mental anxiety transformed into physical symptoms
- Diagnosis can be made once testing is negative for physical ailments
- Both men and women can experience a conversion disorder

Hypochondriasis Disorder

- Excessive fear of illness
- Believes that minor illnesses or medical problems indicate a serious or life threatening disease

Schizophrenia Disorders

Schizophrenia disorders are psychotic in nature and present with disorganization of thought, hallucinations, emotional dysfunction, anxiety, and perceptual impairments. Causative factors include traumatic events, genetic inheritance, biochemical imbalances, and environmental influence.

Catatonic Schizophrenia

- Motor disturbances with rigid posturing
- Patients remain aware during episodes
- Episodes consist of uncontrolled movements
- Medications are required to regulate episodes

Paranoid Schizophrenia

- Delusions of grandeur
- Delusions of persecution
- May believe they possess special powers

Disorganized Schizophrenia

- Usually progressive and irreversible
- Inappropriate emotional responses
- Mumbled talking

Undifferentiated Schizophrenia

- May possess a mix of symptoms
- Does not classify into one category

Personality Disorders

A personality disorder is classified by observing a patient's pattern of behavior, dysfunctional view of society, and level of sadness. Personality disorders are usually ongoing patterns of dysfunctional behavior.

Psychopathic Personality

- Low morality
- Poor sense of responsibility
- No respect for others
- Impulsive behavior for immediate gratification
- High frustration
- Little guilt or remorse for all actions
- Inability to alter behavior even with punishment
- Expert liar

Antisocial Behavior

- Results from particular causes (e.g., need for attention or involvement in a gang)
- Usually have some concern for others
- Blames other institutions (e.g., family, school) for their actions
- Usually begins before 16 years of age
- Violates the rights of others
- Lacks responsibility and emotional stability

Narcissistic Behavior

- Incapable of loving others
- Self-absorbed
- Obsessed with success and power
- Unrealistic perception of self-importance

Borderline Behavior

- Instability in all aspects of life
- Can identify self from others as well as reality
- Uses projection, denial, defensiveness
- Intense and uncontrolled anger
- Chronic feelings of emptiness
- Unpredictable mood or behavior

Pharmacology

Pharmacological Intervention for Psychiatric Management

Neuroleptic Agents

Used for short and long-term treatment of psychosis Used as tranquilizers or for sedation May produce hypotension, abnormal movements, over-sedation, blurred vision, and tics	**Traditional Agents** Chlorpromazine (Thorazine) Prochlorperazine (Compazine) Fluphenazine (Prolixin) Haloperidol (Haldol) Droperidol (Inapsine) Thioridazine (Mellaril) **Atypical Agents** Risperidone (Risperdal) Quetiapine/Fumarate (Seroquel) Clozapine (Clozaril)

Antidepressant Agents

Alleviate depression and/or anxiety; used in obsessive-compulsive disorder, bulimia and anorexia, social phobias, and post-traumatic stress disorders May produce weight gain, sedation, constipation, insomnia, cardiovascular issues, and orthostatic hypotension	**Tricyclic (Tertiary Amine)** Amitriptyline (Elavil) Doxepin (Sinequan) Trimipramine (Surmontil) **Tricyclic (Secondary Amine)** Desipramine (Norpramine) Nortriptyline (Pamelor) **(SSRI)-Selective Serotonin Reuptake Inhibitors** Fluoxetine (Prozac) Paroxetine (Paxil) Sertraline (Zoloft) Escitalopram (Lexapro) Fluvoxamine (Luvox) **Monoamine Oxidase Inhibitors (MAOI)** Phenelzine (Nardil) Tranylcypromine (Parnate) **Other Antidepressants** Maprotiline (Ludiomil) Bupropion (Wellbutrin) Trazodone (Desyrel) Venlafaxine (Effexor)

Sedative-Hypnotic Agents

Alleviate insomnia, frequent awakenings during sleep May become addictive	**Benzodiazepine Agents** Temazepam (Restoril) Triazolam (Halcion) Estazolam (Prosom) Flurazepam (Dalmane) **Nonbenzodiazepine Agents** Zolpidem (Ambien) Trazodone (Desyrel) Diphenhydramine (Benadryl)

Bipolar Disorder Agents

Act as mood stabilizer, controls manic episodes	Lithium carbonate (Lithobid) Sodium dualproex (Depakote) Carbamazepine (Tegretol) Gabepentin (Neurontin) Vigabatrin (Sabril)

Anxiolytic Agents

Alleviate anxiety without significant sedation May produce physical dependence or rebounding anxiety once medication is stopped	**Benzodiazepine Agents** Lorazepam (Ativan) Diazepam (Valium) Alprazolam (Xanax) Chlordiazepoxide (Librium) **Nonbenzodiazepine Agents** Buspirone (BuSpar) Doxepin (Sinequan) Hydroxyzine (Atarax) Propanolol (Inderal)

*selected pharmaceutical drugs and their respective trade names in parentheses, not intended to be a complete listing

Pharmacology-Systems Side Effects

Review of Systems: Side Effects/Subjective Complaints
(In Order of Most Common Occurrence)

Gastrointestinal Distress: dyspepsia, heartburn, nausea, vomiting, abdominal pain, constipation, diarrhea, bleeding

• Salicylates	• Opioids	• ß-Blockers
• Skeletal muscle relaxants	• ACE inhibitors	• Nitrates
• Antiarrhythmic agents	• Neuroleptics	• OCAs
• Theophylline	• NSAIDs	• Corticosteroids
• Calcium-channel blockers	• Diuretics	• Digoxin
• Cholesterol-lowering agents	• Estrogens and progestins	• Antiepileptic agents
• Antidepressants (TCAs and MAOIs, lithium)		

Pulmonary: bronchospasm, shortness of breath, respiratory depression

• Salicylates	• Opioids	• ACE inhibitors
• NSAIDs	• ß-Blockers	

Central Nervous System: dizziness, drowsiness, insomnia, headaches, hallucinations, confusion, anxiety, depression, muscle weakness

• NSAIDs	• Opioids	• ß-Blockers
• Nitrates	• Digoxin	• Antidepressants (TCAs and MAOIs)
• Antiepileptic agents	• Estrogens and progestins	• Skeletal muscle relaxants
• Corticosteroids	• Calcium-channel blockers	• ACE inhibitors
• Antianxiety agents	• Neuroleptics	• OCAs

Dermatologic: skin rash, itching, flushing of face

• NSAIDs	• ß-Blockers	• Calcium-channel blockers
• Nitrates	• Antiarrhythmic agents	• OCAs
• Antiepileptics	• Corticosteroids	• Opioids
• ACE inhibitors	• Cholesterol-lowering agents	• MAOIs and lithium
• Estrogens and progestins		

Musculoskeletal: weakness, fatigue, cramps, arthritis, decreased exercise tolerance, osteoporosis

• Corticosteroids	• Calcium-channel blockers	• Diuretics
• Antianxiety agents	• Antidepressants	• ß-Blockers
• ACE inhibitors	• Digoxin	• Antiepileptic agents
• Neuroleptic agents		

Cardiac: bradycardia, ventricular irritability, AV block, CHF, PVCs, ventricular tachycardia

• Opioids	• ß-Blockers	• Digoxin
• TCAs	• Oral antiasthmatic agents	• Diuretics
• Calcium-channel blockers	• Antiarrhythmic agents	• Neuroleptics

Vascular: claudication, hypotension, peripheral edema, cold extremities

• NSAIDs	• Diuretics	• Calcium-channel blockers
• Nitrates	• Neuroleptics	• Estrogens and progestins
• Corticosteroids	• ß-Blockers	• ACE inhibitors
• Antidepressants (TCAs and MAOIs)	• OCAs	

Genitourinary: sexual dysfunction, urinary retention, urinary incontinence

• Opioids	• ß-Blockers	• Estrogens and progestins
• OCAs	• Diuretics	• Antiarrhythmic agents
• Neuroleptics	• Antidepressants (TCAs and MAOIs)	

HEENT: tinnitus, loss of taste, headache, lightheadedness, dizziness

• Salicylates	• Opioids	• ß-Blockers
• Calcium-channel blockers	• Digoxin	• Antianxiety agents
• Antiepileptic agents	• NSAIDs	• Skeletal muscle relaxants
• Nitrates	• ACE inhibitors	• Antiarrhythmic agents
• Antidepressant (TCAs and MAOIs)		

**Abbreviations: ACE, angiotensin-converting enzyme; MAOIs, monoamine oxidase inhibitors; NSAIDs, nonsteroidal anti-inflammatory drugs; OCAs, oral contraceptive agents; TCAs, tricyclic antidepressants.— From Boissonnault, WG: Examination in Physical Therapy Practice: Screening for Medical Disease. W.B. Saunders Company, Philadelphia 1995, p.350-351, with permission.

Nutrition

Vitamins

Vitamins are essential non-caloric nutrients that are required in small amounts for certain metabolic functions and cannot be manufactured by the body. Vitamins are most often classified as fat-soluble or water-soluble.

Fat-Soluble Vitamins

Fat-soluble vitamins include vitamins A, D, E, and K. After being absorbed by the intestinal tract, the vitamins are stored in the liver and fatty tissues. Fat-soluble vitamins require protein carriers to move through body fluids and excesses are stored in the body. Since they are not water-soluble, it is possible that the vitamins may reach toxic levels.

Vitamin A

Vitamin A is essential to the eyes, epithelial tissue, normal growth and development, and reproduction.

- **Common food sources** containing Vitamin A include green, orange, and yellow vegetables, liver, butter, egg yolks, and fortified margarine.
- **Symptoms of deficiency** include night blindness, rough and dry skin, and growth failure.
- **Symptoms of toxicity** include appetite loss, hair loss, and enlarged liver and spleen.

Vitamin D

Vitamin D increases the blood flow levels of minerals, notably calcium and phosphorus.

- **Common food sources** containing Vitamin D include fortified milk, fish oils, and fortified margarine.
- **Symptoms of deficiency** include faulty bone growth, rickets, and osteomalacia.
- **Symptoms of toxicity** include calcification of soft tissues and hypercalcemia.

Vitamin E

Vitamin E functions as an antioxidant in cell membranes and is especially important for the integrity of cells that are constantly exposed to high levels of oxygen such as the lungs and red blood cells.

- **Common food sources** containing Vitamin E include vegetable oils, wheat germ, nuts, and fish.
- **Symptoms of deficiency** include the breakdown of red blood cells, however, this is relatively rare in adults.
- **Symptoms of toxicity** include decreased thyroid hormone levels and increased triglycerides.

Vitamin K

Vitamin K is necessary for the synthesis of at least two of the proteins involved in blood clotting.

- **Common food sources** containing Vitamin K include dark green leafy vegetables, cheese, egg yolks, and liver.
- **Symptoms of deficiency** include hemorrhage and defective blood clotting.
- **Toxicity** has not been reported.

Water-Soluble Vitamins

Water-soluble vitamins are not stored in the body in any significant amount and therefore need to be included in the diet on a daily basis. Toxicity is less common than with fat-soluble vitamins.

Vitamin B_2 (Riboflavin)

Vitamin B_2 facilitates selected enzymes involved in carbohydrate, protein, and fat metabolism.

- **Common food sources** containing Vitamin B_2 include milk, green leafy vegetables, eggs, and peanuts.
- **Symptoms of deficiency** include inflammation of the tongue, sensitive eyes, and scaling of the skin.
- **Toxicity** has not been reported.

Vitamin B_3 (Niacin)

Vitamin B_3 facilitates several enzymes that regulate energy metabolism.

- **Common food sources** containing Vitamin B_3 include meats, whole grains, and white flour.
- **Symptoms of deficiency** include pellagra and gastrointestinal disturbances.
- **Symptoms of toxicity** include abnormal glucose metabolism, nausea, vomiting, and gastric ulceration.

Vitamin B_6 (Pyridoxine)

Vitamin B_6 is essential in the metabolism of proteins, amino acids, carbohydrates, and fat.

- **Common food sources** containing Vitamin B_6 include liver, red meats, whole grains, and potatoes.
- **Symptoms of deficiency** include peripheral neuropathy, convulsions, and depression.
- **Symptoms of toxicity** include sensory damage, numbness of the extremities, and ataxia.

Vitamin B_{12} (Cobalamin)

Vitamin B_{12} is essential for the functioning of all cells and aids in hemoglobin synthesis.

- **Common food sources** containing Vitamin B_{12} include meats, whole eggs, and egg yolks.
- **Symptoms of deficiency** include pernicious anemia and various psychological disorders.
- **Toxicity** has not been reported.

Vitamin C

Vitamin C assists the body to combat infections and facilitates wound healing. The vitamin is necessary for the development and maintenance of bones, cartilage, connective tissue, and blood vessels.

- **Common food sources** containing Vitamin C include citrus fruits, tomatoes, and cantaloupe.
- **Symptoms of deficiency** include anemia, swollen gums, loose teeth, and scurvy.
- **Symptoms of toxicity** include urinary stones, diarrhea, and hypoglycemia.

Biotin

Biotin is necessary for the action of many enzyme systems.

- **Common food sources** containing biotin include liver, meats, and milk.
- **Symptoms of deficiency** include anemia, depression, and muscle pain.
- **Toxicity** has not been reported.

Choline

Choline is a component of compounds necessary for nerve function and lipid metabolism.

- Choline is synthesized from methionine which is an amino acid.
- **Symptoms of deficiency** only occur when intake of methylamine is low.
- **Toxicity** has not been reported.

Folacin (Folic acid)

Folacin is involved in the formation of red blood cells and in the functioning of the gastrointestinal tract.

- **Common food sources** containing folacin include yeast, dark green leafy vegetables, and whole grains.
- **Symptoms of deficiency** include impaired cell division and alteration of protein synthesis.
- **Toxicity** has not been reported.

Pantothenic acid

Pantothenic acid is an integral component of complex enzymes involved in the metabolism of fatty acids.

- **Common food sources** containing pantothenic acid include liver, eggs, and whole grains.
- **Symptoms of deficiency** include headache, fatigue, and poor muscle coordination.
- **Symptoms of toxicity** include diarrhea.

Minerals

Minerals are organic elements that fulfill essential roles in the metabolic process.

Major Minerals

Calcium (Ca)

Calcium facilitates muscle contraction and relaxation, builds strong bones and teeth, and aids in coagulation.

- **Common food sources** containing calcium include milk, green leafy vegetables, and soy products.
- **Calcium deficiency** may lead to poor bone growth, rickets, osteomalacia, and osteoporosis.
- **Symptoms of toxicity** include kidney stones.

Chloride (Cl)

Chloride facilitates the maintenance of fluid and acid-base balance.

- **Common food sources** containing chloride include table salt, fish, and vegetables.
- **Chloride deficiency** may lead to a disturbance of acid-base balance.
- **Toxicity** has not been reported.

Magnesium (Mg)

Magnesium builds strong bones and teeth, activates enzymes, and helps regulate heartbeat.

- **Common food sources** containing magnesium include raw dark vegetables, nuts, soybeans, milk, and cheese.
- **Symptoms of deficiency** include confusion, apathy, muscle weakness, and tremors.
- **Symptoms of toxicity** include increased calcium excretion.

Phosphorus (P)

Phosphorus strengthens bones, assists in the oxidation of fats and carbohydrates, and aids in maintaining acid-base balance.

- **Common food sources** containing phosphorus include milk and milk products, meats, whole grains, and soft drinks.
- **Symptoms of deficiency** include weakness, stiff joints, and fragile bones.
- **Symptoms of toxicity** include muscle spasms.

Potassium (K)

Potassium maintains fluid and acid-base balance.

- **Common food sources** containing potassium include apricots, bananas, oranges, grapefruit, and milk.
- **Symptoms of deficiency** include impaired growth, hypertension, and diminished heart rate.
- **Symptoms of toxicity** include hyperkalemia and cardiac disturbances.

Sodium (Na)

Sodium facilitates the maintenance of acid-base balance, transmits nerve impulses, and helps control muscle contractions.

- **Common food sources** containing sodium include salt and milk.
- **Deficiency and toxicity** have not been reported.

Sulfur (S)

Sulfur facilitates enzyme activity and energy metabolism.

- **Common food sources** containing sulfur include meat, eggs, milk, and cheese.
- **Deficiency** is extremely rare.
- **Toxicity** has not been reported.

Trace Minerals

Chromium (Cr)

Chromium controls glucose metabolism.

- **Common food sources** containing chromium include whole grains, meats, and cheese.
- **Symptoms of deficiency** include weight loss and central nervous system abnormalities.
- **Symptoms of toxicity** include liver damage.

Cobalt (Co)

Cobalt is an essential component of vitamin B_{12} and functions to activate enzymes.

- **Common food sources** containing cobalt include figs, cabbage, and spinach.
- **Symptoms of deficiency** include pernicious anemia.
- **Symptoms of toxicity** include polycythemia and increased blood volume.

Copper (Cu)

Copper facilitates hemoglobin synthesis and lipid metabolism.

- **Common food sources** containing copper include shellfish, liver, meat, and whole grains.
- **Symptoms of deficiency** include anemia, central nervous system abnormalities, and abnormal electrocardiograms.
- **Symptoms of toxicity** include Wilson's disease.

Fluorine (F)

Fluorine aids in the formation of bones and teeth and prevents osteoporosis.

- **Common food sources** containing fluorine include fish and water.
- **Symptoms of deficiency** include increased susceptibility of dental cavities.
- **Symptoms of toxicity** include fluorosis.

Iodine (I)

Iodine assists with the regulation of cell metabolism and basal metabolic rate.

- **Common food sources** containing iodine include iodized salt and seafood.
- **Symptoms of deficiency** may include goiters.
- **Toxicity** has not been reported.

Iron (Fe)

Iron assists in the oxygen transport and cell oxidation.

- **Common food sources** containing iron include red meats and liver.
- **Symptoms of deficiency** include anemia.
- **Symptoms of toxicity** include hemochromatosis.

Manganese (Mn)

Manganese facilitates proper bone structure and functions as an enzyme component in general metabolism.

- **Common food sources** containing manganese include cereals and whole grains.
- There are no known **symptoms of deficiency**.
- **Toxicity** has not been reported.

Selenium (Se)

Selenium is a synergistic antioxidant with Vitamin E.

- **Common food sources** containing selenium include meat, eggs, milk, seafood, and garlic.
- **Symptoms of deficiency** include Keshan's disease.
- **Symptoms of toxicity** include physical defects of fingernails and toenails, nausea, and abdominal pain.

Molybdenum (Mo)

Molybdenum is a component of three enzymes necessary for normal cell functioning.

- **Common food sources** containing molybdenum include meats, whole grains, and dark green vegetables.
- **Symptoms of deficiency** include vomiting and tachypnea.
- **Toxicity** has not been reported.

Zinc (Zn)

Zinc aids in immune function and cell division.

- **Common food sources** containing zinc include seafood, liver, milk, cheese, and whole grains.
- **Symptoms of deficiency** include depressed immune functions and impaired skeletal growth.
- **Symptoms of toxicity** include anemia, nausea, and vomiting.

Chapter 6

Equipment and Devices; Therapeutic Modalities

Equipment and Devices

Mobility

Preparation for Treatment

In order to create an effective and successful treatment environment the patient must be informed regarding all expectations of the upcoming treatment as well as have all questions answered prior to initiating the actual hands-on intervention. The therapist must obtain informed consent from the patient and document consent in the patient's chart. The therapist must also determine if there are any potential limitations to treatment due to a patient's religious or cultural beliefs. The patient must be notified as to appropriate clothing for therapy, and areas such as draping must also be discussed prior to initiation of therapy in order to ensure a patient's comfort during treatment.

Draping

Draping is a technique utilized by health care providers to ensure the patient's privacy and modesty when treating particular areas of the body. Draping assists to keep the patient warm during treatment, adequately expose the area of treatment, and protect open areas, wounds, scars, and the patient's personal belongings from being soiled or injured during treatment. Draping materials may include gowns, towels, and sheets that must be secured in a manner that will properly expose the area of the body that

requires treatment, while maintaining a patient's modesty and overall level of comfort during treatment.

Bed Mobility Guidelines

✓ A patient that is dependent must be repositioned in bed at least every two hours
✓ Skin should be inspected for redness or breakdown with each position change
✓ A dependent patient must be lifted when changing positions in order to avoid shearing across the bed
✓ Use pillows, towels or blankets when positioning a patient in order to support and maintain a particular position
✓ A patient should always be encouraged to participate in all mobility and positioning
✓ Practice moving segmentally from one side of the bed to the other
✓ Utilize the "bridging" position of hip flexion and knee flexion with feet flat on the surface to assist with movement and rolling
✓ Move from a supine to sitting position by rolling into sidelying and placing the feet over the edge; assist as needed to obtain a sitting position
✓ All components of bed mobility are complete only when the patient ends in a comfortable and safe position

Transfers

Communication During Transfers

The patient should be informed about the transfer itself and their responsibility during the transfer. The explanation should be understood by the patient and should occur prior to performing the transfer.

Commands and counts are used to synchronize the actions of the participants involved in the transfer. The therapist at the head of the patient should give the commands during the transfer when more than one person is involved.

Levels of Physical Assistance

Independent: The patient does not require any assistance to complete the task.

Supervision: The patient requires a therapist to observe throughout completion of the task.

Contact Guard: The patient requires the therapist to maintain contact with the patient to complete the task. Contact guard is usually needed to assist if there is a loss of balance.

Minimal Assist: The patient requires 25% assist from the therapist to complete the task.

Moderate Assist: The patient requires 50% assist from the therapist to complete the task.

Maximal Assist: The patient requires 75% assist from the therapist to complete the task.

Dependent: The patient is unable to participate and the therapist must provide all of the effort to perform the task.

Transfer Guidelines

✓ Evaluate the patient's level of cognition and mobility
✓ When in doubt, utilize a second person to maintain patient/therapist safety
✓ Obtain all appropriate equipment prior to initiating the transfer
✓ Utilize a transfer belt
✓ Educate the patient regarding the expectations and transfer sequence through verbal explanation and demonstration

✓ Instruct the patient in smaller segments of the transfer if necessary prior to performing the entire transfer all at once
✓ Position yourself correctly around the patient and maintain a large base of support; use proper body mechanics throughout the transfer

✓ Vary the amount of assistance as needed
✓ Utilize manual contacts with the patient to direct their participation during the transfer
✓ Complete the transfer with the patient positioned comfortably and safely

Types of Transfers

Dependent Transfers

Three-person carry/lift

The three-person carry or lift is used to transfer a patient from a stretcher to a bed or treatment plinth. Three therapists carry the patient in a supine position; one therapist supports the head and upper trunk, the second therapist supports the trunk, and the third supports the lower extremities. The therapist at the head is usually the one to initiate commands. The therapists flex their elbows that are positioned under the patient and roll the patient on their side towards them. The therapists then lift on command and move in a line to the destination surface, lower, and position the patient properly.

Two-person lift

The two-person lift is used to transfer a patient between two surfaces of different heights or when transferring a patient to the floor. Standing behind the patient, the first therapist should place their arms underneath the patient's axilla. The therapist should grasp the patient's left forearm with their right hand and grasp the patient's right forearm with their left hand. The second therapist places one arm under the mid to distal thighs and the other arm is used to support the lower legs. The therapist at the head usually initiates the command to lift and transfer the patient out of the chair to the destination surface.

Dependent squat pivot transfer

The dependent squat pivot transfer is used to transfer a patient who cannot stand independently, but can bear some weight through the trunk and lower extremities. The therapist should position the patient at a 45-degree angle to the destination surface. The patient places their upper extremities on the therapist's shoulders, but should not be allowed to pull on the therapist's neck. The therapist should position the patient at the edge of the surface, hold the patient around the hips and under the buttocks, and block the patient's knees in order to avoid buckling while standing. The therapist should utilize momentum, straighten his or her legs, and raise the patient or allow the patient to remain in a squatting position. The therapist should then pivot and slowly lower the patient to the destination surface.

Hydraulic lift

The hydraulic lift is a device required for dependent transfers when a patient is obese, there is only one therapist available to assist with the transfer or the patient is totally dependent. The hydraulic lift needs to be locked in position before the transfer. The therapist positions a webbed sling under the patient and attaches the S-ring to the bars on the lift. Once all attachments are checked, the therapist should pump the handle on the device in order to elevate the patient. Once the patient is elevated, the therapist can navigate the lift with the patient to the destination surface. Once transferred, the chains should be removed, however, the webbed sling should remain in place in preparation for the return transfer.

Assisted Transfers

Sliding board transfer

The sliding board transfer is used for a patient who has some sitting balance, some upper extremity strength, and can adequately follow directions. The patient should be positioned at the edge of the wheelchair or bed and should lean to one side while placing one end of the sliding board sufficiently under the proximal thigh. The other end of the sliding board should be positioned on the destination surface. The patient should not hold onto the end of the sliding board in order to avoid pinching the fingers. The patient should place the lead hand four to six inches away from the sliding board and use both arms to initiate a push-up and scoot across the board. The therapist should guard in front of the patient and assist as needed as the patient performs a series of push-ups across the board.

Stand pivot transfer

The stand pivot transfer is used when a patient is able to stand and bear weight through one or both of the lower extremities. The patient must possess functional balance and the ability to pivot. Patients with unilateral weight bearing restrictions or hemiplegia may utilize this transfer and lead with the uninvolved side. The transfer may also be used therapeutically, leading with the involved side for a patient post CVA. A patient should be positioned at the edge of the wheelchair or bed to initiate the transfer.

The therapist can assist the patient to keep their feet flat on the floor while bringing the head and trunk forward. The therapist should assist the patient as needed with their feet. The therapist must guard or assist the patient through the transfer and instruct the patient to reach back for the surface before they begin to sit down. Once the stand pivot is performed, the therapist should assist as needed to ensure control with lowering the patient to the destination surface.

Stand step transfer

The stand step transfer is used with a patient who has the necessary strength and balance to weight shift and step during the transfer. The patient requires guarding or supervision from the therapist and performs the transfer as a stand pivot transfer except the patient actually takes a step to maneuver and reposition his or her feet instead of a pivot.

Wheelchairs

Wheelchair Facts

- Adult standard wheelchair specifications include seat width - 18 inches, seat depth - 16 inches and seat height - 20 inches.
- Hemi-height wheelchairs have decreased seat height (17.5 inches) to allow for propulsion using the unaffected foot.
- Rear wheel axles can be positioned two inches posteriorly from normal for patients with amputations to increase the base of support and to compensate for diminished weight in front of the wheelchair.
- Reclining wheelchairs allow intermittent or constant reclined positioning.
- Tilt-in-space wheelchairs allow for a reclined position without losing the required 90 degrees of hip flexion and 90 degrees of knee flexion. The entire chair reclines without any anatomical changes in positioning.

Patient Considerations

- Physical needs
- Rental versus purchase
- Manual versus power
- Physical abilities
- Cognition
- Coordination
- Level of endurance
- Functional mobility
- Seating systems (support, comfort, pressure relief)

Standard Wheelchair Measurements for Proper Fit

Measurement	Instructions	Average Adult Size
Seat Height Leg Length	Measure from the user's heel to the popliteal fold and add 2 inches to allow clearance of the footrest.	19.5 to 20.5 inches
Seat Depth	Measure from the user's posterior buttock, along the lateral thigh to the popliteal fold; then subtract approximately 2 inches to avoid pressure from the front edge of the seat against the popliteal space.	16 inches
Seat Width	Measure the widest aspect of the user's buttocks, hips or thighs and add approximately 2 inches. This will provide space for bulky clothing, orthoses or clearance of the trochanters from the armrest side panel.	18 inches
Back Height	Measure from the seat of the chair to the floor of the axilla with the user's shoulder flexed to 90 degrees and then subtract approximately 4 inches. This will allow the final back height to be below the inferior angles of the scapulae. (Note: This measurement will be affected if a seat cushion is to be used. The person should be measured while seated on the cushion or the thickness of the cushion must be considered by adding that value to the actual measurement.)	16 to 16.5 inches
Armrest Height	Measure from the seat of the chair to the olecranon process with the user's elbow flexed to 90 degrees and then add approximately 1 inch. (Note: This measurement will be affected if a seat cushion is to be used. The person should be measured while seated on the cushion or the thickness of the cushion must be considered by adding that value to the actual measurement.)	9 inches above the chair seat

From Pierson, FM: Principles and Techniques of Patient Care. W.B. Saunders Company, Philadelphia 2002, p.168, with permission.

Components of a Wheelchair

Footplates/Footrests	Foot loops, Heel loops
Legrests	Stationary Adjustable/removable Swing-away Elevating
Seat	Sling versus solid Gel cushion Air cushion Foam cushion
Armrests	Fixed versus adjustable Stationary versus removable Full-length versus partial Desk top

Wheelchair back	Fixed versus removable
	Sling versus contoured:
	  Gel
	  Foam
	Tall versus low back

Brake options	Pull-to-lock versus push-to-lock Brake extensions
Wheel options	Quick release Axle placement Type of casters Type of tires Rim projections
Restraints	Velcro lap belts and chest belts Airplane seat belts Automobile seat belts
Power control options	Head control Tongue control Puff-n-sip Joystick control Power scanning Microswitching system
Wheelchair frame	Rigid versus folding Narrow versus standard versus large Power versus manual
Other considerations	Lap tray Tilt versus reclining system Anti-tippers Allowance for growth in the system

Ambulation

Assistive Devices

Primary indications for using an assistive device during ambulation include:

- Decreased weight bearing on the lower extremities
- Muscle weakness of the trunk or lower extremities
- Decreased balance or impaired kinesthetic awareness
- Pain

Assistive Device Selection

Parallel Bars

Parallel bars provide maximum stability and security for a patient during the beginning stages of ambulation or standing. Proper fit includes bar height that allows for 20–25 degrees of elbow flexion while grasping on the bars approximately four to six inches in front of the body. A patient must progress out of the parallel bars as quickly as possible to increase overall mobility and decrease dependence using the parallel bars.

Walker

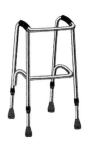

A walker can be used with all levels of weight bearing. The walker has a significant base of support and offers good stability. The walker should allow for 20–25 degrees of elbow flexion to ensure proper fit. The standard walker has many variations including the rolling, hemi, reciprocal, folding, or adjustable walker with brakes, upper extremity attachments and/or a seat platform. The walker is used with a three-point gait pattern.

Axillary Crutches

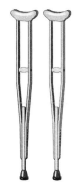

Axillary crutches can be used with all levels of weight bearing, however, require higher coordination for proper use. Proper fit includes positioning with the crutches six inches in front and two inches lateral to the patient. The crutch height should be adjusted no greater than three finger widths from the axilla. The handgrip height should be adjusted to the ulnar styloid process and allow for 20–25 degrees of elbow flexion while grasping the handgrip. A platform attachment can be utilized with this device. The axillary crutches can be used with two-point, three-point, four-point, swing-to, and swing-through gait patterns.

Lofstrand (forearm) Crutches

Lofstrand crutches can be used with all levels of weight bearing, however, require the highest level of coordination for proper use. Proper fit includes 20–25 degrees of elbow flexion while holding the handgrip with the crutches positioned six inches in front and two inches lateral to the patient. The arm cuff should be positioned one to one and one half inches below the olecranon process so it does not interfere with elbow flexion. A platform attachment can be utilized with this device if necessary. The Lofstrand crutches can be used with two-point, three-point, four-point, swing-to, and swing-through gait patterns.

Cane

A cane provides minimal stability and support for patients during ambulation activities. The straight cane provides the least support and is used primarily for assisting with balance. A straight cane should not be utilized for patients that are partial weight bearing. The small base and large base quad canes provide a larger base of support and can better assist with limiting weight bearing on an involved lower extremity and improving balance on unlevel surfaces, curbs, and stairs. Proper fit includes standing the cane at the patient's side and adjusting the handle to the level of the wrist crease at the ulnar styloid. The patient should have 20–25 degrees of elbow flexion while grasping the handgrip. The straight cane can be used with the two-point, four-point, modified two-point, and modified four-point gait patterns.

Levels of Weight Bearing

Non-weight bearing (NWB): A patient is unable to place any weight through the involved extremity and is not permitted to touch the ground or any surface. An assistive device is required.

Toe touch weight bearing (TTWB): A patient is unable to place any weight through the involved extremity, however, may place the toes on the ground to assist with balance. An assistive device is required.

Partial weight bearing (PWB): A patient is allowed to put a particular amount of weight through the involved extremity. The amount of weight bearing is expressed as allowable pounds of pressure or as a percentage of total weight. A therapist must monitor the amount of actual weight transferred through the involved foot during partial weight bearing. An assistive device is required.

Weight bearing as tolerated (WBAT): A patient determines the proper amount of weight bearing based on comfort. The amount of weight bearing can range from minimal to full. An assistive device may or may not be required.

Full weight bearing (FWB): A patient is able to place full weight on the involved extremity. An assistive device is not required at this level, but may be used to assist with balance.

Guidelines for Guarding during Ambulation**

- ✓ A gait belt is recommended
- ✓ Stand to the side (usually the affected side) and slightly behind the patient
- ✓ Grasp the gait belt with one hand; place the other hand on the patient's shoulder
- ✓ Do not grasp the arm, as it will interfere
- ✓ Move your lead foot forward when the patient moves; the assistive device and your back leg should advance as the patient ambulates

**A therapist must always consider the size, weight, and level of impairment of the patient prior to initiating ambulation activities. Guarding guidelines may require modification and/or a second therapist may be required.

Gait Patterns

An appropriate gait pattern is determined by the amount of weight bearing permitted and the severity of the patient's overall condition. Commonly used gait patterns include two-point, three-point, four-point, swing-to, and swing-through.

Two-point gait

This is a pattern in which a patient uses two crutches or canes. The patient ambulates moving the left crutch forward while simultaneously advancing the right lower extremity and vice versa. Each step is one-point and a complete cycle is two-points.

Three-point gait

This pattern can be seen with a walker or crutches. It involves one injured lower extremity that may have decreased weight bearing. The assistive device is advanced followed by the injured lower extremity and then the uninjured lower extremity. The assistive device and each lower extremity are considered separate points.

Four-point gait

This pattern is very similar to the two-point pattern. The primary difference is that the patient does not move the lower extremities simultaneously with the device, but rather waits and advances the opposite leg once the crutch/cane has been advanced. This gait pattern may be prescribed when a patient exhibits impaired coordination, balance or significant strength deficits. Each advancement of the crutch or cane as well as the bilateral lower extremities indicates a single point, thus allowing for a four-point gait pattern.

Swing-to gait

A gait pattern where a patient with bilateral trunk and/or lower extremity weakness, paresis or paralysis, uses crutches or a walker and advances the lower extremities simultaneously only to the point of the assistive device.

Swing-through gait

A gait pattern where the patient performs the same sequence as a swing-to gait pattern, however, advances the lower extremities beyond the point of the assistive device.

Guidelines for Guarding during Stair and Curb Training

- ✓ A gait belt is recommended

- ✓ When ascending stairs or curbs, remain behind the patient (usually towards the weaker side). Place the lead foot on the same step as the patient and the other foot one step lower. Hold the gait belt in one hand and position the other hand on the patient's shoulder. Remain static when the patient is moving, then advance keeping your feet in stride position.

- ✓ When descending stairs or curbs, remain in front of the patient and usually towards the weaker side. Place the lead foot on the step that the patient will step on and the other foot one step lower. Hold the gait belt in one hand and position the other hand on the front of the patient's shoulder. Remain static when the patient is moving, then advance keeping your feet in stride position.

Medical Equipment

Lines, Tubes, and Equipment

Arterial Line

An arterial line is a monitoring device consisting of a catheter that is inserted into an artery and attached to an electronic monitoring system. An arterial line is used to measure blood pressure or to obtain blood samples. The device is considered to be more accurate than traditional measures of blood pressure and does not require repeated needle punctures.

External Catheter

An external catheter is applied over the shaft of the penis and is held in place by a padded strap or adhesive tape.

Foley Catheter

A Foley catheter is an indwelling urinary tract catheter that has a balloon attachment at one end. The balloon which is filled with air or sterile water must be deflated before the catheter can be removed.

Intravenous System

An intravenous system consists of a sterile fluid source, a pump, a clamp, and a catheter to insert into a vein. An intravenous system can be used to infuse fluids, electrolytes, nutrients, and medication. Intravenous lines are most commonly inserted into superficial veins such as the basilic, cephalic or antecubital.

Nasal Cannula

A nasal cannula consists of tubing extending approximately one centimeter into each of the patient's nostrils. The tubing is connected to a common tube that is attached to an oxygen source. This method of oxygen therapy is capable of delivering up to six liters of oxygen per minute.

Nasogastric Tube

A nasogastric tube is a plastic tube inserted through a nostril that extends into the stomach. The device is commonly used for liquid feeding, medication administration or to remove gas from the stomach.

Oximeter

An oximeter is a photoelectric device used to determine the oxygen saturation of blood. The device is most commonly applied to the finger or the ear. Oximetry is often used by therapists to assess activity tolerance.

Suprapubic Catheter

A suprapubic catheter is an indwelling urinary catheter that is surgically inserted directly into the patient's bladder. Insertion of a suprapubic catheter is performed under general anesthesia.

Swan-Ganz Catheter

A Swan-Ganz catheter is a soft, flexible catheter that is inserted through a vein into the pulmonary artery. The device is used to provide continuous measurements of pulmonary artery pressure. Patients utilizing a Swan-Ganz catheter can exercise with the device in place, however, the patient should avoid activities that increase pressure on the catheter's insertion site.

Therapeutic Modalities

Indications for Therapeutic Modalities

Inflammation and Repair: Modalities can alter circulation, chemical reactions, flow of body fluids, and cell function throughout all phases of healing. Modalities enhance and accelerate the healing process and reduce the risk of adverse effects associated with inflammation.

Pain: Modalities can control pain by altering the cause of the pain or altering the process of pain perception.

Restriction in Motion: Thermal agents are used to enhance extensibility of collagen to allow for greater range of motion and tolerance to stretch.

Abnormal Tone: Modalities can influence tonal abnormalities from pain, musculoskeletal or neurological pathology. Alteration in nerve conduction, reduction of pain, and change in muscle biomechanical properties can normalize tone and enhance functional outcome.

Phases of Tissue Healing*

Inflammation Phase

- Lasts one to six days
- Occurs secondary to trauma or disease
- Required for healing to occur
- Presents with calor, rubor, tumor, dolor
- Clot formation and phagocytosis occur

Proliferative Phase

- Lasts from day three through day 20
- Involves connective tissues and epithelial cells
- Epithelialization, collagen production, wound contracture, and neurovascularization occur

Maturation Phase

- Begins at approximately day nine and is ongoing
- This phase is the longest in duration; can last over one year
- Progression towards restoration of the prior function of the injured tissues

- Collagen synthesis and lysis balance
- Collagen fiber orientation

*Phases of tissue healing can overlap

Keloid Scar

A keloid scar can occur during the healing process when collagen production greatly exceeds collagen lysis. A keloid scar extends beyond the original boundaries of an injury and damages healthy tissues.

Hypertrophic Scar

A hypertrophic scar can occur during the healing process when collagen production greatly exceeds collagen lysis. A hypertrophic scar will be raised, but remain within the borders of the original injury.

Principles of Heat Transfer

Conduction: The gain or loss of heat as a result of direct contact between two materials at different temperatures. Examples include hot pack, paraffin, ice massage, and ice pack.

Convection: The gain or loss of heat as a result of air or water moving in a constant motion across the body. Examples include fluidotherapy and whirlpool.

Conversion: The transfer of heat when nonthermal energy (mechanical, electrical) is absorbed into tissue and transformed into heat. Examples include diathermy and ultrasound.

Evaporation: The transfer of heat as a liquid absorbs energy and changes form to a vapor. An example is a vapocoolant spray.

Radiation: The direct transfer of heat from a radiation energy source of higher temperature to one of cooler temperature. Heat energy is directly absorbed without the need for a medium. An example is an infrared lamp.

Types of Pain

ACUTE	CHRONIC	REFERRED
Pain that lasts during the time of healing	Pain that lasts beyond the time of healing	Experience pain in one area with the injury in another area
There is a known causative factor or etiology	Activation of abnormal neurological responses	Can refer joint to joint
Well-localized and defined	Pain continues after noxious stimuli ceases	Can refer from a peripheral nerve to its distal innervation
Pain will last as long as the noxious stimuli persists	Associated with physical, psychological, social dysfunction	Can refer from an organ to outside tissues

Cryotherapy

Therapeutic Effects

- Initial decrease in blood flow to the treated area
- Decrease temperature
- Increase pain threshold
- Decrease metabolism
- Decrease edema
- Initial vasoconstriction
- Decrease nerve conduction velocity
- Reduce spasticity of muscle
- Produce analgesic effects

Indications

- Acute or chronic pain
- Myofascial pain syndrome
- Muscle spasm
- Bursitis
- Acute or subacute inflammation
- Musculoskeletal trauma
- Reduction of spasticity
- Tendonitis

Contraindications

- Area of compromised circulation
- Peripheral vascular disease
- Ischemic tissue
- Cold hypersensitivity
- Raynaud's phenomenon
- Cold urticaria
- Hypertension
- Infection
- Cryoglobulinemia

Stages of Perceived Sensations during Cryotherapy

1. Intense cold within three minutes
2. Aching and/or burning sensation from four to seven minutes
3. Anesthesia to analgesia from eight to 15 minutes
4. Numbness from 15 to 30 minutes

Ice Massage

Ice massage is typically performed by freezing water in paper cups and applying the ice directly to the treatment area. Ice massage is ideal for small or contoured areas, allows for observation, and is inexpensive to use.

Treatment Parameters: Ice massage can be administered using a frozen water popsicle or frozen water in a paper cup. Directly apply ice massage to the area for five to ten minutes.

Cold Pack

A cold pack typically contains silica gel and is available in a variety of shapes and sizes. The cold pack is stored in a refrigeration unit and is usually applied with a moist towel. Cold packs are easy to use, require minimal clinician time, and can cover a large area. Cold packs may not maintain uniform contact with the body and require frequent observation of the skin.

Treatment Parameters: A cold pack requires a temperature of 23 degrees Fahrenheit (–5 degrees Celsius). Apply the cold pack wrapped in a moistened towel to the area for 15 minutes. Application may extend to 30 minutes for reduction in spasticity, however, the skin requires observation every ten minutes. Cold packs can be applied every one to two hours for reduction of inflammation and pain control.

Cold Bath

A cold bath is commonly used for immersion of the distal extremities. A basin or whirlpool is most often used to hold the cold water.

Treatment Parameters: A cold bath requires water temperature ranging from 55 to 64 degrees Fahrenheit (13 to 18 degrees Celsius). A whirlpool or container of water with crushed ice can be used. The body part should be immersed for 5 to 15 minutes to attain the desired therapeutic effects.

Vapocoolant Spray

Vapocoolant sprays are often used in conjunction with passive stretching. Fluori-Methane is a commonly used vapocoolant spray that is typically applied from the proximal to distal muscle attachments. Vapocoolant sprays allow for a short duration of cooling to a very localized area of application, however, may be harmful to the environment and dangerous if inhaled.

Treatment Parameters: Identify the trigger point and make two to five sweeps with the spray in the direction of the muscle fibers. Keep the spray 12 to 18 inches from the skin and apply at a 30-degree angle. Stretching should begin while applying the spray and continue with steady tension and stretch. Repeated applications during the same treatment are safe if the skin is rewarmed between applications. Chlorofluorocarbons are exempt from the Clean Air Act when used for medical purposes, however, may cause environmental and ozone damage.

Superficial Heating Agents

Therapeutic Effects

• Increase temperature	• Vasodilation
• Increase blood flow to the treated area	• Increase nerve conduction velocity
• Decrease nerve conduction latency	• Increase metabolic rate
	• Increase muscle elasticity
• Temporarily decrease muscle strength	• Increase collagen extensibility
• Increase pain threshold	• Decrease tone
• Increase edema	

Indications

• Pain control	• Muscle spasm
• Chronic inflammatory conditions	• Decreased range of motion
• Trigger point	• Desensitization
• Tissue healing	

Contraindications

• Circulatory impairment	• Bleeding or hemorrhage
• Area of malignancy	• Sensory impairment
• Acute musculoskeletal trauma	• Thrombophlebitis
	• Arterial disease

Fluidotherapy

Fluidotherapy consists of a container that circulates warm air and small cellulose particles. The extremity is placed into the container and dry heat is generated through the energy transferred by forced convection. The therapeutic effects include the promotion of tissue healing, skin desensitization, and prevention of edema. Fluidotherapy allows for active movement during treatment and constant treatment temperature, however, is expensive and may require the extremity to be placed in a dependent position.

Treatment Parameters: The body part to be treated should be placed into the fluidotherapy unit prior to turning the machine on. The temperature should be set between 111 to

125 degrees Fahrenheit (44 to 52 degrees Celsius) and the degree of agitation should be adjusted to patient comfort. Treatment time is usually 20 minutes. A protective covering is required for any open area.

Hot Pack

A hot pack consists of a canvas or nylon covered pack filled with a hydrophilic silicate gel that provides a moist heat. The size and shape of the hot pack varies depending on the size and contour of the treatment area. A hot pack is easy to use, inexpensive, and can cover large areas. The main therapeutic effects include soft tissue healing, promoting relaxation, and decreasing pain and stiffness. Disadvantages of a hot pack include the need for close monitoring of the skin, the inability to maintain total contact, and the inability to move during treatment.

Treatment Parameters: A hot pack must be stored in hot water between 158 to 167 degrees Fahrenheit (70 to 75 degrees Celsius). Application requires six to eight layers of towels around the hot pack. The hot pack should be applied on top of the patient. If the patient lies on top of the hot pack additional towels are required. Skin checks are required after five minutes for excess redness or signs of a burn. A patient must have a call device to notify the therapist of discomfort. Hot packs require approximately 20 minutes to achieve the desired effects.

Infrared Lamp (IR)

An infrared lamp produces superficial heating of tissue through radiant heat. This form of heating is usually limited to penetration of less than one to three millimeters. Infrared does not require contact with the area to be treated and allows for constant observation, however, it requires skill to localize a treatment site. The main therapeutic effect is the enhancement of soft tissue healing. The use of infrared is declining due to the limited depth of penetration, dehydrating effects on wounds, and the risk of burns during treatment.

Treatment Parameters: The patient should be positioned approximately 20 inches from the source. A moist towel should be placed over the treatment area and the skin should be monitored intermittently throughout treatment. The standard formula indicates 20 inches in distance should equal 20 minutes of treatment. As the distance decreases, the intensity will increase, and the time of total treatment should decrease.

Paraffin

Paraffin wax is the most commonly used superficial heating agent of the distal extremities. It has the ability to maintain contact over all contoured areas and due to the low specific heat and slower conduction it does not feel as hot as water at the same temperature. Paraffin is easy to use, inexpensive, and can be used at home, however, it cannot be used over open areas.

Treatment Parameters: Temperature of the paraffin mixture should be maintained between 113 and 126 degrees Fahrenheit (45 to 52 degrees Celsius). There are three methods of paraffin application: dip-wrap, dip-reimmersion or paint application. The distal extremities utilize the dip-

wrap or dip-reimmersion methods. The patient's skin should be dry and clean prior to treatment. The patient is required to maintain a static position as the distal extremity dips into the paraffin bath and is removed. Wait a few seconds for the paraffin to harden and redip six to ten times using the dip-wrap method. Next, place a plastic bag over the extremity with a towel around it to insulate and maintain heating for approximately 15 to 20 minutes. Using the dip-reimmersion method place the distal extremity back into the paraffin bath after the initial six to ten dips and allow it to remain for the duration of treatment, up to 20 minutes. The paint method is used for body parts that cannot be immersed into the paraffin bath. A layer of paraffin is painted on the body with a brush. After a few seconds, six to ten additional layers are applied and a plastic wrap is placed over the paraffin with a towel on top to insulate the treatment area. Removal of the paraffin is the same for all forms of application. Paraffin should be peeled off after treatment and placed back into the container to melt or simply be discarded.

Deep Heating Agents

Diathermy

Diathermy is a deep heating agent that converts high frequency electromagnetic energy into therapeutic heat. Electrical energy produces vibration of molecules within a specific tissue, generates heat, and elevates tissue temperature. The main therapeutic effect of diathermy is the enhancement of soft tissue healing. Shortwave diathermy can be delivered in a continuous or pulsed mode. A pulsed mode is typically utilized to attain nonthermal effects while a continuous mode is used for thermal effects. The most common frequency used for shortwave diathermy is 27.12 MHz. Shortwave diathermy can utilize a capacitance technique or inductance technique. Capacitive plate applicators produce a high frequency electrical current that alternates between the plates. The patient becomes part of the electrical circuit and the oscillation of ions increases tissue temperature. Inductive coil applicators utilize a coil that generates alternating electric current, creates a magnetic field perpendicular to the coil, and produces eddy currents within the tissues. Eddy currents cause the oscillation of ions that increases tissue temperature. Inductive coil applicators are bundled as cables that wrap around an extremity or as a drum applicator.

Indications

• Decreased collagen extensibility	• Degenerative joint disease
• Pain	• Joint stiffness
• Tissue healing	• Bursitis
• Chronic inflammatory pelvic disease	• Peripheral nerve regeneration
• Muscle guarding	• Chronic inflammation

Contraindications

• Low back, abdomen, pelvis of a pregnant woman	• Pain and temperature sensory deficits
• Internal and external metal objects	• Moist wound dressing
	• Over hemorrhagic region
• Eyes	• Testes
• Malignant area	• Acute inflammation
• Intrauterine device	• Ischemic tissue
• Cardiac pacemaker	

Therapeutic Effects

• Increase temperature	• Vasodilation
• Altered cell membrane function	• Increase nerve conduction velocity
• Decrease nerve conduction latency	• Increase metabolic rate
• Increase pain threshold	• Increase collagen extensibility
• Increase muscle elasticity	• Alteration of muscle strengths
• Increase edema	

Capacitive Plate Method

- Metal plates encased in a plastic housing
- Field radiation is a strong electrical field and a weaker magnetic field
- Energy is absorbed most within the skin and less into deeper structures
- The heating pattern is superficial
- Application is generally over areas of low-fat content

Inductive Coil Method

- Rigid metal coils encased
- Field radiation is a strong magnetic field and a weaker electrical field
- Energy is absorbed most within the deeper structures; tissues with the highest electrical conductivity such as muscle and synovial fluid
- The heating pattern is deeper
- Application is generally over areas of high water content

Treatment Parameters: A therapist should first select the most appropriate diathermy technique and device based on patient examination. The patient must remove all metal and jewelry in the area surrounding the treatment site. Position the patient and check for clean and dry skin. When using an inductive applicator the therapist must wrap the coils around the extremity that has been covered by a towel. When using a drum the therapist should place the drum directly over the treatment area. When using a capacitive applicator place the two plates over both sides of the treatment area ensuring equal distance from the plates to the skin (two to ten centimeters). The patient must remain in the same position throughout treatment for complete and consistent heating. The patient should have a call bell and should be checked within the first few minutes of treatment. Treatment time varies from 15 to 30 minutes based on diagnosis and desired effects.

Ultrasound

Ultrasound is a common deep heating agent that transfers heat through conversion, elevates tissue temperature to depths up to five centimeters, and uses inaudible acoustic mechanical vibrations of high frequency to produce thermal and nonthermal effects. The piezoelectric crystal transducer converts electrical energy into sound. The main therapeutic effects of ultrasound include enhanced soft tissue healing, decreased inflammatory response, and decreased pain. Therapeutic ultrasound has a frequency between .75 and 3 MHz. Ultrasound requires the use of a coupling agent and can be applied using the stationary or moving technique. Ultrasound can be administered using a pulsed or continuous mode. Continuous mode ultrasound is more effective in elevating tissue temperature where pulsed mode ultrasound conversely minimizes the thermal effects. Duty cycle indicates the portion of treatment time that ultrasound is generated during the entire treatment. For example, continuous ultrasound generates constant ultrasound waves that correlates to a 100% duty cycle and produces thermal effects at a higher intensity and nonthermal effects at a lower intensity. Pulsed ultrasound that generates ultrasound 20% of the treatment time correlates to a 20% duty cycle and will produce nonthermal effects. A frequency setting of 1 MHz is used for heating of deeper tissues (up to five centimeters) where a setting of 3 MHz produces a higher temperature with a depth of penetration of less than two centimeters.

Therapeutic Effects

Thermal	Nonthermal
• Increase extensibility of collagen structures	• Stimulation of tissue regeneration
• Decrease joint stiffness	• Increase macrophage responsiveness
• Pain relief	• Pain relief
• Increase blood flow	• Soft tissue repair
• Decrease muscle spasm	• Increase blood flow
	• Increase skin and cell membrane permeability

Indications

• Soft tissue repair	• Scar tissue
• Contracture	• Pain
• Bone fracture	• Plantar wart
• Trigger point	• Muscle spasm
• Dermal ulcer	

Contraindications

• Over eyes	• Over heart
• Over pregnant uterus	• Over testes
• Over cemented prosthetic joint	• Over epiphyseal areas in children
• Impaired circulation	• Infection
• Thrombophlebitis	• Over malignancy
• Impaired pain or temperature sensory deficits	

Treatment Parameters: Ultrasound can be administered using a stationary or moving technique. For all techniques the therapist should decide the duration, frequency, duty cycle, and intensity of treatment based on diagnosis and desired effects. Apply the coupling medium to the treatment area or place the area to be treated under water if using the immersion technique. Place the transducer on the treatment area or one half-inch parallel to the treatment area under water and then turn on the machine. During the moving technique the transducer should continuously move in a small circular pattern over the treatment area. Maintain contact with the skin and stay within the treatment area. An area two to three times the size of the transducer typically requires a duration of five minutes of treatment. Intensity for continuous ultrasound is normally set between .5 to 2 W/cm^2 for thermal effects. Pulsed ultrasound is normally set between .5 to .75 W/cm^2 with a 20% duty cycle for nonthermal effects.

Beam Nonuniformity Ratio (BNR)

- BNR is the ratio of intensity of the highest peak to the average intensity of all peaks.
- The lower the BNR, the more favorable, since patients will be less likely to experience hot spots and/or discomfort during treatment.
- The BNR of a particular unit is required to be listed on the device for consumer education and awareness.
- The BNR is derived from the intrinsic factors and quality of the piezoelectric transducer. The higher the quality of the transducer, the lower the BNR.
- BNR values should range between 2:1 and 6:1; most devices often fall in the 5:1 or 6:1 range.

Effective Radiating Area (ERA)

The ERA is the area of the transducer that transmits ultrasound energy. The ERA is always smaller than the total size of the transducer head.

Acoustic Cavitation

Acoustic cavitation occurs as a result of the acoustic energy generated by ultrasound that develops into microscopic bubbles causing cavities that surround soft tissues. The microscopic, vapor-filled bubbles expand and contract. There are two types of cavitation that occur:

Stable cavitation: The microscopic bubbles increase and decrease in size, but do no burst. Stable cavitation triggers microstreaming.

Transient (unstable) cavitation: The microscopic bubbles increase in size over multiple cycles and implode. This causes brief moments of local temperature and pressure increases in the area surrounding these bubbles. This process should not occur during therapeutic ultrasound since the intensities required are much higher than 3 W/cm^2.

Microstreaming

Microstreaming is the minute flow of fluid that takes place around the vapor-filled bubbles that oscillate and pulsate.

Acoustic Streaming

Acoustic streaming is the term for the consistent and circular flow of cellular fluids that results from ultrasound. Acoustic streaming is responsible for altering cellular activity and the transport of fluids to different portions of the field.

Phonophoresis

Phonophoresis describes the use of ultrasound for transdermal delivery of medication. Ultrasound enhances the distribution of the medication through the skin, provides a high concentration of the drug directly to the treatment site, and avoids risks that may be involved with injection of medication. Medications regularly used in phonophoresis include anti-inflammatory agents or analgesics. Phonophoresis is effective with both continuous and pulsed techniques.

Hydrotherapy

Hydrotherapy transfers heat through conduction or convection and is administered in tanks of varying size ranging from extremity whirlpools to Olympic size pools. The main therapeutic effects of hydrotherapy include wound care, unloading of weight, and reduction of edema. The specific instrument to be used depends on the treatment objectives and site of the pathology.

Properties of Water

Buoyancy

Archimedes' principle of buoyancy states that there is an upward force on the body when immersed in water equal to the amount of water that has been displaced by the body. The ability to float in water results from the body possessing a specific gravity less than that of water.

Hydrostatic pressure

Water exerts pressure that is perpendicular to the body and increases in proportion with the depth of immersion.

Resistance

Water molecules tend to attract to each other and provide resistance to movement of the body in the water. Resistance by water increases in proportion to speed of motion.

Specific Gravity

The computation for the specific gravity of water is equal to 1. The human body varies based on size and somatotype but typically has a specific gravity of less than 1 (average .974). Therefore, a person will generally float when fully submerged in water.

Specific Heat

The specific heat is the measure of the ability of a fluid to store heat. This is calculated as the amount of thermal energy required to increase the fluid's temperature by one unit. Water can store four times the heat as compared to air. Water's thermal conductivity is approximately 25 times faster than air at the same temperature.

Total Drag Force

The total drag force is comprised of profile drag, wave drag, and surface drag forces. This is a hydromechanic force exerted on a person submerged in water that normally opposes the direction of the body's motion.

Therapeutic Effects

• Increase blood flow	• Vasodilation
• Increase core temperature	• Decrease abnormal tone
• Relaxation	• Wound/debridement
• Pain relief	

Indications

• Burn care	• Wound care
• Superficial heating or cooling	• Decreased range of motion
• Edema control	• Pool therapy/exercise
• Muscle strain	• Sprain
• Arthritis	• Joint stiffness
• Desensitization of residual limb with contrast bath	• Muscle spasm/spasticity
• Pain management	

Contraindications

• Peripheral vascular disease	• Buerger's disease with contrast bath
• Gangrene	• Impaired circulation
• Severe infection	• Renal infection
• Urinary/fecal incontinence	• Bleeding surface area
• Advanced cardiovascular or pulmonary disease	• Diminished sensation

Types of Hydrotherapy

Extremity tank

An extremity tank is used for the distal upper or lower extremity. Approximate dimensions for the extremity tank are a depth of 18 to 24 inches, a length of 28 to 32 inches, and a width of 15 inches. (10-45 gallons)

Lowboy tank

A lowboy tank is used for larger parts of the extremities and permits long sitting with water up to the midthoracic level. Approximate dimensions for the lowboy tank are a depth of 18 inches, a length of 52 to 65 inches, and a width of 24 inches. (90-105 gallons)

Highboy tank

A highboy tank is used for larger parts of the extremities and the trunk and permits sitting in chest-high water with hips and knees flexed. Approximate dimensions for the highboy tank are a depth of 28 inches, a length of 36 to 48 inches, and a width of 20 to 24 inches. (60 - 105 gallons)

Hubbard tank

The Hubbard tank is used for full-body immersion. Approximate dimensions for the Hubbard tank are a depth of four feet, a length of eight feet, and a width of six feet. Contraindications specific to full-body immersion include unstable blood pressure and incontinence. Treatment time ranges between 10 to 20 minutes. Temperature should not exceed 100 degrees Fahrenheit (39 degrees Celsius). (425 gallons)

Therapeutic pool

A therapeutic pool is used for exercising in a water medium. Temperature should range between 79 to 98 degrees Fahrenheit (26 to 37 degrees Celsius) depending on patient age, health status, and goals.

Treatment Temperature Guidelines

Degrees F	Degrees C	Purpose
32 - 79 °F	0 - 26 °C	Acute inflammation of distal extremities
79 - 92 °F	26 - 33 °C	Exercise
92 - 96 °F	33 - 36 °C	Wound care, spasticity
96 - 98 °F	36 - 37 °C	Cardiopulmonary compromise, treatment of burns
99 - 104 °F	37 - 40 °C	Pain management
104 - 110 °F	40 - 44 °C	Chronic rheumatoid or osteoarthritis, increased range of motion

Treatment Parameters for whirlpool: Prior to treatment the therapist should explain the sensations the patient will experience during treatment. Select the water temperature based on diagnosis and goals and assist the patient into a comfortable position. Adjust and turn on the turbine. Monitor the patient's vital signs and level of comfort. Treatment time ranges between 10 and 30 minutes. Exercise can be performed during whirlpool as indicated. After treatment dry and inspect the treated area.

Treatment Parameters for pool therapy: In addition to general contraindications for superficial or deep heating, specific contraindications include incontinence, open areas, fear of water, confusion, and significant respiratory pathology. The therapist should assist the patient as needed into the pool and throughout treatment. The therapist must stay with the patient and monitor vital signs and tolerance to activity. Advantages of pool therapy include decreased weight bearing with the assistance of buoyancy, easier handling by the therapist, control over the amount of resistance during exercise, and diminished risk of falling with activity. Recommended populations for pool therapy include patients with arthritis, musculoskeletal injuries, neurological deficits, spinal cord injury, CVA, multiple sclerosis, and selected cardiopulmonary diagnoses. The tank must be thoroughly cleaned after each use with a disinfectant and antibacterial agent.

Contrast Bath

A contrast bath utilizes alternating heat and cold in order to decrease edema in a distal extremity. The alternating vasodilation and vasoconstriction is theorized to stimulate local circulation and systemic circulation to a lesser degree. The technique provides good contact over irregularly shaped areas, allows for movement during treatment, and assists with pain management. Disadvantages include potential intolerance to cold, dependent positioning, and lack of credible research to support the theory of contrast baths and its effect on edema.

Treatment Parameters: The therapist should position the patient so that both baths are accessible to the patient. The treatment should begin with the patient's distal extremity immersed in the hot whirlpool with a temperature between 100 to 110 degrees Fahrenheit (27 to 40 degrees Celsius) for three to four minutes. The patient should then place the distal extremity into the cold bath with a temperature between 55 to 67 degrees Fahrenheit (13 to 20 degrees Celsius) for one minute. The patient should repeat this hot/cold sequence for 20-30 minutes. The patient should end the treatment in the hot whirlpool and then dry off immediately. Contrast baths are utilized primarily with arthritis of the smaller joints, musculoskeletal sprains and strains, RSD, and to desensitize the residual limb of a patient status post amputation.

Mechanical Agents

Traction

Traction is a modality that applies mechanical forces to the body to separate joint surfaces and decrease pressure. The force can be applied manually by the therapist or mechanically by a machine. Traction is indicated for many diagnoses and allows for variation and adjustment of the established protocol based on individual patient need. Traction affects many of the body's systems and requires ongoing monitoring and reassessment of treatment parameters. Mechanical traction, self-traction, manual traction, and positional traction are commonly utilized techniques.

Therapeutic Effects

• Joint distraction	• Muscle relaxation
• Soft tissue stretching	• Joint mobility
• Reduction of disk protrusion	

Indications

• Nerve impingement	• Joint hypomobility
• Herniated or protruding disc	• Paraspinal muscle spasm
• Subacute joint inflammation	• Degenerative joint disease
• Spondylolisthesis	• Osteophyte formation

Contraindications

• When motion is contraindicated	• Acute inflammatory response
• Joint instability	• Acute sprain
• Tumor	• Osteoporosis
• Pregnancy	• Fracture

Treatment Parameters: Mechanical traction can be performed to the cervical or lumbar spine. All halters and belts should be secured and the patient instructed in what to expect from treatment. The therapist should then set the time of treatment, force of pull, and determine static or intermittent control with hold and relax ratio settings. During treatment the patient should have the ability to stop the machine and call for help. Treatment time varies based on diagnosis and therapeutic goals and falls between five and 20 minutes. To initiate cervical traction the therapist should position the patient in supine with approximately 25-35 degrees of neck flexion or in a sitting position. Cervical traction should start with a force between 10-15 pounds and progress to 7% of the patient's body weight as tolerated for separation of the vertebrae. Application of lumbar traction should be performed in supine or prone. The force of lumbar traction is dependent on the goals of treatment and should be set with a force of less than half of the body weight for the initial treatment. Traction force of 25-50 pounds is recommended when initiating mechanical lumbar traction. Force of up to 50% of the body weight is required for actual separation of the vertebrae.

Compression

Compression is a physical agent that applies a mechanical force to increase pressure on the treated body part. Compression works to keep venous and lymphatic flow from pooling into the interstitial space. Static compression utilizes bandaging and compression garments to shape residual limbs, control edema, prevent abnormal scar formation, and reduce the risk of deep vein thrombosis. Intermittent compression with a pneumatic device is primarily used to reduce chronic or post-traumatic edema and requires adjusting the parameters of inflation pressure, on/off ratio, and total treatment time. Compression has been coupled with therapeutic cold and electrical stimulation.

Therapeutic Effects

• Control of peripheral edema • Shaping of residual limb • Management of scar formation	• Improve lymphatic and venous return • Prevention of deep vein thrombosis

Indications

• Lymphedema • New residual limb • Risk for deep vein thrombosis	• Edema • Stasis ulcers • Hypertrophic scarring

Contraindications

• Malignancy of treated area • Deep vein thrombosis • Unstable or acute fracture • Heart failure	• Infection of treated area • Pulmonary edema • Circulatory obstruction

Treatment Parameters: The therapist must ask the patient to remove all jewelry and ensure appropriate fit of the compression sleeve prior to treatment. The patient should be placed in a comfortable position with the extremity elevated. Blood pressure and girth measurements should be recorded. The therapist should apply the stockinette over the extremity and adjust the compression sleeve. The therapist should set parameters based on desired effect. A 3:1 ratio is generally used for on/off time with inflation between 40 to 100 seconds and deflation between 10 to 35 seconds. Inflation pressure generally ranges from 30 to 80 mm Hg and should not exceed the patient's diastolic blood pressure. Treatment of the upper extremities generally requires between 30 and 60 mm Hg of inflation pressure while treatment of the lower extremities generally requires between 40 and 80 mm Hg of inflation pressure. Treatment time varies based on diagnosis from two to four hours and is utilized from three times per week to three times per day. The patient should have a call bell and should be monitored for comfort and blood pressure readings throughout treatment. When treatment time is complete the therapist should reassess the extremity, girth measurements, and blood pressure readings.

Additional Physical Agents

Ultraviolet (UV)

Ultraviolet light is a form of energy that is used therapeutically and absorbed one to two millimeters into the skin. Ultraviolet is divided into UV-A, UV-B, and UV-C according to wavelength and place on the electromagnetic spectrum. Treatment parameters and application are based on diagnosis, desired effects, and minimal erythemal dose. The most effective use of UV is to treat skin disorders.

Contraindications

• Photosensitive medication • Lupus erythematosus • Tuberculosis • Herpes simplex	• Renal or hepatic pathology • Diabetes mellitus • Pellagra

Therapeutic Effects

• Facilitate healing • Exfoliation • Vitamin D production • Increase pigmentation	• Tanning • Bacteriocidal effects • Thickening of epidermis

Indications

• Acne • Psoriasis • Tetany • Vitamin D deficiency	• Chronic ulcer/wound • Osteomalacia/rickets • Sinusitis

Treatment Parameters: Prior to treatment with UV a therapist must obtain a minimal erythemal dose (MED). This is the time of exposure needed to produce an area of mild redness between eight and 24 hours after treatment. The MED is tested by placing a piece of paper with five one-inch cut outs over a patient's anterior forearm. The patient should have all other non-treatment areas covered as well as wear protective goggles. Once the lamp is warmed up it should be positioned at a 90-degree angle to the area of treatment (for maximum absorption) and at a distance between 24 to 40 inches from the forearm. The squares should be exposed sequentially in 15 second increments for 15, 30, 45, 60, and 75 seconds. Visual inspection after an 8-hour period will determine the MED. Parameters including distance from the lamp, position of the lamp at a 90-degree angle to the treatment site, and the MED must remain consistent over the course of treatment. The treatment time should increase each consecutive treatment day since the skin adapts to UV exposure. The therapist should utilize a stopwatch and continue with ongoing visual inspection during all treatment sessions.

Massage

Massage is a manual therapeutic modality that produces physiologic effects through different types of stroking, rubbing, and pressure. Massage is capable of producing mechanical and reflexive effects.

Massage Techniques

Effleurage: Effleurage is a massage technique that is usually light in stroke and produces a reflexive response. The technique is performed at the beginning and at the end of a massage to allow the patient to relax and should be directed towards the heart. Effleurage can be applied as a deep stroke to produce both a mechanical and a reflexive response.

Friction: Friction is a massage technique that incorporates small circular motions over a trigger point or muscle spasm. This is a deep massage technique that penetrates into the depth of a muscle and attempts to reduce edema, loosen adhesions, and relieve muscle spasm. Friction massage is used quite frequently with chronic inflammation or with overuse injuries.

Petrissage: Petrissage is a massage technique described as kneading where the muscle is squeezed and rolled under the therapist's hands. The goal of petrissage is to loosen adhesions, improve lymphatic return, and facilitate removal of metabolic waste from the treatment area. Petrissage must provide a distal to proximal sequence of kneading over the muscle. Petrissage can be performed with two hands over larger muscle groups or with as few as two fingers over smaller muscles.

Tapotement: Tapotement is a massage technique that provides stimulation through rapid and alternating movements such as tapping, hacking, cupping, and slapping. The primary purpose of tapotement is to enhance circulation and stimulate peripheral nerve endings.

Vibration: Vibration is a massage technique that places the therapist's hands or fingers firmly over an area and utilizes a rapid shaking motion that causes vibration to the treatment area. The therapist initiates this motion from the forearm while maintaining firm contact on the treatment area. Vibration is used primarily for relaxation.

Therapeutic Effects

• Increase lymphatic circulation	• Stimulate reflexive effects
• Improve circulation	• Reduction of edema
• Removal of metabolic waste	• Alters pain transmission
• Decrease muscle atrophy	• Decrease muscle spasm
• Decrease anxiety and tension	• Loosen adhesions
• Facilitate healing	• Relaxation

Indications

• Pain	• Trigger point
• Decreased range of motion	• Muscle spasm and cramping
• Edema	• Scar tissue
• Adhesions	• Bursitis
• Myositis	• Tendonitis
• Lactic acid excess	• Intermittent claudication
• Migraine or general headache	• Raynaud's syndrome

Contraindications

• Infection	• Acute injury
• Arteriosclerosis	• Embolus
• Thrombus	• Cancer
• Cellulitis	

Treatment Parameters: The patient should be comfortable and properly draped prior to the initiation of treatment. The therapist's hands must be clean, dry, and warm. The therapist must be positioned in an efficient posture during treatment and maintain the required pressure and rhythm based on the goals of treatment. The massage should start using the effleurage technique. The amount of time required for each treatment is dependent on the body part and therapeutic goal. Generally, the back requires 15 minutes as opposed to a smaller area or joint that requires eight to ten minutes. The intensity should progressively increase and then decrease, using effleurage again to end the treatment session. Lubricant is indicated with all strokes except friction massage.

Electrotherapy

Electrotherapy is utilized in physical therapy for various reasons including facilitation of skeletal muscle contraction, stimulation of denervated muscle, pain management, to retard muscle atrophy, osteogenesis, driving medications through the skin, and wound management.

Therapeutic Effects

• Relaxation of muscle spasm	• Eliminate disuse atrophy
• Muscle strengthening	• Muscle re-education
• Improve range of motion	• Increase local circulation
• Facilitate wound healing	• Facilitate bone repair
• Decrease edema	• Decrease pain

Indications

• Muscle spasm	• Muscle atrophy
• Muscle weakness	• Open wound/ulcer
• Pain	• Bell's palsy
• Decreased range of motion	• Use with labor and delivery
• Idiopathic scoliosis	• Stress incontinence
• Fracture	• Shoulder subluxation
• Joint effusion	
• Facial neuropathy	

Contraindications

• Cardiac pacemaker	• Malignancy
• Patient with a bladder stimulator	• Use over a pregnant uterus
• Use over carotid sinus	• Cardiac arrhythmia
• Seizure disorders	• Osteomyelitis
• Phlebitis	

Electrode Configuration

Monopolar technique: The stimulating or active electrode is placed over the target area. A second dispersive electrode is placed at another site away from the target area. Typically the active electrode is smaller than the dispersive electrode. This technique is used with wounds, iontophoresis, and in the treatment of edema.

Bipolar technique: Two active electrodes are placed over the target area. Typically the electrodes are equal in size. This technique is used for muscle weakness, neuromuscular facilitation, spasms, and range of motion.

Quadripolar technique: Two electrodes from two separate stimulating circuits are positioned so that the individual currents intersect with each other. This technique is utilized with interferential current.

Electrode Size

When using a smaller electrode it is particularly important to understand that since the current density is quite high compared to a larger electrode, the patient will be more susceptible to pain and potential tissue damage.

Small Electrodes	Large Electrodes
• Increased current density	• Decreased current density
• Increased impedance	• Decreased impedance
• Decreased current flow	• Increased current flow

Waveforms

Direct current

Direct current, also referred to as Galvanic current, is characterized by a constant flow of electrons from the anode to the cathode (for a period of greater than one second) without interruption. Polarity remains constant and is determined by the therapist based on treatment goals. Iontophoresis uses direct current.

Alternating current

Alternating current is characterized by polarity that continuously changes from positive to negative with the change in direction of current flow. Alternating current is biphasic, symmetrical or asymmetrical, and is characterized by a waveform that is sinusoidal in shape. Alternating current is used in muscle retraining, spasticity, and stimulation of denervated muscle.

Interferential current

Interferential current combines two high frequency alternating waveforms that are biphasic. Interferential current attempts to reach deeper tissues using the higher frequencies of each waveform along with the overall shorter pulse widths. Interferential uses a frequency of 50-120 pulses per second and a pulse width of 50-150 microseconds for pain management; and a frequency of 20-50 pulses per second and a pulse width of 100-200 microseconds for muscle contraction.

Indications

• Pain management
• Urinary incontinence
• Edema management
• Osteoarthritic pain
• Migraines

Contraindications

• Malignancy
• With all types of electronic implants
• During the first trimester of pregnancy
• Over lower abdomen/uterus during pregnancy
• Over the anterior transcervical area

Common Methods of Delivery

- Bipolar
- Quadripolar
- Quadripolar with automatic vector scan

Bipolar delivery

Bipolar delivery utilizes two electrodes connected to a single channel with two medium sinusoidal currents. For example, one medium-frequency sinusoidal current produces 3,000 Hz and another medium-frequency sinusoidal current produces 3,050 Hz. The interference between the two currents creates an amplitude modulated interferential current with a beat frequency of 50 bps (beats per second). This is the net difference between the two currents. The bipolar method allows for the interferential current to be modulated prior to delivery of the current to the electrodes.

Quadripolar delivery

Quadripolar delivery utilizes four electrodes with each pair connected to a single channel. The interference between the currents using this method occurs at the level of the treatment area within the targeted tissues (as opposed to the previous method where it occurs prior to the electrode level). When the currents intersect at a 90 degree angle the maximum resultant amplitude occurs halfway between the two lines of current. The current treatment area creates a four-leaf clover shaped treatment field within the area between all four electrodes.

Quadripolar with automatic vector scan

The quadripolar method with automatic vector scan is used when there is a need to increase the size of the field of current that is created by the quadripolar method. One of the circuits is allowed to vary in amplitude and this allows the field pattern to automatically rotate between the two lines of current. The field is circular in shape as opposed to the cloverleaf and allows for the overall larger field of current.

Russian Current

Russian current is a medium frequency polyphasic waveform. The intensity of this form of alternating current is produced in a 50 burst per second interval with a pulse width range of 50-200 microseconds, and an interburst interval of 10 milliseconds. Russian current is a type of NMES or FES and is believed to augment muscle strengthening by depolarizing both sensory and motor nerve fibers resulting in tetanic contractions that are painless and stronger than those made voluntarily by the patient. Since the mode of delivery is theoretically painless, the increased current amplitude allows the deeper motor nerve fibers to depolarize concomitantly.

Indications

- The primary indication is to strengthen the muscle groups of otherwise healthy individuals and athletes.

Contraindications

- Over the abdominal and pelvic area of a pregnant woman
- Over an area of hemorrhage
- Malignancy
- Over the anterior cervical area
- Over electronic implants

Treatment Parameters: Prior to treatment the therapist should ensure that the patient's skin is clean and dry. The electrode orientation should be placed parallel to the muscle fibers along the line of pull of the muscle group. The electrode placement can be monopolar, bipolar, quadripolar, or multipolar in arrangement. Current transmission relies on a coupling gel that is applied to the entire treatment surface area of each electrode. Russian stimulation has an average peak current amplitude of 100 mA, 50 bursts per second, with an on/off time ratio of 10/50. A popular training protocol with Russian current suggests a treatment of 10 evoked contractions with a 10 second contraction and a 50 second rest period between each of the ten contractions.

Neuromuscular Electrical Stimulation (NMES)

Neuromuscular electrical stimulation (NMES) or functional electrical stimulation (FES) is a technique used to facilitate skeletal muscle activity. Stimulation of an innervated muscle occurs when an electrical stimulus of appropriate intensity and duration is administered to the corresponding peripheral nerve. Electrical stimulation of a denervated muscle has been used in an attempt to maintain the muscle, however, there is little documented evidence that supports this treatment option. Neuromuscular electrical stimulation is a commonly used therapeutic technique to facilitate the return of controlled functional muscular activity or to maintain postural alignment until recovery occurs.

Treatment Parameters: The patient should be positioned comfortably. The therapist uses a bipolar electrode placement over the target muscle. An interrupted or surged current is utilized with a range of 20-40 pulses per second and an on time of six to ten seconds followed by an off time of approximately 50-60 seconds in order to avoid immediate motor fatigue. Treatment time ranges from 15 to 20 minutes and can be repeated several times each day.

Transcutaneous Electrical Nerve Stimulation (TENS)

Transcutaneous electrical nerve stimulation is widely used for acute and chronic pain management. Areas of use include obstetrics, temporomandibular joint pain, and post-operative pain. The main therapeutic effects of TENS include pain relief through the gate control theory or the endogenous opiate pain control theory. TENS units are portable and indicated for home use.

Indications

- Post-operative pain
- During labor and delivery
- Bone fractures
- Chronic pain
- Trigeminal neuralgia
- Phantom pain
- For antiemetic effects
- Improved blood flow

Contraindications

- Cardiac pacemakers (relative contraindication)
- Epilepsy
- During the first trimester of pregnancy
- Over lower abdomen/uterus during pregnancy
- Over the anterior transcervical area

**TENS	Frequency	Duration	Amplitude
Conventional	50 – 150 Hz	20 – 100 microseconds	10 – 30 mA
Acupuncture-like (AL)	1 – 4 Hz	100 – 200 microseconds	30 – 80 mA
Pulse burst	70 – 100 Hz / burst	40 – 75 microseconds	30 – 60 mA
Brief intense (high-intensity)	70 – 100 Hz / burst	150 – 200 microseconds	30 – 60 mA

**This chart demonstrates a typical range for each type of TENS, however, there are discrepancies that exist from author to author regarding the appropriate settings for TENS as well as each diagnoses' parameters. Thus, this chart is to be used as a guideline for overall understanding of the mechanism of action behind each type of TENS and its outcome based on those settings.

Treatment Parameters: The waveforms used are monophasic pulsatile current or biphasic pulsatile current with a spiked square, rectangular or sinewave form. Electrode placement may be based on sites of nerve roots, trigger points, acupuncture sites or key points of pain and sensitivity. Net polarity is normally equal to zero. If the waveform is unbalanced there will be an accumulation of charges that will lead to skin irritation under the electrodes. Generally, the parameters when using TENS include a pulse duration that can vary from 20-400 microseconds; pulse frequency that varies in range from 1-200 Hz; and current amplitude from .1-120 mA. Sensory level stimulation requires the patient to experience perceptible tingling.

Iontophoresis

Iontophoresis is the process by which medications are induced through the skin into the body by means of continuous direct current electrical stimulation. The medication is separated into ions based on the polarity of the current.

Acidic reaction: A patient may have an acidic reaction from the iontophoresis treatment that is sclerotic in nature and can cause hardening of the skin over time.

Alkaline reaction: A patient may have an alkaline reaction from the iontophoresis treatment that is sclerolytic in nature and can soften the skin over time, exposing it to the risk of irritation and burn during further treatment.

Buffering: Buffering is a technique used to stabilize the pH of the skin during iontophoresis by placing buffering agents into the electrode pads that cover the designated drug reservoir area within the electrode. This maintains the hydrogen concentration and avoids any significant pH change during treatment.

Electrolysis: Electrolysis is a term used to describe the decomposition of a compound that results from passing an electrical current through it.

Electron exchange: Electron exchange occurs during iontophoresis where there is an exchange between the ions within the solutions and the electrodes.

Redox reaction: A redox reaction is the decomposition of water when an electrical current is passed through it. Water will be reduced to a net accumulation of hydrogen ions (H^+) under the anode and hydroxyl ions (OH^-) under the cathode.

Treatment Parameters: The patient should be positioned comfortably, but should never lie on top of the electrodes. The unit should be set to continuous direct current. Polarity must be set to the same polarity as the ion solution. The ion solution should be massaged into the treatment site or placed into the designated space within the electrode. The therapist must ensure that the conductive surface area of the negative electrode (cathode) is twice the size of the conductive surface area of the positive electrode (anode) regardless of which one is the active electrode. The active electrode should be placed over the target area and the dispersive electrode should be placed as far as possible from the active electrode. The therapist should secure the electrodes and slowly increase the intensity towards a maximum of five milliamperes. Treatment should last 15 to 20 minutes. Additional time is required for treatment at an intensity of less than five milliamperes. The therapist must monitor the patient during treatment to ensure that the skin is not burned under the electrode. Upon completion of treatment the therapist must slowly decrease the intensity, remove the electrodes, and provide the area of skin under the negative electrode with a thorough cleaning followed by the application of lotion to minimize irritation.

Therapeutic Ions and Charge

+ (Positive charge)	– (Negative charge)
• Lidocaine	• Acetate
• Hydrocortisone	• Dexamethasone
• Histamine	• Salicylate
• Lithium	• Iodine
• Magnesium	• Chlorine
• Zinc	• Tap water (+ and –)

High-Voltage Pulsed Current (HVPC)

High-volt pulsed current, also known as high-volt or high-voltage pulsed galvanic current, is a twin-peak (pair of monophasic spike waveforms) monophasic, pulsed current. It is differentiated from other stimulators by the high electromotive forces produced. HVPC has a phase duration of 5-20 microseconds (fixed in most machines), a short pulse duration (includes both spikes and the interspike interval) that ranges between 100-200 microseconds, and voltage greater than 150V to a maximum of 500V. There is one large dispersive pad along with one, two or four active electrodes. The active electrodes can be positive or negative in polarity based on the treatment goals.

Indications

- Wound management
- Pain management
- Soft tissue edema
- Levator ani syndrome
- Muscle spasm
- Muscle weakness
- Bell's palsy

Contraindications

- Cardiac pacemakers (relative contraindication)
- Over heavy scarring tissues
- Malignancy
- Over lower abdomen/uterus during pregnancy
- Over the anterior transcervical area
- Over osteomyelitis
- Anterior cervical region

Treatment Parameters: General treatment parameters are found above. An example of using HVPS for wound healing is as follows: Prepare the patient so the patient is comfortable and the wound is clean from any exudate or foreign materials. The therapist must wash the hands and apply proper protective garments. Secure one electrode over the wound (using a warm sterile gauze and sponge) and the other over healthy skin a minimum of 5 cm from the wound itself. The polarity should be in reversal mode so that it allows for 50% of treatment with negative polarity and 50% of treatment with positive polarity. The frequency is generally 30-200 pps, amplitude 1-500V, and duration of treatment from 10-60 minutes per session. Dermal wounds should be treated five to seven days per week for best results.

Electromyography

Electromyography is the science of evaluating motor units (the anterior horn cell, its axon, neuromuscular junctions and muscle fibers innervated by the unit) through the use of intramuscular needle electrodes or surface electrodes. Surface electrodes are used to monitor larger muscle groups while indwelling electrodes are used for small or deep muscles or when there is a need to record a single motor unit potential.

Muscles at rest: A normal relaxed muscle should exhibit electrical silence (no electrical potentials). Spontaneous potentials during rest are significant abnormal findings.

Abnormal Potentials

Spontaneous

Fibrillation potentials: indicative of lower motor neuron disease

Positive sharp wave: denervated muscle disorders at rest, primary muscle disease such as muscular dystrophy

Fasciculations: irritation/degeneration of anterior horn cell, nerve root compression or muscle spasms

Repetitive discharges: lesions of anterior horn cell and peripheral nerves; and myopathies

Voluntary

Polyphasic potentials: myopathies; muscle or peripheral nerve involvement

Common Muscles used for Insertion of Needle Electrodes

Upper Extremity		Lower Extremity	
C5-6	Lateral deltoid	L4-5	Tibialis anterior
C5-6	Biceps brachii	L5-S1	Peroneus longus
C6-7	Triceps brachii	S1-2	Gastrocnemius
C6-7	Flexor carpi radialis	L2, 3, 4	Vastus medialis
C8-T1	Abductor pollicis brevis	L4-5, S1	Tensor fasciae latae
C8-T1	First dorsal interossei	L5, S1-2	Gluteus maximus
C7-8	Extensor indicis propius	L5, S1-2	Hamstrings

Biofeedback

Biofeedback is a modality that uses an electromechanical device to provide visual and/or auditory feedback. Biofeedback can be utilized to receive information related to motor performance, kinesthetic performance or physiological response. Biofeedback can measure peripheral skin temperature, changes in blood volume through vasodilation and vasoconstriction using finger phototransmission, sweat gland activity, and electrical activity during muscle contraction. Electromyographic biofeedback is the most commonly used biofeedback modality in the clinical setting.

Biofeedback Measures

- Muscle activity
- Heart rate
- Balance
- Skin temperature
- Blood pressure
- Posture
- Abnormal movement
- Normal movement

Types of Biofeedback

- Myoelectric/electromyographic biofeedback
- Position biofeedback
- Blood pressure biofeedback
- Respiratory biofeedback
- Sphincter control biofeedback
- Temperature and blood flow biofeedback
- Electroencephalographic biofeedback

Therapeutic Effects

• Muscle relaxation	• Neuromuscular control
• Improve muscle strength	• Decrease accessory muscle use
• Decrease muscle spasm	• Decrease pain

Indications

• Muscle spasm	• Muscle weakness
• Pain	• Hemiplegia
• Spinal cord injury	• Cerebral palsy
• Urinary incontinence	• Bowel incontinence
• Improve neuromuscular control	• Promote relaxation

Contraindications

• Any condition where muscle contraction is detrimental	• Skin irritation at electrode site

Treatment Guidelines

- ✓ Biofeedback normally uses visual and/or auditory feedback related to the amount of electrical activity detected
- ✓ Biofeedback does not measure muscle contraction but rather the electrical activity associated with muscle contraction
- ✓ Noise is any extraneous electrical activity not produced by the contraction of the muscle
- ✓ Two active electrodes and one ground electrode in a bipolar arrangement best deletes "noise"
- ✓ Surface electrodes with some form of conduction gel are required to adhere to prepared, clean skin
- ✓ The electrodes should be placed parallel to the direction of the muscle fibers
- ✓ Set the level of sensitivity on the device relative to the treatment goals (use low-level sensitivity settings for muscle re-education, use a high-level sensitivity settings for relaxation)

Treatment Parameters: Prior to treatment the therapist should ensure that the patient's skin is clean and dry. The two active electrodes should be placed parallel to the muscle fibers and close to each other. The reference or ground electrode can be placed anywhere on the body, but is often secured between the two active electrodes. The signals are transmitted to a differential amplifier and information is conveyed through visual and audio feedback.

The treatment for muscle re-education should begin with the patient performing a maximal muscle contraction. The sensitivity of the biofeedback unit should be set at a low sensitivity setting and adjusted so that the patient can perform the repetitions at a ratio of two-thirds of the maximal muscle contraction. Isometric contractions should continue for six to ten seconds with relaxation in between each contraction. Treatment duration for a single muscle group is five to ten minutes. The treatment for muscle relaxation requires a high sensitivity setting and a similar electrode placement with active electrodes initially positioned close to each other. As the patient improves with relaxation, the electrodes should be placed further apart and the sensitivity setting increased. During this treatment, the patient may also benefit from adjunct relaxation techniques such as imagery. Treatment duration of 10 to 15 minutes is usually adequate to attain relaxation.

Electrical Equipment Care and Maintenance

The use of electrical equipment can be a potential hazard to both the therapist and the patient. The following is a very abbreviated list of techniques that can minimize the risks of electrical equipment danger.

- Utilize experts to conduct routine inspections to ensure that you meet or exceed all local, state, and federal operation standards.
- Never use a piece of electrical equipment until you have a complete understanding of all aspects of its operation.
- Have routine scheduled service on all electrical equipment at or before the manufacturer's suggested service dates.
- Have repairs performed immediately after the identification of a potential problem.
- Conduct routine inspections of all electrical equipment to identify potential problems.
- Display electrical equipment operation manuals in an accessible location for staff members to use as a resource.

Ground-Fault Circuit Interrupter (GFCI)

A GFCI is a device designed to cut off electrical supply to a piece of equipment if it detects any form of leakage or ground-fault. This prevents a staff member or patient from becoming a ground-fault for electrical current resulting in harmful or deadly injuries.

- All electrical outlets should have the three-prong GFCI outlets
- Ensure all line-powered equipment has a testing seal (maximum leakage of a current < 1 mA)
- Never use extension cord
- Unplug all line-powered equipment at the end of each day
- A sticker should be placed on equipment noting the last inspection/maintenance
- Keep an updated log for all equipment used in the physical therapy department

Electrotherapy Terminology

Accommodation: Accommodation is an occurrence whereby a nerve and muscle membrane's threshold for excitability increases secondary to a stimulation by a pulse that has a slow phase rise time. The quicker the rise time, the less the nerve can accommodate to the impulse.

Alternating current (biphasic): Alternating current allows for the constant change in flow of ions.

Ampere: An ampere is a unit of measure used to describe the rate of current.

Amplitude: Amplitude refers to the magnitude of current. Amplitude controls are often labeled intensity or voltage.

Anode: The anode used during direct current electrotherapy is the positively charged electrode that attracts negative ions.

Biphasic: Biphasic describes a pulse that moves in one direction, returns to baseline, then in the other direction and back to baseline again within a predetermined amount of time.

Types of Biphasic Pulse

Symmetrical: the positive phase is identical to the negative phase

Asymmetrical: the positive phase and the negative phase are not identical in shape

Balanced: the positive phase's electrical charge is equal to the negative phase's electrical charge

Unbalanced: the positive phase and negative phase do not have identical electrical charges

Burst: A burst is an interrupted group of pulses that are delivered in a finite series and a predetermined frequency.

Capacitance: Capacitance is a property of an insulator that allows for the storage of energy when the opposing surfaces of the insulator have an electrical potential difference.

Cathode: The cathode used during direct current electrotherapy is the negatively charged electrode that attracts positive ions.

Chronaxie: Chronaxie is a testing procedure used to measure the amount of time required to produce a small muscle contraction at a particular intensity.

Conductance: Conductance describes the ease at which a particular material will allow current flow (mho).

Current: Current describes the flow of electrons from one place to another.

Direct current (monophasic or Galvanic): Direct current refers to the constant unidirectional flow of ions. The direction of the current is dependent on polarity.

Duration of stimulus/Duration of rest: Duration of stimulus/duration of rest refers to the time period of stimulation and the time period of rest between periods of stimulation. The controls that correspond to the periods of stimulation and rest are labeled on time and off time.

Duty cycle: Duty cycle refers to the percentage of time that electrical current is on in relation to the entire treatment time.

Electrical impedance: Electrical impedance is the resistance of a tissue to electrical current.

Frequency: Frequency determines the number of pulses delivered through each channel per second. Frequency controls are often labeled rate.

High-volt current: High-volt current is characterized by a waveform greater than 150 volts with a short pulse duration. High-volt is intermittent and is used for deeper tissue penetration.

Impedance: Impedance is the property of a substance that provides resistance to the flow of current by offering an alternate current.

Inductance: Inductance describes how easily a certain material will induce an electromotive force (emf) within a circuit.

Interpulse interval: The interpulse interval is the period of time of electrical inactivity between each pulse, usually expressed in microseconds or milliseconds.

Ion: An ion is a positively or negatively charged atom.

Low-volt current: Low-volt current is characterized by a waveform of less than 150 volts and is used for neuromuscular stimulation.

Monophasic: Monophasic describes a pulse that has either a positive or negative polarity and moves in only one direction from a zero baseline and returns to the baseline within a predetermined amount of time.

Negative ion: A negative ion has gained one or more electrons and possesses a negative charge.

Ohm's law: Ohm's law describes the current of an electrical circuit. There is a direct proportional relationship between current and voltage and an indirect proportional relationship between current and resistance.

Positive ion: A positive ion has lost one or more electrons and possesses a positive charge.

Pulse: A pulse is one individual waveform.

Pulse duration: The pulse duration is the amount of time that it takes to complete all phases of a single pulse (which is also termed the positive phase of the waveform). Pulse duration controls are often labeled pulse width.

Pulsed current (interrupted): Pulsed current allows for a non-continuous flow of either alternating or direct current with periods of no electrical activity.

Ramp: Ramp refers to the number of seconds it takes for the amplitude to gradually increase or decrease to the maximum value set by the amplitude control.

Resistance: Resistance describes the ability of a material to oppose the flow of ions through it.

Rheobase: Rheobase is the minimal intensity used with a long current duration that produces a small muscle contraction.

Volt: A volt is a unit of measure of electrical power or electromotive force.

Waveform: A waveform is the consistent pattern of a current measured on an oscilloscope.

Chapter 7

Safety & Professional Roles; Teaching/Learning; Research

Safety & Professional Roles

Ergonomic Guidelines

Workstation Recommendations

- ✓ 18-20 inch monitor
- ✓ Easily adjustable monitor to angle or tilt
- ✓ Split keyboard preferred
- ✓ Adjustable feet for the keyboard
- ✓ Minimum of six feet length for keyboard cord
- ✓ Monitor display should be directed ten degrees below the horizontal
- ✓ Monitor should be placed at least twenty inches away from the eyes
- ✓ Minimum of 30 inches depth for desk surface to accommodate monitor and keyboard
- ✓ Chair should swivel 360 degrees for easy access
- ✓ Wrist rests should match the front edge of the keyboard in order to maximize comfort
- ✓ Hands-free telephone set preferred
- ✓ Use a mouse that contours to the hand and has sufficient cord length
- ✓ 30-second exercise break every hour while at a desk
- ✓ Space under the desk should be at least 30" wide, 19" deep, and 27" in height; there should be 2-3 inches between the top of the thighs and the desk

Workstation Posture

Head: level, facing forward, in line with trunk

Shoulders: relaxed, arms at side

Elbows: remain close to trunk, bent 90-120 degrees

Forearms, wrists, hands: parallel to the floor, straight

Trunk: maintain normal curves of the spine with appropriate lumbar support, shoulders and pelvis are level

Hips, thighs: well supported with contoured seat, parallel to the floor

Knees: maintain a level position with a 90 degree angle of flexion, knees generally at the same height as the hips

Feet: place feet flat on the floor or supported in a slight incline

Body Mechanics

A therapist must consistently use proper body mechanics when treating patients and avoid unnecessary stress and strain by maintaining proper alignment within the musculoskeletal system.

Principles of Proper Body Mechanics

- Use the shortest lever arm possible
- Stay close to the patient when possible
- Use larger muscles to perform heavy work
- Maintain a wide base of support
- Avoid any rotary movement when lifting
- Attempt to maintain the center of gravity of the therapist and patient within the base of support

Lifting Guidelines

- ✓ Always attempt to increase your base of support
- ✓ Maintain a proper lumbar curve as you lift
- ✓ Pivot your feet when lifting; do not twist your back to turn
- ✓ Maintain a slow and consistent speed while lifting
- ✓ Only lift an object as a last resort

Deep Squat Lift

1. Begin with hips below the level of the knees
2. Assume a wide base of support
3. Straddle the object
4. Grasp the object from each side or from beneath
5. The trunk should remain vertical
6. Maintain a lumbar lordosis and anterior pelvic tilt

Half-Kneeling Lift

1. Begin in a half-kneel position
2. The bottom leg should be positioned behind and to the side of the object
3. Maintain a normal lumbar lordosis
4. Lift the object onto the knee and draw it closer to the trunk
5. Continue the lift by holding the object close as you assume a standing position

One Leg Stance Lift

1. Used for lifting light objects that can be lifted with one extremity
2. Face the object in a lunge position
3. Shift weight onto the forward extremity
4. Flex the forward extremity and lower to reach the object
5. The hind leg rises off the ground to counterbalance the shift in weight
6. Maintain a neutral spine throughout the lift

Power Lift

1. Begin with the hips above the level of the knees
2. Assume a wide base of support behind the object with the feet parallel to each other
3. Grasp the object from each side or from underneath
4. The trunk should remain in a vertical position
5. Maintain a lumbar lordosis and anterior tilt

Traditional Lift

1. Begin with the lower extremities in a full squat facing the object
2. The feet should be positioned in an anterior-posterior manner on each side of the object
3. Grasp the object and flex the upper extremities to initiate the lift
4. Use bilateral lower extremities to provide the work of the lift
5. Keep the object close to the trunk during the lift
6. Maintain normal lumbar lordosis
7. Do not lift with the back

Pushing or Pulling an Object

✓ Use a semi-squat position to push or pull
✓ Apply the force parallel to the surface that the object should be moved upon
✓ Exert an initial force that is adequate to overcome the counter force of inertia and friction
✓ Attempt to push, pull, slide or roll the object prior to lifting or carrying an object

Infection Control

Infectious Disease

Infectious disease is defined as a condition where an organism invades a host and develops a parasitic relationship with the host. The invasion and multiplication of the microorganisms produces an immune response with subsequent signs and symptoms.

Potential Symptoms of Infectious Disease

• Fever, chill, malaise	• Headache
• Rash, skin lesion	• Stiff neck
• Bleeding from gums	• Myalgia
• Joint effusion	• Convulsions
• Diarrhea	• Confusion
• Frequency, urgency	• Tachycardia
• Cough, sore throat	• Hypotension
• Nausea, vomiting	

Chain of Transmission for Infection

1. Causative agent, bacteria, pathogen, virus
2. Reservoir of humans, animals, inanimate objects
3. Portal of exit through blood, intestinal tract, respiratory tract, skin/mucous membrane, open lesion, excretions, tears or semen
4. Transmission through airborne, contact, vector, vehicle or droplet modes
5. Portal of entry through non-intact skin, blood, mucous membrane, inhalation, ingestion or percutaneous injection
6. Susceptible host regarding age, health status, nutrition, and environmental status

Standard Precautions

Standard precautions are revised guidelines that update Universal precautions and are designed for the care of all patients in hospitals regardless of infection or diagnosis.

These precautions combine Universal and body substance isolation precautions and apply to all blood/body fluids, secretions, and excretions.

Standard Precautions

Hand washing

✓ Use plain soap for routine hand washing; use an antimicrobial agent for specific incidences based on the infection control policy.

Gloves

✓ Wear gloves when touching all body fluids, blood secretions, excretions, and contaminated items.

✓ Change gloves between tasks with a patient after coming in contact with infectious material. Remove gloves immediately, avoid touching non-contaminated items, and wash hands at that time.

Mask

✓ Wear a mask/eye protection/face shield for protection during activities that are at risk for splashing of any body fluids.

Gown

✓ Wear a gown for protection during activities that are at risk for splashing of any body fluids. Remove gown immediately and wash hands.

Patient Care Equipment

✓ Handle all patient equipment in a manner that prevents transfer of microorganisms.
✓ Ensure that all reusable equipment is properly sanitized prior to reuse.

Occupational Health and Bloodborne Pathogens

✓ Vigilance is required when handling/disposing of sharp instruments. Never recap needles or remove syringes by hand. All sharps disposal should use puncture-resistant containers.
✓ Mouthpieces, resuscitation bags, and ventilation devices should be used as an alternative to mouth-to-mouth resuscitation.

Transmission-based Precautions

Transmission-based precautions are updated guidelines for the particular care of specified patients infected with epidemiologically important pathogens transmitted by airborne, droplet or contact modes. These are additional precautions that should be implemented in addition to standard precautions.

Airborne Precautions

Airborne precautions reduce risk of airborne transmission of infectious agents through evaporated droplets in air or dust particles containing infectious agents

- Private room with monitored air pressure
- Six to twelve air changes within the room per hour
- Room door should remain closed with patient remaining within the room
- Respiratory protection worn when entering room
- Limit patient's transport outside of the room for only essential purposes; patient should wear a mask during transport

Examples:

measles, varicella, tuberculosis

Droplet Precautions

Droplet precautions reduce the risk of droplet transmission of infectious agents through contact of the mucous membranes of the mouth and nose; contact with the conjunctivae, through coughing, sneezing, talking or suctioning. This transmission requires close contact, as the infectious agents do not suspend in the air and travel only three feet or less.

- Private room
- May share a room with a patient that has active infection of the same microorganism
- Maintain at least three feet between the patient and any contact (patient, staff, visitor)
- Room door may remain open
- Wear a mask when working within three feet of the patient
- Limit the patient's transport outside of the room for only essential purposes; patient should wear a mask during transport

Examples:

Bacterial include: Hemophilus influenza (including meningitis, pneumonia, epiglottis, sepsis), Neisseria meningitidis (including meningitis, pneumonia, epiglottis, sepsis), Diphtheria, Mycoplasma pneumonia, Pertussis, Streptococcal (group A)

Viral include: Adenovirus, Influenza, Mumps, Parovirus B19, Rubella

Contact Precautions

Contact precautions reduce the risk of transmission of infectious agents through direct or indirect contact. Direct contact involves skin-to-skin transmission; indirect contact involves a contaminated intermediate object, usually within the patient's environment.

- Private room
- May share a room with a patient that has active infection of the same microorganism
- Use of gloves when entering the room
- Change of gloves after direct contact with infectious material
- Take gloves off prior to leaving the room and perform proper hand washing technique
- Wear a gown if you will have substantial close contact with the patient and remove the gown prior to leaving the room
- Limit patient's transport outside of the room for essential purposes only
- Dedicate non-critical patient care equipment to one patient, do not share between patients or disinfect properly prior to using the equipment again

Examples:

Gastrointestinal, respiratory, skin or wound infections, multi-drug resistant bacteria, Clostridium difficile, Enterohemorrhagic escherichia coli, Shigella, Hepatitis A (for incontinence/diapered), Parainfluenza virus or enteroviral infection (infants/young children), Diphtheria, Herpes simplex virus, Impetigo, Pediculosis, Scabies, Zoster, Viral hemorrhagic infections (Ebola)

Nosocomial Infections

A term used to describe an infection that is acquired during a hospitalization. The primary factor in the prevention of nosocomial infection is proper hand washing. Staff must also follow standard precautions and all infection control procedures at all times.

"The CDC Guidelines for Isolation Precautions in Hospitals" is a document that outlines the guidelines from collaboration between the Centers for Disease Control and Prevention (CDC) and the Hospital Infection Control Practices Advisory Committee (HICPAC). This document describes infection control within the hospital setting and provides strategies for surveillance, prevention, and control of nosocomial infections within the hospital setting.

Application of Sterile Protective Garments

Gowns

- ✓ Hold gown firmly away from the sterile field
- ✓ Shake gown open so it unfolds and keep hands above waist level
- ✓ Touch only the inside of the gown as you place both arms into the sleeves
- ✓ Stop when hands reach the sleeve cuff
- ✓ The gown is tied in back

Sterile Gloves

- ✓ Use the gown's sleeve cuffs as mittens and open the glove pack
- ✓ The sterile glove has a fold at the wrist where the inside (exposed) of the glove is not sterile
- ✓ Grasp the right glove with the left hand (still using the sleeve cuff as a mitten) and pull it on over the open end of the gown sleeve
- ✓ The first three fingers of the right hand should reach under the fold (touching the sterile portion of the left glove) and hold the glove while the left hand positions inside the glove
- ✓ Once both gloves are donned the left glove can unfold the right glove's cuff

Cap and Mask

- ✓ Wash hands
- ✓ Avoid contact with the hair while applying the cap
- ✓ All hair must be contained within the cap
- ✓ Apply a mask, if necessary, by first positioning the mask over the bridge of the nose
- ✓ The mask should form to fit securely over the nose and mouth
- ✓ Secure the upper ties behind the head and the lower ties behind the neck

Sterile Field Guidelines

- ✓ All items on a sterile field must be (and remain) sterile
- ✓ The edges of all packaging of sterile items become non-sterile once the package is opened
- ✓ Sterile gowns are only considered sterile in the front from the waist level upwards, including the sleeves
- ✓ Only the top surface of the table or sterile drape is considered sterile, with the outer one-inch of the field considered non-sterile
- ✓ Avoid all unnecessary activity around the sterile field
- ✓ Do not talk, sneeze or cough, as it will contaminate the sterile field
- ✓ Do not turn your back to a sterile field as the back of the gown is not sterile; constant observation of the sterile field is required
- ✓ If an object on the sterile field becomes contaminated, the field is considered non-sterile and should be discarded
- ✓ Sterile fields should never be left unattended and should be prepared as close to the treatment time as possible in order to further avoid contamination
- ✓ Any item that positions or falls below waist-level is considered contaminated

Infection Control Terminology

Asepsis: The elimination of the microorganisms that cause infection and the creation of a sterile field.

Contamination: A term used to describe an area, surface or item coming in contact with something that is not sterile. Contamination assumes an environment that contains microorganisms.

Hand washing: Hand washing is an important technique for asepsis. Guidelines for acceptable hand washing are as follows:

- ✓ Use warm water
- ✓ Remove all jewelry
- ✓ Wash hands with soap for at least 30 seconds (the time it takes to sing "Happy Birthday" twice)
- ✓ Avoid touching any contaminated surface
- ✓ Rinse thoroughly
- ✓ Use a paper towel barrier when turning off the water

Medical asepsis: A technique that attempts to contain pathogens to a specific area, object or person. A primary goal is to reduce the spread of pathogens. Example: A patient with tuberculosis is hospitalized and kept in isolation.

Personal protective equipment (PPE): Items that are worn and used as barriers to protect someone who is assisting a patient with a potentially infectious disease. Personal protective equipment includes gowns, lab coats, masks, gloves, goggles, spill kits, and mouthpieces.

Sterile field: A sterile field is used to maintain surgical asepsis. A sterile field is a designated area that is considered void of all contaminants and microorganisms. There are standard and required protocols that must be followed in order to develop and maintain a sterile field.

Surgical asepsis: A state in which an area or object is without any microorganisms. Example: A sterile field.

Accessibility

Americans with Disabilities Act

The Americans with Disabilities Act is designed to provide a clear and comprehensive national mandate for the elimination of discrimination. The Americans with Disabilities Act (PL101-336) is federal legislation that was signed into law on July 26, 1990.

The Americans with Disabilities Act is divided into five titles:

Title I	Employment
Title II	Public Services
Title III	Public Accommodations
Title IV	Telecommunications
Title V	Miscellaneous

The Americans with Disabilities Act applies primarily, but not exclusively, to "disabled" individuals. An individual is "disabled" if they meet at least one of the following criteria:

- They have a physical or mental impairment that substantially limits one or more of their major life activities.
- They have a record of such an impairment.
- They are regarded as having such an impairment.

The Employment provisions (Title I) apply to employers of fifteen employees or more. The Public Accommodations provisions (Title III) apply to all businesses, regardless of the number of employees.

Employers are required to make reasonable accommodation for qualified individuals with a disability, who are defined by the Americans with Disabilities Act as individuals who satisfy the job-related requirements of a position held or desired, and who can perform the "essential functions" of such position with or without reasonable accommodation. The Americans with Disabilities Act does not require employers to make accommodations that pose an "undue hardship." "Undue hardship" is defined as significantly difficult or expensive accommodations.

Accessibility Requirements

Ramp	Grade < 8.3% At least 36 inch width Must have handrails on both sides Twelve inches of length for each inch of vertical rise Handrails required for a rise of six inches or more or for a horizontal run of 72 inches or more
Doorway	Minimum 32 inch width Maximum 24 inch depth
Threshold	Less than ¾ inch for sliding doors Less than ½ inch for other doors
Carpet	Requires ½ inch pile or less
Hallway clearance	36 inch width
Wheelchair turning radius (U-turn)	60 inch width 78 inch length
Forward reach in wheelchair	Low reach 15 inches High reach 48 inches

Side reach in wheelchair	Reach over obstruction to 24 inches
Bathroom sink	Not less than 29 inch height Not greater than 40 inches from floor to bottom of mirror or paper dispenser 17 inch minimum depth under sink to back wall
Bathroom toilet	17-19 inches from floor to top of toilet Not less than 36 inch grab bars Grab bars should be 1¼ - 1½ inches in diameter 1½ inch spacing between grab bars and wall Grab bar placement 33-36 inches up from floor level
Hotel	Approximately 2% total rooms must be accessible
Parking space	96 inch width 240 inch length Adjacent aisle must be 60 inches by 240 inches Approximately 2% of the total spaces must be accessible

Sources of Additional Information The Americans with Disabilities Act:

Employment

Equal Opportunity Commission
131 M Street, NE
Fourth Floor, Suite 4NW02F
Washington, DC 20507-0100
(800) 669-4000
(202) 663-4900
www.eeoc.gov

Public Accommodations

Department of Justice
Office on the Americans with Disabilities Act
Civil Rights Division
950 Pennsylvania Ave, NW
Washington, DC 20530
(202) 307-0663
www.usdoj.gov
www.ada.gov

Transportation

Department of Transportation
1200 New Jersey Ave, SE
Washington, DC 20590
(202) 366-4000
www.dot.gov

Accessible Design in New Construction and Alterations

Architectural and Transportation Barriers and Compliance Board
1331 F Street, NW
Suite 1000
Washington, DC 20004-1111
(800) 872-2253
www.access-board.gov

Telecommunications

Federal Communications Commission
445 12th Street SW
Washington, DC 20554
(888) 225-5322
www.fcc.gov

Documentation

Purpose of Documentation

- Communicate with other treating professionals
- Assistance with discharge planning
- Reimbursement
- Assistance with utilization review
- A legal document regarding the course of therapy

Types of Documentation

Record

- An increase in specialization of care and multidisciplinary treatment increases the need for medical records to serve as a means of communication among clinicians.
- Progress notes and referrals related directly to patient care are examples of clinical records.
- Departmental statistics and records are examples of administrative records.

Referral

- Acceptable forms of referral range from a signed prescription form to a highly structured checklist. The referral must include the name of the patient and be signed and dated by the referring physician.
- Referrals commonly include some indication as to the number and frequency of treatments desired and any special precautions or instructions.

Progress Note

- Improvement of patient care is the most important function of progress notes.
- Progress notes allow members of all health services to know what the patient is accomplishing in each given area.
- Progress notes should contain patient identification, the date, and the signature of the therapist.
- Progress notes should be written when the patient's condition changes during the course of treatment.
- Specific frequency of progress notes is usually dictated by department policy.
- Appropriate forms of documentation include diagrams, videotapes, and flow sheets as well as many other less frequently used media.

S.O.A.P. Note

A commonly used record to write daily notes is the S.O.A.P. note. S.O.A.P. stands for:

S: Subjective
O: Objective
A: Assessment
P: Plan

Subjective: Refers to information the patient communicates to the therapist. This could include social or medical history not previously recorded. It could also include the patient's statements or complaints.

Objective: Refers to information the therapist observes. Common examples include range of motion measurements, muscle strength, and functional abilities. It also includes manual techniques and equipment used during treatment.

Assessment: Allows the therapist to express their professional opinion. Short and long-term goals are often expressed in this section as well as changes in the treatment program.

Plan: Includes ideas for future physical therapy sessions. Frequency and expected duration of physical therapy services can also be incorporated into this section.

Discharge Summary

A discharge summary should provide a capsule view of the patient's progress during therapy. The discharge summary is usually conducted on the day of the patient's last therapy session.

Guidelines for Physical Therapy Documentation of Patient/Client Management

Preamble

The American Physical Therapy Association (APTA) is committed to meeting the physical therapy needs of society, to meeting the needs and interests of its members and to developing and improving the art and science of physical therapy, including practice, education, and research. To help meet these responsibilities, the APTA Board of Directors has approved the following guidelines for physical therapy documentation. It is recognized that these guidelines do not reflect all of the unique documentation requirements associated with the many specialty areas within the physical therapy profession. Applicable for both handwritten and electronic documentation systems, these guidelines are intended to be used as a foundation for the development of more specific documentation guidelines in specialty areas, while at the same time providing guidance for the physical therapy profession across all practice settings. Documentation may also need to address additional regulatory or payer requirements.

APTA Position on Documentation

Physical therapy examination, evaluation, diagnosis, prognosis and intervention, shall be documented, dated, and authenticated by the physical therapist that performs the service. Intervention provided by the physical therapist or selected interventions provided by the physical therapist assistant is documented, dated, and authenticated by the physical therapist or, when permissible by law, the physical therapist assistant.

Other notations or flow charts are considered a component of the documented record but do not meet the requirements of documentation in, or of, themselves.

Students in physical therapist or physical therapist assistant programs may document when the record is additionally authenticated by the physical therapist or, when permissible by law, the physical therapist assistant.

Operational Definitions

Guidelines: APTA defines "guidelines" as a statement of advice.

Authentication: The process used to verify that an entry is complete, accurate, and final. Indications of authentication can include original written signatures and computer "signatures" on secured electronic record systems only.

The following describes the main documentation elements of patient/client management: 1. initial examination/ evaluation; 2. visit/encounter; 3. re-examination and 4. discharge/discontinuation summary

Initial Examination/Evaluation: Documentation of the initial encounter is typically called the "initial examination", "initial evaluation" or "initial examination/evaluation." Completion of the initial examination/evaluation is typically completed in one visit, but may occur over more than one visit. Documentation elements for the initial examination/ evaluation include the following:

Examination: Includes data obtained from the history, systems review, and tests and measures.

Evaluation: Evaluation is a thought process that may not include formal documentation. It may include documentation of the assessment of the data collected in the examination and identification of problems pertinent to patient/client management.

Diagnosis: Indicates level of impairment and functional limitation determined by the physical therapist. May be indicated by selecting one or more preferred practice patterns from the Guide to Physical Therapist Practice.

Prognosis: Provides documentation of the predicted level of improvement that might be attained through intervention and the amount of time required to reach that level. Prognosis is typically not a separate documentation element, but the components are included as part of the plan of care.

Plan of care: Typically stated in general terms, includes goals, interventions planned, proposed frequency and duration, and discharge plans.

Visit/Encounter: Documentation of a visit or encounter, often called a progress note or daily note, documents sequential implementation of the plan of care established by the physical therapist, including changes in patient/ client status and variations and progressions of specific interventions used. Also may include specific plans for the next visit or visits.

Reexamination: Documentation of reexamination includes data from repeated or new examination elements and is provided to evaluate progress and to modify or redirect intervention.

Discharge or Discontinuation Summary: Documentation is required following conclusion of the current episode in the physical therapy intervention sequence, to summarize progression toward goals and discharge plans.

General Guidelines

- Documentation is required for every visit/encounter.
- All documentation must comply with the applicable jurisdictional/regulatory requirements.
- All handwritten entries shall be made in ink and will include original signatures. Electronic entries are made with appropriate security and confidentiality provisions.
- Charting errors should be corrected by drawing a single line through the error and initializing/dating the chart or through the appropriate mechanism for electronic documentation that clearly indicates change was made without deletion of the original record.
- All documentation must include adequate identification of the patient and the physical therapist or physical therapist assistant:

  ✓ The patient's/client's full name and identification number, if applicable, must be included on all official documents.
  ✓ All entries must be dated and authenticated with the provider's full name and appropriate designation:

    1. Documentation of examination, evaluation, diagnosis, prognosis, plan of care, and discharge summary must be authenticated by the physical therapist that provided the service.
    2. Documentation of the intervention in a visit/ encounter note must be authenticated by the physical therapist that provided the service.
    3. Documentation by graduates or others pending receipt of an unrestricted license shall be authenticated by a licensed physical therapist.
    4. Documentation by students (SPT/SPTA) in physical therapist or physical therapist assistant programs must be additionally authenticated by the physical therapist or, when permissible by law, documentation by physical therapist assistant students may be authenticated by a physical therapist assistant.

- Documentation should include the referral mechanism by which physical therapy services are initiated. Examples include:

  - Self-referral/direct access
  - Request for consultation from another practitioner
  - Documentation should include indication of no shows and cancellations

Initial Examination/Evaluation

Examination

History: Documentation of history may include the following:

- General demographics
- Social history
- Employment/work
- Growth and development
- Living environment
- General health status
- Social/health habits
- Family history
- Medical/surgical history
- Current condition(s)/chief complaint(s)
- Functional status and activity level
- Medications
- Other clinical tests

Systems Review: Documentation of systems review may include gathering data for the following systems:

Cardiovascular/pulmonary

- Blood pressure
- Edema
- Heart Rate
- Respiratory Rate

Integumentary

- Pliability (texture)
- Presence of scar formation
- Skin color
- Skin integrity

Musculoskeletal

- Gross range of motion
- Gross strength
- Gross symmetry
- Height
- Weight

Neuromuscular

- Gross coordinated movement (e.g., balance, locomotion, transfers, and transition)
- Motor function (motor control, motor learning)

Documentation of systems review may also address communication ability, affect, cognition, language, and learning style:

- Ability to make needs known
- Consciousness
- Expected emotional/behavioral responses
- Learning preferences
- Orientation (person, place, time)

Tests and Measures: Documentation of tests and measures may include findings for the following categories:

Aerobic Capacity/Endurance

Examples of examination findings include:

- Aerobic capacity during functional activities
- Aerobic capacity during standardized exercise test protocols
- Cardiovascular signs and symptoms in response to increased oxygen demand with exercise or activity
- Pulmonary signs and symptoms in response to increased oxygen demand with exercise or activity

Anthropometric Characteristics

Examples of examination findings include:

- Body composition
- Body dimensions
- Edema

Arousal, Attention, and Cognition

Examples of examination findings include:

- Arousal and attention
- Cognition
- Communication
- Consciousness
- Motivation
- Orientation to time, person, place, and situation
- Recall

Assistive and Adaptive Devices

Examples of examination findings include:

- Assistive or adaptive devices and equipment use during functional activities
- Components, alignment, fit, and ability to care for the assistive or adaptive devices and equipment
- Remediation of impairments, functional limitations, or disabilities with use of assistive or adaptive devices and equipment
- Safety during use of assistive or adaptive devices and equipment

Circulation (Arterial, Venous, Lymphatic)

Examples of examination findings include:

- Cardiovascular signs
- Cardiovascular symptoms
- Physiological responses to position change

Cranial and Peripheral Nerve Integrity

Examples of examination findings include:

- Electrophysiological integrity
- Motor distribution of the cranial nerves
- Motor distribution of the peripheral nerves
- Response to neural provocation
- Response to stimuli, including auditory, visual, gustatory, olfactory, pharyngeal, and vestibular
- Sensory distribution of the cranial nerves
- Sensory distribution of the peripheral nerves

Environmental, Home, and Work Barriers

Examples of examination findings include:

- Current and potential barriers
- Physical space and environment

Ergonomics and Body Mechanics

Examples of examination findings for ergonomics include:

- Dexterity and coordination during work
- Functional capacity and performance during work actions, tasks, or activities
- Safety in work environments
- Specific work conditions or activities
- Tools, devices, equipment, and workstations related to work actions, tasks, or activities

Examples of examination findings for body mechanics include:

- Body mechanics during self-care, home management, work, community, or leisure actions, tasks, or activities

Gait, Locomotion, and Balance

Examples of examination findings include:

- Balance during functional activities with or without the use of assistive, adaptive, orthotic, protection, supportive, or prosthetic devices or equipment
- Balance (dynamic and static) with or without the use of assistive, adaptive, orthotic, protective, supportive, or prosthetic devices or equipment
- Gait and locomotion during functional activities with or without the use of assistive, adaptive, orthotic, protective, supportive, or prosthetic devices or equipment
- Gait and locomotion with or without the use of assistive, adaptive, orthotic, protective, supportive, or prosthetic devices or equipment
- Safety during gait, locomotion, and balance

Integumentary Integrity

Examples of examination findings include:

Associated with skin

- Activities, positioning, and postures that produce or relieve trauma to the skin
- Assistive, adaptive, orthotic, protective, supportive, or prosthetic devices and equipment that may produce or relieve trauma to the skin
- Skin characteristics

Wound

- Activities, positioning, or postures that aggravate the wound or scar or that produce or relieve trauma
- Burn
- Signs of infection
- Wound characteristics
- Wound scar tissue characteristics

Joint Integrity

Examples of examination findings include:

- Joint integrity and mobility
- Joint play movements
- Specific body parts

Motor Function

Examples of examination findings include:

- Dexterity, coordination, and agility
- Electrophysiological integrity
- Hand function
- Initiation, modification, and control of movement patterns and voluntary postures

Muscle Performance

Examples of examination findings include:

- Electrophysiological integrity
- Muscle strength, power, and endurance
- Muscle strength, power, and endurance during functional activities
- Muscle tension

Neuromotor Development and Sensory Integration

Examples of examination findings include:

- Acquisition and evolution of motor skills
- Oral motor function, phonation, and speech production
- Sensorimotor integration

Orthotic, Protective, and Supportive Devices

Examples of examination findings include:

- Components, alignment, fit, and ability to care for the orthotic, protective, and supportive devices and equipment
- Orthotic, protective, and supportive devices and equipment use during functional activities
- Remediation of impairments, functional limitations, or disabilities with use of orthotic, protective, and supportive devices and equipment
- Safety during use of orthotic, protective, and supportive devices and equipment

Pain

Examples of examination findings include:

- Pain, soreness, and nociception
- Pain in specific body parts

Posture

Examples of examination findings include:

- Postural alignment and position (dynamic)
- Postural alignment and position (static)
- Specific body parts

Prosthetic Requirements

Examples of examination findings include:

- Components, alignment, fit, and ability to care for prosthetic device
- Prosthetic device use during functional activities
- Remediation of impairments, functional limitations, or disabilities with use of the prosthetic device
- Residual limb or adjacent segment
- Safety during use of the prosthetic device

Range of Motion

Examples of examination findings include:

- Functional ROM
- Joint active and passive movement
- Muscle length, soft tissue extensibility, and flexibility

Reflex Integrity

Examples of examination findings include:

- Deep reflexes
- Electrophysiological integrity
- Postural reflexes and reactions, including righting, equilibrium, and protective reactions
- Primitive reflexes and reactions
- Resistance to passive stretch
- Superficial reflexes and reactions

Self-Care and Home Management

Examples of examination findings include:

- Ability to gain access to home environments
- Ability to perform self-care and home management activities with or without assistive, adaptive, orthotic, protective, supportive, or prosthetic devices and equipment
- Safety in self-care and home management activities and environments

Sensory Integrity

Examples of examination findings include:

- Combined/cortical sensations
- Deep sensations
- Electrophysiological integrity

Ventilation and Respiration

Examples of examination findings include:

- Pulmonary signs of respiration/gas exchange
- Pulmonary signs of ventilatory function
- Pulmonary symptoms

Work (job/school/play), community and leisure integration or reintegration

Examples of examination findings include:

- Ability to assume or resume work (job/school/play), community and leisure activities with or without assistive, adaptive, orthotic, protective, supportive, or prosthetic devices and equipment
- Ability to gain access to work (job/school/play), community and leisure environments
- Safety in work (job/school/play), community and leisure activities and environments

Evaluation

Evaluation is a thought process that may not include formal documentation. However, the evaluation process may lead to documentation of impairments, functional limitations, and disabilities using formats such as:

- A problem list
- A statement of assessment of key factors (e.g., cognitive factors, co-morbidities, social support) influencing the patient/client status.

Diagnosis

Documentation of a diagnosis determined by the physical therapist may include impairment and functional limitations. Examples include:

- Impaired joint mobility, motor function, muscle performance, and range of motion associated with localized inflammation (4E)
- Impaired motor function and sensory integrity associated with progressive disorders of the central nervous system (5E)
- Impaired aerobic capacity/endurance associated with cardiovascular pump dysfunction or failure (6D)
- Impaired integumentary integrity associated with partial-thickness skin involvement and scar formation (7C)

Prognosis

Documentation of the prognosis is typically included in the plan of care. See below.

Plan of Care

Documentation of the plan of care includes the following:

- Overall goals stated in measurable terms that indicate the predicted level of improvement in function
- A general statement of interventions to be used
- Proposed duration and frequency of service required to reach the goals
- Anticipated discharge plans

Visit/Encounter

Documentation of each visit/encounter shall include the following elements:

- Patient/client self-report (as appropriate)
- Identification of specific interventions provided, including frequency, intensity, and duration as appropriate. Examples include:
  - ✓ Knee extension, three sets, ten repetitions, 10# weight
  - ✓ Transfer training bed to chair with sliding board
  - ✓ Equipment provided

- Changes in patient/client impairment, functional limitation, and disability status as they relate to the plan of care
- Response to interventions, including adverse reactions, if any
- Factors that modify frequency or intensity of intervention and progression, including patient/client adherence to patient/client related instructions/consultation
- Communication with providers/patient/client/family/significant other
- Documentation to plan for ongoing provision of services for the next visit(s), which is suggested to include, but not be limited to:
  - ✓ The interventions with objectives
  - ✓ Progression parameters
  - ✓ Precautions, if indicated

Reexamination

Documentation of reexamination shall include the following elements:

- Documentation of selected components of examination to update patient's impairment, function, and/or disability status
- Interpretation of findings and, when indicated, revision of goals
- When indicated, revision of plan of care, as directly correlated with goals as documented

Discharge/Discontinuation Summary

Documentation of discharge or discontinuation shall include the following elements:

- Current physical/functional status
- Degree of goals achieved and reasons for goals not being achieved
- Discharge/discontinuation plan related to the patient/client's continuing care. Examples include:
  - ✓ Home program
  - ✓ Referrals for additional services
  - ✓ Recommendations for follow-up physical therapy care
  - ✓ Family and caregiver training
  - ✓ Equipment provided

From American Physical Therapy Association, 2008.

Top 10 Tips for Defensible Documentation

1. Limit use of abbreviations
2. Date and sign all entries
3. Document legibly
4. Report progress towards goals regularly
5. Document at the time of the visit when possible
6. Clearly identify note types (e.g., progress reports, daily notes)
7. Include all related communications
8. Include missed or cancelled visits
9. Demonstrate skilled care
10. Demonstrate discharge planning through the episode of care

From American Physical Therapy Association, web site 2009.

Top 10 Payer Complaints Regarding Documentation

1. Poor legibility
2. Incomplete documentation
3. No documentation for date of service
4. Abbreviations, too many, cannot understand
5. Does not demonstrate skilled care
6. Documentation does not support the billing code
7. Does not support medical necessity
8. Does not demonstrate progress
9. Repetitious daily notes showing no change in patient status
10. Interventions with no clarification of time, frequency, duration

From American Physical Therapy Association, web site 2009.

Symbols Commonly Used in Clinical Practice

Symbol	Meaning	Symbol	Meaning
=	Equal	±	Very slight trace or reaction, indefinite
≠	Unequal	+	Slight trace or reaction, positive, plus excess, acid reaction
>	Greater than	++	Trace or notable reaction
<	Less than	+++	Moderate amount of reaction
↑	Increase	++++	Large amount or pronounced reaction
↗	Increasing	#	Number, pound, has been given or done
↓	Decrease	→	Yields, leads to
↘	Decreasing	←	Resulting from or secondary to
−	Negative, minus, deficiency, alkaline, reaction	1°, 2°	Primary, secondary

From Miller-Keane: Encyclopedia and Dictionary of Medicine, Nursing, and Allied Health. W.B. Saunders Company, Philadelphia 1997, p.1802, with permission.

Military Time

The 24-hour clock (military time) is used to standardize time in the medical record.

Standard Time	Military Time
Noon	1200 hours
1:00 PM	1300 hours
2:00 PM	1400 hours
3:00 PM	1500 hours
4:00 PM	1600 hours
5:00 PM	1700 hours
6:00 PM	1800 hours
7:00 PM	1900 hours
8:00 PM	2000 hours
9:00 PM	2100 hours
10:00 PM	2200 hours
11:00 PM	2300 hours
Midnight	2400 hours

Measurement

Length

1 cm	= 0.3937 inch
1 m	= 39.37 inches = 3.28 ft = 1.09 yds
1 km	= 0.62 mile
1 inch	= 2.54 centimeters (cm) = 25.4 millimeters (mm) = 0.0254 meters (m)
1 foot	= 30.48 cm = 304.8 mm = 0.304 m
1 mile	= 5280 ft = 1760 yds = 1609.35 m = 1.61 kilometers (km)

Temperature

0°C	= 32°F = 273°K
100°C	= 212°F
°C	= (°F - 32) x 5/9
°F	= (°C x 9/5) + 32

Weight

1 ounce (oz)	= 0.0625 pounds (lb) = 28.35 grams (g) = 0.028 kilograms (kg)
1 pound (lb)	= 16 oz = 454 g = 0.454 kg
1 g	= 0.035 oz = 0.0022 lb = 0.001 kg
1 kg	= 35.27 oz = 2.2 lb = 1000 g

Energy and Work

1 kcal	= 3086 foot-pounds (ft-lbs) = 426.4 kilogram-meter (kg-m) = kilojoules (kJ)
1 kJ	= 1000 joules (J) = 0.23892 kcal
1 liter O_2 consumed	= 5.05 kcal = 15.575 ft-lbs = 2153 kg-m = 21.237 kJ
1 MET	= 3.5 mL O_2/kg-min = 0.0175 kcal/kg = 0.0732 kJ/kg
1 ft-lb	= 0.1383 kg-m
1 kg-m	= 7.23 ft-lbs

Metric versus United States Units of Measure

1 inch	= 2.54 centimeters	1 kilogram	= 2.2 pounds
1 foot	= 30.5 centimeters	1 pound	= 4.45 Newtons
1 mile	= 1.61 kilometers	1 liter	= .2642 gallons
1 meter	= 3.28 feet	1 milliliter	= .0338 once
1 gram	= .0353 ounce	1 gallon	= 3.785 liters
1 ounce	= 28.35 grams	1 calorie	= 4.18 Joule
1 pound	= 454 grams		
°C	= (°F - 32) X 5/9	Boiling	= 212 °F/100°C
°F	= (°C x 9/5) + 32	Freezing	= 32 °F/0 °C

Ethics

"Morality cannot be legislated, but behavior can be regulated. Judicial decrees may
not change the heart, but they can restrain the heartless."   —*Martin Luther King Jr.*

Ethics is a branch of philosophy that emphasizes morality, justice, honesty, right versus wrong, and free will. Ethics is defined as a principle of good conduct or a body of right principles and specific moral choices. We respond to each instance that we face as health care providers based on specific moral choices. These are specific to each person and are based on cultural, religious, environmental, and personal values.

Ethical Principles and Terminology

Autonomy: Requires that the wishes of competent individuals must be honored. Autonomy is often referred to as self-determination.

Beneficence: A moral obligation of health care providers to act for the benefit of others.

Confidentiality: The holding of professional secrets or discussions. Keeping client information within appropriate limits.

Duty: The obligations that individuals have to others in society.

Fidelity: Related to confidentiality and is defined as the moral duty to keep commitments that have been promised.

Justice: The quality of being just and fair; righteousness.

Nonmaleficence: The obligation of health care providers to above all else, do no harm.

Paternalism: A term used when someone fails to recognize another individual's rights and autonomy.

Rights: The ability to take advantage of a moral entitlement to do something or not to do something.

Veracity: Obligation of health care providers to tell the truth.

Ethical Theories and Issues

Teleological theory (consequentialism)

This ethical theory believes that the outcome or consequences of a particular action should come from answering the question "what should I do?" The person judges the good and bad outcome based on answering "which decision would bring the best consequences?" When the decision cannot be made from these questions a person will choose the course of action that brings the most good and least harm. This theory supports paternalistic behavior if no harm is done. The worth of an action is judged by the consequences and the goal will be that the end result justifies the means.

Deontologism theory

This ethical theory does not focus on the consequences of an action, but on the action itself and if the action follows moral principles. The theory believes that a person's obligations should determine the ethical course of action. There is a strict following of the principles of ethics (autonomy, nonmaleficence, beneficence, and justice).

Malpractice

Claims of malpractice usually stem from the theory of negligence. Negligence describes a substandard level of care for the particular profession. Negligence deals with a particular conduct, not state of mind.

In order to prove malpractice through negligence there are four elements:

1. A duty to act in a particular manner
2. Conduct that breaches that particular duty
3. Damage that occurs from that conduct
4. Conduct that is substandard, causing injury

Sexual harassment

This term describes unwanted sexual or gender based behaviors from one person that has formal or informal power over the other.

In order to qualify as sexual harassment, there are three areas that must be satisfied:

1. The behavior is unwelcome or unwanted
2. The behavior is sexual in nature or related to the gender of the person
3. The behavior must occur in a relationship where the person is being harassed by a superior or a peer; someone who has power over the individual in some respect

Four elements that create a sexual harassment case:

1. Submission or rejection of the conduct is used as a factor in obtaining employment
2. Submission or rejection of the conduct is used to determine the status of a person's employment
3. The conduct must substantially interfere with a person's employment
4. The conduct creates a hostile work environment

Professional Behaviors

- ✓ Organization
- ✓ Professional presentation
- ✓ Dependability
- ✓ Initiative
- ✓ Empathy
- ✓ Cooperation
- ✓ Clinical reasoning
- ✓ Written communication
- ✓ Verbal communication

L- Listen

E- Explain

A- Acknowledge

R- Recommend

N- Negotiate

Management

Quality Management Process

- Review selected patient medical records
- Prioritize adverse event outcomes
- Conduct a thorough review of care
- Identify problematic areas of care

- Develop a plan to change identified aspects of care
- Implement the plan
- Monitor the plan
- Determine if the implemented change results in a measurable difference

Quality Improvement

A form of objective self-examination designed to improve the quality of services.

Agencies Responsible for Quality Improvement

- Joint Commission on Accreditation of Healthcare Organizations (JCAHO)
- Professional Standards Review Organization (PSRO)
- Commission of Accreditation of Rehabilitation Facilities (CARF)
- National Committee for Quality Assurance (NCQA)

These measure the structure, process, and outcome of physical therapy care. According to the American Physical Therapy Association structure, process, and outcome are defined as follows:

Structure

A review of structure is an assessment of organization, staffing and staff qualifications, rules and policies governing physical work, records, equipment, and physical facilities. The assessment may include a judgment of the adequacy as well as the presence of the element of structure being examined.

Process

Process assessment is based on the degree or extent to which the therapist conforms to accepted professional practices in providing services. The various approaches to care, their application, efficacy, adequacy, and timeliness are considered. A process review requires that considerable attention be given to developing and specifying the standards to be used in the assessment.

Outcome

Outcome assessment is based on the condition of the patient at the conclusion of care in relation to the goals of treatment. Assessment of outcome provides a means of reviewing the practitioner, the services, and events that led to the results of care. The results of outcome assessment ultimately may lead to the evaluation of the basic treatment procedures and modalities of physical therapy and validation of the approaches to patient care. Outcomes are the ultimate manifestations of effectiveness and quality of care.

Models of Disability

The Nagi Model

This model was originally designed in 1965 by a social worker named Saad Nagi as an alternative to the medical model of disease. It describes health status as a product of the relationship between health and function and is defined by four primary concepts:

Pathology: An interruption or interference in the body's normal processes and the simultaneous efforts of the systems to regain homeostasis. Pathology occurs at the cellular level.

Impairment: The loss or abnormality at the tissue, organ or body system level. This can be of an anatomic, physiologic, mental or emotional nature. Each pathology will present with an impairment, however, impairments can exist without pathology (e.g., congenital defects). Impairments occur at the organ level.

Functional limitation: The inability to perform an action or skill in a normal manner due to an impairment. Functional limitations are at the level of the whole person.

Disability: Any restriction or inability to perform a socially defined role within a social or physical environment due to an impairment. Environmental barriers impose disability.

Example:

A patient with progressive weakness presents with paralysis of the trunk and lower extremities. The patient is diagnosed with a T12 spinal cord tumor. The patient utilizes a wheelchair for mobility and requires assistance with self-care. Prior to hospitalization the patient worked as a delivery man.

Pathology - Spinal cord tumor at T12

Impairment - Loss of motor function below T12

Functional limitation - Unable to ambulate

Disability - Cannot continue to work as a delivery man

The International Classification of Impairment, Disabilities, and Handicaps (ICIDH) Model

The World Health Organization (WHO) developed this model in 1980 with the focus on the long-term impact of non-fatal or chronic diseases. The model is defined by four primary concepts:

Disease: A biomechanical, physiological or anatomical abnormality within the body.

Impairment: The loss or abnormality of psychological, physiological or anatomical structure or function. Impairments occur at the organ level.

Disability: The inability to perform an activity in a normal manner due to an impairment. Disability occurs at the level of the whole person.

Handicap: The inability to perform in a social role due to social or environmental restrictions. Handicap occurs in a person-to-person or person-to-environment level. Handicap clearly separates environmental barriers and the person's ability to interact with the environment.

Example:

A 36-year-old female is diagnosed with multiple sclerosis. The patient resides alone and has recently utilized a wheelchair for mobility secondary to weakness and hypertonicity in her upper and lower extremities. She is no longer able to visit her brother who lives in a second floor apartment two blocks away.

Disease - Demyelination secondary to multiple sclerosis

Impairment - Weakness and tonal abnormalities in lower extremities

Disability - Unable to ambulate

Handicap - Unable to visit her brother who resides in the second floor apartment

Disablement Model

This model was designed by physical therapists appointed by the House of Delegates as the framework for the Guide to Physical Therapist Practice. This model rejects the medical model of disease and focuses on disablement using guidelines from the Nagi model. This model defines three primary concepts as they relate to physical therapy intervention.

Impairment: The loss or abnormality of physiological, psychological or anatomical structure or function.

Functional limitation: A restriction of the ability to perform in a competent manner. This occurs at the level of the whole person.

Disability: The inability to engage in roles in a particular social context and physical environment.

Example:

A 45-year-old right hand dominant female fell down a flight of stairs and sustained a compound fracture of the right humerus. She is currently casted and has difficulty with many self-care skills. She is employed in the data entry department of a local hospital.

Impairment - Fracture of the humerus
Functional limitation - Unable to get dressed
Disability - Cannot use the computer at work

Legal

Elements of a Risk Management Program

- Management involvement
- Risk management organization
- Incident reporting and investigation
- Inspections
- Communications

Recommendations to Avoid Litigation

- Conduct a thorough examination
- Seek consultation when in doubt
- Check the condition of your equipment
- Instruct patients thoroughly
- Keep the referring physician informed
- Obtain proper consent for treatment
- Do not delegate to unqualified individuals
- Keep accurate and timely written records

Legal Terminology

Abandonment: Unacceptable one-sided termination of services by a health care professional without patient consent or agreement.

Administrative law: Administrative agencies at the federal and state level develop rules and regulations to supplement statutes and executive orders.

Common law: Refers to court decisions in the absence of statutory law. Common law often creates legal precedent in areas where statutes have not been enacted.

Constitutional law: Involves law that is derived from the federal Constitution. The United States Supreme Court is responsible for ultimately interpreting and enforcing the Constitution.

Informed consent: The patient is required to sign a document and give permission to the health care professional to render treatment. This should be obtained from the patient in accordance with the standards of practice prior to initiation of treatment. The patient has the right to full disclosure of treatment procedures, risks, expected outcomes, and goals.

Malpractice: The failure to exercise the skills that would normally be exercised by other members of the profession with similar skills and training.

This can include areas of professional negligence, breach of contract issues, and intentional conduct by a health care professional.

Negligence: The failure to do what a reasonable and prudent person would ordinarily have done under the same or similar circumstances for a given situation. In order to prove negligence, the plaintiff must prove all of the following:

- There was a duty owed to the plaintiff by the defendant.

- There was a breach of that duty under conditions that constituted negligence and the negligence was the proximate cause of the breach.

- There was damage to the plaintiff's person or property.

Risk management: The identification, analysis, and evaluation of risks and the selection of the most advantageous method for treating them.

Statutory law: Congress and state legislatures are responsible for enacting statutes. Examples of federal statutes affecting health care include the Americans with Disabilities Act and the Family and Medical Leave Act.

Tort: A private or civil wrong or injury, involving omission and/or commission.

Delegation and Supervision

American Physical Therapy Association Direction, Delegation, and Supervision in Physical Therapy Services

Delegated responsibilities must be commensurate with the qualifications, including experience, education, and training of the individuals to whom the responsibilities are being assigned. When the physical therapist of record delegates patient care responsibilities to physical therapist assistants or other supportive personnel, that physical therapist holds responsibility for supervision of the physical therapy program. Regardless of the setting in which the service is given, the following responsibilities must be borne solely by the physical therapist:

1. Interpretation of referrals when available.

2. Initial examination, evaluation, diagnosis, and prognosis.

3. Development or modification of a plan of care that is based on the initial examination or the re-examination and that includes physical therapy anticipated goals and expected outcomes.

4. Determination of (1) when the expertise and decision making capability of the physical therapist requires the physical therapist to personally render physical therapy interventions and (2) when it may be appropriate to utilize the physical therapist assistant. A physical therapist determines the most appropriate utilization of the physical therapist assistant that will ensure the delivery of service that is safe, effective, and efficient.

5. Re-examination of the patient/client in light of the anticipated goals, and revision of the plan of care when indicated.

6. Establishment of the discharge plan and documentation of discharge summary/status.

7. Oversight of all documentation for services rendered to each patient.

From Guide to Physical Therapist Practice. American Physical Therapy Association, Alexandria 1999, p.1-11, with permission.

Support Personnel Supervised by Physical Therapists

Physical Therapist Assistants

The physical therapist assistant is a technically educated health care provider who assists the physical therapist in the provision of physical therapy. The physical therapist assistant, under the direction and supervision of the physical therapist, is the only paraprofessional who provides physical therapy interventions. The physical therapist assistant is a graduate of a physical therapist assistant associate degree program accredited by the Commission on Accreditation in Physical Therapy Education (CAPTE).

The physical therapist of record is directly responsible for the actions of the physical therapist assistant. The physical therapist assistant may perform specific components of physical therapy interventions, where allowable by law or regulations that have been selected by the supervising physical therapist. The ability of the physical therapist assistant to perform the selected interventions should be assessed on an ongoing basis by the supervising physical therapist. The physical therapist assistant may modify an intervention only in accordance with changes in patient/client status and within the scope of the plan of care that has been established by the physical therapist.

Physical Therapy Aides

Aides are any support personnel who may be involved in the provision of physical therapist directed support services. The physical therapy aide is a non-licensed worker who is specifically trained under the direction and supervision of a physical therapist.

Physical therapist directed support services are limited to those tasks which may include methods and techniques that do not require clinical decision making by the physical therapist or clinical problem solving by the physical therapist assistant. The determination of what tasks are appropriately directed to the aide must be made by the physical therapist or, where allowable by law or regulations, the physical therapist assistant. To make this determination, the physical therapist or physical therapist assistant must have direct contact with the patient/client during each session. The aide may function only with continuous on-site supervision by the physical therapist or, when allowable by law or regulations, the physical therapist assistant.

From Guide to Physical Therapist Practice. American Physical Therapy Association, Alexandria 1999, p.1-10, with permission.

Health Care Professionals

Audiologists

Audiologists assess patients with suspected hearing disorders. The audiologist can educate patients on how to make the best use of their available hearing and assist them in selecting and fitting appropriate aids. Audiologists are required to possess a master's degree or equivalent. The vast majority of states require audiologists to obtain a license to practice.

Chiropractors

Chiropractors diagnose and treat patients whose health problems are associated with the body's muscular, nervous, and skeletal systems. Patient care activities include manually adjusting the spine, ordering and interpreting X-rays, performing postural analysis, and administering various physical agents. Chiropractors are required to complete a four-year chiropractic curriculum leading to the Doctor of Chiropractic degree. All states require chiropractors to obtain a license to practice.

Home Health Aides

Home health aides provide health related services to the elderly, disabled, and ill in their homes. Patient care activities include performing housekeeping duties, assisting with ambulation or transfers, and promoting personal hygiene. A registered nurse, physical therapist, or social worker is often the health care professional that assigns specific duties and supervises the home health aide. The federal government has established guidelines for home health aides whose employers receive reimbursement from Medicare. The National Association for Home Care offers voluntary national certification for home health aides.

Licensed Practical Nurses

Licensed practical nurses care for the sick, injured, convalescent, and disabled under the direction of physicians and registered nurses. Patient care activities include taking vital signs, performing transfers, applying dressings, administering injections, and instructing patients and families. In some states licensed practical nurses can administer prescribed medications or start intravenous fluids. Experienced licensed practical nurses may supervise nursing assistants and aides. Educational programs for licensed practical nurses are approximately one year in length and include classroom study and supervised clinical practice. All states require a license to practice.

Medical Assistants

Medical assistants perform routine administrative and clinical tasks in a medical office. Administrative duties include answering telephones, updating patient files, completing insurance forms, and scheduling appointments. Clinical duties include taking medical histories, measuring vital signs, and assisting the physician during treatment. Educational programs for medical assistants are typically one to two years in length.

Occupational Therapists

Occupational therapists help people improve their ability to perform activities of daily living, work, and leisure skills. The educational preparation of occupational therapists emphasizes the social, emotional, and physiological effects of illness and injury. Occupational therapists most commonly work with individuals who have conditions that are mentally, physically, developmentally or emotionally disabling. Occupational therapists can enter the field with bachelors, masters or doctoral degrees. All states require occupational therapists to obtain a license to practice.

Occupational Therapy Aides

Occupational therapy aides work under the direction of occupational therapists to provide rehabilitation services to persons with mental, physical, developmental or emotional impairments. Occupational therapy aides often prepare materials and assemble equipment used during treatment and may be responsible for a variety of clerical tasks. The majority of training for occupational therapy aides occurs on the job.

Occupational Therapy Assistants

Occupational therapy assistants work under the direction of occupational therapists to provide rehabilitation services to persons with mental, physical, developmental or emotional impairments. Occupational therapy assistants perform a variety of rehabilitative activities and exercises as outlined in an established treatment plan. To practice as an occupational therapy assistant individuals must complete an associate's degree or certificate program from an accredited academic institution. Occupational therapy assistants are regulated in the majority of states.

Physical Therapists

Physical therapists provide services to help restore function, improve mobility, relieve pain, and prevent or limit permanent physical disabilities of patients suffering from injuries or disease. Physical therapists engage in examination, evaluation, diagnosis, prognosis, and intervention in an effort to maximize patient outcomes. Physical therapists can enter the field with a master's or doctorate degree. As of 2002, all physical therapy programs seeking accreditation were required to offer a minimum of a master's degree. All states require physical therapists to obtain a license to practice.

Physical Therapy Aides

Physical therapy aides are considered support personnel who may be involved in support services directed by physical therapists. Physical therapy aides receive on the job training under the direction and supervision of a physical therapist and are permitted to function only with continuous on-site supervision by a physical therapist or in some cases a physical therapist assistant. Support services are limited to methods and techniques that do not require clinical decision making by the physical therapist or clinical problem solving by the physical therapist assistant.

Physical Therapist Assistants

Physical therapist assistants perform components of physical therapy procedures and related tasks selected and delegated by a supervising physical therapist. Physical therapist assistants may modify an intervention only in accordance with changes in patient status and within the established plan of care developed by the physical therapist. Physical therapist assistants are the only paraprofessionals that perform physical therapy interventions. Typically physical therapist assistants have an associate's degree from an accredited physical therapist assistant program. The majority of states require physical therapist assistants to obtain a license to practice.

Physicians

Physicians diagnose illnesses and prescribe and administer treatment for people suffering from injury or disease. The term physician encompasses both the Doctor of Medicine (MD) and the Doctor of Osteopathic Medicine (DO). The role of the MD and DO are very similar, however, the DO tends to place special emphasis on the body's musculoskeletal system, preventive medicine, and holistic patient care. All states require physicians to obtain a license to practice.

Physician Assistants

Physician assistants provide health care services with supervision by physicians. The supervising physician and established state law determine the specific duties of the physician assistant. In the vast majority of states physician assistants may prescribe medication. Physician assistants work with the supervision of a physician. All states with the exception of Mississippi require physician assistants to obtain a license to practice.

Psychologists

Psychologists use various techniques including interviewing and testing to advise people how to deal with problems of everyday life. In the health care setting psychologists may be involved in counseling programs designed to help people achieve goals such as weight loss or smoking cessation. A doctoral degree is usually required for employment as a licensed clinical or counseling psychologist. All states require psychologists to obtain a license to practice.

Recreational Therapists

Recreational therapists provide treatment services and recreation activities to individuals with disabilities or illness. In acute care hospitals and rehabilitation hospitals recreational therapists work closely with other health care professionals to treat and rehabilitate individuals with specific medical conditions. In long-term care settings recreational therapists function primarily by offering structured group sessions emphasizing leisure activities. Recreational therapists are required to have a bachelor's degree in order to be eligible for certification as certified therapeutic recreation specialists.

Registered Nurses

Registered nurses work to promote health, prevent disease, and help patients cope with illness. Patient care activities are extremely diverse including tasks such as assisting physicians during treatments and examinations, administering medications, recording symptoms and reactions, and instructing patients and families. Registered nurse programs include associates, bachelors, and diploma programs. All states require registered nurses to obtain a license to practice.

Respiratory Therapists

Respiratory therapists evaluate, treat, and care for patients with breathing disorders. The vast majority of respiratory therapists are employed in hospitals. Patient care activities include performing bronchial drainage techniques, measuring lung capacities, administering oxygen and aerosols, and analyzing oxygen and carbon dioxide concentrations. Educational programs for respiratory therapists are offered by hospitals, colleges, and universities, vocational-technical institutes, and the military. The vast majority of states require respiratory therapists to obtain a license to practice.

Social Workers

Social workers help patients and their families to cope with chronic, acute or terminal illnesses and attempt to resolve problems that stand in the way of recovery or rehabilitation. A bachelor's degree is often the minimum requirement to qualify for employment as a social worker, however, in the health field the master's degree is often required. All states have licensing, certification or registration requirements for social workers.

Speech-Language Pathologists

Speech-language pathologists evaluate speech, language, cognitive-communication, and swallowing skills of children and adults. The majority of practitioners provide direct clinical services to individuals with communication disorders. Speech-language pathologists are required to possess a master's degree or equivalent. The vast majority of states require speech-language pathologists to obtain a license to practice.

Physical Therapy Practice

The Elements of Patient/Client Management Leading to Optimal Outcomes

Examination: The process of obtaining a history, performing a systems review, and selecting and administering tests and measures to gather data about the patient/client. The initial examination is a comprehensive screening and specific testing process that leads to a diagnostic classification. The examination process also may identify possible problems that require consultation with, or referral to, another provider.

Evaluation: A dynamic process in which the physical therapist makes clinical judgments based on data gathered during the examination. This process also may identify possible problems that require consultation with, or referral to, another provider.

Diagnosis: Both the process and the end result of evaluating examination data, which the physical therapist organizes into defined clusters, syndromes or categories to help determine the prognosis (including the plan of care) and the most appropriate intervention strategies.

Prognosis (including plan of care): Determination of the level of optimal improvement that may be attained through intervention and the amount of time required to reach that level. The plan of care specifies the interventions to be used and their timing and frequency.

Intervention: Purposeful and skilled interaction of the physical therapist with the patient/client and, if appropriate, with other individuals involved in the care of the patient/client, using various physical therapy methods and techniques to produce changes in the condition that are consistent with the diagnosis and prognosis. The physical therapist conducts a re-examination to determine changes in patient/client status and to modify or redirect intervention. The decision to re-examine may be based on new clinical findings or on lack of patient/client progress. The process of re-examination also may identify the need for consultation with, or referral to, another provider.

Outcomes: Results of patient/client management, which include the impact of physical therapy interventions in the following domains: pathology/pathophysiology (disease, disorder or condition); impairments, functional limitations, and disabilities, risk reduction/prevention, health, wellness, and fitness; societal resources; and patient/client satisfaction.

From Guide to Physical Therapist Practice. American Physical Therapy Association, (Phys. Ther. 2001, Vol. 81, Number 1, 43), with permission.

Criteria for Standards of Practice for Physical Therapy

Preamble

The physical therapy profession's commitment to society is to promote optimal health and function in individuals by pursuing excellence in practice. The American Physical Therapy Association attests to this commitment by adopting and promoting the following *Standards of Practice for Physical Therapy*. These *Standards* are the profession's statement of conditions and performances that are essential for provision of high quality professional service to society, and provide a foundation for assessment of physical therapist practice.

I. Ethical/Legal Considerations

A. Ethical Considerations

The physical therapist practices according to the *Code of Ethics* of the American Physical Therapy Association.

The physical therapist assistant complies with the *Standards of Ethical Conduct for the Physical Therapist Assistant* of the American Physical Therapy Association.

B. Legal Considerations

The physical therapist complies with all the legal requirements of jurisdictions regulating the practice of physical therapy.

The physical therapist assistant complies with all the legal requirements of jurisdictions regulating the work of the assistant.

II. Administration of the Physical Therapy Service

A. Statement of Mission, Purposes, and Goals

The physical therapy service has a statement of mission, purposes, and goals that reflects the needs and interests of the patients and clients served, the physical therapy personnel affiliated with the service, and the community.

The statement of mission, purposes, and goals:
- Defines the scope and limitations of the physical therapy service.
- Identifies the goals and objectives of the service.
- Is reviewed annually.

B. Organizational Plan

The physical therapy service has a written organizational plan.

The organizational plan:
- Describes relationships among components within the physical therapy service and, where the service is part of a larger organization, between the service and other components of that organization.
- Ensures that the service is directed by a physical therapist.
- Defines supervisory structures within the service.
- Reflects current personnel functions.

C. Policies and Procedures

The physical therapy service has written policies and procedures that reflect the operation, mission, purposes, and goals of the service, and are consistent with the Association's Code of Ethics.

The written policies and procedures:
- Are reviewed regularly and revised as necessary.
- Meet the requirements for federal and state law and external agencies.

Apply to, but are not limited to:
- Care of patients/clients, including guidelines
- Clinical education
- Clinical research
- Collaboration
- Collection of patient data
- Competency assessment
- Criteria for access to care
- Criteria for initiation and continuation of care
- Criteria for referral to other appropriate health care providers
- Criteria for termination of care
- Documentation
- Environmental safety
- Equipment maintenance
- Fiscal management
- Improvement of quality of care and performance of services
- Infection control
- Job/position descriptions
- Medical emergencies
- Rights of patients/clients
- Personnel-related policies
- Staff orientation

D. Administration

The physical therapist is responsible for the direction of the physical therapy service:
- Ensures compliance with local, state, and federal requirements.
- Ensures compliance with current APTA documents, including Standards of Practice for Physical Therapy and the Criteria, Guide to Physical Therapist Practice, Code of Ethics, Guide for Professional Conduct, Standards of Ethical Conduct for the Physical Therapist Assistant, and Guide for Conduct of the Physical Therapist Assistant.
- Ensures that services are consistent with the mission, purposes, and goals of the physical therapy service.
- Ensures that services are provided in accordance with established policies and procedures.
- Ensures that the process for assignment of physical therapist staff supports the individual therapist responsibility to their patients and meets their needs.
- Reviews and updates policies and procedures.
- Provides training of physical therapy support personnel that ensures continued competence for their job description.
- Provides for continuous inservice training on safety issues and for periodic safety inspection of equipment by qualified individuals.

E. Fiscal Management

The director of the physical therapy service, in consultation with physical therapy staff and appropriate administrative personnel, participates in planning for, and allocation of, resources. Fiscal planning and management of the service are based on sound accounting principles.

The fiscal management plan:
- Includes a budget that provides for optimal use of resources.
- Ensures accurate recording and reporting of financial information.
- Ensures compliance with legal requirements.
- Allows for cost-effective utilization of resources.
- Uses a fee schedule that is consistent with the cost of physical therapy services and that is within customary norms of fairness and reasonableness.
- Considers option of providing pro bono services.

F.   Improvement of Quality of Care and Performance

The physical therapy service has a written plan for continuous improvement of quality of care and performance of services.

The improvement plan:
- Provides evidence of ongoing review and evaluation of the physical therapy service.
- Provides a mechanism for documenting improvement in quality of care and performance.
- Is consistent with requirements of external agencies, as applicable.

G.   Staffing

The physical therapy personnel affiliated with the physical therapy service have demonstrated competence and are sufficient to achieve the mission, purposes, and goals of the service.

The physical therapy service:
- Meets all legal requirements regarding licensure and certification of appropriate personnel.
- Ensures that the level of expertise within the service is appropriate to the needs of the patients/clients served.
- Provides appropriate professional and support personnel to meet the needs of the patient/client population.

H.   Staff Development

The physical therapy service has a written plan that provides for appropriate and ongoing staff development.

The staff development plan:
- Includes self-assessment, individual goal setting, and organizational needs in directing continuing education and learning activities.
- Includes strategies for lifelong learning and professional career development.
- Includes mechanisms to foster mentorship activities.
- Includes knowledge of clinical research methods and analysis.

I.   Physical Setting

The physical setting is designed to provide a safe and accessible environment that facilitates fulfillment of the mission, purposes, and goals of the physical therapy service. The equipment is safe and sufficient to achieve the purposes and goals of the physical therapy.

The physical setting:
- Meets all applicable legal requirements for health and safety.
- Meets space needs appropriate for the number and type of patients/clients served.

The equipment:
- Meets all applicable legal requirements for health and safety.
- Is inspected routinely.

J.   Collaboration

The physical therapy service collaborates with all disciplines as appropriate.

The collaboration when appropriate:
- Uses a team approach for the care of patients/clients.
- Provides instruction to patients/clients and families.
- Ensures professional development and continuing education.

III.   Patient/Client Management

A.   Patient/Client Collaboration

Within the patient/client management process, the physical therapist and the patient/client establish and maintain an ongoing collaborative process of decision making that exists throughout the provision of services.

B.   Initial Examination/Evaluation/ Diagnosis/ Prognosis

The physical therapist performs an initial examination and evaluation to establish a diagnosis and prognosis prior to intervention.

The physical therapist examination:
- Is documented, dated, and appropriately authenticated by the physical therapist who performed it.
- Identifies the physical therapy needs of the patient/client.
- Incorporates appropriate tests and measures to facilitate outcome measurement.
- Produces data that are sufficient to allow evaluation, diagnosis, prognosis, and the establishment of a plan of care.
- May result in recommendations for additional services to meet the needs of the patient/client.

C.   Plan of Care

The physical therapist establishes a plan of care and manages the needs of the patient/client based on the examination, evaluation, diagnosis, prognosis, goals, and outcomes of the planned interventions for the identified impairments, functional limitations, and disabilities.

The physical therapist involves the patient/client and appropriate others in the planning, implementation, and assessment of the plan of care.

The physical therapist, in consultation with appropriated disciplines, plans for discharge of the patient/client taking into consideration achievement of anticipated goals and expected outcomes, and provides for appropriate follow-up or referral.

The plan of care:

- Is based on the examination, evaluation, diagnosis, and prognosis.
- Identifies goals and outcomes.
- Describes the proposed intervention, including frequency and duration.
- Includes documentation that is dated and appropriately authenticated by the physical therapist who established the plan of care.

D. Intervention

The physical therapist provides, or directs and supervises, the physical therapy intervention consistent with the examination, evaluation, diagnosis, prognosis, and plan of care.

The intervention:

- Is based on the examination, evaluation, diagnosis, prognosis, and plan of care.
- Is provided under the ongoing direction and supervision of the physical therapist.
- Is provided in such a way that directed and supervised responsibilities are commensurate with the qualifications and the legal limitations of the physical therapist assistant.
- Is altered in accordance with changes in response or status.
- Is provided at a level that is consistent with current physical therapy practice.
- Is interdisciplinary when necessary to meet the needs of the patient or client.
- Documentation of the intervention is consistent with the Guidelines for Physical Therapy Documentation of Patient/Client Management.
- Is dated and appropriately authenticated by the physical therapist or when permissible by law, by the physical therapist assistant.

E. Re-examination

The physical therapist re-examines the patient/client as necessary during an episode of care to evaluate progress or change in patient/client status and modifies the plan of care accordingly or discontinues physical therapy services.

The physical therapist re-examination:

- Is documented, dated, and appropriately authenticated by the physical therapist who performs it.
- Includes modifications to the plan of care.

F. Discharge/Discontinuation of Intervention

The physical therapist discharges the patient/client from physical therapy when the anticipated goals or expected outcomes for the patient/client have been achieved.

The physical therapist discontinues intervention when the patient/client is unable to continue to progress toward goals or when the physical therapist determines that the patient/client will no longer benefit from physical therapy.

Discharge documentation:

- Includes the status of the patient/client at discharge and the goals and functional outcomes attained.
- Is dated and appropriately authenticated by the physical therapist who performed the discharge.
- Includes, when a patient/client is discharged prior to attainment of goals and functional outcomes, the status of the patient/client and the rationale for discontinuation.

G. Communication/Coordination/Documentation

The physical therapist communicates, coordinates and documents all aspects of patient/client management including the results of the initial examination and evaluation, diagnosis, prognosis, plan of care, interventions, response to interventions, changes in patient/client status relative to the interventions, re-examination, and discharge/discontinuation of intervention and other patient/client management activities.

Physical therapist documentation:

- Is dated and appropriately authenticated by the physical therapist who performed the examination and established the plan of care.
- Is dated and appropriately authenticated by the physical therapist who performed the intervention or, when allowable by law or regulations, by the physical therapist assistant who performed specific components of the intervention as selected by the supervising physical therapist.
- Is dated and appropriately authenticated by the physical therapist who performed the re-examination, and includes modifications to the plan of care.
- Is dated and appropriately authenticated by the physical therapist who performed the discharge, and includes the status of the patient/client and the goals and outcomes achieved.
- Includes, when a patient/client is discharged prior to achievement of goals and outcomes, the status of the patient/client and the rationale for discontinuation.
- As appropriate, records patient data using a method that allows collective analysis.

IV. Education

The physical therapist is responsible for individual professional development. The physical therapist assistant is responsible for individual career development.

The physical therapist and the physical therapist assistant under the direction and supervision of the physical therapist, participate in the education of students.

The physical therapist educates and provides consultation to consumers and the general public regarding the purposes and benefits of physical therapy.

The physical therapist educates and provides consultation to consumers and the general public regarding the roles of the physical therapist and the physical therapist assistant.

The physical therapist:

- Educates and provides consultation to consumers and the general public regarding the roles of the physical therapist, the physical therapist assistant, and other support personnel.

V. Research

The physical therapist applies research findings to practice and encourages, participates in, and promotes activities that establish the outcomes of patient/client management provided by the physical therapist.

The physical therapist:

- Ensures that his or her knowledge of research literature related to practice is current.
- Ensures that the rights of research subjects are protected and the integrity of research is maintained.
- Participates in the research process as appropriate to individual education, experience, and expertise.
- Educates physical therapists, physical therapist assistants, students, other health professionals, and the general public about the outcomes of physical therapist practice.

VI. Community Responsibility

The physical therapist demonstrates community responsibility by participating in community and community agency activities, educating the public, formulating public policy or providing pro bono physical therapy services.

The physical therapist:

- Participates in community and community agency activities.
- Educates the public, including prevention, education, and health promotion.
- Helps formulate public policy.
- Provides pro bono physical therapy services.

BOD S03-06-16-38

From Criteria for Standards of Practice for Physical Therapy. American Physical Therapy Association, with permission.

Code of Ethics

Preamble

This *Code of Ethics* of the American Physical Therapy Association sets forth principles for the ethical practice of physical therapy. All physical therapists are responsible for maintaining and promoting ethical practice. To this end, the physical therapist shall act in the best interest of the patient/client. This *Code of Ethics* shall be binding on all physical therapists.

Principle 1

A physical therapist shall respect the rights and dignity of all individuals and shall provide compassionate care.

Principle 2

A physical therapist shall act in a trustworthy manner toward patients/clients and in all other aspects of physical therapy practice.

Principle 3

A physical therapist shall comply with laws and regulations governing physical therapy and shall strive to effect changes that benefit patients/clients.

Principle 4

A physical therapist shall exercise sound professional judgment.

Principle 5

A physical therapist shall achieve and maintain professional competence.

Principle 6

A physical therapist shall maintain and promote high standards for physical therapy practice, education, and research.

Principle 7

A physical therapist shall seek only such remuneration as is deserved and reasonable for physical therapy services.

Principle 8

A physical therapist shall provide and make available accurate and relevant information to patients/clients about their care and to the public about physical therapy services.

Principle 9

A physical therapist shall protect the public and the profession from unethical, incompetent, and illegal acts.

Principle 10

A physical therapist shall endeavor to address the health needs of society.

Principle 11

A physical therapist shall respect the rights, knowledge, and skills of colleagues and other health care professionals.

HOD S06-00-12-23

From Code of Ethics, American Physical Therapy Association, S06-00-12-23, with permission.

Guide for Professional Conduct

Purpose

This *Guide for Professional Conduct* (Guide) is intended to serve physical therapists in interpreting the *Code of Ethics* (Code) of the American Physical Therapy Association (Association), in matters of professional conduct. The Guide provides guidelines by which physical therapists may determine the propriety of their conduct. It is also intended to guide the professional development of physical therapist students. The Code and the Guide apply to all physical therapists. These guidelines are subject to change as the dynamics of the profession change and as new patterns of health care delivery are developed and accepted by the professional community and the public. This Guide is subject to monitoring and timely revision by the Ethics and Judicial Committee of the Association.

Interpreting Ethical Principles

The interpretations expressed in this Guide reflect the opinions, decisions, and advice of the Ethics and Judicial Committee. These interpretations are intended to assist a physical therapist in applying general ethical principles to specific situations. They should not be considered inclusive of all situations that could evolve.

Principle 1

A physical therapist shall respect the rights and dignity of all individuals and shall provide compassionate care.

1.1 Attitudes of a Physical Therapist

A. A physical therapist shall recognize individual differences and shall respect and be responsive to those differences.
B. A physical therapist shall be guided by concern for the physical, psychological, and socioeconomic welfare of patients/clients.
C. A physical therapist shall not harass, abuse or discriminate against others.

Principle 2

A physical therapist shall act in a trustworthy manner towards patients/clients, and in all other aspects of physical therapy practice.

2.1 Patient/Physical Therapist Relationship

A. To act in a trustworthy manner the physical therapist shall act in the patient/client's best interest. Working in the patient/client's best interest requires knowledge of the patient/client's needs from the patient/client's perspective. Patients/clients often come to the physical therapist in a vulnerable state and normally will rely on the physical therapist's advice, which they perceive to be based on superior knowledge, skill, and experience. The trustworthy physical therapist acts to ameliorate the patient's/client's vulnerability, not to exploit it.
B. A physical therapist shall not exploit any aspect of the physical therapist/patient relationship.

C. A physical therapist shall not engage in any sexual relationship or activity, whether consensual or nonconsensual, with any patient while a physical therapist/patient relationship exists.
D. The physical therapist shall encourage an open and collaborative dialogue with the patient/client.
E. In the event the physical therapist or patient terminates the physical therapist/patient relationship while the patient continues to need physical therapy services, the physical therapist should take steps to transfer the care of the patient to another provider.

2.2 Truthfulness

A physical therapist shall not make statements that he/she knows or should know are false, deceptive, fraudulent or unfair. See Section 8.2.C and D.

2.3 Confidential Information

A. Information relating to the physical therapist/patient relationship is confidential and may not be communicated to a third party not involved in that patient's care without the prior consent of the patient, subject to applicable law.
B. Information derived from peer review shall be held confidential by the reviewer unless the physical therapist who was reviewed consents to the release of the information.
C. A physical therapist may disclose information to appropriate authorities when it is necessary to protect the welfare of an individual or the community or when required by law. Such disclosure shall be in accordance with applicable law.

2.4 Patient Autonomy and Consent

A. A physical therapist shall respect the patient's/client's right to make decisions regarding the recommended plan of care, including consent, modification, or refusal.
B. A physical therapist shall communicate to the patient/client the findings of his/her examination, evaluation, diagnosis, and prognosis.
C. A physical therapist shall collaborate with the patient/client to establish the goals of treatment and the plan of care.
D. A physical therapist shall use sound professional judgment in informing the patient/client of any substantial risks of the recommended examination and intervention.
E. A physical therapist shall not restrict patients' freedom to select their provider of physical therapy.

Principle 3

A physical therapist shall comply with laws and regulations governing physical therapy and shall strive to effect changes that benefit patients/clients.

3.1 Professional Practice

A physical therapist shall comply with laws governing the qualifications, functions, and duties of a physical therapist.

3.2   Just Laws and Regulations

A physical therapist shall advocate the adoption of laws, regulations, and policies by providers, employers, third party payers, legislatures, and regulatory agencies to provide and improve access to necessary health care services for all individuals.

3.3   Unjust Laws and Regulations

A physical therapist shall endeavor to change unjust laws, regulations, and policies that govern the practice of physical therapy. See Section 10.2.

Principle 4

A physical therapist shall exercise sound professional judgment.

4.1   Professional Responsibility

A. A physical therapist shall make professional judgments that are in the patient/client's best interests.
B. Regardless of practice setting, a physical therapist has primary responsibility for the physical therapy care of a patient and shall make independent judgments regarding that care consistent with accepted professional standards. See Section 2.4.
C. A physical therapist shall not provide physical therapy services to a patient/client while his/her ability to do so safely is impaired.
D. A physical therapist shall exercise sound professional judgment based upon his/her knowledge, skill, education, training, and experience.
E. Upon accepting a patient/client for physical therapy services, a physical therapist shall be responsible for: the examination, evaluation, and diagnosis of that individual; the prognosis and intervention; re-examination and modification of the plan of care; and the maintenance of adequate records, including progress reports. A physical therapist shall establish the plan of care and shall provide and/or supervise and direct the appropriate interventions. See Section 2.4 and 6.1.
F. If the diagnostic process reveals findings that are outside the scope of the physical therapist's knowledge, experience, or expertise, the physical therapist shall so inform the patient/client and refer to an appropriate practitioner.
G. When the patient has been referred from another practitioner, the physical therapist shall communicate the findings and/or information to the referring practitioner.
H. A physical therapist shall determine when a patient/client will no longer benefit from physical therapy services. See Section 7.1.D.

4.2   Direction and Supervision

A. The supervising physical therapist has primary responsibility for the physical therapy care rendered to a patient/client.
B. A physical therapist shall not delegate to a less qualified person any activity that requires the unique skill, knowledge, and judgment of the physical therapist.

4.3   Practice Arrangements

A. Participation in a business, partnership, corporation, or other entity does not exempt physical therapists, whether employers, partners, or stockholders, either individually or collectively, from the obligation to promote, maintain and comply with the ethical principles of the Association.
B. A physical therapist shall advise his/her employer(s) of any employer practice that causes a physical therapist to be in conflict with the ethical principles of the Association. A physical therapist shall seek to eliminate aspects of his/her employment that are in conflict with the ethical principles of the Association.

4.4   Gifts and Other Considerations

A. A physical therapist shall not invite, accept, or offer gifts, monetary incentives, or other considerations that affect or give an appearance of affecting his/her professional judgment.
B. A physical therapist shall not offer or accept kickbacks in exchange for patient referrals. See Sections 7.1.F and G and 9.1.D.

Principle 5

A physical therapist shall achieve and maintain professional competence.

5.1   Scope of Competence

A physical therapist shall practice within the scope of his/her competence and commensurate with his/her level of education, training, and experience.

5.2   Self-assessment

A physical therapist has a lifelong professional responsibility for maintaining competence through on-going self-assessment, education, and enhancement of knowledge and skills.

5.3   Professional Development

A physical therapist shall participate in educational activities that enhance his/her basic knowledge and skills. See Section 6.1.

Principle 6

A physical therapist shall maintain and promote high standards for physical therapy practice, education and research.

6.1   Professional Standards

A physical therapist's practice shall be consistent with accepted professional standards. A physical therapist shall continuously engage in assessment activities to determine compliance with these standards.

6.2   Practice

A. A physical therapist shall achieve and maintain professional competence. See Section 5.

B. A physical therapist shall demonstrate his/her commitment to quality improvement by engaging in peer and utilization review and other self-assessment activities.

6.3 Professional Education

A. A physical therapist shall support high quality education in academic and clinical settings.

B. A physical therapist participating in the educational process is responsible to the students, the academic institutions, and the clinical settings for promoting ethical conduct. A physical therapist shall model ethical behavior and provide the student with information about the Code of Ethics, opportunities to discuss ethical conflicts, and procedures for reporting unresolved ethical conflicts. See Section 9.

6.4 Continuing Education

A. A physical therapist providing continuing education must be competent in the content area.

B. When a physical therapist provides continuing education, he/she shall ensure that course content, objectives, faculty credentials, and responsibilities of the instructional staff are accurately stated in the promotional and instructional course materials.

C. A physical therapist shall evaluate the efficacy and effectiveness of information and techniques presented in continuing education programs before integrating them into his or her practice.

6.5 Research

A. A physical therapist participating in research shall abide by ethical standards governing protection of human subjects and dissemination of results.

B. A physical therapist shall support research activities that contribute knowledge for improved patient care.

C. A physical therapist shall report to appropriate authorities any acts in the conduct or presentation of research that appear unethical or illegal. See Section 9.

Principle 7

A physical therapist shall seek only such remuneration as is deserved and reasonable for physical therapy services.

7.1 Business and Employment Practices

A. A physical therapist's business/employment practices shall be consistent with the ethical principles of the Association.

B. A physical therapist shall never place his/her own financial interest above the welfare of individuals under his/her care.

C. A physical therapist shall recognize that third-party payer contracts may limit, in one form or another, the provision of physical therapy services. Third-party limitations do not absolve the physical therapist from making sound professional judgments that are in the patient's best interest. A physical therapist shall avoid under utilization of physical therapy services.

D. When a physical therapist's judgment is that a patient will receive negligible benefit from physical therapy services, the physical therapist shall not provide or continue to provide such services if the primary reason for doing so is to further the financial self-interest of the physical therapist or his/her employer. A physical therapist shall avoid over utilization of physical therapy services. See Section 4.1.H.

E. Fees for physical therapy services should be reasonable for the service performed, considering the setting in which it is provided, practice costs in the geographic area, judgment of other organizations, and other relevant factors.

F. A physical therapist shall not directly or indirectly request, receive, or participate in the dividing, transferring, assigning or rebating of an unearned fee. See Sections 4.4.A and B.

G. A physical therapist shall not profit by means of credit or other valuable consideration, such as an unearned commission, discount, or gratuity, in connection with the furnishing of physical therapy services. See Sections 4.4.A and B.

H. Unless laws impose restrictions to the contrary, physical therapists who provide physical therapy services within a business entity may pool fees and monies received. Physical therapists may divide or apportion these fees and monies in accordance with the business agreement.

I. A physical therapist may enter into agreements with organizations to provide physical therapy services if such agreements do not violate the ethical principles of the Association or applicable laws.

7.2 Endorsement of Products or Services

A. A physical therapist shall not exert influence on individuals under his/her care or their families to use products or services based on the direct or indirect financial interest of the physical therapist in such products or services. Realizing that these individuals will normally rely on the physical therapist's advice, their best interest must always be maintained, as must their right of free choice relating to the use of any product or service. Although it cannot be considered unethical for physical therapists to own or have a financial interest in the production, sale or distribution of products/services, they must act in accordance with law and make full disclosure of their interest whenever individuals under their care use such products/services.

B. A physical therapist may receive remuneration for endorsement or advertisement of products or services to the public, physical therapists, or other health professionals provided he/she discloses any financial interest in the production, sale, or distribution of said products or services.

D. When endorsing or advertising products or services, a physical therapist shall use sound professional judgment and shall not give the appearance of Association endorsement unless the Association has formally endorsed the products or services.

7.3 Disclosure

A physical therapist shall disclose to the patient if the referring practitioner derives compensation from the provision of physical therapy.

Principle 8

A physical therapist shall provide and make available accurate and relevant information to patients/clients about their care and to the public about physical therapy services.

8.1   Accurate and Relevant Information to the Patient

A. A physical therapist shall provide the patient/client information about his/her condition and plan of care. See Section 2.4

B. Upon the request of the patient, the physical therapist shall provide, or make available, the medical record to the patient or a patient-designated third party.

C. A physical therapist shall inform patients of any known financial limitations that may affect their care.

D. A physical therapist shall inform the patient when, in his/her judgment, the patient will receive negligible benefit from further care. See Section 7.1.C.

8.2   Accurate and Relevant Information to the Public

A. A physical therapist shall inform the public about the societal benefits of the profession and who is qualified to provide physical therapy services.

B. Information given to the public shall emphasize that individual problems cannot be treated without individualized examination and plans/programs of care.

C. A physical therapist may advertise his/her services to the public. See Section 2.2.

D. A physical therapist shall not use, or participate in the use of, any form of communication containing a false, plagiarized, fraudulent, deceptive, unfair, or sensational statement or claim. See section 2.2.

E. A physical therapist who places a paid advertisement shall identify it as such unless it is apparent from the context that it is a paid advertisement.

Principle 9

A physical therapist shall protect the public and the profession from unethical, incompetent and illegal acts.

9.1   Consumer Protection

A. A physical therapist shall provide care that is within the scope of practice as defined by the state practice act.

B. A physical therapist shall not engage in any conduct that is unethical, incompetent or illegal.

C. A physical therapist shall report any conduct that appears to be unethical, incompetent, or illegal.

D. A physical therapist may not participate in any arrangements in which patients are exploited due to the referring sources' enhancing their personal incomes as a result of referring for, prescribing, or recommending physical therapy. See Sections 2.1.B, 4, and 7.

Principle 10

A physical therapist shall endeavor to address the health needs of society.

10.1   Pro Bono Services

A physical therapist shall render pro bono publico (reduced or no fee) services to patients lacking the ability to pay for services, as each physical therapist's practice permits.

10.2   Individual and Community Health

A. A physical therapist shall be aware of the patient's health-related needs and act in a manner that facilitates meeting those needs.

B. A physical therapist shall endeavor to support activities that benefit the health status of the community. See Section 3.

Principle 11

A physical therapist shall respect the rights, knowledge, and skills of colleagues and other health care professionals.

11.1   Consultation

A physical therapist shall seek consultation whenever the welfare of the patient will be safeguarded or advanced by consulting those who have special skills, knowledge or experience.

11.2   Patient/Provider Relationships

A physical therapist shall not undermine the relationship(s) between his/her patient and other health care professionals.

11.3   Disparagement

Physical therapists shall not disparage colleagues and other health care professionals. See Section 9 and Section 2.4.A.

Issued by Ethics and Judicial Committee
American Physical Therapy Association
October 1981
Last Amended January 2004

From Guide to Professional Conduct, American Physical Therapy Association, with permission.

Health Insurance

There are three major classifications of health insurance companies. They include private health insurance companies, independent health plans, and government health insurance.

Private Health Insurance Companies

Private health insurance companies include stock companies, mutual companies, and non-profit insurance plans. Reimbursement for physical therapy services is usually on a fee for service basis.

Stock companies: Operated nationally and are owned by independent stockholders.

Mutual companies: Operated nationally and are owned by the individual policyholders.

Non-profit insurance plans: Operate in a specific geographic region and are subject to specific state regulations. They are classified as tax exempt due to their nonprofit status.

Independent Health Plans

Independent health plans are organized into various groups. Health maintenance organizations and self-insurance plans are examples of independent health plans. Reimbursement is typically based on fee-for-service or a predetermined fixed fee.

Managed care: A concept of health care delivery where subscribers utilize health care providers that are contracted by the insurance company at a lower cost. Health maintenance organizations (HMO) and preferred provider organizations (PPO) are two examples of a managed care system. This concept attempts to attain the highest quality of care at the lowest cost.

Health maintenance organization: Subscribers to these insurance plans agree to receive all of their health care services through the predetermined providers of the HMO. The primary physician of the subscriber controls health care access through a referral system. Cost containment is a high priority and subscribers cannot receive care from providers outside of the plan except in an emergency.

Preferred provider organization: Subscribers can choose their health care services from a list of providers that contract with the insurance plan. These contracts provide extreme discounts for health care. Subscribers can use a health care provider that is not associated with the PPO, however, they will absorb a greater portion of the cost.

Consolidated Omnibus Budget Reconciliation Act (COBRA): A law passed that requires an employer to allow an employee to remain under an employer's group plan for a period of time after the loss of a job, death of a spouse, a decrease in hours or a divorce. The employee may be required to pay the employer's portion of the premiums for their insurance coverage as well as their own portion.

Fee for Service versus Managed Care

Fee for Service:	Managed Care:
Payers assume primary financial risk	Providers share in financial risk
Provides enrollees with freedom of choice	Services provided by a specific pool of providers
Unlimited access to specialty providers	Primary care provider serves as a gatekeeper
Co-payments often in the form of 80% / 20%	Provides services for a fixed, prepaid monthly fee
Limited internal/external cost controls	Formal quality assurance and utilization review
Minimal emphasis on health promotion and education	Health education and preventive medicine emphasized

Government Health Insurance

Government health insurance programs such as Medicare and Medicaid are administered by the federal government. The government uses private contractors to manage the payment process of each health plan.

Medicare

Medicare provides health insurance for individuals over 65 years of age and the disabled. Medicare is a nationwide program operated by the Centers for Medicare and Medicaid Services.

Established in 1966, Medicare was the second mandated health insurance program in the United State (Workers' Compensation was the first). In 1972 Medicare coverage was expanded to include certain categories of the disabled, renal dialysis, and transplant patients.

- **Medicare Part A:**

  Provides benefits for care provided in hospitals, outpatient diagnostic services, extended care facilities, hospice, and short-term care at home required by an illness for which the patient is hospitalized.

  Enrollment in Medicare Part A is automatic and funding is through payroll taxes.

- **Medicare Part B:**

  Provides benefits for outpatient care, physician services and services ordered by physicians such as diagnostic tests, medical equipment, and supplies.

  Enrollment in Medicare Part B is voluntary and funding is through premiums paid by beneficiaries and general federal tax revenues.

Cost sharing

The Medicare program requires beneficiaries to share in the costs of health care through deductibles and coinsurance.

- Deductibles require beneficiaries to reach a predetermined amount of personal expenditure each 12-month period before Medicare payment is activated.
- Coinsurance requires that 20% of the costs for hospitalization is covered by the patient.

Medicare sets limits on the total days of hospital care that will be paid based on a lifetime pool of days limit. Medicare payments for post hospital stays in extended care facilities are limited to 100 days.

Providers are reimbursed for Medicare services through intermediaries such as Blue Cross.

Medicaid

Medicaid provides basic medical services to the economically indigent population who qualify by reason of low income or who qualify for welfare or public assistance benefits in the state of their residence. Medicaid is a jointly funded program through the federal and state governments.

Established in 1965, Medicaid is funded through personal income, corporate, and excise taxes. Federal and state support is shared based on the state's per capita income.

Rate setting formulas, procedures, and policies vary widely among states. All state Medicaid operations must be approved by the Centers for Medicare and Medicaid Services. The Medicaid program reimburses providers directly.

The Medicaid program covers inpatient and outpatient hospital services, physician services, diagnostic services, nursing care for older adults, home health care, preventative health screening services, and family planning services.

Workers' Compensation

First designed in 1911 to provide protection for employees that were injured on the job. This legislation provides continued income as well as paid medical expenses for employees injured while working. Workers' compensation is a joint federal and state program that is regulated at the state level. Recently case managers have assisted this process by monitoring the rehabilitation process and controlling potential abuse.

Employers with 10 or more employees or high risk employers must pay a percentage of each employee salary to the worker's compensation board of the state. The exact payment is based on the risk rating of the job or institution.

Reimbursement Coding

Current Procedural Terminology Codes

Current Procedural Terminology (CPT) codes are procedure codes used by physical therapists and other health care professionals to describe the interventions that were provided to a given patient. The majority of codes used by physical therapists are in the CPT 97000 series. Examples of commonly used CPT codes by physical therapists include: 97530 – Therapeutic Activities; 97035 – Ultrasound; 97012 – Traction, mechanical. CPT is a registered trademark of the American Medical Association.

International Classification of Diseases Codes

The International Classification of Diseases (ICD) codes are designed to describe a patient's infirmity through 17 categories based on etiology and affected anatomical systems. The codes consist of five distinct digits (e.g., 755.12). The first three digits indicate the basic diagnosis. The fourth digit and in some cases the fifth digit serve to differentiate the basic diagnosis or anatomical area affected. Physicians are required to make the medical diagnosis, however, in some cases a physical therapist may need to utilize the ICD manual to determine an appropriate ICD code. This action is within a physical therapist's scope of practice and would not be considered equivalent to making a medical diagnosis.

Teaching & Learning

Maslow's Hierarchy of Needs

Maslow's hierarchy of needs hypothesizes that there is a hierarchy of biogenic and psychogenic needs that individuals must progress through. In order to move to a higher level of needs an individual must attain the objectives associated with the previous level. In essence an individual must achieve basic or fundamental needs before moving to upper level needs.

Self-actualization needs: The need to realize one's full potential as a human being.

Esteem needs: The need to feel good about oneself and one's capabilities; to be respected by others, and to receive recognition and appreciation.

Affiliative needs: The need for security, stability, and a safe environment.

Physiological needs: The need for basic things necessary in order to survive such as food, water, and shelter.

Classical Conditioning (Pavlov)

Classical conditioning is a process where learning occurs when an unconditioned stimulus (food) is repeatedly preceded by a neutral stimulus (bell), the neutral stimulus serves as a conditioned stimulus and the learned reaction that results is termed the conditioned response. In order to maintain a conditioned response the conditioned and unconditioned stimuli must occasionally be paired.

Operant Conditioning (B.F. Skinner)

Operant conditioning is a process where learning occurs when an individual engages in specific behaviors in order to receive certain consequences.

Positive reinforcement: Administering desirable consequences to individuals who perform a specific behavior.

Negative reinforcement: Removing undesirable consequences from individuals who perform a specific behavior.

Extinction: Removing selected variables that reinforce a specific behavior.

Punishment: Administering negative consequences to individuals who perform undesirable behaviors.

Reinforcement Frequency and Schedules

Continuous reinforcement: A behavior is reinforced every time it occurs.

Partial reinforcement: A behavior is reinforced intermittently.

Fixed-interval schedule: The period of time between the occurrences of each instance of reinforcement is fixed or set.

Variable-interval schedule: The amount of time between reinforcements varies around a constant average.

Health Behavior Models

Change in behavior is a complex process that is difficult to attain and sustain. There has been significant research that has resulted in many different models for understanding behavior change and specific interventions. The following are a few commonly used models.

Health Belief Model

The Health Belief Model is one of the initial theories for behavior change. It is based on the belief that change in behavior depends upon the following factors:

1. **Perceived susceptibility:** one is at risk for the problem
2. **Perceived severity:** the health problem is serious
3. **Perceived benefit:** changing the behavior will reduce the threat
4. **Perceived barriers:** recognize obstacles required to change a behavior
5. **Cues to action:** strategies to activate readiness for change
6. **Self-efficacy:** the ability to change a behavior

The model provides insight as to why patients make health decisions and outlines a process to encourage change. Limitations of this model may include socioeconomic status, previous experiences, other influences, and cultural factors.

Locus of Control

This model was derived from the Social Learning Theory and is based on the assumption that there is difficulty predicting health behavior from the generalized expectancies. A scale was designed to measure a person's beliefs primarily surrounding the belief that their health is or is not an outcome of their own behavior. The theory is designed to assess the degree to which a patient believes that their health is controlled by internal or external factors.

1. **Internal locus of control:** internal factors are responsible for health status; our choices, personal actions, and decisions have direct bearing on our health.

2. **External locus of control:** powerful others (i.e. doctors) or other factors are responsible for health status; it's out of our personal control
3. **Chance:** fate, luck or chance determines our health status

Through the Health Locus of Control Scale a health care professional can assess the individual's perception of control over their health as well as the success of a health education program.

Social Cognitive Theory (Social Learning Theory)

This theory assesses the cognitive and emotional aspects of behavior for understanding behavioral change. The Social Cognitive Theory also attempts to explain how patients acquire and continue with particular behavioral patterns as well as providing a basis for intervention strategies. According to this theory the environment, personal factors, and behavior are constantly influencing each other. The concepts of the Social Cognitive Theory are below:

- **Behavior capability:** The process of learning how to make a change in behavior. Possessing the knowledge and skill to perform a given behavior; promote mastery learning through skills training.

- **Emotional coping responses:** Strategies or tactics that are used by a person to deal with emotional stimuli. To provide training in problem solving and stress management.

- **Environment:** Factors physically external to the person. The environment provides opportunities and social support.

- **Expectancies:** The value that is placed on the expected results. The values that the person places on a given outcome or incentives. Expectancies also represent present outcomes of change that have functional meaning.

- **Expectations:** Anticipatory outcomes of a behavior. To model positive outcomes of healthful behavior.

- **Observational learning:** Behavioral acquisition that occurs by watching the actions and outcomes of others' behavior. This will include credible role models of the targeted behavior.
- **Reinforcement:** Responses that are either positive or negative consequences of behavior. These are responses to a person's behavior that increase or decrease the likelihood of reoccurrence. Reinforcement promotes self-initiated rewards and incentives.
- **Reciprocal determinism:** The relationship between an individual and their environment. The dynamic interaction of the person, the behavior, and the environment in which the behavior is performed; consider multiple avenues to behavioral change, including environmental, skill, and personal change.
- **Self-control:** Personal regulation of goal-directed behavior or performance. Self-control will provide opportunities for self-monitoring, goal setting, problem solving, and self-reward.
- **Self efficacy:** The belief in one's ability to successfully change a behavior. The person's confidence in performing a particular behavior. Approach behavioral change in small steps to ensure success.
- **Situation:** Perception of the environment; correct misperceptions, and promote healthful forms.

Patient Education

Adult Learning

- Therapists must strive to make patient education sessions practical and useful for the patient.
- Failure to identify the relevance of the presented information will promote disinterest and decrease compliance.

Guidelines to Promote Adult Learning

- Design learning activities that will incorporate the patient's past experiences.
- Encourage the learner to play an active role in their educational program.
- Attempt to demonstrate the relevance of selected learning activities.
- Provide ample opportunities for practice and feedback.
- Recognize skill acquisition or objective improvement in patient performance.

Domains of Learning

Domains of learning are educational terms that describe various aspects of human behavior. The three most commonly recognized domains of learning are the cognitive, psychomotor, and affective domains. Recognizing the various levels of each of the domains can assist therapists to plan appropriate patient learning activities.

It is believed that a patient's reality is formed through the interaction of the environment and a person's cognitions (which change with experience and time). Social comparison of a patient's performance to others is also a strong source of self-efficacy. This theory is used when studying a variety of health pathologies, medical management compliance, alcohol abuse, and other health related issues. A limitation to this theory is that its complexity can make it difficult to use.

Trans-theoretical Model (Stages of Change)

The Trans-theoretical Model is a model of intentional change. It focuses on the decision making process of the individual. The theory differs from many others in its belief that change implies a process over time; not an isolated event. The process of change includes progressing through five stages:

1. **Precontemplation:** not intending to change
2. **Contemplation:** intending to change behavior in the near future
3. **Preparation:** making a plan to change behavior
4. **Action:** implementing the plan to change behavior
5. **Maintenance:** continuation of behavior change

This process for behavior change is not linear as individuals can enter and exit at any point or may repeat stages several times. The model can be useful to health programs and the process of moving a patient through various stages.

Affective domain: The affective domain is primarily concerned with attitudes, values, and emotions.

The domain consists of five specific levels: receiving, responding, valuing, organization, and characterization.

Cognitive domain: The cognitive domain is primarily concerned with knowledge and understanding.

The domain consists of six specific levels: knowledge, comprehension, application, analysis, synthesis, and evaluation.

Psychomotor domain: The psychomotor domain is primarily concerned with physical action or motor skill.

The domain consists of seven specific levels: perception, set, guided response, mechanism, complex overt response, adaptation, and origination.

Learning Style

Therapists can often obtain information related to a patient's preferred learning style by asking a few basic questions.

- Do you prefer to learn new information by observing, reading, listening or experiencing?
- Are you more comfortable learning in an active or passive manner?
- What increases your motivation to learn?

Teaching Methods

Individual

- Therapists most commonly instruct patients on an individual basis.
- The individual approach allows the therapist to focus on the needs of the learner and is the model of choice when the objectives of the session are unique to an individual patient.
- The individual approach allows the therapist to strengthen the patient/therapist bond and provides additional opportunities for specific feedback.

Group

- Therapists often instruct patients in a group.
- Group teaching may occur with patients, family members, staff, and support persons.
- Group teaching can be difficult if patients are not supportive of each other or if the learning needs of the group are diverse.
- Some patients may be intimidated by selected group members and tend to withdraw, while others may attempt to take control of the group.
- Since individuals typically receive less individual attention in a group it is critical for the therapist to regularly assess individual patient progress.
- Group teaching allows participants to support each other in the educational process and permits therapists to effectively use scarce resources such as time or money.
- Patients participating in group activities often feel a sense of camaraderie interacting with others who have similar personal experiences.

Patient Communication

- Verbal commands should focus the patient's attention on specifically desired actions.
- Instruction should remain as simplistic as possible and should not incorporate confusing medical terminology.
- The therapist should describe to the patient the general sequence of events that will occur prior to initiating treatment.
- The therapist should ask the patient questions during treatment in order to establish a rapport with the patient and to provide feedback as to the status of the current treatment.
- The therapist should speak clearly and vary their tone of voice as required by the situation.

Guidelines for Effective Patient Education

- Attempt to establish a positive rapport with the patient.
- Assess the patient's readiness and motivation to learn.
- Attempt to identify the patient's preferred learning style and available resources.

- Identify potential barriers to patient progress.
- Design an individualized education program for the patient based on his/her medical condition and personal goals.
- Coordinate education with the other members of the health care team.
- Focus the majority of available time on the most important concepts.
- Provide clear and succinct communication to the patient.
- Use repetition to improve patient learning.
- Provide frequent feedback to the patient.
- Utilize appropriate teaching resources to facilitate patient learning.
- Assess the effectiveness of patient education.
- Modify the patient education program based on the assessment results.

Principles of Motivation

- Readiness to learn significantly influences motivation.
- Individuals respond differently to selected motivational strategies.
- Success is more motivating than failure.
- Internal motivation has a greater potential to contribute to meaningful and lasting change than external motivation.
- Positive patient/therapist relationship enhances motivation.
- Limited anxiety may serve to motivate, while excessive anxiety may debilitate.
- Affiliation and approval can be motivating.

Cultural Influences

- Understanding cultural differences in patients can assist therapists to function as more effective educators.
- Patient culture is influenced and shaped by society, community, family, personal values, and attitudes.
- Language barriers, nonverbal communication, and limited personal experience can serve as obstacles when educating patients with significant cultural differences.
- Therapists should embrace cultural diversity and avoid efforts to make patients conform to any particular norm or standard.
- Therapists must be cautious when interpreting specific language or behavior and avoid labeling patients as unmotivated or disinterested.
- Therapists should use available resources such as experienced staff members, interpreters or consultants as necessary to achieve desired outcomes.

Designing Effective Patient Education Materials

- Design the materials to convey only the necessary information.
- Emphasize essential information.
- Utilize active instructions such as "you" and avoid passive terms such as "patient."
- Larger print may be more desirable than smaller print.
- Avoid long sentences or complex medical terminology.
- Pictures or graphics should be used where appropriate to complement written information.
- Incorporate answers to frequently asked questions.
- Written materials should flow in a logical sequence.
- Written materials should utilize a reading level appropriate for the target audience.

Teaching Guidelines for Specific Patient Categories

Therapists often vary their approach when educating patients of various ages and ability. It is difficult to develop recommendations that apply to all patients in a given category, however, the following represent general guidelines for therapists to consider when treating selected patient categories.

Infants/Children

- Therapists should try to make therapy sessions with infants/children interactive.
- Sessions should include structured play and should be of relatively short duration.
- Frequent breaks and positive reinforcement will serve to increase the patient's level of participation.

Adolescents

- Therapists should try to assume the role of an advocate when working with adolescents.
- It is important for therapists to establish patients' trust and incorporate patient goals into the plan of care.
- Adolescents prefer to be treated like adults and may resent the presence of parents during therapy sessions.
- Therapists should provide patients with clear and concise instructions and offer frequent positive reinforcement.

Adults

- Therapists should involve adults in determining education outcomes.
- The education program should be compatible with the patient's daily routine and goals.
- Emphasizing the relevance of educational activities will serve to increase patient compliance.
- Therapists should be aware of the available patient support system and identify any barriers to progress.

Elderly

- Therapists may find it necessary to introduce new information gradually when working with the elderly.
- Special attention should be paid to identify signs of hearing loss or visual impairments.
- The elderly population often benefits from the social benefits of group activities.
- Education sessions for the elderly should not be longer in duration, however, the achievement of selected outcomes may require additional sessions.

Terminally Ill

- Therapists should incorporate patient goals as an integral component of any educational session for patients with terminal illness.
- Family members and other support personnel should be encouraged to participate in the educational session, however, it is important to provide the patient with the opportunity to make independent decisions whenever possible.
- Goals for the terminally ill patient often include maximizing function, safety, and comfort.
- Therapists may alter their teaching methods based on the current mental and physical well-being of the patient.

Cognitively Impaired

- The therapist should focus on the education of the caregiver and incorporate the patient whenever possible.
- When incorporating the patient in the session, instructions should be clear and concise and should be summarized through demonstration and pictures.
- Therapists should encourage the patient to compensate for any memory deficit.

Illiteracy

- Therapists should attempt to determine the literacy level of their patients.
- If a patient is determined to be illiterate the therapist may elect to modify language to use basic wording and short sentences.
- Demonstration, repetition, and pictures should be incorporated into educational sessions.
- Therapists may include more detailed written information in educational sessions if the patient has adequate support at home.

Stages of Dying

Elizabeth Kubler-Ross identified five stages in coming to terms with death after interviewing 500 terminally ill patients. The stages Kubler-Ross identified were denial, anger, bargaining, depression, and acceptance.

Denial

The denial stage is characterized by a failure of the individual to believe that his/her condition is terminal. Therapists should attempt to establish trust with a patient in this stage and avoid trying to make the patient accept their condition.

Anger

The anger stage is characterized by frustration and negative emotional feelings often directed at anyone the individual comes in contact with. Individuals often ask "Why me?" Therapists should avoid taking the anger personally and recognize that expressing anger is often a useful step for the individual to move beyond this stage.

Bargaining

The bargaining stage is characterized by the individual trying to negotiate with fate. The individual may try to make a deal with a higher being based on good behavior, compliance with an exercise program or dedication of their life to a specific cause. Therapists should facilitate discussion with the patient and serve as a good listener.

Depression

The depression stage is characterized by the individual expressing the depths of his/her anguish. The individual is often deeply depressed and may show little interest in any form of medical intervention. Therapists should listen to the individual and exhibit a great deal of patience during this stage.

Acceptance

The acceptance stage is characterized by the individual coming to terms with their fate. The individual may attempt to resolve any unfinished business and may experience a sense of inner peace. Therapists should encourage the individual and family to ask questions and attempt to spend meaningful time with the individual.

Education Concepts

Practice

Practice refers to repeated performance of an activity in order to learn or perfect a skill. There are several commonly used terms that describe various types of practice.

Massed practice: The practice time in a trial is greater than the amount of rest between trials.

Distributed practice: The amount of rest time between trials is equal to or is greater than the amount of practice time for each trial.

Constant practice: Practice of a given task under a uniform condition.

Variable practice: Practice of a given task under differing conditions.

Random practice: Varying practice amongst different tasks.

Blocked practice: Consistent practice of a single task.

Whole training: Practice of an entire task.

Part training: Practice of an individual component or selected components of a task.

Feedback

Therapists should provide patients with specific and timely feedback in a manner that will promote attainment of the learning objective.

Summary feedback: Provided at the end of a defined number of activities or at the conclusion of the entire session.

Immediate feedback: Provided at the conclusion of a given activity.

Intrinsic feedback: Provided by the individual's internal sensory system.

Extrinsic feedback: Provided by an external source such as a therapist, spouse or physician.

Team Models

Unidisciplinary: A single discipline provides patient care services.

Multidisciplinary: Several different disciplines are involved in providing patient care, however, the disciplines tend to function independently and communication occurs primarily through the medical record.

Interdisciplinary: Several different disciplines are involved in providing patient care. The disciplines function independently, however, routinely report to each other and may coordinate patient care.

Transdisciplinary: Numerous disciplines function as a collective unit to provide patient care services. Team goals are established rather than individual discipline goals and as a result, discipline specific boundaries tend to erode.

Research & Evidence-Based Practice

Types of Research

Historical research: Investigating, recording, analyzing, and interpreting the events of the past for the purpose of discovering generalizations that are helpful in understanding the past, the present, and to a limited extent, anticipating the future.

Descriptive research: Recording, analyzing, and interpreting conditions that exist. Descriptive research involves some type of comparison or contrast and attempts to discover relationships between existing and non-manipulated variables.

Experimental research: A description of what will result when certain variables are carefully controlled or manipulated. The focus is on variable relationships.

Ethical Considerations

Informed consent: Recruitment of volunteers for experimentation must involve the subject's complete understanding of the procedures, risks, and demands that may be made.

Confidentiality: The researcher must hold all information gathered in an experiment in strict confidence, maintaining the subject's anonymity at all times.

Protection from harm or danger: When using treatments that may have a temporary or permanent effect on a subject, the researcher must take all precautions to preserve the subject's well-being.

Knowledge of outcome: Subjects have a right to receive an explanation for the experimental procedures and the results of the investigation.

Reliability

The degree of consistency that a measuring method or device produces.

Intrarater reliability: The consistency of repeated measurements of the same observation by the same rater.

Interrater reliability: The consistency of repeated measurements of the same observation by different raters.

Validity

Validity is the degree to which data or results of a study are correct or true.

Concurrent validity: The degree to which the measurement being validated agrees with an established measurement standard administered at approximately the same time. Concurrent validity is a form of criterion validity.

Construct validity: The relationship between an instrument and an established theoretical framework. Construct validity is based on theory and not statistical analysis.

Content validity: The degree to which the indicator provides a complete representation of the domain of interest.

Criterion validity: The degree to which a relationship exists between a measurement being validated and other measures.

External validity: The degree to which results of the research study are generalizable.

Internal validity: The degree to which the reported outcomes of the research study are a consequence of the relationship between the independent and dependent variables and not the result of extraneous factors.

Predictive validity: The ability of an instrument to predict the occurrence of a future behavior or event. Predictive validity is a form of criterion validity.

Variables

Independent variable: The factors in a research study that are manipulated by the researcher.

Dependent variable: The factors in a research study used to measure the effect of the independent variable.

Discrete variable: A variable whose measurements are expressed as integers.

Continuous variable: A variable whose measurements can assume any value along a continuum. Values are not limited to integers and instead are only limited by the degree of accuracy of the measuring instrument.

Levels of Measurement

Nominal

This is the weakest level of measurement. Categories are very broad and each participant of the study will fit into only one of the categories. Each category is independent of the other.

Example: male vs. female, yes vs. no

Ordinal

This level of measurement is also known as a ranking scale. Data that is collected will be placed into independent categories, however, the categories have a qualitative relationship regarding the order of ranking. There is not equality between each category.

Example: manual muscle testing, levels of assistance

Interval

A metric measurement scale where the distance between any two numbers is of equal amounts. In this scale the unit of measure and zero are both arbitrary.

Example: Celsius temperature scale, calendar time

Ratio

A metric measurement scale where the unit of measurement is arbitrary, however, there is an absolute zero.

Example: weight and length scales

Sampling

Probability sampling

Probability sampling requires an investigator to identify the parameters of a population. Every member of the population must have the same probability of being selected for the sample. Probability sampling generates smaller sampling error and therefore is often more desirable when an investigator would like to generalize from a specific population to a larger population.

Probability sampling methods:

- **Simple random sampling**
  Subjects have an equal chance of being selected for the sample. The sampling method often relies on a table of random numbers to determine the sample. Sampling can be performed with or without replacement.
- **Systematic sampling**
  Subjects are selected by taking every nth subject from the population. The size of the interval is based on the desired sample size. Systematic sampling is more efficient than simple random sampling and is most commonly employed when a researcher is drawing from a very large sample.
- **Stratified random sampling**
  Subjects are randomly selected from predetermined characteristics related to a particular study. Stratified random sampling enhances the sample representation and lowers sampling error by allowing subgroups to remain homogenous.

Cluster sampling

Subjects are selected based on a random sample of naturally occurring groups. Cluster sampling allows a random sample without a complete listing of each unit. The sampling technique is less costly and more efficient than simple random sampling.

Non-probability sampling

Non-probability sampling does not require the parameters of a population to be identified and there is an absence of randomization. This type of sampling is often utilized in physical therapy due to the increased difficulty of meeting the more rigid requirements of probability sampling.

Non-probability sampling methods:

- **Convenience sampling**
  Subjects are selected as they become available until the desired sample is reached.
- **Purposive sampling**
  Subjects are deliberately selected based on predefined criteria chosen by the investigators.
- **Snowball sampling**
  Subjects are identified by asking existing subjects to identify the names of other potential participants. Snowball sampling is often used when members of a given sample are difficult to identify.

Qualitative and Quantitative Research

Qualitative research

Research that derives data from observation, interviews or verbal interactions and focuses on the meanings and interpretations of the participants.

Quantitative research

Research based on collected objective data that can be subjected to statistical analysis.

	Qualitative Research	Quantitative Research
Purpose	To gain an understanding of underlying reasons and motivations of prevalent trends in thought and opinion. May use generated hypotheses for subsequent quantitative research.	To quantify data and generalize results from a sample to a given population. May later be followed by qualitative research to explore some particular findings further.
Rationale	Human behavior must be bound to the context in which the behavior occurs and therefore must be studied in the manner it occurs, rather than being manipulated.	Social reality can be reduced to variables that when tightly controlled allow researchers to examine how other variables are influenced.
Type of Research Question	Probing, global	Nonprobing, specific
Sample	A small number of subjects.	A large number of subjects representing the population of interest.
Researcher Role	Active participant who becomes immersed in the activity for the purpose of maximizing learning.	Objective observer that does not participate in or influence what is being studied.
Data Analysis	Non-statistical	Statistical
Training of the Researcher	Background is most often in the social sciences with specialized training and skills in interviewing.	Background is most often in statistics and mathematics.
Outcome	Exploratory or investigative. Develop an initial understanding for further decision making. Findings are not conclusive and cannot be used to make generalizations about the population.	Used to recommend a final course of action.

Research Terminology

Hawthorne effect (placebo effect): An untreated subject experiences a change simply from participating in a research study.

Hypothesis: A statement of belief about population parameters.

Level of significance (alpha): Expresses the probability of rejecting the null hypothesis when it is true. Since it is desirable to limit this probability, traditional values for alpha are .05 and .01. Alpha is synonymous with the probability of a type I error.

Null hypothesis: A statement indicating there is no difference between the population mean and the hypothesized value.

One-tailed test: Used when investigators have a prior expectation about the size of a sample mean and want to test whether it is larger or smaller than the population mean.

Parameter: Numerical measurement describing some characteristic of a population.

Population: Group of all elements to be studied.

Sample: Subgroup of elements drawn from a population.

Sensitivity: The percentage of individuals with a particular diagnosis that are correctly identified as positive.

Specificity: The percentage of individuals without a particular diagnosis that are correctly identified as negative.

Statistic: Numerical measurement describing some characteristic of a sample.

Two-tailed test: Used when investigators do not have a prior expectation about the size of a sample mean and want to test whether it is different from the population mean in either direction.

Type I error (alpha error): Rejecting the null hypothesis when it is in fact true. If the level of significance was set at .01, there would be a 1% chance of a type I error occurring.

Type II error (beta error): Accepting the null hypothesis when it is in fact false. An example of a type II error occurs when a researcher concludes that a given intervention did not have a positive outcome on a dependent variable when it actually did. Type I and Type II errors vary inversely.

Statistics

Types of Statistics

Descriptive statistics: Descriptive statistics summarize or describe important characteristics of a known set of population data. Conditions cannot be extended beyond the known set of population data and any similarity to data outside the known set cannot be assumed.

Inferential statistics: Inferential statistics use sample data to make inferences about a population. This form of statistics is often utilized to determine whether there are significant differences between groups.

Measures of Central Tendency

Mean: The results obtained by adding all of the values and dividing by the total number of values that were added.

Median: The point on a distribution at which 50% of the values fell above and below. The median is identified by first rank ordering the values. If the number of values is odd, the median is the middle value. If the number of values is even, the median is found by determining the mean of the two middle values.

Mode: The value that occurs most frequently. A distribution with two modes is termed bimodal. A distribution with more than two modes is termed multimodal.

Measures of Variation

Range: The difference between the highest and lowest value.

Variance: The sum of the squared deviation from the mean divided by the total number of values.

Standard deviation: The average deviation of values around the mean. Standard deviation is based on the distance of sample values from the mean and equals the square root of the mean of the squared deviation. Expressed differently, the standard deviation is the square root of the variance.

Normal Distribution

A bell shaped curve that is symmetrical around its vertical axis with the values tending to cluster around the mean. The mean, median, and mode have the same value. The curve has no boundaries and only a small fraction of the values fall outside of three standard deviations above or below the mean.

- Approximately 68% of all values fall within one standard deviation above or below the mean.
- Approximately 95% of all values fall within two standard deviations above or below the mean.
- Approximately 99% of all values fall within three standard deviations above or below the mean.

Skewness: Refers to the symmetry or lack of symmetry in the shape of a frequency distribution. Negatively skewed or left skewed data is characterized by the mean and median being to the left of the mode. Positively skewed or right skewed data is characterized by the mean and median being to the right of the mode.

Steps in Testing a Statistical Hypothesis

1. State the research question in terms of a statistical hypothesis
    a. null hypothesis
    b. alternative hypothesis
2. Decide on the appropriate test statistic
3. Select the level of significance for the statistical test
4. Determine the value the test statistic must attain to be declared significant
5. Perform the calculations
6. State the conclusion

Parametric Statistics

Parametric statistics assume that samples come from populations that are normally distributed and there is homogeneity of variance. Parametric statistical tests are applied to both interval and ratio level data.

Parametric statistical tests

- **t-test**
  A statistical procedure for comparing a mean with a norm or comparing two means with sample sizes less than or equal to 30.
- **z-test**
  A statistical procedure for comparing a mean with a norm or comparing two means for larger sample sizes greater than 30.
- **Independent t-test**
  A statistical procedure used to compare two independent samples. A sample is independent if the sample selected from one population is not related to the sample selected from the other population.
- **Dependent t-test**
  A statistical procedure used to compare the difference in a numerical variable observed for two paired groups. The test is also used when the same group is subjected to pre-test and post-test measurements.
- **Analysis of variance**
  A statistical procedure used to compare differences between two or more population means by analyzing sample variances.
- **One-way analysis of variance**
  A statistical procedure similar to the independent t-test, however, the test is designed to accommodate two or more population means. One-way refers to the fact that only one independent variable is examined.
- **Two-way analysis of variance**
  A statistical procedure used to compare two or more population means with two or more independent variables.

Nonparametric Statistics

Nonparametric statistics do not assume that samples come from populations that are normally distributed and do not assume homogeneity of variance. Nonparametric statistical tests are most commonly applied to nominal or ordinal level data.

Nonparametric statistical tests

- **Chi Square**
  A statistical procedure used to determine the probability that group differences result from chance. The nonparametric test uses nominal level data.
- **Mann-Whitney test**
  A statistical procedure used to compare two independent samples with ordinal level data. It is the nonparametric alternative of the independent t-test.
- **Kruskal-Wallis test**
  A statistical procedure used to determine if two or more samples come from the same population. It is the nonparametric version of the one-way analysis of variance.
- **Wilcoxon Signed Rank test**
  A statistical procedure used to compare two dependent samples with ordinal level data. It is the nonparametric alternative of the dependent t-test.

Correlation

The relationship between two variables when one is related to the other.

Correlation coefficient:

The correlation coefficient is the measure of the linear relationship between paired variables in a sample.

- A perfect positive correlation indicates that for every unit increase in one variable there is a proportionate unit increase in the other variable. A perfect positive correlation is indicated by +1.0.
- A perfect negative correlation indicates that for every unit increase in one variable there is a proportionate unit decrease in the other variable. A perfect negative correlation is indicated by −1.0.

Pearson product moment correlation (r):

The Pearson product moment correlation is a type of correlation statistic that requires interval level data. The test yields a value between −1.0 and +1.0.

Spearman rho:

The Spearman rho is a type of correlation statistic that requires ordinal level data. The test yields a value between −1.0 and +1.0. When interpreting a correlation coefficient it is important to remember that the coefficient does not imply a cause and effect relationship between variables. Attempt to avoid using rates or averages since this type of data reduces variation and may result in an inflated correlation coefficient.

Graphs

Histogram: A graphical display of a frequency distribution. A histogram typically includes the measurement of interest along the x-axis and the number or percentage of observations along the y-axis.

Dotplots: A graphical display in which each piece of data is plotted as a dot along a horizontal scale. When values occur more than once at a given point on the horizontal scale the dots are stacked vertically.

Stem and leaf plots: A graphical display which enables the reader to observe the entire distribution of data without losing any information. Most commonly this is done by organizing data into categories (e.g., 20-29, 30-39), and then dividing a number into two digits. The first digit is placed to the left side of a vertical line (stem) and the second digit is placed on the right side of the vertical line (leaves). The first digit within a category (stem) does not need to be repeated, however, the second digit (leaves) should be repeated.

Scatterplot: A graphical display that illustrates the relationship between two measures or variables measured on a numeric scale. Each value is represented by a point or dot on the scatterplot. A scatterplot should not be used to determine if a relationship is significant or occurs due to chance.

Box and whisker plot: A graphical display constructed based on the information in a stem and leaf plot. The graph illustrates both the frequencies and the distribution of the data and is commonly used to illustrate certain locations in the distribution.

Evidence-Based Medicine

Evidence-based medicine is the integration of best research evidence with clinical expertise and patient values. Evidence-based medicine functions as a framework for decision making in health care. The goal is to help clinicians make sense of knowledge derived from research and use the information as a basis for making health care decisions. The increased availability of affordable, user-friendly methods to critically appraise the literature has resulted in wide spread diffusion of evidence-based medicine. Utilizing the wealth of information available still requires a selected skill set and in many areas of clinical practice there remains a relative scarcity of high quality evidence. It is important to remember that the patient remains a critical component of decision making when practicing evidence-based medicine. Clinicians must be aware of the concerns, preferences, and expectations of each patient.

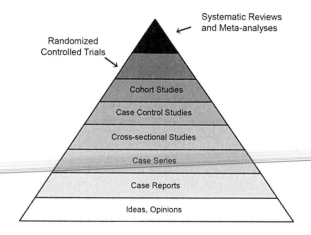

Stages of Evidence-Based Medicine Implementation

1. Identify a problem or area of uncertainty

2. Formulate a concise clinical question from a specific patient problem

3. Search the literature for relevant clinical articles

4. Critically appraise the identified evidence for its validity and usefulness

5. Implement relevant findings in clinical practice

6. Assess the outcomes of the selected action

7. Summarize findings for future reference

Hierarchy of Evidence

The hierarchy of evidence refers to how different types of evidence are ranked in terms of importance when decisions need to be made about clinical interventions. To evaluate the strength of the different types of clinical evidence, studies or clinical trials are ranked from those with the least amount of bias to those with the potential for the greatest amount of bias.

The base of the pyramid is where ideas typically start and basic research activities begin. As a user moves up the pyramid the amount of available literature decreases, but the relevance to the clinical setting dramatically increases. In many cases it is not possible to find the best level of evidence to answer a particular research question. In these

instances a clinician will need to consider moving down the pyramid to other types of studies, however, clinicians must be aware of the limitations incurred as the strength of the evidence diminishes.

Types of Clinical Evidence

Systematic Review

A systematic review is a comprehensive survey of a topic in which all of the primary studies of the highest level of evidence have been systematically identified, appraised, and then summarized according to an explicit and reproducible methodology. Each trial found is assessed by independent reviewers and the results combined and discussed using specific criteria to assess their quality before inferences can be made. A Cochrane Systematic Review is a type of review aimed at providing evidence specifically in the health care setting.

Meta-analysis

A meta-analysis is a specific statistical strategy for deriving a single numerical estimate from the results of several randomized controlled trials. This strategy can minimize the problem of small sample size since the pooling of trials increases the overall sample size. There are two potential limitations of meta-analysis that are most often cited. The first is that the results of different studies rarely precisely agree and in most cases the number of subjects in a single study is not large enough to come up with a definitive undisputable conclusion. The second is that if authors are interested in supporting a particular conclusion, they can include studies that are favorable to their conclusion and omit studies that are not.

Randomized Controlled Trial

A randomized controlled trial (RCT) is a type of research normally used to assess the relative effect of a specific intervention. Patients are randomized and split into two groups with one group receiving the intervention and the other serving as the control group. The control group receives either no treatment or a standard default treatment. Ideally, the two patient groups will be identical except for the intervention they have been randomized to receive. Assigning patients at random reduces the risk of bias and increases the probability that differences between the groups can be attributed to the intervention.

Cohort Study

A cohort study is an observational study of subjects with a specific condition and/or are receiving a particular treatment. The subjects are followed over a period of time and compared with another group who are not affected by the condition under investigation. Limitations of cohort studies include the excessive length of time a study can take and the influence of other lifestyle variables that invariably result in the two groups being uniquely different. As a result, cohort studies are not as reliable as randomized controlled trials. They are, however, generally preferred to case control studies since there are fewer statistical problems and they tend to produce more reliable answers.

Case Control Study

A case control study involves patients who already have a particular disease being matched with controls, but rather than following the subjects into the future, data on past exposure to possible causal agents are collected (e.g., by searching through medical records or interviewing subjects). Histories are then compared. Patients with the condition would be matched with patients without the condition in order to determine what risk factors might be linked to the development of the condition. This type of research will produce results faster than cohort studies, but is not as reliable. In some cases a new medical conclusion will be suggested based on a case control study which will then be followed by a researcher attempting to confirm the results with a RCT or a cohort study.

Cross-sectional Study

A cross-sectional study examines the frequency and characteristics of a disease or specific condition in a population at a particular point in time "snapshot." This type of research is often used to assess the prevalence of acute or chronic conditions in a population. Unlike time series, cross-sectional analysis relates to how variables affect each other at the same time.

Case Report or Case Series

A case report describes the medical history of a single patient in the form of a story and a case series consists of a collection of similar reports. They are most often used to record and alert other health professionals to rare occurrences. Since there is no control group, case reports and case series are not valid statistically and are therefore considered a source of anecdotal information.

Research Questions and Associated Types of Clinical Evidence

Question Type	Purpose	Study Design
Prognosis	How to estimate the patient's likely clinical course over time and anticipate likely complications	Cohort Study, Case Control Study, Case Series
Diagnosis	How to select and interpret diagnostic tests	Cross-Sectional Study
Therapy	How to select interventions that do more good than harm and are cost effective	Systematic Reviews, Meta- Analyses, Randomized Controlled Trials
Screening	How to assess the effectiveness of procedures performed to detect the presence of a specific disease or condition	Randomized Controlled Trials
Etiology/Harm	How to identify causes for a disease or specific condition	Cohort Study, Case Control Study, Case Series

Research Design Terminology

Controls: A trial that is controlled indicates that the treatment group is compared with another group. The two most common forms of control include placebo and active.

Placebo: Patients receive an "inactive treatment" which will look and feel like the active intervention given to the treatment group.

Active: The control is a treatment that is already in use because the use of a placebo (inactive treatment) may be unethical. For example, it would be unethical to attempt to measure the effect of smoking on health by asking one group to smoke two packs a day and ask another group to abstain given the known health risks of smoking.

Trial Groups: In most trials, subjects will be split into different groups, also called "arms." RCTs usually have two arms (i.e., control and treatment), but may have more. Other terms used to describe grouping are:

Parallel Groups: Subjects are randomized to one of two different interventions, usually for the entire trial and then the two groups are compared.

Matching/pairing: Investigators identify pairs of subjects who have identical characteristics (i.e., weight, age, race) before randomizing them so that each one receives a different intervention. This will reduce the influence of other factors on the results.

Cross Over: Each patient receives two sequential interventions (e.g., treatment and control) in random order separated by a period of no treatment. This design feature will "allow within subject differences" to be investigated. Because the same subject is used there is no need for matching.

Factorial: A study with a factorial design allows the effects of treatments used in combination as well as separately to be investigated.

Randomization: In a RCT patients are randomized to either the intervention or the control group. The method of randomization is important with the most robust method being the use of computer generated numbers or the use of random number tables.

Blinding: A term used to describe conditions that are imposed to keep groups of individuals from knowing which subjects have or have not received an intervention. Sometimes called masking, blinding is used to reduce bias and the placebo effect. There are several different types of blinding.

Single blind: The patients do not know which intervention they receive.

Double blind: Neither the patient nor the investigators know who was receiving which treatment.

Triple blind: Neither the patient nor the investigators nor the data analyzers know who was receiving which treatment.

Non-blind: Patients know which interventions they receive.

Practice Guidelines

Practice guidelines have been developed in many health professions to assist health care providers to make decisions based on the best available evidence. When developing practice guidelines organizations often use panels of experts to analyze the current research and make recommendations. The recommendations are usually accompanied by information about the consensus reached (or not reached) by the panel, called categories of consensus. Rigorously developed evidence-based guidelines assist health care providers to make the best decision about treatment for a particular patient. They also serve to limit potential harm, however, are only one option to improve the quality of patient care.

For example, a specific intervention may be recommended or not recommended based on an established Evidence Classification Schema. The following represents a specific example of an Evidence Classification Schema.

Evidence Classification Schema

Recommendation	Description	Example
Recommended for practice	Effectiveness is demonstrated by strong evidence from rigorously designed studies. Expected benefits exceed expected harms.	Two multi-site randomized controlled trials of more than 100 subjects. Panel of expert recommendations based on extensive literature search, quality rating, and synthesis of evidence.
Effectiveness not established for practice	Data currently are insufficient or are of inadequate quality.	Well conducted case control study. Conflicting evidence or statistically insignificant results.

Goals of Practice Guidelines

1. Improve the diagnosis and treatment of a particular condition
2. Reduce variation in clinical practice, thereby improving the quality of patient care
3. Encourage future research

Barriers to Evidence-based Medicine

1. A shortage of coherent and consistent scientific evidence associated with many clinical conditions.
2. Limited outcome data demonstrating that evidence-based medicine is in fact a superior method of practice.
3. Many clinicians need to develop new skills to effectively integrate evidence-based medicine into their daily practice.
4. Resources necessary to practice evidence-based medicine (e.g., online access) still do not exist in many clinical settings.
5. Relatively small incentives to change the status quo combined with extremely high productivity expectations of practicing clinicians.
6. Limited availability of mentors to assist practicing clinicians with adopting evidence-based medicine.

Advantages and Limitations of Various Forms of Data Collection

Form of Data	Advantages	Potential Limitations
Observation	Provides detailed, context related information Permits collection of information on items not mentioned in an interview May be particularly effective to collect behavioral data May be time consuming	Confidentiality issues Potential for observer bias Potential for the presence of the observer to influence the observed situation Controls must be used to limit environmental influences from skewing data Recordings of the observations must be systematic and standardized
Interview	Permits clarification of answers Higher response rate than written questionnaires Suitable for literate and illiterate subjects High labor costs	Presence of the interviewer can influence responses Interviewers may require special training
Using existing information	Cost effective since data already exists Allows examination of trends over time	Confidentiality issues Information may be incomplete or imprecise Data is not always accessible or in a complete form Available records may not accurately represent sample
Written questionnaire	Permits anonymity and therefore may result in more valid responses Less expensive than more labor intensive data collection techniques such as interviewing Able to minimize bias by phrasing questions differently with different respondents Provides a form of standardization	Cannot be used with illiterate subjects Low response rates Questions may be misinterpreted Need homogenous group if response rate is low

Outcome Measurement Tools

Outcome is the term used to qualitatively describe the end result of a particular intervention including changes (good or bad) that occurred to the health of a person, group or community. Factors that influence outcome include: primary diagnosis, co-morbidities, medical stability, prior physical status, current physical status, age and gender, beliefs, and attitudes.

Measuring outcome data is imperative to continually improve intervention strategies. Outcome data is also a powerful tool for positive feedback for the clinical staff and patient. The measuring tool must be both valid and reliable and the staff administering the tool must be familiar and qualified to do so in order to obtain meaningful and reliable results.

Balance

Berg Balance Scale

A tool designed to assess a patient's risk for falling. There are fourteen tasks, each scored on an ordinal scale from 0-4. These tasks include static, transitional, and dynamic activities in sitting and standing positions. The maximum score is a 56 with a score less than 45 indicating an increased risk for falling. This tool is used as a one-time examination or as an ongoing tool to monitor a patient who may be at risk for falls.

Functional Reach Test

A single task screening tool used to assess standing balance and risk of falling. A person is required to stand upright with a static base of support. A yardstick is positioned to measure the forward distance that a patient can reach without moving the feet. Three trials are performed and averaged together. The following are age related standard measurements for functional reach:

> 20 - 40 years – 14.5 - 17 inches
>
> 41 - 69 years – 13.5 - 15 inches
>
> 70 - 87 years – 10.5 - 13.5 inches

A patient that falls below the age appropriate range for functional reach has an increased risk for falling. The outcome measure demonstrates high test-retest correlation and intrarater reliability.

"Get Up and Go" Test

A functional performance screening tool used to assess a person's level of mobility and balance. The person initially sits in a supported chair with a firm surface, transfers to a standing position, and walks a few feet. The patient must then turn around without external support, walk back towards the chair, and return to a sitting position. The patient is scored based on amount of postural sway, excessive movements, reaching for support, side stepping, or other signs of loss of balance. The 5-point ordinal rating scale designates a score of one as normal and a score of five as severely abnormal. In an attempt to increase overall reliability the use of time was implemented. Patients who require over 20 seconds to complete the process may be at an increased risk for falling.

Romberg Test

An assessment of balance that positions the patient in unsupported standing, feet together, upper extremities folded, and eyes closed. A patient receives a grade of "normal" if they are able to maintain the position for 30 seconds.

Tinetti Performance Oriented Mobility Assessment

A tool used to screen patients and identify if there is an increased risk for falling. The first section assesses balance through sit to stand and stand to sit from an armless chair, immediate standing balance with eyes open and closed, tolerating a slight push in the standing position, and turning 360 degrees. A patient is scored from 0-2 in most categories with a maximum score of 16. The second section assesses gait at normal speed and at a rapid, but safe speed. Items scored in this section include initiation of gait, step length and height, step asymmetry and continuity, path, stance during gait, and trunk motion. A patient is scored either 0 to 1 or 0 to 2 with a maximum score of 12. The tool has a combined maximum total of 28 with the risk of falling increasing as the total score decreases. A total score less than 19 indicates a high risk for a fall.

Cognitive Assessment

Mini Mental State Examination

A tool designed to screen patients for cognitive impairment, psychoses or affective disorders. Each of the five sections: orientation, registration, attention and calculation, recall and language, and motor skills have multiple questions that receive one point for the correct answer or zero for the incorrect answer. There is a maximum score of 30 with a progressive level of cognitive impairment noted when a score of 24 or less is obtained.

Short Portable Mental Status Questionnaire

A ten item screening tool used to assess cognitive impairment primarily in the geriatric population. Orientation, short and long-term memory, practical skills, and mathematical tasks are tested. The maximum score is ten with a score below eight indicating cognitive impairment. The lower the score below eight the more significant the cognitive impairment.

Coordination and Manual Dexterity

Frenchay Arm Test

A tool used to assess coordination and dexterity by performing five activities based on functional movement patterns. The activities include stabilizing and drawing lines with a ruler, manipulating a cylinder without dropping it, drinking from a glass, placing and removing a clothespin, and combing hair. A patient receives three attempts to complete each task. A score of one is noted for successful completion; a score of zero is noted for failure to complete the task.

Jebsen Hand Function Test

A tool designed to assess hand function using seven timed activities. These activities include writing a 24-letter sentence, turning cards, placing six small objects into a container, using a teaspoon to pick up five small items, stacking items, moving large lightweight items, and large heavy objects. Each activity is timed and the results are compared to normative data.

Peg Test

There are multiple tools that utilize a pegboard to assess dexterity including the Purdue Pegboard test, the nine-hole peg test, and the ten-hole peg test. These tools use the element of time for completion of the task and compare results to normative data.

Endurance

Borg's Rating of Perceived Exertion Scale

A tool designed to measure perceived exertion, dyspnea, and exercise intensity. The original scale measures 6 to 20 points and the revised scale measures 0 to 10 points. The patient is instructed that a 6 (original) or 0 (new) corresponds to walking at a normal pace without fatigue. A score of 20 (original) or 10 (new) indicates high intensity exercise that cannot be completed due to exhaustion. After an activity a patient's score can indicate cardiopulmonary fatigue versus muscle fatigue. The score correlates with exercise intensity, heart rate, oxygen consumption, and blood lactate levels. Cardiopulmonary training effects can be seen with exercise intensity beginning at a 14 (original) or 4 to 5 (new) respectively. The scale is commonly used for patients with cardiovascular impairments.

Dyspnea Levels

A tool designed by Rancho Los Amigos Medical Center that attempts to rate the intensity and level of dyspnea that a patient experiences with activity. This ordinal scale consists of ratings from 0 to 4. A patient at level 0 is able to perform an activity and count to 15 without any additional breaths required. Levels 1, 2, and 3 require progressive extra breaths to count to 15. Level 4 indicates that the patient is unable to count while performing an activity. The test has not been shown to be valid, however, can be used to measure progress or decline during a course of rehabilitation.

Six-Minute Walk Test

A tool used to determine a patient's functional exercise capacity. The patient walks as far as he or she can for a timed six minutes with rest periods permitted as necessary. The tool is commonly used upon admission, discharge, and to monitor progress or decline throughout physical therapy. It allows for observation of heart rate and oxygen consumption during activity. This tool is administered to various populations including those with cardiac impairments, pulmonary disease, geriatrics with chronic conditions, and patients recovering from orthopedic surgical procedures.

Motor Recovery

Fugl-Meyer Assessment

An ordinal scale used to measure recovery post CVA. The framework is based on Brunnstrom's sequence of recovery. The five areas of assessment are joint movement and pain, balance, upper extremity motor function, sensation, and lower extremity motor function. Each item tested within an area is assigned a score from 0-3. The maximum combined score for upper extremity and lower extremity motor function is 100 and can be interpreted as a percentage of motor recovery. A score of 63 indicates approximately 63% return of motor function. This tool utilizes cumulative scoring for the entire assessment.

Montreal Evaluation

A tool that determines a patient's level of mobility by examining six specific areas in the following order: mental clarity, muscle tone, reflex activity, voluntary movement, automatic reactions, and pain. The construction of this tool utilized Bobath's NDT approach to neurological recovery. An ordinal scale of 0 to 3 is used for each item in each category. Muscle tone and active movements are examined separately, but scoring is cumulative for all areas. Each scored item includes multiple factors for a single score. This makes comparison of the individual scored items difficult.

Rivermead Motor Assessment

A tool based on the NDT approach to neurological recovery. The Rivermead Motor Assessment is divided into three major sections: gross function, leg and trunk, and arm. Each section is comprised of a subscale of tasks. These tasks increase in difficulty and are graded with a score of one for completion or zero for inability to perform the activity. The assessment possesses a high level of sensitivity when examining higher level patients and is reliable within one point.

Pain

McGill Pain Questionnaire

A pain assessment tool that is divided into four parts with a total of 70 questions.

Part 1 Patient marks on a drawing of the body to indicate area and type of pain (internal or external)

Part 2 Patient chooses one word that best describes the pain from each of the twenty categories

Part 3 Patient describes pattern of pain, factors that increase and relieve pain

Part 4 Patient rates the intensity of pain on a scale of zero to five

This tool can be used to establish a baseline, evaluate particular treatment regimens, and monitor progress. It is valid, reliable, and the most widely used pain assessment scale.

Numerical Rating Scale

A tool used to assess pain intensity by rating pain on a scale of 0-10 or 0-100. The 0 represents no discernable pain and the 10 or 100 represent the worst pain ever. The information is used as a baseline and should be reassessed at regular intervals in order to monitor progress. This scale is easy to administer, assess, and monitor.

Visual Analogue Scale

A tool used to assess pain intensity using a 10-15 cm line with the left anchor indicating "no pain" and the right anchor indicating "the worst pain you can have." The level of perceived pain is indicated on the line and is reassessed frequently over the course of physical therapy to record changes and progress, and to predict patient outcome. This scale can be highly sensitive if small increments such as millimeters are used to measure the patient's point of pain on the scale. The visual analogue scale is a valid tool if measurements are taken accurately.

Self-Care and ADL

Barthel Index

A tool designed to measure the amount of assistance needed to perform ten different activities with a total maximum score of 100. These activities include bowel management, bladder management, grooming, toilet use, feeding, transfers, mobility, dressing, stairs, and bathing. A score of 75-95 denotes mild impairment, 50-70 moderate impairment, 20-45 severe impairment, and below 20 indicates a very severe impairment. The index does not account for cognitive or safety issues and is not sensitive to higher level patients regarding their level of disability. It remains one of the oldest and most widely used tools that is reliable and possesses predictive validity.

Functional Independence Measure (FIM)

A tool that is primarily used in rehabilitation hospitals in order to determine a patient's level of disability and burden of care. This tool is part of the Uniform Data System for Medical Rehabilitation (UDS). A seven-point scale is utilized to examine 18 areas, which include self-care, sphincter control, transfers, locomotion, communication, and social cognitive activities. These items were designed based on the World Health Organization's Model of Disability. Scoring between a 1 and 5 denotes a level of dependence and between 6 and 7 a level of independence for a specific item. This tool is both valid and reliable and is used as a predictor of disability for the CVA population. The FIM is utilized on a larger scale to assess change within rehabilitation programs over time.

Katz Index of Activities of Daily Living

A nominal scale index used to identify self-care problems and the level of assistance required with the six areas of bathing, dressing, toileting, transfers, continence, and feeding. The score for each area is combined and the total score correlates with a letter grade scale (A through G). Each letter represents a level of ability with "A" representing independence in all six areas, the following letters representing increasing dependence, and "G" representing dependence in all six areas. This tool was originally intended only for inpatient and nursing home settings, however, it is now utilized with patients that require outpatient and community based services. It is a simple and quick assessment tool used to efficiently gather self-care information and predict outcome and need for ongoing assistance.

Pediatric Assessment Tools

Instrument	Purpose	Other
Alberta Infant Motor Scale	Identify components of motor development Measure gross motor acquisition and skill maturation over time	Use from birth to walking Piper
Bayley Scale of Infant Development II	Assessment of current developmental status using a mental scale, motor scale, and behavioral scale Includes special populations	Use from one month to 42 months Bayley
Denver II	Screen of four domains: personal-social, fine motor adaptive, language, and gross motor Screens for developmental delay and need for further evaluation	Use from two weeks to six years Frankenburg
Functional Independence Measure for Children (WeeFIM)	Assesses and notes progression of functional independence A measure of disability Requires consistent performance of a skill	Use from six months to seven years Utilized by Uniform Data System (UDS)
Milani-Comparetti Motor Development Screening Test	Measures functional motor skills and related reflexes Demonstrates age appropriate responses through profile Neuromotor delay	Use from birth to two years Milani-Comparetti, Gidoni
Movement Assessment of Infants	Focus on infants that were treated in neonatal intensive care Categories include muscle tone, reflexes, automatic reactions, and volitional movements Identifies motor dysfunction and establishes baseline	Use from birth to 12 months Chandler, Swanson
Neonatal Behavioral Assessment	Focus on interactive behavior, competence, and neurological status Predictor of further neurological problems	Use from three days to four weeks Brazelton
Peabody Developmental Motor Scales	Provides detailed assessment with instruction programming Gross and fine motor scales Identifies emergency skills Does not require verbal language	Use from birth to 83 months Folio, Fewell
Pediatric Evaluation of Disability Inventory (PEDI)	Assessment of functional skills Designed for rehabilitation use Includes areas of self care, mobility, social skills, level of assistance, and use of adaptive equipment	Use from six months to 7.5 years Haley

Unit 3

Clinical Application Templates

The clinical application template allows candidates to explore many of the elements of patient/client management for a wide variety of medical conditions. Although candidates have been exposed to a variety of medical conditions during their clinical education experiences it is unlikely they have been exposed to the vast number of medical conditions commonly encountered on the examination. By utilizing clinical application templates students can broaden their experience base and as a result be better prepared to answer examination questions.

This section contains an executive summary of selected information associated with 60 different clinical application templates followed by an expansive two page summary of each medical condition. Candidates are encouraged to review the templates and carefully reflect on the presented information. Candidates should attempt to make this activity an active learning exercise and resist the urge to simply read each of the templates. For example, let's assume that a candidate was reviewing a clinical application template on an anterior cruciate ligament sprain. In each category of the clinical application template candidates should assess their knowledge by asking specific questions. Two specific examples for the tests and measures section are listed below:

When reviewing range of motion, candidates should ask themselves the following:
- What is normal range of motion at the knee?
- Which type of end-feel would be considered normal for knee flexion and extension?
- Where should the axis, moving arm, and stationary arm of the goniometer be aligned when measuring range of motion?
- Where should the therapist stabilize when conducting the measurement?

When reviewing joint integrity and mobility, candidates should ask themselves the following:
- Which special test or tests would be the most appropriate to assess the ligamentous integrity of the anterior cruciate ligament?
- Describe the process for administering the special test?
- What finding would be indicative of a positive test?

By engaging in this type of active learning exercise, candidates are able to further assess their level of preparedness for the examination. Although some candidates may be quite comfortable reviewing selected clinical application templates, many candidates learn that they lack necessary content in many others. For example, do you feel adequately prepared to discuss the patient/client management of each of the following diagnoses: amyotrophic lateral sclerosis, cystic fibrosis, cerebrovascular accident, and rotator cuff tendonitis? Prior to taking the actual examination candidates should have some reasonable level of comfort discussing each of the 60 clinical application templates included in this unit.

Candidates should not rely solely on the presented clinical application templates and instead should utilize the template format to review a variety of other medical conditions. This type of active learning is best performed by a small group of candidates with a given candidate acting as the facilitator. In this manner students can share their individual clinical experience with the group and at the same time benefit from the knowledge of their classmates.

*The clinical application template was adapted from a document by the Academy of Specialty Boards entitled "Preparing Items that Measure More than Recall." The document was originally designed to help item writers develop sample questions for the Physical Therapy Specialty Examinations.

Clinical Application Templates

Clinical Application Templates (continued)

Clinical Application Templates (continued)

Clinical Application Template Executive Summary

Achilles Tendon Rupture

- Typically occurs within one to two inches above the tendinous insertion on the calcaneus
- Incidence is greatest between 30-50 years of age without history of calf or heel pain
- Patients with an Achilles tendon rupture will typically be unable to stand on their toes and tend to exhibit a positive Thompson test

Adhesive Capsulitis

- Occurs more in the middle-aged population with females having a greater incidence than males
- Arthrogram can assist with diagnosis by detecting decreased volume of fluid within the joint capsule
- Range of motion restriction typically in a capsular pattern (lateral rotation, abduction, medial rotation)

Alzheimer's Disease

- Progressive neurological disorder that results in deterioration and irreversible damage within the cerebral cortex and subcortical areas of the brain
- Disease is initially noted by a change in higher cortical functions characterized by subtle changes in memory, impaired concentration, and difficulty with new learning
- Typical course of the disease averages between 7-11 years with death resulting from infection or dehydration

Amyotrophic Lateral Sclerosis

- Risk is higher in males than females and usually occurs between 40-70 years of age
- Clinical presentation may include both upper and lower motor neuron involvement with weakness occurring in a distal to proximal progression
- Average course of the diagnosis is two to five years with 20-30% of patients surviving longer than five year

Ankylosing Spondylitis

- Systemic condition characterized by inflammation of the spine and the larger peripheral joints
- Males are at two to three times greater risk than females with peak onset observed between 20-40 years of age
- Clinical presentation initially includes recurrent and insidious onset of back pain, morning stiffness, and impaired spinal extension

Anterior Cruciate Ligament Sprain - Grade III

- Injury most commonly occurs during hyperflexion, rapid deceleration, hyperextension or landing in an unbalanced position
- Females involved in selected athletic activities have significantly higher ligament injury rates compared to males
- Approximately two-thirds of complete anterior cruciate ligament tears have an associated meniscal tear

Bicipital Tendonitis

- Increased incidence of injury is associated with selected athletic activities such as baseball pitching, swimming, rowing, gymnastics, and tennis
- Characterized by subjective reports of a deep ache directly in front and on top of the shoulder made worse with overhead activities or lifting
- Examination may reveal a positive Speed's test or Yergason's test

Breast Cancer

- May spread to the lymphatic system and commonly metastasizes to the brain, lungs, bones, adrenals, and liver
- Breast cancer makes up 30% of all female cancers and is the second leading cause of death for females in the United States
- Prognosis and ten-year survival rates for women are over 85% for stage I; 66% for stage II; 36% for stage III; and 7% for stage IV disease

Carpal Tunnel Syndrome

- Incidence is higher in females than males with the most common age being from 35-55 years of age
- Muscle atrophy is often noted in the abductor pollicis brevis muscle and later in the thenar muscles
- Electromyography studies, Tinel's sign, and Phalen's test can be used to assist with confirming the diagnosis

Central Cord Syndrome

- An incomplete spinal cord lesion that most often results from a cervical hyperextension injury
- Clinical presentation involves motor loss that is greater in the upper extremities than the lower extremities
- Most common incomplete spinal cord lesion accounting for approximately 30% of all incomplete forms of tetraplegia

Cerebral Palsy

- Spastic cerebral palsy involves upper motor neuron damage; athetoid cerebral palsy involves damage to the cerebellum, cerebellar pathways or both
- Clinical presentation includes motor delays, abnormal muscle tone and motor control, reflex abnormalities, poor postural control, and balance impairments
- Mental retardation and epilepsy are present in 50-60% of children diagnosed with cerebral palsy

Cerebrovascular Accident (CVA)

- Types of CVA include ischemic stroke (thrombus, embolus, lacunar) and hemorrhagic stroke (intracerebral, subdural, subarachnoid)
- Left CVA may present with weakness or paralysis to the right side, impaired processing, heightened frustration, aphasia, dysphagia, and motor apraxia
- Right CVA may present with weakness or paralysis to the left side, poor attention span, impaired awareness and judgment, spatial deficits, memory deficits, emotional lability, and impulsive behavior

Congenital Torticollis

- Causes the neck to involuntarily contract to one side secondary to contraction of the sternocleidomastoid muscle
- The head is laterally flexed toward the contracted muscle, the chin faces the opposite direction, and there may be facial asymmetries
- Studies indicate that between 85-90% of patients with congenital torticollis respond to conservative treatment and passive stretching within the first year of life

Congestive Heart Failure (CHF)

- Common etiologies contributing to CHF include arrhythmia, pulmonary embolism, hypertension, valvular heart disease, myocarditis, unstable angina, renal failure, and severe anemia
- Left-sided heart failure is generally associated with signs of pulmonary venous congestion; right-sided heart failure is associated with signs of systemic venous congestion
- Diminished cardiac output causes compensatory changes including an increase in blood volume, cardiac filling pressure, heart rate, and cardiac muscle mass

Cystic Fibrosis
- Causes the exocrine glands to overproduce thick mucus which causes subsequent obstruction
- Autosomal recessive genetic disorder (both parents are carriers of the defective gene) located on the long arm of chromosome seven
- A terminal disease, however, the median age of death has increased to 35 years of age due to early detection and comprehensive management

Degenerative Spondylolisthesis
- Caused by the weakening of joints that allows for forward slippage of one vertebral segment on the one below due to degenerative changes
- Most common site of degenerative spondylolisthesis is the L4-L5 level
- William's flexion exercises may be indicated to strengthen the abdominals and reduce lumbar lordosis

Diabetes Mellitus (Type 1)
- Insulin is functionally absent due to the destruction of the beta cells of the pancreas; where the insulin would normally be produced
- Starts in children ages four years or older, with the peak incidence of onset coinciding with early adolescence and puberty
- Common symptoms include polyuria, polydipsia, polyphagia, nausea, weight loss, fatigue, blurred vision, and dehydration

Down Syndrome
- Clinical manifestations include hypotonia, flattened nasal bridge, Simian line (palmar crease), epicanthal folds, enlargement of the tongue, and developmental delay
- Detection occurs in approximately 60-70% of women tested that are carrying a baby with Down syndrome
- Exercise is essential for a child with Down syndrome in order to avoid inactivity and obesity

Duchenne Muscular Dystrophy
- X-linked recessive trait manifesting in only male offspring while female offspring become carriers
- Clinical presentation includes waddling gait, proximal muscle weakness, toe walking, pseudohypertrophy of the calf, and difficulty climbing stairs
- There is usually rapid progression of this disease with the inability to ambulate by ten to twelve years of age with death occurring as a teenager or less frequently in the 20's

Emphysema
- Results from a long history of chronic bronchitis, recurrent alveolar inflammation or from genetic predisposition of a congenital alpha 1-antitrypsin deficiency
- Clinical presentation may include barrel chest appearance, increased subcostal angle, rounded shoulders secondary to tight pectorals, and rosy skin coloring
- Symptoms of emphysema worsen with the progression of the disease and include a persistent cough, wheezing, difficulty breathing especially with expiration, and an increased respiration rate

Erb's Palsy
- Muscles affected are supplied by cervical roots C5 and C6 which result in a loss of function of the rotator cuff, deltoid, brachialis, coracobrachialis, and biceps brachii
- Brachial plexus injury in a newborn usually occurs during a difficult delivery, due to a large baby, a breech presentation with a prolonged labor or with the use of forceps
- Results in flaccid paralysis nicknamed the "Waiter's tip deformity" (characterized by a loss of shoulder function, loss of elbow flexion, loss of forearm pronation, and the hand positioned in a pinch grip manner)

Fibromyalgia Syndrome

- Nonarticular rheumatic condition with pain caused by tender points within muscles, tendons, and ligaments
- Greater incidence in females (almost 75% of the cases) potentially affecting any age
- Widespread history of pain that exists in all four quadrants of the body (above and below the waist), axial pain is present, and there is pain in at least 11 of 18 standardized "tender point" sites

Full-Thickness Burn

- Burn causes immediate cellular and tissue death and subsequent vascular destruction
- Eschar forms from necrotic cells and creates a dry and hard layer that requires debridement
- Absent sensation and pain due to destruction of free nerve endings, however, there may be pain from adjacent areas that experience partial-thickness burns

Guillain-Barre Syndrome

- Results in motor weakness in a distal to proximal progression, sensory impairment, and possible respiratory paralysis
- Etiology of the disease is unknown, however, it is hypothesized to be an autoimmune response to a previous respiratory infection, influenza, immunization or surgery
- Majority of patients experience full recovery, 20% have remaining neurologic deficits, and 3-5% of patients die from respiratory complications

Human Immunodeficiency Virus (HIV)

- Primary risk factors for contracting HIV include unprotected sexual relations, intravenous drug use or mother to fetus transmission
- Patients may actually be "symptom free" for one to two years post infection or may exhibit flu-like symptoms including rash and fever
- Leading cause of death for patients with the virus is kidney failure secondary to the extended drug therapies

Huntington's Disease

- Chronic progressive genetic disorder that is fatal within 15 to 20 years after clinical manifestation
- Characterized by degeneration and atrophy of the basal ganglia (specifically the striatum) and cerebral cortex within the brain
- Clinical presentation includes enlarged ventricles secondary to atrophy of the basal ganglia, mental deterioration, speech disturbances, and ataxic gait

Juvenile Rheumatoid Arthritis (JRA)

- Autoimmune disorder found in children less than 16 years of age that occurs when the immune cells mistakenly begin to attack the joints and organs causing local and systemic effects throughout the body
- Girls have a higher incidence of JRA and are most commonly diagnosed as toddlers or in early adolescence
- Clinical symptoms include persistent joint swelling, pain, and stiffness

Lateral Epicondylitis "Tennis Elbow"

- Characterized by inflammation or degenerative changes at the common extensor tendon that attaches to the lateral epicondyle of the elbow
- Repeated overuse of the wrist extensors, particularly the extensor carpi radialis brevis can produce tensile stress and result in microscopic tearing and damage to the extensor tendon
- Clinical symptoms include difficulty holding or gripping objects and insufficient forearm functional strength

Lymphedema Post-Mastectomy
- Caused by an excess load of lymph fluid or inadequate transport capacity within the lymphatic system secondary to the loss of homeostasis
- Primary contributing factor in the development of lymphedema following a mastectomy is the damage and/or removal of the axillary lymph nodes and vessels
- Intervention should focus on manual lymph drainage, short stretch compression bandages, retrograde massage, exercise, compression therapy, and use of a mechanical pump

Medial Collateral Ligament Sprain – Grade II
- Grade II injury is characterized by partial tearing of the ligament's fibers resulting in joint laxity when the ligament is stretched
- Mechanism of injury is usually a blow to the outside of the knee joint causing excess force to the medial side of the joint
- Return to previous functional level should occur within four to eight weeks following the injury if no other associated structures are involved

Multiple Sclerosis
- Characterized by demyelination of the myelin sheaths that surround nerves within the brain and spinal cord resulting in plaque development, decreased nerve conduction velocity, and eventual failure of impulse transmission
- Clinical symptoms may include visual problems, paresthesias, sensory changes, clumsiness, weakness, ataxia, balance dysfunction, and fatigue
- Intervention includes regulation of activity level, relaxation and energy conservation techniques, normalization of tone, balance activities, gait training, and core stabilization

Myocardial infarction (MI)
- Myocardial infarction occurs when there is poor coronary artery perfusion, ischemia, and subsequent necrosis of the cardiac tissue usually due to thrombus, arterial blockage or atherosclerosis
- Risk factors include patient or family history of heart disease, smoking, physical inactivity, stress, hypertension, elevated cholesterol, diabetes mellitus, and obesity
- Clinical presentation may include deep pain or pressure in the substernal area with or without pain radiating to the jaw or into the left arm or the back

Osteoarthritis
- Degenerative process primarily involving articular cartilage resulting from excessive loading of a healthy joint or normal loading of an abnormal joint
- Typically diagnosed based on the results of a clinical examination and x-ray findings
- Prevalence is higher among women than men with approximately 80-90% of individuals older than 65 years of age demonstrating evidence of osteoarthritis

Osteogenesis Imperfecta
- Classified into four types with a wide range of clinical presentations ranging from normal appearance with mild symptoms to severe involvement that can be fatal during infancy
- Bone densitometry may be used to measure bone mass and estimate the risk of fracture for specific sites within the body
- Children with osteogenesis imperfecta often have delayed developmental milestones secondary to ongoing fractures with immobilization, hypermobility of joints, and poorly developed muscles

Osteoporosis

- Metabolic bone disorder where the rate of bone resorption accelerates while the rate of bone formation slows down
- Patients may complain of low thoracic or lumbar pain and experience compression fractures of the vertebrae
- Bone mineral density test accounts for 70% of bone strength and is the easiest way to determine osteoporosis

Parkinson's Disease

- Degenerative disorder characterized by a decrease in production of dopamine (neurotransmitter) within the corpus striatum portion of the basal ganglia
- Clinical presentation may include hypokinesia, difficulty initiating and stopping movement, festinating and shuffling gait, bradykinesia, poor posture, and "cogwheel" or "lead pipe" rigidity
- Medical management includes dopamine replacement therapy (Levodopa, Sinemet, Madopar) which is designed to minimize bradykinesia, rigidity, and tremor

Patellofemoral Syndrome

- Causes damage to the articular cartilage of the patella ranging from softening to complete cartilage destruction resulting in exposure of subchondral bone
- Etiology is unknown, however, it is extremely common during adolescence, is more prevalent in females than males, and has a direct association with activity level
- Management includes controlling edema, stretching, strengthening, improving range of motion, and activity modification

Peripheral Vascular Disease

- Characterized by narrowing of the lumen of blood vessels causing a reduction in circulation usually secondary to atherosclerosis
- Risk factors include phlebitis, injury or surgery, autoimmune disease, diabetes mellitus, smoking, hyperlipidemia, inactivity, hypertension, positive family history, increased age, and obesity
- Patient education is paramount regarding the disease process, limb protection, foot and skin care, and risk factor reduction (smoking cessation, avoid cold exposure)

Plantar Fasciitis

- Chronic overuse condition that develops secondary to repetitive stretching of the plantar fascia through excessive foot pronation during the loading phase of gait
- Characterized by severe pain in the heel when first standing up in the morning (when the fascia is contracted, stiff, and cold)
- Intervention consists of ice massage, deep friction massage, heel insert, orthotic prescription, activity modification, and gentle stretching program of the Achilles tendon and plantar fascia

Pressure Ulcer

- Unrelieved pressure deprives the tissues of oxygen which causes ischemia, subsequent cell death, and tissue necrosis
- High risk areas for pressure ulcers include the occiput, heels, greater trochanters, ischial tuberosities, sacrum, and epicondyles of the elbow
- Impaired cognition, poor nutrition, altered sensation, incontinence, decreased lean body mass, and infection contribute to the development of a pressure ulcer

Reflex Sympathetic Dystrophy

- Increase in sympathetic activity causes a release of norepinephrine in the periphery and subsequent vasoconstriction of blood vessels resulting in pain and an increase in sensitivity to peripheral stimulation
- Affects all age groups, but is most likely found in individuals 35-60 years of age with females being three times more likely to be affected than males
- Patients experience intense burning and chronic pain in the affected extremity that eventually spreads in a proximal direction

Restrictive Lung Disease

- Classification of disorders caused by a pulmonary or extrapulmonary restriction that produces impairment in lung expansion and an abnormal reduction in pulmonary ventilation
- Pulmonary restriction of the lungs can be caused by tumor, interstitial pulmonary fibrosis, scarring within the lungs, pleural effusion, chest wall stiffness, structural abnormality, and respiratory muscle weakness
- Pathogenesis includes a decrease in lung and chest wall compliance, decrease in lung volumes, and an increase in the work of breathing

Rheumatoid Arthritis

- Systemic autoimmune disorder of the connective tissue that is characterized by chronic inflammation within synovial membranes, tendon sheaths, and articular cartilage
- Incidence is three times greater in females than males and is diagnosed most frequently between 30-50 years of age
- Blood work assists with the diagnosis of rheumatoid arthritis through evaluation of the rheumatoid factor, white blood cell count, erythrocyte sedimentation rate, hemoglobin, and hematocrit values

Rotator Cuff Tendonitis

- Caused by an inability of a weak supraspinatus muscle to adequately depress the head of the humerus in the glenoid fossa during elevation of the arm
- Participating in activities that require excessive overhead activity such as swimming, tennis, baseball, painting, and other manual labor activities increase the risk of rotator cuff tendonitis
- Patient may experience a feeling of weakness and identify the presence of a painful arc of motion most commonly occurring between 60 and 120 degrees of active abduction

Sciatica Secondary to a Herniated Disk

- The sciatic nerve experiences an inflammatory response and subsequent damage secondary to compression from the herniated disk
- Sciatica is characterized by low back and gluteal pain that typically radiates down the back of the thigh along the sciatic nerve distribution
- Pain will increase in a sitting position or when lifting, forward bending or twisting

Scoliosis

- Curvature is usually found in the thoracic or lumbar vertebrae and can be associated with kyphosis or lordosis
- A patient with scoliosis that ranges between 25 and 40 degrees requires a spinal orthosis and physical therapy intervention for posture, flexibility, strengthening, respiratory function, and proper utilization of the spinal orthosis
- Scoliosis does not usually progress significantly once bone growth is complete if the curvature remains below 40 degrees at the time of skeletal maturity

Spina Bifida – Myelomeningocele

- Classifications include occulta (incomplete fusion of the posterior vertebral arch with no neural tissue protruding), meningocele (incomplete fusion of the posterior vertebral arch with neural tissue/meninges protruding outside the neural arch), and myelomeningocele (incomplete fusion of the posterior vertebral arch with both meninges and spinal cord protruding outside the neural arch)
- Approximately 75% of vertebral defects are found in the lumbar/sacral region most often at L5-S1
- Prenatal testing of alpha-fetoprotein (AFP) in the blood will show an elevation in levels that indicate a probable neural tube defect at approximately week 16 of gestation

Spinal Cord Injury – Complete C7 Tetraplegia

- Clinical presentation includes impaired cough and ability to clear secretions, altered breathing pattern, and poor endurance
- Outcomes at this level include independence with feeding, grooming, dressing, self-range of motion, independent manual wheelchair mobility, independent transfers, and independent driving with an adapted automobile
- The triceps, extensor pollicis longus and brevis, extrinsic finger extensors, and flexor carpi radialis will remain the lowest innervated muscles

Spinal Cord Injury – Complete L3 Paraplegia

- Patients possess at least partial innervation of the gracilis, iliopsoas, quadratus lumborum, rectus femoris, and sartorius with full upper extremity use
- Additional findings that can exist include sexual dysfunction, a nonreflexive bladder, the need for a bowel program, urinary tract infections, muscle contractures, and pressure sores
- Patients with L3 paraplegia should be able to live independently with education regarding the management of their disability

Spondylolisthesis

- Characterized by forward slippage of one vertebral body with respect to the vertebral body below it
- Patients participating in gymnastics, wrestling, football, and weight lifting are at greater risk for spondylolisthesis
- X-ray oblique views can show the pars as having the appearance of a "Scottie dog with a collar" when a spondylolysis is present

Systemic Lupus Erythematosus

- Connective tissue disorder caused by an autoimmune reaction in the body
- Females are at greater risk than males with the most common age group ranging from 15-40 years of age
- Clinical presentation includes a red butterfly rash across the cheeks and nose, a red rash over light exposed areas, arthralgias, alopecia, pleurisy, kidney involvement, seizures, and depression

Temporomandibular Joint Dysfunction

- Females are at greater risk than males with the most common age ranging from 20-40 years of age
- Clinical presentation includes pain (persistent or recurring), muscle spasm, abnormal or limited jaw motion, headache, and tinnitus
- Intervention includes patient education, posture retraining, and modalities such as moist heat, ice, biofeedback, ultrasound, electrostimulation, TENS, and massage

Thoracic Outlet Syndrome

- Results from compression and damage to the brachial plexus nerve trunks, subclavian vascular supply, and/or the axillary artery
- Contributing factors in the development of the condition include the presence of a cervical rib, an abnormal first rib, postural deviations, hypertrophy or spasms of the scalene muscles, and an elongated cervical transverse process
- Females are at two to three times greater risk than males with the most common age ranging from 30-40 years of age

Total Hip Arthroplasty

- Patients are typically over 55 years of age and have experienced consistent pain that is not relieved through conservative measures which serve to limit the patient's functional mobility
- Posterolateral approach allows the abductor muscles to remain intact, however, there may be a higher incidence of post-operative joint instability due to the interruption of the posterior capsule
- Cemented hip replacement usually allows for partial weight bearing initially, while a noncemented hip replacement requires toe touch weight bearing for up to six weeks

Total Knee Arthroplasty

- Primary indication for total knee arthroplasty is the destruction of articular cartilage secondary to osteoarthritis
- Post-operative care may include a knee immobilizer, elevation of the limb, cryotherapy, intermittent range of motion using a continuous passive motion (CPM) machine, and initiation of knee protocol exercises
- Patient education may include items such as avoiding excessive stress to the knee, avoid squatting, avoid quick pivoting, avoid using pillows under the knee while in bed, and avoid low seating

Total Shoulder Arthroplasty

- Surgical candidates typically have irreparable damage, deterioration, and destruction to the humeral head and the glenoid fossa within the shoulder complex
- Surgical complications include mechanical loosening of the prosthesis, instability, rotator cuff tear, implant failure, heterotopic ossification, and intraoperative fracture
- Life expectancy is longer for the shoulder compared to the knee or hip since the shoulder is a non-weight bearing joint

Transfemoral Amputation due to Osteosarcoma

- Osteosarcoma is a highly malignant cancer that begins in the medullary cavity of a bone and leads to the formation of a mass
- A patient status post transfemoral amputation may present with fatigue, loss of balance, phantom pain or sensation, hypersensitivity of the residual limb, and psychological issues regarding the loss of the limb
- Lying in a prone position is beneficial to decrease the incidence of a hip flexion contracture

Transtibial Amputation due to Arteriosclerosis Obliterans

- Arteriosclerosis obliterans results in ischemia and subsequent ulceration of the affected tissues
- A patient status post transtibial amputation may have a decrease in cardiovascular status depending on the frequency of intermittent claudication experienced prior to the amputation
- Preprosthetic intervention should focus on strength, range of motion, functional mobility, use of assistive devices, desensitization, and patient education for care of the residual limb

Traumatic Brain Injury

- Occurs due to an open head injury where there is penetration through the skull or closed head injury where the brain makes contact with the skull secondary to a sudden, violent acceleration or deceleration
- Brain injury may include swelling, axonal injury, hypoxia, hematoma, hemorrhage and changes in intracranial pressure
- High risk groups include males between 15-24 years of age, individuals over 65 years of age, and children between 1-2 years of age

Urinary Stress Incontinence

- Occurs during activities where there is an increase in abdominal pressure through straining, sneezing, coughing or lifting
- Risk factors include pregnancy, vaginal delivery, episiotomy, prostate or pelvic surgery, aging, diabetes mellitus, central nervous system dysfunction, and recurrent urinary infection
- Accounts for 50-60% of all incontinence cases and is manifested solely by the involuntary loss of urine with any form of exertion or increased abdominal pressure

Achilles Tendon Rupture

Diagnosis:

What condition produces a patient's symptoms?

Rupture of the Achilles tendon normally occurs within one to two inches above its tendinous insertion on the calcaneus. A patient will present with symptoms secondary to the rupture and discontinuity of the Achilles tendon.

An injury was most likely sustained to which structure?

The Achilles tendon is the largest and strongest tendon in the human body and is formed from the tendinous portions of the gastrocnemius and soleus muscles coalescing above the insertion on the calcaneal tuberosity. Theories suggest that an Achilles tendon rupture usually occurs in an Achilles tendon that has undergone degenerative changes. The degenerative changes will begin with hypovascularity in the Achilles tendon area. The impaired blood flow in combination with repetitive microtrauma creates degenerative changes within the tendon and as a result makes the tendon more susceptible to injury.

Inference:

What is the most likely contributing factor in the development of this condition?

An Achilles tendon rupture occurs most frequently when pushing off of a weight bearing extremity with an extended knee, through unexpected dorsiflexion while weight bearing or with a forceful eccentric contraction of the plantar flexors. Participation in sports that require quick-changing footwork such as softball, tennis, basketball, and football are high-risk activities. Other contributing factors include poor stretching routine, tight calf muscles, improper shoe wear during high risk activities, and altered biomechanics at the foot during activities (such as a flattened arch). A person over 30 years of age is at a higher risk for rupture secondary to the decrease in blood flow to the area of the tendon associated with aging. A person with a history of corticosteroid injections to the tendon may also have a predisposition for rupture. The highest incidence for rupture is in individuals between 30 and 50 years of age that usually have no history of calf or heel pain and commonly participate in recreational activities.

Confirmation:

What is the most likely clinical presentation?

A patient with an Achilles tendon rupture will present with swelling over the distal tendon, a palpable defect in the tendon above the calcaneal tuberosity, and pain and weakness with plantar flexion. The patient may limp and will often complain that during the injury there was a snap or a pop that was associated with the severe pain. A patient will not be able to stand on their toes and in a prone position will not demonstrate any passive plantar flexion with squeezing of the affected calf muscle (the Thompson test). A complete rupture will result in a palpable gap in the tendon prior to the insertion.

What laboratory or imaging studies would confirm the diagnosis?

Confirmation of an Achilles tendon rupture should utilize x-ray to rule out an avulsion fracture or bony injury. MRI can be used to locate the presence and severity of the tear or rupture.

What additional information should be obtained to confirm the diagnosis?

Diagnosis of an Achilles tendon rupture relies on patient history of the event and a positive Thompson's test. Patient history usually reveals a popping sound and a release from the back of the ankle. Physical examination and palpation reveal a discontinuity within the tendon. The O'Brien needle test may be used by the physician to confirm the rupture.

Examination:

What history should be documented?

Important areas to explore include mechanism of present injury, past medical history, medications, current health status, social history and habits, occupation, living environment, and social support system.

What test/measures are most appropriate?

Anthropometric characteristics: circumferential measurements for edema, palpation to determine ankle effusion

Arousal, attention, and cognition: examine mental status, learning ability, memory, motivation

Assistive and adaptive devices: potential utilization of crutches

Gait, locomotion, and balance: safety with/without an assistive device during gait; biomechanics of gait

Integumentary integrity: assessment of sensation

Joint integrity and mobility: special tests such as Thompson's test

Muscle performance: strength assessment, characteristics of muscle contraction

Pain: pain perception assessment scale

Range of motion: active and passive range of motion

Sensory integration: proprioception and kinesthesia

Self-care and home management: assessment of functional capacity

What additional findings are likely with this patient?

An Achilles tendon rupture is more common in men and in individuals that do not consistently exercise, but are the "weekend warriors." There are risks and benefits to both philosophies of treatment (non-operative and operative) and the physician usually determines the course of treatment on a patient-by-patient basis accounting for the patient's age, activity level, and co-morbidities.

Management:

What is the most effective management of this patient?

Medical management of a ruptured Achilles tendon incorporates immobilization through casting or a surgical approach for repair or reconstruction. Pharmacological intervention is not necessary for this condition except to relieve pain through NSAIDs, acetaminophen or narcotics depending on physician preference, and patient profile. Non-surgical treatment includes serial casting for approximately ten weeks followed by the use of a heel lift to ensure maximal healing without stress on the tendon for three to six months. Physical therapy begins when the cast is removed. If a patient requires surgical intervention then a cast or a brace is required for six to eight weeks. Physical therapy intervention is primarily the same for surgical and non-surgical patients and includes range of motion, stretching, icing, assistive device training, endurance programming, gait training, strengthening, plyometrics, and skill specific training. Modalities, pool therapy, and other cardiovascular equipment may assist in the recovery of functional motion and endurance.

What home care regimen should be recommended?

A home care regimen is vital to the success of a patient's recovery. A program must be based on a patient's post-operative impairments and follow the physician's post-surgical protocol. A home program generally incorporates icing and elevation early in the rehabilitation process. A patient is required to continue a home program throughout the six to seven months of rehabilitation. Other areas of focus include range of motion, strengthening, gait, endurance activities, and high-level skill and sport specific tasks.

Outcome:

What is the likely outcome of a course in physical therapy?

Physical therapy should begin after surgical intervention or when the cast is removed from a non-surgical patient. Assuming an unremarkable recovery, a patient should return to their previous functional level within six to seven months.

What are the long-term effects of the patient's condition?

A patient that manages the Achilles tendon rupture without surgery and allows the tendon to heal on its own has a higher rate of rerupture (40% rerupture the tendon) compared to a patient that has surgical repair of the tendon (0-5% rerupture the tendon). An advantage to non-surgical management is a reduced risk of infection from surgery. However, it may result in an incomplete return of functional performance. A patient that has surgical intervention has a decreased risk for reinjury and a higher rate of return to athletic activities.

Comparison:

What are the distinguishing characteristics of a similar condition?

Achilles tendonitis can be an acute or chronic condition due to repetitive microtrauma that builds scar tissue in the area over time. A patient initially feels an aching sensation after activity and progresses to pain with walking. There may be localized tenderness and swelling in the area. In the acute stage a patient should utilize anti-inflammatory medications, rest for 2-3 weeks and use a heel lift. In the chronic stage the symptoms and pain may last beyond six weeks. Examination often reveals a thickened and nodular Achilles tendon. Surgical intervention may be warranted at this stage.

Clinical Scenarios:

Scenario One

A 32-year-old female is playing soccer in a recreational league. A therapist that assists the team observes her kick the ball and then fall to the ground. The therapist examines the patient in the training room and finds that the patient has some plantar flexion in a non-weight bearing position, but is unable to plantar flex the foot while weight bearing. The patient states that something popped while running and palpation indicates a separation in the Achilles tendon.

Scenario Two

A 46-year-old male is referred to physical therapy status post surgical reconstruction of a left Achilles tendon rupture. The patient has been casted for one week and has been using axillary crutches for household mobility. The patient has no significant past medical history. He is employed as a truck driver and resides in a one-story home. The patient sustained the injury while playing tennis.

Adhesive Capsulitis

Diagnosis:

What condition produces a patient's symptoms?

Adhesive capsulitis (also known as "frozen shoulder") is an enigmatic shoulder disorder characterized by inflammation and fibrotic thickening of the anterior joint capsule of the shoulder. The inflamed capsule becomes adherent to the humeral head and undergoes contracture. This condition is characterized by the symptoms of limitation in glenohumeral motion and pain.

An injury was most likely sustained to which structure?

Adhesive capsulitis is classified as primary or secondary. Primary adhesive capsulitis occurs spontaneously and secondary adhesive capsulitis results from an underlying condition. Inflammation within the joint capsule causes fibrous adhesions to form and the capsule to thicken. A decrease in space within the capsule leads to a decrease of synovial fluid and further irritation to the glenohumeral joint.

Inference:

What is the most likely contributing factor in the development of this condition?

Primary adhesive capsulitis has no known etiology, however, it is associated with conditions such as diabetes mellitus, hypothyroidism or cardiopulmonary conditions. Secondary adhesive capsulitis can result from trauma, immobilization, reflex sympathetic dystrophy, rheumatoid arthritis, abdominal disorders, and psychogenic disorders. Orthopedic intrinsic disorders that may initiate this process include supraspinatus tendonitis, partial tear of the musculotendinous cuff, and bicipital tendonitis. Adhesive capsulitis occurs more in the middle-aged population with females having a greater incidence than males.

Confirmation:

What is the most likely clinical presentation?

Data regarding the prevalence and incidence of adhesive capsulitis is lacking. According to a published study adhesive capsulitis occurs in 2% of the population within the United States and in 11% of individuals that are diagnosed with diabetes mellitus. A small percentage of patients (10-15%) develop bilateral adhesive capsulitis. Adhesive capsulitis is characterized by restricted active and passive range of motion at the glenohumeral joint. Characteristics of the acute phase include pain that radiates below the elbow and awakens the patient at night. Passive range of the shoulder is limited during this phase due to pain and guarding. During the chronic phase pain is usually localized around the lateral brachial region, the patient is not awakened by pain, and passive range is limited due to capsular stiffness. Pain is present with a loss of glenohumeral motion, restricted elevation, and lateral rotation.

What laboratory or imaging studies would confirm the diagnosis?

An arthrogram can assist with the diagnosis of adhesive capsulitis by detecting a decreased volume of fluid within the joint capsule. The glenohumeral joint normally holds approximately 16-20 ml of fluid, however, adhesive capsulitis decreases the size of the capsule so it holds only 5-10 ml of fluid. Other tests should only be performed for differential diagnosis.

What additional information should be obtained to confirm the diagnosis?

The diagnosis of adhesive capsulitis is confirmed from clinical evaluation and past medical history. The patient may present with the greatest restriction of glenohumeral motion in abduction and lateral rotation but all planes of motion are usually affected. There is tightness within the anteroinferior joint capsule, pain with stretching, and restriction with passive and active range of motion.

Examination:

What history should be documented?

Important areas to explore include past medical and surgical history, medications, family history, current symptoms, current health status, social history and habits, occupation, leisure activities, and social support system.

What test/measures are most appropriate?

Anthropometric characteristics: circumferential measurements of bilateral upper extremities
Arousal, attention, and cognition: examine mental status, learning ability, memory, motivation
Community and work integration: analysis of community, work, and leisure activities
Cranial nerve integrity: assessment of muscle innervation by the cranial nerves, dermatome assessment
Environmental, home, and work barriers: analysis of current and potential barriers or hazards
Integumentary integrity: skin assessment, assessment of sensation
Joint integrity and mobility: assessment of hyper- and hypomobility of a joint, soft tissue swelling and inflammation
Muscle performance: strength assessment, muscle tone assessment
Pain: pain perception assessment scale, visual analog scale, assessment of muscle soreness
Posture: analysis of resting and dynamic posture
Range of motion: active and passive range of motion
Self-care and home management: assessment of functional capacity

What additional findings are likely with this patient?

A patient with adhesive capsulitis may encounter muscle spasms around the shoulder secondary to muscle guarding. A loss of reciprocal arm swing may be seen and disuse muscle atrophy may occur over time. A thorough examination must be completed to rule out concomitant systemic, rheumatologic, inflammatory, metastatic or infectious disorders.

Management:

What is the most effective management of this patient?

Medical management varies with adhesive capsulitis. Adhesive capsulitis is a self-limiting process that can take over 12 months in its course. Pharmacological intervention should emphasize the control of pain through acetaminophen, longer acting analgesics, NSAIDs or narcotics. A physician may inject the shoulder with corticosteroids to assist with recovery of motion. Surgical intervention to break up adhesions or release muscles adhered to the capsule is a last resort if conservative management fails. Physical therapy intervention during the acute phase includes icing or superficial heat, gentle joint mobilization, progressive strengthening, pendulum exercises, and isometric strengthening. During the chronic phase physical therapy intervention and goals may also include ultrasound, grade III and IV mobilization, increasing the extensibility of the joint capsule, and techniques such as PNF to restore painless functional range of motion.

What home care regimen should be recommended?

A home care regimen during the acute phase should include some self-stretching but avoid abduction secondary to the risk of damage to subacromial tissue. Once the patient enters the chronic phase the program should emphasize self-stretching, progressive exercises, posture management, PNF and other exercises such as pendulum exercises and "wall climbing" to assist with improving range of motion.

Outcome:

What is the likely outcome of a course in physical therapy?

Physical therapy is usually prescribed on an outpatient basis for three to five months after diagnosis. Adhesive capsulitis usually follows a nonlinear pattern of recovery. Spontaneous recovery is said to take 12-24 months in duration.

What are the long-term effects of the patient's condition?

Most patients are able to fully recover over time, but an estimated 7-14% of patients experience some permanent loss of range of motion at the shoulder joint. This loss is frequently asymptomatic and may not impair a patient's functional ability.

Comparison:

What are the distinguishing characteristics of a similar condition?

Acute bursitis is characterized by pain that is intense and sometimes throbbing over the lateral brachial region. This condition may arise secondary to calcific tendonitis. Active and passive motion in all directions is limited by pain. Abduction greater than 60 degrees and flexion greater than 90 degrees usually produces severe pain. Acute bursitis lasts for only a few days and unlike adhesive capsulitis this condition will usually resolve itself within a few weeks.

Clinical Scenarios:

Scenario One

A 29-year-old was diagnosed with primary adhesive capsulitis and referred to outpatient physical therapy. The patient is self-employed as an artist and enjoys outdoor activities. Past medical history includes diabetes mellitus since age six and a femur fracture 11 months ago. The patient noticed reduced range of motion and an increase in pain over the last few weeks.

Scenario Two

A 53-year-old female fell off her bike six months ago while cycling in a road race and sustained an injury to her shoulder complex. The patient attempted to immobilize her arm in a sling for two weeks. The patient states that she was unable to regain functional motion in her shoulder once she stopped using the sling. She saw a physician who diagnosed her with "frozen shoulder." The patient is limited to 10 degrees lateral rotation and 95 degrees of shoulder flexion.

Alzheimer's Disease

Diagnosis:

What condition produces a patient's symptoms?

Alzheimer's disease is a progressive neurological disorder that results in deterioration and irreversible damage within the cerebral cortex and subcortical areas of the brain. The loss of neurons results from the breakdown of several processes that would normally sustain the brain cells.

An injury was most likely sustained to which structure?

Neurons that are normally involved with acetylcholine transmission deteriorate within the cerebral cortex of the brain. Postmortem biopsy reveals neurofibrillary tangles within cytoplasm, amyloid plaques, and cerebral atrophy. Amyloid plaques contain fragmented axons, altered glial cells, and cellular waste that result in an inflammatory response that provides further damage to the nervous system. Amyloid can also cause atrophy of the smooth muscle of the arteries of the brain, predisposing them to rupture.

Inference:

What is the most likely contributing factor in the development of this condition?

The exact etiology of Alzheimer's disease is unknown, however, hypothesized causes include lower levels of neurotransmitters, higher levels of aluminum within brain tissue, genetic inheritance, autoimmune disease, abnormal processing of the substance amyloid, and virus. Approximately 4.5 million individuals are living with Alzheimer's disease in the United States. The risk of developing Alzheimer's disease increases with age and there is a higher incidence in women. The prevalence of Alzheimer's disease is 6% of individuals over 65 and 20% of individuals over 80 years of age.

Confirmation:

What is the most likely clinical presentation?

Alzheimer's disease is initially noted by a change in higher cortical functions characterized by subtle changes in memory, impaired concentration, and difficulty with new learning. These symptoms progress in the early stages and there is a loss of orientation, word finding difficulties, emotional lability, depression, poor judgment, and impaired ability to perform self-care skills. During the middle stages of Alzheimer's disease the patient will develop behavioral and motor problems characterized by neurological symptoms such as aphasia, apraxia, perseveration, agitation, and violent or socially unacceptable behavior that can include wandering. Eventually all ability to learn is lost and long-term memory also disappears. End-stage Alzheimer's disease is characterized by severe intellectual and physical destruction. Patients in this stage will present with vegetative symptoms

including incontinence, functional dependence, the inability to speak, and seizure activity.

What laboratory or imaging studies would confirm the diagnosis?

Alzheimer's disease presently cannot be confirmed until a postmortem biopsy reveals the neurofibrillary tangles and amyloid plaques. MRI can be used to assess any abnormalities or signs of atrophy within the brain that is associated with Alzheimer's disease or to rule out other medical conditions. Single photon emission computed tomography (SPECT) may be used to determine brain activity and predict potential for Alzheimer's disease. Blood work, urine, and spinal fluid may be required to rule out other diseases that may cause signs of dementia.

What additional information should be obtained to confirm the diagnosis?

A physical examination, neurological examination, and neuropsychological testing are required for diagnosis of probable Alzheimer's disease. The patient must demonstrate at least two deficits of cognition, memory, and related cognitive functioning with the absence of all other brain disease or disturbances in consciousness that may contribute to the identified deficits. Family history and symptoms may provide insight into the expected speed of progression of the disease.

Examination:

What history should be documented?

Important areas to explore include past medical history, family history, history of current symptoms, current health status, living environment, social history and habits, occupation, and social support system.

What test/measures are most appropriate?

Aerobic capacity and endurance: assessment of vital signs at rest and with activity

Arousal, attention, and cognition: examine mental status, learning ability, memory, motivation, Mini-Mental State Examination, level of consciousness

Assistive and adaptive devices: analysis of components and safety of a device

Environmental, home, and work barriers: analysis of current and potential barriers or hazards

Gait, locomotion, and balance: static and dynamic balance in sitting and standing, safety during gait with/without an assistive device, Functional Ambulation Profile, Berg Balance Scale

Motor function: equilibrium and righting reactions, coordination, physical performance scales

Muscle performance: strength assessment

Posture: analysis of resting and dynamic posture

Range of motion: active and passive range of motion
Reflex integrity: assessment of deep tendon and pathological reflexes (e.g., Babinski, ATNR)
Self-care and home management: assessment of functional capacity, Functional Independence Measure (FIM), Barthel Index

What additional findings are likely with this patient?

A patient with end-stage Alzheimer's disease is at high risk for infection and pneumonia. These patients may experience complications from a persistent vegetative state such as contractures, decubiti, fracture, and pulmonary compromise.

Management:

What is the most effective management of this patient?

Medical management of Alzheimer's disease may include pharmacological intervention during the early stages of the disease process. Medications are administered to inhibit acetylcholinesterase, alleviate cognitive symptoms, and control behavioral changes. Drug therapies are usually short-term in effect lasting six to nine months. Tacrine (Cognex), donepezil (Aricept), and rivastigmine (Exelon) are common pharmacological agents used to treat Alzheimer's disease, however, the side effects can be substantial. Physical therapy management should focus on maximizing the patient's remaining function and providing family and caregiver education. The therapist should attempt to create an emotional and physical environment that provides the patient with the opportunity to experience success. Modifying the layout of the patient's living space in order for the patient to easily find items is one example of creating an environment that encourages success. Safety with functional mobility and gait training may be indicated in the early stages of the disease. Later stages may require ongoing caregiver education regarding assistance with mobility, range of motion, and positioning. Many patients require a long-term care facility that specializes in Alzheimer's disease secondary to personality changes, aggressive behavior, and end-stage complications.

What home care regimen should be recommended?

During the early stages of Alzheimer's disease a patient should continue with activity as tolerated and utilize a memory book or other compensatory strategies at home. As the disease progresses, a patient will rely on caregiver support to assist with a daily exercise program. The patient should be encouraged to exercise, ambulate, and participate in everyday activities such as folding laundry, making beds, and assisting with dinner in order to avoid restlessness and wandering.

Outcome:

What is the likely outcome of a course in physical therapy?

Physical therapy may be indicated intermittently throughout the course of the disease, however, the therapy will not alter or cease the progression of the disease process.

What are the long-term effects of the patient's condition?

Alzheimer's disease is a chronic and progressive disorder and is the fourth leading cause of death in adults. The typical course of the disease averages between seven and eleven years. The leading cause of death of a patient with Alzheimer's disease is infection or dehydration.

Comparison:

What are the distinguishing characteristics of a similar condition?

Multi-infarct dementia produces symptoms in a step-like manner secondary to ongoing cerebral infarcts. This form of dementia is usually found in patients that are over 70 years of age and is more common in males. Hypertension is a primary risk factor and depression is common. A patient may also experience neurological deficits such as hemiplegia and emotional lability.

Clinical Scenarios:

Scenario One

A 65-year-old female is referred to physical therapy for gait disturbances. The patient resides alone and drives on a regular basis. During the initial examination the patient reveals that she is sometimes confused when driving. The patient complains that she has difficulty managing her time around the house and requires an extended amount of time to get ready in the morning.

Scenario Two

A 79-year-old male is seen by a therapist in an Alzheimer's residential facility. The physician recommends gait training with a walker. The patient enjoys walking around the unit, however, he has fallen several times within the last month.

Amyotrophic Lateral Sclerosis

Diagnosis:

What condition produces a patient's symptoms?

Amyotrophic lateral sclerosis (ALS) is a chronic degenerative disease that produces both upper and lower motor neuron impairments. Demyelination, axonal swelling, and atrophy within the cerebral cortex, premotor areas, sensory cortex, and temporal cortex cause the symptoms of ALS.

An injury was most likely sustained to which structure?

Rapid degeneration and demyelination occur in the giant pyramidal cells of the cerebral cortex and affect areas of the corticospinal tracts, cell bodies of the lower motor neurons in the gray matter, anterior horn cells, and areas within the precentral gyrus of the cortex. The rapid degeneration causes denervation of muscle fibers, muscle atrophy, and weakness.

Inference:

What is the most likely contributing factor in the development of this condition?

The exact etiology of ALS is unknown (90% of all cases), however, there are multiple theories of causative factors that include genetic inheritance as an autosomal dominant trait, a slow acting virus, metabolic disturbances, and theories of toxicity of lead and aluminum. Familial ALS occurs in 5-10% of all cases. Risk for ALS is higher in men and usually occurs between 40 to 70 years of age.

Confirmation:

What is the most likely clinical presentation?

Early clinical presentation of ALS may include both upper and lower motor neuron involvement. Early lower motor neuron signs include asymmetric muscle weakness, cramping, and atrophy that are usually found within the hands. Muscle weakness due to denervation eventually causes significant fasciculations, atrophy and wasting of the muscles. The weakness spreads throughout the body over the course of the disease and generally follows a distal to proximal path. Upper motor neuron symptoms occur due to the loss of inhibition of the muscle. Incoordination of movement, spasticity, clonus, and a positive Babinski reflex are some of the indicators of upper motor neuron involvement. Bulbar involvement is characterized by dysarthria, dysphagia, and emotional lability. Initially a person may have either upper or lower motor neuron involvement, but eventually both categories are affected. A patient with ALS will exhibit fatigue, oral motor impairment, fasciculations, spasticity, motor paralysis, and eventual respiratory paralysis.

What laboratory or imaging studies would confirm the diagnosis?

There are multiple tests used to assist with diagnosing ALS. Electromyography assesses fibrillation and muscle fasciculations. Muscle biopsy verifies lower motor neuron involvement rather than muscle disease and a spinal tap may reveal a higher protein content in some patients with ALS. CT scan will appear normal until late in the disease process.

What additional information should be obtained to confirm the diagnosis?

Diagnosis relies heavily on symptoms that determine both upper and lower motor neuron involvement. A patient that presents with motor impairment without sensory impairment is a primary indicator of ALS. Definitive diagnosis also first requires a physician to rule out other neurological conditions such as multiple sclerosis, spinal cord tumors, progressive muscular dystrophy, Lyme disease, and syringomyelia. In 1990 the World Federation of Neurology established four categories for diagnosis of ALS: Suspected ALS, Possible ALS, Probable ALS, and Definite ALS. Each category has specific criteria for diagnosis.

Examination:

What history should be documented?

Important areas include past medical history, family history, history of current symptoms, current health status, living environment, social history and habits, occupation, and social support system.

What test/measures are most appropriate?

Aerobic capacity and endurance: assessment of vital signs at rest and with activity, perceived exertion scale
Anthropometric characteristics: weight and height
Arousal, attention, and cognition: examines mental status, learning ability, memory, motivation
Assistive and adaptive devices: analysis of components and safety of a device
Environmental, home, and work barriers: analysis of current and potential barriers or hazards
Gait, locomotion, and balance: static and dynamic balance in sitting and standing, safety during gait with/without an assistive device
Motor function: motor assessment scales, coordination, equilibrium and righting reactions
Muscle Performance: strength assessment, muscle endurance, muscle tone assessment, muscle atrophy
Neuromotor development and sensory integration: analysis of reflex movement patterns, assessment of involuntary movements, sensory integration tests, gross and fine motor skills
Posture: analysis of resting and dynamic posture
Range of motion: active and passive range of motion

Reflex integrity: assessment of deep tendon and pathological reflexes (e.g., Babinski, ATNR)
Self-care and home management: Barthel Index
Ventilation, respiration, and circulation: respiratory muscle strength, accessory muscle utilization, assessment of cough

What additional findings are likely with this patient?

During the initial stages of ALS there are various effects on the body. Progression of the disease allows for significant deterioration within the brain and spinal cord and a patient may exhibit paralysis of vocal cords, swallowing impairment, contractures, decubiti, and breathing difficulty that requires ventilatory support. Throughout the course of ALS, however, sensation, eye movement, and bowel and bladder function remain preserved.

Management:

What is the most effective management of this patient?

Effective management of ALS is based on supportive care and symptomatic therapy. Pharmacological intervention may include riluzole (Rilutek). This drug appears to have an effect on the progression of the disease process, however, its long-term effects are unknown. Symptomatic therapy may include anticholinergic, antispasticity, and antidepressant medications. Physical, occupational, speech, respiratory, and nutritional therapies may be warranted. Physical therapy intervention should focus on the quality of life and should include a low-level exercise program, range of motion, mobility training, assistive/adaptive devices, wheelchair prescription, bronchial hygiene, and energy conservation techniques. Patient, family, and caregiver training are very important as the disease continues to progress.

What home-care regimen should be recommended?

A home care regimen for a patient with ALS must consider the rate of disease progression and level of respiratory involvement. Goals should focus on maximizing the patient's functional capacity. A low-level exercise program may be indicated as long as the patient does not exercise to fatigue and promote further weakness. Family involvement is encouraged to support the patient through the course of the disease and assist with mobility, pacing skills, energy conservation techniques, and overall safety. During the later part of the disease the family and caregivers must be competent with positioning, bronchial hygiene, range of motion, and assistance with mobility.

Outcome:

What is the likely outcome of a course in physical therapy?

Physical therapy intervention may assist with current issues, however, therapy does not hinder progression of ALS. Therapeutic goals will consider disease progression and focus on teaching for the patient and caregivers.

What are the long-term effects of the patient's condition?

ALS is usually a rapidly progressing neurological disease with an average course of two to five years with 20-30% of patients surviving longer than five years. Research indicates that although there is no structured course of this disease process, if a patient is diagnosed before 50 years of age the disease is usually longer in course. Death usually occurs from respiratory failure.

Comparison:

What are the distinguishing characteristics of a similar condition?

Muscular dystrophy (MD) is the term for a group of inherited disorders that are progressive and exhibit degeneration of muscles without sensory or neural impairment. Progressive weakness occurs to the muscle fibers secondary to the absence of dystrophin within the skeletal muscles. This group of disorders presents early in life and usually shortens life expectancy. Disuse atrophy, muscle deterioration, contractures, and cardiac and respiratory weakness are common characteristics of this disease process. A patient with MD usually dies from respiratory/cardiac complications secondary to the primary disease process.

Clinical Scenarios:

Scenario One

A 56-year-old male is diagnosed with ALS and presents with mild atrophy of the hand. The patient owns his own business as a painter and wants to continue working for as long as he can. The patient is referred to physical therapy for a home exercise program.

Scenario Two

A 60-year-old female is referred to physical therapy secondary to a left CVA. The patient was also diagnosed with ALS two years ago, requires the use of a wheelchair for mobility, and occasionally chokes while eating. The patient has assistance at home from her husband who is in good health.

Ankylosing Spondylitis

Diagnosis:

What condition produces a patient's symptoms?

Ankylosing spondylitis (AS), also known as Marie-Strumpell disease, is a systemic condition that is characterized by inflammation of the spine and larger peripheral joints. The chronic inflammation causes destruction of the ligamentous-osseous junction with subsequent fibrosis and ossification of the area.

An injury was most likely sustained to which structure?

AS primarily affects the sacroiliac joint, intervertebral disks, spine, costovertebral and apophyseal joints, connective tissue, and larger peripheral joints (hips, knees, and shoulders). Ossification can occur within all affected joints resulting in pain and deformity.

Inference:

What is the most likely contributing factor in the development of this condition?

AS is a progressive systemic disorder with uncertain etiology. Research supports the possibility of genetic inheritance combined with environmental influence. Gender, race, age, and family history are all factors to consider regarding risk for developing AS. A person born with a histocompatibility antigen HLA-B27 has a high risk for the disease. Approximately 80-90% of patients with AS are HLA-B27 positive, but only 2% of individuals that are HLA-B27 positive develop AS. HLA-B27 is found in 8.5% of Caucasians and only 2.5% of African Americans. Men are at a two to three time greater risk than women and onset is typically seen between twenty and forty years of age.

Confirmation:

What is the most likely clinical presentation?

A patient with early AS will present with recurrent and insidious episodes of low back pain, morning stiffness, impaired spinal extension, and limited range of motion in the affected joints for over a three-month period of time. As the disease progresses pain will become severe, consistent, and extending to the midback, and sometimes towards the neck. The natural lumbar curve will eventually flatten due to muscle spasms. Other manifestations include fixed flexion at the hips, spinal kyphosis, fatigue, weight loss, and peripheral joint involvement. If the costovertebral joints are affected a patient will present with impaired chest mobility, compromised breathing, and decreased vital capacity.

What laboratory or imaging studies would confirm the diagnosis?

X-ray of the spine may be negative in the initial stage of AS but with progression will reveal areas of erosion, demineralization, calcification, and syndesmophyte formation (ossification of the outside of the intervertebral disks). In the later stages of the disease x-ray will reveal fusion of the sacroiliac joint, calcification of apophyseal joints and spinal ligaments, and a bamboo appearance of the spine. Blood work can be used to rule out other diseases and assists with the diagnosis since the majority of patients with AS possess the HLA-B27 antigen and approximately 40% have an elevated erythrocyte sedimentation rate.

What additional information should be obtained to confirm the diagnosis?

Physical examination may reveal joint tenderness, pain, and/or limitation of the sacroiliac joint and the spine. Family inheritance and a thorough history of a patient's symptoms assist with the diagnosis of AS.

Examination:

What history should be documented?

Important areas to explore include past medical history, medications, current health status, family inheritance, living environment, occupation, leisure activities, social history and habits, and social support system.

What test/measures are most appropriate?

Anthropometric characteristics: baseline height measurement, circumferential chest measurements during inspiration

Arousal, attention, and cognition: examine mental status, learning ability, memory, motivation

Assistive and adaptive devices: analysis of components and safety of a device

Community and work integration: analysis of community, work, and leisure activities

Environmental, home, and work barriers: analysis of current and potential barriers or hazards

Ergonomics and body mechanics: analysis of dexterity and coordination

Gait, locomotion, and balance: assessment of static and dynamic balance in sitting and standing, safety during gait, Functional Ambulation Profile, analysis of wheelchair management

Joint integrity and mobility: assess hypomobility and limitation of a joint, Wright-Schober test for spinal mobility

Muscle performance: strength assessment

Pain: pain perception assessment scale

Posture: analysis of resting and dynamic posture

Range of motion: active and passive range of motion

Reflex integrity: assessment of deep tendon and pathological reflexes (e.g., Babinski, ATNR)

Self-care and home management: assessment of functional capacity

Sensory integrity: assessment of sensation

Ventilation, respiration, and circulation: analysis of thoracolumbar movement and chest expansion during breathing, measurement of vital capacity

What additional findings are likely with this patient?

Long-term AS will present with progressive symptoms and multiple complications. Iritis, uveitis, osteoporosis, fracture, atlantoaxial subluxation, and complete spinal fusion can occur in severe long-standing cases of AS. Pericarditis, cardiac pathology, pulmonary fibrosis, cardiac arrhythmias, amyloidosis, and aortic insufficiency have also been noted as potential complications.

Management:

What is the most effective management of this patient?

The goals of medical management are to reduce inflammation, maintain functional mobility, and relieve pain. Pharmacological intervention may include NSAIDs, disease-modifying drugs such as methotrexate, analgesics, and specifically Indomethacin to relieve pain. Physical therapy intervention should include postural exercises emphasizing extension, general range of motion, pain management, and energy conservation techniques. Low-impact and aerobic exercise with emphasis on extension and rotation are appropriate for a patient with AS. High-impact and flexion exercises are contraindicated. Patient education should include posture retraining, positioning for sleeping, and lifting techniques. Excessive exercise should be avoided as it can increase the inflammatory response and injury. Swimming is a highly recommended activity. Surgical intervention is rarely indicated to correct or stabilize a musculoskeletal deformity.

What home care regimen should be recommended?

A home care regimen for a patient with AS should include a daily low-impact therapeutic exercise program. Range of motion should focus on spinal movement in all directions. The patient requires a firm sleeping surface and competence with proper positioning and use of pillows to maintain optimal alignment. Ongoing breathing exercises and posture retraining will assist with overall level of function.

Outcome:

What is the likely outcome of a course in physical therapy?

Physical therapy cannot modify the progression of AS, however, it may assist to alleviate pain and improve a patient's functional capacity. A patient may require physical therapy on an intermittent basis for secondary complications throughout the disease process.

What are the long-term effects of the patient's condition?

AS progresses slowly over a fifteen to twenty-five year period and may remain isolated to the spine and sacroiliac joint or spread to larger peripheral joints. Stiffness and joint limitation are common long-term effects of AS that can negatively impact a patient's functional mobility. The extent of disability varies greatly with only 1% of patients experiencing complete remission. Normal course includes periods of exacerbations and remissions. Hip disease with AS is a marker for a severe form of AS and is more likely to occur in a patient that is diagnosed at a young age.

Comparison:

What are the distinguishing characteristics of a similar condition?

Sjogren's syndrome, like AS, is classified as a spondylarthropathy. Sjogren's is a chronic arthritis and autoimmune disease that also can affect several organs. Lymphocytes attack healthy tissues and organs and are usually found in combination with RA or lupus. Postmenopausal women are affected most often with over two to four million individuals in the United States living with the disease. It does not have a cure, but can be managed through medications, exercise, and proper nutrition. Exercise should follow general guidelines for the treatment of RA.

Clinical Scenarios:

Scenario One

A 28-year-old male is seen in physical therapy shortly after being diagnosed with AS. The patient complains of sacroiliac pain and tenderness. The patient has a negative family history and is currently employed as a high school maintenance technician.

Scenario Two

A 60-year-old female is seen in physical therapy with advanced AS. The patient has bilateral hip flexion contractures and kyphosis. The patient resides alone and receives daily assistance from her two sisters who live locally. The patient has previously refused recommendations to utilize an assistive device for ambulation.

Anterior Cruciate Ligament Sprain – Grade III

Diagnosis:

What condition produces a patient's symptoms?

The anterior cruciate ligament (ACL) extends from the anterior intracondylar region of the tibia to the medial aspect of the lateral femoral condyle in the intracondylar notch. The ligament prevents anterior translation of the tibia on the fixed femur and posterior translation of the femur on the fixed tibia. The ACL is a broad cord that has long collagen strands that permits up to 500 pounds of pressure prior to rupture. The ligament has a poor blood supply and does not have the ability to heal a complete tear. Injuries to the ACL most commonly occur during hyperflexion, rapid deceleration, hyperextension or landing in an unbalanced position.

An injury was most likely sustained to which structure?

A grade III ACL sprain refers to a complete tear of the ligament with excessive laxity. Tears of the anterior cruciate ligament most often occur in the midsubstance of the ligament and not at the ligament's attachment on the femur or tibia. Laxity rarely occurs solely in a straight plane and instead is often classified as anterolateral or anteromedial.

Inference:

What is the most likely contributing factor in the development of this condition?

Participation in athletic activities requiring high levels of agility (soccer, basketball, volleyball) and contact sports increases the incidence of an ACL injury. Recent studies indicate that women involved in selected athletic activities experienced significantly higher ACL injury rates (estimated two to eight times higher) than their male counterparts. There are many hypothesized reasons for this finding but to date a definitive answer has not been identified. Causative factors for ACL disruption include body movement and positioning, muscle strength, joint laxity, Q angle, and a narrow intercondylar notch.

Confirmation:

What is the most likely clinical presentation?

Epidemiological studies estimate that approximately 1:3000 individuals sustain an ACL injury annually in the United States with the peak incidence occurring between 14 and 29 years of age. This age group corresponds to an overall higher activity level, which increases the risk of injury. A grade III ACL sprain is characterized by significant pain, effusion, and edema that significantly limits range of motion. The patient may be unable to bear weight on the involved extremity resulting in dependence on an assistive device. Ligamentous testing reveals visible laxity in the knee and may exacerbate the patient's pain level.

What laboratory or imaging studies would confirm the diagnosis?

MRI is the preferred imaging tool to identify the presence of an ACL tear and possible disruption of other soft tissue structures such as ligaments and menisci. X-rays may be used to rule out a fracture.

What additional information should be obtained to confirm the diagnosis?

Subjective reports such as hearing a loud pop or feeling as though the knee buckled is often associated with a complete tear of the anterior cruciate ligament. Special tests such as the Lachman, anterior drawer, and pivot shift test can be used to confirm the diagnosis. It is important to perform all special tests bilaterally.

Examination:

What history should be documented?

Important areas to explore include mechanism of present injury, current symptoms, past medical history, medications, living environment, social history and habits, and social support system.

What test/measures are most appropriate?

Anthropometric characteristics: knee effusion and lower extremity circumferential measurements

Arousal, attention, and cognition: examine mental status, learning ability, memory, motivation

Assistive and adaptive devices: analysis of components and safety of a device, potential utilization of crutches

Gait, locomotion, and balance: safety during gait with an assistive device

Integumentary integrity: assessment of sensation (pain, temperature, tactile), skin assessment

Joint integrity and mobility: special tests for ligaments and menisci, Lachman and reverse Lachman test, anterior drawer test, palpation of structures, joint play, soft tissue restrictions, joint pain

Muscle performance: strength and active movement assessment, resisted isometrics, muscle contraction characteristics, muscle endurance

Orthotic, protective, and supportive devices: utilization of bracing, taping or wrapping, foot orthotic assessment

Pain: pain perception assessment scale

Range of motion: active and passive range of motion

Self-care and home management: assessment of functional capacity

Sensory integrity: proprioception and kinesthesia

What additional findings are likely with this patient?

Approximately two-thirds of the time the ACL is torn there is an accompanying meniscal tear. The collateral ligaments can also be involved although not as commonly as the menisci. When all three structures (ACL, MCL, and medial meniscus) are damaged it is referred to as the "unhappy triad."

Management:

What is the most effective management of this patient?

Management of a patient following a grade III ACL sprain includes controlling edema, increasing range of motion, strengthening, and improving the fluidity of gait. For patients electing to have surgery the patellar tendon is the most commonly utilized graft for intra-articular reconstruction. Patients often initially present with a knee immobilizer and crutches to protect the reconstructed ligament. Specific parameters are difficult to identify since many orthopedic surgeons utilize very specific protocols. Physical therapy management in the initial post-operative phase includes protecting the integrity of the graft, controlling edema, and improving range of motion. Specific intervention activities include pain modulation, patellar mobility, active range of motion exercises, gait activities, and quadriceps exercises. As patients progress in their rehabilitation program treatment begins to focus on strengthening activities emphasizing closed-chain exercises and selected functional activities. Closed-chain exercises are considered more desirable than open-chain exercises since they minimize anterior translation of the tibia. Patients should be required to complete a functional progression prior to returning to unrestricted athletics. For patients opting for a conservative (non-operative) approach, it is necessary to begin an aggressive strengthening program once the acute phase of the injury has subsided.

What home care regimen should be recommended?

The home care regimen should consist of range of motion, strengthening, palliative care, and functional activities as warranted based on the results of the patient examination and course (operative versus non-operative) of treatment.

Outcome:

What is the likely outcome of a course in physical therapy?

It is possible that with an aggressive strengthening program and/or activity modification patients may be able to participate in light to moderate athletic activities without formal surgical reconstruction. Patients electing to have surgery can expect to return to their previous functional level in four to six months.

What are the long-term effects of the patient's condition?

Patients that sustain a complete tear of the ACL and elect not to have reconstructive surgery will likely be at increased risk for instability and subsequent deterioration of joint surfaces.

Comparison:

What are the distinguishing characteristics of a similar condition?

A grade III posterior cruciate ligament (PCL) sprain is less common than an ACL sprain. The most common mechanism of injury for a PCL sprain is a "dashboard" injury or forced knee hyperflexion as the foot is plantar flexed. A grade III PCL injury will typically produce effusion, posterior tenderness, and a positive posterior drawer test. Knee extension is often limited due to the effusion and stretching of the posterior capsule and gastrocnemius. The rehabilitation program typically emphasizes strengthening of the quadriceps muscles. Individuals with an isolated PCL sprain may not exhibit any functional performance limitations and as a result, surgical intervention is far less common than with an ACL sprain. A PCL sprain alters the arthrokinematics of the knee joint and as a result a patient will be susceptible to degenerative changes such as arthritis.

Clinical Scenarios:

Scenario One

A 16-year-old gymnast sustains a grade I ACL injury after landing awkwardly on her left leg during a vault. The patient is two days status post injury and has mild effusion in the involved knee. The patient is a competitive gymnast and needs to compete in a regional meet in slightly less than four weeks.

Scenario Two

A 35-year-old male is referred to physical therapy after injuring his knee in a softball game. The patient reports tearing the ACL ten years ago in a skiing accident. The patient is active, however, reports more recent episodes of instability. The physician notes significant arthritic changes in the involved knee including diminished joint space.

Bicipital Tendonitis

Diagnosis:

What condition produces a patient's symptoms?

Bicipital tendonitis is an inflammatory process of the tendon of the long head of the biceps. Impingement or an inflammatory injury can result in symptoms of shoulder pain. Repeated full abduction and lateral rotation of the humeral head can lead to irritation that produces inflammation, edema, microscopic tears within the tendon, and degeneration of the tendon itself.

An injury was most likely sustained to which structure?

Continuous or repetitive shoulder motions can cause overuse of the biceps tendon. Damaged cells within the tendon do not have time to heal, leading to tendonitis. This is common in sports or work activities that require frequent and repeated use of the upper extremities, especially when the motion is performed overhead. Athletes who throw, swim or swing a racquet or club are at greatest risk. Years of shoulder wear and tear can cause the biceps tendon to become inflamed. Degeneration in a tendon causes a loss of the normal arrangement of the collagen fibers that join together to form the tendon. Some of the individual strands of the tendon become intertwined due to the degeneration, while allowing other fibers to break and the tendon to lose strength.

Inference:

What is the most likely contributing factor in the development of this condition?

Bicipital tendonitis is often caused through repetitive overhead activity and motion. There is usually direct trauma to the tendon as the shoulder motion approaches excessive abduction and lateral rotation. Examples of high risk athletes include baseball pitchers, tennis players, gymnasts, rowers, and swimmers. Bicipital tendonitis can also be caused secondary to other shoulder pathology including rotator cuff disease, impingement syndrome or intra-articular pathology such as labral tears.

Confirmation:

What is the most likely clinical presentation?

Patients generally report the feeling of a deep ache directly in the front and on the top of the shoulder. The ache may spread down into the biceps muscle and is usually made worse with overhead activities or lifting heavy objects. Resting the shoulder typically reduces the pain. A catching or slipping sensation of the biceps muscle may indicate a tear of the transverse humeral ligament. Bicipital tendinopathy, pain to palpation over the anterior shoulder in the area of the bicipital groove, pain with the biceps resistance test (i.e., shoulder flexion against resistance with elbow extended and forearm supinated), and a positive Yergason's or Speed's test (i.e., pain with resisted supination of the forearm or with the elbow flexed at 90° and the arm adducted against the body) are positive indicators for bicipital tendonitis.

What laboratory or imaging studies would confirm the diagnosis?

There are no laboratory tests to assist with the diagnosis of bicipital tendonitis. Plain x-rays do not diagnose bicipital tendonitis, but may show calcification in the groove or subacromial spurring. Other x-rays of the neck and elbow may be indicated to rule out referred shoulder pain. MRI can view the tendon, but is expensive and not usually used unless the patient is not responding to conservative treatment.

What additional information should be obtained to confirm the diagnosis?

Testing such as the biceps resistance test, Speed's test, and Yergason's test may be performed in conjunction with a full physical examination.

Examination:

What history should be documented?

Important areas to explore include past medical history, medications, current health status, nutritional status, social history and habits, occupation, living environment, and social support system.

What test/measures are most appropriate?

Arousal, attention, and cognition: examine mental status, learning ability, memory, motivation

Community and work integration: analysis of community, work, and leisure activities

Environmental, home, and work barriers: analysis of current and potential barriers or hazards

Ergonomics and body mechanics: analysis of dexterity and coordination

Joint integrity and mobility: assessment of hyper- and hypomobility of a joint, soft tissue swelling and inflammation

Muscle performance: strength assessment, muscle tone assessment

Pain: pain perception assessment scale, visual analog scale, assessment of muscle soreness

Posture: analysis of resting and dynamic posture

Range of motion: active and passive range of motion, Speed's test, Yergason's test

Reflex integrity: assessment of deep tendon reflexes

Self-care and home management: assessment of functional capacity

Sensory integrity: assessment of proprioception and kinesthesia

What additional findings are likely with this patient?

Patients with long-term chronic tendonitis may experience shoulder instability and subluxation secondary to biceps degeneration. Bicipital tendonitis will also frequently accompany impingement syndrome, rotator cuff tendonitis, and forms of glenohumeral instability.

Management:

What is the most effective management of this patient?

The primary goal of medical management is to relieve pain, reduce inflammation, and regain full available range of motion. Rest and/or immobilization using a splint or a removable brace may be indicated initially for a brief period of time. Generally, the patient should avoid all overhead movement, reaching, and lifting of objects. Pharmacological intervention may include nonsteroidal anti-inflammatory medications (NSAIDs) which will reduce both pain and inflammation. Active physical therapy is not often initiated immediately, however, the patient may be referred for instruction in general education of the pathology, guidelines for restrictions, pendulum exercises, and the use of TENS. The application of heat or cold to the affected area can also assist with relief of pain. The patient may benefit from the use of iontophoresis or phonophoresis. As the patient progresses out of the acute phase, physical therapy should focus on an exercise program that stretches and strengthens the affected muscle groups. This can restore the tendon's ability to function properly, improve healing, and prevent future injury. Surgical intervention is only recommended for patients that have not progressed with conservative treatment over a six month period of time. The typical procedure includes arthroscopic decompression and acromioplasty with anterior acromionectomy.

What home care regimen should be recommended?

Patients with bicipital tendonitis are recommended to always perform warm-up activities prior to vigorous exercises, consistently perform passive selective stretching and strengthening, use proper body mechanics, and avoid any painful activity. The ongoing focus of a home program should be on strengthening and endurance surrounding the tendon. Patients will have to consistently participate in an ongoing home exercise program to prevent the risk of recurrence.

Outcome:

What is the likely outcome of a course in physical therapy?

The goal of physical therapy is to restore full available range of motion without pain. Once the patient does not experience pain or discomfort with activity they may slowly return to their previous level of activity. Most patients are successful with conservative treatment and are able to return to their activities after an average of six to eight weeks of physical therapy and rehabilitation.

What are the long-term effects of the patient's condition?

Although the overall prognosis depends on the level of involvement, most patients have a positive long-term outcome and are able to return to their previous level of functioning. Statistically, there are approximately 10% of patients that do not achieve a positive outcome and have further deterioration or a rupture of the tendon.

Comparison:

What are the distinguishing characteristics of a similar condition?

The glenoid labrum is a fibrocartilage rim that surrounds the glenoid cavity, attaches to the glenoid cavity of the scapula to increase its depth, and protects the edge of the bone within the joint capsule. A labral tear is most susceptible with anterior damage or subluxation. A Bankart lesion is the name given to the avulsion of the labral ligamentous complex from the anteroinferior aspect of the glenoid. This is the most common lesion resulting in anterior joint instability. A CT scan can diagnose the tear and surgical intervention is normally successful for repair.

Clinical Scenarios:

Scenario One

A 27-year-old male is referred to physical therapy by his primary care physician for "probable bicipital tendonitis." He went to see his doctor secondary to pain when performing overhead activities and lifting objects of varying weight. He works as an auto mechanic 50 hours per week. He was trying to "work through the pain" but it has worsened over the last month. He resides with his wife and twin girls in a ranch style home.

Scenario Two

A 56-year-old tennis instructor has noticed an increase in pain through a particular arc of motion at her shoulder. She was diagnosed with impingement syndrome years ago, but has not had any recurrence or discomfort again until now. She states that her goal is to return to teaching tennis.

Breast Cancer

Diagnosis:

What condition produces a patient's symptoms?

Breast cancer's primary symptom is a painless mass within the breast tissue. This mass is composed of malignant altered cells that proliferate and spread without control. A malignancy can occur anywhere within the breast tissue, however, the lump is usually found directly behind the areola in men and is usually located behind the areola or in the outer upper quadrant of the breast in women. There may or may not be generalized discomfort in the area of the mass.

An injury was most likely sustained to which structure?

Injury occurs initially at the cellular level within the breast tissue. Breast cancer either begins in the lobules which are the milk producing glands or in the ducts that bring the milk to the nipples. Breast cancer can spread into the lymphatic system and will commonly metastasize to the brain, lungs, bones, adrenals, and liver.

Inference:

What is the most likely contributing factor in the development of this condition?

The etiology of breast cancer is unknown, however, estrogen is believed to have some relationship to the disease process. Risk factors include gender, age, young menarche, late menopause, family history of breast cancer, high alcohol intake, high fat diet, radiation exposure, and past history of cancer. Breast cancer can occur in both males and females, however, males account for less then 1% of all breast cancer cases.

Confirmation:

What is the most likely clinical presentation?

Breast cancer has a median and mean age between 60 and 61 years of age. Breast cancer makes up approximately 30% of all female cancers and is the second leading cause of death in female cancers within the United States. Approximately 70% of all breast cancer occurs in women over the age of 50. A patient with breast cancer will present with a lump in the breast that is noticed by a physician (10%) or by the patient through self-examination (90%). Breast cancer is initially otherwise asymptomatic. As the disease progresses the breast may become painful, change shape, bleed from the nipple, and dimple over the area of the mass. Symptoms associated with metastases may include bone pain, upper extremity edema, and weight loss.

What laboratory or imaging studies would confirm the diagnosis?

Mammography is used to detect the location and growth of a mass, however, definitive diagnosis of breast cancer is made only after microscopic examination of a suspected mass by needle or excision biopsy. Ultrasound can also be used to detect if a lump is filled with fluid or a solid mass. Sentinel lymph node mapping is used upon diagnosis to identify exact lymph node involvement.

What additional information should be obtained to confirm the diagnosis?

Additional information such as family history of cancer, past medical history, and history of self-examination is helpful in support of a definitive diagnosis. This information is usually obtained prior to mammography and biopsy.

Examination:

What history should be documented?

Important areas to explore include past medical history, family history of cancer, medications, current health status, social history and habits, hand dominance, occupation, living environment, and social support system.

What test/measures are most appropriate?

Aerobic capacity and endurance: assessment of vital signs at rest and with activity
Anthropometric characteristics: upper extremity circumferential measurements
Arousal, attention, and cognition: examine mental status, learning ability, memory, motivation
Community and work integration: analysis of community, work, and leisure activities
Gait, locomotion, and balance: assess static/dynamic balance in sitting and standing, safety during gait
Integumentary integrity: assessment for potential infection of surgical incision
Muscle performance: strength assessment
Pain: pain perception assessment scale, visual analog scale
Range of motion: active and passive range of motion
Self-care and home management: assessment of self-care and home management skills, assessment of functional capacity, Barthel Index
Sensory integrity: assessment of superficial and combined sensations, proprioception, and kinesthesia

What additional findings are likely with this patient?

Additional findings are dependent on the stage of the cancer (I, II, III, IV) and course of treatment. If a patient has undergone surgical resection or mastectomy the patient may experience pain, edema, fatigue, and psychological issues. Patients that are diagnosed with advanced breast cancer may experience pleural effusion, pathological fractures, and spinal compression.

Management:

What is the most effective management of this patient?

The medical management of breast cancer is based on the size and the stage of the mass and corresponding involvement of the lymph nodes. Surgical management may range from excision of the mass (lumpectomy) to total radical mastectomy with axillary dissection. Chemotherapy, radiation therapy, and hormone therapies may be used in isolation or after a surgical procedure. Physical therapy may be indicated to assist with lymphedema management, post-surgical breathing exercises, positioning, pain management, strengthening and endurance activities, range of motion exercises, massage, intermittent compression, and patient education.

What home care regimen should be recommended?

A home care regimen should include education, positioning, and techniques to manage lymphedema. Range of motion exercises, energy conservation techniques, as well as general exercise and endurance activities should continue on a regular basis at home.

Outcome:

What is the likely outcome of a course in physical therapy?

Physical therapy may be indicated for post-surgical management to assist with impairments and promote independence with self-care and functional skills.

What are the long-term effects of the patient's condition?

The long-term effects of breast cancer are varied. The risk of recurrence is always present and should be monitored closely. Post-surgical lymphedema may persist and require ongoing home management. Overall prognosis and ten-year survival rates for women are over 85% for stage I disease; 66% for stage II; 36% for stage III; and 7% for stage IV disease. The survival rate decreases as the tumor progresses and lymph nodes become involved. Overall mortality has decreased 1-2% annually within the United States secondary to changes in lifestyle, improved self-examination, earlier diagnosis, and better treatment.

Comparison:

What are the distinguishing characteristics of a similar condition?

Fibrocystic breast disease (mammary dysplasia) usually occurs in both breasts and is characterized by nodular lumps within the breast tissue. The cysts are benign and become tender immediately prior to menstruation. Fibrocystic breast disease is the most common breast disorder occurring in 89 per 100,000 women. Other symptoms include aching and burning within the breast. Symptoms normally disappear after menstruation is over. Although benign, fibrocystic breast disease increases a patient's risk for breast cancer later in life.

Clinical Scenarios:

Scenario One

A 65-year-old female is seen by a therapist 24 hours after total mastectomy. The patient was active prior to the surgery and walked for exercise two miles everyday. The patient's past medical history is positive for fibrocystic breast disease, diabetes mellitus, and skin cancer. The patient reports pain with coughing. The patient resides alone in a retirement village and lost her husband to cancer last year. She has three supportive children that reside in the local area.

Scenario Two

A 45-year-old female is referred to outpatient physical therapy with lymphedema secondary to stage III breast cancer and radical mastectomy three months ago. The patient is fatigued and anxious about the increased size of her arm and limitation in range of motion. The patient runs a daycare center out of her home and is active in her church. Past medical history includes endometriosis and pharmacological treatment for depression.

Carpal Tunnel Syndrome

Diagnosis:

What condition produces a patient's symptoms?

The carpal tunnel is created by the transverse carpal ligament, the scaphoid tuberosity and trapezium, the hook of the hamate and pisiform, and the volar radiocarpal ligament and volar ligamentous extensions between the carpal bones. The median nerve, four flexor digitorum profundus tendons, four flexor digitorum superficialis tendons, and the flexor pollicis longus tendon pass through the carpal tunnel. Carpal tunnel syndrome (CTS) occurs as a result of compression of the median nerve where it passes through the carpal tunnel.

An injury was most likely sustained to which structure?

The median nerve is injured by compression within the carpal tunnel at the wrist. Normal tissue pressure within the tunnel is seven to eight mm Hg but CTS can result in pressure above 30 mm Hg, which further increases with flexion and extension of the wrist. The increase in pressure produces ischemia in the nerve. This results in sensory and motor disturbances in the median nerve distribution of the hand.

Inference:

What is the most likely contributing factor in the development of this condition?

Any condition such as edema, inflammation, tumor or fibrosis may cause compression of the median nerve within the carpal tunnel and result in ischemia. The exact etiology of CTS is unclear, however, conditions that produce inflammation of the carpal tunnel that can contribute to CTS include repetitive use, rheumatoid arthritis, pregnancy, diabetes, trauma, tumor, hypothyroidism, and wrist sprain or fracture. Other etiologies include a congenital narrowing of the tunnel and vitamin B6 deficiency.

Confirmation:

What is the most likely clinical presentation?

Approximately five million individuals in the United States are diagnosed with CTS. Most patients are diagnosed between 35 and 55 years of age with prevalence in women. A patient with CTS will initially present with sensory changes and paresthesia along the median nerve distribution in the hand. It may also radiate into the upper extremity, shoulder, and neck. Symptoms include night pain, weakness of the hand, muscle atrophy, decreased grip strength, clumsiness, and decreased wrist mobility. Initially, muscle atrophy is often noted in the abductor pollicis brevis muscle and progresses to the thenar muscles.

What laboratory or imaging studies would confirm the diagnosis?

Electromyography and electroneurographic studies can be used to diagnose a motor conduction delay along the median nerve within the carpal tunnel. MRI is sometimes used to identify inflammation of the median nerve, altered tendon or nerve positioning within the tunnel or thickening of the tendon sheath.

What additional information should be obtained to confirm the diagnosis?

Physical examination, history, and review of symptoms are extremely important when diagnosing CTS. Provocation testing such as a positive Tinel's sign, a positive Phalen's test, and a positive tethered median nerve stress test along with the other symptoms will assist to confirm the diagnosis.

Examination:

What history should be documented?

Important areas to explore include past medical history, medications, history of symptoms, current health status, occupation, living environment, social history and habits, leisure activities, and social support system.

What test/measures are most appropriate?

Anthropometric characteristics: wrist and hand circumferential measurements

Arousal, attention, and cognition: examine mental status, learning ability, memory, motivation

Community and work integration: analysis of community, work, and leisure activities

Environmental, home, and work barriers: analysis of current and potential barriers or hazards

Ergonomics and body mechanics: analysis of dexterity and coordination

Integumentary integrity: skin and nailbed assessment, assessment of sensation

Joint integrity and mobility: assessment of hypomobility of a joint, assessment of soft tissue swelling/inflammation, Tinel's sign, Phalen's test, tethered median nerve stress test

Muscle performance: strength assessment including hand musculature

Orthotic, protective, and supportive devices: potential utilization of bracing or splinting

Pain: pain perception assessment scale

Range of motion: active and passive range of motion

Self-care and home management: assessment of functional capacity

What additional findings are likely with this patient?

Advanced CTS can present with muscle atrophy of the hand, radiating pain in the forearm and shoulder, and nerve damage with motor and sensory loss. Unrelieved compression creates initial neurapraxia with some demyelination of the axons. This results in eventual axonotmesis and wallerian degeneration within the nerve distribution. The patient may present with ape hand deformity caused by atrophy of the thenar musculature and first two lumbricals. Research indicates that approximately 50% of cases include bilateral involvement.

Management:

What is the most effective management of this patient?

A patient with CTS will initially receive conservative management including local corticosteroid injections, splinting, and physical therapy management. Recent pharmacological intervention has included Methylprednisolone injected proximally to the tunnel. Research indicates a 77% relief of symptoms from this method after 30 days. Physical therapy is one aspect of conservative management and includes splinting, carpal mobilization, and gentle stretching. Biomechanical analysis and adaptation of a patient's occupation, work place, leisure activities, and living environment may be necessary. If conservative treatment fails the patient may require surgery to release the carpal ligament and decompress the median nerve. Newer surgical techniques allow for smaller incisions, less manipulation of the nerve, and are highly successful for long-term relief of symptoms. Post-surgical physical therapy intervention should include the use of moist heat with electrical stimulation, iontophoresis, cryotherapy, gentle massage, desensitization of the scar, tendon gliding exercises, and active range of motion. A patient should initially avoid wrist flexion and a forceful grasp. After four weeks a patient can progress with active wrist flexion, gentle stretching, putty exercises, light progressive resistive exercise, and continued modification of body mechanics. Radial deviation against resistance should be avoided due to the tendency for irritation and inflammation. Post-surgical rehabilitation usually lasts six to eight weeks.

What home care regimen should be recommended?

A home care regimen should consist of continued stretching and strengthening exercises. The patient must be competent and compliant regarding the use of a splint and follow all work and leisure modifications.

Outcome:

What is the likely outcome of a course in physical therapy?

Physical therapy intervention should improve a patient's condition and decrease symptoms of CTS within four to six weeks. If conservative treatment fails and the patient requires surgical intervention, rehabilitation may last six to eight weeks.

What are the long-term effects of the patient's condition?

CTS can have minor effects on some patients while having debilitating effects on others. The overall long-term effects are dependent on the degree of involvement, the amount of permanent damage, and the level of success with conservative or surgical management. It is possible to have no long-term effects from this condition if the patient responds positively to physical therapy and the rehabilitation process. Other patients may be left with permanent motor and sensory impairments along the median nerve distribution.

Comparison:

What are the distinguishing characteristics of a similar condition?

Compression in the tunnel of Guyon occurs with inflammation to the ulnar nerve between the hook of the hamate and the pisiform. This condition occurs from tasks such as leaning during extended handwriting, leaning on bike handles while riding, repetitive gripping activities or trauma. The patient will present with paresthesias along the ulnar distribution, weakness and atrophy of the hypothenar musculature, decreased mobility of the pisiform, and impaired grip strength. This condition can be treated with conservative management or surgical intervention.

Clinical Scenarios:

Scenario One

A 26-year-old female is seen in physical therapy with a diagnosis of bilateral CTS. The patient has not been treated previously for this syndrome and is employed as a telephone sales specialist. The patient complains of pain in her hands, numbness when sleeping and while performing at work, and muscle soreness in both hands.

Scenario Two

A 45-year-old male with CTS is referred to physical therapy ten days after surgical decompression. The patient's post-operative routine includes resting the hand, using a splint, icing, and elevation. Minimal edema is noted at the wrist. The patient is anxious to return to work.

Central Cord Syndrome

Diagnosis:

What condition produces a patient's symptoms?

Central cord syndrome (CCS) is an incomplete spinal cord lesion that most often results from a cervical hyperextension injury. Symptoms are secondary to damage to the central aspect of the spinal cord. CCS usually occurs from a fall but can occur from other forms of trauma such as a motor vehicle accident.

An injury was most likely sustained to which structure?

The spinal cord sustains bleeding into the central gray matter that causes damage to the centrally located cervical tracts. Injury is caused by a ligamentum flavum (hyperextension) injury or otherwise from anterior compression of the cord due to osteophyte formation. Studies often reveal axonal disruption in the lateral columns at the level of injury with preservation of the gray matter.

Inference:

What is the most likely contributing factor in the development of this condition?

The most common mechanism of injury for CCS is a hyperextension injury of the cervical spine. Other potential contributing factors in the development of CCS include cervical spondylosis, narrowing or congenital defect of the spinal canal, tumor, rheumatoid arthritis or syringomyelia. CCS predominantly affects the population over 50 years of age with a greater incidence in men.

Confirmation:

What is the most likely clinical presentation?

CCS presents with motor loss that is greater in the upper extremities than the lower extremities and is most severe distally in the upper extremities. This presentation is due to the damage that occurs within the central location of the spinal cord. Sensory loss found below the level of the lesion is usually limited but can be variable. Lumbar, thoracic, and cervical components proceed medially in order towards the center of the spinal cord. Sacral segments are usually unaffected since they are located laterally within the spinal cord. Bowel and bladder functions resolve in 55-85% of patients with CCS after six months.

What laboratory or imaging studies would confirm the diagnosis?

MRI is used to assess spinal cord impingement from bone or disk. CT scan of the spine will assess spinal canal compromise and the degree of impingement. X-rays can be utilized to assess potential fractures, dislocations, and degree of spondylolitic deterioration.

What additional information should be obtained to confirm the diagnosis?

Diagnosis is made using results of MRI, CT scan, and X-ray findings. Information may be obtained from past medical history and mechanism of injury that usually supports the diagnosis of CCS.

Examination:

What history should be documented?

Important areas to explore include past medical history, medications, family history, current symptoms, mechanism of injury, social history and habits, occupation, leisure activities, and social support system.

What test/measures are most appropriate?

Aerobic capacity and endurance: autonomic responses to positional changes, assessment of vital signs at rest/activity

Arousal, attention, and cognition: examine mental status, learning ability, memory, motivation

Assistive and adaptive devices: analysis of components and safety of a device, wheelchair prescription

Community and work integration: analysis of community, work, and leisure activities

Environmental, home, and work barriers: analysis of current and potential barriers or hazards

Gait, locomotion, and balance: static and dynamic balance in sitting and standing, safety during gait with/without an assistive device, Berg Balance Scale, Tinetti Performance Oriented Mobility Assessment, wheelchair management

Integumentary integrity: skin assessment, American Spinal Injury Association (ASIA)-Standard Neurological Classification of Spinal Cord Injury Sensory Examination

Motor function: equilibrium and righting reactions, posture and balance in sitting

Muscle performance: ASIA-Standard Neurological Classification of Spinal Cord Injury Motor Examination, muscle tone examination

Neuromotor development and sensory integration: analysis of reflex movement patterns

Pain: assessment of neuropathic pain

Posture: analysis of resting and dynamic posture

Range of motion: active and passive range of motion

Reflex integrity: assessment of deep tendon and pathological reflexes (e.g., Babinski, ATNR)

Self-care and home management: assessment of functional capacity, Functional Independence Measure (FIM), Barthel Index

Ventilation, respiration, and circulation: breathing patterns, auscultation of the lungs and heart

What additional findings are likely with this patient?

Each patient with CCS will present differently based on location and extent of injury to the spinal cord. Potential side effects and complications include autonomic dysreflexia, spasticity, neurogenic bladder and bowel, allodynia, and pressure ulcers.

Management:

What is the most effective management of this patient?

Rehabilitation services are initiated once the patient is medically stable. Medical management should include physiatry, physical therapy, occupational therapy, vocational counseling, and social services. Methylprednisolone should be administered within eight hours of injury to assist with neurologic recovery. Other pharmacological intervention may include blood pressure medication to combat autonomic dysreflexia, antispasticity medication for treatment of spasticity, anticonvulsants for treatment of neurogenic pain, prophylactic anticoagulants, and antidepressants if warranted. Physical therapy intervention should include patient and caregiver education, range of motion, strengthening, endurance activities, balance retraining, proximal stabilization exercises, and functional mobility based on the patient's current functional status. Adaptive devices may be required to assist with overall mobility. If a patient ambulates, a platform attachment walker may initially be indicated since hand function is usually poor for grasp. Surgical intervention is rare but may be indicated if compression within the spinal cord persists or progress ceases without cause.

What home care regimen should be recommended?

A home care regimen should include a continuation of exercise, endurance, and functional mobility training based on the patient's current functional abilities. Outpatient physical therapy may be warranted and should modify the home program as necessary.

Outcome:

What is the likely outcome of a course in physical therapy?

Physical therapy can assist a patient with CCS to attain maximum functional outcome based on level and extent of injury. Overall outcome, however, is based on age, motivation, compliance, and extent of injury.

What are the long-term effects of the patient's condition?

CCS is the most common incomplete spinal cord lesion and accounts for approximately 30% of overall incomplete tetraplegia. Statistics indicate 77% of patients with CCS

will ambulate, 53% will gain bowel and bladder control, and 42% regain some hand function. Older patients do not tend to recover as well as younger ones. Favorable long-term prognostic factors for a good outcome include early hand function, improvement of strength in all extremities during the inpatient stay, and little to no lower extremity involvement.

Comparison:

What are the distinguishing characteristics of a similar condition?

Anterior cord syndrome (ACS) normally affects two-thirds of the spinal cord and can occur from a cervical flexion injury or anterior spinal artery embolization. There is a complete loss of motor function as well as pain and temperature below the level of the lesion due to damage of the spinothalamic and corticospinal tracts. Preservation of the posterior columns allow for intact vibration and proprioception. ACS has the worst prognosis for all the spinal cord syndromes with only 10-15% of patients achieving functional recovery.

Clinical Scenarios:

Scenario One

A 22-year-old female is admitted to the rehabilitation floor with CCS secondary to a MVA. She has some motion in her lower extremities, shoulders, and trace motion at the elbows. She only wants to practice walking and refuses therapy for any other treatment. She also is currently refusing any form of adaptive equipment for use during ambulation and with dressing. The patient is currently living with her friend and planned to move out of state in six weeks. She is employed as a teacher assistant at a local middle school.

Scenario Two

A 79-year-old male is diagnosed with CCS after being admitted through the emergency room secondary to a fall down his basement steps. He complains of severe neck pain and currently is not able to initiate movement in all four extremities. He is anxious and wants to return home to his second floor apartment as soon as he can. He misses his wife of 60 years who he has cared for since her stroke three years ago.

Cerebral Palsy

Diagnosis:

What condition produces a patient's symptoms?

Cerebral palsy (CP) is an umbrella term used to describe a group of non-progressive movement disorders that result from brain damage. CP has an incidence of 2-4:1,000 births and is the most common cause of permanent disability in children.

An injury was most likely sustained to which structure?

There is a wide variety of neurological damage that can occur with injury. Autopsy reports have indicated lesions that include hemorrhage below the lining of the ventricles, damage to the central nervous system that caused neuropathy and anoxia, and hypoxia that caused encephalopathy. Hypoxic and ischemic injuries disrupt normal metabolism that results in global damage to the developing fetus. CP is classified by neurological dysfunction and extremity involvement. Spastic CP involves upper motor neuron damage; athetoid CP involves damage to the cerebellum, cerebellar pathways or both.

Inference:

What is the most likely contributing factor in the development of this condition?

The etiology may be multifactorial and is sometimes unknown. Risk factors are categorized as prenatal (80%) or perinatal and postnatal (20%) cases. Prenatal risk factors include Rh incompatibility, maternal malnutrition, hypothyroidism, infection, diabetes, and chromosome abnormalities. Perinatal factors include multiple or premature births, breech delivery, low birth weight, prolapsed cord, placenta abruption, and asphyxia. Postnatal factors include CVA, head trauma, neonatal infection, and brain tumor. The most common causative factor of CP is prenatal cerebral hypoxia.

Confirmation:

What is the most likely clinical presentation?

CP is the second most common neurological impairment seen in children (following mental retardation). CP is a neuromuscular disorder of posture and controlled movement, however, clinical presentation is highly variable based on the area and extent of CNS damage. A child may present with high tone, low tone or athetoid movement. CP is classified as monoplegia (one involved extremity), hemiplegia (unilateral involvement of the upper and lower extremities), and quadriplegia (involvement of all extremities). CP is also classified as mild, moderate, and severe. General characteristics include motor delays, abnormal muscle tone and motor control, reflex abnormalities, poor postural control, high risk for hip dislocations, and balance impairments. Intellect, vision, hearing, and perceptual

skills are usually altered in conjunction with CP. All other characteristics of CP are classification dependent.

What laboratory or imaging studies would confirm the diagnosis?

If CP is suspected through clinical findings, including seizures, an electroencephalography (EEG) may be performed. X-ray of the hip may rule out hip dislocation; blood and urine tests can be used to investigate a metabolic cause of CP. Observation usually will diagnose CP secondary to the observed outward characteristics.

What additional information should be obtained to confirm the diagnosis?

Diagnosis of CP is regularly confirmed through an extensive neurological evaluation, patient observation, and patient history including developmental progress, and the presence of pathological reflexes. Differential diagnosis is performed to rule out other potential disorders.

Examination:

What history should be documented?

Important areas to explore include past medical history, risk factors, maternal course of pregnancy, medications, family history, current characteristics, social history, and social support system.

What test/measures are most appropriate?

Aerobic capacity and endurance: assessment of vital signs at rest and with activity, auscultation of the lungs
Arousal, attention, and cognition: examine mental status, learning ability, memory, motivation
Assistive and adaptive devices: analysis of components and safety of a device
Environmental, home, and work barriers: analysis of current and potential barriers or hazards
Gait, locomotion, and balance: static/dynamic balance
Integumentary integrity: skin assessment, assessment of sensation
Joint integrity and mobility: assessment of hyper- and hypomobility of a joint
Motor function: equilibrium and righting reactions, coordination, posture and balance, sensorimotor integration, Barthel Index, Bayley Scale of Infant Development, Bruininks-Oseretsky Test of Motor Proficiency, Alberta Infant Motor Scale, Pediatric Evaluation of Disability Inventory
Muscle performance: muscle tone assessment, strength assessment if appropriate
Neuromotor development and sensory integration: analysis of reflex movement patterns, assessment of involuntary movements, sensory integration tests, gross and fine motor skills, developmental milestones
Orthotic, protective, and supportive devices: analysis of components of a device

Pain: adapted pain scale
Posture: analysis of resting and dynamic posture
Range of motion: active and passive range of motion, assessment of contractures
Reflex integrity: assessment of deep tendon and pathological reflexes (e.g., Babinski, ATNR, Moro)
Sensory integrity: proprioception and kinesthesia
Ventilation, respiration, and circulation: breathing patterns, respiratory strength, accessory muscle utilization

What additional findings are likely with this patient?

Specific additional findings are dependent on the classification and extent of CP. Generally, complications can include aspiration, pneumonia, contractures, scoliosis, and constipation. Mental retardation and epilepsy are present in 50-60% of children diagnosed with CP. Common co-morbidities include learning disabilities, seizure disorders, vision and hearing impairments, bowel and bladder dysfunction, microcephalus, and hydrocephalus. Secondary impairments may include psychosocial issues for the patient and family members.

Management:

What is the most effective management of this patient?

Effective medical management of CP requires a life-long team approach. Pharmacological intervention may require antianxiety, antispasticity, and anticonvulsant medications. Physical therapy for CP often uses neurodevelopmental treatment and sensory integration techniques. Treatment should include normalization of tone, patient and caregiver education, motor learning, developmental milestones, positioning, stretching, strengthening, balance, and mobility skills. Adaptive equipment, specialized wheelchair seating, and orthotic prescription may be indicated. Surgical management may be required and include hip correction, contracture release, motor point block, dorsal rhizotomy or correction of scoliosis.

What home care regimen should be recommended?

A home care regimen for a patient with CP is also a life-long process that will require ongoing modification to meet the progression of goals. Family and caregiver involvement is vital for patients with moderate to severe CP. A home program may include patient and caregiver education, exercise, positioning, stretching, mobility training, and strengthening.

Outcome:

What is the likely outcome of a course in physical therapy?

Physical therapy will attempt to maximize a patient's level of current function and prevent secondary loss. If a patient is going to ambulate, this will usually occur by the age of eight. The ability or inability to ambulate will have a large impact on the direction and goals of therapeutic intervention.

What are the long-term effects of the patient's condition?

CP is a non-progressive, but permanent condition. The long-term effects and overall functional outcome depend on the extent of injury, associated impairments, and caregiver support. Prognosis for mild to moderate CP is a near normal lifespan. Fifty percent of children with severe CP die by the age of ten.

Comparison:

What are the distinguishing characteristics of a similar condition?

Arthrogryposis multiplex congenita (AMC) occurs in utero and is also considered to be non-progressive. AMC is considered a neuromuscular syndrome and is classified into three forms. The infant is born with multiple contractures and may have fibrous bands that developed in place of muscle. A patient with AMC should have a normal life expectancy and is usually of normal intelligence. It is usually difficult for these individuals to live independently due to their level of physical disability.

Clinical Scenarios:

Scenario One

A two-year-old female diagnosed with moderate spastic quadriplegia is seen in physical therapy. She is delayed in developmental milestones and beginning to acquire contractures. The parents are very supportive and the child appears happy and cooperative. The child's chart indicates normal intelligence.

Scenario Two

A nine-year-old male is seen in physical therapy at the request of his parents. The patient is diagnosed with moderate low tone quadriplegia, has minimal impairments with intelligence, and has acquired a 30-degree left thoracic scoliosis. The parents requested the evaluation since the child remains nonambulatory.

Cerebrovascular Accident

Diagnosis:

What condition produces a patient's symptoms?

Cerebrovascular accident (CVA) occurs when there is an interruption of cerebral circulation that results in cerebral insufficiency, destruction of surrounding brain tissue, and subsequent neurological deficit. The ischemia occurs from either a stroke in evolution (the infarct slowly progresses over one to two days) or as a completed stroke (an abrupt infarct with immediate neurological deficits).

An injury was most likely sustained to which structure?

CVA results from prolonged ischemia to an artery within the brain. This condition can cause subsequent neurological damage relative to the size and location of the infarct. Disruption of blood flow to a certain artery will lead to damage of a specific area of the brain and its functions. There are different types of CVA that include ischemic stroke (thrombus, embolus, lacunar) and hemorrhagic stroke (intracerebral, subdural, subarachnoid).

Inference:

What is the most likely contributing factor in the development of this condition?

The primary risk factors for CVA are classified as modifiable and non-modifiable. Modifiable factors include hypertension, atherosclerosis, heart disease, diabetes, elevated cholesterol, smoking, and obesity. Hypertension is the most prevalent modifiable cause of CVA. Non-modifiable risk factors include age, race, family history, and sex. Age constitutes the greatest risk for CVA, in fact 73% of patients sustaining a stroke are greater than 65 years of age.

Confirmation:

What is the most likely clinical presentation?

The incidence for an initial CVA is 114:100,000 persons or 750,000 individuals that have a first CVA in the United States per year. It is estimated there are four million stroke survivors living today. The clinical presentation of a CVA is determined by the location and extent of the infarct. Typical characteristics can include hemiplegia or hemiparesis, sensory, visual, and perceptual, impairments, balance abnormalities, dysphagia, aphasia, cognitive deficits, incontinence, and emotional lability.

What laboratory or imaging studies would confirm the diagnosis?

Computed tomography can confirm an area of infarct in the brain and its vascular origin, however, it can present as negative for up to a few days after the event. MRI allows for the diagnosis of ischemia within the brain almost immediately after onset. Positron emission tomography (PET)

can provide information regarding cerebral perfusion and cell function. Ultrasonography identifies areas of diminished blood flow in vessels and angiography may identify a clot and determine if surgical intervention is necessary.

What additional information should be obtained to confirm the diagnosis?

A chest x-ray may be warranted to rule out lung disease, while an electrocardiogram is used to examine potential cardiac abnormalities. Diagnosis is usually based upon patient history, physical and neurological examinations, symptoms, and diagnostic testing.

Examination:

What history should be documented?

Important areas to explore include past medical history, medications, risk factor profile, current health status, social history and habits, occupation, living environment, and social support system.

What test/measures are most appropriate?

Arousal, attention, and cognition: examine mental status, learning ability, memory, motivation, Mini-Mental State Exam, Boston Diagnostic Aphasia Examination

Assistive and adaptive devices: analysis of components and safety of a device

Gait, locomotion, and balance: static and dynamic balance in sitting and standing, safety during gait with an assistive device, Berg Balance Scale, Tinetti Performance Oriented Mobility Assessment, Functional Ambulation Profile

Integumentary integrity: skin and sensation assessment

Motor function: equilibrium and righting reactions, coordination, motor assessment scales

Muscle performance: muscle tone assessment, assessment of active movement, Stroke Rehabilitation Assessment of Movement (STREAM)

Neuromotor development and sensory integration: assess involuntary movements, sensory integration, gross and fine motor skills, reflex movement patterns

Orthotic, protective, and supportive devices: analysis of components of a device, analysis of movement while wearing a device

Posture: analysis of resting and dynamic posture

Pain: pain perception assessment scale

Range of motion: active and passive range of motion

Reflexes: assessment of pathological reflexes (e.g., Babinski, ATNR)

Self-care and home management: assessment of functional capacity, Rankin Scale, NIH Stroke Scale, Functional Independence Measure (FIM)

Sensory integrity: proprioception and kinesthesia

What additional findings are likely with this patient?

A patient with a left CVA may present with weakness or paralysis to the right side, impaired processing, heightened frustration, aphasia, dysphagia, motor apraxia, and right hemianopsia. A patient with a right CVA may present with weakness or paralysis to the left side, poor attention span, impaired awareness and judgment, spatial deficits, memory deficits, left inattention, emotional lability, impulsive behavior, and left hemianopsia. Coma and death are the most severe consequences of a CVA. It is common for patients post CVA to have residual complications and deficits that persist.

Management:

What is the most effective management of this patient?

Medical management will initially include medically stabilizing the patient through medication and surgical intervention. Pharmacological intervention can include thrombolytic agents, anticoagulants (contraindicated for hemorrhagic CVA), diuretics, antihypertensives, and potential long-term use of aspirin. Respiratory care must also be a priority during acute rehabilitation. Physical therapy during the acute phase focuses on positioning, pressure relief, sensory awareness and integration, ROM, weight bearing, facilitation, muscle re-education, balance, and postural control. The therapist is responsible for implementing the most appropriate therapeutic strategies based on the degree of impairment. There are many approaches to neurological rehabilitation that include, but are not limited to Bobath's Neuromuscular Developmental Treatment (NDT), motor control, Brunnstrom's Movement Therapy in Hemiplegia, Rood, and Kabat, Knott, and Voss' Proprioceptive Neuromuscular Facilitation (PNF). Many therapists integrate facets from multiple approaches based on the patient's response to selected interventions.

What home care regimen should be recommended?

Approximately 75% of patients that have experienced a CVA return home at various levels of functional mobility. The majority of patients require ongoing therapy services part of their home care regimen. A therapeutic program should be designed for a patient to continue at home independently or with the required level of assistance. Fall prevention, control of spasticity, endurance training, and optimizing functional mobility are important components of a successful home program.

Outcome:

What is the likely outcome of a course in physical therapy?

A patient that experiences neurological deficits due to a CVA may require physical therapy to assist with motor re-education, sensory stimulation, and functional mobility. The outcome is dependent on the patient's overall health, level of cognition and motivation, motor recovery, residual deficits, and family support.

What are the long-term effects of the patient's condition?

The effects of a CVA can be quite diverse ranging from spontaneous recovery to permanent disability requiring compensatory strategies and techniques in order to function. The first three months of recovery typically reveals the most measurable neurologic recovery and is usually a good indicator of the long-term outcome. Long-term outcome is based on several factors including the site and extent of CVA, premorbid status, age, potential for plasticity of the nervous system, and motivation. Research indicates that a patient can continue to improve the control of movement and show progress for an average of two to three years post CVA.

Comparison:

What are the distinguishing characteristics of a similar condition?

A transient ischemic attack (TIA) is also characterized by diminished blood supply to the brain, however, it is transient. Although the patient may present with similar symptoms of a CVA, the symptoms last for only a brief period of time. Unlike a CVA, the TIA does not cause permanent residual neurological deficits. A TIA is an indication, however, of future risk for a CVA.

Clinical Scenarios:

Scenario One

A 43-year-old male is diagnosed with a left hemorrhagic CVA due to an aneurysm of the middle cerebral artery. The patient resides with his wife and two teenage sons.

Scenario Two

A 79-year-old female is diagnosed with a right CVA involving the anterior cerebral artery. The patient was unconscious for two days and is functioning at a very low-level. The patient was residing in an independent living facility where she had meals provided for her in the dining area.

Congenital Torticollis

Diagnosis:

What condition produces a patient's symptoms?

Torticollis is a condition that causes the neck to involuntarily unilaterally contract to one side secondary to contraction of the sternocleidomastoid muscle. The head is laterally flexed toward the contracted muscle, the chin faces the opposite direction, and there may be facial asymmetries. The word torticollis means twisted neck. It is a disease, but also a symptom of many conditions.

An injury was most likely sustained to which structure?

Congenital torticollis is not usually seen immediately at birth. Muscle injury may be due to birth trauma, breech position in utero or other forms of intrauterine malpositioning. Infants born with torticollis appear healthy at delivery, however, over days or weeks they develop swelling over the injured sternocleidomastoid.

Inference:

What is the most likely contributing factor in the development of this condition?

The exact etiology of congenital torticollis is unknown, however, congenital torticollis may be caused by local trauma to the soft tissues of the neck just before or during delivery. The most common hypothesis is that birth trauma with resultant hematoma formation results in muscular contracture. Typically children with congenital torticollis have had breech or difficult forceps delivery. The fibrosis that develops in the muscle may be due to venous occlusion and pressure on the neck in the birth canal secondary to skull and neck position. Another theory includes malpositioning in utero resulting in intrauterine compartment syndrome.

Confirmation:

What is the most likely clinical presentation?

Congenital torticollis occurs in approximately 0.4-1.9% of newborns. The patient's head is laterally flexed towards the shortened muscle's side and the chin is pointed toward the opposite shoulder. Intermittent painful spasms of the sternocleidomastoid, trapezius, and other neck muscles may occur. The neck movements vary from jerky to smooth. The first sign may be a firm nontender enlargement of the sternocleidomastoid muscle visible at birth or within the infant's first few weeks of life. This mass, which is usually localized near the clavicular attachment of the sternocleidomastoid muscle, enlarges during the first few weeks of life, and then gradually decreases in size. Usually, the mass disappears by the sixth month of life and the only remaining clinical finding is the contracture of the sternocleidomastoid muscle that creates the torticollis posturing.

What laboratory or imaging studies would confirm the diagnosis?

Cervical spine x-rays are used to assess potential fracture or subluxation. A CT scan or MRI of the cervical spine can identify the presence of a potential neck mass. Electromyography (EMG) study may be useful in defining the degree of muscle or nerve involvement.

What additional information should be obtained to confirm the diagnosis?

The presence of the mass over the sternocleidomastoid along with the classic posturing will confirm the presence of congenital torticollis.

Examination:

What history should be documented?

Important areas to explore include history of labor and delivery, family history, medications, current health status, and social support system.

What test/measures are most appropriate?

Arousal, attention, and cognition: examine level of consciousness and alertness
Cranial nerve integrity: assessment of muscle innervation by the cranial nerves, dermatome assessment
Environmental, home, and work barriers: analysis of current and potential barriers or hazards in the home
Integumentary integrity: skin assessment, assessment of sensation
Joint integrity and mobility: assessment of hyper- and hypomobility of a joint, soft tissue swelling and inflammation
Motor function: motor assessment scales, coordination, Barthel Index, Bayley Scale of Infant Development, Denver II Scale, Neonatal Behavioral Assessment, Alberta Infant Motor Scale
Neuromotor development and sensory integration: analysis of reflex movement patterns, assessment of involuntary movements, sensory integration tests
Posture: analysis of resting and dynamic posture
Range of motion: active and passive range of motion
Reflex integrity: assessment of deep tendon and pathological reflexes (e.g., Babinski, ATNR)

What additional findings are likely with this patient?

Up to 20% of children with congenital torticollis have congenital dysplasia of the hips. In many instances, these infants will also present with facial asymmetries and plagiocephaly or flattening of the skull.

Management:

What is the most effective management of this patient?

Congenital torticollis is usually treated with non-operative intervention for 12-24 months before considering surgical intervention. Pharmacological intervention may include nonsteroidal anti-inflammatory drugs (NSAIDs), benzodiazepines and other muscle relaxants, anticholinergics, and local intramuscular injections of botulinum toxin or phenol. Physical therapy includes family/caregiver education and teaching, passive stretching exercises to the sternocleidomastoid and upper trapezius muscles, massage, local heat, analgesics, sensory biofeedback, and transcutaneous electrical nerve stimulation (TENS). Active range of motion with subsequent strengthening is also indicated to correct the infant's positioning of their head. Family training is extremely beneficial if there is consistency with handling and proper positioning during feeding and sleeping in order to promote stretch and active motion of the sternocleidomastoid muscle. If conservative treatment fails, surgical intervention will consist of unipolar sternocleidomastoid release, bipolar sternocleidomastoid release or selective denervation. Physical therapy is indicated after surgery and should include manual stretching of the neck to maintain the overcorrected position. Manual stretching should be continued three times daily for 3-6 months. A cervical collar may be used for the first 6-12 weeks after surgery.

What home care regimen should be recommended?

The family must continue with the stretching program and the correct handling techniques that are recommended by the therapist. The family will need to include proper positioning for the infant's sleep and alert times in order to maximize the benefits of the intervention.

Outcome:

What is the likely outcome of a course in physical therapy?

Studies indicate that between 85 - 90% of patients with congenital torticollis respond to conservative treatment and passive stretching within the first year of life. The best results for conservative management require the child to have had conservative treatment prior to the age of one. If surgical intervention is required, physical therapy will be required after surgery with an expected positive outcome for the patient.

What are the long-term effects of the patient's condition?

If a child is left untreated, congenital torticollis could have detrimental effects including the impairment of normal growth and development. The vast majority of children with congenital torticollis that receive conservative management are expected to fully recover and live a normal life.

Comparison:

What are the distinguishing characteristics of a similar condition?

Torticollis can also be acquired at an older age and presents in different forms. Acute wryneck is a term to describe a common type of torticollis that develops overnight without provocation. It is a self-limiting process and usually the symptoms subside within one to two weeks. Infectious torticollis may occur when the surrounding tissues become infected such as with a retropharyngeal abscess, nasopharyngeal abscess, tonsillitis, and sinusitis.

Clinical Scenarios:

Scenario One

A three-week-old infant is referred to outpatient physical therapy with a moderate right torticollis. There is a mass felt over the sternocleidomastoid muscle belly. The parents are concerned with this diagnosis and are very eager to assist with the infant's program. The mother is at home during the day and they have three other children at home.

Scenario Two

A child is referred to physical therapy status post unipolar sternocleidomastoid release two weeks ago. The child is 18 months old and was unsuccessful with conservative treatment for a significant left torticollis. The child resides with his foster mother in a studio apartment. The mother works full-time and the child participates in full-time daycare.

Congestive Heart Failure

Diagnosis:

What condition produces a patient's symptoms?

Congestive heart failure (CHF) occurs when the heart can no longer meet the metabolic demands of the body. The heart's inability to pump a sufficient amount of blood occurs when there is insufficient or defective cardiac filling and/or impaired contraction and emptying of the heart. The impairment in cardiac output causes the body to compensate for this deficit and this results in an increase in blood volume, cardiac filling pressure, heart rate, and cardiac muscle mass.

An injury was most likely sustained to which structure?

CHF is not an independent disease process but rather a symptom of pathology within the heart muscle itself or in the cardiac valves. Injury within the heart can be left-sided, right-sided or both. The abnormal retention of fluids and diminished blood flow causes further stress and injury to the cardiac system.

Inference:

What is the most likely contributing factor in the development of this condition?

There are many pathologies (reversible and irreversible) that can contribute to CHF. Common etiologies shown to contribute to CHF include arrhythmia (e.g., atrial fibrillation), pulmonary embolism, hypertension, valvular heart disease, myocarditis, unstable angina, renal failure, medication-induced problems, high salt intake, and severe anemia. CHF occurs when there is a decrease in cardiac output, abnormalities in skeletal muscle metabolism, impaired left ventricular function or all of the above.

Confirmation:

What is the most likely clinical presentation?

A patient with CHF will initially show signs of tachycardia. Other signs include venous congestion, high catecholamine levels, and finally impaired cardiac output. As the severity of CHF increases, signs of venous congestion usually become apparent. Left-sided heart failure is generally associated with signs of pulmonary venous congestion; right-sided heart failure is associated with signs of systemic venous congestion. Impairment to either ventricle can affect the other, leading to both systemic and pulmonary venous congestion. A patient may present with pulmonary edema, nocturnal dyspnea, orthopnea, S3 gallop, dry cough, exertional dyspnea with low level exercise, sudden weight gain, possible cyanotic extremities, cardiac hypertrophy, and shortness of breath.

What laboratory or imaging studies would confirm the diagnosis?

Lab tests including urinalysis and a CBC count that includes electrolyte, thyroid stimulating hormone, blood urea nitrogen [BUN], and serum creatinine levels should be performed. A chest x-ray, electrocardiogram, and echocardiogram are also recommended. A Doppler echocardiogram can determine systolic and diastolic performance, the cardiac output (ejection fraction), and pulmonary artery and ventricular filling pressures.

What additional information should be obtained to confirm the diagnosis?

A patient history and administration of cardiac questionnaires will assist with diagnosis of CHF. In the Framingham classification system, the diagnosis of CHF requires that either two major criteria or one major and two minor criteria be present concurrently. The New York Heart Association functional capacity classification also classifies heart disease based on symptomology as it relates to physical activity.

Examination:

What history should be documented?

Important areas to explore include past medical history, medications, current health status, nutritional status, social history and habits, occupation, living environment, and social support system.

What test/measures are most appropriate?

Aerobic capacity and endurance: assessment of vital signs at rest and with activity, perceived exertion scale, pulse oximetry, auscultation of the lungs
Anthropometric characteristics: circumferential measurements
Arousal, attention, and cognition: examine mental status, learning ability, memory, motivation
Community and work integration: analysis of community, work, and leisure activities
Environmental, home, and work barriers: analysis of current and potential barriers or hazards
Gait, locomotion, and balance: static and dynamic balance in sitting and standing, safety during gait with/without an assistive device
Integumentary integrity: skin assessment
Muscle performance: strength assessment
Pain: pain perception assessment scale, VAS
Range of motion: active and passive range of motion
Self-care and home management: assessment of functional capacity, Functional Independence Measure
Sensory integrity: proprioception and kinesthesia
Ventilation, respiration, and circulation: assessment of cough and clearance of secretions, breathing patterns, vital capacity, perceived exertion scale, pulse oximetry, palpation of pulses, auscultation of the lungs and heart

What additional findings are likely with this patient?

Diagnoses such as left ventricular infarction, aortic or mitral valve disease, and hypertension create pulmonary congestion that may result in left-sided CHF. Over time, however, fluid accumulation spreads and ankle edema, congestive hepatomegaly, ascites, and pleural effusion occur. This leads the patient to develop right-sided CHF as well. Later stages of CHF are characterized by symptoms of low cardiac output.

Management:

What is the most effective management of this patient?

A patient with CHF will be treated based on the root cause of the heart failure. Medical management includes the use of diuretics, nitrates, analgesics, and angiotensin-converting enzyme inhibitor agents. Medications play a vital role in the optimal management of this disease process. Therapists must be aware of the potential side effects such as digitalis toxicity when treating this population. The patient may be referred to physical therapy for generalized conditioning and mobility. Primary goals include improving exercise tolerance and increasing knowledge of the disease process. Therapeutic intervention has to be individualized by each patient since the etiology, current medications, and overall health play a role in the plan of care. Walking is commonly used to initiate an exercise program with cardiac patients. Patients can progress their overall endurance following their own heart rate and perceived exertion guidelines. Caregiver education and instruction may also be appropriate. Psychosocial support, nutritional counseling (no salt diet and no alcohol), and caretaker education are also important components of the plan of care.

What home care regimen should be recommended?

A patient will usually follow a similar program at home once they are discharged from the hospital or in addition to their outpatient therapy. The patient should continue energy conservation and pacing techniques with all activities. The family and patient must be fully educated as to the signs and symptoms of concern as well as potential medication toxicity.

Outcome:

What is the likely outcome of a course in physical therapy?

A patient can live with CHF and should benefit from physical therapy in order to improve endurance and strength after a decline in function from hospitalization or bed rest. Physical therapy will improve skeletal muscle function, blood flow, metabolic capacity, and overall exercise tolerance. Physical therapy, however, will not cure CHF or its cause.

What are the long-term effects of the patient's condition?

CHF is a common disorder. Approximately 4.6 million Americans are being treated for CHF, and over 500,000 new cases are diagnosed each year. The prevalence of CHF increases significantly with age, occurring in 1-2% of persons aged 50-59 years and in up to 10% of persons older than 75 years. Despite the heart's compensatory mechanisms, the ability of the heart to contract and relax progressively worsens and eventually fails. Thirty-year data from the Framingham heart study demonstrated a median survival of 3.2 years for males and 5.4 years for females after diagnosis.

Comparison:

What are the distinguishing characteristics of a similar condition?

Cor pulmonale is a form of right-sided heart failure but is normally seen as a consequence of chronic obstructive pulmonary disease. Sustained hypoxia produces an increase in pulmonary artery pressure that leads to right ventricular hypertrophy and finally, right-sided heart failure. When the right side fails, the left side does not receive adequate amounts of blood and then cannot sustain a normal cardiac output. This is not congestive in nature, however, as there is no fluid build up within the lungs. The right-sided heart failure also does not present with an audible S3 gallop.

Clinical Scenarios:

Scenario One

A 69-year-old male has been hospitalized for five days with congestive heart failure. He was diagnosed last year with the condition and has been doing well on medication. He started having shortness of breath and noted a six pound weight gain. His medications have been adjusted and he is motivated to get home to his wife. The physician requests a physical therapy consult for baseline data and a home exercise program.

Scenario Two

An 82-year-old female resides in a nursing home since her husband who cared for her passed away last summer. She was diagnosed with a left CVA three years ago that resulted in moderate weakness of her right upper extremity and as a result she requires assistance for ADLs. She requires a quad cane and supervision for ambulation. She has been in bed for the last month due to pneumonia and she currently has been diagnosed with CHF.

Cystic Fibrosis

Diagnosis:

What condition produces a patient's symptoms?

Cystic fibrosis (CF) is an inherited disease that affects the ion transport of the exocrine glands resulting in impairment of the hepatic, digestive, respiratory, and reproductive systems. The disease causes the exocrine glands to overproduce thick mucus (that causes subsequent obstruction), overproduce normal secretions or overproduce sodium and chloride.

An injury was most likely sustained to which structure?

CF affects multi-systems within the body, however, the respiratory and gastrointestinal systems are usually the most involved in the disease process. There is an underlying impermeability of epithelial cells to chloride that results in viscosity of mucous gland secretions within the lungs, sweat glands, pancreas, and intestines. CF creates an elevation of sodium chloride and pancreatic enzyme insufficiency.

Inference:

What is the most likely contributing factor in the development of this condition?

CF is an autosomal recessive genetic disorder (both parents are carriers of the defective gene) and is located on the long arm of chromosome seven. This disorder creates an abnormality in the CF transmembrane conductance regulator (CFTR) protein. CFTR normally is involved with the process that allows for chloride to pass through the plasma membrane of epithelial cells. It is estimated that 5% of the population carry a recessive gene for CF.

Confirmation:

What is the most likely clinical presentation?

CF is the most common lethal genetic disorder affecting Caucasian children in the United States. Incidence is estimated at 1:2,500 births for Caucasians compared to 1:17,000 births for African Americans. CF can be diagnosed shortly after birth, however, it is sometimes not diagnosed for years. The most consistent symptom is the finding of high concentrations of sodium and chloride in the sweat. Parents will notice a salty taste when kissing their child. Other symptoms vary depending on the systems that are affected by the disease and the course of progression. These systems include pulmonary, gastrointestinal, digestive (liver, intestinal, pancreatic), genitourinary, and musculoskeletal impairments. Early symptoms may include a persistent cough, salty skin, sputum production, wheezing, poor weight gain, and recurrent infections.

What laboratory or imaging studies would confirm the diagnosis?

Neonates' meconium can be tested as a screening tool for increased albumin. The quantitative pilocarpine iontophoresis sweat test is the sole diagnostic tool in determining the presence of CF. Sodium and chloride amounts greater than 60 mEq/l (standard value is 40 mEq/l) is a positive diagnosis for CF. The sweat test should be performed twice to ensure accuracy.

What additional information should be obtained to confirm the diagnosis?

Additional information in the diagnosis of CF is found through a positive family history, genetic screening of the parents, a previous diagnosis of failure to thrive, and in the manifestation of symptoms.

Examination:

What history should be documented?

Important areas to explore include past medical history (if diagnosed after birth), medications, current health status, developmental milestones, living environment, and social support system.

What test/measures are most appropriate?

Aerobic capacity and endurance: assessment of vital signs at rest and with activity, perceived exertion scale
Arousal, attention, and cognition: examine mental status, learning ability, memory, motivation
Assistive and adaptive devices: analysis of components and safety of a device
Integumentary integrity: skin assessment, sweat test findings, clubbing of the digits
Muscle performance: active motion, strength assessment
Posture: analysis of resting and dynamic posture, especially thorax and shoulder girdle
Range of motion: active and passive range of motion, chest wall mobility
Self-care and home management: functional capacity
Ventilation, respiration, and circulation: assess cough and clearance of secretions, pulmonary function testing (FEV$_1$ and FVC), pulse oximetry, auscultation of the lungs, accessory muscle utilization and vital capacity

What additional findings are likely with this patient?

The most common complication of CF is an exacerbation of obstructive pulmonary disease. Pulmonary function testing results in a decreased forced expiratory volume (FEV_1) and forced vital capacity (FVC). The functional residual capacity (FRC) and residual volume (RV) become increased. Hypoxemia and hypercapnia develop due to the alteration in perfusion. Chronic pulmonary infections and poor absorption often lead to barrel chest, pectus carinatum, and kyphosis deformities. Approximately 90% of patients have pancreatic enzyme deficiency, degeneration, and eventual progressive fibrosis of the pancreas. This process interferes with digestion and absorption of nutrients. Airway obstruction can cause pulmonary hypertension, atelectasis, pneumonia, and lung abscess. Severe complications can include cirrhosis, diabetes mellitus, pneumothorax, cardiac pathology, pancreatitis, cor pulmonale, and intestinal obstruction.

Management:

What is the most effective management of this patient?

Medical management of CF is a multidisciplinary approach that should focus on the quality of life, providing emotional and psychosocial support, and controlling symptoms. Nutritional support is necessary throughout the patient's life to ensure adequate nutrition. Pharmacological intervention is required to treat infections, thin mucus secretions, replace pancreatic enzymes, reduce inflammation, and assist with breathing. Psychological counseling is indicated as needed. Gene therapy is experimental and attempts to correct the defect in CF cells. Physical therapy intervention is essential for management of the disease. Chest physical therapy should be performed several times per day and includes bronchial drainage, percussion, vibration, breathing and assistive cough techniques, and ventilatory muscle training. Posture training, mobilization of the thorax, and breathing exercises must be incorporated into the overall program. A patient may also be trained to use autogenic drainage, a positive expiratory pressure (PEP) device or Flutter valve therapy to assist with independent bronchial drainage. General exercise and stretching are indicated to optimize overall function. Family and patient education are vital to the survival of the patient.

What home care regimen should be recommended?

A home care regimen for a patient with CF requires an ongoing routine performing postural drainage and chest physical therapy several times each day. Family members are trained to provide this ongoing support at home. Mechanical percussors may be used to ease the time and energy spent on manual percussion by the care provider. Mechanical percussors also offer the patient control and independence with treatment. Physical conditioning including exercise and endurance training are indicated except with severe lung disease. Exercise programs may improve pulmonary function, increase maximal work capacity, improve mucus expectoration, and increase self-esteem.

Outcome:

What is the likely outcome of a course in physical therapy?

A patient with CF will require intermittent physical therapy throughout his or her life. The goals of physical therapy are to maximize secretion clearance from the lungs, optimize pulmonary function, and maximize the patient's quality of life.

What are the long-term effects of the patient's condition?

CF is a terminal disease, however, the median age of death has increased to 35 years of age due to early detection and comprehensive management. The most common cause of death for patients with CF remains respiratory failure. A child that initially presents with gastrointestinal symptoms generally has a good clinical course whereas a child that initially presents with pulmonary symptoms is more likely to clinically deteriorate at a faster pace. Males generally have a better prognosis than females.

Comparison:

What are the distinguishing characteristics of a similar condition?

There is no other respiratory disease that is similar to the etiology of CF, however, chronic obstructive pulmonary disease (COPD) has similar lung characteristics. COPD is characterized by altered pulmonary function tests, difficulty with expiration, cough, sputum production, and physical damage to specific portions of the lungs. Chest physical therapy and pharmacological intervention are indicated for moderate to advanced COPD.

Clinical Scenarios:

Scenario One

A four-week-old infant is referred to physical therapy after being diagnosed with CF. The infant has a pleasant disposition and does not have any observable discomfort, however, the parents are very anxious. The patient has three siblings that do not have CF disease.

Scenario Two

A 26-year-old female with CF is referred to physical therapy with a severe respiratory infection. The patient recently moved into an apartment with her boyfriend and works 30 hours per week in a hair salon. Prior to the infection the patient was living at home and was able to manage the disease with occasional assistance from family members. The physical therapy referral is for chest physical therapy.

Degenerative Spondylolisthesis

Diagnosis:

What condition produces a patient's symptoms?

Spondylolisthesis is the forward slippage of one vertebra on the vertebra below. There are several types of spondylolisthesis classified by the actual cause for the slippage. Classifications include congenital, isthmic, degenerative, post-traumatic, and pathologic spondylolisthesis. Degenerative spondylolisthesis (DS) is caused by the weakening of joints that allows for forward slippage of one vertebral segment on the one below due to degenerative changes. These changes include segmental ligamentous instability and hypertrophic subluxating facet joints which can result in stenosis of the spinal canal.

An injury was most likely sustained to which structure?

The most common site of DS is the L4-L5 level. The slippage causes cauda equina symptoms secondary to stenosis of the canal. It is theorized that ischemia and poor nourishment secondary to the stenosis deprives the associated spinal nerves and results in pain. The L5 nerve root is compressed in an L4-L5 olisthesis. Other structures that can be irritated include the intervertebral disk, posterior and anterior longitudinal ligaments, and vertebral periosteum and bone.

Inference:

What is the most likely contributing factor in the development of this condition?

DS is caused by arthritis and degenerative changes in the spine. The intervertebral disk looses some of its ability to resist motion and as a result the vertebral facets increase in size and develop bone spurs to compensate. This condition can actually produce spinal stenosis and weaken the spine itself resulting in the slippage of a vertebrae. Since all structures of the spine remain intact the slippage is usually limited due to the secondary bony restraints of the spine.

Confirmation:

What is the most likely clinical presentation?

DS usually affects individuals over 50 years of age. It is more common with African Americans and women also have a higher incidence of occurrence than men. Back pain is a primary symptom that is said to increase with exercise, lifting overhead, prolonged standing, getting out of bed or a car, walking up stairs or an incline, and positioning in extension. The pain may be severe and radiate depending on the area of stenosis secondary to the vertebral slippage. Sensory and motor loss may be significant and follow a myotomal and/or dermatomal distribution. Most patients do not have significant neurologic deficits, however, a few do experience severe changes.

What laboratory or imaging studies would confirm the diagnosis?

Plain radiographs of the vertebral column are adequate to confirm the diagnosis of DS. CT scan or MRI may be indicated to rule out any other contributing conditions or to further assess nerve impingement.

What additional information should be obtained to confirm the diagnosis?

Physical and neurological examinations in combination with a full medical history usually provide adequate information for probable diagnosis, however, X-rays are required for definitive diagnosis of DS.

Examination:

What history should be documented?

Important areas to explore include past medical history and previous testing, medications, family history, current symptoms, current health status, social history and habits, occupation, leisure activities, and social support system.

What test/measures are most appropriate?

Arousal, attention, and cognition: examine mental status, learning ability, memory, motivation
Assistive and adaptive devices: analysis of components and safety of a device
Community and work integration: analysis of community, work, and leisure activities
Environmental, home, and work barriers: analysis of current and potential barriers or hazards
Ergonomics and body mechanics: analysis of dexterity and coordination, evaluation of proper lifting techniques
Gait, locomotion, and balance: static and dynamic balance in sitting and standing, safety during gait with/without an assistive device, Functional Ambulation Profile
Joint integrity and mobility: assessment of hyper- and hypomobility of a joint, soft tissue swelling and inflammation
Muscle performance: strength assessment
Pain: pain perception assessment scale, visual analog scale, assessment of muscle soreness
Posture: analysis of resting and dynamic posture
Range of motion: active and passive range of motion
Reflex integrity: assessment of deep tendon and pathological reflexes (e.g., Babinski, ATNR)
Self-care and home management: assessment of functional capacity
Sensory integrity: assessment of sensation

What additional findings are likely with this patient?

A patient with DS may or may not have additional slippage of the vertebra over time. If the slippage of the vertebra worsens it does not necessarily correspond to an increase in symptoms. Symptoms may increase with or without marked degenerative changes and vice versa. A patient that does experience ongoing neurological deficits will require surgical intervention regardless of the amount of slippage.

Management:

What is the most effective management of this patient?

Medical management of a patient diagnosed with DS should initially include education, medication, activity modification, and physical therapy intervention. Pharmacological intervention should include NSAIDs to decrease acute inflammation. Corticosteroids may be indicated for severe symptoms. Epidural steroid injections and selective nerve root injections are sometimes indicated if oral medications fail. Activity modification and rest should be instituted to further allow inflammation to subside and improve overall symptoms. Long-term bed rest, however, should be avoided. Once the acute phase has subsided physical therapy should begin. William's flexion exercises should be performed to strengthen the abdominals and reduce lumbar lordosis. Back school, modalities, postural education, and other exercises that provide core stabilization and increase flexibility should be included in the patient's program. External support such as bracing or wearing of a corset may relieve intradiscal pressure. Surgical intervention is only indicated if conservative treatment fails, the pain becomes disabling or significant neurological impairment exists. Surgical intervention usually involves decompression with or without spinal fusion.

What home care regimen should be recommended?

A patient with DS should initially take NSAIDs and decrease overall activities to allow for a reduction in the acute symptoms. Once a patient is able to tolerate physical therapy the home care regimen should include prescribed exercises to improve abdominal strength and core stabilization, flexibility exercises, and proper positioning. Goals for the home program are to alleviate pain and improve function. A patient should only modify the home program per therapist instruction.

Outcome:

What is the likely outcome of a course in physical therapy?

The majority of patients with DS are successful with conservative treatment that may include physical therapy, home program, bracing, and use of NSAIDs as needed.

What are the long-term effects of the patient's condition?

The long-term effects of DS vary based on progression and advancement of the slipped vertebrae and/or progression of symptoms. Some patients may be able to manage pain and maintain function without any further associated pathology. If symptoms continue to progress, then surgical intervention may be required.

Comparison:

What are the distinguishing characteristics of a similar condition?

Congenital spondylolisthesis is the slippage of one vertebra on the vertebra below due to an anomaly or defect in the fusion of the neural arch. This usually occurs in the upper sacral vertebral arches or at the L5 level. The condition is usually diagnosed during the growth spurts between 12 and 16 years of age. Patients are normally pain free prior to this point and begin to express complaints of back pain, "sciatica" pain, and other symptoms. There is a strong genetic association found in this type of spondylolisthesis.

Clinical Scenarios:

Scenario One

A 65-year-old female is seen in physical therapy with a diagnosis of L5 degenerative spondylolisthesis. She complains of pain in her back that can occasionally radiate down her left leg. She resides with her husband in their two-story home and works part-time at a grocery store as a clerk. She also enjoys gardening but has been having a difficult time with all activities in the last eight weeks secondary to pain.

Scenario Two

A 74-year-old male two weeks status post spinal fusion is examined in a nursing home. The patient was diagnosed six months ago with DS, shortly after he began to exhibit neurological symptoms. The physician prescribes physical therapy daily to improve strength and functional independence.

Diabetes Mellitus (Type I)

Diagnosis:

What condition produces a patient's symptoms?

Type I diabetes mellitus (DM) is a multi-system disease with both biochemical and anatomical consequences. There is persistent hyperglycemia due to diminished or absent production of insulin. In type I DM, insulin is functionally absent due to the destruction of the beta cells of the pancreas where the insulin would normally be produced.

An injury was most likely sustained to which structure?

Type I DM is characterized as an autoimmune disease in which circulating insulin is very low or absent, plasma glucose is elevated, and the pancreatic beta cells fail to respond to all insulin producing stimuli. The pancreas shows lymphocytic infiltration and destruction of insulin-secreting cells of the islets of Langerhans, causing insulin deficiency. Patients need exogenous insulin to reverse this catabolic condition, prevent ketosis, decrease hyperglycemia, and normalize lipid and protein metabolism.

Inference:

What is the most likely contributing factor in the development of this condition?

The exact etiology of type I DM is unknown, however, there are several theories. It is an autoimmune process with a strong genetic component. It is also believed that the genetic predisposition in combination with an unknown factor, potentially environmental, triggers the ongoing cycle of destruction of the beta cells of the pancreas.

Confirmation:

What is the most likely clinical presentation?

Type I DM usually starts in children ages 4 years or older, with the peak incidence of onset at 11-13 years of age, coinciding with early adolescence and puberty. Also, a relatively high incidence exists in people in their late 30s and early 40s, when it tends to present in a less aggressive manner. The most common symptoms of type I DM are polyuria, polydipsia, and polyphagia, along with nausea, weight loss, fatigue, blurred vision, and dehydration. A fasting glucose reading of 126 mg/dl is also a sign of DM. The disease onset is usually sudden or within a short period of time. It is not unusual for type I DM to present with ketoacidosis.

What laboratory or imaging studies would confirm the diagnosis?

A test of blood glucose levels will be necessary. In asymptomatic patients, physicians use the American Diabetes Association (ADA) recommendation of two different fasting plasma glucose levels of greater than 125 mg/dl. In symptomatic patients, a random glucose of 200 mg/dl suggests DM. Other testing includes urinalysis for glucose, ketones, and protein and a white blood cell count as well as blood and urine cultures to rule out infection.

What additional information should be obtained to confirm the diagnosis?

A detailed history and exam should provide the physician with confirmation of the previously mentioned symptoms that present with type I DM. Diagnosis is based on one of the subsequent factors: fasting glucose levels, two-hour post-load glucose levels or symptoms of DM.

Examination:

What history should be documented?

Important areas to explore include past medical history, medications, current health status, history of incontinence, recent polyuria, polydipsia, nocturia or weight loss, nutritional status, social history and habits, occupation, living environment, and social support system.

What test/measures are most appropriate?

Arousal, attention, and cognition: examine mental status, learning ability, memory, motivation
Community and work integration: analysis of community, work, and leisure activities
Environmental, home, and work barriers: analysis of current and potential barriers or hazards
Gait, locomotion, and balance: static and dynamic balance in sitting and standing, safety during gait
Integumentary integrity: skin assessment, assessment of sensation
Motor function: equilibrium and righting reactions, coordination, posture and balance in sitting
Muscle performance: strength assessment, muscle tone assessment
Posture: analysis of resting and dynamic posture
Range of motion: active and passive range of motion
Self-care and home management: assessment of functional capacity, Functional Independence Measure

What additional findings are likely with this patient?

Complications of type I DM include hypoglycemia and hyperglycemia, diabetic ketoacidosis, increased risk of infections, cardiovascular and peripheral vascular disease, retinopathy, nephropathy, impotence, and acceleration of atherosclerosis. DM is the major cause of blindness in adults aged 20-74 years, as well as the leading cause of non-traumatic lower extremity amputation and end-stage renal disease.

Management:

What is the most effective management of this patient?

Patients with type I DM require insulin therapy to control initial hyperglycemia and maintain serum electrolytes and hydration. At times, the first incidence of ketoacidosis is followed by a symptom-free period where patients do not need treatment. Pharmacological intervention includes the use of exogenous insulin per physician orders. Insulin can be administered through oral medication, intramuscular injections or through a continuous subcutaneous insulin infusion pump (requires surgical implantation). Medical management should also include regular self-monitoring of blood glucose levels through finger stick samples and urine testing. Patient education and counseling is appropriate for nutritional components, weight loss if obese, the disease process, complications, medications, and long-term effects. Physical therapy may be indicated for a home exercise program and the patient may be seen intermittently for change and update of their program. Exercise is an important aspect in management of DM. Patients should be taught general exercise and strengthening, stretching, and self-monitoring of their cardiac status. The therapist should coordinate exercise sessions around the patient's meal schedule in order to avoid hypoglycemia and optimize exercise tolerance. Patients should exercise at 50-60% of their predicted maximum heart rate unless directed by a physician otherwise.

What home care regimen should be recommended?

A patient with type I DM requires a good nutritional program, regular self-monitoring of blood glucose levels, and adequate and consistent daily exercise.

Outcome:

What is the likely outcome of a course in physical therapy?

Type I DM is the most common metabolic disease of childhood, with a yearly incidence of 15 cases per 100,000 people less than 18 years of age. Approximately one million Americans have type I DM, and physicians diagnose 10,000 new cases every year. Physical therapy may be indicated initially for a patient with goals of optimizing exercise endurance and implementing a home exercise program. Otherwise, patients are usually seen in physical therapy for co-morbidities or due to complications from DM. Physical therapy attempts to maximize patients' functional and health status, but cannot alter the disease process.

What are the long-term effects of the patient's condition?

Type I DM is associated with a high morbidity and premature mortality due to complications. As a result of these complications, people with diabetes have an increased risk of developing ischemic heart disease, cerebral vascular disease, peripheral vascular disease (that sometimes leads to amputation), chronic renal disease, reduced visual acuity and blindness, and autonomic and peripheral neuropathy.

Comparison:

What are the distinguishing characteristics of a similar condition?

Type II DM is more common in the United States than type I. Type II usually involves a defect in the insulin release sites within the pancreas or a resistance to the insulin due to impairment of the receptor sites in the peripheral tissues. In contrast to type I, type II is usually diagnosed in a patient older than 40 years of age. This form of DM is significantly linked to a person's lifestyle, weight, and age. A patient with type II can present with the symptoms of type I, but can also include paresthesias, visual changes, recurrent infections, inadequate wound healing, and cold extremities. In most cases, oral hypoglycemics are used instead of insulin injections.

Clinical Scenarios:

Scenario One

A three-year-old girl is seen in physical therapy that has just been diagnosed with type I DM. She also has a greenstick fracture of the left tibia secondary to an auto accident, but otherwise is in good health. Her mother has stated that her blood sugar levels were not yet regulated and it has been difficult for the physician to find the correct amount and timing of insulin.

Scenario Two

A 35-year-old male was just diagnosed with type I DM after he visited his physician for a routine check-up. He did note polyuria, polydipsia, and visual changes over the last six months time. He is referred to physical therapy for a home exercise program. The physician also recommended a nutritional consult as the patient is approximately 40 pounds overweight.

Down Syndrome

Diagnosis:

What condition produces a patient's symptoms?

Down syndrome (trisomy 21) occurs when there is an error in cell division either through nondisjunction (95%), translocation (4%) or mosaicism (1%) and the cell nucleus results in 47 chromosomes. Nondisjunction occurs when faulty cell division results in three specific chromosomes instead of two and extra chromosomes are then replicated for every cell. Translocation occurs when part of a chromosome breaks off during cell division and attaches to another chromosome. The total number of chromosomes remains 46 but Down syndrome exists. Mosaicism occurs right after fertilization when nondisjunction occurs in the initial cell divisions. This results in a mixture of cells with 46 and 47 chromosomes.

An injury was most likely sustained to which structure?

The pair of 21st chromosomes is responsible for Down syndrome when nondisjunction, translocation or mosaicism occurs during cell division.

Inference:

What is the most likely contributing factor in the development of this condition?

The exact etiology of Down syndrome is currently unknown. Some theories suggest that an increase in maternal age (and age of the oocyte) may cause predisposition to errors in meiosis. Environmental factors such as virus, paternal age, medical exposure, reproductive medications, and intrinsic predispositions have been associated with Down syndrome.

Confirmation:

What is the most likely clinical presentation?

Down syndrome occurs once in every 800-1,000 live births. In the United States there are approximately 350,000 individuals living with Down syndrome. Down syndrome is the most common cause of mental retardation. Other clinical manifestations include hypotonia, flattened nasal bridge, almond-shaped eyes, abnormally shaped ears, Simian line (palmar crease), epicanthal folds, enlargement of the tongue, congenital heart disease, developmental delay, and a variety of musculoskeletal disorders.

What laboratory or imaging studies would confirm the diagnosis?

During pregnancy a female can be tested for Alpha-fetoprotein, human chorionic gonadotropin, and unconjugated estrogen levels (the triple screen). Three diagnostic studies include chorionic villus sampling, amniocentesis or percutaneous umbilical blood sampling. Detection of Down syndrome occurs in approximately 60-70% of the women tested that are carrying a baby with Down syndrome. After birth a chromosome analysis called a karyotype can be performed to confirm the suspected diagnosis.

What additional information should be obtained to confirm the diagnosis?

In most cases diagnosis of Down syndrome is made through the physical attributes that are present at birth. Chromosomal testing is also used to determine the exact chromosomal pathogenesis.

Examination:

What history should be documented?

Important areas to explore include past medical history including cardiac status, family history, history of seizures, current health status, physical attributes, developmental delay, and social support system.

What test/measures are most appropriate?

Arousal, attention, and cognition: mental status, learning ability, memory, intelligence testing
Environmental, home, and work barriers: analysis of current and potential barriers or hazards
Ergonomics and body mechanics: analysis of dexterity and coordination
Gait, locomotion, and balance: static and dynamic balance in sitting and standing, safety during gait with/without an assistive device
Integumentary integrity: skin and sensation assessment
Joint integrity and mobility: assessment of hyper- and hypomobility of a joint, ligamentous laxity
Motor function: equilibrium and righting reactions, motor assessment scales, coordination, posture and balance in sitting, assessment of sensorimotor integration, Peabody Developmental Motor Scales
Muscle performance: strength and tone assessment
Neuromotor development and sensory integration: analysis of reflex movement patterns, assessment of involuntary movements, sensory integration tests, gross and fine motor skills, Bayley Scales of Infant Development
Posture: analysis of resting and dynamic posture
Range of motion: active and passive range of motion
Reflex integrity: assessment of deep tendon and pathological reflexes (e.g., Babinski, ATNR)
Self-care and home management: assessment of functional capacity, WEE-FIM
Ventilation, respiration, and circulation: assessment of cough and clearance of secretions, breathing patterns, respiratory muscle strength, accessory muscle utilization and vital capacity, perceived exertion scale, pulse oximetry, palpation of pulses, pulmonary function testing, auscultation of the lungs and heart

What additional findings are likely with this patient?

There are many associated impairments that a child with Down syndrome may inherit. Potential manifestations and secondary complications that are associated with Down syndrome include atlantoaxial instability, sensory, hearing, and visual impairments, umbilical hernia, respiratory compromise, and Alzheimer's disease. Persons with Down syndrome also have an increased incidence of celiac disease, epilepsy, constipation, as well as blood, dermatologic, and musculoskeletal disorders.

Management:

What is the most effective management of this patient?

Medical management of Down syndrome is a team approach that requires life long intervention and should be directed toward the specific medical and developmental goals. The overall goal of treatment is to achieve maximum potential and level of function. Pharmacological intervention is based on a particular characteristic or complication such as leukemia or a seizure disorder. Physical therapy intervention plays an important role in the treatment of Down syndrome. Developmental delay, hypotonia, laxity of the ligaments, and poor strength are key areas for the focus of physical therapy treatment. A child with Down syndrome will also require learning strategies based on his or her level of mental retardation. Children with Down syndrome regularly have significant verbal-motor impairments when they verbally respond to a stimulus. Physical therapy will not accelerate developmental milestones, but help the patient avoid compensatory patterns with static positioning and mobility.

What home care regimen should be recommended?

A home care regimen should be multifaceted with caregivers being proficient with all aspects of care. A routine of exercise is highly important for a child with Down syndrome in order to avoid inactivity and obesity. Positioning and handling are key components in order to maximize proper alignment and to minimize pathological reflexes, malalignment, and instability.

Outcome:

What is the likely outcome of a course in physical therapy?

Physical therapy will assist a child by teaching optimal movement patterns during developmental activities and by improving strength. Physical therapy will be indicated on an intermittent basis based on level of function and secondary complications. Strengthening and endurance activities should be encouraged within a home program.

What are the long-term effects of the patient's condition?

Individuals with Down syndrome today have a longer life expectancy secondary to advances in medical care, however, it is still less than standard life expectancy. Higher mortality results from issues such as congenital heart defects and gastrointestinal anomalies. Immune system dysfunction, repeated respiratory infections, onset of leukemia, pulmonary hypertension, and complications from Alzheimer's disease all contribute to a higher overall mortality rate compared to the general population. Approximately 80% of patients with Down syndrome reach the age of 55.

Comparison:

What are the distinguishing characteristics of a similar condition?

Prader-Willi syndrome is a genetic disorder that occurs when there is a partial deletion of chromosome 15. Characteristics include hypotonia, difficulties with feeding during infancy, short stature, excessive appetite, and obesity through childhood. Learning disabilities also exist.

Clinical Scenarios:

Scenario One

A six-month-old boy with Down syndrome is evaluated for outpatient physical therapy. Moderate hypotonia exists and the child does not roll or sit with support. The child's chart indicates atlantoaxial instability with minimal subluxation between C1 and C2. The boy's parents are supportive but both work full-time and are concerned about the competence of the daycare provider.

Scenario Two

A 12-year-old-girl with Down syndrome is seen in physical therapy two times per week at her school. The child is status post right femur fracture and the cast was taken off two weeks ago. The physician orders strengthening and cardiovascular endurance activities. The child has mild scoliosis and minimal learning deficits. The child is moderately obese and complains of pain consistently during treatment.

Duchenne Muscular Dystrophy

Diagnosis:

What condition produces a patient's symptoms?

Duchenne muscular dystrophy (DMD) is a progressive neuromuscular degenerative disorder that manifests symptoms once fat and connective tissue begin to replace muscle that has been destroyed by the disease process. The mutation of the dystrophin gene causes the symptoms of DMD.

An injury was most likely sustained to which structure?

A patient with DMD is born with a mutation in the dystrophin gene Xp21 that normally codes for the muscle membrane protein dystrophin. This gene is found on the X-chromosome and since it is a recessive trait, only males are affected while females are carriers. The lack of dystrophin allows for damage within the sarcolema with contraction of the muscle. The mutated gene causes weakening of cell membranes, destruction of myofibrils, and loss of muscle contractility. The destroyed muscle cells are replaced with fatty deposits.

Inference:

What is the most likely contributing factor in the development of this condition?

The etiology of DMD is inheritance as an X-linked recessive trait. The mother is the silent carrier of this disorder. Since it is a recessive trait, only male offspring will manifest the disorder while female offspring become carriers.

Confirmation:

What is the most likely clinical presentation?

The incidence of DMD in the United States is 20-35:100,000 live male births. Diagnosis of DMD usually occurs between two and five years of age. The first symptoms include a waddling gait, proximal muscle weakness, clumsiness, toe walking, excessive lordosis, pseudohypertrophy of the calf and other muscle groups, and difficulty climbing stairs. DMD primarily affects the shoulder girdle musculature, pectorals, deltoids, rectus abdominis, gluteals, hamstrings, and calf muscles, and is initially identified when a child begins to have difficulty getting off the floor, needing to use the Gowers' maneuver. During this technique a patient uses his hands to stabilize and walk up his legs in order to attain an upright posture. Approximately one-third of patients have some form of learning disability secondary to the dystrophin abnormalities. The disabilities usually present as subtle cognitive and/or behavioral deficits. There is usually rapid progression of this disease with the inability to ambulate by ten to twelve years of age.

What laboratory or imaging studies would confirm the diagnosis?

Electromyography is used to examine the electrical activity within the muscles. A muscle biopsy can be performed to determine the absence of dystrophin and evaluate the muscle fiber size. DNA analysis and high serum creatinine kinase levels in the blood also assist with confirming the diagnosis.

What additional information should be obtained to confirm the diagnosis?

Clinical examination, current symptoms, and family history are used to assist in the diagnosis, the type, and progression of the disease. Definitive diagnosis is made from clinical findings along with EMG and muscle biopsy results.

Examination:

What history should be documented?

Important areas to explore include past medical history, family history, medications, current symptoms, current health status, living and school environment, and social support system.

What test/measures are most appropriate?

Anthropometric characteristics: circumferential measurements to monitor muscle atrophy

Aerobic capacity and endurance: assessment of vital signs at rest and with activity

Arousal, attention, and cognition: examine mental status, learning ability, memory, motivation

Assistive and adaptive devices: analysis of components and safety of a device

Environmental, home, and work barriers: analysis of current and potential barriers or hazards

Gait, locomotion, and balance: static and dynamic balance in sitting and standing, safety during gait with/without an assistive device

Joint integrity: assessment of hypermobility and hypomobility of a joint, assessment of deformity

Muscle performance: assessment of active movement

Orthotic, protective, and supportive devices: analysis of components of a device, analysis of movement while wearing a device

Pain: pain perception assessment scale

Posture: analysis of resting and dynamic posture

Range of motion: active and passive range of motion, contracture assessment

Ventilation, respiration, and circulation: breathing patterns, respiratory muscle strength, accessory muscle utilization, pulmonary function testing

What additional findings are likely with this patient?

Additional findings occur with progression of the disease. Disuse atrophy, contractures, scoliosis, inability to ambulate, weight gain/obesity, cardiac and respiratory impairments, musculoskeletal deformity, and gastrointestinal dysfunction are the most common findings. Respiratory problems and scoliosis progress once the child is utilizing a wheelchair.

Management:

What is the most effective management of this patient?

Medical management of DMD focuses on maintaining function of the unaffected musculature for as long as possible. Pharmacological intervention may include glucocorticoids and immunosuppressant medications. Physical therapy intervention is initially indicated to assist a young child with progression through the developmental milestones. Once a child presents with impairments, physical therapy should focus on maintaining available strength, encouraging mobility, adapting to the loss of function, and promoting family involvement in a home program. Manual muscle testing and range of motion should be evaluated on a consistent basis to determine the pattern and rate of disability. Orthotic prescription, adaptive devices, and wheelchair prescription are areas that will require attention during the course of the disease. Respiratory care will also become a vital part of the plan of care as the patient weakens and strength diminishes. As DMD progresses, treatment will include range of motion, prevention of contracture/deformity, positioning, pain management, breathing exercises and postural drainage, and the use of a wheelchair or adaptive equipment. Ongoing emotional support for the child/family is necessary.

What home care regimen should be recommended?

A home care regimen relies on family involvement for a successful home program. Proper positioning, range of motion, submaximal exercise, and breathing exercises are all important aspects that assist a child to maintain function for as long as possible.

Outcome:

What is the likely outcome of a course in physical therapy?

Physical therapy is an important aspect in the care of a child with DMD, however, it will not alter the degenerative process of the disease. The goals of physical therapy throughout the course of the disease are to maintain present function, adapt to the progressive loss of mobility skills, and educate the patient and family. It is the role of the therapist to ensure that full and proper training has been completed on all aspects of a patient's care to ensure the highest level of function.

What are the long-term effects of the patient's condition?

DMD is a progressive disorder that occurs early in childhood and progresses rapidly. DMD usually affects the cardiac muscle in the later stages of the disease. Death occurs primarily from cardiopulmonary complications due to cardiac muscle involvement or respiratory muscle dysfunction. Death usually takes place by the time a patient is a teenager or less frequently into their 20's.

Comparison:

What are the distinguishing characteristics of a similar condition?

Facioscapulohumeral dystrophy (FSHD), also known as Landouzy-Dejerine dystrophy, is a form of muscular dystrophy that is also inherited but the exact genetic origin is unclear. This disease presents later in a child's life, usually between seven and twenty years of age. Characteristics include facial and shoulder girdle weakness, weakness lifting the arms over the head, and difficulty closing the eyes. This disease is more common in males than females. The females tend to be carriers of the disorder. Lifespan remains normal.

Clinical Scenarios:

Scenario One

A three-year-old male was recently diagnosed with DMD. The mother reports that the child can ambulate, but prefers to be carried. The child crawls up the stairs and has been falling more frequently. The patient has two sisters at home and resides in a two-story home. At present, both parents work full-time and the child is enrolled in a home daycare.

Scenario Two

A 12-year-old male diagnosed with DMD is referred to physical therapy secondary to increased weakness and frequent falls. The patient is currently ambulating with bilateral Lofstrand crutches. There is evidence of pseudohypertrophy and a mild plantar flexion contracture. The patient's mother is concerned that he is at risk for serious injury while ambulating at school.

Emphysema

Diagnosis:

What condition produces a patient's symptoms?

Emphysema is the condition of pathologic accumulation of air in the lungs found with chronic obstructive pulmonary disease (COPD). There are three classifications of emphysema that include centrilobular emphysema, panlobular emphysema, and paraseptal emphysema. Emphysema results from a long history of chronic bronchitis, recurrent alveolar inflammation or from genetic predisposition of a congenital alpha 1-antitrypsin deficiency.

An injury was most likely sustained to which structure?

Emphysema results from a non-reversible injury and destruction of elastin protein within the alveolar walls. This process causes permanent enlargement of the air spaces distal to the terminal bronchioles within the lungs. Anatomical changes include loss of elastic recoil, excessive airway collapse during exhalation, and chronic obstruction of airflow. Progression of the disease includes further destruction of the alveolar walls, collapse of the peripheral bronchioles, and impaired gas exchange. Emphysema causes pockets of air to form between the alveolar spaces, (known as blebs), and within the lung parenchyma (known as bullae). This results in an increase in dead space within the lungs that diminishes gas exchange.

Inference:

What is the most likely contributing factor in the development of this condition?

The primary risk factors for the development of emphysema include chronic bronchitis, lower respiratory infections, cigarette smoking, and genetic predisposition. Environmental influence includes air pollution and other airborne toxins. The risk of acquiring emphysema increases with age.

Confirmation:

What is the most likely clinical presentation?

COPD is the second leading cause of disability in individuals under 65 years of age worldwide. There are two million individuals in the United States diagnosed with emphysema (and another 14 million with some form of COPD). Emphysema can be asymptomatic until middle age and is most often diagnosed between 55 and 60 years of age. Centrilobular emphysema usually destroys the bronchioles in the upper lungs while the alveolar sacs usually remain intact. Panlobular emphysema destroys the air spaces of the acinus and is usually found in the lower lungs. Paraseptal emphysema destroys the alveoli in the lower lobes resulting in blebs along the lung periphery. Symptoms of emphysema worsen with the progression of the disease and include a persistent cough, wheezing, difficulty breathing especially with expiration, and an increased respiration rate. Advanced disease symptoms include increased use of accessory muscles, severe dyspnea, cor pulmonale, and cyanosis.

What laboratory or imaging studies would confirm the diagnosis?

X-ray is utilized to visually evaluate the shape and spacing of the lungs. Other imaging studies include a planogram to detect bullae and a bronchogram to evaluate mucus ducts and detect possible enlargement of the bronchi. Arterial blood gases may indicate a decreased PaO_2.

What additional information should be obtained to confirm the diagnosis?

A physical examination, thorough patient history (including cigarette smoking), and pulmonary function tests are required for diagnosis. Pulmonary function testing will result in impaired forced expiratory volume (FEV_1), vital capacity (VC), and forced vital capacity (FVC). Total lung capacity (TLC), residual volume (RV), and functional residual capacity (FRC) will be increased.

Examination:

What history should be documented?

Important areas to explore include past medical history, history of smoking, medications, current health status, social history and habits, occupation, living environment, and social support system.

What test/measures are most appropriate?

Aerobic capacity and endurance: assessment of vital signs at rest and with activity, perceived exertion scale, Six-Minute Walk Test, Three-Minute Step Test

Arousal, attention, and cognition: examine mental status, learning ability, memory, motivation

Assistive and adaptive devices: analysis of components and safety of a device

Environmental, home, and work: analysis of current and potential barriers or hazards

Gait, locomotion, and balance: static and dynamic balance in sitting and standing, safety during gait with/without an assistive device

Muscle performance: strength assessment, assessment of active movement and muscle endurance

Posture: analysis of resting and dynamic posture

Self-care and home management: functional capacity

Ventilation, respiration, and circulation: assessment of thoracoabdominal movement, auscultation of vesicular sounds/potential rhonchi, pulse oximetry, pulmonary function testing, accessory muscle utilization

What additional findings are likely with this patient?

A patient with emphysema may present with a barrel chest appearance, an increased subcostal angle, rounded shoulders secondary to tight pectorals, rosy skin coloring, and may utilize pursed-lip breathing to assist with ventilation. Patients will also have high rates of anxiety associated with difficulty breathing and may present with claustrophobia, insomnia, and depression. Complications such as the formation and rupture of bullae and blebs can lead to pneumothorax. Cor pulmonale is a serious complication that can occur with advanced emphysema.

Management:

What is the most effective management of this patient?

Medical management of a patient with emphysema includes pharmacological intervention, oxygen therapy, and physical therapy. Pharmacological intervention promotes bronchodilation, improved oxygenation, and ventilation. Drugs such as oral/inhaled bronchodilators, anti-inflammatory agents, mucolytic expectorants, mast cell membrane stabilizers, and antihistamines may be used in the treatment of emphysema. Preventative immunizations against influenza and pneumonia are also recommended. Physical therapy intervention is based on the severity of the disease process and can include general exercise and endurance training, breathing exercises including pursed-lip breathing, ventilatory muscle strengthening, chest wall exercises, and patient education on posture, airway secretion clearance, and energy conservation techniques. Pulse oximetry should be used to monitor a patient's oxygen saturation during activities and exercise. This will assist with patient education and deter the effects of hypoxemia. Chest physical therapy is required during advanced stages of emphysema.

What home care regimen should be recommended?

The home care regimen should include breathing strategies and exercises, energy conservation, pacing techniques, and general strength and endurance training.

Outcome:

What is the likely outcome of a course in physical therapy?

A patient with emphysema may require physical therapy intermittently as the disease progresses. The goals of physical therapy are to maximize the patient's functional abilities and optimize pulmonary function.

What are the long-term effects of the patient's condition?

Emphysema is a chronic progressive disease process. Patients require ongoing medical care and intermittent physical therapy intervention. Life expectancy decreases to less than five years with severe expiratory slowing measured at a rate of <1L of air during forced expiratory volume (FEV_1).

Comparison:

What are the distinguishing characteristics of a similar condition?

Bronchiectasis is inherited or acquired and is characterized by chronic inflammation and dilation of bronchi and destruction of the bronchial walls. This disease is associated with chronic bacterial infections and is an extreme form of bronchitis. Incidence within the United States is low. Bronchiectasis has a higher risk for development in patients with cystic fibrosis, sinusitis, Kartagener's syndrome, and endobronchial tumors. Characteristics include a chronic cough with sputum, hemoptysis, wheezing, dyspnea, and recurrent respiratory infections. Primary treatment includes physical therapy, bronchodilators, and antibiotics.

Clinical Scenarios:

Scenario One

A 65-year-old male is referred to physical therapy after recently being diagnosed with emphysema. The patient works in an oil refinery part-time and manages a small dairy farm. The patient's past medical history is negative for smoking and consists of recurrent respiratory infections and chronic cough. The patient complains of shortness of breath with exertion, however, pulmonary function testing indicates only minimal impairment in lung volumes.

Scenario Two

A 75-year-old female requires physical therapy for management of emphysema. The patient has a history of smoking cigarettes for over 40 years and continues to smoke approximately one pack per day. The patient has an oxygen saturation rate of 94% at rest and requires two liters of oxygen with exertion. The patient has moderate impairment in pulmonary function testing and a persistent cough. The patient presently resides in a two-story home and assists with the care of her disabled husband.

Erb's Palsy

Diagnosis:

What condition produces a patient's symptoms?

Erb's palsy is a term used to denote an upper brachial plexus injury or palsy that usually results from a difficult birth. The type of injury is the most common palsy related to the brachial plexus. It primarily affects the muscles of the shoulder and elbow.

An injury was most likely sustained to which structure?

The brachial plexus is damaged with the most common avulsion located at Erb's point (which is an area in the anterolateral neck). This damages the nerves supplying the ipsilateral upper limb and shoulder. The muscles affected are those supplied by cervical roots C5 and C6; axillary, lateral pectoral, upper and lower subscapular, suprascapular and partial paralysis of the long thoracic and the musculocutaneous nerves. The result is loss of rotator cuff, deltoid, brachialis, coracobrachialis, and biceps brachii function.

Inference:

What is the most likely contributing factor in the development of this condition?

A brachial plexus injury in a newborn usually occurs during a difficult delivery, due to a large baby, a breech presentation, with a prolonged labor or with the use of forceps. One side of the baby's neck is stretched which damages the nerves. If the upper nerves are affected the condition is termed Erb's palsy. One theory suggests that congenital chicken pox or amniotic bands may also produce this condition. When it occurs in adults the cause typically is an injury that has caused stretching, tearing or other trauma to the upper brachial plexus network.

Confirmation:

What is the most likely clinical presentation?

There are four types of brachial plexus injury: avulsion, rupture, neuroma, (the nerve is torn and scar tissue has developed), and neuropraxia (the most common form of injury where the nerve has been damaged, but remains intact). The clinical presentation is a flaccid paralysis that is nicknamed the "Waiter's tip deformity", characterized by a loss of shoulder function, loss of elbow flexion, forearm pronation, and the hand positioned in a pinch grip manner.

What laboratory or imaging studies would confirm the diagnosis?

An x-ray or magnetic resonance imaging (MRI) may be performed to see if there is any damage to the bones and joints of the neck and shoulder. The physician may also use an electromyogram (EMG) or nerve conduction studies (NCS) to see if any nerve signals are present in the upper extremity muscles. In complete injuries, motor and sensory nerve conduction studies of median, ulnar, and radial nerves may be conducted.

What additional information should be obtained to confirm the diagnosis?

A complete history from the patient or parent should be taken regarding upper extremity weakness. Other testing that will assist with diagnosis may include the active movement scale, Gilbert shoulder classification, and the Pediatric Outcomes Data Collection Instrument.

Examination:

What history should be documented?

Important areas to explore include past medical history including labor and delivery (infant patients), mechanism of injury (adult patients), medications, current health status, nutritional status, social history, occupation, living environment, and support system.

What test/measures are most appropriate?

Anthropometric characteristics: circumferential measurements of the extremities
Cranial nerve integrity: assessment of muscle innervation by the cranial nerves, dermatome assessment
Environmental, home, and work barriers: analysis of current and potential barriers or hazards (adult cases)
Integumentary integrity: assessment of sensation
Joint integrity and mobility: assessment of hyper- and hypomobility of a joint
Motor function: equilibrium and righting reactions, motor assessment scales, coordination, posture and balance in sitting, assessment of sensorimotor integration, physical performance scales
Muscle performance: strength assessment, muscle tone assessment
Neuromotor development and sensory integration: analysis of reflex movement patterns, assessment of involuntary movements, sensory integration tests, gross and fine motor skills
Posture: analysis of resting and dynamic posture
Range of motion: active and passive range of motion
Reflex integrity: assessment of deep tendon and pathological reflexes (e.g., Babinski, ATNR)
Self-care and home management: assessment of functional capacity
Sensory integrity: proprioception and kinesthesia

What additional findings are likely with this patient?

The child may exhibit characteristics such as an underdeveloped extremity or deformed area if amniotic bands were the congenital cause for the brachial plexus injury. The patient may also experience glenohumeral subluxation or dislocation, skeletal deformity, poor bone growth, and a learned pattern of non-use of the upper extremity. Overall, the chance of a child having a brachial plexus palsy is equally distributed according to gender, gestational age, and race. It occurs frequently in perfectly normal and healthy infants. The reported incidence of brachial plexus palsies is approximately 1 in every 1,000 live births.

Management:

What is the most effective management of this patient?

Physical therapy is recommended for a patient with Erb's palsy with the goal of developing a program that focuses on increasing active and passive movement and promoting use of the weak upper extremity for functional activities. Occupational and physical therapies are usually indicated immediately when the patient is diagnosed. The length of treatment will depend on the patient's recovery of active movements. If a patient has spontaneous recovery (full active movements) within three to four months, the caregivers are usually given a home program before discharge in order to continue the program at home. However, if spontaneous recovery does not occur within that time frame, the patient may continue in therapy with close monitoring of progress. If conservative management fails, surgery may be indicated, but will not restore normal function and does not usually assist infants over one-year-old. After surgery, the infant will wear a splint for approximately three to four weeks. Caregiver education is very important regarding positioning to avoid any further traction during the child's daily activities. Other treatment techniques may include adaptation of developmental milestones and other functional activities, tapping, weight bearing activities, and other sensory techniques.

What home care regimen should be recommended?

The patient's caregivers must be competent with all aspects of the home program and must perform the program in a consistent fashion. The program should include AROM, PROM, general strengthening, functional activities and integration of the weakened upper extremity into all functional activities.

Outcome:

What is the likely outcome of a course in physical therapy?

The therapeutic management of a patient with Erb's palsy must begin in infancy (or immediately) in order to achieve optimal functional return. Nerve regeneration remains at a constant speed, however, physical therapy intervention can assist with overall strength and function during recovery. The chance of an infant having a brachial plexus palsy is equally distributed according to gender, gestational age, and race and occurs frequently in normal healthy infants.

What are the long-term effects of the patient's condition?

Approximately nine out of ten infants with brachial plexus palsy can recover with conservative treatment. The final functional outcome will depend on the degree of damage to the nerves and the caregiver's ability to maintain their motion and their level of interest towards the affected upper extremity during the initial first few months of life. Since nerves grow at a rate of one inch per month, it may take several months or even years for nerves repaired at the cervical spine to reach the muscles of the hand.

Comparison:

What are the distinguishing characteristics of a similar condition?

Klumpke palsy is the name for the brachial plexus palsy where there is an injury from childbirth affecting the spinal nerves C7, C8, and T1. It is uncommon and can be contrasted to Erb's palsy, which affects C5 and C6. Classically, it produces flexion and supination of the elbow, extension of the wrist, hyper-extension of the metacarpophalangeal joints, and flexion of the interphalangeal joints allowing for a "claw hand" posture. The mechanism of injury is traction of the upper extremity while in an abducted position.

Clinical Scenarios:

Scenario One

A six-week-old infant girl is seen in outpatient physical therapy with a recent diagnosis of Erb's palsy. The mother has taken a leave of absence from her job in order to assist her infant. She also has a set of three-year-old twins and her husband has been deployed for 12 months for duty in Iraq.

Scenario Two

A 56-year-old farmer was admitted to the hospital with a humeral fracture and traction injury to the upper brachial plexus. The injuries were sustained while the farmer was using a piece of faulty equipment. He cannot use the muscles in the C5-C6 distribution and is very anxious to return to work.

Fibromyalgia Syndrome

Diagnosis:

What condition produces a patient's symptoms?

Fibromyalgia syndrome (FMS) is classified as a rheumatology syndrome or a nonarticular rheumatic condition. Pain is the primary symptom caused by tender points within muscles, tendons, and ligaments.

An injury was most likely sustained to which structure?

The exact etiology of FMS is unknown. Theories suggest potential biochemical, metabolic or immunologic pathology. Researchers believe it to be multifactorial in origin and suggest a link to a dysfunction within the stress system, autonomic nervous system, immune system and/or reproductive and hormone systems.

Inference:

What is the most likely contributing factor in the development of this condition?

Since the exact etiology of FMS is unknown there is speculation linking many factors to the development of this condition. Factors include diet, sleep disorders, viral infections, psychological distress, occupational and environmental factors, hypothyroidism, trauma, and potential hereditary links. Many individuals diagnosed with FMS note multiple causative factors, however, there are individuals diagnosed with FMS that possess none of the theorized causative factors.

Confirmation:

What is the most likely clinical presentation?

The American College of Rheumatology's data indicates that there are approximately six million individuals living with FMS making it the most common musculoskeletal disorder in the United States. FMS has a greater incidence in females (almost 75% of the cases) and can affect any age but most frequently is diagnosed between 14 and 68 years of age. FMS is diagnosed when a patient exhibits the criteria authored by the American College of Rheumatology. There is a widespread history of pain that exists in all four quadrants of the body (above and below the waist), axial pain is present, and there is pain in at least 11 of 18 standardized "tender point" sites. These sites include the occiput, low cervical area, trapezius, supraspinatus, second rib, lateral epicondyle, gluteal area, greater trochanter, and the knee. The patient may also complain of fatigue, memory and visual impairment, sleep disturbances, irritable bowel syndrome, headaches, and anxiety/depression.

What laboratory or imaging studies would confirm the diagnosis?

FMS has been commonly misdiagnosed as myofascial pain, systemic lupus erythematosus, fibrocytis, and chronic fatigue syndrome. There are no specific tests used to diagnose FMS. Radiographs are negative and blood work often appears normal except for a possible alteration in the levels of substance P. This substance is a chemical involved with pain transmission. Image studies and other lab testing are performed only for differential diagnosis.

What additional information should be obtained to confirm the diagnosis?

FMS is diagnosed according to the criteria from the American College of Rheumatology. A dolorimeter is used for reliability when testing the tender points by providing a consistent pressure (4 kg/cm2). If the patient meets the criteria and has experienced symptoms for greater than three months then a patient may be diagnosed with FMS. Diagnostic written tools that can assist with diagnosis include the Beck Depression Inventory and the Fibromyalgia Impact Questionnaire.

Examination:

What history should be documented?

Important areas to explore include past medical history, medications, family history, current symptoms, current health status, social history and habits, occupation, leisure activities, and social support system.

What test/measures are most appropriate?

Aerobic capacity and endurance: assessment of vital signs at rest and with activity, perceived exertion scale, pulse oximetry, auscultation of the lungs

Arousal, attention, and cognition: examine mental status, learning ability, memory, motivation

Community and work integration: analysis of community, work, and leisure activities

Environmental, home, and work barriers: analysis of current and potential barriers or hazards

Ergonomics and body mechanics: analysis of dexterity and coordination

Gait, locomotion, and balance: static and dynamic balance in sitting and standing, safety during gait

Integumentary integrity: skin assessment, assessment of sensation

Joint integrity and mobility: assessment of hyper- and hypomobility of a joint, effusion, edema

Muscle performance: strength assessment, muscle tone assessment

Neuromotor development and sensory integration: analysis of reflex movement patterns, assessment of involuntary movements, sensory integration tests, gross and fine motor skills

Pain: pain perception assessment scale, visual analog scale, assessment of muscle soreness and tender points

Posture: analysis of resting and dynamic posture

Range of motion: active and passive range of motion

Self-care and home management: assessment of functional capacity

What additional findings are likely with this patient?

The aforementioned symptoms can progress over time. Certain symptoms intensify and cause the patient to lose functional independence secondary to increased pain, decreased range of motion, and severe fatigue.

Management:

What is the most effective management of this patient?

FMS is best treated with a multidisciplinary approach including education, medical management, and exercise. Medical management will attempt to normalize various dysfunctions of the autonomic nervous system, hormonal imbalances, and metabolic abnormalities. Physicians must address sleep disorders (which can be common) and pharmacological intervention based on symptoms. Psychotherapy may be warranted for anxiety or depression and must incorporate stress management and coping strategies into the plan of care. Physical therapy intervention may include relaxation techniques, energy conservation, gentle stretching, moist heat, ultrasound, posture and body mechanics, biofeedback, and exercise to tolerance. Aquatic therapy is recommended to improve a patient's fitness level and an ergonomic evaluation should be performed at the patient's work place. This population should not work through pain. They require short exercise sessions initially (three to five minutes) due to a low tolerance for exertion.

What home care regimen should be recommended?

A home care regimen should include short duration exercise, aquatic therapy (if indicated), energy conservation strategies, the use of proper positioning, proper body mechanics, and gentle stretching. Patient education is the key to success. Exercises that strain muscles such as weight lifting should be avoided. A comprehensive plan should also include lifestyle management, nutritional support, and stress management.

Outcome:

What is the likely outcome of a course in physical therapy?

A patient with FMS may benefit from multidisciplinary intervention. Patient compliance with a home program increases the overall success rate. In many cases symptoms can remain unchanged even with intervention and patient compliance. A percentage of patients will report improvement in areas of fatigue, sleep, and self-reported pain.

What are the long-term effects of the patient's condition?

FMS is presently not "curable." Many patients that have mild symptoms do not require multidisciplinary intervention and have a good long-term outcome. The majority of patients diagnosed with FMS exhibits moderate levels of symptoms and usually continue to experience these symptoms for years or even their entire lifetime.

Comparison:

What are the distinguishing characteristics of a similar condition?

Myofascial pain syndrome (MPS) is often misdiagnosed for FMS. MPS is characterized by trigger points rather than tender points and lacks associated symptoms. MPS is a localized musculoskeletal condition that is specific to a muscle. FMS on the other hand is a systemic condition. MPS is usually caused by overuse, reduced muscle activity or repetitive motions.

Clinical Scenarios:

Scenario One

A 32-year-old female recently diagnosed with FMS is seen in physical therapy. Her chief complaints are fatigue, pain throughout her body, and difficulty with sleeping which has effected her employment as a mail carrier. She has been on disability for the last six months and under a physician's care for depression.

Scenario Two

A 45-year-old construction worker is referred to physical therapy with diagnosis of FMS. His history reveals mild symptoms for the last year. He has seen specialists and was diagnosed last week by a rheumatologist. He is positive for 12 tender points and denies any sleep disturbances or other medical history. He is currently working and appears motivated for therapy.

Full-Thickness Burn

Diagnosis:

What condition produces a patient's symptoms?

Full-thickness burns can be caused by thermal (fire, hot fluids, steam), chemical (acid, alkalis, vesicants) or electrical (lightning, high voltage, faulty wiring) agents. This severe burn causes immediate cellular and tissue death and subsequent vascular destruction. The patient will experience primary and secondary symptoms secondary to the extent and area of injury.

An injury was most likely sustained to which structure?

A full-thickness burn indicates complete destruction of the epidermis, dermis, hair follicle, and nerve endings within the dermis; and also affects the subcutaneous fat layer and underlying muscles, resulting in red blood cell destruction. There is irreversible damage sustained to all epithelial elements.

Inference:

What is the most likely contributing factor in the development of this condition?

The National Burn Information Exchange indicates that 75% of burns are a direct result of the patient's actions. There are approximately two million individuals burned annually with 70,000 hospitalized and 6,000-7,000 deaths. There is higher risk for burns in children between one and five years of age as well as individuals over 70 years of age. Burns are currently the third leading cause of accidental death in all age categories with males having a higher overall frequency of injury.

Confirmation:

What is the most likely clinical presentation?

A full-thickness burn is characterized by a variable appearance of deep red, black or white coloring. Eschar forms from necrotic cells and creates a dry and hard layer that requires debridement. Edema is present at the site of injury and in surrounding tissues. Hairs within the region of the burn are easily pulled from the follicle due to the destruction. An area of full-thickness burn does not have sensation or pain due to destruction of free nerve endings, however, there may be pain from adjacent areas that experience partial-thickness burns. During the initial stages the patient will experience thermoregulation impairment, shortness of breath, electrolyte disturbances, poor urine output, and variation in level of consciousness.

What laboratory or imaging studies would confirm the diagnosis?

Blood work should include a complete blood count, electrolytes, blood urea nitrogen, creatinine, bilirubin, and arterial blood gases. This will indicate baseline data, systemic changes, level of shock, and metabolic complications. Bronchoscopy and pulmonary function tests may be indicated to assess airway damage and pulmonary insufficiency.

What additional information should be obtained to confirm the diagnosis?

Diagnosis is primarily based on observation and assessment regarding the extent and depth of the burn. The rule of nines and the Lund-Browder charts grossly approximate the percentage of the body affected by a burn.

Examination:

What history should be documented?

Important areas to explore include past medical history, mechanism of injury, medications, family history, type and percentage of burn, current symptoms and health status, social history and habits, occupation, leisure activities, and social support system.

What test/measures are most appropriate?

Aerobic capacity and endurance: assessment of vital signs, perceived exertion scale, pulse oximetry
Anthropometric characteristics: circumferential measurements of affected areas
Arousal, attention, and cognition: examine mental status, learning ability, memory, motivation
Cranial nerve integrity: dermatome assessment
Gait, locomotion, and balance: static and dynamic balance in sitting and standing
Integumentary integrity: sensation assessment, assessment of burn, size, color, eschar, hair follicle integrity, wound mapping
Joint integrity and mobility: assessment of contracture, hypomobility of joints, soft tissue swelling
Muscle performance: strength and tone assessment
Pain: pain perception assessment scale, visual analog scale to the area of the burn and surrounding tissues
Posture: analysis of resting and dynamic posture
Range of motion: active and passive range of motion
Reflex integrity: assessment of deep tendon and pathological reflexes (e.g., Babinski, ATNR)
Self-care and home management: functional capacity, Functional Independence Measure (FIM)
Ventilation, respiration, and circulation: cough and clearance of secretions, auscultation of the lungs, breathing patterns, respiratory muscle strength, accessory muscle utilization, vital capacity, pulse oximetry and palpation, pulmonary function testing

What additional findings are likely with this patient?

A patient with a full-thickness burn will present with multiple secondary effects based on the mechanism of the burn, size of the burn, and location of the burn. Infection, hypertrophic scarring, and contractures are the most common complications. Other secondary damage may include impairments of the cardiovascular system, renal system, gastrointestinal system, respiratory system and/or immune system. Damage to these vital areas can result in metabolic disorders, acidosis, sepsis, and dehydration.

Management:

What is the most effective management of this patient?

The initial management includes medically stabilizing the patient followed by a full assessment of primary and secondary damage. This emergent phase lasts 48-72 hours and concludes with regaining capillary permeability and hemodynamic stability. An autograft procedure is usually required for full-thickness burns. The rehabilitation phase is a long-term commitment that includes all aspects of functional recovery. Physical therapy intervention begins immediately following skin grafting and includes wound care, pulmonary exercises, positioning, splinting, and immobilization for the first three to five days. A therapist will also provide education regarding skin care, positioning, and contracture prevention. Early ambulation and mobility activities should be incorporated as soon as possible in order to decrease complications such as atelectasis, pneumonia, and contracture. Continued physical therapy management will involve edema control, monitoring of any elastic garments, massage, stretching, hydrotherapy, ROM, debridement, relaxation techniques, progressive exercise, ambulation, and functional mobility training.

What home care regimen should be recommended?

A patient must continue with the established splinting and positioning schedule at home. Physical therapy may initially be warranted for continued pulmonary management, stretching, and functional mobility. A home program is vital to the patient's continued success and should include strengthening exercises, massage, scar management, positioning, and stretching. As the patient progresses, participation in wound management, activities of daily living, and functional activities should be incorporated into the daily routine.

Outcome:

What is the likely outcome of a course in physical therapy?

Patient outcome is dependent on location, extent, and secondary complications of the burn. Physical therapy will provide the patient with education for an ongoing therapeutic program. Therapeutic exercise, stretching, compression garments, and other modalities will enhance the probability of a positive outcome.

What are the long-term effects of the patient's condition?

The mortality rate has decreased over the last two decades due to improvement in burn care, prevention of infection, and advances in grafting procedures. Mortality rates are highest for children under four and adults over 65 years of age. Overall prognosis is dependent on factors such as cardiac pathology, alcoholism, peripheral vascular disease, and obesity. Other factors that also require consideration are depression, social and emotional shock, and level of difficulty reintegrating into a daily routine (with employment, spouse, children, community). Long-term outcome is also based on the extent of secondary effects such as scarring and contractures. Garments may be worn up to two years after injury. Without significant complications a patient should achieve independence within a few months post injury.

Comparison:

What are the distinguishing characteristics of a similar condition?

A partial-thickness burn damages the epidermis and the papillary layer of the dermis (the dermis remains largely intact). This burn presents with blister formation, bright red coloring, intact blanching, moderate edema, and pain. The burn will heal without surgical intervention within 14-21 days with minimal to no scarring noted.

Clinical Scenarios:

Scenario One

A 32-year-old female six weeks status post full-thickness burns to 50% of her right arm and 70% of her right leg is referred to physical therapy. She wears compression garments and has decreased range of motion. She resides alone in a two-story home and is employed as a cook.

Scenario Two

A three-year-old boy is referred to physical therapy 48 hours after an autograft for a full-thickness burn on the left side of his thorax. The chart review notes the mechanism of injury as pulling a cup of coffee off a table. Other medical history includes developmental delay, seizures, and hydrocephaly.

Guillain-Barre Syndrome

Diagnosis:

What condition produces a patient's symptoms?

Guillain-Barre syndrome (GBS) or acute polyneuropathy is a temporary inflammation and demyelination of the peripheral nerves' myelin sheaths, potentially resulting in axonal degeneration. GBS results in motor weakness in a distal to proximal progression, sensory impairment, and possible respiratory paralysis.

An injury was most likely sustained to which structure?

The autoantibodies of GBS attack segments of the myelin sheath of the peripheral nerves. The infecting organism is of similar structure to molecules found on the surface of myelin sheaths. The antibodies produced attack both the organism of infection as well as the Schwann cells due to the similar structure. This decreases nerve conduction velocity and results in weakness or paralysis of the involved muscles. The demyelination that is initiated at Ranvier's nodes occurs secondary to macrophage response and inflammation, and as a result, destruction of the myelin. The body responds to this process and attempts to repair the damage through Schwann cell division and myelinization of the damaged nerves. Motor fibers are predominantly affected.

Inference:

What is the most likely contributing factor in the development of this condition?

The exact etiology of GBS is unknown, however, it is hypothesized to be an autoimmune response to a previous respiratory infection, influenza, immunization or surgery. Viral infections, Epstein-Barr syndrome, cytomegalovirus, bacterial infections, surgery, and vaccinations have been associated with the development of GBS.

Confirmation:

What is the most likely clinical presentation?

GBS can occur at any age, however, there is a peak in frequency in the young adult population and again in adults that are between their fifth and eighth decades. Incidence is slightly greater in males than females and in Caucasians than African Americans with an overall incidence of 1.7:100,000 within the United States. A patient with GBS will initially present with distal symmetrical motor weakness and will likely experience mild distal sensory impairments and transient paresthesias. The weakness will progress towards the upper extremities and head. The level of disability usually peaks within two to four weeks after onset. Muscle and respiratory paralysis, absence of deep tendon reflexes, and the inability to speak or swallow may also occur. GBS can be life threatening if there is respiratory involvement. There are multiple subtypes of GBS, but the classic type involves acute onset of symptoms with peak impairment within four weeks, followed by a two to four week static period and gradual recovery that can take months to years.

What laboratory or imaging studies would confirm the diagnosis?

GBS can be diagnosed through a cerebrospinal fluid sample that contains high protein levels and little to no lymphocytes. Electromyography will result in abnormal and slowed nerve conduction.

What additional information should be obtained to confirm the diagnosis?

A physical and neurological examination, strength testing, and a review of relevant medical history are all important in the diagnosis of GBS. The National Institute of Neurologic and Communicative Disorders and Stroke has established criteria to assist with the diagnosis of GBS.

Examination:

What history should be documented?

Important areas to explore include past medical, family, and surgical history, recent illness, medications, immunizations, current symptoms and health status, social history and habits, occupation, living environment, and social support system.

What test/measures are most appropriate?

Aerobic capacity and endurance: vital signs at rest/activity, responses to positional changes

Arousal, attention, and cognition: examine mental status, learning ability, memory, motivation

Assistive and adaptive devices: analysis of components and safety of a device

Cranial nerve integrity: assessment of muscles innervation by the cranial nerves, dermatome assessment

Community and work integration: analysis of community, work, and leisure activities

Gait, locomotion, and balance: static and dynamic balance in sitting and standing, safety during gait with/without an assistive device, Berg Balance Scale, Tinetti Performance Oriented Mobility Assessment, analysis of wheelchair management

Integumentary integrity: skin and sensation assessment

Motor function: equilibrium and righting reactions, coordination, motor assessment scales

Muscle performance: strength and tone assessment

Orthotic, protective, and supportive devices: potential utilization of bracing

Pain: pain perception assessment scale

Range of motion: active and passive range of motion

Reflex integrity: assessment of deep tendon and pathological reflexes

Self-care and home management: assessment of functional capacity

Ventilation, respiration and circulation: pulmonary function tests, assessment of cough and secretions

What additional findings are likely with this patient?

The extent of impairment for each patient depends on the clinical course of the GBS. The patient may also experience bladder weakness, deep muscle pain, and autonomic nervous system involvement including arrhythmia, tachycardia, postural hypotension, heart block, and absent reflexes. Up to 30% of patients require mechanical ventilation during the acute stage. Respiratory assistance can last as long as 50-60 days.

Management:

What is the most effective management of this patient?

Medical management of a patient with GBS may require hospitalization for treatment of symptoms. Pharmacological intervention often includes immunosuppressive and analgesic/narcotic medications. Corticosteroids are controversial and usually contraindicated. Cardiac monitoring, plasma exchange (through plasmapheresis), and mechanical ventilation may be required. A tracheostomy may be performed for ventilation. Physical, occupational, and speech therapies are indicated to facilitate neurological rehabilitation. Physical therapy should be initiated upon admission to the hospital with focus on passive range of motion, positioning, and light exercise. During the acute stage a therapist must limit overexertion and fatigue to avoid exacerbation of symptoms. As the patient progresses, intervention may include orthotic, wheelchair or assistive device prescription, exercise and endurance activities, family teaching, functional mobility and gait training, and progressive respiratory therapy. The therapeutic pool may be indicated to initiate movement without the effects of gravity.

What home-care regimen should be recommended?

A home care regimen should include breathing exercises and incentive spirometry for respiratory involvement. A patient, along with the caregiver, must continue with therapeutic exercise, ongoing functional mobility training, and endurance activities as tolerated.

Outcome:

What is the likely outcome of a course in physical therapy?

Physical therapy may assist with recovery, but it cannot alter the course of the disease. Physical therapy intervention may be required on an ongoing basis to assist with recovery that can last from 3-12 months.

What are the long-term effects of the patient's condition?

GBS is an autoimmune response that varies in severity from person to person. Recovery is slow and can last up to two years after onset. Although most patients experience full recovery, statistics indicate that 20% have remaining neurologic deficits, and 3-5% of patients die from respiratory complications.

Comparison:

What are the distinguishing characteristics of a similar condition?

Polyneuropathy is a progressive condition that affects the nerves. The most common etiology is metabolic conditions such as diabetes mellitus. Polyneuropathy develops slowly, bilaterally, and symmetrically. The first symptom is often sensory impairment of the distal lower extremities. Pain, diminished deep tendon reflexes, and motor loss are other symptoms of this condition that is marked by exacerbations and remissions. Medical management will focus on stabilizing the underlying metabolic condition.

Clinical Scenarios:

Scenario One

A 25-year-old female has been hospitalized for one week with a diagnosis of GBS. The patient's strength assessment reports 3-/5 bilateral hip strength, 2+/5 bilateral knee strength, and 2-/5 bilateral ankle strength. The patient is anxious to improve and is eager to begin physical therapy. The patient resides alone in a second floor apartment and works as a bank teller.

Scenario Two

A 43-year-old male was admitted to the hospital one month ago with GBS. The patient had significant paralysis and was ventilator dependent. The patient began to improve two weeks ago and was taken off the ventilator. The patient was in good health prior to admission and worked as an independent international sales representative. The patient is diabetic and has a history of alcoholism. He is divorced with no children.

Human Immunodeficiency Virus

Diagnosis:

What condition produces a patient's symptoms?

The human immunodeficiency virus (HIV) is a retrovirus that initially invades and destroys cells within the immune system; specifically CD4+ T-lymphocytes (T-cells). This virus also affects monocytes, macrophages, and B-cells. Once the T-cells decrease beyond a specific level a patient will begin to demonstrate symptoms of the HIV infection.

An injury was most likely sustained to which structure?

HIV infects T-cells within the immune system. Other cells that eventually house HIV include monocytes, macrophages, microglia, cervical cells, and epithelial cells of the GI tract. HIV uses and destroys these cells that possess the antigen CD4 on their surface in order to replicate HIV, and as a result the immune system becomes weaker and unable to function.

Inference:

What is the most likely contributing factor in the development of this condition?

HIV is transmitted through contact with blood, semen, vaginal secretions, and breast milk. Contact can be sexual, perinatal or through contact with blood or body fluids that carry infected cells. Risk factors for contracting HIV include unprotected sexual relations, intravenous drug use or mother to fetus transmission. The top three largest risk factors for contracting HIV are homosexual male sex (46% of HIV cases), intravenous drug use (25% of HIV cases), and heterosexual sex (11%).

Confirmation:

What is the most likely clinical presentation?

The incidence of newly diagnosed cases of HIV is approximately 40,000 per year within the United States (decreased from 150,000 new cases yearly during the mid-1980s). A patient will not immediately present with any symptoms after the initial transmission of the infection. A patient may actually be "symptom free" for one to two years post infection or may exhibit flu-like symptoms including rash and fever. HIV immediately begins a latent phase where replication of the virus is minimal. The three phases of this disease process include asymptomatic HIV, symptomatic HIV, and acquired immunodeficiency syndrome (AIDS). The T-cell count will begin to decrease during the "asymptomatic" phase, however, symptoms will not appear until the count decreases to a certain level. Manifestations of HIV may lead to other infections, malignancies, neurological dysfunction, dementia, and cardiac pathologies.

What laboratory or imaging studies would confirm the diagnosis?

HIV is diagnosed through various blood tests such as the enzyme-linked immunosorbent test or Western blot test. Once diagnosed the lab results can also assist with classifying the stage of HIV infection.

What additional information should be obtained to confirm the diagnosis?

Definitive diagnosis is made through blood tests, however, the physician should ascertain accurate medical and social history. Accurate drug use and sexual partner history will allow for appropriate patient education in order to cease the spread of the virus. A positive diagnosis will allow the patient to notify others at risk.

Examination:

What history should be documented?

Important areas to explore include past medical history, medications, family history, current symptoms, current health status, social history and habits, occupation, leisure activities, and social support system.

What test/measures are most appropriate?

Aerobic capacity and endurance: assessment of vital signs, perceived exertion scale, auscultation of the lungs

Arousal, attention, and cognition: examine mental status, learning ability, memory, and level of motivation

Community and work integration: analysis of community, work, and leisure activities

Environmental, home, and work barriers: analysis of current and potential barriers or hazards

Gait, locomotion, and balance: static and dynamic balance in sitting and standing, safety during gait with/without an assistive device, Tinetti Performance Oriented Mobility Assessment, analysis of wheelchair management

Integumentary integrity: skin assessment and sensation assessment

Motor function: equilibrium and righting reactions, motor assessment scales, coordination, posture and balance in sitting, assessment of sensorimotor integration, physical performance scales

Muscle performance: strength assessment, muscle tone assessment

Pain: pain perception assessment scale

Range of motion: active and passive range of motion

Reflex integrity: assessment of deep tendon and pathological reflexes (e.g., Babinski, ATNR)

Self-care and home management: assessment of functional capacity

Ventilation, respiration, and circulation: pulmonary function testing, breathing patterns, perceived exertion scale, assessment of cough

What additional findings are likely with this patient?

The Centers for Disease Control classifies HIV into three categories based on the T-cell count. Symptoms and secondary illnesses occur as the T-cell count decreases. The onset of AIDS occurs when the T-cell count falls below 200 cells per mm3 (normal ranges 650-1,200 cells) or when one of 26 specific AIDS defining disorders is present or both. A patient may experience musculoskeletal, neuromuscular, cardiopulmonary, integumentary, and other impairments secondary to HIV.

Management:

What is the most effective management of this patient?

Early detection is important so that pharmacological intervention can be initiated and slow progression of the virus. There is no cure for HIV, however, proper medical intervention can allow this virus to remain a manageable chronic condition. Medical management will institute antiretroviral therapy (HAART) when T-cells drop below 500 mm3. The goal of drug therapy is to significantly decrease the virus' ability to replicate, and therefore, decrease the progression of the disease. Drugs may include nucleoside analogs, protease inhibitors, and non-nucleoside reverse transcriptase inhibitors. Physical therapy intervention may be indicated during the course of HIV/AIDS due to secondary impairments. Physical therapy goals and intervention would include the promotion of optimal fitness, flexibility, energy conservation, stress management, ADL equipment, relaxation, aquatic therapy, modalities, positioning, pain management, breathing exercises, and neurological rehabilitation.

What home care regimen should be recommended?

A patient with HIV must follow a home regimen including medication, proper nutrition and sleep, and fitness in order to remain as healthy as possible. A physical therapy home program can also minimize the negative effects on functional ability and improve the overall independence and quality of life.

Outcome:

What is the likely outcome of a course in physical therapy?

Physical therapy may be warranted for periods of time throughout the progression of HIV/AIDS. Physical therapy cannot alter the progression of the virus, but can foster improvement in functional mobility, conditioning, and overall independence.

What are the long-term effects of the patient's condition?

There are currently 42 million individuals around the world living with HIV/AIDS. There is presently no cure for HIV/AIDS, however, with early combination therapies patients are surviving longer and living more productive lives. Studies indicate that psychosocial factors influence progression of the virus as well as survival. Presently, the leading cause of death is kidney failure secondary to the extended drug therapies.

Comparison:

What are the distinguishing characteristics of a similar condition?

Hepatitis B (HBV) is a form of viral hepatitis that produces inflammation and damage to the liver. Like HIV, hepatitis B is transmitted parenterally through intravenous drug use, sexual relations, blood transfusions, perinatal transmission or dialysis. A vaccine is available for prevention and blood tests are used for diagnosis. Approximately 95% of those infected with HBV fully recover, however, 10% of these become carriers. Some of the carriers develop chronic liver disease and may die prematurely.

Clinical Scenarios:

Scenario One

A 19-year-old female is seen in outpatient physical therapy secondary to weakness and balance impairments. She was diagnosed with HIV two years ago but the physician believes that she was infected at least one to two years prior to diagnosis by IV drug use. Her T-cell count is 404 mm3 using HIV drug therapies.

Scenario Two

A 58-year-old male was diagnosed with AIDS one year ago and has lost significant weight. He presents with general muscle atrophy and is having difficulty with ambulation and ADLs. The patient is referred to physical therapy for adaptive and assistive devices. He lives with his partner in a ranch style home and is on medical disability.

Huntington's Disease

Diagnosis:

What condition produces a patient's symptoms?

Huntington's disease (HD), also known as Huntington's chorea, is a neurological disorder of the CNS and is characterized by degeneration and atrophy of the basal ganglia (specifically the striatum) and cerebral cortex within the brain.

An injury was most likely sustained to which structure?

HD affects the basal ganglia and cerebral cortex of the brain. The ventricles of the brain become enlarged secondary to atrophy of the basal ganglia and there is extensive loss of small and medium sized neurons. There appears to be an overall decrease in the quantity and activity of gamma-aminobutyric acid (GABA) and acetylcholine neurons that are produced in these areas. The identified neurotransmitters become deficient and are unable to modulate movement. Loss of neurons creates dysfunction in inhibition that results in the symptoms of chorea, bradykinesia, and rigidity. The thalamus is also believed to contribute to the movement disorders associated with the disease process.

Inference:

What is the most likely contributing factor in the development of this condition?

HD is genetically transmitted as an autosomal dominant trait with the defect linked to chromosome four and to the gene identified as IT-15. The disease is usually perpetuated by a person that has children prior to the normal onset of symptoms and without knowledge that he/she possesses the defective gene. Genetic testing is able to identify the defective gene for HD prior to the onset of symptoms.

Confirmation:

What is the most likely clinical presentation?

The prevalence of HD is approximately 4-8:100,000 in North America with 25,000 individuals diagnosed with HD in the United States. The average age for developing symptoms ranges between 35 and 55 years, however, symptoms can develop at any age. HD is a disease that produces a movement disorder, affective dysfunction, and cognitive impairment. The patient will initially present with involuntary choreic movements and a mild alteration in personality. Unintentional facial expressions such as a grimace, protrusion of the tongue, and elevation of the eyebrows are common. As the disease progresses gait will become ataxic and a patient will experience choreoathetoid movement of the extremities and the trunk. Speech disturbances and mental deterioration are common. Late stage HD is characterized by a decrease in IQ, dementia, depression, dysphagia, incontinence, inability to ambulate or transfer, and progression from choreiform movements to rigidity.

What laboratory or imaging studies would confirm the diagnosis?

Magnetic resonance imaging (MRI) or computed tomography (CT scan) may indicate atrophy or abnormalities within the cerebral cortex as well as the basal ganglia. Positron-emission tomography (PET) may be used to augment other testing and obtain information regarding blood flow, oxygen uptake, and metabolism of the brain. A DNA marker study may be administered to determine if the autosomal dominant trait is present for HD.

What additional information should be obtained to confirm the diagnosis?

A physical examination, review of symptoms, and family history are important components in the diagnosis of HD.

Examination:

What history should be documented?

Important areas to explore include past medical history, medications, family history, current symptoms, health status, social history/habits, occupation, living environment, and social support system.

What test/measures are most appropriate?

Aerobic capacity and endurance: assessment of vital signs at rest and with activity

Arousal, attention, and cognition: examine mental status, learning ability, memory, motivation

Gait, locomotion, and balance: static/dynamic balance in sitting/standing, safety during gait, Functional Reach Test, Tinetti Performance Oriented Mobility Assessment, Functional Ambulation Profile

Motor function: equilibrium/righting reactions, coordination

Muscle performance: strength and tone assessment, tremor assessment, testing for dysdiadochokinesia

Neuromotor development and sensory integration: analysis of reflex movement patterns, assessment of involuntary movements

Posture: analysis of resting and dynamic posture

Range of motion: active and passive range of motion

Self-care and home management: assessment of functional capacity, Functional Independence Measure (FIM), Barthel Index

What additional findings are likely with this patient?

Dementia and other psychological changes usually occur after neurological symptoms appear. The emotional disorder worsens with progression and may require admission to a psychiatric facility for severe depression and/or suicidal attempts. Secondary complications that can occur from symptoms of HD include loss of range of motion, deformity, pain, communication breakdown, aspiration and choking, and fatigue and weakness from weight loss.

Management:

What is the most effective management of this patient?

Medical management of HD requires a team approach including genetic, psychological, and social counseling for the patient and family. Education regarding disease process, coping strategies, and genetic consequences should initiate immediately following diagnosis. Medical treatment will focus on symptoms and pharmacological management for HD is usually initiated once choreiform movement impairs a patient's functional capacity. Drug classes such as anticonvulsants and antipsychotics may assist as these block dopamine transmission, however, have very serious side effects. Commonly utilized drugs include Perphenazine, Haloperidol (Haldol), and Reserpine. Physical, occupational, and speech therapy interventions may be warranted intermittently throughout the course of the disease and should focus on current problems with mobility and self-care skills. Physical therapy should maximize endurance, strength, balance, postural control, and functional mobility. Intervention should focus on motor control and utilize techniques including coactivation of muscles, trunk stabilization, the use of biofeedback, and relaxation in attempt to maintain a patient's functional status. Patient education should include prone lying, stretching, prevention of deformity and contracture, and safety with mobility. As the disease progresses, the degree of dementia will influence treatment and goals. The therapist must continue to emphasize family involvement and caregiver teaching. As the patient continues to lose function the caregiver will require education regarding posture, seating, assistance with transfers, mobility, and the use of adaptive equipment.

What home care regimen should be recommended?

A home care regimen should include an exercise routine, functional mobility skills, relaxation techniques, range of motion, stretching exercises, and endurance activities. Participation in a home care regimen can assist to maintain the optimal quality of life during the progression of the disease process.

Outcome:

What is the likely outcome of a course in physical therapy?

Physical therapy is recommended on an intermittent basis throughout the course of the disease. Physical therapy will not prevent further degeneration, however, it will maximize the patient's functional potential and safety. The goal of physical therapy is to attain an optimal functional outcome within the limitations of the disease process.

What are the long-term effects of the patient's condition?

HD is a chronic progressive genetic disorder that is fatal within 15 to 20 years after clinical manifestation. Late stages of the disease result in total physical and mental incapacitation. The patient usually requires an extended care facility due to the burden of care and physical, cognitive, and emotional dysfunction.

Comparison:

What are the distinguishing characteristics of a similar condition?

Athetoid (dyskinetic) cerebral palsy is a non-progressive motor disorder caused by central nervous system damage specifically to the basal ganglia. Clinical manifestations include slow and involuntary movements, choreiform movements, severe dysarthria, and an increased risk of aspiration pneumonia. The involuntary movements will increase with stress and fatigue and subside with sleep. Physical therapy intervention should focus on motor control and mobility deficits in order to attain the highest level of functioning.

Clinical Scenarios:

Scenario One

A 48-year-old attorney is referred for physical therapy home services. The patient was diagnosed with HD two years ago and resides in a two-story home. The patient has a significant other and they reside together. The patient's primary complaint is a loss of balance while ambulating. The patient refuses to utilize an assistive device.

Scenario Two

A 45-year-old female is referred to physical therapy. She was diagnosed with HD seven years ago and has recently fallen multiple times. According to family members the patient is short-tempered, irritable, and occasionally demonstrates poor judgment. The physician requests physical therapy for an evaluation and home program.

Juvenile Rheumatoid Arthritis

Diagnosis:

What condition produces a patient's symptoms?

Juvenile rheumatoid arthritis (JRA) is a form of arthritis found in children less than 16 years of age. JRA causes inflammation and stiffness to multiple joints for a period of greater than six weeks. The inflammatory process affects the tissues surrounding the affected synovial joints causing symptoms of JRA.

An injury was most likely sustained to which structure?

JRA, like adult rheumatoid arthritis, is an autoimmune disorder that occurs when the immune cells mistakenly begin to attack the joints and organs causing local and systemic effects throughout the body. The severity of ongoing injury is based on the specific classification and subtype of the disease.

Inference:

What is the most likely contributing factor in the development of this condition?

The etiology for JRA is currently unknown. Research postulates that JRA develops in children with a genetic predisposition for the disease. The predisposition may be triggered by environmental factors or a viral or bacterial infection. Girls have a higher incidence of JRA and it is found to begin most commonly in the toddler or adolescent.

Confirmation:

What is the most likely clinical presentation?

JRA is an umbrella term for three specific classifications and subtypes of childhood arthritis. Classification is based on the number of joints involved, symptoms, presence of the rheumatoid factor (RF) or antinuclear antibody (ANA), and systemic involvement. General symptoms include persistent joint swelling, pain, and stiffness. Pauciarticular JRA involves four or less joints, is asymmetric, and is usually a mild form of JRA. This is the most common form of JRA and accounts for 50% of the cases, with girls under eight most likely to develop this subtype. ANA can also be found in 20-30% of patients and correlates with eye disease. Polyarticular JRA involves more than four joints, is usually symmetrical, involves the joints of the hands and feet as well as larger joints, and has potential for severe destruction. This subtype accounts for 30-40% of the cases and children may have the IgM rheumatoid factor (RF) similar to adult RA. Systemic JRA accounts for 10-20% of the cases and is otherwise known as Still's disease. Onset includes a high fever, chills, and a rash that may last for weeks, followed by severe myalgia and polyarthritis. This form presents with severe extraarticular manifestations including anemia, hepatosplenomegaly, lymphadenopathy, pericarditis, and myocarditis. Most children in this subtype are negative for RF or ANA antibodies. About 25% experience severe and unremitting arthritis.

What laboratory or imaging studies would confirm the diagnosis?

There is not a single test to identify the presence of JRA. Blood tests may include serum evaluation to measure inflammation and detect RF, ANA or HLAB27 (human leukocyte antigen). Only a small percentage of patients with JRA possess RF or ANA. An erythrocyte sedimentation rate (ESR or "sed rate") may also indicate rheumatic disease. Other tests or procedures may be used to rule out other conditions such as Lyme disease, lupus, infection, and cancers.

What additional information should be obtained to confirm the diagnosis?

Diagnosis is made largely through physical examination, a patient's past and present medical status, and meeting the criteria set forth by the American Rheumatoid Association regarding the diagnosis and classification of JRA.

Examination:

What history should be documented?

Important areas to explore include past medical history, medications, family history, current symptoms, current health status, social history and habits, leisure activities, and social support system.

What test/measures are most appropriate?

Aerobic capacity and endurance: vital signs at rest and with activity, timed walk, aerobic endurance, VO2 max

Anthropometric characteristics: circumferential measurements of all affected joints

Arousal, attention, and cognition: examine mental status, learning ability, memory, motivation

Assistive and adaptive devices: analysis of components and safety of a device

Environmental and home barriers: analysis of current and potential barriers or hazards

Ergonomics and body mechanics: analysis of dexterity and coordination

Gait, locomotion, and balance: static/dynamic balance in sitting and standing, visual inspection of gait with and without shoes, timed walk, gait over level and unlevel surfaces, footprint analysis and videography

Integumentary integrity: skin and sensation assessment

Joint integrity and mobility: active joint count, joint effusion, articular tenderness

Motor function: equilibrium and coordination

Muscle performance: break testing of isometric contractions, manometer method of strength testing, dynamic muscle strength using repetition maximum (only if pain free)

Neuromotor development and sensory integration: analysis of reflex movement patterns, assessment of involuntary movements, sensory integration tests, gross and fine motor skills
Orthotic, protective, and supportive devices: analysis of components and movement using a device
Pain: Pediatric Pain Questionnaire (PPQ), visual analog scale
Posture: analysis of resting and dynamic posture, scoliosis screening
Range of motion: active/passive range of motion for extremities, active motion only for cervical spine, angular deformities and joint play assessments
Self-care and home management: Pediatric Evaluation of Disability Inventory (PEDI), Child Health Assessment Questionnaire (CHAQ), Juvenile Arthritis Functional Status Index (JASI)

What additional findings are likely with this patient?

Potential complications are dependent on the subtype of JRA and the presence (or absence) of RF or ANA. Joint swelling, stiffness, and pain are the most common symptoms. Eye inflammation and development of iritis/uveitis can be a significant complication. Some patients have periods of exacerbations and remissions while other patient's symptoms will persist.

Management:

What is the most effective management of this patient?

A pediatric rheumatologist is ideal to direct a multidisciplinary team in the complex care of JRA. Primary goals of treatment are to maintain a high level of physical functioning and quality of life. Pharmacological intervention may include NSAIDS, immunosuppressive medications, disease-modifying antirheumatic drugs, and corticosteroids. Physical therapy intervention is a key component and should include range of motion, exercise, and pain control. Functional mobility, strengthening, endurance, and aerobic training will assist a patient in overall function. Range of motion exercises, modalities, splints and orthotics, patient/family education, and the integration of recreational activities should optimize the quality of life. Surgical intervention is sometimes warranted for severe contractures or irreversible joint destruction. Soft tissue release, supracondylar osteotomy, and arthroplasty are the most common surgical procedures.

What home care regimen should be recommended?

A home care regimen should provide an individualized exercise program. The program should be simple and take no more than 20 minutes to complete in order to optimize compliance. Swimming is also a beneficial activity for a child with JRA.

Outcome:

What is the likely outcome of a course in physical therapy?

Physical therapy may be indicated periodically throughout a patient's childhood based on symptoms and complications. Ongoing education and revision of a home program is vital to promote patient compliance. Physical therapy outcome is variable depending on the severity of the patient's symptoms.

What are the long-term effects of the patient's condition?

Long-term effects of JRA are dependent on subtype, symptoms, and any complications encountered. Some patients "outgrow" JRA and are not affected as adults while others experience pain and other manifestations of the disease on a consistent and long-term basis.

Comparison:

What are the distinguishing characteristics of a similar condition?

Infectious bacterial arthritis most often develops within a joint secondary to systemic corticosteroid use, trauma, HIV or alcohol/drug abuse. If treated immediately, long-term prognosis is good. If left uncontrolled, toxemia and septicemia can be fatal. Inflammation and pannus within the synovium erodes articular cartilage. There is an acute onset of swelling, tenderness, and loss of range of motion. A child will usually not bear weight through the involved joint.

Clinical Scenarios:

Scenario One

A 12-year-old boy diagnosed with systemic JRA is seen in physical therapy two days status post soft tissue release of the bilateral heel cords. The patient primarily uses a wheelchair for mobility.

Scenario Two

A six-year-old girl is seen in physical therapy shortly after diagnosis of pauciarticular JRA two months ago. The patient's primary complaint is pain in the right ankle with any weight bearing activity. The patient enjoys playing outside and participates in soccer in the fall.

Lateral Epicondylitis

Diagnosis:

What condition produces a patient's symptoms?

Lateral epicondylitis (tennis elbow) is characterized by inflammation or degenerative changes at the common extensor tendon that attaches to the lateral epicondyle of the elbow. The primary symptom of this condition is pain.

An injury was most likely sustained to which structure?

Repeated overuse of the wrist extensors, particularly the extensor carpi radialis brevis can produce tensile stress and result in microscopic tearing and damage to the extensor tendon. Other muscles that can be affected include the extensor digitorum, extensor carpi radialis longus, and extensor carpi ulnaris.

Inference:

What is the most likely contributing factor in the development of this condition?

The exact etiology is uncertain, however, repetitive wrist action against resistance during extension and supination appear to produce this condition. Over time inflammation of the periosteum may develop with formation of adhesions. The continued microtrauma does not allow for proper healing and will continue to injure the tissues. This pattern is best seen while hitting a backhand in tennis, however, overuse with painting, hand tools, gardening, and any repeated activity that involves forceful wrist extension can result in lateral epicondylitis. Men are more likely to develop lateral epicondylitis and it is also more common for individuals in their late 30's and 40's secondary to the normal loss of the extensibility of connective tissue with age.

Confirmation:

What is the most likely clinical presentation?

A typical patient with lateral epicondylitis is usually between the third and fifth decades of life and has unilateral involvement of the elbow. Lateral epicondylitis presents with pain along the lateral aspect of the elbow especially over the lateral epicondyle that sometimes radiates into the dorsum of the hand. The pain will increase with wrist flexion with elbow extension, resisted wrist extension, and resisted radial deviation. The patient may also have difficulty holding or gripping objects and insufficient forearm functional strength. Range of motion of the elbow usually remains normal, however, may be limited in severe cases. The patient will have localized tenderness over the lateral epicondyle and may present with localized swelling. The pain usually increases with activity and is noted at night.

What laboratory or imaging studies would confirm the diagnosis?

No lab or imaging studies are required to diagnose lateral epicondylitis. X-ray or MRI may be used to rule out other conditions. Electrodiagnostic tests are only beneficial if there is radial nerve involvement.

What additional information should be obtained to confirm the diagnosis?

Lateral epicondylitis is usually diagnosed based on history, physical examination of the extremity, and several manual maneuvers that specifically identify the presence of lateral epicondylitis. An increase in pain at the lateral epicondyle with resisted wrist extension confirms the pathology of the extensor carpi radialis brevis.

Examination:

What history should be documented?

Important areas to explore include past medical history, medications, family history, current symptoms, current health status, social history and habits, occupation, leisure and sport activities, and social support system.

What test/measures are most appropriate?

Anthropometric characteristics: circumferential measurements of the forearm
Arousal, attention, and cognition: examine mental status, learning ability, memory, motivation
Community and work integration: analysis of community, work, and leisure activities
Environmental, home, and work barriers: analysis of current and potential barriers or hazards
Integumentary integrity: skin assessment, assessment of sensation
Joint integrity and mobility: assessment of hyper- and hypomobility of a joint, soft tissue swelling and inflammation, quality of movement of the elbow complex, provocative tests for lateral epicondylitis including Cozen's/ test 1, Mills/test 2, Tennis Elbow test
Muscle performance: strength assessment, muscle tone assessment, grip test dynamometer
Orthotic, protective, and supportive devices: potential utilization of bracing, splinting
Pain: pain perception assessment scale, visual analog scale, assessment of muscle soreness
Posture: analysis of resting and dynamic posture
Range of motion: active and passive range of motion of bilateral upper extremities
Reflex integrity: assessment of deep tendon reflexes
Self-care and home management: assessment of functional capacity

What additional findings are likely with this patient?

If the patient is involved in tennis or some other potential overuse activity there should be remediation and modification in training, technique, and equipment to minimize the chance of recurrence.

Management:

What is the most effective management of this patient?

Medical management initially treats the pain and inflammation through protection, rest, ice, compression, and elevation. During the initial phase the patient should avoid all activities that aggravate the injury. Pharmacological intervention should include NSAIDs to alleviate pain and inflammation. Modalities may also be used such as phonophoresis with hydrocortisone or iontophoresis with dexamethasone. On occasion, resting splints may be used during the acute stage to relieve tension of the involved muscles. Physical therapy intervention should initiate stretching and strengthening to improve flexibility and increase functional activities. All exercise must remain pain free. Other modalities including electrical stimulation and cryotherapy may be beneficial. Strengthening should include elbow, wrist, and hand exercises. As a patient progresses resistive, isokinetic, and sport-specific exercises should be introduced. Counter-force bracing in the form of a forearm band may be indicated to reduce the degree of tension in the region of the muscular attachment. A patient should wean from the brace, prior to the completion of rehabilitation so the patient does not depend on it or use it as a replacement for rehabilitation.

What home care regimen should be recommended?

A home care regimen should include the same therapeutic program the patient performs during physical therapy. Patient education should include modification of all activities that exacerbate the symptoms. It is imperative that the patient not rush or advance beyond the parameters of the home program as it will exacerbate the condition. A patient must avoid all activities that produce pain and use ice, elevation, and rest as needed.

Outcome:

What is the likely outcome of a course in physical therapy?

Physical therapy may be indicated for one to three months with goals of regaining appropriate strength, flexibility, and endurance while reducing inflammation and pain of the involved muscles. Overall outcome is favorable and a patient should be able to return to all previous functional activities without restrictions.

What are the long-term effects of the patient's condition?

Lateral epicondylitis will commonly recur, however, continued stretching and exercise will decrease the risk of future recurrence. If conservative treatment does not improve symptoms after two to three months surgical intervention may be indicated.

Comparison:

What are the distinguishing characteristics of a similar condition?

Medial epicondylitis (golfer's or swimmer's elbow) results from repeated microtrauma to the flexor carpi radialis and/or the humeral head of the pronator teres during pronation and wrist flexion. There is pain with resisted wrist flexion and resisted pronation and point tenderness over the medial epicondyle. Treatment is similar in protocol to lateral epicondylitis, however, is directed at the appropriate location. Complete immobilization is never recommended, however, counter-force bracing or splinting may be indicated.

Clinical Scenarios:

Scenario One

A 27-year-old tennis player is seen in physical therapy diagnosed with right lateral epicondylitis. The patient plays in a competitive league and recently changed his instructor and increased the number of games played per week. He complains of pain and point tenderness over the lateral epicondyle. He is very frustrated, as this pain has had a large impact on his ability to win games.

Scenario Two

A 42-year-old female diagnosed with right lateral epicondylitis has been seen in physical therapy for four weeks. She has a past medical history that includes reflex sympathetic dystrophy two years ago in the right upper extremity and status post hysterectomy three months ago. She has not had any relief of pain and states that she cannot hold anything in her right hand. She enjoys gardening and works at a vegetable farm, but does not want to decrease any of her current activities.

Lymphedema Post-Mastectomy

Diagnosis:

What condition produces a patient's symptoms?

Lymphedema following a mastectomy is termed secondary lymphedema and is the result of damage to the lymphatic nodes and vessels during surgery. Excessive accumulation of lymph fluid within the soft tissues is caused by an excess load of lymph fluid or inadequate transport capacity within the lymphatic system secondary to the loss of homeostasis.

An injury was most likely sustained to which structure?

The lymphatic system is damaged as a result of the mastectomy, the surgical removal of the breast, whereby the lymphatic nodes and vessels are removed or damaged. The lymph system is unable to compensate, the lymph vessels dilate, and the valve flaps are not able to fully stop lymph flow. This allows for backflow of lymph into the tissues. This chain reaction causes further injury, chronic inflammation and progression including fibrosis, hypoxia within the tissues, and an increase risk of infection.

Inference:

What is the most likely contributing factor in the development of this condition?

The most likely contributing factor in the development of lymphedema following a mastectomy is the damage and/or removal of the axillary lymph nodes and vessels in an attempt to prevent the spread of breast cancer. If the lymphatic nodes have not been removed but have received radiation they may stop functioning due to chronic inflammation, fibrosis, and scarring. Globally, the parasitic infection called filariasis is the most common cause of secondary lymphedema. The virus is carried by mosquitoes in regions such as Africa, India, and Malaysia. Other causes include severe infection, crush injuries, burns or repeated pregnancies. There are an estimated three million new cases of secondary lymphedema each year with approximately 30% of breast cancer survivors affected by this condition. Primary lymphedema statistics indicate 15% of cases present at birth and 75% of the cases are acquired from adolescence through midlife years. Females are affected more than males with a 4:1 ratio.

Confirmation:

What is the most likely clinical presentation?

The clinical presentation of lymphedema includes edema in an affected area/extremity that increases with dependent positioning. The patient usually does not experience pain but rather a tight or heavy sensation. Lymphedema is classified into three stages that present differently based on the severity of the condition. Stage I is characterized by pitting edema that reduces with elevation overnight and does not exhibit any fibrotic changes. Stage II is identified by some fibrotic changes that begin to occur and increase in non-pitting edema that does not reduce with elevation. Stage III is characterized with skin changes, frequent infections, and severe edema that is non-pitting and fibrotic.

What laboratory or imaging studies would confirm the diagnosis?

Diagnosis is confirmed through history, observation, and several diagnostic tools to rule out other potential disorders. A Doppler study of the affected area is able to rule out a deep vein thrombosis. A CT scan or MRI may be performed before treatment of lymphedema is initiated to rule out malignancy. A lymphoscintigram is a nuclear medicine procedure that tests the function of the lymphatic system.

What additional information should be obtained to confirm the diagnosis?

A medical evaluation should include a thorough history including all illnesses, hospitalizations, and surgeries. History should be noted regarding the current edema and its course. Date of onset, progression, and symptoms associated with the edema are important to attain and note in the patient's record.

Examination:

What history should be documented?

Important areas to explore include past medical history and surgical history, medications, history of swelling, family history, current symptoms, current health status, living environment, social history and habits, occupation, and social support system.

What test/measures are most appropriate?

Aerobic capacity and endurance: assessment of vital signs at rest and with activity, perceived exertion scale, pulse oximetry, auscultation of the lungs

Anthropometric characteristics: circumferential and volumetric measurements of involved areas, skinfold measurements

Arousal, attention, and cognition: examine mental status, learning ability, memory, motivation

Community and work integration: analysis of community, work, and leisure activities

Environmental, home, and work barriers: analysis of current and potential barriers or hazards

Gait, locomotion, and balance: static and dynamic balance in sitting and standing, safety during gait with/ without an assistive device

Integumentary integrity: skin assessment, assessment of sensation, nailbed assessment

Joint integrity and mobility: soft tissue swelling and inflammation

Muscle performance: strength and tone assessment

Pain: pain perception assessment scale
Range of motion: active and passive range of motion
Self-care and home management: assessment of functional capacity
Ventilation, respiration, and circulation: assessment of brachial and radial pulses, capillary refill assessment

What additional findings are likely with this patient?

Additional findings are based on the etiology, stage, and progression of the lymphedema. Complications can include ulcer formation, increased risk for fungal and bacterial infections, loss of range, fatigue, and fibrotic edema with atrophic skin changes. If left untreated a patient could progress to stage III "lymphostatic elephantiasis."

Management:

What is the most effective management of this patient?

Effective medical management of secondary lymphedema may involve pharmacological intervention or natural substances that increase proteolysis and macrophage activity, however, there is no particular class of drugs that can "cure" lymphedema. Surgery is used in the treatment of severe lymphedema but only achieves limited results since the cause remains unchanged. Physical therapy intervention usually follows a treatment approach termed combined decongestive physiotherapy (CDP). The philosophy of lymphatic management includes patient education in skin care, hygiene, bandaging, self-massage, and exercise. Therapeutic intervention should focus on manual lymph drainage, short stretch compression bandages, retrograde massage, exercise, compression therapy, and use of a mechanical pump. Care must be taken, however, not to exceed 45 mm Hg during compression therapy since a greater pressure can damage or collapse the lymphatic walls.

What home care regimen should be recommended?

A home care regimen is vital to the success of the CDP treatment of lymphedema. A patient must understand and comply with skin care, bandaging, self-massage, lymphatic drainage techniques, compression therapy, and an exercise program. Each patient must also understand the lifetime precautions that can increase lymphedema such as sunburn, air travel, excessive exercise, poor nutrition, and obesity.

Outcome:

What is the likely outcome of a course in physical therapy?

Comprehensive lymphedema intervention such as CDP has shown significant reduction in lymphedema during treatment and continued reduction with an ongoing home program over time.

What are the long-term effects of the patient's condition?

Lymphedema is progressive if left untreated but can be managed through intervention and education. Patients must comply with a home program and must remain aware of all activities that place the patient at an increased risk for lymphedema.

Comparison:

What are the distinguishing characteristics of a similar condition?

Lipedema is a condition where there appears to be swelling throughout the bilateral lower extremities from the hips to the ankle joints. This swelling is actually subcutaneous adipose tissue. This condition is sometimes confused with lymphedema but does not affect the lymphatic system. It most often occurs in women with hormonal disorders and is believed to have a family history in approximately 20% of the cases. Medical management treats the hormonal imbalance and assists with nutritional guidance to allow for effective weight management.

Clinical Scenarios:

Scenario One

A 39-year-old female post right mastectomy secondary to malignancy develops lymphedema in her right arm four months after surgery. She resides alone and is employed as a web design consultant. She complains of heaviness in the arm, but denies pain. She was referred by her oncologist for outpatient physical therapy.

Scenario Two

A 68-year-old male is seen in physical therapy with stage II lymphedema in his right lower extremity. He underwent a total hip replacement two months ago and states immediate swelling and discomfort. His history includes multiple abdominal surgeries with edema present after each surgery. He presents with non-pitting edema that does not reduce with elevation.

Medial Collateral Ligament Sprain – Grade II

Diagnosis:

What condition produces a patient's symptoms?

The medial collateral ligament (MCL) connects the medial epicondyle of the femur to the medial tibia and as a result resists medially directed force at the knee. The MCL is the primary stabilizer of the medial side of the knee against valgus force and lateral rotation of the tibia (especially during knee flexion). This extra-articular ligament is a thick and flat band which attaches proximally on the medial femoral condyle and extends to the medial surface of the tibia approximately six centimeters below the joint line. A common mechanism of injury is a direct blow against the lateral surface of the knee causing valgus stress and subsequent damage to the medial aspect of the knee.

An injury was most likely sustained to which structure?

The medial collateral ligament is comprised of two parts. A deep part of the ligament attaches to the cartilage meniscus and the superficial part attaches further down the joint. A grade II injury of the MCL is characterized by partial tearing of the ligament's fibers resulting in joint laxity when the ligament is stretched. Often the medial capsular ligament is involved in a grade II sprain of the MCL.

Inference:

What is the most likely contributing factor in the development of this condition?

Individuals participating in contact activities requiring a high level of agility are particularly susceptible to a MCL injury. Mechanism of injury is usually a blow to the outside of the knee joint causing excess force to the medial side of the joint. The MCL can also be injured by a twisting of the knee. Muscle weakness resulting in poor dynamic stabilization may also increase the incidence of this type of injury.

Confirmation:

What is the most likely clinical presentation?

A patient with a grade II MCL injury will likely present with an inability to fully extend and flex the knee, pain and significant tenderness along the medial aspect of the knee, possible decrease in strength, potential loss of proprioception, and an antalgic gait. There is typically discernable laxity with valgus testing, instability of the joint, and slight to moderate swelling around the knee. More severe swelling may be indicative of meniscus or cruciate ligament involvement.

What laboratory or imaging studies would confirm the diagnosis?

MRI is a non-invasive imaging technique that can be utilized to view soft tissue structures such as ligaments. The imaging technique is extremely expensive and therefore m[...] commonly employed on an individual with a susp[...]ed injury without other extenuating circumstances.

What additional information should be obtained to confirm the diagnosis?

A valgus stress test is a technique designed to detect medial instability in a single plane. The examiner applies a valgus stress at the knee while stabilizing the ankle in slight lateral rotation. The test is often performed initially in full extension and then in 30 degrees of flexion. A patient with a grade II MCL sprain may exhibit 5-15 degrees of laxity with valgus stress at 30 degrees of flexion.

Examination:

What history should be documented?

Important areas to explore include mechanism of present injury, current symptoms, past medical history, medications, living environment, occupation, social history and habits, and social support system.

What test/measures are most appropriate?

Anthropometric characteristics: palpation to determine knee effusion, lower extremity circumferential measurements

Arousal, attention, and cognition: examine mental status, learning ability, memory, motivation

Assistive and adaptive devices: analysis of components and safety of a device, potential utilization of crutches

Community and work integration: analysis of community, work, and leisure activities

Environmental, home, and work barriers: analysis of current and potential barriers or hazards

Gait, locomotion, and balance: safety during gait with an assistive device

Integumentary integrity: assessment of sensation (pain, temperature, tactile), skin assessment

Joint integrity and mobility: special tests for ligaments and menisci, valgus stress test, palpation of structures, joint play, soft tissue restrictions, joint pain

Muscle performance: strength assessment, assessment of active movement, resisted isometrics, muscle contraction characteristics, muscle endurance

Orthotic, protective, and supportive devices: potential utilization of bracing, taping or wrapping

Pain: pain perception assessment scale, visual analog scale

Range of motion: active and passive range of motion

Self-care and home management: assessment of functional capacity

Sensory integrity: assessment of proprioception and kinesthesia

What additional findings are likely with this patient?

Anterior cruciate ligament and/or meniscal damage often accompanies a grade II MCL injury. As a result it is often prudent to perform special tests directed at these particular structures. The MCL normally has a good secondary support system with weight bearing forces compressing the medial side of the joint and adding to the overall stability of the joint. This allows the structures to be protected after injury along with use of a brace.

Management:

What is the most effective management of this patient?

Medical management for a grade II MCL sprain usually involves conservative management including R.I.C.E. (rest, icing, compression, and elevation). Pharmacological intervention is directed towards pain management through acetaminophen or NSAIDs. The patient may utilize a full-length knee immobilizer or a hinge brace and crutches to limit weight bearing through the involved lower extremity for initial rehabilitation. Physical therapy intervention should be directed towards increasing range of motion in the involved extremity and beginning light resistive exercises. Range of motion exercises may include heel slides or stationary cycling without resistance. Resistive exercises should be directed towards the quadriceps and may include isometrics and closed kinetic chain exercises. Functional activities such as gait and stair climbing should be incorporated into the treatment program. Superficial modalities and electrical stimulation may be utilized to combat pain and inflammation. Transverse friction massage may be applied to the healing ligament so it does not adhere to surrounding and adjacent structures. Care must be taken not to massage the proximal attachment of the MCL due to potential bony periosteal disruption. A patient should be required to complete a functional progression prior to returning to unrestricted activity.

What home care regimen should be recommended?

The home care regimen should consist of range of motion, strengthening, palliative care, and functional activities as warranted based on the results of the patient examination. The use of crutches should continue until the patient can adequately extend the knee joint.

Outcome:

What is the likely outcome of a course in physical therapy?

A grade II MCL sprain should progress fairly quickly if no other structures (ACL or meniscus) are involved. A patient should be able to return to their previous functional level within four to eight weeks following the injury.

What are the long-term effects of the patient's condition?

Proper healing time and rehabilitation management should allow the patient to return to all forms of activity once the patient demonstrates full range of motion, ambulation without a limp, no visual swelling, and competence with all agility testing. If the patient has residual laxity from the injury the patient may be susceptible to reinjury.

Comparison:

What are the distinguishing characteristics of a similar condition?

A grade II lateral collateral ligament injury differs from a MCL injury in several ways. The lateral collateral ligament attaches proximally on the lateral femoral condyle and runs distally and posteriorly to insert on the head of the fibula. Lateral collateral ligament injuries are far less common than MCL injuries. Management should focus on the same general goals (range of motion, strengthening, palliative care, and functional activities) as those outlined for the MCL injury.

Clinical Scenarios:

Scenario One

A 17-year-old male is diagnosed with a left grade III MCL sprain and a small tear in the medial meniscus. The patient was playing football when he was tackled and hit at the knee. The patient has no significant past medical history and plans to participate in football at the collegiate level.

Scenario Two

A 20-year-old college field hockey player complains of knee pain after being diagnosed with a grade I MCL sprain. The patient is mildly tender to palpation over the medial joint line and exhibits trace effusion. The patient has no significant past medical history and would like to return to athletic competition as soon as possible.

Multiple Sclerosis

Diagnosis:

What condition produces a patient's symptoms?

Multiple sclerosis (MS) produces patches of demyelination that decreases the efficiency of nerve impulse transmission. Symptoms vary based on the location and the extent of demyelination.

An injury was most likely sustained to which structure?

Multiple sclerosis is characterized by demyelination of the myelin sheaths that surround nerves within the brain and spinal cord. Myelin breakdown results in plaque development, decreased nerve conduction velocity, and eventual failure of impulse transmission. Lesions are scattered throughout the central nervous system and do not follow a particular pattern.

Inference:

What is the most likely contributing factor in the development of this condition?

The exact etiology of MS is unknown. Genetics, viral infections, and environment all have a role in the development of MS. It is theorized that a slow acting virus initiates the autoimmune response in individuals that have environmental and genetic factors for the disease. The incidence of MS is higher in Caucasians between the ages of 20 and 35 years and is nearly twice as common in women as in men. There is also a higher incidence of MS in temperate climates.

Confirmation:

What is the most likely clinical presentation?

The prevalence of MS differs by geographic area, sex, and race. In the United States the prevalence is 30-80:100,000 with 250,000-350,000 current cases. The highest incidence is 20-35 years of age, however, MS can occur at any age. MS can be classified as relapsing-remitting MS (85%), secondary-progressive MS, primary-progressive MS or progressive-relapsing MS. The clinical presentation varies based on the type of disease, the location, extent of demyelination, and degree of sclerosis. Initial symptoms can include visual problems, paresthesias and sensory changes, clumsiness, weakness, ataxia, balance dysfunction, and fatigue. The clinical course usually consists of periods of exacerbations and remissions, however, the degree of neurologic dysfunction and subsequent recovery will follow typical patterns of the specific type of MS. The frequency and intensity of exacerbations may indicate the speed/course of the disease process.

What laboratory or imaging studies would confirm the diagnosis?

There is not a single testing procedure to diagnose MS early in the disease. MRI may assist with observation and establishing a baseline for lesions, evoked potentials may demonstrate slowed nerve conduction, and cerebrospinal fluid can be analyzed for an elevated concentration of gamma globulin and protein levels.

What additional information should be obtained to confirm the diagnosis?

Clinical presentation and reliable patient history of symptoms are vital in the diagnosis of MS. Guidelines indicate that a clinically definitive diagnosis of MS can be made if a person experiences two separate attacks and shows evidence of two separate lesions. Other diagnoses (having specific criteria) include laboratory-supported definite MS, clinically probable MS, and laboratory-supported probable MS.

Examination:

What history should be documented?

Important areas to explore include past medical history, history of symptoms, medications, current health status, social history, occupation, living environment, and social support system.

What test/measures are most appropriate?

Aerobic capacity and endurance: assessment of vital signs at rest and with activity

Arousal, attention and cognition: examine mental status, learning ability, memory, and motivation, Mini-Mental State Examination

Assistive and adaptive devices: analysis of components and safety of a device

Community and work integration: analysis of community, work, and leisure activities

Gait, locomotion, and balance: static/dynamic balance in sitting/standing, Tinetti Performance Oriented Mobility Assessment, Berg Balance Scale

Motor function: assessment of dexterity and coordination; assessment of postural, equilibrium, and righting reactions; gross and fine motor skills

Muscle performance: strength and tone assessment, tremor assessment, muscle endurance, Modified Fatigue Impact Scale

Neuromotor development and sensory integration: analysis of reflex movement patterns

Pain: pain perception assessment scale

Posture: resting/dynamic posture, potential contracture

Range of motion: active and passive range of motion

Self-care and home management: Barthel Index, assessment of functional capacity and safety, Kurtzke Expanded Disability Status Scale

What additional findings are likely with this patient?

A low percentage of patients experience benign MS and have little to no long-term disability. The majority experience progressive degeneration through periods of exacerbations and remissions. As the disease advances exacerbations leave greater ongoing disability and the length of remissions decrease. Ongoing symptoms can include emotional lability, depression, dementia, psychological problems, spasticity, tremor, weakness, paralysis, sexual dysfunction, and loss of bowel and bladder control.

Management:

What is the most effective management of this patient?

Management of MS includes pharmacological, medical, and therapeutic intervention. The goal of medical treatment of MS is to lessen the length of exacerbations and maximize the health of the patient. Pharmacological intervention is quite complex and can include ABC drugs (approved in the treatment of MS) that are classified as immunomodulatory medications. Physical, occupational, and speech therapies are indicated throughout the clinical course of the disease and well as nutritional and psychological counseling. Physical therapy intervention includes regulation of activity level, relaxation and energy conservation techniques, normalization of tone, balance activities, gait training, core stabilization and control, and adaptive/assistive device training. Patient and caregiver education regarding safety, energy conservation, patterns of fatigue, and the use of adaptive devices is vital to the quality of life.

What home care regimen should be recommended?

A home care regimen should include a submaximal exercise/ endurance program. Exercise in the morning when the patient is rested is advisable to avoid fatigue. The patient may need frequent rest periods throughout the day and may benefit from breaking a task into smaller steps to avoid fatigue. Ongoing ambulation and mobility activities are important to maintain endurance and prevent disuse atrophy. Aquatic therapy may also be indicated as it is beneficial to this population.

Outcome:

What is the likely outcome of a course in physical therapy?

Physical therapy is indicated intermittently throughout the clinical course of MS with the goal of maximizing functional capacity and the quality of life. Physical therapy will not alter the progression of the disease process but rather treat the current symptoms and assist the patient to attain the highest level of function. Factors that influence exacerbations include heat, stress, infection, trauma, and pregnancy.

What are the long-term effects of the patient's condition?

MS is generally a progressive degenerative disease process that creates permanent damage and disability. Factors that influence exacerbations include heat, stress, and trauma. Most patients live with MS for many years and die from secondary complications such as disuse atrophy, pressure sores, contractures, pathological fractures, renal infection, and pneumonia. If left untreated 50% of patients will require a wheelchair within 15 years post diagnosis. Overall mortality rate and long-term outcome correlates to age at diagnosis, number of attacks and exacerbations, frequency and duration of remissions, and type of MS. Suicide is also seven times greater when compared to the same age control group without MS.

Comparison:

What are the distinguishing characteristics of a similar condition?

Dystonia is a neurologic syndrome that presents with involuntary and sustained muscle contractions that cause repetitive movements. Idiopathic dystonia has a genetic basis and accounts for two-thirds of all cases. Secondary dystonia usually results from brain damage or CNS damage. There are no definitive tests to diagnose dystonia. Treatment is based on current symptoms and includes pharmacological intervention, physical therapy, and occasional surgical intervention. Prognosis is based on age of onset and spontaneous remission occurs in 25-30% of the cases.

Clinical Scenarios:

Scenario One

A 28-year-old female has had visual difficulty, urinary urgency, tingling, and upper extremity weakness on two separate occasions recently. The patient has an aunt with MS, however, has no other significant medical history. The patient was referred to physical therapy by her primary physician.

Scenario Two

A 42-year-old male with MS is referred to physical therapy. The patient has experienced several exacerbations and remissions with full recovery in the past. The patient presently appears to have an exacerbation of symptoms including excessive fatigue. He lives alone and works in a library.

Myocardial Infarction

Diagnosis:

What condition produces a patient's symptoms?

Myocardial infarction (MI) occurs when there is poor coronary artery perfusion, ischemia, and subsequent necrosis of the cardiac tissue usually due to thrombus, arterial blockage or atherosclerosis. The location and severity of the infarct will determine symptoms and the overall acute clinical picture.

An injury was most likely sustained to which structure?

A MI produces ischemia and subsequent necrosis to a portion of the myocardium. The extent of the damage to the myocardium is dependent on the duration of ischemia and on the thickness of the tissue involved. A transmural MI involves the full-thickness of the myocardium while a nontransmural MI involves the subendocardial area (inner third of the myocardium). The myocardium has three zones that form concentric circles around the point of infarct termed zone of infarct, zone of hypoxic injury, and zone of ischemia. Thrombosis of the anterior descending branch of the left coronary artery is the most common location of infarct and affects the left ventricle. A right coronary artery thrombosis can result in an infarct of the posteroinferior portion of the left ventricle and potentially affect the right ventricular myocardium.

Inference:

What is the most likely contributing factor in the development of this condition?

The primary risk factors for MI include patient or family history of heart disease, smoking, physical inactivity, stress, hypertension, elevated cholesterol, diabetes mellitus, and obesity. The use of cocaine, aortic stenosis or coronary artery dissection may also cause a MI. It has been documented that a MI will occur more frequently in the morning hours and during the November to December holiday season.

Confirmation:

What is the most likely clinical presentation?

MI occurs in 1.5 million individuals each year within the United States with a mortality rate of 500,000 deaths annually. Approximately two-thirds of patients experience prodromal symptoms days to weeks before the event, including unstable angina, shortness of breath, and fatigue. A patient that is experiencing a MI will initially present with deep pain or pressure in the substernal area. The pain may or may not radiate to the jaw and down the left arm or to the back. The patient cannot alleviate the pain with rest or nitroglycerin and the pain may last for hours. The patient is usually anxious, pale, sweating, fatigued, and may present with nausea and vomiting. Symptoms of a MI frequently do not follow a typical pattern, especially in females. There are also instances of a silent MI where no symptoms are noted.

What laboratory or imaging studies would confirm the diagnosis?

The primarily tool to detect a MI is a 12-lead electrocardiogram. An inverted T wave indicates myocardial ischemia, elevated ST segment indicates acute infarction, and a depressed ST segment indicates a pending subendocardial or transmural infarction. A blood serum analysis can be utilized to determine the level of selected cardiac enzymes. The level of selected enzymes such as creatine phosphokinase (CPK), aspartate transferase (AST), and lactic dehydrogenase (LDH) can be dramatically altered during and after a MI. A complete blood count (CBC), chest radiograph, radionuclide imaging, and amylase level may be ordered to assist with the diagnosis.

What additional information should be obtained to confirm the diagnosis?

Additional information in the diagnosis of a MI is found through the manifestation of symptoms (see clinical presentation) and clinical examination including a thorough past medical history and history of current symptoms.

Examination:

What history should be documented?

Important areas to explore include past medical history, family history, medications, current health status, living environment, social history and habits, occupation, and social support system.

What test/measures are most appropriate?

Aerobic capacity and endurance: vital signs at rest and during activity, palpation of pulses, perceived exertion scale, electrocardiogram analysis, auscultation of the heart and lungs, pulse oximetry

Arousal, attention, and cognition: examine mental status, learning ability, memory, motivation

Assistive and adaptive devices: analysis of components and safety of a device

Environmental, home, and work: analysis of current and potential barriers or hazards

Gait, locomotion, and balance: assessment of static and dynamic balance in sitting and standing, safety during gait with/without an assistive device

Muscle performance: strength assessment through active movement only (no manual muscle testing)

Pain: pain perception scale, visual analog scale

Posture: analysis of resting and dynamic posture

Self-care and home management: assessment of functional capacity, Barthel Index

Ventilation, respiration, and circulation: ventilation, respiration, and circulation; assessment of pulses

What additional findings are likely with this patient?

A patient status post MI is at risk for complications that include arrhythmias, hypotension, pericarditis, impaired cardiac output, pulmonary edema, congestive heart failure, pericarditis, cardiogenic shock, recurrent infarction and sudden death. Arrhythmias occur in 90% of patients post MI and are caused by ischemia, ANS impairment, electrolyte imbalances, conduction defects, and other chemical imbalances.

Management:

What is the most effective management of this patient?

Initial medical management of a MI is to stabilize the patient and initiate pharmacological intervention to hinder the evolution of the MI. Anticoagulants, beta-blockers, thrombolytic agents, angiotensin-converting enzyme inhibitors, vasodilators, and estrogen (in women) may be used. Once stable, the patient is managed through a cardiac rehabilitation program. Surgical intervention including angioplasty, stenting, endarterectomy, and bypass grafting may be indicated based on the underlying cause of the MI. Exercise testing is performed within three days of the MI in order to establish baseline guidelines for patients that are cleared to exercise and do not exhibit any arrhythmias or angina. Physical therapy intervention usually follows a multi-phase cardiac rehabilitation program and continues in an outpatient setting once the patient is discharged from the hospital. Low-level therapeutic exercise, functional activities, relaxation, breathing techniques, endurance training, and continuous monitoring of vital signs are key components this program. Patient education regarding reduction of risk factors, return to activity, and commitment to fitness and health are also important to the success of physical therapy intervention.

What home care regimen should be recommended?

A home care regimen should follow the guidelines indicated for each phase of cardiac rehabilitation. A patient must continue with safe exercise, and integration of risk factor reduction. Symptom recognition and nutritional strategies are also important in a daily routine.

Outcome:

What is the likely outcome of a course in physical therapy?

Cardiac rehabilitation is recommended status post MI. The patient should start in the coronary care unit (CCU) and progress through each of the phases of cardiac rehabilitation. The goal is successful completion of a cardiac rehabilitation program allowing the patient to resume all activities of daily living and recreational pursuits. Upon completion the patient should possess self-management skills associated with symptoms/risk factors of heart disease.

What are the long-term effects of the patient's condition?

A patient that has experienced a MI may be able to return to all previous activities after successful completion of a cardiac rehabilitation program. A patient must continue to reduce the modifiable risk factors and maintain an appropriate level of exercise in order to limit a possible subsequent MI. Long-term outcome is dependent on prior functional ability, the extent and damage to the heart, and factors that negatively affect prognosis such as age, cardiovascular disease, hypotension, the presence of co-morbidities, and an abnormal treadmill exercise test.

Comparison:

What are the distinguishing characteristics of a similar condition?

Angina pectoris is a myocardial ischemic disorder that occurs when there is an oxygen deficit to the coronary arteries. Coronary artery disease accounts for 90% of all cases of angina. Angina is classified as stable, post-infarction, Prinzmetal's, resting, unstable, nocturnal or variant. Symptoms often occur during exertion and include chest pain that may radiate. Rest or nitroglycerin normally provides relief of the symptoms. Treatment of the underlying cause is essential to prevent further damage to the heart.

Clinical Scenarios:

Scenario One

A 51-year-old male is referred to a phase I cardiac rehabilitation program after a transmural MI two days ago. The patient has hypertension, high cholesterol, smokes, and is obese. The patient currently supervises a local automobile dealership. The patient is divorced and lives in a two-story home.

Scenario Two

A 78-year-old female is status post nontransmural MI. The patient is very active and plays golf. The patient's past medical history includes treatment for a cardiac arrhythmia, obesity, and diabetes mellitus. The physician referred the patient for cardiac rehabilitation.

Osteoarthritis

Diagnosis:

What condition produces a patient's symptoms?

Osteoarthritis (OA) is a heterogeneous group of conditions resulting in common physiological changes. The most common type of joint disease, OA is a degenerative chronic disorder resulting from the biochemical breakdown of articular cartilage in the synovial joints. Although theories indicate that OA is due to excessive wear and tear, secondary inflammatory changes may also affect the involved joints. OA has been divided into primary and secondary forms.

An injury was most likely sustained to which structure?

The progression of OA begins with degenerative alterations primarily in the articular cartilage. This degenerative process is usually a result of excessive loading of a healthy joint or normal loading of an abnormal joint. External forces create the breakdown of the chondrocytes and cause disruption of the cartilaginous matrix. Loss of cartilage results in the loss of the joint space. Through this process, reactive new bone forms, usually at the margins and subchondral areas of the joint.

Inference:

What is the most likely contributing factor in the development of this condition?

The etiology of primary OA is idiopathic occurring within intact joints with no history that supports the initiation of this condition. Primary OA is related to the aging process and typically occurs in older individuals. Secondary OA refers to degenerative disease of the synovial joints that results from some predisposing condition (i.e., trauma) that has adversely altered the articular cartilage and/or subchondral bone of the affected joints. Secondary OA often occurs in relatively young individuals. General risk factors include age, obesity, female gender, trauma, infection, repetitive microtrauma, genetic factors, inflammatory arthritis, neuromuscular and metabolic disorders.

Confirmation:

What is the most likely clinical presentation?

Potential sites for primary OA include joints of the hands specifically the distal interphalangeal joints (DIP), proximal interphalangeal joints (PIP), and joints at the base of the thumb, knees, hips, and the spine. Bilateral symmetry is often seen in cases of primary OA, particularly when the hands are affected. Primary OA occurs most commonly in the hands. A patient with OA may experience a decrease in range of motion accompanied by crepitus within the affected joints. The patient will frequently complain of deep and aching joint pain exacerbated by prolonged activity and use. Heberden's nodes consist of palpable osteophytes in the

DIP joints and are usually seen in women, but not men. Pain is the main reason patients seek medical attention. Initially, patients have pain during activity that is alleviated by rest and they usually respond to analgesics. Morning stiffness in the affected joints usually occurs with progression of the disease, resulting in an increased pain level even at rest that may not respond to analgesics. Erythema or warmth over the joints is not usually present, but effusion may exist. Malalignment and limitation of the joint may occur as the disease progresses in severity. The patient may also present with a deviated gait pattern, atypical movement patterns, and muscle atrophy.

What laboratory or imaging studies would confirm the diagnosis?

OA is typically diagnosed on the basis of clinical examination and x-ray findings. Laboratory tests will not diagnose OA.

What additional information should be obtained to confirm the diagnosis?

Visual inspection of the affected joints, a thorough examination, and a history of the condition will normally support the diagnosis.

Examination:

What history should be documented?

Important areas to explore include past medical history, medications, current health status, nutritional status, social history and habits, occupation, living environment, and social support system.

What test/measures are most appropriate?

Aerobic capacity and endurance: assessment of vital signs at rest and with activity, perceived exertion scale, pulse oximetry, auscultation of the lungs

Anthropometric characteristics: circumferential measurements

Arousal, attention, and cognition: mental status exam

Assistive and adaptive devices: analysis of components and safety of a device

Community and work integration: analysis of community, work, and leisure activities

Environmental, home, and work barriers: analysis of current and potential barriers or hazards

Ergonomics and body mechanics: analysis of dexterity and coordination

Gait, locomotion, and balance: static and dynamic balance in sitting and standing, safety during gait with/ without an assistive device, Berg Functional Balance Scale, Functional Ambulation Profile

Integumentary integrity: assessment of sensation

Joint integrity and mobility: hyper- and hypomobility of a joint, soft tissue swelling and inflammation

Motor function: equilibrium and righting reactions, motor assessment scales, coordination
Muscle performance: strength assessment
Pain: pain perception assessment scale, VAS
Posture: analysis of resting and dynamic posture
Range of motion: active and passive range of motion
Self-care and home management: assessment of functional capacity, Functional Independence Measure
Sensory integrity: proprioception and kinesthesia

What additional findings are likely with this patient?

In patients greater than 55 years old, the prevalence of OA is higher among women than men. DIP and PIP joint involvement resulting in Heberden's and Bouchard's nodes is also more common in women. Disease progression characteristically is slow, occurring over several years or decades. Pain is usually the initial and principal source of morbidity in OA. The patient can become progressively inactive leading to additional co-morbidities including weight gain. There is also an increased incidence of strains and sprains around joints affected with OA.

Management:

What is the most effective management of this patient?

Medical management of a patient with OA is usually multifaceted based on symptoms and the specific affected joints. Long-term management would include pharmacological intervention using acetaminophen or other NSAIDs to alleviate the pain. Glucocorticoid intra-articular injections may also be prescribed to improve a patient's symptoms, however, must be used sparingly due to the long-term negative effects. Nutritional education and weight reduction may be indicated to reduce the stress on the affected joints. Physical therapy may be indicated intermittently in order to preserve joint motion and flexibility. Other treatment may include posture retraining, work site evaluation, general strengthening, relaxation and endurance activities, icing or heat for pain management, hydrotherapy, modalities, patient education, aquatic therapy, and functional activities. If conservative treatment fails, a patient may be a candidate for joint replacement surgery with the goal of pain relief.

What home care regimen should be recommended?

A home care regimen for OA should include general strengthening to tolerance, AROM exercises, endurance activities, continued use of relaxation techniques, and supportive or assistive devices that would decrease pain and improve functional ability. It is very important that the patient avoid overexertion and fatigue.

Outcome:

What is the likely outcome of a course in physical therapy?

Physical therapy can assist the patient during periods of exacerbation of the disease process, however, cannot change the ultimate outcome of the condition. OA is a progressive and chronic condition. Physical therapy can assist in minimizing the effects of the process and allow for as much independence as allowed by patient tolerance during functional activities.

What are the long-term effects of the patient's condition?

Approximately 80-90% of individuals older than 65 years have evidence of primary OA. The degree of disability also depends on the site(s) of involvement and rate of progression. Usually, the pain slowly worsens over time, but it may stabilize. OA of the knee is a leading cause of disability in elderly persons.

Comparison:

What are the distinguishing characteristics of a similar condition?

Psoriatic arthritis is a rheumatic condition characterized by inflammatory arthritis and is often seen in combination with psoriatic skin lesions. Symptoms include silver or grey scaly spots on the scalp, elbows, knees and spine, pitting of fingernails and toenails, pain and swelling in one or more joints, and swelling of the fingers and toes. Psoriatic arthritis affects men and women of all races and usually occurs between the ages of 20 and 50 but can occur at any age. The etiology is unknown but theories suggest a relationship to genetic inheritance, psoriasis, and environmental factors.

Clinical Scenarios:

Scenario One

A 71-year-old female is referred to physical therapy with significant OA in her hands, knees, and hips. She is approximately 35 pounds overweight and has lost mobility. She rates her pain as an eight out of ten and wants to have surgery to "fix" her legs. She resides in a two-story home with her husband.

Scenario Two

A 39-year-old male has developed secondary OA as a result of a 15-year career in semi-professional football. The patient lives a very active lifestyle, however, has a significant amount of pain in both knee joints. The patient is currently married and working full-time.

Osteogenesis Imperfecta

Diagnosis:

What condition produces a patient's symptoms?

Osteogenesis Imperfecta (OI) is a rare congenital disorder of collagen synthesis that affects all connective tissue in the body. The genetic defect affects collagen-producing genes and reduces production of collagen from 20-50%. There are many mutations identified and various underlying causes that combine to produce the phenotypic expression of OI in a patient.

An injury was most likely sustained to which structure?

The genes for type I collagen production (COL1A1 and COL1A2) have been identified as the genes that become mutated and result in OI. Since collagen production is vital throughout the body, bones and all forms of connective tissue are compromised. OI can also compromise growth, hearing, cardiopulmonary function, and joint integrity.

Inference:

What is the most likely contributing factor in the development of this condition?

Most children inherit OI from parents as either an autosomal dominant or autosomal recessive trait. Twenty-five percent of the time the genetic defect occurs by spontaneous mutation of the genes. Statistics estimate that 30 to 50 thousand individuals are living with OI in the United States.

Confirmation:

What is the most likely clinical presentation?

OI is classified into four types and has a wide range of clinical presentations ranging from normal appearance with mild symptoms to severe involvement that is fatal during infancy. Type I is the mildest form where a child has near normal growth and appearance with frequency of fractures usually ceasing after puberty. The patient experiences mild or moderate fragility, but most times without deformity. This patient will usually present with blue sclera, easy bruising, triangular face, and possible hearing loss. Type II is the most severe form where a child dies in utero or by early childhood. This child has significant fragility of connective tissue, experiences multiple fractures with extreme deformities, and has a soft skull. Type III is severe but these children present with greater ossification of the skull. Type III characteristics include significant growth, retardation, progressive deformities, ongoing fractures, severe osteoporosis, triangular face, blue sclera, and significant limitations with functional mobility. Type IV is usually a milder course that involves mild to moderate fragility and osteoporosis (but greater than type I). The patient will experience fractures easily prior to puberty, but some children improve at that time. Type IV may or may not have a shorter stature, will have bowing of long bones, a barrel shape of their rib cage, possible hearing loss, brittle

teeth, and will present with near normal sclera. These children have a near normal life expectancy.

What laboratory or imaging studies would confirm the diagnosis?

A skin biopsy is used to examine the collagen and determine what type of OI is present. X-rays and bone scans may be used for evidence of deformities and old fractures. Bone densitometry may also be used to measure bone mass and estimate the risk of fracture for specific sites within the body. The diagnosis is made through these tests and in combination with the examination and history.

What additional information should be obtained to confirm the diagnosis?

Diagnosis should be determined based on physical examination, family and personal medical history, and testing described in the above paragraph.

Examination:

What history should be documented?

Important areas to explore include past medical history including falls, medications, family history, current symptoms and health status, and social support system.

What test/measures are most appropriate?

Arousal, attention, and cognition: examine mental status, learning ability, memory, motivation
Environmental, home, and work barriers: analysis of current and potential barriers or hazards
Ergonomics and body mechanics: analysis of dexterity and coordination
Gait, locomotion, and balance: static/dynamic balance in sitting/standing, safety during gait with/without an assistive device, analysis of wheelchair management
Integumentary integrity: skin and sensation assessment
Joint integrity and mobility: assessment of hyper- and hypomobility of a joint
Muscle performance: strength assessment of active motion, muscle tone assessment
Neuromotor development and sensory integration: reflex movement patterns and involuntary movements, sensory integration tests, gross/fine motor skills
Orthotic, protective, and supportive devices: analysis of components of a device, analysis of movement while wearing a device
Pain: pain perception assessment scale, visual analog scale, assessment of muscle soreness
Posture: analysis of resting and dynamic posture, scoliosis assessment
Range of motion: active range of motion only
Self-care and home management: assessment of functional capacity

What additional findings are likely with this patient?

Children with OI often have delayed developmental milestones secondary to ongoing fractures with immobilization, hypermobility and laxity of joints, and poorly developed muscles. Most Type I children are community ambulators, approximately 57% of Type IV are household ambulators and 26% are community ambulators, and only 26% of Type III become household ambulators.

Management:

What is the most effective management of this patient?

Medical management is directed at controlling the symptoms of OI. General goals include maximizing independence with mobility, improving optimal bone mass and muscle strength, and prevention of fractures and deformities. Pharmacological interventions have been studied, but have not shown any strong effect. Children should not be given steroids since it may deplete bone and increase fragility. Nutritional counseling and strong dental care are important in the management of OI. Lightweight orthotics may be indicated early to support the extremities, assist with ambulation, encourage weight bearing, and prevent fractures. Physical therapy intervention initially focuses on parent handling techniques, recognition of fractures, positioning, and activities that facilitate safe movement. Treatment of a child with OI should incorporate developmental activities, strengthening, positioning, weight bearing, and the use of mobility aids (scooters, riding toys or wheelchair). Swimming is also a good alternative for strengthening and exercise. All strengthening exercises should avoid rotational forces, placing weights/resistance near a joint, and using long lever arms. Surgical procedures known as "rodding" may also be indicated if a child has more than two fractures to the same bone within six months or if the angle of the long bone would not allow for stable ambulation.

What home care regimen should be recommended?

A home care regimen will be successful if parents are competent with many of the relevant aspects of care. Handling techniques, recognition of fractures, precautions and contraindications, standing program, and exercise through activities are all key components of a home program for a child with OI. A child needs to continue to move and exercise in a safe fashion in order to optimize strength and bone mass.

Outcome:

What is the likely outcome of a course in physical therapy?

Physical therapy may be required intermittently over the course of the patient's childhood depending on the severity of OI and the secondary complications. Physical therapy must also update a home program for optimal therapeutic results. Physical therapy may be in an outpatient setting or through the school system. The therapist should work closely with the physician and caregivers for comprehensive care.

What are the long-term effects of the patient's condition?

A patient with OI has outcome potential based on the type of disorder, symptoms, and secondary complications encountered. A strong predictor of a child's ability to ambulate in the future also lies in the child's ability to sit by ten months of age. Some children live normal lives with minimal involvement while others use power wheelchairs for mobility and experience multiple secondary complications.

Comparison:

What are the distinguishing characteristics of a similar condition?

Arthrogryposis multiplex congenita (AMC) is a non-progressive neuromuscular disorder that results from multiple conditions that ultimately limit fetal movement in an intact skeleton and cause multiple congenital contractures at birth. Children are also born with muscle atrophy and weakness, and articular rigidity. Primary forms of AMC include contracture syndromes, amyoplasia, and distal arthrogryposis. Some children will ambulate and others will require wheelchairs for mobility.

Clinical Scenarios:

Scenario One

A nine-month-old boy is seen in physical therapy with Type IV OI. He currently has a cast on his left lower extremity due to a femur fracture. His mother wants to learn activities in sitting and handling techniques that would help her son.

Scenario Two

A 12-year-old female is seen by a school therapist. She underwent intramedullary rod placement in her right femur six weeks ago. She has type III OI and uses a wheelchair. She also presents with a 45 degree thoracic scoliosis and bowing in her upper extremities.

Osteoporosis

Diagnosis:

What condition produces a patient's symptoms?

Osteoporosis is a metabolic bone disorder where the rate of bone resorption accelerates while the rate of bone formation slows down; osteoclast activity exceeds osteoblast activity. This reduction of bone mass decreases the overall bone density and strength. Primary osteoporosis includes classifications such as idiopathic osteoporosis, involutional (senile) osteoporosis, and postmenopausal osteoporosis. Secondary osteoporosis occurs due to a primary disease process or as a result of taking certain medications.

An injury was most likely sustained to which structure?

Osteoporosis primarily affects trabecular bone in a postmenopausal patient, however, is primarily seen in both trabecular and cortical bone in the geriatric population. Impaired bone formation due to declining osteoblast function in addition to the loss of calcium and phosphate salts within the bone structure cause brittle and porous bones that easily fracture. All bones can be affected with fractures of the vertebrae, distal radius/ulna, and femoral neck being the most common.

Inference:

What is the most likely contributing factor in the development of this condition?

The exact cause of primary osteoporosis is unknown, however, there are risk factors that include inadequate dietary calcium, smoking, excessive caffeine, high intake of alcohol or salt, small stature, Caucasian race, inactive lifestyle, family history or history of chronic disease. Secondary osteoporosis may be caused by prolonged drug therapies of heparin or corticosteroid use, endocrine disorders, malnutrition, and other disease processes. Postmenopausal osteoporosis targets women approximately 50-60 years of age. Involutional (senile) osteoporosis usually targets men and women >70 years of age. Idiopathic osteoporosis can occur in both genders at all ages.

Confirmation:

What is the most likely clinical presentation?

Osteoporosis is the most frequently seen metabolic bone disease that affects approximately 10 million individuals within the United States. The prevalence is expected to increase with the increase in the aging population. A patient diagnosed with osteoporosis may complain of low thoracic or lumbar pain, experience compression fractures of the vertebrae, and complain of back pain. Vertebral and other crush fractures may occur with little to no trauma. Pain is acute and increases with weight bearing and palpation. A patient may also present with deformities such as kyphosis, Dowager's hump, a decrease in height, and other postural changes.

What laboratory or imaging studies would confirm the diagnosis?

There is not an accurate measure of overall bone strength or standards for routine screening that have been established, however, X-rays are taken to investigate the amount of degeneration and the decrease in density of a particular area. A bone mineral density test accounts for 70% of bone strength and is the easiest way to determine osteoporosis. A photon absorptiometry is used to measure bone mass particularly of the vertebrae, hips, and extremities. Quantitative CT scans may be used to aid diagnosis by examining the bone density of the spine.

What additional information should be obtained to confirm the diagnosis?

Differential diagnosis including lab testing and urinalysis must exclude other disease processes through examination and testing. A patient's past medical history, current symptoms, and type and location of pain all play a role in diagnosing osteoporosis.

Examination:

What history should be documented?

Important areas to explore include past medical history, medications, family history, current symptoms, current health status, social history and habits, occupation, leisure activities, and social support system.

What test/measures are most appropriate?

Aerobic capacity and endurance: assessment of vital signs at rest and with activity, perceived exertion scale
Arousal, attention, and cognition: examine mental status, learning ability, memory, motivation
Assistive and adaptive devices: analysis of components and safety of a device
Environmental, home, and work barriers: analysis of current and potential barriers or hazards
Ergonomics and body mechanics: analysis of dexterity and coordination
Gait, locomotion, and balance: static and dynamic balance in sitting and standing, safety during gait with/without an assistive device, Berg Balance Scale, functional capacity evaluation
Integumentary integrity: skin and sensation assessment
Motor function: coordination, posture/balance in sitting
Muscle performance: strength of active range of motion only
Pain: pain perception scale, visual analog scale
Posture: analysis of resting and dynamic posture
Range of motion: active range of motion
Self-care and home management: assessment of functional capacity

What additional findings are likely with this patient?

Once osteoporosis progresses in severity it can affect areas other than weight bearing bones such as the skull, long bones, and ribs. Spontaneous fractures and skeletal deformities may increase due to the continuing bone loss. A single fracture significantly increases the risk for subsequent fractures and skeletal deformities such as kyphosis.

Management:

What is the most effective management of this patient?

Effective management of osteoporosis includes vitamin and pharmaceutical supplements, proper nutrition, education and physical therapy intervention. Hormone replacement therapy is recommended for postmenopausal patients. Calcium supplements, vitamin D, Raloxifene, and Fosamax (prevents bone resorption) may be recommended in the treatment of osteoporosis. Physical therapy intervention should include patient education regarding exercise, positioning, pain management, nutrition, and fall prevention. Physical therapy should include an exercise program that emphasizes weight bearing activities as tolerated. A patient may require a corset or lumbar support if at risk for vertebral fractures and many patients will require training with an assistive device. Aquatic therapy will assist with conditioning, however, should not replace weight bearing activities. Surgical intervention may be indicated for a patient requiring fracture stabilization.

What home care regimen should be recommended?

The home care regimen for osteoporosis includes a consistent home exercise program that combines exercise, walking, and other activities within a patient's tolerance. Exercise is crucial to slowing the bone resorption process and increasing bone development. Patients should be educated to avoid heavy resistive exercise, excessive flexion during exercise or household activities, and the use of ballistic movements. Light resistance such as small dumbbells or Theraband can be used with caution after consulting with the physician.

Outcome:

What is the likely outcome of a course in physical therapy?

Physical therapy should prescribe an exercise program that the patient can follow independently. Patient education should allow for independent decision making regarding proper nutrition and activities that incorporate precautions and fall prevention techniques. This level of patient competency should assist in decreasing the risk of fractures and other complications. Physical therapy cannot cease the process, but can empower the patient to effectively manage this bone disorder.

What are the long-term effects of the patient's condition?

Osteoporosis will create thin and porous bones that will fracture easily and result in direct and indirect complications. Deformity and pain can become long-term effects of osteoporosis. Early detection and management of osteoporosis is important to the long-term effects of the disease.

Comparison:

What are the distinguishing characteristics of a similar condition?

Paget's disease (osteitis deformans) is a chronic bone disease of unknown etiology where there is thickened, spongy, and abnormal bone formation. Large multinucleated osteoblasts, fibrous tissue, and thickened lamellae and trabeculae form and create weak and brittle bones. Bone pain, headache, hearing loss, fatigue, and stiffness are some early characteristics of Paget's disease. Progression of the disease includes bowing of long bones, an increase in skull size, bone deformities, and fractures (especially of the vertebrae).

Clinical Scenarios:

Scenario One

A 63-year-old female is seen in outpatient physical therapy for a home exercise program. She is postmenopausal and does not take hormone replacement therapy. She has been recently diagnosed with osteoporosis and X-rays revealed three old vertebral fractures. The patient's major complaints are pain and stiffness.

Scenario Two

A 92-year-old male was admitted to the hospital for internal fixation of a femoral neck fracture. The patient's history reveals osteoporosis, diabetes, and anxiety. He wants to be discharged home to care for his cat. The physician orders are for physical therapy two times per week with the goal of returning home alone.

Parkinson's Disease

Diagnosis:

What condition produces a patient's symptoms?

Parkinsonism syndrome is used to describe a group of disorders within subcortical gray matter of the basal ganglia that produces a similar disturbance of balance and voluntary movements. This syndrome occurs as a secondary effect or disorder from another disease process. Parkinson's disease is a primary degenerative disorder and is characterized by a decrease in production of dopamine (neurotransmitter) within the corpus striatum portion of the basal ganglia. The degeneration of the dopaminergic pathways creates an imbalance between dopamine and acetylcholine. This process produces the symptoms of Parkinson's disease.

An injury was most likely sustained to which structure?

Injury occurs to the subcortical gray matter within the basal ganglia, specifically the substantia nigra and the corpus striatum. The basal ganglia stores the majority of dopamine and is responsible for modulation and control of voluntary movement. A patient with Parkinson's disease exhibits degeneration of dopaminergic neurons that results in depletion of dopamine production within the basal ganglia. Change in the neurochemical production damages the complex loop between the basal ganglia and the cerebrum.

Inference:

What is the most likely contributing factor in the development of this condition?

Primary Parkinson's disease has an unknown etiology and accounts for the majority of patients with Parkinsonism. Contributing factors that can produce symptoms of Parkinson's disease include genetic defect, toxicity from carbon monoxide, excessive manganese or copper, carbon disulfide, vascular impairment of the striatum, encephalitis, and other neurodegenerative diseases such as Huntington's disease or Alzheimer's disease.

Confirmation:

What is the most likely clinical presentation?

There are approximately 500,000 individuals affected by Parkinsonism and about 42% of these are diagnosed specifically with Parkinson's disease. The risk for developing Parkinson's disease increases with age and 1:100 are affected over the age of 75. The majority of patients are between 50 and 79 years of age and approximately 10% are diagnosed before 40 years. The majority of patients with Parkinson's disease will initially notice a resting tremor in the hands (sometimes called a pill-rolling tremor) or feet that increases with stress and disappears with movement or sleep. Early in the disease process a patient may attribute symptoms to "old age" such as balance disturbances, difficulty rolling over and rising from bed, and impairment

with fine manipulative movements seen in writing, bathing and dressing. A patient's symptoms slowly progress and often include hypokinesia, sluggish movement, difficulty with initiating (akinesia) and stopping movement, festinating and shuffling gait, bradykinesia, poor posture, dysphagia, and "cogwheel" or "lead pipe" rigidity of skeletal muscles. Patients may also experience "freezing" during ambulation, speech, blinking, and movements of the arms. A patient with Parkinson's disease will also have a mask-like appearance with no facial expression.

What laboratory or imaging studies would confirm the diagnosis?

There are no laboratory or imaging studies that initially diagnose Parkinson's disease. CT scan or MRI may be used to rule out other neurodegenerative diseases and obtain a baseline for future comparison.

What additional information should be obtained to confirm the diagnosis?

Definitive diagnosis is difficult during the early stages of the disease. Parkinson's disease is believed to progress slowly over 25 to 30 years prior to the onset of pharmacological intervention. Diagnosis is made from patient history, history of symptoms, and differential diagnosis to rule out other potential disorders. There are evaluation tools that are utilized to classify a patient by stage of the disease process.

Examination:

What history should be documented?

Important areas to explore include past medical history, medications, current symptoms, current health status, social history and habits, occupation, living environment, and social support system.

What test/measures are most appropriate?

Aerobic capacity and endurance: assessment of vital signs at rest and with activity
Arousal, attention, and cognition: examine mental status, learning ability, memory, motivation, and Mini-Mental State Examination
Environmental, home, and work barriers: analysis of current and potential barriers or hazards
Gait, locomotion, and balance: static and dynamic balance in sitting and standing, Functional Reach Test, Tinetti Performance Oriented Mobility Assessment, Berg Balance Scale, outcome measurement tools, safety with/without an assistive device during gait
Joint integrity and mobility: analysis of quality of movement, examine joint hypermobility and hypomobility
Motor function: assessment of dexterity, coordination and agility, assessment of postural, equilibrium, and righting reactions
Muscle performance: strength assessment, muscle tone assessment, and tremor assessment

Posture: analysis of resting and dynamic posture
Range of motion: active and passive range of motion
Self-care and home management: functional capacity, Barthel Index, safety assessments, Parkinson's disease Questionnaire (PDQ-39)
Sensory integration: assessment of combined sensation, assessment of proprioception and kinesthesia
Ventilation, respiratory, and circulation: assessment of chest wall mobility, expansion, and excursion

What additional findings are likely with this patient?

Since Parkinson's disease is a progressive condition there are ongoing physical and cognitive impairments. A patient may develop a stooped posture and an increased risk for falling. Progression of the disease may result in dysphagia, difficulty with speech, and pulmonary impairment. Greater attention is required for skin care once nutrition and mobility are further compromised. Many patients with Parkinson's disease die from complications of bronchopneumonia.

Management:

What is the most effective management of this patient?

The medical management of Parkinson's disease relies heavily on pharmacological intervention. Dopamine replacement therapy, (Levodopa, Sinemet, Madopar) is the most effective treatment in reducing the symptoms of Parkinson's disease such as movement disorders, bradykinesia, rigidity, and tremor. Antihistamines, anticholinergics, and antidepressants are also utilized. Physical, occupational, and speech therapies may be warranted intermittently throughout the course of the disease. Physical therapy intervention should include maximizing endurance, strength, and functional mobility. Verbal cueing and oral/visual feedback are effective tools to use with this population. Family teaching, balance activities, gait training, stretching, trunk rotation activities, assistive device training, relaxation techniques, and respiratory therapy are all important components in the treatment of Parkinson's disease. Psychological and nutritional counseling are recommended.

What home care regimen should be recommended?

A home care regimen should include an exercise routine, functional mobility skills, the use of relaxation techniques, range of motion and stretching exercises, and endurance activities. A competent caretaker is vital to the success of the home program and must continuously motivate the patient to continue with mobility and endurance activities in order to avoid deleterious effects of the disease process.

Outcome:

What is the likely outcome of a course in physical therapy?

Physical therapy is recommended on an intermittent basis throughout the course of the disease and will focus on current symptoms that arise. Physical therapy will not prevent further degeneration or cure the movement disorder, however, it will assist the patient to maximize their level of function and quality of life.

What are the long-term effects of the patient's condition?

Parkinson's disease does not significantly alter a patient's lifespan if the patient is diagnosed with a generalized form between 50 and 60 years of age. As the disease progresses, however, there will be an exacerbation of all symptoms and significant loss of mobility. The inactivity and deconditioning allows for complications and eventual death.

Comparison:

What are the distinguishing characteristics of a similar condition?

Wilson's disease is inherited as an autosomal recessive trait and causes a defect in the metabolism of copper. The accumulation of copper within erythrocytes, the liver, the brain, and kidneys produces the associated degenerative changes. The patient presents with hepatic insufficiency, tremor, choreoathetoid movements, dysarthria, and progressive rigidity.

Clinical Scenarios:

Scenario One

A 35-year-old female is sent to physical therapy shortly after being diagnosed with Parkinson's disease. She is presently having difficulty maintaining a grasp on items from an assembly line at work and complains of frequently tripping.

Scenario Two

A 42-year-old male was diagnosed with Parkinson's disease four years ago. The patient requires physical therapy to reassess gait and prescribe an assistive device. The son states that the patient sits a great deal at home and lacks motivation to engage in exercise.

Patellofemoral Syndrome

Diagnosis:

What condition produces a patient's symptoms?

Patellofemoral syndrome is caused by an abnormal tracking of the patella between the femoral condyles. The tracking problem places increased and misdirected forces between the patella and femur. This most commonly occurs when the patella is pulled too far laterally during knee extension.

An injury was most likely sustained to which structure?

Patellofemoral syndrome causes damage to the articular cartilage of the patella. The damage can range from softening of the cartilage to complete cartilage destruction resulting in exposure of subchondral bone.

Inference:

What is the most likely contributing factor in the development of this condition?

The exact etiology of patellofemoral syndrome is unknown, however, it is extremely common during adolescence, is more prevalent in females than males, and has a direct association with the activity level of the patient. In an older population patellofemoral syndrome is often associated with osteoarthritis. Additional factors associated with patellofemoral syndrome include patella alta, insufficient lateral femoral condyle, weak vastus medialis obliquus, excessive pronation, excessive knee valgus, and tightness in lower extremity muscles (the iliotibial, hamstrings, gastrocnemius, and vastus lateralis).

Confirmation:

What is the most likely clinical presentation?

A patient with patellofemoral syndrome often describes a gradual onset of anterior knee pain following an increase in physical activity. The pain is characteristically located behind the patella (retropatellar pain) and may be exacerbated with activities that increase patellofemoral compressive forces (stair climbing, jumping) and also with prolonged static positioning (sitting with the knee flexed at 90 degrees as in a car, plane, theatre). Point tenderness is common over the lateral border of the patella and crepitus may be elicited when the patella is manually compressed into the trochlear groove. Visible quadriceps atrophy may be noted in the involved lower extremity particularly along the vastus medialis obliquus. The patient may also complain of burning pain when sitting for prolonged periods of time or when ascending stairs.

What laboratory or imaging studies would confirm the diagnosis?

Laboratory or imaging studies are not commonly used to diagnose patellofemoral syndrome. X-rays are often used to rule out a fracture, examine the configuration of the patellofemoral joint, and identify potential osteophytes, joint space narrowing, patella alta, and arthritic changes. Arthrogram and arthroscopy can be used to examine the articular cartilage.

What additional information should be obtained to confirm the diagnosis?

Special tests such as Clarke's sign can be useful when attempting to confirm the diagnosis. The test is performed by applying pressure immediately proximal to the upper pole of the patient's patella. The physician/therapist then asks the patient to isometrically contract the quadriceps. A positive test is indicated by a failure to fully contract the quadriceps or by the presence of retropatellar pain. The test should be performed at varying degrees of flexion and extension. It is helpful to determine the patient's Q angle and examine the alignment of the patient's feet, as these factors can contribute to the causative factors.

Examination:

What history should be documented?

Important areas to explore include past medical history, medications, current symptoms and health status, social history, occupation/recreational activities, living environment, and social support system.

What test/measures are most appropriate?

Anthropometric characteristics: knee effusion, lower extremity circumferential measurements

Arousal, attention, and cognition: examine mental status, learning ability, memory, motivation

Assistive and adaptive devices: components and safety of a device, potential utilization of crutches

Environmental, home, and work barriers: analysis of current and potential barriers or hazards

Gait, locomotion, and balance: safety during gait with an assistive device

Integumentary integrity: assessment of sensation (pain, temperature, tactile), skin assessment

Joint integrity and mobility: Clarke's sign, patella grind test (active and passive), dynamic patella tracking, patella glide test, palpation of structures, joint play, soft tissue restrictions, joint pain

Muscle performance: strength assessment, assessment of active movement, resisted isometrics, muscle contraction characteristics, muscle endurance

Orthotic, protective, and supportive devices: potential utilization of bracing, taping or wrapping

Pain: pain perception assessment scale

Range of motion: active and passive range of motion

Self-care and home management: functional capacity

Sensory integrity: proprioception and kinesthesia

What additional findings are likely with this patient?

Patients diagnosed with patellofemoral syndrome often have an increased Q angle. The normal Q angle is 13 degrees in males and 18 degrees in females. The Q angle is measured using the anterior superior iliac spine, the midpoint of the patella, and the tibial tubercle. Differential diagnosis should rule out other problems such as referred pain from the hip, Osgood-Schlatter syndrome, neuroma, patellar tendonitis, plica syndrome, and infection of the knee joint.

Management:

What is the most effective management of this patient?

Medical management of patellofemoral syndrome is usually successful with conservative measures, surgical intervention is rare. Pharmacological intervention may include acetaminophen, NSAIDs, and steroid injections into the joint. Physical therapy management includes controlling edema, stretching, strengthening, improving range of motion, and activity modification. Mobilization activities to increase medial glide can be beneficial to increase the flexibility of the lateral fascia. Strengthening activities emphasizing the vastus medialis obliquus in non-weight bearing and weight bearing positions are recommended. Biofeedback can be a useful tool in order to selectively train the muscle. Stretching activities should emphasize the hamstrings, iliotibial band, tensor fasciae latae, and rectus femoris. Strengthening activities may include quadriceps setting exercises, straight leg raising and mini-squats incorporating the hip adductors. Exercises such as deep squats should be avoided since they will tend to aggravate the patient's condition. Patellar taping to improve the position and tracking of the patella during dynamic activities can be useful to limit irritation.

What home care regimen should be recommended?

The home care regimen should consist of range of motion, strengthening, stretching, palliative care, and functional activities. An active patient must decrease their level of activities to relieve the additional stress placed on the patellofemoral joint. A patient must also comply with recommendations for proper footwear and orthotics to improve alignment and lessen aggravation of symptoms, specifically knee pain.

Outcome:

What is the likely outcome of a course in physical therapy?

A patient with patellofemoral syndrome that undergoes conservative management may be able to return to their previous functioning within four to six weeks.

What are the long-term effects of the patient's condition?

Prognosis for a full recovery is good with successful conservative management, however, failure to adequately address the cause of the patellofemoral syndrome will likely result in a patient's condition further deteriorating. The patient may experience increased irritation of the patellofemoral joint that further impacts their ability to participate in activities of daily living. Periodic exacerbations of the condition most commonly due to an increased activity level may require further physical therapy intervention.

Comparison:

What are the distinguishing characteristics of a similar condition?

Patellar tendonitis is an overuse condition characterized by inflammatory changes of the patellar tendon. The condition is most prevalent in athletes who participate in activities requiring repetitive jumping skills. The primary complaint is often pain over the anterior portion of the superior tibia with activities such as jumping or ascending/descending stairs. Patients may also experience pain after prolonged sitting and often exhibit point tenderness at the superior pole of the patella tendon. Management of patellar tendonitis incorporates many of the same interventions as patellofemoral syndrome such as range of motion, stretching, and palliative care.

Clinical Scenarios:

Scenario One

A 14-year-old female is referred to physical therapy with patellofemoral syndrome. The patient has mild edema and is sensitive to light touch over the anterior surface of the knee. The patient reports gaining ten pounds and expresses that she is willing to do "anything" to improve her present condition.

Scenario Two

A 45-year-old male is referred to physical therapy after experiencing anterior knee pain for the last week. The patient is 19 weeks status post ACL reconstruction and has recently returned to a softball league. The patient reports an insidious onset of pain and insists that he has been faithful to his home program. A note from the referring physician confirms that the integrity of the graft is fine and he suspects patellofemoral syndrome.

Peripheral Vascular Disease

Diagnosis:

What condition produces a patient's symptoms?

Peripheral vascular disease (PVD) is a condition where there has been narrowing of the lumen of blood vessels causing a reduction in circulation usually secondary to atherosclerosis. This can be compounded by either emboli or thrombi.

An injury was most likely sustained to which structure?

PVD, also known as arteriosclerosis obliterans, is primarily the result of atherosclerosis. Damage can occur to the walls of both arteries and veins from fatty plaque buildup that creates hard and narrow vessels. The atherosclerotic process will gradually progress to significant or complete occlusion of medium and large arteries.

Inference:

What is the most likely contributing factor in the development of this condition?

The primary factor for developing PVD is atherosclerosis. Other etiologies and risk factors that have been associated with the development of PVD may include phlebitis, injury or surgery, autoimmune disease, diabetes mellitus, smoking, hyperlipidemia, inactivity, hypertension, positive family history, increased age, and obesity.

Confirmation:

What is the most likely clinical presentation?

Symptoms and clinical presentation will differ depending on which vessel or blood flow has been compromised. During the early stages of PVD intermittent claudication may be the only manifestation. Symptoms are precipitated by walking a predictable distance and are normally relieved by rest. Claudication also may present as buckling or "giving out" of the lower extremity after a certain period of exertion and may not demonstrate the typical symptom of pain on exertion. Other symptoms may include tingling and numbness of the affected extremities, pain at rest and during sleep, slowed healing, changes in skin coloring, a decrease in skin temperature, absence of hair on the extremity, and a weak or absent pulse.

What laboratory or imaging studies would confirm the diagnosis?

Routine blood tests generally are indicated and include CBC, BUN, creatinine, and electrolytes studies. Doppler ultrasound studies are used to determine flow status. MRI, angiogram or arteriogram can also be used to assist with the diagnosis.

What additional information should be obtained to confirm the diagnosis?

The ankle-brachial index (ABI) can be used to provide a ratio of systolic blood pressure of the lower extremity compared to the upper extremity. An ABI above 0.90 is normal; 0.70-0.90 indicates mild peripheral vascular disease; 0.50-0.70 indicates moderate disease; and less than 0.50 indicates severe peripheral vascular disease. A rubor of dependency test, transcutaneous oximetry, and treadmill exercise test may also assist with baseline information and diagnosis of insufficiency.

Examination:

What history should be documented?

Important areas to explore include past medical history, medications, current health status, nutritional status, social history and habits, occupation, living environment, and social support system.

What test/measures are most appropriate?

Aerobic capacity and endurance: assessment of vital signs at rest and with activity, perceived exertion scale, pulse oximetry, auscultation of the lungs
Arousal, attention, and cognition: examine mental status, memory, motivation
Assistive and adaptive devices: analysis of components and safety of a device
Community and work integration: analysis of community, work, and leisure activities
Environmental, home, and work barriers: analysis of current and potential barriers or hazards
Gait, locomotion, and balance: static and dynamic balance in sitting and standing, safety during gait with/without an assistive device, Functional Ambulation Profile
Integumentary integrity: skin assessment, assessment of sensation
Muscle performance: strength assessment
Pain: pain perception assessment scale, visual analog scale, assessment of muscle soreness
Posture: analysis of resting and dynamic posture
Range of motion: active and passive range of motion
Self-care and home management: assessment of functional capacity, Functional Independence Measure
Sensory integrity: proprioception and kinesthesia
Ventilation, respiration, and circulation: palpation of pulses, pulse oximetry, ABI, capillary refilling test

What additional findings are likely with this patient?

Ischemic rest pain can occur from the combination of PVD and inadequate perfusion. It is fairly common for a patient with PVD to be diagnosed with coronary artery disease or diabetes mellitus. There is a higher risk for complications such as deep vein thrombosis, insufficiency ulcers, gangrene, and amputation.

Management:

What is the most effective management of this patient?

The medical management of a patient with PVD should include a physician, psychiatrist or psychologist, nurse, nutritionist, occupational therapist, physical therapist, vocational therapist, and case manager. Pharmacological intervention may be utilized to reduce morbidity and prevent complications. Anticoagulants such as heparin, antiplatelet agents and thrombolytics may be indicated. Patient education is paramount regarding the disease process, limb protection, foot and skin care, and risk factor reduction (smoking cessation, avoid cold exposure). Physical therapy is an important component in the treatment of PVD. A walking program will initially have the patient walk until near maximal pain and then rest until the pain is relieved. The goal is to have the patient achieve longer walking periods with less rest, eventually walking for 30 minutes continuously. Non-weight bearing exercises such as swimming or stationary cycling can supplement the program. After 4-6 weeks of therapy including isometric and active range exercises, the patient should tolerate the implementation of resistive exercise. Physical rehabilitation, involving dynamic aerobic exercise and resistance training improves cardiovascular endurance and demonstrates a positive impact on patient function and independence. In more severe cases, surgical intervention may be required. Common procedures include balloon angioplasty, endarterectomy, stent implantation or bypass surgery.

What home care regimen should be recommended?

A patient must continue with their walking program and a generalized exercise program to tolerance. They should perform skin and foot inspections daily and continue with smoking cessation and a low cholesterol diet. For patients with pain at rest, particularly at night, the head of the bed should be elevated 4-6 inches, which should improve lower extremity perfusion by the effects of gravity on blood flow.

Outcome:

What is the likely outcome of a course in physical therapy?

Physical therapy can be instrumental in managing PVD through education of the disease process, implementing a walking program that allows for the development of collateral circulation, and designing an exercise program that allows the patient to gain strength and endurance for activities. The patient must have the desire, discipline, and motivation to continue with habit modification and maintain their exercise regimen in order to be successful.

What are the long-term effects of the patient's condition?

PVD can be controllable with pharmacological treatment, risk factor reduction, and in some cases, surgical intervention. Patients with PVD are at a higher risk overall for complications such as permanent numbness, tingling or weakness in lower extremities and/or feet, permanent sensory changes such as burning or aching pain, gangrene, and amputation of the affected body part. Patients with PVD are also at higher risk of heart attack and stroke. Symptomatic PVD has at least a 30% risk of death within five years and approximately 50% in ten years, secondary to MI or cerebrovascular disease.

Comparison:

What are the distinguishing characteristics of a similar condition?

Coronary artery disease (CAD) is the narrowing or blockage due to fatty build up (cholesterol) within the artery walls reducing the overall blood flow to the cardiac muscle. Patient symptoms will vary based on the location and severity of blockage. Patients range from asymptomatic to symptoms at rest. These symptoms can include nausea, vomiting, heartburn, shortness of breath, and profuse sweating. Risk factors include hypertension, smoking, obesity, stress, elevated cholesterol, and sedentary lifestyle. Electrocardiograms and angiograms are typically used to diagnose CAD.

Clinical Scenarios:

Scenario One

A 66-year-old male is seen in physical therapy with a new diagnosis of PVD. The patient's past medical history consists of L5 disc herniation with surgical stabilization and type II diabetes mellitus. The patient complains of increasing lower extremity pain with ambulation while at his job as a surveyor. The patient lives alone and has two dogs.

Scenario Two

An 82-year-old female is seen in physical therapy in an acute care hospital with orders for whirlpool secondary to an ulcer on her right lower extremity. The patient has moderate to severe PVD affecting both lower extremities. She presents with sensory loss and significant pain with ambulation greater than 20 feet. She also complains of pain at night. She resides with her husband in a first floor apartment.

Plantar Fasciitis

Diagnosis:

What condition produces a patient's symptoms?

The plantar fascia is a thin layer of tough connective tissue that supports the arch of the foot. Plantar fasciitis is an inflammatory process of the plantar fascia (or aponeurosis) at its origin on the calcaneus. Plantar fasciitis is a chronic overuse condition that develops secondary to repetitive stretching of the plantar fascia through excessive foot pronation during the loading phase of gait. This results in stress at the calcaneal origin of the plantar fascia.

An injury was most likely sustained to which structure?

Injury can occur to the plantar fascia itself and cause microtearing, inflammation, and pain. The abductor hallucis, flexor digitorum brevis, and quadratus plantae muscles share the same origin on the medial tubercle of the calcaneus and may also become inflamed and irritated.

Inference:

What is the most likely contributing factor in the development of this condition?

Factors that contribute to the development of plantar fasciitis include excessive pronation during gait, tightness of the foot and calf musculature, obesity, and possessing a high arch. A person participating in endurance sports such as running and dancing or a person with an occupation that requires prolonged walking or standing has an increased risk for plantar fasciitis. It is believed that development of plantar fasciitis results from a combination of predisposing factors. Although it is more common in the middle-age population, it also occurs in younger individuals, but usually in combination with calcaneal apophysitis.

Confirmation:

What is the most likely clinical presentation?

A patient with plantar fasciitis presents with severe pain in the heel when first standing up in the morning (when the fascia is contracted, stiff, and cold). This pain has also been reported to radiate proximally up the calf and/or distally to the toes. This is the most common symptom that relates directly to the diagnosis of plantar fasciitis and in one study was expressed in over 84% of cases. Pain typically subsides for a few hours during the day, but increases with prolonged activity or when the patient has been non-weight bearing and resumes a weight bearing posture. Pain has also been described by patients as "pain that moves around." A patient will typically experience point tenderness and pain with palpation over the calcaneal insertion of the plantar fascia. There may be bony growths in the plantar fascia near its insertion. Plantar fasciitis is usually unilateral and tightness in the Achilles tendon is found in the majority of the patients.

What laboratory or imaging studies would confirm the diagnosis?

Plantar fasciitis is initially treated based on symptoms and physical examination. If pain persists after six to eight weeks of physical therapy intervention, MRI may be used to confirm the diagnosis. Other diagnostic tools may include x-ray and bone scan to rule out a stress fracture, rheumatology work up to rule out systemic etiology, and EMG testing to rule out nerve entrapment.

What additional information should be obtained to confirm the diagnosis?

A thorough history and biomechanical assessment of the foot, observation of the fat pad, examination for Achilles tendon tightness, analysis of footwear, and gait disturbances all assist in diagnosing plantar fasciitis.

Examination:

What history should be documented?

Important areas to explore include mechanism of current injury, training routine, past medical history, medications, social history and habits, occupation, living environment, and social support system.

What test/measures are most appropriate?

Anthropometric characteristics: circumferential measurements of affected area or extremity

Arousal, attention, and cognition: examine mental status, learning ability, memory, motivation

Community and work integration: analysis of community, work, and leisure activities

Environmental, home, and work barriers: analysis of current and potential barriers or hazards

Gait, locomotion, and balance: biomechanical analysis of gait during walking and running (if appropriate), footprint analysis, dynamic plantar pressure distribution

Integumentary inspection: assessment of sensation, skin assessment

Joint integrity and mobility: assessment of swelling, inflammation, and joint restriction

Muscle performance: strength assessment, muscle endurance

Pain: pain perception scale, visual analog scale

Orthotic, protective, and supportive devices: potential utilization of taping or use of cushions

Posture: analysis of resting and dynamic posture

Range of motion: active and passive range of motion

Sensory integrity: assessment of proprioception and kinesthesia

Self-care and home management: assessment of functional capacity

What additional findings are likely with this patient?

Bony hypertrophy can occur at the origin of the plantar fascia resulting in a heel spur. Plantar fasciitis is a relative of heel spur syndrome, but is not the same condition. Heel spurs develop initially as calcium deposits that form due to the repetitive stress and inflammation in the plantar fascia.

Management:

What is the most effective management of this patient?

Medical and pharmacological management of a patient with plantar fasciitis usually requires local corticosteroid injections or anti-inflammatory medications to reduce inflammation within the plantar fascia. Physical therapy intervention consists of ice massage, deep friction massage, shoe modification, heel insert application, foot orthotic prescription, modification of activities to include non-weight bearing endurance activities, and a gentle stretching program of the Achilles tendon and plantar fascia. Muscle strengthening exercises for the intrinsic and extrinsic muscles should be implemented once the acute symptoms have subsided. During the acute phase the patient must also modify activities and rest the affected foot. Heel cup prescription and casting may also be indicated.

What home care regimen should be recommended?

A home care regimen for a patient with plantar fasciitis should include ongoing strengthening and stretching exercises (especially stretching of the gastrocnemius and medial fascial band in the morning and prior to and after exercise), maintenance of a fitness program, the use of proper footwear, and the use of foot orthotics and heel inserts if warranted. Night tension splints may be indicated if symptoms persist.

Outcome:

What is the likely outcome of a course in physical therapy?

Conservative physical therapy intervention on an outpatient basis in combination with a consistent home program should allow the patient to return to a more functional level within eight weeks. Total resolution of symptoms can take up to twelve months. Physical therapy, orthotic prescription, splinting, pharmacological injections, and physician follow-up are all components of the treatment program that may be required for a positive outcome.

What are the long-term effects of the patient's condition?

A patient previously diagnosed with plantar fasciitis is at an increased risk for recurrence, however, successful conservative management, compliance with a home program, and proper footwear will decrease the incidence of any negative long-term effects. If conservative management fails the patient may require surgical intervention, however, this option is relatively rare. Approximately 10% of patients can develop persistent, chronic, and disabling symptoms.

Comparison:

What are the distinguishing characteristics of a similar condition?

The tarsal tunnel is the region where the tibial nerve passes between the medial malleolus and the calcaneus. The tibial nerve splits into the medial and lateral plantar nerves while still traversing in the tunnel along with other nerves in this region. Tarsal tunnel syndrome is characterized by pain that is experienced with weight bearing, but not with direct palpation to the plantar fascia. Characteristics of tarsal tunnel syndrome include complaints of numbness, burning pain, tingling, and paresthesias at the heel. Etiology consists of entrapment and compression of the posterior tibial nerve or plantar nerves within the tarsal tunnel due to inflammation or thickening of the flexor retinaculum.

Clinical Scenarios:

Scenario One

A 19-year-old male athlete is referred to physical therapy with bilateral heel pain. The physician has ruled out systemic disorders and diagnosed bilateral mechanical plantar fasciitis. The athlete is a swimmer and began running cross-country last fall. The patient is otherwise healthy, but wants to return to athletic activities as soon as possible.

Scenario Two

A 56-year-old female is referred to physical therapy with left plantar fasciitis. The patient is mildly obese and works the night shift at a paper mill. She stands at her station throughout the shift and is required to walk between the two buildings every hour. The patient has a history of mild asthma and a cardiac murmur. She is anxious to obtain relief from her symptoms since she feels that her employment may be jeopardized.

Pressure Ulcer

Diagnosis:

What condition produces a patient's symptoms?

A pressure ulcer is a type of ulcer or wound caused by unrelieved pressure to a specific area that results in damage to the underlying tissues. The unrelieved pressure deprives the tissues of oxygen, which causes ischemia to the site, subsequent cell death, and tissue necrosis. A definition of unrelieved pressure is >32 mm Hg of pressure to an area for more than two hours.

An injury was most likely sustained to which structure?

A pressure ulcer can affect different structures based on the degree or staging of the ulcer. Damage can be contained to only the epidermis in stage I ulcers, while stage IV ulcers will include damage to the epidermis, dermis, the fascia and deeper, potentially damaging muscles, ligaments, tendons and/or bones. The most high risk areas for pressure ulcers include the occiput, heels, greater trochanters, ischial tuberosities, sacrum, and epicondyles of the elbow.

Inference:

What is the most likely contributing factor in the development of this condition?

A pressure ulcer can occur at any time secondary to unrelieved pressure, but there are certain populations and risk factors that are associated with its development. Immobility is a leading factor and is seen with populations such as spinal cord injury, other paralysis, and hemiplegia. Impaired cognition, poor nutrition, altered sensation, incontinence, decreased lean body mass, and infection are other contributing factors in the development of a pressure ulcer. At the cellular level, the interface pressure, shear and/or friction are the contributing factors in the development of a pressure ulcer.

Confirmation:

What is the most likely clinical presentation?

A patient will usually develop a pressure ulcer over a bony prominence with common sites including the greater trochanter, ischium, sacrum, and heel. A stage I pressure ulcer is classified as an area of nonblanchable erythema of intact skin. There may also be an increase in warmth to the site or altered coloration. Stage II is classified as a partial thickness wound involving the epidermis, dermis or both. This ulcer does not extend through the entire dermis. Stage III is classified as an ulcer that has extended into subcutaneous tissue, but not through fascia. Stage IV is classified as an ulcer that extends through the fascia and deeper. It is a full thickness wound that may damage muscles, bones, ligaments and/or tendons. Pressure ulcers will vary in color, odor, drainage, and volume.

What laboratory or imaging studies would confirm the diagnosis?

A diagnosis is made from visual inspection, however, blood studies such as a CBC, electrolyte, and protein levels, as well as tests for bacteremia or sepsis may be indicated. Urinalysis and stool samples may be indicated to determine contributing factors in the development of the ulcer. Coagulation studies and tissue sampling may also be indicated.

What additional information should be obtained to confirm the diagnosis?

Extensive examination and photography of the site are necessary for accurate baseline data. A patient's history and current status are also important factors in designing the plan of care. Diagnosis of staging of the ulcer requires the use of the Braden Scale, Gosnell Scale or Norton Scale along with baseline measurements of size and depth of the ulcer.

Examination:

What history should be documented?

Important areas to explore include past medical history, medications, current health status, history of incontinence, nutritional status, social history, living environment, occupation, and social support system.

What test/measures are most appropriate?

Aerobic capacity and endurance: assessment of vital signs at rest and with activity
Arousal, attention, and cognition: examine mental status, learning ability, memory and motivation
Environmental, home, and work barriers: analysis of current and potential barriers or hazards
Gait, locomotion, and balance: static and dynamic balance in sitting and standing, safety during gait with/without an assistive device
Integumentary integrity: skin assessment, assessment of sensation, Braden Scale, Norton Scale, photography of ulcer, eschar, granulation formation, Gosnell Scale
Joint integrity and mobility: assessment of hyper- and hypomobility of a joint, soft tissue swelling and inflammation
Muscle performance: strength assessment
Pain: pain perception assessment scale, VAS
Posture: analysis of resting and dynamic posture
Range of motion: active and passive range of motion
Sensory integrity: proprioception and kinesthesia

What additional findings are likely with this patient?

Complications that may prevent healing of the ulcer include infection, osteomyelitis, sepsis, pain, spasticity, malnutrition, incontinence, and depression. Patients at high risk may also develop multiple ulcers at once.

Management:

What is the most effective management of this patient?

Patient and caregiver education for the prevention of subsequent pressure ulcers is very important and should include skin inspection, positioning, and pressure relief techniques. The use of pressure reducing devices such as seat cushions, multipodus boots or specialized mattresses is also an important aspect to the overall care of ulcers. Pharmacological intervention may include antimicrobials and antibiotics to fight infection and allow for proper healing. Dressings for the ulcer may include nonocclusive or occlusive types of dressings. Nonocclusive dressings include dry to dry, wet to wet, wet to dry or composite dressings. Occlusive dressings include semipermeable films, hydrocolloids, hydrogels, semipermeable foams, and alginates. The ulcer may require cleansing agents, and/or debridement (enzymatic, mechanical non-selective or sharp). Mobility training and proper positioning for the patient will also be vital in order to decrease forces of shear and friction upon the site of the ulcer. A general exercise program should be initiated as well as mobility training to tolerance. Skin inspection should be provided daily and photography should be documented regularly to track the progress of healing. Patients should avoid the use of hot water and the use of massage surrounding the site. The therapist should promote proper positioning techniques (such as positioning of the bed at less than a 45 degree angle) in order to decrease friction and shear forces.

What home care regimen should be recommended?

The home care regimen is dependent on the size and staging of the pressure sore. The patient should continue with the appropriate schedule for dressings and follow physician orders. The patient should maintain an appropriate activity level, use correct positioning, and receive adequate protein and calorie intake to assist with the healing process. The patient should use a mild cleansing agent, dry and wrinkle free sheets for their bed, and appropriate moisturizers.

Outcome:

What is the likely outcome of a course in physical therapy?

The care of ulcers is estimated to cost $6 billion dollars annually which makes this diagnosis the most costly preventable injury. Approximately 60,000 patients die annually due to secondary complications from ulcers. However, many people that develop a pressure ulcer completely recover with no residual impairments.

What are the long-term effects of the patient's condition?

Treatment of a pressure ulcer should provide a normal path of recovery without any residual deficits. If there is infection or complications to healing, the patient may have to undergo additional treatment such as further pharmacological intervention or surgical procedures. If the patient is in a high risk group for skin breakdown the patient may require the ongoing use of a pressure relief seating system or air mattress for the bed.

Comparison:

What are the distinguishing characteristics of a similar condition?

A neuropathic ulcer is an ulcer that develops due to the lack of neural function, which occurs commonly in patients with diabetes mellitus. Other high risk groups include spinal cord injury, stroke, spina bifida, sensory neuropathies, and tumors. The feet are the prime region for neuropathic ulcers in the diabetic patient. These ulcers occur in areas of weight bearing where there are mechanical shear forces such as under the metatarsal heads. These ulcers are usually round in shape and are not painful. It is believed that these ulcers occur not only due to motor neuropathy, but also impairment of the sensory and autonomic systems. Approximately 15% of patients with diabetes mellitus will develop a foot ulcer. Treatment is usually the same as with a pressure ulcer, but care must be taken to continually assess progress since there is usually motor and sensory damage surrounding the ulcer site.

Clinical Scenarios:

Scenario One

A 31-year-old male has been in the hospital for four weeks secondary to a motor vehicle accident. He was in a coma for ten days and was required to stay in bed due to multiple fractures for three of the four weeks. He developed a stage two pressure ulcer on his right heel and has orders for whirlpool treatment. He is being discharged home alone in two weeks to his two-story home and is currently NWB on the right lower extremity and WBAT on the left lower extremity.

Scenario Two

An 85-year-old female is admitted to the hospital due to a stage four pressure ulcer on her sacrum. She had been cared for at home by her husband since her stroke four months ago. The husband states that the wife remained in bed most of the time, has lost over 30 pounds, and presents with some mild cognitive deficits.

Reflex Sympathetic Dystrophy

Diagnosis:

What condition produces a patient's symptoms?

Reflex sympathetic dystrophy (RSD), also known as complex regional pain syndrome type I (occurring subsequent to trauma) or complex regional pain syndrome type II (associated with peripheral nerve injury) is usually found in an extremity that has experienced some form of trauma. Symptoms result from a disturbance in the functioning of the sympathetic nervous system. The increase in sympathetic activity causes a release of norepinephrine in the periphery and subsequent vasoconstriction of blood vessels. This results in pain and an increase in sensitivity to peripheral stimulation.

An injury was most likely sustained to which structure?

RSD results from injured sensory nerve fibers at one somatic level that initiates sympathetic efferent activity that affects many segmental levels. The extremity of origin sustains injury as well as areas adjacent to the extremity.

Inference:

What is the most likely contributing factor in the development of this condition?

The exact etiology of RSD is unknown, however, predisposing factors include trauma, surgery, CVA, TBI, repetitive motion disorders, and lower motor neuron and peripheral nerve injuries. RSD is reported to occur following 5% of all injuries. While many cases of RSD resolve, others progress and become a disabling disorder. RSD can affect all age groups but is most likely found in the age group of 35-60 years with females three times more likely to be affected by RSD than males.

Confirmation:

What is the most likely clinical presentation?

A patient with RSD will experience intense, burning, and chronic pain in the affected extremity that will eventually spread proximally. Early in the syndrome the degree of pain is greater than expected based on the amount of trauma that the tissue sustained. Edema, thermal changes, discoloration, stiffness, and dryness are seen during stage I (acute stage) of RSD. Progression to stage II (dystrophic stage) is characterized by worsening and constant pain, continued edema, and trophic skin changes. X-rays may reveal bone loss, osteoporosis, and subchondral bone erosion in the affected extremity. Stage III (atrophic stage) is characterized by pain that continues to spread, hardened edema, decreased limb temperature, and atrophic changes to fingertips or toes. X-rays at this stage may reveal demineralization and ankylosis. Motor disorders such as tremor, spasms, and atrophy may also be present throughout each stage of RSD.

What laboratory or imaging studies would confirm the diagnosis?

Imaging studies that can assist with the diagnosis of RSD include X-rays, thermographic studies, a three-phase bone scan, and laser Doppler flowmetry.

What additional information should be obtained to confirm the diagnosis?

RSD is diagnosed primarily through a complete physical examination and a patient's complete medical history including a history and course of illness.

Examination:

What history should be documented?

Important areas to explore include past medical history, medications, family history, current symptoms, current health status, social history and habits, occupation, leisure activities, and social support system.

What test/measures are most appropriate?

Anthropometric characteristics: circumferential measurements of affected area or extremity
Arousal, attention, and cognition: examine mental status, learning ability, memory, motivation
Environmental, home, and work barriers: analysis of current and potential barriers or hazards
Gait, locomotion, and balance: static and dynamic balance in sitting and standing, safety during gait
Integumentary integrity: skin assessment, assessment of sensation, skin temperature changes
Joint integrity and mobility: assessment of hyper- and hypomobility of a joint, soft tissue swelling
Motor function: motor assessment scales, assessment of sensorimotor integration, physical performance scales
Muscle performance: strength assessment, muscle tone assessment
Pain: pain perception scale, visual analog scale, assessment of muscle soreness, McGill Pain Questionnaire
Reflex integrity: assessment of deep tendon and pathological reflexes
Posture: analysis of resting and dynamic posture
Range of motion: active and passive range of motion
Sensory integrity: assessment of proprioception and kinesthesia
Self-care and home management: assessment of functional capacity

What additional findings are likely with this patient?

RSD will affect a patient's function throughout the progression of this neurovascular syndrome. RSD may progress to the point of bone demineralization and joint ankylosis (seen in stage III). Muscle atrophy, contractures, spasms, and incoordination will also contribute to functional decline. Depression and anxiety are also frequently seen and require medical attention. Malingering for secondary gain has been documented in some cases and should be monitored by the rehabilitation team.

Management:

What is the most effective management of this patient?

RSD requires prolonged medical management. Treatment is based on identifying the underlying cause and stage of RSD at the time of diagnosis. Pharmacological intervention may include NSAIDs and corticosteroids for pain relief in early stages. Amitriptyline may be used for sleep and calcium channel blockers used for increasing peripheral circulation. Baclofen has been used as a long-term intervention to assist motor function. Biphosphonate administration is warranted in later stages to combat bone loss. Surgical interventions such as sympathetic blocks or a sympathectomy are used to alleviate pain. Physical therapy intervention is a key component in the management of RSD. Pain control, patient education, skin care, joint mobilization, desensitization, and functional activity training are vital to the program. Modalities, pool therapy, relaxation training, and a home program all assist a patient with management of this syndrome.

What home care regimen should be recommended?

A home program is vital to the management of RSD. Stretching and ROM, light weight bearing activities, ice and/or heat, TENS, and light exercise for conditioning are all key components of a home program. The patient must be educated and encouraged to use the involved extremity as tolerated. Edema management using a pump or compression garments may be indicated. Functional activities must also be encouraged.

Outcome:

What is the likely outcome of a course in physical therapy?

Overall prognosis is better for a patient that begins treatment early in the cycle of the disease process. Physical therapy attempts to break the pain cycle and allows for a patient to continue with functional activities. Outcome is also dependent on a patient's motivation to maintain all aspects of a home program.

What are the long-term effects of the patient's condition?

RSD can spontaneously resolve or can continue with ongoing symptoms that can last for years or follow a pattern of remissions and recurring symptoms that develop from subsequent injuries. A patient's long-term outcome is dependent on how early the RSD was detected and treated. Research indicates a better prognosis if treatment is initiated within the first six months of the disease process.

Comparison:

What are the distinguishing characteristics of a similar condition?

Sympathetically maintained pain (SMP) is a pain syndrome that is maintained by sympathetic efferent activity and is caused by a partial peripheral nerve lesion. SMP occurs less than RSD and is characterized by pain that is produced by a non-painful stimulus, vasomotor disturbances, and trophic changes. These symptoms remain localized to the affected nerve and the pain can usually be temporarily alleviated by sympathetic nerve block. Physical therapy intervention is warranted to assist with pain control through the use of modalities.

Clinical Scenarios:

Scenario One

A 39-year-old female is seen in physical therapy with stage I (acute) RSD. The patient complains of burning pain in her left arm and presents with mild edema. The patient injured her shoulder two months ago. Past medical history includes being diagnosed with fibromyalgia two years ago. She is a team manager for a photography company and works approximately 50 hours per week.

Scenario Two

A 62-year-old female is evaluated in physical therapy. She was diagnosed with RSD 13 months ago. She complains of significant pain in her right lower extremity and cannot walk without a walker. She has both hip and knee flexion contractures and significant swelling of the affected lower extremity.

Restrictive Lung Disease

Diagnosis:

What condition produces a patient's symptoms?

Restrictive lung disease (RLD) is a classification of disorders caused by a pulmonary or extrapulmonary restriction that produces impairment in lung expansion and an abnormal reduction in pulmonary ventilation. There are multiple conditions that can cause restrictive lung disease. Many symptoms are common regardless of the underlying etiology and other symptoms are disease-specific.

An injury was most likely sustained to which structure?

Pulmonary restriction of the lungs can be caused by tumor, interstitial pulmonary fibrosis, scarring within the lungs, and pneumonia. Extrapulmonary restrictions of the lungs include pleural effusion, chest wall stiffness, structural abnormality, postural deformity, respiratory muscle weakness, and central nervous system injury.

Inference:

What is the most likely contributing factor in the development of this condition?

There are varying etiologies for the group of disorders that cause restrictive lung disease. Musculoskeletal etiology includes scoliosis, pectus excavatum or other chest wall deformity, rib fractures, ankylosing spondylitis, and kyphosis. Pulmonary etiology includes idiopathic pulmonary fibrosis, pneumonia, pleural effusion, sarcoidosis, hyaline membrane disease, and tumor within the lungs. Other etiologies include inhalation of toxic fumes, drug therapy, asbestos, rheumatoid arthritis, systemic lupus erythematosus, muscular dystrophy, spinal cord injury, obesity, neurologic, and neuromuscular diseases.

Confirmation:

What is the most likely clinical presentation?

The clinical presentation varies based on the underlying cause or disease process. The pathogenesis of RLD includes a decrease in lung and chest wall compliance, decrease in lung volumes and an increase in the work of breathing. Generally, restrictive lung disease is characterized by a reduction of lung volumes (total lung capacity, vital capacity, inspiratory reserve volume, tidal volume, expiratory reserve volume, and inspiratory capacity) due to impaired lung expansion. A patient with restrictive lung disease will present with decreased chest mobility, decreased breath sounds, shortness of breath, hypoxemia, a rapid and shallow respiratory pattern (tachypnea), respiratory muscle weakness, ineffective cough, and increased use of accessory muscles.

What laboratory or imaging studies would confirm the diagnosis?

A chest radiograph is utilized to evaluate lung structure and evidence of fibrosis, infiltrates, tumor, and deformity. Arterial blood gas analysis may indicate a decrease in PaO_2.

What additional information should be obtained to confirm the diagnosis?

Pulmonary function testing will result in impaired vital capacity (VC), forced vital capacity (FVC), and total lung capacity (TLC). The patient will usually present with normal residual volume (RV) and expiration flow rates. Expiratory reserve volume (ERV) and functional residual capacity (FRC) are often decreased. Arterial blood gas analysis examines the presence of hypoxemia and hypocapnia.

Examination:

What history should be documented?

Important areas to explore include past medical history, medications, current health status, social history and habits, occupation, living environment, and social support system.

What test/measures are most appropriate?

Aerobic capacity and endurance: assessment of vital signs at rest and with activity, perceived exertion scale, pulse oximetry, auscultation of the lungs

Arousal, attention, and cognition: examine mental status, learning ability, memory, motivation

Assistive and adaptive devices: analysis of components and safety of a device

Environmental, home, and work barriers: analysis of current and potential barriers or hazards

Gait, locomotion, and balance: static and dynamic balance in sitting and standing, safety during gait with/without an assistive device, Berg Balance Scale, Tinetti Performance Oriented Mobility Assessment, Functional Ambulation Profile

Motor function: assessment of dexterity, coordination and agility, assessment of postural, equilibrium, and righting reactions

Muscle performance: strength assessment, active movement

Posture: analysis of resting and dynamic posture

Range of motion: active and passive range of motion

Self-care and home management: assessment of functional capacity

Ventilation, respiration, and circulation: auscultation of breath sounds, thoracoabdominal movement, pulmonary function testing, perceived exertion scale, assessment of cough and clearance of secretions

What additional findings are likely with this patient?

A patient with restrictive lung disease may become incapable of deep inspiration due to poor lung expansion. As restrictive lung disease progresses respiratory muscle fatigue will lead to impaired alveolar ventilation and carbon dioxide retention. A patient will initially present with exertional dyspnea and progress to dyspnea at rest if the restriction progresses. Hypoxemia, pulmonary hypertension, cor pulmonale, severe decrease in oxygenation, and ventilatory failure are complications and outcomes of advanced restrictive lung disease.

Management:

What is the most effective management of this patient?

Medical management of restrictive lung disease includes treatment of the underlying cause through pharmacological intervention, physical therapy, and potential surgical intervention. Physical therapy intervention is based on the severity of the condition, but is consistently oriented toward the goals of maximizing gas exchange and obtaining maximal functional capacity. Physical therapy intervention may include body mechanics, posture training, diaphragm and ventilatory muscle strengthening, relaxation and energy conservation techniques, and the use of these techniques during functional mobility. Breathing exercises, coughing techniques, and airway secretion clearance are often components of a comprehensive care plan.

What home care regimen should be recommended?

A home care regimen should include breathing strategies and exercises, proper positioning, energy conservation and pacing techniques, general strengthening and endurance activities, and postural awareness with mobility. Low-level general strengthening and endurance training are indicated as tolerated.

Outcome:

What is the likely outcome of a course in physical therapy?

Physical therapy intervention is specific to the underlying cause of the restrictive lung disease. Outcome is based on the etiology of the restrictive lung disease and patient response to physical therapy intervention. Treatment goals should include improving oxygenation and obtaining the maximal level of functioning.

What are the long-term effects of the patient's condition?

Long-term effects from restrictive lung disease are also specific to the underlying cause. Some disorders require surgical intervention that alleviates the condition while other conditions are progressive and irreversible. Some

patients with end-stage disease may be candidates for lung transplantation, however, most eventually progress to ventilatory failure. Idiopathic pulmonary fibrosis is a restrictive lung disease that has a high mortality rate within four to six years of diagnosis whereas many conditions that cause restrictive lung disease are alleviated through appropriate management.

Comparison:

What are the distinguishing characteristics of a similar condition?

Tuberculosis is an infectious and inflammatory systemic disease that can result in restrictive lung disease. The disease is a chronic pulmonary and extrapulmonary disease that causes fibrosis within the lungs. It is caused by the mycobacterium tuberculosis (tubercle bacillus) and transmitted through infected airborne droplets that are inhaled. Pulmonary symptoms include fatigue, weakness, an initial non-productive cough, and dyspnea with exertion. The disease also can affect other systems within the body including the lymph nodes and organs. Pharmacological intervention is the primary means of treating a patient with tuberculosis.

Clinical Scenarios:

Scenario One

A 32-year-old male shows signs of restrictive lung disease. The patient is slightly short of breath with activity, has difficulty with deep inspiration, and complains of a non-productive cough. The patient had prolonged exposure to asbestos at his last place of employment and is under a physician's care. The physician referred the patient to physical therapy to improve the patient's general pulmonary status.

Scenario Two

A 65-year-old female is seen in physical therapy for restrictive lung disease secondary to the removal of a benign tumor from the left lung. The patient reports having difficulty breathing, limited inhalation capability, and a productive cough. The patient has not been able to perform self-care and home activities secondary to breathing difficulties and relies solely on her 72-year-old husband.

Rheumatoid Arthritis

Diagnosis:

What condition produces a patient's symptoms?

Rheumatoid arthritis (RA) is a systemic autoimmune disorder of the connective tissue that is characterized by chronic inflammation within synovial membranes, tendon sheaths, and articular cartilage. The acute and chronic inflammatory changes produce the symptoms of this condition.

An injury was most likely sustained to which structure?

Smaller peripheral joints are usually the first to be affected by RA, however, all connective tissue may become involved. Inflammation is present within the synovial membrane and granulation tissue forms as a result of the synovitis. The granulation tissue and protein degrading enzymes erode articular cartilage resulting in destruction, adhesions, and fibrosis within the joint.

Inference:

What is the most likely contributing factor in the development of this condition?

The etiology of RA is unknown, however, there appears to be evidence of genetic predisposition with viral or bacterial triggers. Approximately 80% of individuals diagnosed with RA possess a positive rheumatoid factor (RF). RF represents the presence of autoantibodies that conflict with immunoglobulin antibodies found in the blood. The incidence of RA in women is three times greater than the incidence in men.

Confirmation:

What is the most likely clinical presentation?

RA affects approximately 1-2% of the population within the United States or two million individuals (1.5 million women, 600,000 men). This condition is characterized by periods of exacerbations and is diagnosed most frequently between 30 and 50 years of age. RA will vary in onset and progression from patient to patient. Onset of RA may be sudden or develop over a period of weeks. Early characteristics include fatigue, bilateral involvement, tenderness of smaller joints, and low-grade fever. Patients often experience pain with motion, stiffness including prolonged morning stiffness, and progression of symptoms to larger synovial joints. In late stages of the disease the heart can become affected and deformities, subluxations, and contractures can occur.

What laboratory or imaging studies would confirm the diagnosis?

Blood work assists with the diagnosis of RA through evaluation of the rheumatoid factor (RF), white blood cell count, erythrocyte sedimentation rate, hemoglobin, and hematocrit values. A synovial fluid analysis evaluates the content of synovial fluid within a joint. X-rays can be used to evaluate the joint space and the extent of decalcification.

What additional information should be obtained to confirm the diagnosis?

Physical examination and patient history of symptoms are required to confirm the diagnosis. The American Rheumatoid Association has designed diagnostic criteria for RA that can be used as a guide to determine a definite, possible, probable or classic diagnosis.

Examination:

What history should be documented?

Important areas to explore include past medical history, family history, medications, current symptoms and health status, living environment, social history and habits, occupation, and social support system.

What test/measures are most appropriate?

Aerobic capacity and endurance: assessment of vital signs at rest and with activity, timed walk, VO2 max

Anthropometric characteristics: circumferential measurements of all affected joints

Arousal, attention, and cognition: examine mental status, learning ability, memory, motivation

Community and work integration: analysis of community, work, and leisure activities

Ergonomics and body mechanics: analysis of dexterity and coordination

Environmental, home, and work barriers: analysis of current and potential barriers or hazards

Gait, locomotion, and balance: safety during gait with/without an assistive device, Functional Ambulation Profile, gait over level/unlevel surfaces, visual inspection of gait with and without shoes

Integumentary integrity: skin and sensation assessment

Joint integrity and mobility: assessment of joint hypomobility, soft tissue inflammation, presence of deformity, active joint count, articular tenderness

Motor function: equilibrium and righting reactions, motor assessment scales, coordination, posture and balance in sitting, physical performance scales

Muscle performance: break testing of isometric contractions, manometer method of strength testing

Orthotic, protective, and supportive devices: potential utilization of bracing, analysis of movement while wearing a device

Pain: pain perception assessment scale

Range of motion: active and passive range of motion

Self-care and home management: assessment of functional capacity

Sensory integrity: assessment of sensation, proprioception, and kinesthesia

What additional findings are likely with this patient?

Extraarticular manifestations with RA can include pericarditis, anemia, tearing of tendons and musculature, osteoporosis, swan neck and/or boutonniere deformities, compression neuropathies, peripheral neuropathies, depression, pleurisy, skin changes, and anorexia.

Management:

What is the most effective management of this patient?

Early medical management of a patient with RA is critical to improve the long-term outcomes of the disease. Medical treatment will focus on pain relief, reduction of edema, and preservation of joint integrity. Pharmacological intervention is required to decrease inflammation and retard the progression of the disease. NSAIDs, corticosteroids, and disease-modifying medications such as methotrexate are indicated. Physical therapy management during the acute stage or exacerbation includes patient education regarding regular rest, pain relief, relaxation, positioning, joint protection techniques, splinting, energy conservation, and body mechanics. Treatment may include gentle massage, hydrotherapy, hot pack, paraffin or cold modalities, gentle isometrics, and instruction in the use of assistive devices. Treatment during the acute stage should avoid resistive exercise, deep heating modalities, and any form of active stretching since these activities will further exacerbate the arthritis. Physical therapy management during the chronic stage or remission focuses on improving overall functional capacity, endurance, and strength. Treatment consists of low-impact conditioning through swimming or the stationary bicycle. Gentle stretching may be indicated to maintain available range of motion, however, aggressive stretching is contraindicated.

What home care regimen should be recommended?

A home care regimen for a patient with RA must maintain a delicate balance between activity and rest. The patient should perform low-level exercise, utilize relaxation and energy conservation techniques, and use splints as needed. The patient should recognize when total rest is indicated due to an acute exacerbation.

Outcome:

What is the likely outcome of a course in physical therapy?

Physical therapy cannot halt the progression of RA, however, it can improve a patient's ability to function. Physical therapy may be indicated intermittently throughout the disease process with goals that focus on pain relief, relaxation, improving motion, and preventing deformity.

What are the long-term effects of the patient's condition?

RA is a chronic disease process that currently does not have a known cure, progresses at a varied rate, creates irreversible damage and deformity, and results in disability. As the disease progresses there is bilateral and symmetrical involvement of joints. Systemic effects include insomnia, fatigue, and organ involvement including the heart and lungs.

Comparison:

What are the distinguishing characteristics of a similar condition?

Osteoarthritis is a chronic degenerative condition that usually develops secondary to repetitive trauma, disease or obesity. The hyaline cartilage in the joint softens and breaks apart allowing bone-to-bone contact that results in joint deformity, crepitus, impaired range of motion, and pain. Pain typically increases with prolonged activity. Joints become swollen and tender and joint deformity develops. Women have a slightly greater risk for OA than men. Surgical procedures including osteotomy and joint replacement may be indicated if conservative treatment is unsuccessful.

Clinical Scenarios:

Scenario One

A 38-year-old female diagnosed with RA is seen in an outpatient clinic. The patient history reveals fatigue and malaise for two to three weeks and pain in the fingers and wrists. The patient has difficulty caring for herself at home and is on medical leave from her job. The patient does not have any other significant past medical history and resides alone.

Scenario Two

A 74-year-old male diagnosed with RA is treated by a therapist. The patient presents with multi-joint involvement, deformities of the hands and feet, poor endurance, stiffness, and pain. The patient is ambulatory, however, is currently in a wheelchair secondary to pain from an exacerbation. The patient is oriented and has a history of COPD.

Rotator Cuff Tendonitis

Diagnosis:

What condition produces a patient's symptoms?

Repetitive overhead activities can produce impingement of the supraspinatus tendon immediately proximal to the greater tubercle of the humerus. The impingement is caused by an inability of a weak supraspinatus muscle to adequately depress the head of the humerus in the glenoid fossa during elevation of the arm. As a result the humerus translates superiorly due to the disproportionate action of the deltoid muscle. Primary impingement occurs from intrinsic or extrinsic factors within the subacromial space. Secondary impingement describes symptoms that occur from poor mechanics or instability at the shoulder joint.

An injury was most likely sustained to which structure?

The supraspinatus muscle has the most commonly involved tendon in rotator cuff tendonitis. The muscle originates on the supraspinatus fossa of the scapula and inserts on the greater tubercle of the humerus. Bicipital and infraspinatus tendonitis as well as bursitis may also coexist as other contributing factors.

Inference:

What is the most likely contributing factor in the development of this condition?

Individuals participating in activities that require excessive overhead activity such as swimming, tennis, baseball, painting, and other manual labor activities are at increased risk for rotator cuff tendonitis. Excessive use of the upper extremity following a prolonged period of inactivity also can produce this condition. Statistically individuals from 25-40 years of age are the most likely to develop this condition.

Confirmation:

What is the most likely clinical presentation?

A patient with rotator cuff tendonitis often reports difficulty with overhead activities and a dull ache following periods of activity. The patient may experience a feeling of weakness and identify the presence of a painful arc of motion most commonly occurring between 60 and 120 degrees of active abduction. The patient usually presents with pain with palpation of the musculotendinous junction of the involved muscle and/or with stretching or resisted contraction of the muscle. Pain often increases at night resulting in difficulty sleeping on the affected side. The patient will often have difficulty with dressing and repetitive shoulder motions such as lifting, reaching, throwing, swinging or pushing and pulling with the involved upper extremity.

What laboratory or imaging studies would confirm the diagnosis?

Magnetic resonance imaging can be used to identify the presence of rotator cuff tendonitis, however, due to the high cost it is not commonly employed prior to the initiation of formal treatment. X-rays with the shoulder laterally rotated can be used to identify the presence of calcific deposits or other bony abnormalities.

What additional information should be obtained to confirm the diagnosis?

A number of specific special tests including the empty can test, Jobe test, Neer impingement test, and Hawkins-Kennedy impingement test can be used to confirm the presence of rotator cuff tendonitis or impingement.

Examination:

What history should be documented?

Important areas to explore include past medical history, family history, medications, history of symptoms, current health status, living environment, social history and habits, occupation, and social support system.

What test/measures are most appropriate?

Anthropometric characteristics: upper extremity circumferential measurements
Arousal, attention, and cognition: examine mental status, learning ability, memory, motivation
Assistive and adaptive devices: analysis of components and safety of a device
Community and work integration: analysis of community, work, and leisure activities
Integumentary integrity: skin assessment, assessment of sensation
Joint integrity and mobility: soft tissue swelling and inflammation, assessment of joint play, palpation of the joint, empty can test, Neer impingement test, Hawkins-Kennedy impingement test
Motor function: posture and balance
Muscle performance: strength assessment
Pain: pain perception assessment scale
Posture: analysis of resting and dynamic posture
Range of motion: active and passive range of motion
Reflex integrity: assessment of deep tendon reflexes
Self-care and home management: assessment of functional capacity

What additional findings are likely with this patient?

Rotator cuff tendonitis often presents in association with impingement syndrome. Impingement syndrome typically involves the supraspinatus tendon, glenoid labrum, long head of the biceps, and subacromial bursa. It is extremely difficult to determine through examination the level of involvement of each of the identified structures.

Management:

What is the most effective management of this patient?

Medical management of acute rotator cuff tendonitis usually includes pharmacological intervention and physical therapy. Pharmacological intervention will focus on pain relief through analgesics and NSAIDs. Acute physical therapy intervention guidelines should include cryotherapy, activity modification, range of motion, and rest. As the acute phase subsides the patient is often instructed in strengthening exercises. Since the rotator cuff muscles are dependent on adequate blood supply and oxygen tension it is essential that all range of motion and strengthening exercises are pain free. Range of motion exercises using a pulley system or a cane can serve as an effective intervention. Strengthening exercises are initiated with the arm at the patient's side in order to prevent the possibility of impingement. Elastic tubing or handheld weights are often the preferred equipment of choice. It is important for the entire rotator cuff to be strong prior to initiating overhead activities. Shoulder shrugs and push-ups with the arms abducted to 90 degrees can effectively be used to strengthen the upper trapezius and serratus anterior. This type of activity promotes elevation of the acromion without direct contact with the rotator cuff.

What home care regimen should be recommended?

The home care regimen should consist of range of motion, strengthening, palliative care, and functional activities as warranted based on the results of the patient examination.

Outcome:

What is the likely outcome of a course in physical therapy?

A patient with rotator cuff tendonitis should be able to return to their previous level of functioning with conservative management within four to six weeks. Outcome can be dependent, however, on the patient's classification of stage I, II or III impingement syndrome. Stage I is usually found in the population less than 25 years of age and consists of localized inflammation, edema and minimal bleeding around the rotator cuff. Stage II represents progressive deterioration of the tissues surrounding the rotator cuff and is common in 25 to 40-year-old patients. Stage III represents the end-stage and is usually found in patients over 40 years of age. There is usually disruption and/or rupture of numerous soft tissue structures.

What are the long-term effects of the patient's condition?

Failure to adequately treat rotator cuff tendonitis may necessitate significant activity modification or more aggressive surgical management such as subacromial decompression. Prolonged inflammation of the rotator cuff tendon may facilitate eventual tearing of the rotator cuff musculature.

Comparison:

What are the distinguishing characteristics of a similar condition?

A rotator cuff tear is usually the result of repetitive microtrauma but can also result suddenly from a single traumatic event. Partial tears often occur in a younger population while complete tears more commonly occur in older individuals. The mechanism of injury is often a fall on an outstretched arm or a sudden strain applied to the shoulder during pushing or pulling activities. Diagnosis is made through MRI to identify the tear. Surgical repair of the rotator cuff is often required and may be done with arthroscopy or through a traditional open technique. The shoulder is usually protected by a sling and small abduction pillow for the first six weeks post surgery. Rehabilitation and return to full function can take upwards of six months, heavy lifting may be restricted for six to twelve months following surgery.

Clinical Scenarios:

Scenario One

A 23-year-old female diagnosed with rotator cuff tendonitis is referred to physical therapy after experiencing pain while swimming the breaststroke in a competitive swim meet one week ago. The patient participates on a school swim team and a private club and practices four to six times a week. A few days after experiencing the shoulder pain the patient was back in the pool, however, was unable to return to her previous training regimen.

Scenario Two

A 45-year-old male employed as a pipe fitter is referred to physical therapy after subacromial decompression. The patient is one week status post surgery and is anxious to "test" his involved shoulder. Prior to surgery the patient was placed on "light duty." It has been six months since the patient was able to perform his job without restrictions. The patient presently denies any pain in the involved shoulder.

Sciatica Secondary to a Herniated Disk

Diagnosis:

What condition produces a patient's symptoms?

A herniated disk is an intervertebral disk that bulges and protrudes posterolaterally against a nerve root. Sciatica is the diagnosis of compression of the sciatic nerve (L4, L5, S1, S2, S3) secondary to a herniated disk causing a patient's symptoms. Other causes for sciatica include tumor, infection, spondylolisthesis, narrowing of the canal, and blood clots.

An injury was most likely sustained to which structure?

As a patient gets older there are natural and significant alterations in the composition of the intervertebral disks and supporting structures. In a herniated disk the nucleus pulposus has bulged posterolaterally secondary to a weakening of the outer annulus fibrosis and posterior longitudinal ligament. The sciatic nerve experiences an inflammatory response and subsequent damage secondary to the compression from the herniated disk.

Inference:

What is the most likely contributing factor in the development of this condition?

The most common contributing factor for this condition is the natural aging process. Each decade the composition of the annulus fibrosus and nucleus pulposus is altered and decreases in overall stability. Once there is adequate structural breakdown within the disk a patient becomes a high risk for injury. A "normal mechanical load on a normal disk" is now an "excessive load on a compromised disk." As expected, sciatica secondary to a herniated disk is most often seen in patients between 40 and 60 years of age.

Confirmation:

What is the most likely clinical presentation?

Sciatica is characterized by low back and gluteal pain that typically radiates down the back of the thigh along the sciatic nerve distribution. Sciatic pain occurs from nerve root compression and can be dull, aching or sharp. Pain may have a sudden onset or develop gradually over time. Early sciatica may involve discomfort or pain limited to the low back and gluteal region. Leg pain can become greater than the back pain and can radiate the entire length of the nerve to the toes. The patient may also experience intermittent numbness and tingling localized to the dermatomal distribution, limited thoracolumbar range of motion in all planes, tenderness to palpation at the segment of herniation, and muscle guarding.

What laboratory or imaging studies would confirm the diagnosis?

Radiologic testing of the spine and electrophysiologic studies are initially performed to assist with diagnosis. Other imaging may include myelogram, discography, CT scan or MRI. Blood work may assist with differential diagnosis.

What additional information should be obtained to confirm the diagnosis?

A full examination should be performed that includes history (trauma, osteoporosis, corticosteroid use), functional assessment, inspection, palpation, and special tests. The straight leg raise test will reproduce symptoms in the case of a herniated disk. The exam should also include testing for non-organic back pain to rule out psychological factors.

Examination:

What history should be documented?

Important areas to explore include past medical history and treatment, history of trauma and accidents, medications, family history, current symptoms, current health status, social history and habits, occupation, leisure activities, and social support system.

What test/measures are most appropriate?

Arousal, attention, and cognition: examine mental status, learning ability, memory, motivation

Assistive and adaptive devices: analysis of components and safety of a device

Community and work integration: analysis of community, work, and leisure activities

Environmental, home, and work barriers: analysis of current and potential barriers or hazards

Ergonomics and body mechanics: analysis of dexterity and coordination

Gait, locomotion, and balance: static and dynamic balance in sitting and standing, Functional Ambulation Profile

Integumentary integrity: skin assessment, assessment of sensation, dermatome testing of the lower extremities

Joint integrity and mobility: assessment of hyper- and hypomobility of a joint, soft tissue swelling and inflammation

Muscle performance: strength assessment, resisted isometrics, straight leg raise testing

Pain: Oswestry Function Test, McGill Pain Questionnaire, visual analog scale

Posture: analysis of resting and dynamic posture

Range of motion: active and passive movement of the spine, combined movements, segmental mobility testing

Reflex integrity: assessment of deep tendon and pathological reflexes (clonus)

Self-care and home management: assessment of functional capacity, Functional Independence Measure

What additional findings are likely with this patient?

Sciatica will produce pain that increases with certain positions due to an increase in intradiskal pressure. Pain will increase in a sitting position or when lifting, forward bending or twisting. Sneezing and coughing can also exacerbate the pain. Although a patient may want to stop all activity to relieve pain, prolonged bed rest is contraindicated and will not relieve pain on a long-term basis.

Management:

What is the most effective management of this patient?

Medical management of sciatica due to a herniated disk includes short-term bed rest, overall reduction of intradiskal pressure, patient education, physical therapy, medications, and in rare instances surgical intervention. Pharmacological intervention will incorporate NSAIDs initially to relieve pain followed by epidural injections of cortisone and local anesthetics that may be indicated for temporary relief, however, do not alter the root of the problem. Physical therapy intervention should include patient education on positioning and biomechanics, pain management, traction, heat, lumbar stabilization exercises, McKenzie exercises, stretching, and endurance activities. Swimming, stationary bicycling and walking are indicated within tolerance. Lifting, squatting, and climbing are contraindicated due to the significant increase in intradiskal pressure. Most herniations will spontaneously decrease in size with conservative treatment. Research indicates that the majority of patients improve with two to four months of conservative treatment, however, approximately 2% of patients undergo surgery. Common surgical intervention may include laminectomy, discectomy, chemonucleolysis, laser discectomy or laminotomy.

What home care regimen should be recommended?

A home care regimen should include ongoing caution regarding positioning and constant effort to decrease intradiskal pressure. A home exercise program including stabilization exercises is indicated as well as other aerobic/endurance activities to tolerance.

Outcome:

What is the likely outcome of a course in physical therapy?

Most patients improve with conservative treatment over a two to four month period. Physical therapy intervention combined with a consistent home program will provide the patient with the necessary tools to relieve pain and improve function.

What are the long-term effects of the patient's condition?

Sciatica secondary to a herniated disk can be corrected through rest and physical therapy intervention. Healing of the disk can also occur and scarring can reinforce the posterior aspect and annular fibers so that it is protected from further protrusion. Restoration of functional mobility is plausible, however, surgical intervention may be required if neurological symptoms increase or no progress is made with conservative measures.

Comparison:

What are the distinguishing characteristics of a similar condition?

Spinal stenosis is another condition that can be a causative factor of sciatica. Symptoms that would indicate spinal stenosis include lower extremity weakness with or without sciatica, back and leg pain after ambulating a short distance, increasing symptoms with continued ambulation, and relief of symptoms through flexion. Radiologic results reveal disk narrowing and degenerative spondylolisthesis. Surgery is only recommended as a last resort when conservative treatment fails.

Clinical Scenarios:

Scenario One

A 42-year-old female is referred to physical therapy with an L5 herniated disk and sciatica. The patient injured her back skiing three months ago. She presently works 50 hours per week at a daycare facility. Current symptoms include radiating pain down the left leg, a "feeling of weakness," and an inability to sleep at night due to pain.

Scenario Two

A 65-year-old male has been seen in physical therapy for three months with sciatica secondary to a L4 herniated disk. The patient states that he experiences constant pain. The therapist questions the patient's overall compliance with his established home exercise program. The physician orders are prescribed as physical therapy three times per week.

Scoliosis

Diagnosis:

What condition produces a patient's symptoms?

A patient with scoliosis presents with a lateral curvature of the spine. The curvature is usually found in the thoracic or lumbar vertebrae and can be associated with kyphosis or lordosis. The curvature of the spine may be towards the right or towards the left and rotation of the spine may or may not occur. Typically, the rotation will occur towards the convex side of the major curve.

An injury was most likely sustained to which structure?

The injury or deformity begins when the vertebrae of the spine deviate from the normal vertical position. The curvature disrupts normal alignment of the ribs and muscles and can create compensatory curves that attempt to keep the body in proper alignment. The vertebral column, rib cage, supporting ligaments, and muscles are all affected by a scoliosis of the spine.

Inference:

What is the most likely contributing factor in the development of this condition?

Idiopathic scoliosis, termed for its unknown etiology, accounts for approximately 80% of all cases. Upwards of 1:10 children are affected by some form of scoliosis with 1:4 requiring treatment for the curvature. The age of onset determines the subset of classification as infantile (0 to 3), juvenile (four to puberty), adolescent (12 for girls and 14 for boys) or adult (skeletal maturation) scoliosis. Non-structural scoliosis is a reversible curve that can change with repositioning. This type of curve is non-progressive and is usually caused by poor posture or leg length discrepancy. Structural scoliosis cannot be corrected with movement and can be caused by congenital, musculoskeletal, and neuromuscular reasons. Contributing factors of a structural curve include altered development of the spine in utero, association with neuromuscular diseases (cerebral palsy, muscular dystrophy, congenital defect of the vertebrae), and inheritance as an autosomal dominant trait. Research indicates a predisposition for scoliosis with a multifactorial etiology.

Confirmation:

What is the most likely clinical presentation?

A patient with a structural curve will present with asymmetries of the shoulders, scapulae, pelvis, and skinfolds. Juvenile idiopathic scoliosis is characterized by a thoracic curve with convexity towards the right. This curve may progress quickly and develop compensatory curves above and below. As the curve progresses there will be a rib hump posteriorly over the thoracic region on the convex side of the curve. The patient does not typically experience pain or

other subjective symptoms until the curve has progressed. Adolescent scoliosis of greater than 30 degrees is seen more in females than males (10:1). Adult scoliosis affects approximately 500,000 adults in the United States. Curves that are less than 20 degrees rarely cause a person to experience significant problems or impairments.

What laboratory or imaging studies would confirm the diagnosis?

X-rays should be taken in an anterior and lateral view with the patient standing and with the patient bending over. A device called a scoliometer can be used to measure the angle of trunk rotation. The Cobb method can be used to determine the angle of curvature. A bone scan or MRI can be used to determine and rule out conditions such as infections, neoplasms, spondylolysis, disk herniations or compression fractures.

What additional information should be obtained to confirm the diagnosis?

Physical examination allows visual inspection of the curvature and physical asymmetries. A scoliometer can assist with measurement and the examiner can determine if the curve is non-structural or structural.

Examination:

What history should be documented?

Important areas to explore include past medical history, family history, medications, current health status, living environment, school activities, and social support system.

What test/measures are most appropriate?

Aerobic capacity and endurance: assessment of vital signs at rest and with activity, perceived exertion scale

Arousal, attention, and cognition: examine mental status, learning ability, memory, motivation

Ergonomics and body mechanics: analysis of dexterity and coordination

Integumentary integrity: skin and sensation assessment

Gait, locomotion, and balance: static and dynamic balance in sitting and standing, safety during gait with/ without an assistive device, analysis of wheelchair management

Joint integrity and mobility: assessment of hyper- and hypomobility of a joint

Muscle performance: strength assessment

Orthotic, protective, and supportive devices: analysis of components of a device, analysis of movement while wearing a device

Pain: assessment of muscle soreness

Posture: analysis of resting and dynamic posture

Range of motion: active and passive range of motion

Self-care and home management: assessment of functional capacity

What additional findings are likely with this patient?

Common postural findings with scoliosis include increased spacing between the elbow and trunk during standing, leg length discrepancy, uneven shoulder and hip heights, and prominence on one side of the pelvis or breast (due to rotation of the curve). If a progressive scoliosis is untreated the deformity can increase to an angle in excess of 60 degrees and cause pulmonary insufficiency, significant pain, impairment in lung capacity, and degenerative changes including arthritis and disk pathology. Early screening, detection and treatment are necessary to control the curvature and avoid surgical intervention.

Management:

What is the most effective management of this patient?

Medical management of scoliosis is based on the type and severity of the curve, patient age, and previous management. Patients with scoliosis may utilize electrical stimulation to alleviate pain and biofeedback for education with proper posture and positioning. A patient with scoliosis that is less than 25 degrees should be monitored every three months. Breathing exercises and a strengthening program for the trunk and pelvic muscles are indicated. A patient with scoliosis that ranges between 25 and 40 degrees requires a spinal orthosis and physical therapy intervention for posture, flexibility, strengthening, respiratory function, and proper utilization of the spinal orthosis. A patient with scoliosis that is greater than 40 degrees usually requires surgical spinal stabilization. One method to surgically correct scoliosis is through posterior spinal fusion and stabilization with a Harrington rod. Physical therapy intervention after surgical fusion is indicated for breathing exercises, posture, flexibility, general strengthening, and respiratory muscle strengthening.

What home care regimen should be recommended?

A home care regimen is based on the type and severity of the curve. Exercise, stretching, posture, and flexibility are important components of an exercise program.

Outcome:

What is the likely outcome of a course in physical therapy?

Physical therapy intervention should improve a patient's condition through patient education and therapeutic exercise. Physical therapy may be indicated for implementation of a home program, pain management, posture retraining, orthotic training or following surgical stabilization.

What are the long-term effects of the patient's condition?

Prognosis for structural scoliosis is based on the age of onset and the severity of the curve. Early intervention results in the best possible outcome. Scoliosis does not usually progress significantly once bone growth is complete if the curvature remains below 40 degrees at the time of skeletal maturity. If the curvature is over 50 degrees there likely will be ongoing progression of the curve each year of life.

Comparison:

What are the distinguishing characteristics of a similar condition?

Torticollis is a deformity of the neck that is caused by shortened or spastic sternocleidomastoid muscles. The patient presents with a bending of the neck towards the affected side and rotation of the head towards the unaffected side. Causative factors include damage to the sternocleidomastoid muscle, malpositioning in utero, spasms secondary to central nervous system impairment or psychogenic origin. Conservative treatment for acquired torticollis includes heat, traction, massage, stretching, positioning, and bracing. Surgical intervention may be indicated if conservative management fails.

Clinical Scenarios:

Scenario One

An 11-year-old female is seen in physical therapy with diagnosis of a 30-degree right thoracic scoliosis. The physician has prescribed a spinal orthosis and physical therapy. The patient denies any pain, but states that she has soreness in her back. The patient is in the marching band and plays basketball. There is no past medical history and her parents are very supportive.

Scenario Two

A seven-year-old boy is referred to physical therapy with a 12-degree right thoracic scoliosis. The physical therapy prescription requests evaluation for a home exercise program. The patient has insulin-dependent diabetes and a low I.Q. The mother is present for the evaluation and appears to be supportive.

Spina Bifida – Myelomeningocele

Diagnosis:

What condition produces a patient's symptoms?

Spina bifida is a congenital neural tube defect that generally occurs in the lumbar spine but can also occur at the sacral, cervical, and thoracic levels. Spina bifida has three classifications that include spina bifida -occulta (incomplete fusion of the posterior vertebral arch with no neural tissue protruding), spina bifida -meningocele (incomplete fusion of the posterior vertebral arch with neural tissue/meninges protruding outside the neural arch), and spina bifida -myelomeningocele (incomplete fusion of the posterior vertebral arch with both meninges and spinal cord protruding outside the neural arch).

An injury was most likely sustained to which structure?

Spina bifida - myelomeningocele is characterized by a sac or cyst that protrudes outside the spine and contains a herniation of meninges, cerebrospinal fluid, and the spinal cord through the defect in the vertebrae. The cyst may or may not be covered by skin. Spina bifida results from failure of neural tube closure by day 28 of gestation when the spinal cord is expected to form. Approximately 75% of vertebral defects are found in the lumbar/sacral region, typically L5-S1 with injury to the structures at that level and below. Defects can also occur in the cervical or thoracic spine, however, this is rare.

Inference:

What is the most likely contributing factor in the development of this condition?

The Centers for Disease Control estimates the incidence for neural tube defects to be five per 10,000 live births within the United States. The incidence varies by socioeconomic status, geographic area, and ethnic background. The overall incidence is declining due to improved prenatal care. The exact etiology for spina bifida - myelomeningocele has not been identified, however, causative and risk factors include genetic predisposition, environmental influence (certain solvents, lead, herbicides, glycol ethers), insulin-dependent diabetes, low-levels of maternal folic acid, alcohol, maternal hyperthermia, and certain classifications of drugs (teratogenic exposure and vitamin A toxicity). Theories suggest that the cause is multifactorial rather than a single source of etiology. Prenatal care including recommended amounts of folic acid, especially in the first six weeks of pregnancy, appears to be the most effective way to prevent neural tube defects.

Confirmation:

What is the most likely clinical presentation?

Myelomeningocele is a severe condition that is characterized by a sac that is seen on an infant's back protruding from a specific area of the spinal cord. Impairments associated with myelomeningocele include motor and sensory loss below the vertebral defect, hydrocephalus, Arnold-Chiari Type II malformation, clubfoot, scoliosis, bowel and bladder dysfunction, and learning disabilities. The higher the neural lesion the worse the prognosis is for survival. The infant will require surgical intervention to close the lesion and in 90% of the cases a shunt is required for hydrocephalus. Approximately two-thirds of children with myelomeningocele and shunted hydrocephalus have normal intelligence and the other third demonstrate only mild retardation. Regardless of intelligence, children with myelomeningocele exhibit difficulties with perceptual abilities, attention, problem solving, and memory.

What laboratory or imaging studies would confirm the diagnosis?

Prior to birth a fetal ultrasound may identify the myelomeningocele defect in the spine. Prenatal testing of alpha-fetoprotein (AFP) in the blood will show an elevation in levels that indicate a probable neural tube defect at approximately week 16 of gestation. At birth an obvious sac will be present over the spinal defect. Spinal films and CT scan can evaluate for the presence of defects and hydrocephalus.

What additional information should be obtained to confirm the diagnosis?

Diagnosis is confirmed through prenatal testing or upon visual observation at birth. Past medical history of the mother, history of the pregnancy, and family history of neural tube defects may be noted.

Examination:

What history should be documented?

Important areas to explore with the parents include past medical history, current symptoms and health status, medications, past surgical procedures, living environment, and social support system.

What test/measures are most appropriate?

Aerobic capacity and endurance: assessment of vital signs at rest and with activity
Arousal, attention, and cognition: examine mental status, learning ability, memory, motivation
Assistive and adaptive devices: use of appropriate devices, analysis of components/safety of a device
Ergonomics and body mechanics: analysis of dexterity and coordination
Gait, locomotion, and balance: developmental milestones assessment, static/dynamic balance in prone and sitting, analysis of wheelchair management, standing with frame, gait with assistive device
Integumentary integrity: skin and sensation assessment
Motor function: equilibrium and righting reactions, motor assessment scales, balance in sitting

Muscle performance: assessment of active movement, muscle tone assessment
Orthotic, protective, and supportive devices: analysis of components of a device, analysis of movement while wearing a device
Range of motion: active and passive range of motion
Reflex integrity: assessment of deep tendon and pathological reflexes (e.g., Babinski, ATNR)

What additional findings are likely with this patient?

Immediately after birth, an infant with myelomeningocele has an increased risk of meningitis, hemorrhage, and hypoxia, however, surgical intervention may significantly reduce the risks. Ongoing additional findings with myelomeningocele include hydrocephalus, clubfoot, neuropathic fracture, visual problems, osteoporosis, kyphosis, hip dislocations, and latex allergy.

Management:

What is the most effective management of this patient?

Medical management of a patient with myelomeningocele begins with immediate surgical intervention to repair and close the defect and for placement of a shunt to alleviate hydrocephalus. Orthopedic surgical intervention may be warranted throughout a patient's life to correct deformities such as clubfoot, hip dysplasia, and scoliosis. Pharmacological intervention may include medications that assist in the management of bowel and bladder dysfunction. Physical and occupational therapies are important components in the management of myelomeningocele. Physical therapy is initiated immediately and focuses on family education regarding positioning, handling techniques, range of motion, and therapeutic play. Long-term physical therapy attempts to maximize functional capacity and may include range of motion, facilitation of developmental milestones, therapeutic exercise, skin care, strengthening, balance, and mobility training. Physical therapy will also assist with wheelchair prescription, assistive and adaptive device selection, and the use of orthotics and splinting.

What home care regimen should be recommended?

A home care regimen should include a formal exercise program, range of motion, and mobility training. Family and caregiver involvement are important in assisting a patient through their exercise program. The home program will require modification as the child matures and goals change.

Outcome:

What is the likely outcome of a course in physical therapy?

Physical therapy initially evaluates and documents the baseline information regarding the patient's motor and sensory function and level of ability. Physical therapy is ongoing through adolescence and is based on the severity of impairments and the needs of the child. Physical therapy is usually initiated based on symptoms, functional problems, and disability.

What are the long-term effects of the patient's condition?

A patient with myelomeningocele has a near normal life expectancy as long as the patient receives consistent and thorough health care. Functional outcome of the patient depends on the level of injury, the amount of associated impairments, and the caregiver support that is provided.

Comparison:

What are the distinguishing characteristics of a similar condition?

Anencephaly is a condition that is characterized by failed closure of the cranial end of the neural tube. The cerebral hemispheres do not form and some neural tissue may protrude through the defect. This type of neural tube defect cannot be repaired. Many infants with this condition are stillborn, while others only survive a short time after birth.

Clinical Scenarios:

Scenario One

A six-month-old boy is seen in physical therapy after revision of a ventriculoperitoneal shunt. The parents state that the child has been responsive at home and has been doing well. The child can position himself in prone on elbows and is able to sit with support.

Scenario Two

An 11-year-old girl with a T12 spinal cord lesion is seen in outpatient physical therapy. The patient presently uses a wheelchair for mobility, however, indicates that her goal is to walk in her home. The patient's upper body strength is good and intellect is normal.

Spinal Cord Injury – Complete C7 Tetraplegia

Diagnosis:

What condition produces a patient's symptoms?

The majority of traumatic spinal cord injuries result from compression, flexion or extension of the spine with or without rotation. Spinal cord injuries are classified as a concussion, contusion or laceration, and injury results in primary and secondary neural destruction. Traumatic injury to the spinal cord produces a physiological and biochemical chain of events that results in vascular impairment and permanent tissue and nerve damage.

An injury was most likely sustained to which structure?

A patient sustains primary damage to the spinal cord and surrounding tissues at the C7 level through disruption of the membrane, displacement or compression of the spinal cord, and subsequent hemorrhage and vascular damage. Secondary damage occurs beyond the level of injury due to biochemicals that are released as a result of the initial damage. This process destroys adjacent cells and neural tracts due to the acute inflammation and can last for days or even weeks. After injury, C7 is the most distal segment of the spinal cord that both the motor and sensory components remain intact.

Inference:

What is the most likely contributing factor in the development of this condition?

There is an estimated 190,000 to 230,000 persons living with SCI within the United States. Statistics from the National Spinal Cord Injury Database (NSCID) indicate that motor vehicle accidents, violence, and falls are the top causes of traumatic spinal cord injury. Statistics also indicate a higher ratio of injury in men (approximately 80%) and Caucasians. The highest incidence of age of injury (over 50%) occurs between 15 to 30 years of age.

Confirmation:

What is the most likely clinical presentation?

Spinal shock, which is the total depression of all nervous system function below the level of lesion, occurs immediately following injury and may last for days. Presentation includes total flaccid paralysis and loss of all reflexes and sensation. Surgical intervention may be required after injury in order to stabilize the spinal cord through decompression and fusion at the site of injury. A Halo device is commonly used with cervical injuries to stabilize the spine. As spinal shock subsides, a patient will experience an increase in muscle tone below the level of lesion and neurologic reflexes reappear. Spasticity will evolve and may become problematic. Autonomic dysreflexia and loss of thermoregulation are other impairments that occur secondary to autonomic nervous system dysfunction. A patient with C7 tetraplegia will also present with impaired cough and ability to clear secretions, altered breathing pattern, and poor endurance. The patient is at high risk for contractures and impaired skin integrity.

What laboratory or imaging studies would confirm the diagnosis?

X-rays of the cervical spine observe the positioning and damage of the involved vertebrae. The results of imaging determine subsequent medical intervention including stabilization of the spine. A myelogram or tomogram may be useful to confirm the extent of surrounding damage at the level of the injury.

What additional information should be obtained to confirm the diagnosis?

Other information commonly obtained in order to support the diagnosis includes physician conducted interviews regarding the mechanism of injury as well as a full neurological examination.

Examination:

What history should be documented?

Important areas to explore include past medical history, medications, mechanism of injury, precautions, current health status, social history and habits, occupation or school responsibilities, living environment, and social support system.

What test/measures are most appropriate?

Aerobic capacity and endurance: autonomic responses to positional changes, vital signs at rest/activity

Arousal, attention, and cognition: examine mental status, learning ability, memory, motivation

Assistive and adaptive devices: analysis of components and safety of a device, wheelchair prescription, adaptive devices, environmental controls

Integumentary integrity: skin assessment, American Spinal Injury Association (ASIA) - Standard Neurological Classification of Spinal Cord Injury Sensory Examination

Motor function: posture and balance in sitting

Muscle performance: ASIA - Standard Neurological Classification of Spinal Cord Injury Motor Examination, muscle tone assessment

Neuromotor development and sensory integration: analysis of reflex movement patterns

Pain: dysesthetic pain (deafferentation pain), nerve root pain, musculoskeletal pain

Posture: positioning, resting and dynamic posture

Range of motion: active and passive range of motion

Reflex integrity: assessment of deep tendon reflexes and pathological reflexes

Sensory integrity: proprioception and kinesthesia

Ventilation, respiration, and circulation: assessment of cough and clearance of secretions, breathing patterns, respiratory muscle strength, accessory muscle utilization, pulmonary function tests

What additional findings are likely with this patient?

There are many additional findings that can exist with a C7 injury, but the most common complications include orthostatic hypotension, pressure sores, spasticity, heterotopic ossification, and autonomic dysreflexia. Autonomic dysreflexia is considered a medical emergency and requires immediate attention to remove the noxious stimuli and lower the blood pressure or the patient will be at risk for subarachnoid hemorrhage. Other findings that require management include sexual dysfunction, respiratory complications, and pain management (neurogenic, central cord, peripheral nerve or musculoskeletal pain).

Management:

What is the most effective management of this patient?

Medical management of a SCI injury has both an acute and rehabilitation phase. The acute phase begins at injury and includes medically stabilizing the patient. Pharmacological intervention is started immediately using Methylprednisolone (corticosteroid), lipid peroxidation inhibitors, and drugs that block opiate receptors. These drugs appear to control the amount of secondary damage and improve the neurological damage. Once a patient is medically stable, inpatient rehabilitation, which is typically six to eight weeks, should initially focus on range of motion, positioning in bed, and respiratory management such as cough, clearance of secretions, bronchial drainage, and incentive spirometry. Compensatory techniques, strengthening, muscle substitution, the use of momentum, and the head-hips relationship should be utilized during all activities. Ongoing intervention should include mat and endurance activities, pressure relief training, wheelchair skills, self-range of motion, transfer skills, and community reintegration.

What home care regimen should be recommended?

A home care regimen should include breathing exercises, incentive spirometry, stretching, and mobility skills. Physical therapy intervention may be indicated for continuation of community skills and furthering the patient's independence within the boundaries of the physical limitations.

Outcome:

What is the likely outcome of a course in physical therapy?

A patient diagnosed with C7 tetraplegia will require extensive physical therapy with projected outcomes based upon the C7 level of motor and sensory innervation. Typical outcomes at this level include independence with feeding, grooming, and dressing, self-range of motion, independent manual wheelchair mobility, independent transfers, and independent driving with an adapted automobile. Independent living with adaptive equipment is possible.

What are the long-term effects of the patient's condition?

At this time there is no cure for a complete spinal cord injury, therefore a patient with a complete C7 injury will not regain innervation below this level. The triceps, extensor pollicis longus and brevis, extrinsic finger extensors, and flexor carpi radialis will remain the lowest innervated muscles. There will be ongoing musculoskeletal and cardiopulmonary deficits that can increase the risk for other health issues. The latest research suggests, however, that approximately 40% of the spinal cord injured population have a life expectancy over 45 years of age.

Comparison:

What are the distinguishing characteristics of a similar condition?

Brown-Sequard's syndrome is a condition that results from injury to one side of the spinal cord. Motor function, proprioception, and vibration are lost ipsilateral to the lesion and vibration, pain, and temperature are absent contralateral to the lesion.

Clinical Scenarios:

Scenario One

A patient is diagnosed with T12 paraplegia after a motor vehicle accident. Neurological examination reveals no active movement or sensation below T12. The patient is a chemistry teacher and coaches basketball. He is otherwise in good health.

Scenario Two

A 25-year-old male was injured when he was hit from behind. The blow produced cervical hyperextension and bleeding within the central gray matter of the spinal cord. The patient was diagnosed with central cord syndrome and referred to physical therapy. The patient resides alone in a second floor apartment and is a full-time graduate student.

Spinal Cord Injury – Complete L3 Paraplegia

Diagnosis:

What condition produces a patient's symptoms?

The majority of traumatic spinal cord injuries result from compression, flexion or extension of the spine with or without rotation. Spinal cord injuries are classified as a concussion, contusion or laceration, and injury results in primary and secondary neural destruction. Traumatic injury to the spinal cord produces a physiological and biochemical chain of events that results in vascular impairment and permanent tissue and nerve damage.

An injury was most likely sustained to which structure?

The forces responsible for spinal fractures are compression, flexion, extension, rotation, shear or distraction forces or a combination of these. A patient sustains primary damage to the spinal cord and surrounding tissues at the L3 level through the disruption of the membrane, displacement or compression of the spinal cord, and subsequent hemorrhage and vascular damage. Secondary damage occurs beyond the level of injury due to biochemicals that are released as a result of the initial damage. This process destroys adjacent cells and neural tracts due to the acute inflammation that can last for days or even weeks. After a complete injury at this level, L3 is the most distal segment of the spinal cord that both the motor and sensory components remain intact.

Inference:

What is the most likely contributing factor in the development of this condition?

There is an estimated 190,000 to 230,000 persons living with SCI within the United States. Statistics from the National Spinal Cord Injury Database (NSCID) indicate that motor vehicle accidents, violence, and falls are the top causes of traumatic spinal cord injury. Statistics also indicate a higher ratio of injury in men (approximately 80%) and Caucasians. The highest incidence of age of injury (over 50%) occurs between 15 to 30 years of age. It is also reported that 40% of spinal injuries are caused by motor vehicle accidents.

Confirmation:

What is the most likely clinical presentation?

Spinal shock occurs immediately after the injury and can last for days. Surgical intervention may be required for stabilization of the spine. The patient is usually required to wear a spinal orthosis to maintain stability. As spinal shock subsides, a patient will experience an increase in muscle tone below the level of lesion and neurologic reflexes reappear. Spasticity will evolve and may become problematic. Patients specifically with a complete lesion at the L3 level typically have at least partial innervation of the gracilis, iliopsoas, quadratus lumborum, rectus femoris, and sartorius. Patients have full use of their upper extremities and have hip flexion, adduction, and knee extension.

What laboratory or imaging studies would confirm the diagnosis?

The evaluation of a patient with an acute lumbar spine fracture should include routine laboratory tests, such as CBC, and electrolytes. X-rays, CT scan, and MRI allows for bony and ligamentous injury diagnosis.

What additional information should be obtained to confirm the diagnosis?

A detailed neurological evaluation should include evaluation of sensory level, posterior column function, normal and abnormal reflexes, and examination of rectal tone and perianal sensation. The cutaneous abdominal reflex, bulbocavernosus reflex, and the presence of the Babinski sign also should be examined.

Examination:

What history should be documented?

Important areas to explore include past medical history, medications, mechanism of injury, precautions, current health status, nutritional status, social history, living environment occupation, and social support system.

What test/measures are most appropriate?

Aerobic capacity and endurance: autonomic responses to positional changes, vital signs at rest/activity
Arousal, attention, and cognition: examine mental status, memory, motivation, level of consciousness
Assistive and adaptive devices: analysis of components and safety of a device, wheelchair prescription, adaptive devices, environmental controls
Community and work integration: analysis of community, work, and leisure activities
Environmental, home, and work barriers: analysis of current and potential barriers or hazards
Gait, locomotion, and balance: static and dynamic balance in sitting, analysis of wheelchair management
Integumentary integrity: skin assessment, American Spinal Injury Association (ASIA) – Standard Neurological Classification of Spinal Cord Injury Sensory Examination
Motor function: equilibrium and righting reactions, posture and balance in sitting
Muscle performance: ASIA – Standard Neurological Classification of Spinal Cord Injury Motor Examination, muscle tone assessment
Neuromotor development and sensory integration: analysis of reflex movement patterns
Orthotic, protective, and supportive devices: analysis of components of a device and movement with a device
Pain: dysesthetic pain (deafferentation pain), nerve root pain, musculoskeletal pain

Range of motion: active and passive range of motion
Reflex integrity: assessment of deep tendon and pathological reflexes
Self-care and home management: assessment of functional capacity, Functional Independence Measure
Sensory integrity: proprioception and kinesthesia

What additional findings are likely with this patient?

There are many additional findings that can exist with a L3 injury including sexual dysfunction, a nonreflexive bladder, and the need for a bowel program. These patients usually present with flaccid paralysis below the level of lesion and are at risk for pain, urinary tract infections, muscle contractures, and pressure sores.

Management:

What is the most effective management of this patient?

Medical emergency management of a patient with a L3 SCI is initiated by stabilization of the patient's airway in order to secure adequate oxygenation. As soon as the patient is stabilized all patients with spinal cord injuries should immediately receive intravenous methylprednisolone since it has proven to control the amount of secondary damage and improve the neurological outcome. The patient may be placed in a thoracolumbar orthosis (TLSO) with restriction of activities or undergo stabilization surgery followed by the use of a TLSO. Once the patient's spine is stable, rehabilitation should be initiated on an inpatient basis for approximately four to eight weeks. Rehabilitation management may include physical, occupational, vocational therapies, physiatry, nutritional consult, counseling services, and case management. Physical therapy should initially focus on mobility including transfers, bed mobility, and wheelchair mobility. Range of motion and selective strengthening programs, endurance activities, and balance activities should be performed on an ongoing basis in order to optimize functional outcomes. Orthotic prescription (KAFOs or AFOs) is recommended once the patient has gained strength to assist with ambulation using crutches. Community reintegration must be a component of the overall rehabilitation program.

What home care regimen should be recommended?

A home care regimen for a patient with L3 SCI should include continued selective strengthening, selective stretching, endurance activities, balance and postural control training, and continued use of all orthotics and assistive/adaptive devices. The patient must continue with a home program in order to attain and maintain the highest level of functioning and endurance.

Outcome:

What is the likely outcome of a course in physical therapy?

A patient with L3 SCI will usually participate in four to eight weeks of inpatient rehabilitation immediately after injury and stabilization. The patient should be able to function independently from a wheelchair level and ambulation level. Outcome is based on the degree of injury, the patient's mental capacity, outside support, emotional stability, motivation, and co-morbidities.

What are the long-term effects of the patient's condition?

There are approximately 12,000 persons that sustain a spinal cord injury each year and nearly 5,000 of these cases are diagnosed with paraplegia. Patients with SCI are always at a greater risk for osteoporosis, pressure ulcers, hypertension, and heterotopic ossification. The leading cause of death at present is pneumonia, followed by nonischemic heart disease and sepsis. Patients with L3 paraplegia should be able to live independently with education regarding the management of their disability.

Comparison:

What are the distinguishing characteristics of a similar condition?

There are various outcomes from spinal cord injuries that occur in the lumbosacral region. Fractures of the thoracolumbar junction can produce a mixture of cord and root syndromes caused by lesions of the conus medullaris and lumbar nerve roots. Complete damage of the conus medullaris presents with no motor function or sensation below L1. Patients with complete damage to the sacral portion of the cord have no control of bowel and bladder function and sacral motor paralysis.

Clinical Scenarios:

Scenario One

A 16-year-old male involved in a MVA sustained a complete L4 injury that required surgery to stabilize his spine. He has just been transferred to rehabilitation and has a TLSO for support. His parents are divorced and he lives between their two homes.

Scenario Two

A 23-year-old male sustained a conus medullaris injury in a MVA. He was admitted to the acute care hospital and has been having complications regulating his blood glucose level. The patient was diagnosed with type I diabetes mellitus when he was seven years old. The patient resides in a two-story condominium.

Spondylolisthesis

Diagnosis:

What condition produces a patient's symptoms?

Spondylolisthesis is a descriptive term referring to forward slippage of one vertebral body with respect to the vertebral body below it. The patient's symptoms will vary based on the type and degree of the slippage.

An injury was most likely sustained to which structure?

Spondylolisthesis may not produce collateral injury to other structures, but in many cases there can be symptoms that range from localized or radiating pain to significant nerve compression, radiculopathy or neurogenic claudication.

Inference:

What is the most likely contributing factor in the development of this condition?

Spondylolysis is a term used to describe a defect in the pars interarticularis that may produce the forward slippage of a vertebrae as found with spondylolisthesis. There are several etiologies (all are multifactorial) that can produce a spondylolisthesis. All categories ultimately lead to a loss in stability of the locking mechanism of the articular processes with subsequent slippage. The etiologies can be classified as congenital (a defect at birth in the upper sacrum or sacral facet joints); isthmic (results from a defect in the pars interarticularis which allows for increased stress and subsequent fracture); degenerative (usually found later in life as a result of degenerative changes primarily through facet arthropathy or discopathy); traumatic (can occur at any age from acute fracture of the pars or facets that results in listhesis); and pathologic (results secondary to bone disease that compromises the joint). High risk activities include gymnastics, wrestling, football, and weight lifting.

Confirmation:

What is the most likely clinical presentation?

The presentation of spondylolisthesis is dependent on the causative factors and age of the patient. Pain is the most common symptom of spondylolysis and spondylolisthesis. Pain may originate in the area of lysis or may arise from other structures that have been affected by secondary changes of lysis or spondylolisthesis. These include degenerative changes in the disk, facet arthropathy, and ligamentous sprain or strain. If the patient is young, pain is usually confined to the area of slippage and may occasionally radiate. Progression involves neurological, motor, sensory and reflex changes. Pain is usually provoked with activity especially when it involves extension of the spine. The patient may also present with a palpable step-off over the spine, hamstrings tightness, lumbar spasm, trunk shortening, and gait abnormalities due to a shortened stride length. The most common location of isthmic spondylolisthesis is at L5-S1, while degenerative spondylolisthesis most commonly occurs at L4-L5.

What laboratory or imaging studies would confirm the diagnosis?

Lateral and anteroposterior plain x-rays of the lumbar spine should be obtained. The oblique view can show the pars as having the appearance of a "Scottie dog with a collar" when a spondylolysis is present. Other studies may include a bone scan, CT scan and myelogram. Laboratory studies will not assist with diagnosis.

What additional information should be obtained to confirm the diagnosis?

Once a spondylolisthesis is diagnosed, it should also be graded. Meyerding's scale is used frequently and measures the degree of slippage as Grade 1 through 5. The slippage is measured as the percentage of distance that the vertebral body has moved anteriorly over the superior end plate of the vertebral body below it. Grade 1=1-25%; grade 2= 26-50%; grade 3= 51-75%; grade 4= 76-100%; and grade 5= greater than 100%.

Examination:

What history should be documented?

Important areas to explore include past medical history, medications, current health status, history of illness, nutritional status, social history and habits, occupation, living environment, and social support system.

What test/measures are most appropriate?

Assistive and adaptive devices: analysis of components and safety of a device
Community and work integration: analysis of community, work, and leisure activities
Cranial nerve integrity: dermatome assessment, assessment of muscle innervation by the cranial nerves
Environmental, home, and work barriers: analysis of current and potential barriers or hazards
Ergonomics and body mechanics: analysis of dexterity and coordination
Gait, locomotion, and balance: static and dynamic balance in sitting and standing, safety during gait with/without an assistive device
Integumentary integrity: assessment of sensation
Joint integrity and mobility: assessment of hyper- and hypomobility of a joint, assessment of sprain
Muscle performance: strength assessment, muscle tone assessment
Orthotic, protective, and supportive devices: analysis of components of a device, analysis of movement while wearing a device
Pain: pain perception assessment scale, visual analog scale, assessment of muscle soreness
Posture: analysis of resting and dynamic posture
Range of motion: active and passive range of motion
Reflex integrity: assessment of deep tendon reflexes
Self-care and home management: assessment of functional capacity, Functional Independence Measure

What additional findings are likely with this patient?

Spondylolysis has a 2:1 male-to-female predominance compared to all forms of spondylolisthesis, which indicate a female-to-male predominance of 2:1 (congenital) and 5:1 (degenerative). Overall, females tend to be more prone to progressive spondylolisthesis and require surgery more often than males. Most patients are diagnosed with isthmic type by the age of 15 with a significant increase in symptoms during puberty whereas patients diagnosed with degenerative type are usually over 40 when diagnosed.

Management:

What is the most effective management of this patient?

Patients with spondylolisthesis are initially treated conservatively regardless of the type or causative factors. Medical management may initially include rest if the spondylolisthesis is acute in nature. Pharmacological intervention may include NSAIDs, acetaminophen, hydrocodone, and/or vicodin. Steroid injections may be used to assist with radicular pain or neurogenic claudication. Physical therapy is indicated with emphasis on activity modification, patient education regarding disease process, bracing, and therapeutic stretching and strengthening. Exercise protocols should include exercise and activity that reduces stress with spinal extension. Bracing (typically a thoracolumbosacral spinal orthosis) may be prescribed to increase spinal stability and reduce symptoms. Conservative treatment is very successful especially with the younger patient, however, surgery may be indicated for unsuccessful patients or patients that present with neurological deficits secondary to the spondylolisthesis. Goals of surgery would include decompression of neural impingement and stabilization of the unstable segments of the spinal cord.

What home care regimen should be recommended?

A home care regimen should include a stretching program, posture exercises, and compliance with a wearing schedule if bracing is indicated.

Outcome:

What is the likely outcome of a course in physical therapy?

Physical therapy can play a vital role in the rehabilitation process, however, outcome is also based on the type and amount of slippage present, age, and comorbidities. Generally, the higher the grade of the slippage, the more variable the outcome becomes.

What are the long-term effects of the patient's condition?

Spondylolisthesis can be asymptomatic or can cause significant neurological deficits due to compression of the neural components surrounding the slippage. Conservative management is effective for many people, especially those with an isthmic type of spondylolisthesis. The degenerative type may continue with some persistent low back pain. Surgical intervention is warranted for patients with significant pain, failed conservative treatment, and/or neurological involvement. Surgery provides most patients with a relief of symptoms and improvement in function.

Comparison:

What are the distinguishing characteristics of a similar condition?

Retrolisthesis is a slippage in the posterior direction (opposite of anterolisthesis) or the relative posterior displacement of vertebra on the one below it that usually results from degenerative factors. Initially treatment incorporates activity modification and pharmacological intervention for pain control. If the pain worsens or a progressive neurologic deficit develops despite treatment, surgery may be indicated.

Clinical Scenarios:

Scenario One

A 14-year-old gymnast is seen in physical therapy shortly after she was diagnosed with a grade 2 spondylolisthesis. She is highly motivated to return to her physical activity, but has pain in the low back that will frequently go down her leg. She resides with her parents and younger sister in a two-story home.

Scenario Two

A 50-year-old male that works construction is seen in physical therapy after two months on medical leave for back pain. The patient just underwent surgical fusion of L4-L5 due to degenerative spondylolisthesis. He needs to work to provide for his family and wants to get back to his activity as soon as possible. He still complains of back pain and has some residual neurological deficits. He resides in a three-story townhouse with his wife and four children.

Systemic Lupus Erythematosus

Diagnosis:

What condition produces a patient's symptoms?

Systemic lupus erythematosus (SLE) is a connective tissue disorder caused by an autoimmune reaction in the body. The primary manifestation of the condition is the production of destructive antibodies that are directed at the individual's own body. The chronic inflammatory disorder produces a variety of symptoms depending on the severity and extent of involvement.

An injury was most likely sustained to which structure?

SLE is an autoimmune disorder that creates high levels of autoantibodies (antinuclear antibodies) that attack various cells and tissues within the body. The autoantibodies form immune complexes that produce an inflammatory response and cause further tissue destruction. Proliferation of immune complexes precipitates inflammation responses that in turn destroy cells, tissues, and organs. Specific injury is organ or system dependent depending on which areas of the body are affected by SLE.

Inference:

What is the most likely contributing factor in the development of this condition?

The exact etiology of SLE is unknown, however, it is described as an immunoregulatory disturbance from genetic, environmental, viral, and hormonal contributing factors. Environmental factors associated with SLE include ultraviolet light exposure, infection, antibiotics (specifically penicillin and sulfa drugs), extreme stress, immunization, and pregnancy. SLE can occur at any age, but the most common age group is 15 to 40 years of age. The disorder is 10-15 times more common in women.

Confirmation:

What is the most likely clinical presentation?

There are an estimated 1.4 million individuals diagnosed with SLE in the United States. A patient with SLE will have diverse symptoms based on the involvement of the connective tissue throughout the body. Symptoms will appear with exacerbations and disappear with remissions throughout the course of the disease. Symptoms such as arthralgias, malaise, and fatigue may persist even during a remission period. A patient may initially see a physician for symptoms that include fever, malaise, rash, arthralgias, headache, and weight loss. Common clinical presentation throughout the course of SLE includes a red butterfly rash across the cheeks and nose, a red rash over light exposed areas, arthralgias, alopecia, pleurisy, kidney involvement, seizures, depression, fibromyalgia, and cardiac involvement. SLE can affect the skin, joints, kidneys, lungs, heart, and other organs and tissues within the body. Patients can also have CNS

involvement that can lead to neuropsychiatric manifestations that present with depression, irritability, emotional instability, and seizures.

What laboratory or imaging studies would confirm the diagnosis?

Microscopic fluorescent techniques are indicated to detect the presence of the antinuclear antibody (ANA) within the blood. A positive ANA test warrants an additional test for antideoxyribonucleic acid antibodies. These two tests in combination with the physical presentation support the presence of SLE. Other testing including erythrocyte sedimentation rate, complete blood count, and urinalysis.

What additional information should be obtained to confirm the diagnosis?

The American Rheumatism Association has designated criteria to confirm the diagnosis of SLE. A patient requires at least four of fourteen characteristics that occur during the same period of time. A patient evaluation including a thorough history and current symptoms assists with confirming a diagnosis of SLE.

Examination:

What history should be documented?

Important areas to explore include past medical and family history, medications, current symptoms and health status, living environment, social history and habits, occupation, and social support system.

What test/measures are most appropriate?

Aerobic capacity and endurance: assessment of vital signs at rest/activity, auscultation of the lungs/heart
Arousal, attention, and cognition: examine mental status, learning ability, memory, motivation
Assistive and adaptive devices: analysis of components and safety of a device
Community and work integration: analysis of community, work, and leisure activities
Environmental, home, and work barriers: analysis of current and potential barriers or hazards
Ergonomics and body mechanics: analysis of dexterity and coordination
Gait, locomotion, and balance: static/dynamic balance in sitting and standing, safety during gait, Tinetti Performance Oriented Mobility Assessment, Berg Balance Scale, Functional Ambulation Profile
Integumentary integrity: skin assessment, assessment of sensation, presence and assessment of rash
Joint integrity and mobility: soft tissue swelling and inflammation, presence of deformity
Motor function: posture and balance
Muscle performance: strength assessment

Neuromotor development and sensory integration: analysis of reflex movement patterns, sensory integration tests, gross and fine motor skills
Orthotic, protective, and supportive devices: potential utilization of bracing
Pain: pain perception assessment scale
Range of motion: active and passive range of motion
Self-care and home management: assessment of functional capacity

What additional findings are likely with this patient?

SLE can produce skeletal deformities such as ulnar deviation and subluxed interphalangeal joints. Kidney involvement and cardiovascular impairments such as endocarditis, myocarditis, and pericarditis can occur during an exacerbation. Patients that experience nephritis, myocarditis or neurological implications have a poor prognosis. Modifiable risk factors for exacerbation include high stress, limited emotional and social support, and psychological distress.

Management:

What is the most effective management of this patient?

Medical management of SLE focuses on reversing the autoimmune response in order to avoid complications and exacerbations of symptoms. Pharmacological intervention for a patient with mild SLE will include salicylates, Indomethacin or NSAIDs. Antimalarial medications, corticosteroids, and immunosuppressive therapy may be used. General management of SLE includes good nutrition, ongoing medical supervision, and avoidance of ultraviolet exposure. Physical therapy intervention is usually indicated after a period of exacerbation and includes a slow resumption of physical activity, energy conservation techniques, gradual endurance activities and significant patient education regarding skin care, pacing, exercise, and strengthening to tolerance.

What home care regimen should be recommended?

A home care regimen during an acute exacerbation of SLE should include relaxation and energy conservation techniques, stress reduction strategies, therapeutic exercise as tolerated, and pain management.

Outcome:

What is the likely outcome of a course in physical therapy?

Physical therapy cannot cease or alter the clinical course of SLE, however, it may assist in controlling the debilitating effects during an acute phase/exacerbation of the disease. Goals include focus on pain relief, relaxation, strengthening, and preventing deformity.

What are the long-term effects of the patient's condition?

The clinical course of SLE is highly unpredictable. A patient may only exhibit symptoms for skin and joint involvement or may exhibit multi-system involvement. Periods of remission may last years and the prognosis depends on the severity and the extent of the disease process. The overall prognosis for SLE is good, although in rare cases the disease process can remain acute and become fatal within a short period of time. There is a high ten-year survival rate with SLE. Death is usually attributed to kidney failure or secondary infections.

Comparison:

What are the distinguishing characteristics of a similar condition?

Scleroderma, also termed progressive systemic sclerosis, is a chronic disease that primarily affects the skin, but can involve articular structures and internal organs. There is long-term hardening and shrinking of the affected connective tissues. The two subtypes of this disease are systemic scleroderma and localized scleroderma. Etiology is unknown and the disease varies in course (months, years or a lifetime) and progression.

Clinical Scenarios:

Scenario One

A 25-year-old female is referred to physical therapy for a therapeutic exercise program. The patient was diagnosed last year with SLE and has not exercised since that time. The patient is currently taking corticosteroids and antimalarial medications to manage a recent exacerbation.

Scenario Two

A 43-year-old female was seen in outpatient physical therapy to assist with pain management. The patient was diagnosed five years ago with SLE and has recently experienced increased difficulty using her hands secondary to deformity and pain. The patient's goal is to reduce the pain in her hands.

Temporomandibular Joint Dysfunction

Diagnosis:

What condition produces a patient's symptoms?

The temporomandibular joint (TMJ) is a complex joint that is classified as a condylar, hinge, and synovial joint. The TMJ contains fibrocartilaginous surfaces and articular discs. Temporomandibular joint dysfunction (TMD) occurs due to a change in the joint structure that can cause multiple symptoms and a limitation in function. In many instances inflammation and muscle spasm surrounding the joint produces symptoms for the patient with TMD.

An injury was most likely sustained to which structure?

TMD results from injury, derangement or incongruence of the TMJ itself, intra-articular disks, and/or supporting surrounding structures. Over time the meniscus of the TMJ becomes compressed and torn allowing for the bony portion of the joint (the ball and socket) to deteriorate secondary to the grinding of bone on bone.

Inference:

What is the most likely contributing factor in the development of this condition?

TMD can be classified by three primary etiological factors: predisposing factors, triggering factors, and perpetuating/sustaining factors. TMD can occur secondary to multiple causative factors including injury or trauma to the joint, congenital abnormalities, internal derangement of joint structure, arthritis, dislocation, disk degeneration, metabolic conditions or stress. Risk factors include chewing on one side, eating tough food, clenching, and grinding of teeth. Habits of gum chewing and nail biting may increase the incidence of injury to the TMJ. Patients are typically between 20 to 40 years of age with a greater incidence in women. Research indicates a possible link between gender-specific hormones and the risk for TMD.

Confirmation:

What is the most likely clinical presentation?

The National Institute of Dental and Craniofacial Research indicates that approximately 10.8 million individuals have TMD within the United States and 90% of the individuals that are seeking treatment are women in their childbearing years. A patient with TMD will present with symptoms that include pain (persistent or recurring), muscle spasm, abnormal or limited jaw motion, headache, and tinnitus. These symptoms can be unilateral or bilateral. The patient will often complain of feeling and hearing a "clicking or popping" sound with motion at the TMJ. Clinical manifestation of symptoms relates to the actual cause of the TMD.

What laboratory or imaging studies would confirm the diagnosis?

Procedures used in diagnosing TMD and its origin may include X-ray, MRI, mandibular kinesiography, CT scan, and a dental examination.

What additional information should be obtained to confirm the diagnosis?

A physical examination, upper quarter screening, TMJ loading, condyle-meniscus relationship, review of symptoms, and past medical history are all important components in the diagnosis of TMD. An occlusion examination may be indicated to evaluate a patient's bite.

Examination:

What history should be documented?

Important areas to explore include past medical history, medications, family history, current symptoms, current health status, diet, social history and habits, occupation, leisure activities, and social support system.

What test/measures are most appropriate?

Arousal, attention, and cognition: examine mental status, learning ability, memory, motivation
Community and work integration: analysis of community, work, and leisure activities
Cranial nerve integrity: assessment of muscle innervation by the cranial nerves, dermatome assessment
Integumentary integrity: skin assessment, assessment of sensation
Joint integrity and mobility: assessment of hyper- and hypomobility of a joint, soft tissue swelling and inflammation, joint play
Muscle performance: strength assessment including mastication, tongue, and lips; upper quarter screening
Pain: pain perception assessment scale, visual analog scale, assessment of muscle soreness
Posture: analysis of resting and dynamic posture
Range of motion: active and passive range of motion
Self-care and home management: assessment of functional capacity
Ventilation, respiration, and circulation: breathing patterns, respiratory muscle strength, accessory muscle utilization

What additional findings are likely with this patient?

TMD produces a general clinical presentation that includes pain, headache, muscle spasms, and tinnitus. Specific findings result from the specific cause of the TMD. Other findings can include popping and clicking when opening the mandible, locking of the TMJ, restriction of movement of the unaffected side, and/or pulling of the mandible towards the affected side. Common underlying causes include arthritis, fracture, congenital abnormalities, dislocations, and tension-relieving habits (chewing gum, bruxism, clenching or grinding the teeth).

Management:

What is the most effective management of this patient?

Medical management of TMD may include pharmacological intervention, the use of splinting, physical therapy treatment, and possible surgical intervention. Pharmacological treatment of TMD may include analgesics, NSAIDs, muscle relaxants, and antianxiety medications. A patient may also benefit from a splint to assist with realignment of the joint and a guard or bite plate to maintain proper positioning and avoid grinding of the teeth throughout the night. Specific physical therapy intervention is based on the exact etiology of the TMD. Generally, physical therapy intervention includes patient education regarding habits such as nail biting, posture retraining, the use of modalities such as moist heat, ice, biofeedback, ultrasound, electrostimulation, TENS, and massage. Soft tissue manipulation, joint mobilization, ROM, stretching, occlusal appliance prescription, and relaxation techniques are also appropriate. If conservative treatment fails or the exact etiology warrants surgical intervention, (approximately 5% of cases) the patient may require a condylectomy, osteotomy, arthrotomy, arthroscopy, reduction of subluxation or joint debridement.

What home care regimen should be recommended?

A home care regimen for a patient with TMD should include relaxation techniques, self-stretching, posture retraining exercises, and progressive ROM. A patient should avoid all foods and activities (such as gum chewing) that aggravate and stress the TMJ. The patient should continue with the proper use of an occlusal appliance if indicated. In order to maintain progress the patient must have ongoing consistency with the home program.

Outcome:

What is the likely outcome of a course in physical therapy?

Physical therapy intervention should improve a patient's condition and decrease the symptoms of the TMD. Physical therapy is usually conducted on an outpatient basis with focus on maximizing function and alleviating pain.

What are the long-term effects of the patient's condition?

A patient previously diagnosed with TMD is at an increased risk of recurrence, however, with successful management, ongoing compliance with the home program, and use of an indicated appliance, the patient may not have any long-term effects. If conservative management fails the patient may require surgical intervention for the underlying cause in order to alleviate the TMD.

Comparison:

What are the distinguishing characteristics of a similar condition?

Myofascial pain dysfunction (MPD) syndrome is a nonarticular disorder that affects the area surrounding the TMJ, however, symptoms are produced secondary to muscle spasm. MPD occurs more in females and can be of psychophysiologic origin. Habits such as grinding and jaw clenching increase tension in the muscles of mastication and create spasm. MPD can mimic the symptoms of TMD, however, differential diagnosis will rule out true TMJ involvement.

Clinical Scenarios:

Scenario One

A 12-year-old female is referred to physical therapy with a diagnosis of TMD secondary to condylar hyperplasia. The patient required a condylectomy with post-operative orders for physical therapy. The female is motivated and she has very supportive parents.

Scenario Two

A 30-year-old male is referred to physical therapy with a diagnosis of TMD. The physician referral notes inflammation, muscle spasm, and poor posture. The patient states that he will feel clicking when he eats certain foods. The patient has a history of childhood scoliosis that was controlled with exercise and short-term bracing. The patient is a stockbroker and spends a great deal of time talking on the phone.

Thoracic Outlet Syndrome

Diagnosis:

What condition produces a patient's symptoms?

Thoracic outlet syndrome is a term used to describe a group of disorders that presents with symptoms secondary to neurovascular compression of fibers of the brachial plexus. This usually occurs between the points of the interscalene triangle and the inferior border of the axilla. Compression of the nerves and blood supply can also occur as they pass over the first rib.

An injury was most likely sustained to which structure?

Thoracic outlet syndrome results from compression and damage to the brachial plexus nerve trunks, subclavian vascular supply, and/or the axillary artery. Nerve injury can result in neurapraxia with segmental degeneration and progress to axonotmesis due to continued and unrelieved compression.

Inference:

What is the most likely contributing factor in the development of this condition?

Contributing factors in the development of thoracic outlet syndrome include the presence of a cervical rib, an abnormal first rib, postural deviations or changes, body composition, chronic hyperabduction of the arm, hypertrophy or spasms of the scalene muscles, degenerative disorders, and an elongated cervical transverse process.

Confirmation:

What is the most likely clinical presentation?

A patient with thoracic outlet syndrome will present with symptoms based on nerve and/or vascular compression. Typical symptoms include diffuse pain in the arm most often at night, paresthesias in the fingers and through the upper extremities, weakness and muscle wasting, poor posture, edema, and discoloration. If the upper plexus is involved, pain will be reported in the neck that may radiate to the face and may follow the lateral aspect of the forearm into the hand. If the lower plexus is involved, pain is reported in the back of the neck and shoulder, which will radiate over the ulnar distribution to the hand. A patient's symptoms are usually enhanced with behaviors that aggravate the symptoms such as poor posture, lifting activities, and movements overhead.

What laboratory or imaging studies would confirm the diagnosis?

X-ray will confirm the presence of a cervical rib or other bony abnormality. Nerve conduction velocity testing may be valuable if a neuropathy exists. Otherwise, diagnosis relies solely on a thorough history of patient symptoms, provocative testing, and a physical examination. Other testing should be used for differential diagnosis to rule out cervical radiculopathy, RSD, myofascial pain syndrome, tumor, carpal tunnel syndrome, brachial plexus injury, ulnar never compression, and angina.

What additional information should be obtained to confirm the diagnosis?

A patient can be diagnosed with thoracic outlet syndrome following a thorough history of symptoms, physical examination, and provocative testing that includes Adson maneuver, Wright test, Roo's test, Halstead maneuver, Allen test, and the costoclavicular and hyperabduction tests.

Examination:

What history should be documented?

Important areas to explore include past medical history, family history, medications, history of symptoms, current health status, living environment, social history and habits, occupation, and social support system.

What test/measures are most appropriate?

Anthropometric characteristics: upper extremity circumferential measurements
Arousal, attention, and cognition: examine mental status, learning ability, memory, motivation
Community and work integration: analysis of community, work, and leisure activities
Cranial nerve integrity: assessment of muscles innervation by the cranial nerves, dermatome assessment
Environmental, home, and work barriers: analysis of current and potential barriers or hazards
Ergonomics and body mechanics: analysis of dexterity and coordination
Integumentary integrity: skin assessment, assessment of sensation
Joint integrity and mobility: soft tissue swelling and inflammation, assessment of joint play, palpation of the joint
Motor function: posture and balance; upper quarter screening
Muscle performance: strength assessment
Pain: pain perception assessment scale, assessment of interscalene triangle point tenderness
Posture: analysis of resting and dynamic posture
Range of motion: active and passive range of motion
Reflex integrity: assessment of deep tendon and pathological reflexes (e.g., Babinski, ATNR)
Self-care and home management: assessment of functional capacity

What additional findings are likely with this patient?

A patient with thoracic outlet syndrome may have difficulty sleeping due to excessive pillows or malpositioning of the arm. The patient may have difficulty at work with carrying items on the affected side or with driving a car. Thoracic outlet most commonly affects the population between 30 and 40 years of age with women being affected two to three times more than men.

Management:

What is the most effective management of this patient?

Initial medical management of thoracic outlet syndrome takes a conservative approach. If conservative management fails, it is followed by surgical intervention. A patient with thoracic outlet syndrome requires physical therapy intervention to assist with modification of posture, breathing patterns, positioning in bed and at the work site, and gentle stretching. Physical therapy should focus on pain management, strengthening (especially the trapezius, levator scapulae, and rhomboids), joint mobilization, body mechanics, flexibility, and postural awareness. A therapist may utilize modalities such as transcutaneous nerve stimulation, ultrasound, and biofeedback to attain goals. Work site analysis and subsequent activity modification may be necessary to relieve the pain and other symptoms. A patient may benefit from anti-inflammatory agents in combination with physical therapy. If physical therapy management fails, the patient may require surgical decompression of bony or fibrotic abnormalities. The exact type of surgical intervention and approach is chosen by the surgeon based on symptoms and current damage.

What home care regimen should be recommended?

A home care regimen for a patient with thoracic outlet syndrome should include stretching, strengthening, and postural awareness. The patient should utilize these strategies on an ongoing basis at work and with recreational activities in order to promote pain free movement and limit undesirable symptoms associated with the condition.

Outcome:

What is the likely outcome of a course in physical therapy?

Most patients with thoracic outlet syndrome have positive results from physical therapy intervention and are able to return to their previous level of function within four to eight weeks.

What are the long-term effects of the patient's condition?

If a patient has positive results from physical therapy intervention, there will not be any long-term impairments, however, if the patient's symptoms persist for three to four months surgical intervention may be warranted. Approximately 75% of patients post surgery have a positive response, however, complications from surgery can include winging of the scapula, pneumothorax, and nerve compression. Research indicates no significant long-term difference between surgical resection of the first rib and successful conservative management.

Comparison:

What are the distinguishing characteristics of a similar condition?

A radial nerve lesion may be caused by direct trauma, excessive traction, entrapment or compression. A patient presents with an inability to extend the wrist, thumb, and fingers. The patient will also present with impaired grip strength and coordination. Splinting is recommended to maintain proper positioning. Passive range of motion is necessary to prevent secondary impairments such as contractures within the hand.

Clinical Scenarios:

Scenario One

A 35-year-old female is seen in physical therapy secondary to pain and paresthesias throughout the left upper extremity. The patient's work history reveals that she is employed as a telemarketer and is required to hold the phone between her ear and shoulder throughout her shift. The patient carries a five-pound brief case with a shoulder strap as she walks one-half mile to work. The patient has a one-year-old child.

Scenario Two

A 45-year-old female is referred to physical therapy secondary to pain when reaching overhead and carrying objects. The patient recently complains of waking up during the night with pain and paresthesias in the involved arm. The patient is very anxious and concerned because she is required to carry items and place them above her head as part of her job at a local production mill.

Total Hip Arthroplasty

Diagnosis:

What condition produces a patient's symptoms?

A total hip arthroplasty (THA) may be warranted secondary to progressive and severe osteoarthritis or rheumatoid arthritis in the hip joint, developmental dysplasia of the hip, tumors, failed reconstruction of the hip or other hip conditions that produce incapacitating pain and disability. A THA may also be required secondary to trauma, avascular necrosis or a nonunion fracture.

An injury was most likely sustained to which structure?

Arthritis causes the hip joint to undergo a degenerative process including destruction of articular cartilage that results in bone-to-bone contact. Degenerative changes are usually apparent in both the acetabulum and the femoral head requiring a THA, however, if the acetabulum does not exhibit degenerative changes then only the femoral head will be replaced in a hemiarthroplasty procedure.

Inference:

What is the most likely contributing factor in the development of this condition?

Intra-articular disease or the destruction of articular cartilage may come from arthritis, repetitive microtrauma, obesity, nutritional imbalances, falls or abnormal joint mechanics. Indications for THA include osteoarthritis, rheumatoid arthritis, avascular necrosis, developmental dysplasia, osteomyelitis, failed fixation of a fracture, ankylosing spondylitis, and failed conservative management.

Confirmation:

What is the most likely clinical presentation?

A patient that requires a THA will present with decreased range of motion, impaired mobility skills, and persistent pain that increases with motion and weight bearing. The patient is usually over 55 years of age and has experienced consistent pain that is not relieved through conservative measures and limits the patient's functional mobility on a regular basis.

What laboratory or imaging studies would confirm the diagnosis?

X-ray, computed tomography, and magnetic resonance imaging procedures may be used to view the integrity of the joint. These procedures are also used to rule out a fracture or a tumor.

What additional information should be obtained to confirm the diagnosis?

Patient history, current functional status, and level of pain and disability are important factors in determining the need for surgical intervention. A standardized pain assessment scale and the Arthritis Impact Measurement tool may be used to establish an objective baseline. Relative or absolute contraindications must be considered prior to the recommendation for a THA. Contraindications may include but are not limited to active infection, severe obesity, arterial insufficiency, neuromuscular disease, and certain mental illness.

Examination:

What history should be documented?

Important areas to explore include past medical history, family history, medications, current symptoms, current health status, living environment, social history and habits, occupation, and social support system.

What test/measures are most appropriate?

Aerobic capacity and endurance: assessment of vital signs at rest and with activity, perceived exertion scale

Anthropometric characteristics: hip circumferential measurements, leg length measurements

Arousal, attention, and cognition: examine mental status, learning ability, memory, motivation

Assistive and adaptive devices: analysis of components and safety of a device

Environmental, home, and work barriers: analysis of current and potential barriers or hazards

Gait, locomotion, and balance: safety during gait with/without an assistive device, Functional Ambulation Profile

Joint integrity and mobility: soft tissue swelling and inflammation

Muscle performance: strength assessment, assessment of active movement

Pain: pain perception assessment scale

Range of motion: active and passive range of motion

Self-care and home assessment: assessment of functional capacity, Barthel Index

Sensory integrity: assessment of sensation

What additional findings are likely with this patient?

A patient that requires a THA may also have arthritis in other areas of the body. The patient may present with low endurance and may be deconditioned secondary to inactivity from the effects of arthritis. Post-surgical complications may include nerve injury, vascular damage, dislocation, pulmonary embolism, myocardial infarction, and CVA. The prosthesis is also at risk for loosening, infection, heterotopic ossification, and fracture.

Management:

What is the most effective management of this patient?

Medical management includes choosing a surgical approach that meets the patient's needs and level of activity. A THA that utilizes a posterolateral approach allows the abductor muscles to remain intact, however, there may be a higher incidence of post-operative joint instability due to the interruption of the posterior capsule. This type of surgical approach requires a patient to avoid excessive hip flexion greater than 90 degrees, hip adduction, and hip medial rotation. A patient with a THA that utilizes an anterolateral approach should avoid hip flexion and lateral rotation. A direct lateral approach leaves the posterior portion of the gluteus medius attached to the greater trochanter and the posterior capsule left intact. This method is preferred for patients that may be noncompliant in order to avoid posterior dislocation. Pharmacological intervention status post THA will require anticoagulant therapy and pain medication. The patient's post-operative care includes hip precautions, use of an abduction pillow (with posterolateral approach), initiation of hip protocol exercises, and physical therapy intervention. The hip protocol exercises usually include ankle pumps, quadriceps sets, gluteal sets, heel slides, and isometric abduction. Physical therapy should emphasize patient education regarding hip precautions and weight bearing status, scar management, and soft tissue mobilization. At the time of hospital discharge the patient should be able to extend the hip to neutral and flex the hip to 90 degrees. A cemented hip replacement usually allows for partial weight bearing initially and a noncemented hip replacement requires toe touch weight bearing for up to six weeks. Physical therapy encourages early ambulation training in order to avoid deconditioning and the risk of deep vein thrombosis. A patient must practice all mobility skills using the proper hip precautions. Outpatient physical therapy may be indicated to assist with progression to a cane.

What home care regimen should be recommended?

The patient should be instructed in a home care regimen that includes range of motion, strengthening, and progressive ambulation. The patient must adhere to the hip precaution guidelines for a minimum of three months or until a physician determines that the hip demonstrates adequate stability.

Outcome:

What is the likely outcome of a course in physical therapy?

A patient status post THA will benefit from physical therapy and should attain an improved functional outcome. The patient should have diminished to no pain, increased strength and endurance, and improved mobility within six to eight weeks after surgery.

What are the long-term effects of the patient's condition?

A THA is a highly successful surgical procedure. The current lifespan of the prosthesis is less than 20 years and as a result some patients may require a subsequent replacement. Studies indicate pain relief and improved function with good to excellent results in 85-95% of the patients at 15 to 20 years post THA. Validated scoring systems such as the Harris Hip Scoring System or the Special Surgery Rating system are measures used to determine the quality of life after the THA.

Comparison:

What are the distinguishing characteristics of a similar condition?

A hemiarthroplasty of the hip is a replacement of the femoral head due to a subcapital fracture of the femur or degeneration of the femoral head. This type of surgical intervention is sometimes used as an alternative to a THA for elderly patients that sustain a hip fracture or patients that have a shortened expected lifespan.

Clinical Scenarios:

Scenario One

A patient is seen in physical therapy after THA surgery. The surgeon performed an anterolateral approach and used a noncemented prosthesis. The patient is mildly obese and has a lengthy cardiac history. The patient has osteoarthritis and had progressive pain and difficulty with mobility prior to surgery. The patient complains of soreness in the hip and is anxious to get home.

Scenario Two

A 75-year-old male is seen in physical therapy status post reduction of a dislocated right hip prosthesis. The patient had a THA three weeks ago and dislocated the hip two days ago while bending over to tie his shoes. The patient is currently using a walker for mobility and is toe touch weight bearing. The patient resides alone in a garden apartment and does not have any family in the area.

Total Knee Arthroplasty

Diagnosis:

What condition produces a patient's symptoms?

A total knee arthroplasty (TKA) may be warranted secondary to progressive and disabling pain within the knee joint. The pain is most often due to severe degenerative osteoarthritic destruction and deformity that can occur within the knee.

An injury was most likely sustained to which structure?

Arthritis causes the knee joint to undergo a degenerative process that includes destruction of articular cartilage and resultant bone-to-bone contact within the joint. The knee presents with decreased joint space and osteophyte formation. Injury occurs to the femoral condyles, tibial articulating surface, and the dorsal side of the patella.

Inference:

What is the most likely contributing factor in the development of this condition?

The destruction of articular cartilage secondary to osteoarthritis is the most common indication for a TKA. A patient with a history of participation in high-impact sports or has experienced trauma to the knee is at a higher risk for arthritis and subsequent TKA. Obesity, varus/valgus deformity, previous mechanical derangement, infection, rheumatoid arthritis, hemophilia, crystal deposition diseases, avascular necrosis or bone dysplasia at the knee are some other contributing factors that may warrant a TKA.

Confirmation:

What is the most likely clinical presentation?

Approximately 130,000 TKAs are performed each year within the United States. A patient that requires a TKA will present with severe knee pain that worsens with motion and weight bearing, impaired range of motion, possible deformity of the knee, and impaired mobility skills. Night pain is common and may include localized or diffuse pain. Other symptoms may include stiffness, swelling, locking, and giving way of the affected knee. Patients often attempt conservative treatment measures to address the condition with only limited success.

What laboratory or imaging studies would confirm the diagnosis?

X-ray, computed tomography, and magnetic resonance imaging are used to determine the extent of deterioration and bony abnormalities within the knee joint. Radiographic images can be utilized post-operatively to ensure proper fit and obtain baseline information.

What additional information should be obtained to confirm the diagnosis?

Patient history, current functional status, and level of pain and disability are important factors in determining the need for surgical intervention. A pain assessment scale and the Arthritis Impact Measurement tool may be used to establish an objective baseline.

Examination:

What history should be documented?

Important areas to explore include past medical history, family history, medications, current symptoms, living environment, social history and habits, occupation, current functional status, and social support system.

What test/measures are most appropriate?

Aerobic capacity and endurance: assessment of vital signs at rest and with activity, perceived exertion scale
Anthropometric characteristics: knee circumferential measurements
Arousal, attention, and cognition: examine mental status, learning ability, memory, motivation
Assistive and adaptive devices: analysis of components and safety of a device
Environmental, home, and work barriers: analysis of current and potential barriers or hazards
Gait, locomotion, and balance: safety during gait/stairs with device, Functional Ambulation Profile
Joint integrity and mobility: soft tissue swelling and inflammation
Muscle performance: strength/active movement assessment
Pain: pain perception assessment scale
Range of motion: active and passive range of motion
Self-care and home assessment: assessment of functional capacity, Barthel Index
Sensory integrity: assessment of sensation

What additional findings are likely with this patient?

A patient that requires TKA may have arthritis in other joints, previous replacement surgeries or previous trauma to the knee joint. Patients with significant osteoarthritis and severe pain may exhibit sleep disorders or depression due to the disease process. Relative or absolute contraindications must be considered prior to the recommendation for a TKA. Contraindications may include but are not limited to active infection of the knee, severe obesity, significant genu recurvatum, arterial insufficiency, neuropathic joint, and certain mental illnesses. Post-surgical complications after a TKA include infection, vascular damage, patellofemoral instability, fracture surrounding the prosthesis, pulmonary embolism, nerve damage, loosening of the prosthesis, and arthrofibrosis.

Management:

What is the most effective management of this patient?

Medical management of a patient requiring a TKA includes choosing of the appropriate surgical procedure based on the patient's symptoms and level of activity. Pharmacological intervention status post TKA will require anticoagulant therapy and pain medications. The patient's post-operative care includes a knee immobilizer, elevation of the limb, cryotherapy, intermittent range of motion using a continuous passive motion (CPM) machine, and initiation of knee protocol exercises. A cemented knee prosthesis allows for either partial weight bearing or weight bearing as tolerated post surgery based on the individual physician's discretion. A noncemented knee prosthesis requires toe touch weight bearing for up to six weeks to allow for the bone to grow and affix to the prosthesis. Physical therapy should focus on mobility training with the proper weight bearing status using an appropriate assistive device. Early ambulation training is encouraged in order to avoid deconditioning and the risk of deep vein thrombosis. Physical therapy intervention should emphasize ankle pumps, quad sets, and hamstrings sets as well as range of motion and stretching. A goal of 90 degrees of knee flexion and 0 degrees knee extension is often established prior to discharge from the hospital or rehabilitation facility. The following precautions should be used for several months after surgery to avoid excessive stress to the knee: avoid squatting, avoid quick pivoting, do not use pillows under the knee while in bed, and avoid low seating. Outpatient therapy may be recommended to progress the patient from an assistive device. Once the physician progresses the patient to weight bearing as tolerated, physical therapy intervention should include strengthening with closed-chain exercises and functional activities.

What home care regimen should be recommended?

A home care regimen would typically include range of motion, strengthening, and progressive ambulation exercises. The patient must adhere to precautions, use of an immobilizer, and proper weight bearing status until a physician determines that the knee joint demonstrates adequate stability.

Outcome:

What is the likely outcome of a course in physical therapy?

A patient status post TKA will benefit from physical therapy and should attain an improved functional capacity. The patient should experience relief of pain that will allow for a full return to previous functional activities within eight to twelve weeks after surgery depending on a cemented or noncemented prosthesis and potential complications that were encountered.

What are the long-term effects of the patient's condition?

A TKA is a highly successful surgical procedure that should significantly reduce pain and increase function. After finishing a rehabilitation protocol, a patient may have only minor limitations in knee range of motion. A knee replacement may loosen over time and require revision, however, the life expectancy of the knee prosthesis is between 15 and 20 years.

Comparison:

What are the distinguishing characteristics of a similar condition?

A patellectomy (surgical removal of the patella) is a surgical procedure that is indicated for a comminuted facture of the patella that cannot be repaired with internal fixation. A patellectomy can include the entire patella or just the inferior or superior pole of the patella. The retinaculum and extensor mechanism are repaired with the surgical procedure and the patient is immobilized for six to eight weeks. Once rehabilitation is initiated the patient starts with range of motion and closed-chain exercises.

Clinical Scenarios:

Scenario One

An 80-year-old female in an acute care hospital is two days status post left TKA. The patient presents with partial hearing loss and moderate dementia. The patient's past medical history includes a right CVA with no residual impairment and hypertension that is controlled by medication. The patient resides with her sister in a ranch style home with three steps to enter.

Scenario Two

A 49-year-old male is referred to outpatient physical therapy seven weeks after surgery. The patient received a noncemented knee prosthesis and has recently advanced to weight bearing as tolerated. The patient's range of motion in the involved knee is 10-85 degrees. The patient is otherwise independent with axillary crutches. No significant past medical history is noted.

Total Shoulder Arthroplasty

Diagnosis:

What condition produces a patient's symptoms?

A patient that is a candidate for a total shoulder arthroplasty (TSA) will have severe pain and impaired shoulder motion due to deterioration of the glenohumeral joint. These candidates have undergone conservative treatment measures that have failed to improve their condition.

An injury was most likely sustained to which structure?

TSA candidates will have irreparable damage, deterioration, and destruction to the humeral head and the glenoid fossa within the shoulder complex. The joint surfaces are severely damaged or destroyed by wear and tear, inflammation, injury or previous surgery.

Inference:

What is the most likely contributing factor in the development of this condition?

Indications for a TSA include severe glenohumeral degenerative joint disease, pain and limited range of motion secondary to osteoarthritis, rheumatoid arthritis, avascular necrosis, fracture or rotator cuff arthropathy. Other patients that may require a TSA would include a patient with a bone tumor, Paget's disease or with recurrent dislocations. A patient will be considered for TSA if conservative treatment of the underlying cause fails.

Confirmation:

What is the most likely clinical presentation?

A patient will exhibit impaired range of motion at the shoulder, may lack independence with functional mobility and ADLs, and will experience severe pain. It is this unremitting pain (with failed conservative treatment) that is the primary indication for the TSA. A TSA performed secondary to arthritis is usually performed on patients between 55 and 70 years of age while TSA performed secondary to irreparable damage from dislocation or avascular necrosis is usually performed on patients between 40 and 50 years of age.

What laboratory or imaging studies would confirm the diagnosis?

X-ray will reveal the level of degeneration within the shoulder complex. MRI or CT scan will allow the physician to assess the integrity of the rotator cuff and deltoid muscles surrounding the joint as well as the overall integrity of the shoulder complex.

What additional information should be obtained to confirm the diagnosis?

A full medical history along with a physical examination is a key component that is required in determining if a patient is a candidate for a TSA. The patient must possess motivation, realistic expectations, and appropriate goals regarding outcome.

Examination:

What history should be documented?

Important areas to explore include past medical and family history, medication, current symptoms, surgical precautions/contraindications, rehabilitation protocol, social history and habits, occupation, leisure activities, and social support system.

What test/measures are most appropriate?

Aerobic capacity and endurance: assessment of vital signs at rest and with activity
Anthropometric characteristics: circumferential measurements of the affected upper extremity
Arousal, attention, and cognition: examine mental status, learning ability, memory, motivation
Community and work integration: analysis of community, work, and leisure activities
Environmental, home, and work barriers: analysis of current and potential barriers or hazards
Integumentary integrity: skin assessment, assessment of sensation
Joint integrity and mobility: assessment of hyper- and hypomobility of a joint, soft tissue swelling and inflammation
Muscle performance: strength assessment except for surgical extremity
Pain: pain perception assessment scale, visual analog scale, assessment of muscle soreness
Range of motion: passive range of motion within limits of physician protocol for involved shoulder, active and passive range of motion for all other extremities
Self-care and home management: assessment of functional capacity, Functional Independence Measure (FIM)
Sensory integrity: assessment of proprioception and kinesthesia

What additional findings are likely with this patient?

Surgical complications post TSA include mechanical loosening of the prosthesis, instability, rotator cuff tear, implant failure, heterotopic ossification and intraoperative fracture. Risk for complication is dependent on the type of prosthesis (unconstrained, semiconstrained, constrained), surgical skill in reproducing proper alignment, use of cemented prosthesis versus press-fit prosthesis, and integrity of rotator cuff musculature.

Management:

What is the most effective management of this patient?

A patient status post TSA will remain hospitalized for an average of two to five days. Medical management of the patient will rely on a team approach including nursing, physician services, and rehabilitation therapies. The success of the TSA will rely on the style of the implant, the quality of the soft tissue, bone, and the rehabilitation program. A CPM may be prescribed by the surgeon for use during the patient's hospitalization. Pharmacological intervention includes anticoagulation and pain medications. Physical therapy is initiated the day after surgery and should follow the shoulder rehabilitation protocol designed by the surgeon. The shoulder usually remains immobilized using a sling during initial rehabilitation. The Neer shoulder protocol advocates initiating isometric shoulder exercises approximately three weeks after surgery and active shoulder exercises approximately six weeks after surgery. PROM and AAROM are indicated but AROM at the shoulder is contraindicated during the first phase of rehabilitation. Physical therapy intervention includes pain management, prevention of adhesions, functional activities, PROM/AAROM/AROM, therapeutic exercise, edema management, patient education in self-ROM and wand/pendulum exercises, and the use of modalities.

What home care regimen should be recommended?

The home care regimen should include a range of motion and therapeutic exercise program that follows the surgeon's shoulder rehabilitation protocol. During initial recovery, pendulum and wand exercises are appropriate as well as self-ROM. A patient must not perform any form of medial rotation or lateral rotation beyond 35 to 40 degrees during the first two to three weeks post surgery. Controlled motion and return to functional activity are incorporated into the home program as directed by the physician protocol. A patient must also continue to manage edema and follow other physician orders regarding precautions.

Outcome:

What is the likely outcome of a course in physical therapy?

The goal of a TSA is to relieve pain and regain functional motion. Physical therapy should assist the patient to meet these goals unless hindered by post-surgical or other complications.

What are the long-term effects of the patient's condition?

Since the shoulder is a non-weight bearing joint there is a longer life expectancy for the prosthesis than for the knee or hip. There is a high success rate for long-term results with a TSA. Patients should avoid activities such as heavy lifting, chopping wood or contact sports since these can increase the risk of fracture, loosening or rotator cuff tear.

Comparison:

What are the distinguishing characteristics of a similar condition?

A shoulder hemiarthroplasty is a similar surgery that involves the replacement of the head and neck of the humerus leaving the glenoid fossa of the scapula intact. This surgery is indicated when the humeral head has deteriorated or fractured without healing. This procedure may also be performed if the patient does not have enough bone density to support the glenoid component or when there are significant rotator cuff deficiencies that exist.

Clinical Scenarios:

Scenario One

A 60-year-old female is 14 days status post left TSA and is currently attending outpatient therapy three days per week. The patient's rehabilitation is complicated by right upper extremity paralysis secondary to a CVA two years ago. The patient is motivated, cooperative, and does not have any residual cognitive deficits.

Scenario Two

A 58-year-old male is one-month status post TSA and has been attending outpatient therapy three days per week. His wife states that he complains of significant pain during his home exercise program. He appears to be progressing otherwise. He has no significant medical history other than the rheumatoid arthritis that created the need for the TSA.

Transfemoral Amputation due to Osteosarcoma

Diagnosis:

What condition produces a patient's symptoms?

Osteosarcoma (osteogenic sarcoma) is the second most common primary bone tumor and accounts for 15-20% of bone tumors. Osteosarcoma is a highly malignant cancer that begins in the medullary cavity of a bone and leads to the formation of a mass. It usually affects bones with an active growth phase such as the femur or tibia and is often located in the metaphysis. Amputation may be necessary to remove the tumor and surrounding tissues to avoid metastatic disease.

An injury was most likely sustained to which structure?

The cancer cells are found in osteoblasts within the primitive mesenchymal cells of the medullary cavity of a bone. The cancer rapidly proliferates, replaces normal bone, and causes tissue destruction. Osteosarcoma will also metastasize to the lungs very early in the disease process.

Inference:

What is the most likely contributing factor in the development of this condition?

Osteosarcomas can occur as a primary or secondary cancer and the etiology remains unknown. This form of tumor primarily affects young children (especially males), adolescents, and young adults under 30 years of age. A peak time for incidence is during a growth spurt as an adolescent. Risk factors associated with secondary osteosarcoma include Paget's disease, osteoblastoma, giant cell tumor or chronic osteomyelitis. Environmental and genetic factors have been associated with the disease. In many instances amputation is required to cease the disease process.

Confirmation:

What is the most likely clinical presentation?

Osteosarcoma can be found most often in the long bones especially at the site of the most active epiphyseal growth plate, the distal femur, proximal tibia, proximal humerus and pelvis. The knee region accounts for approximately 50% of osteosarcomas. Patients that require amputation secondary to an osteosarcoma will present with a mass often found in the tibia or femur. The most common symptoms of osteosarcoma are pain and swelling within the extremity. Pain may worsen at night or with exercise and a lump may develop in the extremity sometime after the onset of pain. The osteosarcoma may weaken the involved extremity leading to a fracture. In some cases, a fracture may be the first sign of the osteosarcoma. Metastases appear in the lungs early in 90% of the cases.

What laboratory or imaging studies would confirm the diagnosis?

X-ray, MRI, and scintigraphy allow the physician to determine the presence, location, and size of a tumor. The "Codman's triangle" can be seen on x-ray indicating reactive bone at the site where the periosteum has been elevated by the neoplasm. Definitive diagnosis for an osteosarcoma is made through tissue biopsy of the tumor.

What additional information should be obtained to confirm the diagnosis?

Diagnosis of osteosarcoma is confirmed solely through biopsy. The course of treatment and the need for surgical amputation is determined by the size, location of the tumor, and progression of the malignancy.

Examination:

What history should be documented?

Important areas to explore include past medical history, medications, family history, current symptoms and health status, social history and habits, occupation, leisure activities, and social support system.

What test/measures are most appropriate?

Aerobic capacity and endurance: assessment of vital signs at rest and with activity, auscultation of the lungs, palpation of pulses

Anthropometric characteristics: residual limb circumferential measurements, length of limb

Arousal, attention, and cognition: examine mental status, learning ability, memory, motivation

Assistive and adaptive devices: analysis of components and safety of a device

Community and work integration: analysis of community, work, and leisure activities

Gait, locomotion, and balance: analysis of wheelchair mobility, static and dynamic balance in sitting and standing, safety during gait with an assistive device

Integumentary integrity: skin assessment, assessment of sensation, temperature of limb

Muscle performance: strength and tone assessment

Pain: phantom pain, pain perception assessment scale

Prosthetic requirements: analysis and safety of the prosthesis; alignment, efficiency, and fit of the prosthesis with the residual limb

Range of motion: active and passive range of motion

Self-care and home management: assessment of functional capacity, Barthel Index, Functional Independence Measure (FIM),

Sensory integrity: proprioception and kinesthesia

What additional findings are likely with this patient?

A patient status post transfemoral amputation secondary to an osteosarcoma may present with fatigue, loss of balance, phantom pain or sensation, hypersensitivity of the residual limb, and psychological issues regarding the loss of the limb. The patient may also have associated symptoms from chemotherapy that can include anemia, abnormal bleeding, infection, and kidney impairment. The presence of these findings can have a negative influence on a patient's ability to utilize a prosthesis.

Management:

What is the most effective management of this patient?

Medical management will focus on adjunctive therapies to treat the osteosarcoma. Pharmacological intervention may include pain medication and other medication to deter effects from cancer treatment. Physical and occupational therapies should begin immediately after the transfemoral amputation. Preprosthetic intervention should focus on range of motion, positioning, strengthening, desensitization, residual limb wrapping, functional mobility, gait training, and patient education for care of the residual limb. Patients with a transfemoral amputation should lie prone for a period of time each day to prevent a hip flexion contracture. Modalities may be used to improve range of motion and decrease pain. Serial casting may be indicated if a contracture develops. Without complication the patient should be able to return home with support and receive short-term physical therapy for prosthetic training.

What home care regimen should be recommended?

A home care regimen for a patient status post transfemoral amputation should include limb desensitization, stretching, proper positioning, and prone lying. The patient must be independent with residual limb care, skin inspection, and proper wrapping. Endurance activities, strengthening, and mobility with an assistive device are necessary as a precursor to prosthetic training.

Outcome:

What is the likely outcome of a course in physical therapy?

Physical therapy is necessary for both preprosthetic and prosthetic training. A patient should be able to achieve the established goals and function with a prosthesis for all mobility including ambulation, balance, transfers, and stair activities. The general health, cognition, motivation, and social support system of the patient will influence the patient's functional outcome.

What are the long-term effects of the patient's condition?

The survival rate for a patient status post osteosarcoma has increased in recent years to a five-year cure rate of 70-80% with treatment that may include amputation, radiation, and chemotherapy. The transfemoral amputation should not permanently impair the patient's independence with mobility, self-care or ambulation using a prosthesis. The patient's long-term outcome is dependent on the status of the cancer.

Comparison:

What are the distinguishing characteristics of a similar condition?

Ewing's sarcoma is a malignant nonosteogenic primary bone tumor that infiltrates the bone marrow and usually affects children and adolescents under 20 years of age. A patient will present with pain of increasing severity, swelling, and fever. This tumor is not found consistently in a specific location within the bone and is extremely malignant with a high frequency of metastases. Ewing's sarcoma requires aggressive treatment that may include amputation and adjunctive chemotherapy. The five-year survival rate is approximately 70%.

Clinical Scenarios:

Scenario One

A 10-year-old female is seen in physical therapy after a right transfemoral amputation. The patient was diagnosed with osteosarcoma four months ago. The patient is in good spirits and is anxious to receive "a new leg" and begin walking. Her parents are supportive and are eager to assist her during rehabilitation.

Scenario Two

A 16-year-old male is seen for the first time in physical therapy since a left transfemoral amputation. The boy states that his leg had bothered him for a few weeks and the pain got worse everyday. He also stated that he was told that the cancer was now also found in his lungs. He wants to start an exercise program so that he will be ready for his prosthesis when his residual limb heals.

Transtibial Amputation due to Arteriosclerosis Obliterans

Diagnosis:

What condition produces a patient's symptoms?

Arteriosclerosis obliterans, also known as peripheral arterial disease (PAD), is a form of peripheral vascular disease that produces thickening, hardening, and eventual narrowing and occlusion of the arteries. Arteriosclerosis obliterans results in ischemia and subsequent ulceration of the affected tissues. The affected area may become necrotic, gangrenous, and require amputation.

An injury was most likely sustained to which structure?

Injury will occur to all structures that receive blood supply from vessels that have become occluded. Prolonged ischemia results in tissue death and infection. Arteriosclerosis obliterans is the most common arterial occlusive disease and accounts for approximately 95% of the cases of vascular disease.

Inference:

What is the most likely contributing factor in the development of this condition?

Risk factors associated with arteriosclerosis obliterans include age, diabetes, sex, hypertension, high serum cholesterol and low-density lipid levels, smoking, impaired glucose tolerance, obesity, and sedentary lifestyle. Unsuccessful management of peripheral vascular disease may ultimately lead to uncontrolled infection, gangrene, necrosis, and amputation. Males have an overall higher incidence of arteriosclerosis than female counterparts.

Confirmation:

What is the most likely clinical presentation?

The patient that requires a transtibial amputation secondary to arteriosclerosis obliterans is typically an individual over 45 years that smokes (75-90%) and will present with intermittent claudication that produces cramps and pain in the affected areas. Intermittent claudication will typically present in the gastrocnemius-soleus complex, secondary to its high oxygen demand. Other characteristics include resting pain, decreased pulses, ischemia, pallor skin, and decreased skin temperature.

What laboratory or imaging studies would confirm the diagnosis?

Arteriosclerosis obliterans can be diagnosed using Doppler ultrasonography, MRI or arteriography. These diagnostic tests examine the degree of blood flow throughout the extremities. A patient with arteriosclerosis obliterans would typically demonstrate poor results including blockage, tissue damage, and tissue death.

What additional information should be obtained to confirm the diagnosis?

The physician should examine the limb for temperature, skin condition, the presence of hair, sensation, and palpable pulses when determining the need for amputation. The physician may perform a selected non-invasive test such as a claudication test that examines the presence of intermittent claudication that can occur with prolonged ambulation. The ankle-brachial index, segmental limb pressures or pulse volume recordings may also be used to assist with the diagnosis.

Examination:

What history should be documented?

Important areas to explore include past medical history, medications, current health status, social history and habits, occupation, living environment, and social support system.

What test/measures are most appropriate?

Aerobic capacity and endurance: palpation of pulses, pulse oximetry, assessment of vital signs at rest and with activity

Anthropometric characteristics: residual limb circumferential measurements, length of limb

Arousal, attention, and cognition: examine mental status, learning ability, memory, motivation

Assistive and adaptive devices: analysis of components and safety of a device

Gait, locomotion, and balance: analysis of wheelchair mobility, static and dynamic balance in sitting and standing, safety during gait with an assistive device

Integumentary integrity: examine presence of hair growth, color, temperature, assessment of sensation

Muscle performance: strength assessment, muscle tone assessment

Pain: phantom pain, pain perception assessment scale

Prosthetic requirements: (when appropriate) analysis and safety of the prosthesis; assessment of alignment, efficiency, and fit of the prosthesis; assessment of residual limb with the prosthesis

Range of motion: active and passive range of motion

Self-care and home management: assessment of functional capacity, Barthel Index, Functional Independence Measure (FIM)

Sensory integrity: assessment of proprioception and kinesthesia

What additional findings are likely with this patient?

A patient status post transtibial amputation may have a decrease in cardiovascular status depending on the frequency of intermittent claudication the patient experienced prior to the amputation. The patient may initially experience diminished balance secondary to the loss of the limb. Other issues that directly affect the residual limb include phantom pain, decreased range of motion, poor skin integrity, and hypersensitivity. The presence of any of these findings can have a negative influence on a patient's ability to utilize a prosthesis.

Management:

What is the most effective management of this patient?

A patient should be a candidate for inpatient physical therapy services immediately after the transtibial amputation. Preprosthetic intervention should focus on strength, range of motion, functional mobility, use of assistive devices, desensitization, and patient education for care of the residual limb. Intervention should focus on proper positioning in order to avoid the risk of contractures, especially a knee flexion contracture. If the patient does not experience complications they should be able to return home either independently or with support. The patient may receive continued short-term physical therapy for prosthetic intervention once the residual limb has fully healed.

What home care regimen should be recommended?

A home care regimen for a patient status post transtibial amputation should include exercises, limb desensitization, proper positioning, and stretching. Since ambulation with a prosthesis increases the energy cost, the patient should be encouraged to perform cardiovascular activities on a frequent basis. In order to be successful, the patient will need to consistently monitor the residual limb and wrap the limb to ensure proper shaping until the prosthesis is tolerated.

Outcome:

What is the likely outcome of a course in physical therapy?

Physical therapy for both preprosthetic and prosthetic intervention is typically necessary. A patient should be able to achieve the established goals and function with a prosthesis and an assistive device if warranted. The general health, cognition, motivation, and social support system of the patient will influence the patient's functional outcome.

What are the long-term effects of the patient's condition?

Arteriosclerosis obliterans is a chronic disease that a patient should continue to manage. The current transtibial amputation should not permanently alter a patient's level of functional mobility. The patient should be able to manage all aspects of self-care and functional mobility after prosthetic training with the permanent prosthesis unless hindered by other ailments. Approximately 20% of all individuals with arteriosclerosis obliterans have a myocardial infarction or CVA at some point after diagnosis.

Comparison:

What are the distinguishing characteristics of a similar condition?

There will be many similar characteristics regardless of the level of amputation to the lower or upper extremity. Intervention will include desensitization, phantom pain education, proper compression and shaping, strength improvement, proper positioning, and self-care and mobility with all patients. In most cases patients and therapists share the common goal of functional prosthetic utilization.

Clinical Scenarios:

Scenario One

A two-year-old female born with congenital malformation of the ankle joint and without a foot is referred to physical therapy for a pre-operative evaluation. The child is in good health, active, and has no other past medical history. The child has become increasingly frustrated with her alternate means of mobility. Her parents are supportive and carry her for community mobility. She prefers to scoot and crawl around the house since she cannot bear weight through the affected lower extremity. She is scheduled for a Syme's amputation in one week.

Scenario Two

An 83-year-old male, status post right transtibial amputation secondary to insulin-dependent diabetes mellitus, is admitted to a skilled nursing facility for rehabilitation. The patient is obese and presents with cardiopulmonary insufficiency. The patient previously resided alone with intermittent home health care and requires two liters of oxygen with activity.

Traumatic Brain Injury

Diagnosis:

What condition produces a patient's symptoms?

Traumatic brain injury (TBI) occurs due to an open head injury where there is penetration through the skull or closed head injury where the brain makes contact with the skull secondary to a sudden, violent acceleration or deceleration impact. Traumatic brain injury can also occur secondary to anoxia as with cardiac arrest or near drowning.

An injury was most likely sustained to which structure?

Any structure within the brain is vulnerable to injury; however, primary damage will occur at the site of impact. Secondary damage occurs as a result of metabolic and physiologic reactions to the trauma. Brain injury may include swelling, axonal injury, hypoxia, hematoma, hemorrhage and changes in intracranial pressure (ICP).

Inference:

What is the most likely contributing factor in the development of this condition?

Statistics from the Brain Injury Association indicate that motor vehicle accidents (45-60%) and falls (25%) are the two leading causes of TBI. Statistics reveal that 92% of all children diagnosed with severe brain injuries were involved in motor vehicle accidents. Males between 15-24 years have the highest incidence of injury. Individuals over 65 years of age and children between 1-2 years of age are also in a higher risk group.

Confirmation:

What is the most likely clinical presentation?

The incidence of head injury is close to two million individuals per year with an estimated five million individuals living with a brain injury. The clinical presentation of a TBI varies due to the type, area, extent of injury, and secondary damage within the brain. Characteristics of a TBI may include altered consciousness (coma, obtundity, delirium), cognitive and behavioral deficits, changes in personality, motor impairments, alterations in tone, and speech and swallowing issues.

What laboratory or imaging studies would confirm the diagnosis?

Diagnostic imaging such as CT scan or MRI should be performed immediately in order to rule out hemorrhage, infarction, and swelling. X-rays taken of the cervical spine can be used to rule out fracture and potential for subluxation. An electroencephalogram (EEG), positron emission tomography (PET), and cerebral blood flow mapping (CBF) may also be utilized for diagnosis and baseline data.

What additional information should be obtained to confirm the diagnosis?

A full neurological evaluation by a physician should include a mental examination, cranial nerve assessment, tonal assessment and papillary reactivity assessment. The physician will classify the patient using the Glasgow Coma Scale and indicate severe (coma), moderate or mild brain injury. The Rancho Los Amigos Levels of Cognitive Functioning can also be used to classify injury and assist with developing an appropriate plan of care.

Examination:

What history should be documented?

Important areas to explore include past medical history, medications, family history, current symptoms, level of cognitive functioning, social history and habits, occupation, leisure activities, and social support system.

What test/measures are most appropriate?

Aerobic capacity and endurance: vital signs at rest/activity, pulse oximetry, auscultation of lungs

Arousal, attention, and cognition: using Rancho Los Amigos levels of cognitive functioning

Assistive and adaptive devices: analysis of components and safety of a device

Cranial nerve integrity: muscle innervation by the cranial nerves, dermatome assessment

Environmental, home, and work barriers: analysis of current and potential barriers or hazards

Gait, locomotion, and balance: static and dynamic balance in sitting and standing, safety during gait with/without an assistive device, Berg Balance Scale, Tinetti Performance Oriented Mobility Assessment, analysis of wheelchair management

Integumentary integrity: skin and sensation assessment

Joint integrity and mobility: assessment of hyper- and hypomobility of a joint

Motor function: equilibrium and righting reactions, motor assessment scales, coordination, posture and balance in sitting, assessment of sensorimotor integration, physical performance scales

Muscle performance: strength assessment, muscle tone assessment

Neuromotor development and sensory integration: analysis of reflex movement patterns, assessment of involuntary movements, sensory integration tests, gross and fine motor skills

Orthotic, protective, and supportive devices: analysis of components and movement while wearing a device

Pain: pain perception assessment scale, visual analog scale, assessment of muscle soreness

Posture: analysis of resting and dynamic posture
Range of motion: active and passive range of motion
Reflex integrity: assessment of deep tendon and pathological reflexes (e.g., Babinski, ATNR)
Self-care and home management: assessment of functional capacity, Functional Independence Measure (FIM), Barthel Index, Rankin Scale, Rivermead Motor Assessment

What additional findings are likely with this patient?

There are multiple impairments that can develop secondary to TBI. Intracranial pressure must be monitored initially since it is at risk to increase or develop hemorrhage. A patient can develop heterotopic ossification, contractures, skin breakdown, seizures, and deep vein thrombosis. A patient with a severe TBI may remain in a persistent vegetative state.

Management:

What is the most effective management of this patient?

Medical management is initiated at the site of injury or in the emergency room for life preserving measures. The initial goal is to stabilize the patient, control intracranial pressure, and prevent secondary complications. Surgical intervention may be required in attempt to regain homeostasis within the brain secondary to hemorrhage or fracture. Once a patient is medically stable, physical therapy rehabilitation is initiated. Treatment of a patient with TBI usually includes a team approach with goals based on the patient's level of injury. Pharmacological intervention may include cerebral vasoconstrictive agents, psychotropic agents, hypertensive agents, antispasticity agents and medication to assist with cognition and attention. Physical therapy will focus on sensory stimulation and PROM for a comatose patient or pathfinding and high-level balance activities for a patient with a mild injury. Physical therapy may include functional mobility training, behavior modification, serial casting, compensatory strategies, vestibular rehabilitation, task specific activities, wheelchair seating, and pulmonary intervention.

What home care regimen should be recommended?

A home care regimen should include ongoing therapeutic activities that focus on goals associated with the patient's current Rancho Los Amigos level. Consistency is vital to the success of a home program. The patient may also participate in a community re-entry based program for the TBI population if warranted by their level of current function.

Outcome:

What is the likely outcome of a course in physical therapy?

A patient diagnosed with TBI does not have a specific projected outcome. Outcome is based on the degree of primary and secondary damage and the extent of cognitive and behavioral impairments. Physical therapy should continue in all settings until the patient has attained all realistic goals.

What are the long-term effects of the patient's condition?

TBI affects approximately two million Americans each year. Recent statistics state 80,000 Americans experience the onset of long-term disability secondary to TBI. Over 50,000 die each year as a result of TBI. Long-term effects are determined by the extent of injury and impairments resulting from the TBI. Many patients experience life long deficits that do not allow them to return to their pre-injury lifestyle.

Comparison:

What are the distinguishing characteristics of a similar condition?

Meningitis is a bacterial or viral infection that spreads through the cerebrospinal fluid to the brain. The meninges of the brain become inflamed as well as the meningeal membranes. The patient will have a headache and may complain of stiffness in the neck. The patient may also show symptoms of confusion, fatigue, and irritability. As the virus progresses the patient may experience seizures and may progress into a coma. Medical treatment varies based on the causative strain of the virus/bacteria. Mortality ranges from 5-25% and approximately 30% have some degree of permanent neurological impairment.

Clinical Scenarios:

Scenario One

A 22-year-old male with TBI is admitted to an inpatient rehabilitation hospital. The patient is presently classified as Rancho Los Amigos Level IV. The patient required surgical decompression after the TBI. The patient's parents are with the patient almost constantly.

Scenario Two

A 42-year-old female sustained a severe TBI in a motor vehicle accident and is presently classified as Rancho Los Amigos Level II. The accident was two weeks ago. Prior to admission the patient was healthy and worked full-time. She has a supportive husband.

Urinary Stress Incontinence

Diagnosis:

What condition produces a patient's symptoms?

Urinary incontinence is the involuntary loss of urine. There are four classifications that include functional incontinence, stress incontinence, urge incontinence, and overflow incontinence. Urinary stress incontinence may occur during activities when there is an increase in abdominal pressure through straining, sneezing, coughing or lifting.

An injury was most likely sustained to which structure?

Urinary stress incontinence usually occurs from loss of strength and/or integrity of the contractile and noncontractile tissues that maintain bladder control. Urinary stress incontinence is caused by weakness of the pelvic floor musculature (pubococcygeus muscle), damage of the pudendal nerve, weakness of the urogenital diaphragm muscles, malposition of the urethra and/or urethral sphincter incompetence.

Inference:

What is the most likely contributing factor in the development of this condition?

Risk factors for the development of urinary stress incontinence include pregnancy, vaginal delivery, episiotomy, prostate or pelvic surgery, aging, diabetes mellitus, central nervous system and peripheral system dysfunction, and recurrent urinary infection. A prolapsed bladder, uterus or bowel may contribute to leakage and is seen in women that have had multiple vaginal deliveries. Medications that treat other illnesses can sometimes contribute to incontinence especially with the older population. Obesity is another risk factor that is believed to increase the risk of stress incontinence due to increased intra-abdominal pressure and the effect of obesity on the neuromuscular function of the genitourinary tract.

Confirmation:

What is the most likely clinical presentation?

It is estimated that approximately 10 million adults experience some form of urinary incontinence. Urinary stress incontinence accounts for 50-60% of all incontinence cases and is manifested solely by the involuntary loss of urine with any form of exertion or increased abdominal pressure. The amount of urine that leaks is typically less than 50 milliliters with coughing, sneezing or straining. Physical activity or exercise can also produce leakage due to exertion with these activities. Other manifestations may include dribbling of urine, urgency, frequency, nocturia, and a weak stream while voiding.

What laboratory or imaging studies would confirm the diagnosis?

Cystometry is used to evaluate bladder capacity, control, contractility, and sensation. During this procedure provocative stress testing will be performed when stress incontinence is suspected. Urodynamic testing observes the stability of the bladder and electromyography observes bladder contractions. Urinalysis is used for differential diagnosis to rule out infection, diabetes, and other conditions.

What additional information should be obtained to confirm the diagnosis?

Urinary stress incontinence can be determined through history, pelvic examination, and noted loss of urine with straining activities. The Marshall-Marchetti test utilizes finger elevation of the paraurethral vaginal tissues at the neck of the bladder in order to stop the leakage of urine during coughing, sneezing or straining. Baseline exam should include the amount of time that a patient can hold urine, repetitions performed of a holding contraction, and the amount of pelvic floor contractions a patient can perform.

Examination:

What history should be documented?

Important areas to explore include past medical history, childbirth history, medications, current health status, fluid intake, social history, occupation, living environment, and social support system.

What test/measures are most appropriate?

Aerobic capacity and endurance: assessment of vital signs at rest and with activity, perceived exertion scale
Arousal, attention, and cognition: examine mental status, learning ability, memory, motivation, Urge Impact scale
Community and work integration: analysis of community, work, and leisure activities
Environmental, home, and work barriers: analysis of current and potential barriers or hazards
Ergonomics and body mechanics: analysis of dexterity and coordination, assessment of lifting techniques (intra-abdominal pressure)
Integumentary integrity: skin assessment, examination of the pelvic floor
Muscle performance: strength assessment of the pelvic floor muscles, muscle tone assessment
Pain: pain perception assessment scale
Posture: analysis of resting and dynamic posture
Range of motion: active and passive range of motion
Self-care and home management: assessment of functional capacity

What additional findings are likely with this patient?

A patient with urinary stress incontinence may be at increased risk for a urinary tract infection with subsequent skin breakdown. Pelvic floor weakness, uterine prolapse, and kidney infection may all relate to urinary stress incontinence. A patient that has poor diet and nutrition, constipation, and inadequate hydration will further promote incontinence.

Management:

What is the most effective management of this patient?

Medical management of urinary incontinence usually consists of conservative measures (physical therapy) as a first line of defense followed by pharmacological and surgical interventions depending on the underlying cause and response to conservative treatment. Physical therapy intervention for pelvic floor muscle weakness that is tested as 0/5 – 2/5 includes biofeedback, electrical stimulation, bladder retraining, and therapeutic exercise. Pelvic floor muscle strengthening at this level includes facilitation and tapping of the pelvic floor muscles, overflow exercises using the buttocks, adductors, and lower abdominals, and implementation of Kegel exercises. Physical therapy intervention for pelvic floor muscle weakness that is tested as 3/5 – 5/5 includes continued biofeedback and bladder retraining, weighted vaginal cones for resistance training, and implementation of pelvic floor muscle exercise during activities.

What home care regimen should be recommended?

A home care regimen for a patient with urinary stress incontinence should emphasize an active exercise program that includes pelvic floor strengthening in order to regain control of the flow of urine. Patients are encouraged to perform the recommended exercises throughout the day and integrate the pelvic exercises during activities that may trigger an increase in abdominal pressure within their daily routine.

Outcome:

What is the likely outcome of a course in physical therapy?

Outpatient physical therapy for urinary stress incontinence should alleviate pelvic floor weakness and involuntary leakage of urine within eight to twelve weeks. If a patient requires surgical intervention or presents with multiple impairments then physical therapy may be warranted for a longer period of time to assist with gaining bladder control.

What are the long-term effects of the patient's condition?

The long-term effects of urinary stress incontinence depend on the exact cause for the incontinence and the responsiveness to therapeutic intervention. Some patients do not have any long-term effects upon successful completion of physical therapy while other patients do not benefit from physical therapy intervention and require surgical intervention for the underlying cause. Compliance with the home exercise program is required when the underlying cause is weakness of the pelvic floor musculature. Research indicates that in an older population approximately 50% of all admissions to skilled nursing facilities have a direct relationship to unresolved urinary incontinence and impairments.

Comparison:

What are the distinguishing characteristics of a similar condition?

Bowel incontinence can occur from birth defects, trauma to the rectum, spinal cord injuries, fecal impaction, and tumor. Conservative treatment is preferred and includes diet, pharmacological agents, and strengthening of the sphincter muscles through exercise, electrical stimulation, and biofeedback. Surgical intervention may be warranted.

Clinical Scenarios:

Scenario One

A 32-year-old female is referred to physical therapy with a diagnosis of incontinence. The patient gave birth to her fourth child six weeks ago. The patient reports involuntary leakage of urine with exertion. The patient has no significant past medical history; however, reports that she is very anxious about participating in physical therapy.

Scenario Two

A 68-year-old female complains to her doctor during her annual examination that she has difficulty controlling her bladder since a kidney infection six months ago. The patient states that she is unable to hold her urine if she sneezes or coughs and cannot perform any activity of exertion without wearing feminine pads due to leakage. The physician referred the patient to physical therapy for Kegel exercises.

Unit 4

Study Concepts

A Comprehensive Study Plan

The inclusion of Study Concepts in *PTEXAM: The Complete Study Guide* serves to remind candidates that preparing for the National Physical Therapy Examination requires more than simply reviewing academic content and taking sample examinations.

Each of the presented Study Concepts provides candidates with an idea or concept to potentially integrate into their comprehensive study plan. For example, perhaps a candidate has a strong learning style preference where they tend to favor active learning over passive learning. To date their study plan has consisted of purely passive activities such as reading the academic review section of a review book and reviewing class notes. Not surprisingly, the candidate has experienced a great deal of difficulty moving through the academic review and class notes and has serious doubts about how much of the material they have retained. In addition, the candidate finds they are unable to concentrate after approximately 90 minutes of studying and typically discontinues the study session at this point.

The presented Study Concept entitled "Learning Styles" offers a number of practical suggestions to assist candidates to identify their own unique learning style and to design study sessions to incorporate these preferences. Study plans that are designed to address decided learning preferences yield a much greater return on investment than generic study plans.

As a second example, consider the Study Concept entitled "Golden Rules." This item explores whether it is possible to develop specific rules that allow candidates to differentiate between two or more plausible options on multiple-choice questions used on the National Physical Therapy Examination. A potential rule would be something like the following: "When choosing between a number of acceptable interventions, always select the most conservative option in an effort to minimize any potential safety risk to the patient."

Potential rules like this are very tempting since they provide candidates with a means to make questions more objective and therefore less amorphous. The problem, however, is that the National Physical Therapy Examination is designed to assess a candidate's ability to make clinical decisions rather than to rely on memorization or simply apply a set of standardized rules. The Study Concept presents a variety of potential rules and walks candidates through a number of clinical scenarios demonstrating why rules are better used as only loose guidelines to consider when answering multiple-choice questions.

Study Concepts

Study Concept 1	**Learning Styles**
Study Concept 2	**Time Management**
Study Concept 3	**Levels of Knowledge and Understanding**
Study Concept 4	**Golden Rules**
Study Concept 5	**Automaticity**
Study Concept 6	**Truths and Myths**
Study Concept 7	**Blood Pressure**
Study Concept 8	**Lines, Tubes, and Equipment**
Study Concept 9	**Emergent Conditions**
Study Concept 10	**Assessment**

In truth, many questions on the examination require candidates to make unique judgments based on the exact circumstances presented in the two to four sentences that make up the question stem. Candidates who develop the flexibility to apply clinical information in a wide variety of scenarios are well poised to be successful on the National Physical Therapy Examination.

Enjoy each of the presented Study Concepts and use the notes section to make observations of your present performance related to each of these unique topics.

Study Concept 1: Learning Styles

Studying for a comprehensive examination such as the National Physical Therapy Examination can be a significant challenge for any candidate. Given the volume of information required to be reviewed or relearned, it is critical for candidates to be as efficient as possible as they move through their established study plan. In order to maximize the efficiency of established study sessions, candidates should consider their preferred learning channels.

Perhaps the most critical question to answer relates to your preferred learning style for input and processing. Is your preferred learning style for input and processing more active or passive? Here is a brief description of each style that may assist you to label your individual preference.

Active learning style – when exposed to new material a learner who likes to hear it, see it, say it, question it, interact with it, and then keep on doing this. Learners with this style tend to be multisensoral (visual, auditory, tactile/kinesthetic).

Passive learning style – when exposed to new material a learner who likes to hear it or read it and then keep on doing this. Learners with this style tend to determine the relationship to known material after input and before processing.

It is important to recognize that one learning style is not better than another, but each learning style can come with particular strengths and weaknesses. For example, a candidate who is active for both input and processing may be able to focus intently on the application and utility of ideas, however, may consider details boring and have a short attention span. Conversely, a candidate who is passive for both input and processing may be effective at sequential thinking and focusing on details, but may miss the "big picture."

Please recognize that an individual's learning style varies depending on the situation, however, it is equally important to recognize that most candidates have decided learning style preferences that when harnessed can result in greater efficiency of study sessions.

General Recommendations for Specific Learning Styles

Active learning style

Study sessions should consist of 60-90 minute sessions of interactive study. Study sessions should take place as frequently as possible. Group studying is recommended since multisensory stimulation is difficult to achieve alone. Learning tools should include items such as discussions, simulations, hands-on practice, and role playing.

Passive learning style

Study sessions should be two to three hours in length and focus on large pieces of material. Study sessions should take place three to five times per week. Group studying is recommended periodically with members who are application driven. Learning tools should include items such as lectures, briefings, observations, handouts, texts, and notes.

Awareness of one's learning style will not make an unqualified candidate qualified, however, it can significantly increase the rate of new learning, reviewing, and relearning. A well conceived study plan combined with an awareness of learning style is a powerful one-two combination that can pay significant dividends for candidates on the National Physical Therapy Examination.

Notes:

Study Concept 2: Time Management

Physical therapy students by definition tend to have strong time management skills, however, these skills are severely tested when preparing for the National Physical Therapy Examination. The majority of students take the National Physical Therapy Examination shortly after graduation which can be a very anxious and unsettled time. Candidates are often actively seeking employment or are attempting to adjust to a new job. They may have relocated to a different residence or perhaps moved to another part of the country.

The thought of preparing for an examination that represents a minimum of three years of graduate study makes it critical that available study time is spent in areas that will yield the highest return on investment. To illustrate this point consider the relative systems weighting of the current examination.

System	Percentage
Musculoskeletal System	18.0%
Neuromuscular & Nervous Systems	17.0%
Cardiac, Vascular, & Pulmonary Systems	11.5%
Integumentary System	7.0%
Other Systems	16.0%
Non-Systems	30.5%

For example, on a typical examination a candidate will have 36 musculoskeletal system questions and 14 integumentary system questions. The number of questions is determined by multiplying the percentage of questions specified in each system area by two since the National Physical Therapy Examination consists of a total of 150 scored items. Given the relative weighting of these areas, a typical candidate should spend more than three times the amount of time studying musculoskeletal content compared to integumentary content. The actual percentage of time spent in each area may vary from candidate to candidate, but the relative weighting of the system on the examination should always remain an important variable to consider when determining the necessary breadth and depth in each area. Fortunately there are a number of specific strategies candidates can utilize to ensure that they make meaningful progress in their study sessions.

Strategy: Master Study Schedule

Develop a master schedule for studying which emphasizes the relative weighting of the Systems and Non-Systems areas on the National Physical Therapy Examination.

Step One – Create a monthly calendar that identifies specific study days and the anticipated duration of each session.

Step Two – Allocate more frequent study sessions and therefore additional study time to systems that are more heavily weighted on the National Physical Therapy Examination.

Step Three – Integrate weekly activities that are designed to maintain a balance in life. These areas may address emotional, intellectual, physical, and social needs.

Step Four – Reassess your progress on a weekly basis and make any necessary changes to the master schedule.

PTEXAM: The Complete Study Guide offers a great deal of additional information on the National Physical Therapy Examination Blueprint. The blueprint specifies the relative weighting of the Systems and Non-Systems areas and introduces the Content Outline.

Notes:

Study Concept 3: Levels of Knowledge and Understanding

The National Physical Therapy Examination has evolved into an examination that requires candidates to demonstrate their ability to make clinical decisions rather than purely recall factual information. Candidates need to demonstrate solid didactic knowledge of entry-level physical therapy concepts, however, they also need to be able to apply the information in diverse clinical scenarios usually presented in multiple-choice questions of two to four sentences. Candidates who can effectively integrate physical therapy concepts into the various presented scenarios and make informed clinical decisions tend to perform strongly on the examination, while candidates who struggle with this skill tend to perform poorly.

When reviewing academic content it is important that candidates familiarize themselves with the content at multiple levels of breadth and depth. The following table depicts a hierarchy of knowledge and understanding.

Typically within a physical therapy academic program students acquire the information in a hierarchical progression beginning with the lower cognitive levels (i.e., vocabulary level, literal level) and progress over time to higher cognitive levels (i.e., interpretive level and applied level). As candidates begin to prepare for the National Physical Therapy Examination it is likely that the majority of candidates are comfortable at the vocabulary and literal level, however,

there is far greater variability in comfort level at the interpretive and applied levels. Varying levels of comfort may result from exposure or lack thereof to specific subject matter on clinical education experiences or opportunities to develop competence with applied learning activities in the classroom. Regardless of where a candidate is on this spectrum, it is critical that candidates constantly challenge themselves to explore higher level cognitive knowledge as they progress through their academic review.

The presented hierarchy of knowledge and understanding can also be useful for candidates when answering multiple-choice questions. After reading the stem of a given examination question it may be beneficial for candidates to ask themselves what the question is specifically asking. In this manner candidates can ensure that their interpretation of the question is consistent with the intended meaning of each question. Failure to interpret the specific meaning of a question often results in a candidate selecting an incorrect response to a multiple-choice item. Test taking mistakes can be extremely harmful on the examination since once this occurs a candidate's examination score is no longer consistent with their true ability. As a candidate's score moves further away from their true ability there is a greater risk of failing the examination.

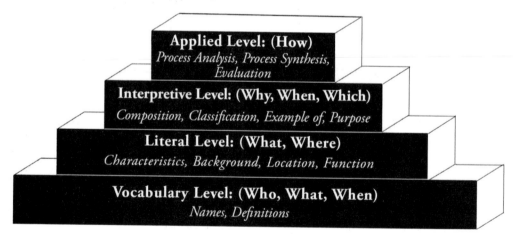

Applied Level: (How)
Process Analysis, Process Synthesis, Evaluation

Interpretive Level: (Why, When, Which)
Composition, Classification, Example of, Purpose

Literal Level: (What, Where)
Characteristics, Background, Location, Function

Vocabulary Level: (Who, What, When)
Names, Definitions

Notes:

Study Concept 4: Golden Rules

We have all used certain rules to help us move through our education such as "I before E, except after C." When preparing for the National Physical Therapy Examination candidates often look for similar rules that can assist them to make important distinctions between two or more plausible options to a given question. Unfortunately these types of rules do not exist on the National Physical Therapy Examination since every question relies on the nuances of a particular scenario that is typically conveyed in two to four sentences. Perhaps this is best demonstrated by stating a possible rule and then providing several examples to explore the rule in more detail.

Hypothetical Golden Rule Number One: When confronted with a situation where patient safety is potentially compromised, always contact the referring physician.

Rule Buster: Candidates must be vigilant to identify and act on any potential threat to patient safety, but this does not mean that it is always necessary to contact the referring physician. In some cases it would be appropriate for a physical therapist to minimize the threat to safety themselves. For example, consider the situation where a patient has a sudden and dramatic drop in their systolic blood pressure while working on vertical positioning. In this case it may only be necessary for the physical therapist to lower the patient toward the horizontal, in other cases contact with the physician would undoubtedly be necessary.

New Rule: It depends.

Hypothetical Golden Rule Number Two: When choosing between a number of acceptable interventions, always select the most conservative option in an effort to minimize any potential safety risk to the patient.

Rule Buster: Patient safety is a critical component on the National Physical Therapy Examination, but in many cases it is equally important to weigh the relative benefit of a selected option to achieving a desired patient outcome. How aggressive a therapist should be in a particular situation can only be determined after carefully weighing the relative risk versus the relative reward of each option. It is also important to recognize that all interventions have some degree of risk. If each of the available options to a given question offered no tangible difference in patient outcome, but were considered to be very different in terms of the relative degree of risk, it would then be sensible to select the safest or most conservative option.

New Rule: It depends.

Hypothetical Golden Rule Number Three: Physical therapist assistants should always contact the supervising physical therapist prior to changing any aspect of a patient's therapy session.

Rule Buster: Physical therapist assistants are licensed personnel in the vast majority of states and tend to have a fairly standardized list of acceptable work activities. Communication between a physical therapist and physical therapist assistant is strongly encouraged, however, in some instances it may not always be necessary. For example, what about the case where a physical therapist assistant wants to change the sequence of resistive exercises or needs to increase or decrease a weight on an existing progressive resistive exercise. In this case formal communication with the physical therapist would typically not be necessary since physical therapist assistants are able to engage in ongoing assessment. In other instances formal communication would be necessary. For example, a physical therapist assistant may want to introduce a new intervention that falls outside the current established plan of care or perhaps identifies several findings that indicate a relevant change in a patient's medical status.

New Rule: It depends.

As you can see the only safe rule to rely on is "it depends." Stated differently, the answer to a given question is always dependent on the specific terms and conditions presented in each clinical scenario. Candidates should attempt to inform future clinical decision making based on their experiences with previous sample examination items, but should avoid becoming inflexible or attempting to develop general rules that apply to all situations.

Notes:

Study Concept 5: Automaticity

On occasion candidates attempt to complete an academic review by simply taking sample examinations and then reviewing and memorizing the correct answers. This strategy, although potentially helpful, is at best a scattered approach since the scope of the review is dependent solely on the questions asked.

For example, a given series of sample examinations may have a total of eight questions on ultrasound, but it is possible that the questions do not address necessary subject matter such as ultrasound using the underwater technique or explore important concepts such as beam nonuniformity ratio or effective radiating area. This example emphasizes the need for a thorough academic review which allows candidates access to the vast majority of didactic content potentially encountered on the National Physical Therapy Examination.

Consider another example dealing with accessibility standards such as a ramp. Most candidates would quickly recall that the ratio of rise:run is 1:12 or stated differently; each inch of rise requires a minimum of 12 inches of run. Although candidates are likely to be familiar with this concept they may not be prepared to handle each of the various ways this concept could be tested on the National Physical Therapy Examination. Consider each of the following:

An examination item could require a candidate to:

- Determine the minimum length of a ramp after being given a specific height in inches or feet

- Determine the minimum height of a ramp after being given a specific length in inches or feet

- Determine if a ramp violates the minimum ada requirements given a height and length in inches or feet

- Determine a given maximum percentage grade for a ramp (using rise:run formula)

- Determine if a ramp violates the maximum percentage grade given a height and length in inches or feet

- Determine the minimum length of a ramp in inches or feet given the need to safely traverse a height the equivalent of a given number of standard size steps

The example illustrates both the need to be familiar with specific didactic content and the need to apply the information in different scenarios. In truth, each of the listed examination items related to ramps relies on the same basic formula (i.e., rise:run), but a candidate's ability to answer the question correctly will depend on their ability to recognize this and in some cases utilize related information (i.e., the relationship of percentage grade to rise:run and the size of a standard step).

Candidates who have this skill are demonstrating automaticity. Automaticity is a test taking term that describes the ability to quickly recall relevant facts, procedures, and routines and apply this information within the context of a clinically-oriented multiple-choice question. As candidates become increasingly comfortable with the academic knowledge and the ability to apply the information via multiple-choice questions, they tend to score higher on sample examinations.

When reviewing completed sample examination items, candidates greatly benefit from considering other possible scenarios related to the same subject matter or topic being tested. In many cases the incorrect options for a question are often correct for a variation of the question. For example, a question may ask specifically about the testing procedure for a given cranial nerve. In this case a candidate may identify option 1 as being correct, but upon reviewing the question later may recognize that options 2, 3, and 4 are also correct for different cranial nerves. Given that there are literally thousands of potential questions that could be asked on the National Physical Therapy Examination, candidates who possess greater flexibility with particular subject matter have a greater probability of answering the item correctly.

Notes:

Study Concept 6: Truths and Myths

There are a variety of popular myths that exist in regard to the National Physical Therapy Examination. Most of the myths are simply misinformation that becomes perpetuated over time. The following section addresses some of the more common myths about the current examination and then sets the record straight.

Truths and Myths Number One: The National Physical Therapy Examination has several different forms (i.e., versions), each which has a particular emphasis in terms of systems weighting. For example, a given form may emphasize the musculoskeletal system while another may emphasize the neuromuscular and nervous system.

Answer: False

Explanation: There are several different forms of the National Physical Therapy Examination that are available concurrently, however, the relative weighting of the examination by system specific and content outline area remain consistent. The Federation of State Boards of Physical Therapy publicly disseminates a blueprint that provides detailed information on the current examination.

Truths and Myths Number Two: When studying for the examination it is critical to be familiar with multiple academic resources for a selected topic since a given question could require knowledge from a specific resource.

Answer: False

Explanation: An examination question would not require a candidate to differentiate between multiple academic sources. For example, different academic resources sometimes have subtle differences in select subject matter such as dermatomes or temperature ranges for physical agents. Instead of focusing on this level of detail a candidate should become comfortable with a given source and have confidence that if this information is encountered on the examination their answer will be correct.

Truths and Myths Number Three: The 50 questions on the National Physical Therapy Examination that are considered pre-test items are clearly identifiable from scored items on the examination.

Answer: False

Explanation: The 50 pre-test items are intermingled with 200 scored items to make up the 250 question National Physical Therapy Examination. The pre-test items are not distinguishable from scored items and exist in each of the five sections of the examination.

Truths and Myths Number Four: Candidates have exactly one hour to complete each of the five sections of the National Physical Therapy Examination.

Answer: False

Explanation: Candidates have a total of five sections, each with 50 questions, to complete on the National Physical Therapy Examination, however, they are not timed independently. The examination clock will begin at five hours and count down from this value regardless of the rate at which each of the sections is completed. The examination will conclude when the candidate submits their final section or when the five hours has elapsed.

Truths and Myths Number Five: A score of 75% correct or 150 of 200 scored items is necessary to pass the National Physical Therapy Examination in most states.

Answer: False

Explanation: Each form of the examination has an individual criterion-referenced passing score. The passing score may differ by a relatively small amount from form to form. If a particular form was determined to be slightly more difficult than another form, the more difficult form would have a slightly lower criterion-referenced passing score. Individual states do not have the ability to determine passing scores in their respective jurisdictions and instead rely on the established national criterion-referenced passing scores. Recently criterion-referenced passing scores have been below 150 or 75% of the questions answered correctly.

Truths and Myths Number Six: Scores on subsequent attempts of sample examinations are good indicators of success on the National Physical Therapy Examination.

Answer: False

Explanation: Scores on subsequent attempts of a given sample examination are usually better indicators of memory and less accurate as predictors of future performance. Candidates should always review correct and incorrect answers from a given sample examination, however, should resist the urge to retake the same examination for the purpose of assessing performance.

Notes:

Study Concept 7: Blood Pressure

Vital signs serve as an important screening tool for physical therapists and should be formally measured for all examinations and then periodically thereafter based on the particular medical diagnosis and specific physical therapy interventions. Given the obvious safety implications associated with measuring and interpreting the results of vital signs, it is critical that candidates have in-depth knowledge of this particular content. This section will present a variety of detailed information related to blood pressure.

- Systolic pressure measures the force exerted against the arteries during the ejection cycle, while diastolic pressure measures the force exerted against the arteries during rest.

- Blood pressure is directly related to cardiac output and peripheral vascular resistance and therefore is an effective non-invasive performance measure of the pumping mechanism of the heart.

- Systolic pressure increases with exertion in a linear progression, often at a rate of 8-12 mm Hg per metabolic equivalent, however, with sustained activity no further increases typically occur. If systolic pressure does not rise with increasing workload it may indicate that the functional reserve capacity of the heart has been exceeded.

- Diastolic pressure may increase or decrease a maximum of 10 mm Hg due to adaptive dilation of peripheral vasculature. In a typical clinical setting the exercise session should be terminated if the systolic pressure exceeds 210 mm Hg or if the diastolic pressure exceeds 110 mm Hg.

- Pulse pressure, which is the difference between systolic and diastolic pressure, generally increases in direct proportion to the intensity of exercise since systolic pressure increases with exercise and diastolic pressure tends to stay the same. In a healthy adult it is common to see a 40-50 mm Hg change in systolic pressure with intense exercise. Excessive pulse pressure may be indicative of stiffening of the aorta secondary to atherosclerosis.

- Normally systolic blood pressure in the legs is 10-20% higher than the pressure in the arms (brachial artery). This is why in some cases an ankle-brachial index value of greater than 1.0 is still considered to be normal. Blood pressure readings that are lower in the legs as compared to the arms are abnormal and may be indicative of peripheral vascular disease.

- Blood pressure increases during dynamic resistance exercise such as free weights, machines or isokinetics and continues to increase as an exercise set progresses. Blood pressure response is higher during weight training that incorporates a concentric and eccentric phase compared to isokinetic exercise. Blood pressure tends to be higher during the concentric phase of the repetition or when the Valsalva maneuver is used.

- With advancing age the same amount of blood fills the ventricles, but the pumping mechanism is less effective. As a result, the body compensates by increasing blood pressure in an attempt to maintain homeostasis.

- During exercise testing, a systolic blood pressure that fails to increase or decrease with increasing workloads may signal a plateau or decrease in cardiac output.

- Systolic blood pressure normally decreases promptly with the cessation of exercise. As a general guideline, the three-minute post exercise systolic blood pressure should be less than the 90% of the systolic blood pressure at peak exercise.

Notes:

Study Concept 8: Lines, Tubes and Equipment

The National Physical Therapy Examination is designed to protect consumers from unqualified practitioners. Given the purpose of the examination, it is inevitable that candidates will encounter a variety of questions that deal with patients with significantly compromised medical status.

This section presents information on various types of lines, tubes, and equipment. The purpose is to remind physical therapists of some of the more critical elements to consider when treating patients using these devices. Please remember that this is not an all-inclusive list and additional detail will be provided on the vast majority of items throughout **PTEXAM: The Complete Study Guide.**

Lines

Arterial Lines (A line)

- Avoid applying a blood pressure cuff above the infusion site
- Grasp the IV line support pole so the infusion site is at heart level
- Avoid activities that require the infusion site to be above the level of the heart for a prolonged period
- Exercise is possible with the line, but avoid disturbing the apparatus

Swan-Ganz Catheters (Pulmonary Artery Catheters), Central Venous Pressure Catheters, Indwelling Right Atrial Catheters

- Exercise is possible with the line, but mobility may need to be restricted near the catheter insertion

Total Parenteral Nutrition, Hyperalimentation Devices (Intravenous Feeding)

- Alarm sound indicates the fluid source is empty or the system has become unbalanced
- Disruption or disconnection may result in an air embolus
- Shoulder motion on the side of the infusion site may be restricted primarily in flexion and abduction
- Exercise is possible with the line, but mobility may need to be restricted near the catheter insertion

Intracranial Monitoring

- Isometric exercise and the Valsalva maneuver should be avoided since these activities increase intracranial pressure
- Avoid neck flexion, hip flexion greater than 90 degrees, and lying down in a prone position
- Venous drainage is maximal with the head of the bed elevated 30 degrees
- Momentary elevation of intracranial pressure is normal, but sustained increases are not and therefore should be reported

Tubes

Nasogastric Tube (NG Tube)

- Patient will not be able to eat food or drink fluids by mouth while the nasogastric tube is in place
- Enteral feedings can be disconnected temporarily for mobility
- Exercise requiring movements of the head and neck should be avoided, especially forward bending

Gastrostomy Tube (G tube)

- Distal tubing can inadvertently become caught on items such as furniture and be pulled out
- Enteral feedings should be turned off temporarily prior to and during treatment
- Enteral feedings can be disconnected temporarily for mobility

Urinary Catheters

- Tubes should be placed below the region being drained since the devices rely on gravity
- The collection bag should not be raised above the level of the bladder for any sustained period
- Avoid disrupting, stretching, disconnecting or occluding the tube during exercise

Chest Tubes

- When ambulating, collection bottles should be kept below the level of the inserted tube location
- Monitor the patient for changes in breath sounds before and after intervention
- Avoid pressing directly on the chest tube during mobility activities

Equipment

Mechanical Ventilation

- Alarm may indicate disconnected tube, coughing or change in respiratory pattern
- Develop nonverbal means of communication with the patient
- Patient is at greater risk for developing contractures, skin ulcers, and deconditioning

Supplemental Oxygen Delivery System

- Be aware of signs of respiratory distress (i.e., dyspnea, cyanosis, cramping)
- Monitor SaO_2, PaO_2, and hemodynamics prior to, during, and after physical therapy intervention
- Exercise is possible, but avoid disturbing the tubing

Notes:

Study Concept 9: Emergent Conditions

According to the Federation of State Boards of Physical Therapy, the National Physical Therapy Examination is designed to assess basic entry-level competence of the licensure candidate who has graduated from an accredited program. The primary purpose of the examination is therefore to protect the public from unqualified practitioners. Given the purpose of the examination, it is reasonable to expect that a high percentage of examination items will deal with safety related issues including the identification and management of potentially emergent conditions. When encountering this type of question it is critical that candidates are armed with the necessary knowledge to make informed clinical decisions.

The following provides relevant information on three commonly encountered emergent conditions.

Pulmonary Embolism

Description: A blockage of the pulmonary artery or one of its branches, usually precipitated by a blood clot from a vein (venous thrombus) becoming dislodged from its site of formation. The dislodged blood clot then travels to the arterial blood supply of one of the lungs.

Clinical presentation: Difficulty breathing, chest pain that often mimics a heart attack, rapid pulse; in more severe cases circulatory instability and death

Risk factors: Surgery, long periods of inactivity, increased levels of clotting factor in the blood, and abnormal factors in the vessel wall

Diagnosis: Pulmonary angiography is the most accurate method to diagnose pulmonary embolism, however, because the procedure carries inherent risks to the patient, other diagnostic procedures such as chest x-ray, lung scan, and spiral computerized tomography scan are more commonly utilized.

Treatment: Anticoagulant medication such as Heparin and Warafarin

Notes: Pulmonary embolism remains the leading cause of hospital death in the United States.

Hypovolemic Shock

Description: A life threatening condition caused by insufficient circulating blood volume. Primary causes include hemorrhage or severe burns.

Clinical presentation: Hypotension due to lack of circulating volume, anxiety, altered mental state, cool and clammy skin, rapid and thready pulse, thirst, and fatigue due to inadequate oxygenation

Risk factors: Exposure to severe trauma or burns

Diagnosis: Primarily through the identification of the described clinical presentation

Treatment: Management of suspected shock includes activating the emergency medical system. Positional management includes lying in supine with the legs elevated approximately 12 inches in situations where it is tolerated. Management of confirmed shock includes controlling bleeding and attempting to restore blood volume by providing infusions of balanced salt solutions or blood in more severe cases.

Notes: There are several other common forms of shock including cardiogenic, septic, and anaphylactic. Cardiogenic shock is characterized by failure of the heart to pump effectively. Management includes oxygen therapy and administering cardiac medications. Septic shock is characterized by an overwhelming infection leading to vasodilation. Management includes restoring intravascular volume and identifying and controlling the source of infection. Anaphylactic shock is characterized by a severe and sometimes fatal reaction to an allergen, antigen or drug which causes vasodilation leading to hypotension and increased capillary permeability. Management includes identifying and removing the causative antigen and administering counter-mediators such as anti-histamine.

Autonomic Dysreflexia

Description: A massive sympathetic discharge that can occur in association with a spinal cord injury or disease. The condition is triggered by a variety of noxious stimuli including bladder distention, urinary tract infection, skin ulcers, and bowel impaction.

Clinical presentation: Sweating above the level of the lesion, flushing of the skin above the level of the lesion, elevated blood pressure, blurred vision

Risk factors: Patients with spinal cord injuries at and above the T6 level

Diagnosis: Primarily through the identification of the described clinical presentation

Treatment: Management of autonomic dysreflexia includes immediate determination and removal of the triggering stimuli. Positional management includes sitting the patient upright to lower the elevated blood pressure below dangerous levels. Tight clothing and stockings should also be removed. If the noxious stimuli cannot be identified, medical management may include vasodilators to assist with symptomatic relief.

Notes: Prevalence rates for autonomic dysreflexia have been reported ranging from 48-90% of all individuals with spinal cord injuries at T6 and above. The occurrence of autonomic dysreflexia is increased as an individual moves out of spinal shock.

Notes:

Study Concept 10: Assessment

Candidates must carefully assess their examination performance when taking sample examinations. Each of the sample examinations in **PTEXAM: The Complete Study Guide** offers candidates the opportunity to view their performance according to six system specific and five content outline categories. The shaded areas in the tables below will be used in the performance analysis section to express the number of questions answered correctly in each category, the total number of questions in the category, and the percentage of questions correct.

System Specific Summary

Musculoskeletal System	
Neuromuscular & Nervous Systems	
Cardiac, Vascular, & Pulmonary Systems	
Integumentary System	
Other Systems	
Non-Systems	

Content Outline Summary

Clinical Application of Physical Therapy Principles and Foundational Sciences	
Examination	
Foundations for Evaluation, Differential Diagnosis, & Prognosis	
Interventions	
Equipment & Devices; Therapeutic Modalities	
Safety & Professional Roles; Teaching/ Learning; Evidence-Based Practice	

Candidates should use this information to develop remedial plans to improve performance on sample examinations. Candidates must be familiar with the content contained in each system specific and content outline category and carefully assess how their performance changes over time.

The academic review section of **PTEXAM: The Complete Study Guide** is arranged according to the exact categories used in the system specific summary and therefore serves as an excellent resource for candidates to utilize when initially remediating deficient areas. In some instances, a candidate may determine that it is necessary to access a more formal academic resource such as a textbook to locate information not covered in the review book. In these situations it is important for candidates to stay focused and avoid purely exploring the textbook since often candidates do not emerge for several hours.

The content outline is less intuitive than the system specific categories since the content outline is not system based, however, is still very useful given the detailed information available on the National Physical Therapy Examination Blueprint. For example, a candidate may find that they tend to perform very well on questions within the "Clinical Application of Foundational Sciences" category, but have more difficulty on questions within the "Examination" category. By consulting the National Physical Therapy Examination Blueprint a candidate will quickly realize that the "Clinical Application of Foundational Sciences" category deals primarily with anatomy and physiology, pharmacology, and effects of activity and exercise, while the "Examination" category deals primarily with tests/measures and movement analysis. The information from the content outline combined with the system specific information allows candidates to gain greater insight toward their current performance and should assist them to be more specific when selecting appropriate remedial activities.

Candidates are encouraged to look for general trends in their scoring when taking sample examinations and avoid making a definitive statement on their level of competence in any given category based on the results of a single sample examination. This is especially true in a category where there is a smaller number of questions such as the integumentary system. As the number of questions in each category diminishes the category becomes less accurate as a predictor of actual performance. In some instances candidates will have a few glaring areas of deficiency (e.g., "Musculoskeletal" and "Other Systems"), while in other cases candidates will demonstrate more consistency. Consistency can be a very good thing if the scores are consistent at a very high level (i.e., a high percentage of questions answered correctly in the majority of areas) or more problematic if the scores are consistent at a very low level (i.e., a low percentage of questions answered correctly in the majority of areas).

In summary, studying for the examination is analogous to developing a plan of care for a patient; the more specific the plan of care is for the particular needs of the patient, the better the patient outcome. In terms of preparing for the examination, the more specific a remedial plan is to the particular needs of a given candidate, the better the candidate's outcome.

Notes:

Unit 5

National Physical Therapy Examination Blueprint

Perhaps the most valuable piece of information a candidate can utilize when preparing for the National Physical Therapy Examination is the National Physical Therapy Examination Blueprint. The blueprint provides a detailed analysis of each of the content areas of the National Physical Therapy Examination. A thorough understanding of the content outline and system specific weighting will streamline a candidate's preparation. Less time will be spent covering topics that are not clinically relevant to the actual examination and as a result, more time will be available for reviewing and relearning.

This Unit will explore the examination in detail according to the content outline and system specific areas. Each of the sample examinations in **_PTEXAM: The Complete Study Guide_** offers candidates the opportunity to view their performance according to six system specific and six content outline categories. Candidates must be familiar with the content contained in each system specific and content outline category and use this information to develop remedial plans to improve performance on sample examinations. We will begin with an exploration of the National Physical Therapy Examination Content Outline.

Content Outline Summary

Content	Percentage	Questions
Clinical Application of Foundational Sciences	14.5%	29
Examination	13.0%	26
Foundations for Evaluation, Differential Diagnosis, & Prognosis	23.5%	47
Interventions	18.5%	37
Equipment & Devices; Therapeutic Modalities	11.0%	22
Safety & Professional Roles; Teaching/Learning; Research	19.5%	39
	100.0%	**200**

Clinical Application of Foundational Sciences (29 Questions)

Clinical Application of Foundational Sciences: This category refers to the essential scientific principles that serve as the foundation for understanding system involvement in the treatment of patients/clients across the lifespan.

More detailed information on each of the systems is available in the System Specific Summary.

Physical Therapist NPTE Test Content Outline, Federation of State Boards Physical Therapy, www.fsbpt.org

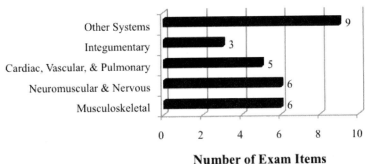

Clinical Application of Foundational Sciences

Other Systems — 9
Integumentary — 3
Cardiac, Vascular, & Pulmonary — 5
Neuromuscular & Nervous — 6
Musculoskeletal — 6

0   2   4   6   8   10

Number of Exam Items

The nine questions labeled "Other Systems" in this section are from the following systems:

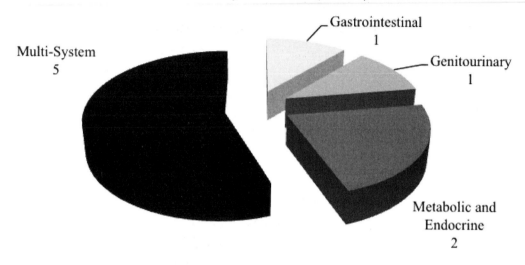

Other Systems (n=9)

Multi-System 5

Gastrointestinal 1

Genitourinary 1

Metabolic and Endocrine 2

Examination (26 Questions)

Examination: This category refers to the types and applications of system tests and measures and their relevance to information collected during the history and systems review. The category also includes the reaction of a specific system to tests and measures, and the mechanics of body movement as related to the system. Information covered in these areas supports appropriate and effective patient/client management across the lifespan.

More detailed information on each of the systems is available in the System Specific Summary.

Physical Therapist NPTE Test Content Outline, Federation of State Boards Physical Therapy, www.fsbpt.org

Examination

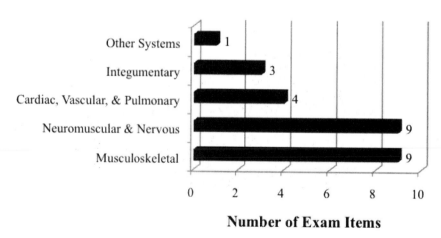

Other Systems   1
Integumentary   3
Cardiac, Vascular, & Pulmonary   4
Neuromuscular & Nervous   9
Musculoskeletal   9

0   2   4   6   8   10

Number of Exam Items

The one question labeled "Other Systems" in this section is from the Metabolic and Endocrine

Foundations for Evaluation, Differential Diagnosis, & Prognosis (47 Questions)

Foundations for Evaluation, Differential Diagnosis, and Prognosis: This category refers to the interpretation of knowledge about the diseases and conditions of a specific system in order to ensure the appropriate and effective patient/client treatment and management decisions across the lifespan.

More detailed information on each of the systems is available in the System Specific Summary.

Physical Therapist NPTE Test Content Outline, Federation of State Boards Physical Therapy, www.fsbpt.org

Foundations for Evaluation, Differential Diagnosis, & Prognosis

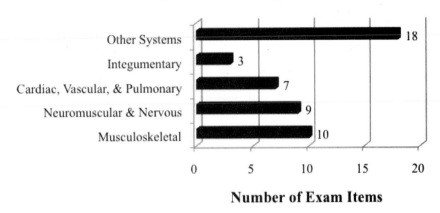

The 18 questions labeled "Other Systems" in this section are from the following systems:

Other Systems (n=18)

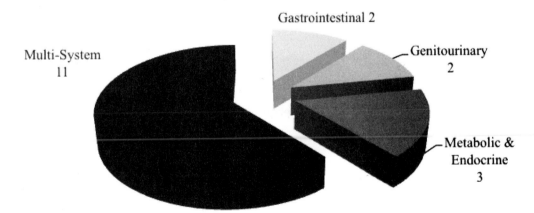

Interventions (37 Questions)

Interventions: This category refers to specific system interventions (including types, applications, responses, and potential complications) as well as the impact on the specific system of interventions performed on other systems in order to support patient/client management across the lifespan.

More detailed information on each of the systems is available in the System Specific Summary.

Physical Therapist NPTE Test Content Outline, Federation of State Boards Physical Therapy, www.fsbpt.org

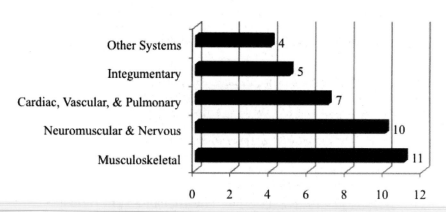

Interventions

System	Number of Exam Items
Other Systems	4
Integumentary	5
Cardiac, Vascular, & Pulmonary	7
Neuromuscular & Nervous	10
Musculoskeletal	11

Number of Exam Items

The four questions labeled "Other Systems" in this section are from the following systems:

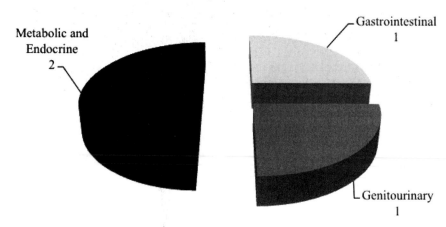

Other Systems (n=4)

Metabolic and Endocrine 2

Gastrointestinal 1

Genitourinary 1

Equipment & Devices; Therapeutic Modalities (22 Questions)

Equipment & Devices: This category refers to the different types of equipment and devices, use requirements and/or contextual determinants, as well as any other influencing factors involved in the selection and application of equipment and devices in order to support patient/client treatment and management decisions across the lifespan.

- Assistive and adaptive devices
- Prosthetic devices
- Orthotic devices
- Protective devices
- Supportive devices
- Gravity-assisted devices
- Bariatric equipment and devices

Therapeutic Modalities: This category refers to the underlying principles for the use of therapeutic modalities as well as the justification for the selection and use of the variety of types of therapeutic modalities employed to support patient/client treatment and management decisions across the lifespan.

- Indications, contraindications, and precautions of therapeutic modalities
- Physical agents (e.g., athermal agents, cryotherapy, hydrotherapy, light agents, sound agents, thermotherapy)
- Mechanical modalities (e.g., compression therapies, mechanical motion devices, traction devices)
- Electrotherapeutic delivery of medications (e.g., iontophoresis)
- Electrical stimulation (e.g., Functional Electrical Stimulation (FES), High Voltage Pulsed Current (HVPC), Neuromuscular Electrical Stimulation (NES), TENS)

More detailed information on each of the systems is available in the System Specific Summary.

Physical Therapist NPTE Test Content Outline, Federation of State Boards Physical Therapy, www.fsbpt.org

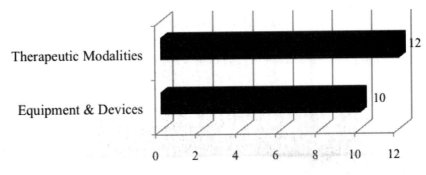

Equipment & Devices; Therapeutic Modalities

Number of Exam Items

Safety & Professional Roles; Teaching/Learning; Research (39 Questions)

Safety, Protection, & Professional Roles: This category refers to the critical issues involved in patient/client safety and protection and the responsibilities of health care providers to ensure that patient/client management and health care decisions take place in a secure and trustworthy environment.

- Factors influencing patient/client safety (e.g., fall risk, use of restraints, use of equipment, environmental factors)
- Emergency preparedness (e.g., CPR, first aid, disaster response)
- Proper body mechanics
- Injury prevention
- Infection control procedures (e.g., standard/universal precautions)
- Legal obligations for reporting abuse and neglect
- Patient/client rights (e.g., ADA, IDEA, HIPAA)
- Human resource legal issues (e.g., OSHA, sexual harassment)
- Standards of documentation
- Risk guidelines (e.g., documentation, policies and procedures, incident reports)
- Roles and responsibilities of other health care professionals and support staff

Teaching & Learning: This category refers to the principles and theories of teaching and learning required to create a learning environment in which information is effectively communicated to patients/clients to ensure that they receive appropriate instruction designed to support patient/client management decisions.

- Teaching and learning strategies, theories, and techniques (e.g., cognitive, motor, models of education)
- Health behavior change models
- Communication skills

Research & Evidence-Based Practice: This category refers to the application of measurement principles and research methodology to make reasoned and appropriate assessment and interpretation of information sources and practice research to support patient/client management decisions fundamental to evidence-based practice.

- Research design and interpretation (e.g., qualitative, quantitative)
- Measurement science (e.g., reliability, validity, common statistical methods)
- Outcome measures (e.g., suitability, applications)
- Data collection techniques (e.g., surveys, direct observation)
- Hierarchy of evidence (e.g., randomized control, case studies, anecdotal observation)

More detailed information on each of the systems is available in the System Specific Summary.

Physical Therapist NPTE Test Content Outline, Federation of State Boards Physical Therapy, www.fsbpt.org

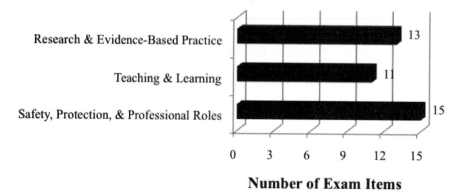

Safety & Professional Roles; Teaching/Learning; Research

Research & Evidence-Based Practice — 13
Teaching & Learning — 11
Safety, Protection, & Professional Roles — 15

0   3   6   9   12   15

Number of Exam Items

System Specific Summary

Systems (139)	Percentage	Questions
Musculoskeletal System	18.0%	36
Neuromuscular & Nervous Systems	17.0%	34
Cardiac, Vascular, & Pulmonary Systems	11.5%	23
Integumentary System	7.0%	14

Other Systems
 	
    Gastrointestinal (4)
    Genitourinary (4)
    Metabolic and Endocrine (8)
    Multi-System (16)
	16.0%	32

Non-Systems (61)

	Percentage	Questions
Equipment & Devices; Therapeutic Modalities		
Equipment & Devices	5.0%	10
Therapeutic Modalities	6.0%	12
Safety & Professional Roles; Teaching/Learning; Research		
Safety, Protection, & Professional Roles	7.5%	15
Teaching & Learning	5.5%	11
Research & Evidence-Based Practice	6.5%	13
	100.0%	**200**

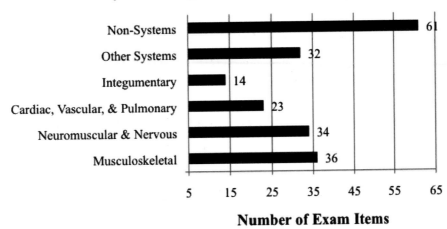

System Specific Summary

Number of Exam Items

Musculoskeletal System (36 Questions)

Clinical Application of Foundational Sciences: This category refers to the essential scientific principles that serve as the foundation for understanding musculoskeletal system involvement in the treatment of patients/clients across the lifespan.

- Anatomy, physiology and pathophysiology of the muscular and skeletal systems
- Pharmacology as related to the musculoskeletal system
- Physiological response to environmental factors and characteristics (e.g., air temperature, humidity, water temperature, water depth, buoyancy, altitude)
- Effects of activity and exercise on the musculoskeletal system
- Joint structure
- Joint functionality and mobility

Examination: This category refers to the types and applications of musculoskeletal system tests and measures and their relevance to information collected during history and systems review. The category also includes the reaction of the musculoskeletal system to tests and measures, and the mechanics of body movement as related to the musculoskeletal system. Information covered in these areas supports appropriate and effective patient/client management across the lifespan.

- Appropriate types of musculoskeletal system tests/measures and their applications
- Physiological response of the musculoskeletal system to various types of tests/measures
- Movement analysis including applications of kinesiology/kinematics as related to the musculoskeletal system (e.g., gait analysis)

Foundations for Evaluation, Differential Diagnosis, and Prognosis: This category refers to the diseases and conditions of musculoskeletal system in order to ensure the appropriate and effective patient/client treatment and management decisions across the lifespan.

- Diseases/conditions of the muscular and skeletal systems
- Diseases/conditions of the connective tissue
- Differential diagnoses related to pathologies of the muscular and skeletal systems
- Differential diagnoses related to pathologies of the connective tissue
- Diseases or conditions of the muscular and skeletal systems in order to make effective treatment decisions
- Diseases or conditions of the connective tissue in order to make effective treatment decisions
- Diagnostic imaging of the musculoskeletal system
- Medical management of the musculoskeletal system (e.g., surgical procedures, medical tests)

Interventions: This category refers to the features (e.g., types, applications, responses, and potential complications) of musculoskeletal system interventions as well as the impact on the musculoskeletal system of interventions performed on other systems in order to support patient/client management across the lifespan.

- Appropriate types of musculoskeletal system interventions and their applications
- Physiological response of the musculoskeletal system to various types of interventions
- Secondary effects or complications from interventions on the musculoskeletal system
- Secondary effects or complications on the musculoskeletal system from interventions used on other systems

Physical Therapist NPTE Test Content Outline, Federation of State Boards Physical Therapy, www.fsbpt.org

Neuromuscular & Nervous Systems (34 Questions)

Clinical Application of Foundational Sciences: This category refers to the essential scientific principles that serve as the foundation for understanding neuromuscular/nervous system involvement in the treatment of patients/clients across the lifespan.

- Anatomy, physiology and pathophysiology of the neuromuscular system
- Anatomy, physiology and pathophysiology of the nervous system (CNS, PNS, ANS)
- Pharmacology as related to the neuromuscular/nervous system
- Physiological response to environmental factors and characteristics (e.g., air temperature, humidity, water temperature, water depth, buoyancy, altitude)
- Effects of activity and exercise as related to the neuromuscular/nervous system
- Motor control as related to the neuromuscular/nervous system
- Motor learning as related to the neuromuscular/nervous system
- Neurological functioning (e.g., cognition, affect, arousal, memory)

Examination: This category refers to awareness of the types and applications of neuromuscular/nervous system tests and measures and their relevance to information collected during history and systems review. The category also includes the reaction of the neuromuscular/nervous system to tests and measures, and the mechanics of body movement as related to the neuromuscular/nervous system. Information covered in these areas supports appropriate and effective patient/client management across the lifespan.

- Appropriate types of neuromuscular/nervous system tests/measures and their applications
- Physiological response of the neuromuscular/nervous system to various types of test/measures
- Movement analysis including application of kinesiology/kinematics as related to the neuromuscular/nervous system (e.g., gait analysis, balance assessment)

Foundations for Evaluation, Differential Diagnosis, and Prognosis: This category refers to the diseases and conditions of neuromuscular/nervous system in order to ensure the appropriate and effective patient/client treatment and management decisions across the lifespan.

- Diseases/conditions of the nervous system (CNS, PNS, ANS)
- Differential diagnoses related to pathologies of the nervous system (CNS, PNS, ANS)
- Diseases or conditions of the nervous system (CNS, PNS, ANS) in order to make effective treatment decisions
- Diagnostic imaging of the neuromuscular/nervous system
- Medical management of the neuromuscular/nervous system (e.g., surgical procedures, medical tests)

Interventions: This category refers to the features (e.g., types, applications, responses, and potential complications) of neuromuscular/nervous system interventions as well as the impact on the neuromuscular/nervous system of interventions performed on other systems in order to support patient/client management across the lifespan.

- Appropriate types of neuromuscular/nervous system interventions and their applications
- Physiological response of the neuromuscular/nervous system to various types of interventions
- Secondary effects or complications from interventions on the neuromuscular/nervous system
- Secondary effects or complications on the neuromuscular/nervous system from interventions used on other systems
- Motor control as related to the neuromuscular/nervous system interventions
- Motor learning as related to the neuromuscular/nervous system interventions

Physical Therapist NPTE Test Content Outline, Federation of State Boards Physical Therapy, www.fsbpt.org

Cardiac, Vascular, & Pulmonary Systems (23 Questions)

Clinical Application of Foundational Sciences: This category refers to the essential scientific principles that serve as the foundation for understanding the involvement of the cardiac, vascular, and pulmonary systems in the treatment of patients/clients across the lifespan.

- Anatomy, physiology and pathophysiology of the cardiac, vascular, and pulmonary systems
- Anatomy, physiology and pathophysiology of the lymphatic system
- Pharmacology as related to the cardiovascular/pulmonary system
- Physiological response to environmental factors and characteristics (e.g., air temperature, humidity, water temperature, water depth, buoyancy, altitude)
- Effects of activity and exercise on the cardiovascular/pulmonary system (including the physiological response of the cardiovascular/pulmonary system to various types of test/measures and interventions)

Examination: This category refers to awareness of the types and applications of cardiac, vascular, and pulmonary systems tests and measures and their relevance to information collected from the history and systems review. The category includes the reaction of the cardiac, vascular, and pulmonary systems to tests and measures, and the mechanics of body movement as related to the cardiac, vascular, and pulmonary systems. Information covered in these areas supports appropriate and effective patient/client management across the lifespan.

- Appropriate types of cardiovascular/pulmonary system tests/measures and their applications
- Movement analysis as related to the cardiovascular/pulmonary system (e.g., rib cage excursion)

Foundations for Evaluation, Differential Diagnosis, and Prognosis: This category refers to the interpretation of knowledge about the diseases and conditions of cardiac, vascular, and pulmonary systems in order to ensure the appropriate and effective patient/client treatment and management decisions across the lifespan.

- Diseases/conditions of the cardiac, vascular, and pulmonary systems
- Diseases/conditions of the lymphatic system
- Differential diagnoses related to pathologies of the cardiac, vascular, and pulmonary systems
- Differential diagnoses related to pathologies of the lymphatic system
- Diseases or conditions of the cardiac, vascular, and pulmonary systems in order to make effective treatment decisions
- Diseases or conditions of the lymphatic system in order to make effective treatment decisions
- Diagnostic imaging of the cardiovascular/pulmonary system
- Medical management of the cardiovascular/pulmonary system (e.g., surgical procedures, medical tests)

Interventions: This category refers to the cardiac, vascular, and pulmonary systems interventions (including types, applications, responses, and potential complications) as well as the impact on the cardiac, vascular, and pulmonary systems of interventions performed on other systems in order to support patient/client management across the lifespan.

- Appropriate types of cardiovascular/pulmonary system interventions and their applications
- Secondary effects or complications from interventions on the cardiovascular/pulmonary system
- Secondary effects or complications on the cardiovascular/pulmonary system from interventions used on other systems

Physical Therapist NPTE Test Content Outline, Federation of State Boards Physical Therapy, www.fsbpt.org

Integumentary System (14 Questions)

Clinical Application of Foundational Sciences: This category refers to the essential scientific principles that serve as the foundation for understanding integumentary system involvement in the treatment of patients/clients across the lifespan.

- Anatomy, physiology and pathophysiology of the integumentary system
- Pharmacology as related to the integumentary system
- Physiological response to environmental factors and characteristics (e.g., air temperature, humidity, water temperature, water depth, buoyancy, altitude)
- Effects of activity and exercise on the integumentary system

Examination: This category refers to awareness of the types and applications of integumentary system tests and measures and their relevance to information collected during history and systems review. The category also includes the reaction of the integumentary system to tests and measures. Information covered in these areas supports appropriate and effective patient/client management across the lifespan.

- Appropriate types of integumentary system tests/measures and their applications
- Physiological response of the integumentary system to various types of tests/measures
- Movement analysis as related to the integumentary system (e.g., friction, shear, pressure, and scar).

Foundations for Evaluation, Differential Diagnosis, and Prognosis: This category refers to the diseases and conditions of integumentary system in order to ensure the appropriate and effective patient/client treatment and management decisions across the lifespan.

- Diseases/conditions of the integumentary system
- Differential diagnoses related to pathologies of the integumentary system
- Diseases or conditions of the integumentary system in order to make effective treatment decisions
- Medical management of the integumentary system (e.g., surgical procedures, medical tests)

Interventions: This category refers to the features (e.g., types, applications, responses, and potential complications) of integumentary system interventions as well as the impact on the integumentary system of interventions performed on other systems in order to support patient/client management across the lifespan.

- Appropriate types of integumentary system interventions and their applications
- Physiological response of the integumentary system to various types of interventions
- Secondary effects or complications from interventions on the integumentary system
- Secondary effects or complications on the integumentary system from interventions used on other systems
- Wound management techniques (e.g., selective debridement, nonselective debridement, dressings, topical agents)

Physical Therapist NPTE Test Content Outline, Federation of State Boards Physical Therapy, www.fsbpt.org

Other Systems (Overview)

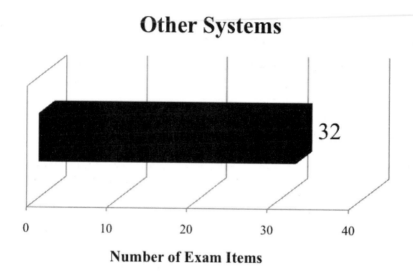

This category consists of the following systems:

- Metabolic & Endocrine Systems
- Gastrointestinal System
- Genitourinary System
- Multi-System

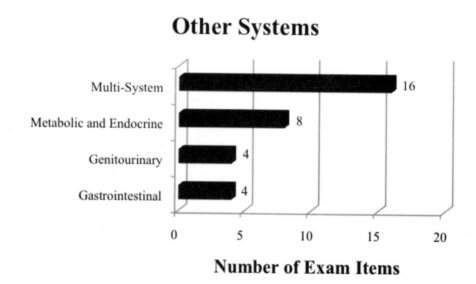

Gastrointestinal System (4 Questions)

Clinical Application of Foundational Sciences: This category refers to the essential scientific principles that serve as the foundation for understanding gastrointestinal system involvement in the treatment of patients/clients across the lifespan.

- Anatomy, physiology and pathophysiology of the gastrointestinal system
- Effects of activity and exercise on the gastrointestinal system

Foundations for Evaluation, Differential Diagnosis, and Prognosis: This category refers to the interpretation of knowledge of diseases and conditions of gastrointestinal system in order to ensure the appropriate and effective patient/client treatment and management decisions across the lifespan.

- Diseases/conditions of the gastrointestinal system
- Diseases or conditions of the gastrointestinal system in order to make effective treatment decisions

Interventions: This category refers to the features (e.g., types, applications, responses, and potential complications) of gastrointestinal system interventions and their relevance to information collected during history and systems review and examination. It also includes the impact on the gastrointestinal system of interventions performed on other systems in order to support patient/client management across the lifespan.

- Appropriate types of gastrointestinal system interventions and their applications (e.g., positioning for reflux, positioning for bowel programs)
- Physiological response of the gastrointestinal system to various types of interventions
- Secondary effects or complications from interventions on the gastrointestinal system
- Secondary effects or complications on the gastrointestinal system from interventions used on other systems

Genitourinary System (4 Questions)

Clinical Application of Foundational Sciences: This category refers to the essential scientific principles that serve as the foundation for understanding genitourinary system involvement in the treatment of patients/clients across the lifespan.

- Anatomy, physiology, and pathophysiology of the genitourinary system
- Effects of activity and exercise on the genitourinary system
- Motor control as related to the genitourinary system
- Motor learning as related to the genitourinary system

Foundations for Evaluation, Differential Diagnosis, and Prognosis: This category refers to the diseases and conditions of genitourinary system in order to ensure the appropriate and effective patient/client treatment and management decisions across the lifespan.

- Diseases/conditions of the genitourinary system
- Diseases or conditions of the genitourinary system in order to make effective treatment decisions

Interventions: This category refers to the features (e.g., types, applications, and potential complications) of genitourinary system interventions as well as the impact on the genitourinary system of interventions performed on other systems in order to support patient/client management across the lifespan.

- Appropriate types of genitourinary system interventions and their applications (e.g., positioning for bladder programs, biofeedback, pelvic floor retraining)
- Secondary effects or complications from interventions on the genitourinary system
- Secondary effects or complications on the genitourinary system from interventions used on other systems

Metabolic & Endocrine Systems (8 Questions)

Clinical Application of Foundational Sciences: This category refers to the essential scientific principles that serve as the foundation for understanding metabolic and endocrine systems' involvement in the treatment of patients/clients across the lifespan.

- Anatomy of the endocrine system
- Physiology and pathophysiology of the metabolic and endocrine systems
- Pharmacology as related to the metabolic and endocrine systems

- Physiological response to environmental factors and characteristics (e.g., air temperature, humidity, water temperature, water depth, buoyancy, altitude)
- Effects of activity and exercise on the metabolic and endocrine systems

Examination: This category refers to awareness of the types and applications of metabolic and endocrine tests and measures and their relevance to information collected during history and systems review. The category also includes the reaction of the metabolic and endocrine systems to tests and measures. Information covered in these areas supports appropriate and effective patient/client management across the lifespan.

- Appropriate types of metabolic and endocrine systems tests/measures and their applications
- Physiological response of the metabolic and endocrine systems to various types of tests/measures

Foundations for Evaluation, Differential Diagnosis, and Prognosis: This category refers to the diseases and conditions of metabolic and endocrine systems in order to ensure the appropriate and effective patient/client treatment and management decisions across the lifespan.

- Diseases/conditions of the metabolic and endocrine systems
- Differential diagnoses related to pathologies of the metabolic and endocrine systems
- Diseases or conditions of the metabolic and endocrine systems in order to make effective treatment decisions
- Medical management of the metabolic and endocrine systems (e.g., surgical procedures, medical tests)

Interventions: This category refers to the features (e.g., types, applications, responses, and potential complications) of metabolic and endocrine systems interventions as well as the impact on the metabolic and endocrine systems of interventions performed on other systems in order to support patient/client management across the lifespan.

- Appropriate types of metabolic and endocrine systems interventions and their applications
- Physiological response of the metabolic and endocrine systems to various types of interventions
- Secondary effects or complications from interventions on the metabolic and endocrine systems
- Secondary effects or complications on the metabolic and endocrine systems from interventions used on other systems

Multi-System (16 Questions)

Clinical Applications of Foundational Sciences: This category refers to the essential scientific principles that serve as the foundation for understanding multi-system involvement in the treatment of patients/clients across the lifespan.

- Normal interrelationships among multiple systems
- Polypharmacy as it relates to multi-system involvement
- Physiological response to environmental factors and characteristics (e.g., air temperature, humidity, water temperature, water depth, buoyancy, altitude)

Foundations for Evaluation, Differential Diagnosis, and Prognosis: This category refers to the interpretation of knowledge of multiple system involvement in order to ensure the appropriate and effective patient/client treatment and management decisions.

- Diseases/conditions affecting multiple systems (e.g., cancer, pregnancy, morbid obesity)
- Differential diagnoses related to pathologies of multi-system involvement
- Diseases or conditions of multiple systems in order to make effective patient/client management decisions
- Medical management of multiple systems (e.g., surgical procedures, medical tests, diagnostic imaging)
- Impact of co-morbidities on patient/client management (e.g., diabetes and hypertension, obesity, arthritis)
- Impact of coexisting conditions on patient/client management (e.g., hip fracture, dementia)
- Psychological and psychiatric conditions that impact patient/client management (e.g., depression, schizophrenia)

Physical Therapist NPTE Test Content Outline, Federation of State Boards Physical Therapy, www.fsbpt.org

Non-Systems

Equipment & Devices; Therapeutic Modalities (22 Questions)

Equipment & Devices: This category refers to the different types of equipment and devices, use requirements and/or contextual determinants, as well as any other influencing factors involved in the selection and application of equipment and devices in order to support patient/client treatment and management decisions across the lifespan.

- Assistive and adaptive devices
- Prosthetic devices
- Orthotic devices
- Protective devices
- Supportive devices
- Gravity-assisted devices
- Bariatric equipment and devices

Therapeutic Modalities: This category refers to the underlying principles for the use of therapeutic modalities as well as the justification for the selection and use of the variety of types of therapeutic modalities employed to support patient/client treatment and management decisions across the lifespan.

- Indications, contraindications, and precautions of therapeutic modalities
- Physical agents (e.g., athermal agents, cryotherapy, hydrotherapy, light agents, sound agents, thermotherapy)
- Mechanical modalities (e.g., compression therapies, mechanical motion devices, traction devices)
- Electrotherapeutic delivery of medications (e.g., iontophoresis)
- Electrical stimulation (e.g., Functional Electrical Stimulation (FES), High Voltage Pulsed Current (HVPC), Neuromuscular Electrical Stimulation (NES), TENS)

Physical Therapist NPTE Test Content Outline, Federation of State Boards Physical Therapy, www.fsbpt.org

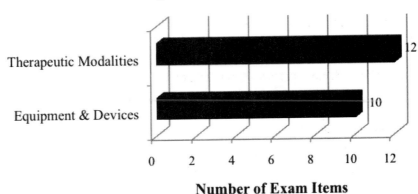

Equipment & Devices; Therapeutic Modalities

Therapeutic Modalities — 12

Equipment & Devices — 10

0   2   4   6   8   10   12

Number of Exam Items

Safety & Professional Roles; Teaching/Learning; Research (39 Questions)

Safety, Protection, & Professional Roles: This category refers to the critical issues involved in patient/client safety and protection and the responsibilities of health care providers to ensure that patient/client management and health care decisions take place in a secure and trustworthy environment.

- Factors influencing patient/client safety (e.g., fall risk, use of restraints, use of equipment, environmental factors)
- Emergency preparedness (e.g., CPR, first aid, disaster response)
- Proper body mechanics
- Injury prevention
- Infection control procedures (e.g., standard/universal precautions)
- Legal obligations for reporting abuse and neglect
- Patient/client rights (e.g., ADA, IDEA, HIPAA)
- Human resource legal issues (e.g., OSHA, sexual harassment)
- Standards of documentation
- Risk guidelines (e.g., documentation, policies and procedures, incident reports)
- Roles and responsibilities of other health care professionals and support staff

Teaching & Learning: This category refers to the principles and theories of teaching and learning required to create a learning environment in which information is effectively communicated to patients/clients to ensure that they receive appropriate instruction designed to support patient/client management decisions.

- Teaching and learning strategies, theories, and techniques (e.g., cognitive, motor, models of education)
- Health behavior change models
- Communication skills

Research & Evidence-Based Practice: This category refers to the application of measurement principles and research methodology to make reasoned and appropriate assessment and interpretation of information sources and practice research to support patient/client management decisions fundamental to evidence-based practice.

- Research design and interpretation (e.g., qualitative, quantitative)
- Measurement science (e.g., reliability, validity, common statistical methods)
- Outcome measures (e.g., suitability, applications)
- Data collection techniques (e.g., surveys, direct observation)
- Hierarchy of evidence (e.g., randomized control, case studies, anecdotal observation)

Physical Therapist NPTE Test Content Outline, Federation of State Boards Physical Therapy, www.fsbpt.org

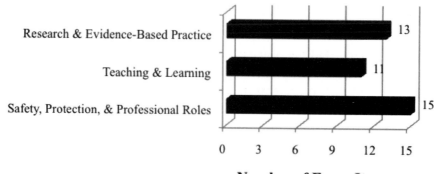

Safety & Professional Roles; Teaching/Learning; Research

Research & Evidence-Based Practice — 13
Teaching & Learning — 11
Safety, Protection, & Professional Roles — 15

Number of Exam Items

Unit 6

Computer-Based Examinations

The section contains three, 200 question sample examinations located on a CD-ROM attached to the inside of the back cover of the text. Candidates who are exposed to sample examinations have several distinct opportunities that otherwise may not be available.

- Candidates have the opportunity to refine their test taking skills with sample questions that are similar in design and format to actual examination questions.
- Candidates have the opportunity to assess their current level of preparedness prior to the actual examination.

The sample examinations on the CD-ROM include questions representative of each of the categories and subcategories of the current content outline of the National Physical Therapy Examination. A sophisticated performance analysis section offers candidates detailed feedback on their examination performance according to six system specific areas and six content outline areas.

System Specific Summary

Musculoskeletal System
Neuromuscular & Nervous Systems
Cardiac, Vascular, & Pulmonary Systems
Integumentary System
Other Systems
Non-Systems

Content Outline Summary

Clinical Application of Foundational Sciences
Examination
Foundations for Evaluation, Differential Diagnosis, & Prognosis
Interventions
Equipment & Devices; Therapeutic Modalities
Safety & Professional Roles; Teaching/Learning; Research

An answer key located in this section includes the correct answer, explanations supporting the correct answer and each of the incorrect answers, a cited resource with page number, and the system specific and content outline area classification. A complete index for the sample examinations is included at the conclusion of the unit. The index allows candidates to identify the location of specific subject matter within each of the sample examinations.

There are a number of indicators that must be closely examined after completing each sample examination in order to assess a candidate's performance. Perhaps the most obvious indicator is the number of questions a candidate answers correctly. Candidates should attempt to answer 75% or more of the questions correctly. Although this is a relatively lofty goal 75% was selected since the score is safely above a typical criterion-referenced score and therefore would likely be considered a passing score.

There are a number of less obvious indicators that can offer candidates feedback as they prepare for the National Physical Therapy Examination. These indicators often are best examined by answering several specific questions.

- Were you able to maintain the same level of concentration throughout the entire examination?
- Did you have adequate time to complete the examination?
- Did you effectively incorporate test taking strategies?
- Did you misinterpret or fail to identify what selected questions were asking?
- Did the questions that were answered incorrectly exhibit any similar characteristics?
- Did you make any careless mistakes?

Candidates should attempt to integrate this information in conjunction with the performance analysis summary to accurately identify current strengths and weaknesses and develop appropriate remedial strategies. The computer-based examinations include a number of helpful tools to assist candidates to integrate this information. Candidates should avoid becoming overly excited or depressed based on the results of a given sample examination and use the number of questions answered correctly only as a general indicator of their current level of preparedness. Studying for the examination is much closer to running a marathon than running a sprint. By engaging in meaningful self-assessment activities candidates can gather valuable information to improve future examination performance.

Physical Therapy
Exam One

STRATEGY

"Good fortune is what happens when opportunity meets preparation." - Thomas Edison

Candidates need to have a strategy or plan to prepare for the National Physical Therapy Examination. An important component of any comprehensive study plan involves answering multiple-choice questions and carefully analyzing the results. Identifying strengths and weaknesses in the various system specific and content outline areas can be a useful activity to direct remedial activities.

Exam One: Question 1

A note in a patient's medical record indicates a specific drug is taken through enteral administration. Which of the following is an example of enteral administration?

1. inhalation
2. injection
3. topical
4. **oral**

> **Correct Answer: 4** (Ciccone p. 13)

Enteral administration of drugs involves the esophagus, stomach, and small and large intestines. The most common routes of enteral administration are oral, sublingual, and rectal.

1. Drugs that are in a gaseous or volatile state or that can be suspended as tiny droplets in an aerosol form can be administered through inhalation. Examples are general anesthetics and anti-asthmatic drugs.
2. Injection allows drugs to be introduced systemically or locally. Common types of injection include intravenous, intra-arterial, subcutaneous, intramuscular, and intrathecal. Examples are insulin and narcotic analgesics.
3. Topical administration refers to the application of drugs topically to the surface of the skin or mucous membranes. Topical administration is most often used to treat the outer layer of the skin and not other areas since most medications are absorbed poorly through the epidermis and into the systemic circulation.
4. **Oral administration is considered the easiest form of taking medication when self-medication is required and is relatively safe since drugs enter the system in a fairly controlled manner.**

System Specific: Other Systems
Content Outline: Clinical Application of Foundational Sciences

Exam One: Question 2

A patient is positioned in supine with the hips flexed to 90 degrees and the knees extended. As the patient slowly lowers her extended legs toward the horizontal, there is an increase in lordosis of the low back. This finding is indicative of weakness of the:

1. hip flexors
2. back extensors
3. hip extensors
4. **abdominals**

> **Correct Answer: 4** (Kendall p. 212)

Muscle testing is often a standard component of a physical examination and can be useful in differential diagnosis and the treatment of musculoskeletal and neuromuscular conditions. Physical therapists should be aware of standard methods of assessing muscle strength and interpreting the results.

1. The strength of the hip flexors is assessed with the patient in short sitting. The patient is asked to raise their leg toward the ceiling. The physical therapist stabilizes the iliac crest of the test leg while placing a resistive downward force at the distal end of the femur. Weakness would be indicated by inability to maintain the leg off of the table or attempted substitution.
2. The strength of the back extensors is assessed with the patient in prone. The patient is asked to raise their trunk off of the surface of the table while clasping their hands behind the buttocks or behind the head. The physical therapist stabilizes by providing a downward force to the legs so that they remain firmly on the table. Resistance is provided by gravity. Weakness would be indicated by an inability to maintain the trunk off of the surface of the table or attempted substitution.
3. The strength of the hip extensors, as a group, is assessed in prone. The patient is asked to raise the leg off of the surface of the table, toward the ceiling. The physical therapist stabilizes the pelvis of the test leg while placing a resistive downward force at the distal end of the femur. Weakness would be indicated by an inability to maintain the leg off of the surface of the table.
4. **The supplied description of the resistive test in the question is a standard method to assess the strength of the lower abdominal muscles. Failure to maintain the low back flat on the surface of the table as the legs are lowered is indicative of muscle weakness.**

System Specific: Musculoskeletal System
Content Outline: Examination

Exam One: Question 3

In a clinical trial, patient height is measured in centimeters and weight is measured in kilograms. What inference can the physical therapist make about the scale of measurement for height and weight?

1. **Height and weight are measurements on the ratio scale.**
2. Height and weight are measurements on the ordinal scale.
3. Height and weight are measurements on the nominal scale.
4. Height and weight are measurements on the interval scale.

> **Correct Answer: 1** (Portney p. 71)

The four scales of measurement – nominal, ordinal, interval, and ratio – have different characteristics and a special set of rules for manipulating and interpreting numerical data.

1. **Measurements on the ratio scale have an absolute zero point, meaning a score of 0 represents a total absence of the property being measured. Length in centimeters and mass in kilograms are examples of ratio scale measurements because the numbers represent the actual amount of the attributes being measured. All mathematical and statistical operations can be performed on ratio level measurements.**
2. Measurements on an ordinal scale are rank-ordered according to an operationally defined characteristic or property. The measurements exhibit a greater than – less than relationship. Ordinal scale measurements are common in physical therapy. For example, scales of sensation (normal > impaired > absent), spasticity (none < minimal < moderate < severe), balance (good > fair > poor), and manual muscle test scores (trace < poor < fair < good < normal).
3. In the nominal scale or classification scale, elements are assigned to mutually exclusive categories according to some criterion. The categories may be coded by a name, number or symbol, which are used as labels for identification, but have no quantitative value. Gender, blood type, and diagnosis are examples of nominal variables. Counting the frequency or determining the percentages of elements within each category are the only permissible mathematical operations with nominal measurements.
4. The interval scale has the same rank-order characteristics as an ordinal scale, but also demonstrates known and equal distances or intervals between the units of measurement. Unlike the ratio scale, the interval scale has no true zero point. Temperature measured on the Celsius and Fahrenheit scales are examples of interval measurements.

System Specific: Non-Systems
Content Outline: Safety & Professional Roles; Teaching/Learning; Research

Exam One: Question 4

A physical therapist attempts to select an appropriate intervention to treat a patient with a 10 degree limitation in knee extension. Which of the following mobilization techniques would be indicated?

1. lateral glide of the patella
2. caudal glide of the patella
3. posterior glide of the tibia
4. **anterior glide of the tibia**

> **Correct Answer: 4** (Kisner p. 696)

The patellofemoral articulation consists of a convex patella articulating with the concave femoral condyles. The tibiofemoral articulation consists of a concave tibial plateau articulating with the convex femoral condyles.

1. A lateral glide of the patella may be used to improve accessory motion of the patellofemoral joint, but would not be useful to improve knee extension.
2. A caudal glide refers to a downward glide (i.e., inferior) toward the feet. A caudal glide would not be useful to improve knee extension range of motion since the patella slides superiorly in knee extension.
3. A posterior glide of the tibia on the femur would be used to increase knee flexion range of motion.
4. **An anterior glide of the tibia on the femur would be used to increase knee extension range of motion.**

System Specific: Musculoskeletal System
Content Outline: Interventions

Exam One: Question 5

A patient with a right radial head fracture is examined in physical therapy. The patient's involved elbow range of motion begins at 15 degrees of flexion and ends at 90 degrees of flexion. The physical therapist should record the patient's elbow range of motion as:

1. 0 - 15 - 90
2. 15 - 0 - 90
3. **15 - 90**
4. 0 - 90

Correct Answer: 3 (Norkin p. 31)

Physical therapists must accurately record the results of goniometric measurements in a manner that is easily interpreted by all health care providers. Any recording of range of motion must include the beginning of the range as well as the end of range.

1. This style of recording is not acceptable since it is not possible to have two distinct values to the right of the "0".
2. The use of "0" between the starting and ending value indicates the patient has 15 degrees of elbow hyperextension. The total available degrees of movement would be 105 degrees.
3. **The recording depicts a patient who begins in 15 degrees of elbow flexion and ends in 90 degrees of elbow flexion. The total available degrees of movement would be 75 degrees.**
4. The recording depicts a patient who is able to fully extend the elbow and flex the elbow to 90 degrees. The total available degrees of movement would be 90 degrees.

System Specific: Musculoskeletal System
Content Outline: Examination

Exam One: Question 6

A physical therapist attempts to improve a patient's lower extremity strength. Which proprioceptive neuromuscular facilitation technique would be the MOST appropriate to achieve the therapist's goals?

1. contract-relax
2. **repeated contractions**
3. rhythmic stabilization
4. hold-relax

Correct Answer: 2 (Sullivan p. 71)

There are a wide variety of proprioceptive neuromuscular facilitation techniques. Each technique is designed with a specific purpose and therapeutic objective. Repeated contractions is designed to initiate movement and promote strength while the other listed options are designed to increase range of motion or promote stability.

1. Contract-relax is a technique used to increase range of motion. As the extremity reaches the point of limitation the patient performs a maximal contraction of the antagonistic muscle group. The therapist resists the movement followed by relaxation and passive movement into newly gained range of motion.
2. **Repeated contractions are used to initiate movement and sustain a contraction through the range of motion. The therapist provides a quick stretch followed by isometric or isotonic contractions. Providing resistance at the point of weakness can enhance the effectiveness of repeated contractions.**
3. Rhythmic stabilization is a technique used to increase range of motion and coordinate isometric contractions. The technique requires isometric contractions of all muscles around a joint against progressive resistance.
4. Hold-relax uses isometric contractions to increase range of motion. The contractions are facilitated for all muscle groups at the limiting point within the range of motion. Relaxation occurs and the extremity moves through the newly acquired range to the next point of limitation.

System Specific: Neuromuscular & Nervous Systems
Content Outline: Interventions

Exam One: Question 7

A physical therapist instructs a patient diagnosed with rotator cuff tendonitis in transverse plane resistive exercises. Which motions would be appropriate based on the given information?

1. abduction and adduction
2. flexion and extension
3. **medial and lateral rotation**
4. pronation and supination

Correct Answer: 3 (Norkin p. 4)

Motions are described as occurring around three cardinal planes of the body (frontal, sagittal, transverse). Movement in the cardinal planes occurs around three corresponding axes (anterior-posterior, medial-lateral, vertical).

1. Abduction and adduction occur in the frontal (coronal) plane. The frontal plane divides the body into anterior and posterior sections. Motions in the frontal plane occur around an anterior-posterior axis.
2. Flexion and extension occur in the sagittal plane. The sagittal plane divides the body into left and right halves. Motions in the sagittal plane occur around a medial-lateral axis.
3. **Medial and lateral rotation occur in the transverse plane. The transverse plane divides the body into upper and lower sections. Motions in the transverse plane occur around a vertical axis.**
4. Pronation and supination occur in the transverse plane with the patient positioned in the anatomical position. With the patient positioned in short sitting with the elbow flexed to 90 degrees, the motion occurs in the frontal plane around an anterior-posterior axis.

System Specific: Musculoskeletal System
Content Outline: Clinical Application of Foundational Sciences

Test Taking Tip: A candidate may have experienced difficulty deciding between options three and four since each of the listed motions can occur in the transverse plane. Although this is accurate, given the diagnosis it is far more likely the answer would relate directly to the shoulder complex instead of the elbow and forearm.

Exam One: Question 8

A patient is limited in passive ankle dorsiflexion when the knee is extended, but is not limited when the knee is flexed. The MOST logical explanation is:

1. **the gastrocnemius is responsible for the limitation**
2. the soleus is responsible for the limitation
3. the popliteus is responsible for the limitation
4. the gastrocnemius and soleus are both responsible for the limitation

Correct Answer: 1 (Kendall p. 375)

The gastrocnemius muscle consists of a medial and lateral head innervated by the tibial nerve. The medial head originates on the proximal and posterior part of the medial condyle and adjacent part of the femur and capsule of the knee joint. The lateral head originates on the lateral condyle and posterior surface of the femur, and capsule of the knee joint. The muscle inserts on the middle part of the posterior surface of the calcaneus.

1. **The gastrocnemius is a two-joint muscle that crosses both the knee and ankle joints. When the knee is flexed, the muscle is placed on slack which allows for normal ankle range of motion. A limitation in ankle range of motion when the knee is extended may indicate a restriction in the gastrocnemius and possibly the plantaris.**
2. The soleus is a one-joint muscle that plantar flexes the ankle joint and is innervated by the tibial nerve. The muscle's length would not be influenced by the position of the knee.
3. The popliteus muscle medially rotates the tibia on the femur and flexes the knee joint in non-weight bearing. The muscle acts to laterally rotate the femur on the tibia and flexes the knee joint in weight bearing. The popliteus muscle is also a one-joint muscle.
4. The gastrocnemius and soleus work together to plantar flex the ankle. The length of the gastrocnemius would be affected based on the position of the knee, however, the length of the soleus would not be affected since it is a one-joint muscle.

System Specific: Musculoskeletal System
Content Outline: Clinical Application of Foundational Sciences

Exam One: Question 9

A patient employed in a machine shop is referred to physical therapy with a diagnosis of carpal tunnel syndrome. The patient indicates that he is scheduled for a diagnostic test that may help to confirm the diagnosis. Which of the following electrodiagnostic tests would be the MOST appropriate?

1. electroencephalography
2. evoked potentials
3. **nerve conduction velocity**
4. electromyography

Correct Answer: 3 (Tan p. 45)

Carpal tunnel syndrome results from repetitive compression of the median nerve where it passes through the carpal tunnel at the wrist. Nerve conduction velocity is commonly used to diagnose carpal tunnel syndrome. Less formal methods to assist in identifying carpal tunnel syndrome include Phalen's test and Tinel's sign.

1. Electroencephalography is the recording of the electrical activity of the brain. The electrical activity is collected by examining the difference between the electrical potential of two electrodes placed at different locations on the scalp. Electroencephalography is used to assess seizure activity, metabolic disorders, and cerebellar lesions.
2. An evoked potential refers to electrical activity recorded from the presentation of a stimulus. Signals can be recorded from the cerebral cortex, brain stem, spinal cord, and peripheral nerves. Evoked potentials can be used to determine how quickly and completely nerve signals reach the brain and can be used to assist with the diagnosis of several medical conditions including multiple sclerosis.
3. **Nerve conduction velocity refers to the speed by which an action potential travels down a peripheral nerve. The measure is recorded in meters per second. Nerve conduction velocity can be used to diagnose conditions such as carpal tunnel syndrome, peripheral neuropathy, and Guillain-Barre syndrome.**
4. Electromyography is the recording of the electrical activity of a selected muscle or muscle group at rest and during voluntary contraction. Electromyography is performed by inserting a needle electrode percutaneously into a muscle or through the use of surface electrodes. The test is commonly used to assess peripheral nerve injuries and to differentiate between various neuromuscular disorders.

System Specific: Neuromuscular & Nervous Systems
Content Outline: Foundations for Evaluation, Differential Diagnosis, & Prognosis

Exam One: Question 10

A physical therapist uses iontophoresis over the anterior knee of a patient with patellar tendonitis. Assuming the therapist's goal is to reduce the patient's present pain level, the MOST appropriate solution to utilize is:

1. acetic acid
2. **lidocaine**
3. sodium chloride
4. zinc oxide

Correct Answer: 2 (Cameron p. 224)

Iontophoresis refers to the transcutaneous delivery of ions into the body for therapeutic purposes using an electrical current. Physical therapists must possess an in-depth awareness of the most appropriate ions to treat specific conditions.

1. Acetate, a derivative of acetic acid, is a negatively charged ion used to treat calcific deposits.
2. **Lidocaine, a derivative of xylocaine, is a positively charged ion used to treat pain and inflammation associated with acute inflammatory conditions.**
3. Chlorine, a derivative of sodium chloride, is a negatively charged ion used to treat scar tissue, keloids, and burns.
4. Zinc, a derivative of zinc oxide, is a positively charged ion used to promote healing, most often with open lesions and ulcerations.

System Specific: Non-Systems
Content Outline: Equipment & Devices; Therapeutic Modalities

Exam One: Question 11

A physical therapist performs the talar tilt test on a 22-year-old female rehabilitating from an inversion ankle sprain. Which ligament does the talar tilt test examine?

1. anterior talotibial
2. **calcaneofibular**
3. deltoid
4. posterior talotibial

Correct Answer: 2 (Magee p. 890)

The talar tilt test requires the patient to be positioned in supine or sidelying with the knee flexed to 90 degrees. The physical therapist stabilizes the distal tibia with one hand while grasping the talus with the other hand. The foot is maintained in a neutral position. The therapist tilts the talus into abduction and adduction. A positive test is indicated by excessive adduction and may be indicative of a calcaneofibular ligament sprain.

1. The anterior talotibial ligament extends from the tip of the medial malleolus to the anterior aspect of the medial surface of the talus. The ligament is extremely strong and resists abduction of the talus when it is in plantar flexion and eversion.
2. **The calcaneofibular ligament is a round cord that passes posteroinferiorly from the tip of the lateral malleolus to the lateral surface of the calcaneus. The integrity of the ligament can be assessed using the talar tilt test.**
3. The deltoid ligament refers to the collective medial ligaments of the ankle. The ligament as a whole attaches proximally to the medial aspect of the medial malleolus and fans out to the various distal attachments.
4. The posterior talotibial ligament extends from the medial malleolus to the medial side of the talus and the medial tuberosity of the talus. The ligament resists ankle dorsiflexion and lateral translation and external rotation of the talus.

System Specific: Musculoskeletal System
Content Outline: Examination

Exam One: Question 12

A physical therapist completes a developmental assessment on a seven-month-old infant. Assuming normal development, which of the following reflexes would NOT be integrated?

1. asymmetrical tonic neck reflex
2. Moro reflex
3. **Landau reflex**
4. symmetrical tonic neck reflex

Correct Answer: 3 (Ratliffe p. 30)

Integration of a reflex refers to the period of time when a reflex is no longer present despite an appropriate stimulus.

1. The asymmetrical tonic neck reflex is stimulated when the head is turned to one side. The response is a fencing posture (arm and leg on face side are extended, arm and leg on scalp side are flexed). The normal age of the response is from birth to 6 months.
2. The Moro reflex is stimulated when an infant's head is suddenly dropped into extension for a few inches. The response is that the arms abduct with fingers open, then cross the trunk into adduction; often followed immediately by crying. The normal age of the response is from 28 weeks of gestation to 5 months.
3. **The Landau reflex is an equilibrium response that occurs when a child responds to prone suspension by aligning their head and extremities in line with the plane of the body. Although the response begins around three months of age, it is not fully integrated until the child's second year.**
4. The symmetrical tonic neck reflex is stimulated by the head moving into flexion or extension. When the head is in flexion, the arms are flexed and the legs are extended. When the head is in extension, the arms are extended and the legs are flexed. The normal age of the response is from 6-8 months.

System Specific: Neuromuscular & Nervous Systems
Content Outline: Examination

Exam One: Question 13

A physical therapist examines a patient with limited cervical range of motion. As part of the examination, the therapist attempts to screen the patient for possible vertebral artery involvement, but is unable to position the patient's head and neck in the recommended test position. The MOST appropriate action is to:

1. complete the vertebral artery test with the head and neck positioned in approximately 50 percent of the available cervical range of motion
2. **complete the vertebral artery test as far into the available cervical range of motion as tolerated**
3. avoid completing the vertebral artery test until the patient has full cervical range of motion
4. avoid all direct cervical treatment techniques until the vertebral artery test can be assessed at the limits of normal cervical range of motion

Correct Answer: 2 (Dutton p. 1239)

The vertebral artery test is performed with the patient positioned in supine. The therapist places the patient's head in extension, lateral flexion, and rotation to the ipsilateral side. A positive test is indicated by dizziness, nystagmus, slurred speech or loss of consciousness and may be indicative of compression of the vertebral artery.

1. The vertebral artery test should be administered using the available cervical range of motion and as a result it would not make sense to utilize only a portion of the available range of motion.
2. **The physical therapist should perform the test and clear the patient's vertebral artery for their available range of motion. As the patient gains additional range of motion the test can be readministered.**
3. The vertebral artery test can be performed on patients that possess less than full cervical range of motion.
4. Direct cervical treatment techniques are often employed on patients with less than full cervical range of motion. In many cases it is still necessary to clear the vertebral artery using the patient's available cervical range of motion.

System Specific: Neuromuscular & Nervous Systems
Content Outline: Examination

Test Taking Tip: In some cases two options express different ways of saying the exact same thing. When this happens the options mutually exclude each other since it would be impossible for one of the respective options to be correct and the other to be incorrect. In this particular question, option 3 and option 4 imply that the vertebral artery test, and therefore direct cervical treatment techniques, cannot be performed until the patient possesses full cervical range of motion. Regardless of a candidate's knowledge in this particular area it would be possible to eliminate options 3 and 4.

Exam One: Question 14

A 42-year-old female is admitted to a rehabilitation hospital after sustaining a stroke. During the examination the physical therapist identifies significant sensory deficits in the anterolateral spinothalamic system. Which sensation would be MOST affected?

1. barognosis
2. kinesthesia
3. graphesthesia
4. **temperature**

Correct Answer: 4 (O'Sullivan p. 138)

Sensory information enters the spinal cord through the dorsal roots and is delivered to higher centers through the spinothalamic system or the dorsal columns. The spinothalamic system is involved with the transmission of nondiscriminative sensations which are activated by mechanoreceptors, thermoreceptors, and nociceptors.

1. Barognosis refers to the recognition of weight. Barognosis is tested by asking a patient to identify the comparative weight of similar sized objects presented in a series. This type of sensory information is transmitted through the dorsal columns.
2. Kinesthesia refers to the ability to identify the direction and extent of movement of a joint or body part. This type of sensory information is transmitted through the dorsal columns.
3. Graphesthesia refers to the ability to recognize symbols, letters or numbers traced on the skin. This type of sensory information is transmitted through the dorsal columns.
4. **Temperature information is transmitted through the spinothalamic system. The system consists of small diameter and relatively slow conducting afferent fibers. Conversely, the dorsal columns consist of large diameter, rapidly conducting afferent fibers.**

System Specific: Neuromuscular & Nervous Systems
Content Outline: Clinical Application of Foundational Sciences

Exam One: Question 15

A 13-year-old girl discusses the possibility of anterior cruciate ligament reconstruction with an orthopedic surgeon. The girl injured her knee while playing soccer and is concerned about the future impact of the injury on her athletic career. Which of the following factors would have the GREATEST influence on her candidacy for surgery?

1. anthropometric measurements
2. hamstrings/quadriceps strength ratio
3. **skeletal maturity**
4. somatotype

> **Correct Answer: 3** (Hertling p. 518)

Physical therapists should possess a general idea of how specific factors such as normal growth and development influence a candidate's eligibility for selected medical and surgical procedures.

1. Common anthropometric measurements used for adults include height, weight, body mass index (BMI), waist-to-hip ratio, and percentage of body fat. These measures are then compared to reference standards to assess items such as weight status and the risk for various diseases.

2. Hamstrings/quadriceps strength ratio is a general measure of the relative strength of the hamstrings compared to the relative strength of the quadriceps. Strength is an important factor both prior to and post surgery, however, it is unlikely that this would influence candidacy for surgery.

3. **Due to the potential impact on future bone growth, lack of skeletal maturity can be a contraindication to anterior cruciate ligament reconstruction surgery.**

4. Somatotype is a term used to classify a system of body typing. The most common classifications of somatotype include endomorph, mesomorph, and ectomorph.

System Specific: Musculoskeletal System
Content Outline: Foundations for Evaluation, Differential Diagnosis, & Prognosis

Exam One: Question 16

A physical therapist identifies a bluish discoloration of the skin and nailbeds of a 55-year-old male referred to physical therapy for pulmonary rehabilitation. What does this objective finding indicate?

1. hyperoxemia
2. hyperoxia
3. hypokalemia
4. **hypoxemia**

> **Correct Answer: 4** (Paz p. 70)

Individuals whose blood is deficient in oxygen tend to have a bluish discoloration of their skin called cyanosis. Cyanosis is most noticeable in mucous membranes and nailbeds.

1. Hyperoxemia refers to increased acidity of the blood.

2. Hyperoxia refers to increased oxygen in the blood.

3. Hypokalemia refers to severe potassium depletion in the circulating blood. The condition is commonly manifested by episodes of muscular weakness or paralysis and postural hypotension.

4. **Hypoxemia refers to a decreased oxygen concentration in the blood measured by arterial oxygen partial pressure (PaO_2) values. A PaO_2 less than 80 mm Hg constitutes hypoxemia.**

System Specific: Other Systems
Content Outline: Examination

Exam One: Question 17

A manager develops a policy on physical therapy utilization of continuing education resources. Which of the following would be the MOST appropriate action to enhance the quality of patient care?

1. offer continuing education resources to senior therapists in relation to their years of experience
2. divide the continuing education resources evenly among therapy staff
3. establish a committee to review requests for continuing education resources
4. **prioritize requests for continuing education resources based on established patient care standards**

Correct Answer: 4 (Nosse p. 226)

Continuing education resources should be allocated in a manner that advances the established goals of the physical therapy department.

1. Providing resources to therapists based on experience would not specifically address the needs of all therapists. This type of continuing education strategy may be more effective as a method to retain experienced therapists.
2. Individual therapists have diverse interests that may or may not be compatible with the established goals of the physical therapy department. As a result, some form of oversight or prioritization would likely be necessary to ensure a meaningful impact on the quality of patient care.
3. Establishing a committee to review requests for continuing education resources provides necessary oversight and may be useful to enhance the quality of patient care, however, the strategy does not provide any specific insight as to how the established committee will enhance the quality of patient care.
4. **Prioritizing requests for continuing education resources based on established patient care standards is a specific strategy that will allocate resources directly toward educational opportunities which are consistent with established patient care standards. This type of allocation sends a strong message to all therapists about the priorities of the department and reinforces efforts to improve the quality of patient care.**

System Specific: Non-Systems
Content Outline: Safety & Professional Roles; Teaching/Learning; Research

Exam One: Question 18

A physical therapist uses the body mass index scale as a means of assessing a patient's total body composition. The therapist determines the body mass index by dividing the body weight in kilograms by height in meters squared. Which of the following values would be the MOST representative of a healthy male or female?

1. 14 kg/m^2
2. **22 kg/m^2**
3. 28 kg/m^2
4. 37 kg/m^2

Correct Answer: 2 (American College of Sports Medicine p. 267)

The body mass index (BMI) is used to assess weight relative to height and is calculated by dividing body weight (kilograms) by height (meters squared). A BMI of greater than 30 is associated with an increased risk of hypertension, hypercholesterolemia, coronary disease, and mortality. A BMI of less than 18.5 also increases the risk of cardiovascular disease.

1. A BMI of 14 is considered underweight since any value less than 18.5 is classified as underweight.
2. **A BMI from 18.5 – 24.9 is considered normal.**
3. A BMI of 28 is considered overweight since any value between 25.0 - 29.9 is classified as overweight.
4. A BMI of 37 is considered Obesity, Class II since any value between 35.0 - 39.9 is classified as obesity, Class II.

System Specific: Other Systems
Content Outline: Examination

Exam One: Question 19

A patient diagnosed with patellofemoral syndrome discusses his past medical history with a physical therapist. The patient reports having anterior cruciate ligament reconstruction surgery on his right knee two years ago, however, the therapist is not able to identify a scar over the anterior surface of the right knee. Assuming the surgeon utilized an autograft for the reconstruction, which of the following would be the MOST likely graft site?

1. semitendinosus and semimembranosus
2. **semitendinosus and gracilis**
3. semimembranosus and gracilis
4. semitendinosus and biceps femoris

> **Correct Answer: 2** (Brotzman p. 185)

Anterior cruciate ligament (ACL) reconstruction refers to the use of a graft to replace a damaged anterior cruciate ligament. The graft is placed through drilled holes in the femoral and tibial tunnels and then anchored with a fixation device. The most common grafts used are the patellar tendon or the tendons of the semitendinosus and gracilis.

1. The semitendinosus and semimembranosus both function as medial hamstrings muscles. The muscles are innervated by the tibial branch of the sciatic nerve (L5-S1). The semimembranosus is not used as a graft for ACL reconstruction.
2. **The semitendinosus and gracilis tendons are commonly used together as a graft for anterior cruciate ligament reconstruction. The grafts result in a decreased incidence of post-operative patellofemoral knee pain, however, provide weaker initial fixation. The gracilis functions as a hip adductor and is innervated by the obturator nerve (L2-L4).**
3. The semimembranosus is not used as a graft for ACL reconstruction.
4. The semitendinosus and biceps femoris are hamstrings muscles. The semitendinosus is considered a medial hamstrings muscle and the biceps femoris is a lateral hamstrings muscle. The biceps femoris is not used as a graft for ACL reconstruction.

System Specific: Musculoskeletal System
Content Outline: Foundations for Evaluation, Differential Diagnosis, & Prognosis

Exam One: Question 20

A physical therapist assesses a one-month-old infant. During the treatment session the therapist strokes the cheek of the infant causing the infant to turn its mouth towards the stimulus. This action is utilized to assess the:

1. Moro reflex
2. **rooting reflex**
3. startle reflex
4. righting reflex

> **Correct Answer: 2** (Ratliffe p. 26)

Primitive reflexes begin in utero and are typically integrated within the first year. Many of the primitive reflexes initially provide a useful purpose and the presence of the reflexes indicates normal functioning of the nervous system.

1. The Moro reflex is a primitive reflex that is normally present at 28 weeks gestation through five months of age. The reflex is stimulated by the head suddenly dropping into extension for a few inches. The response is abduction of the arms with the fingers open, followed by the arms crossing the trunk into adduction, and crying.
2. **The rooting reflex is a primitive reflex that is normally present from 28 weeks of gestation through three months of age. The reflex assists the mother when feeding an infant.**
3. The startle reflex is a primitive reflex that is normally present at 28 weeks gestation through five months of age. The reflex is stimulated by a loud, sudden noise. The response is similar to the Moro reflex, but the elbows remain flexed and the hands closed.
4. The righting reflex is a general term used to describe a group of reflexes that are responsible for the development of upright posture and smooth transitional movements. Equilibrium reactions occur in response to a change in body position or surface support to maintain body alignment.

System Specific: Neuromuscular & Nervous Systems
Content Outline: Examination

A physical therapist elects to use mechanical lumbar traction for a patient rehabilitating from a back injury. The therapeutic goals of the session include decreasing the patient's muscle spasm. The MOST appropriate force based on the stated objective would be:

1. 10% of body weight
2. 15% of body weight
3. **25% of body weight**
4. 50% of body weight

Correct Answer: 3 (Prentice – Therapeutic Modalities p. 471)

The optimal amount of force when using traction depends on the patient's clinical presentation, the goals of the treatment, and the position selected. There are, however, some general guidelines that physical therapists can use. Guidelines are often expressed in percentages of total body weight instead of strictly an amount of force in pounds or kilograms since this method accommodates for patients of varying sizes.

1. Ten percent of the patient's body weight would be far less than the amount of force needed to accomplish the identified goal of decreasing the patient's muscle spasm.
2. Fifteen percent of the patient's body weight would be less than the amount of force needed, although it is possible that this amount of force could be used as a trial to determine how the patient will tolerate traction. Assuming the patient tolerates fifteen percent, the therapist could then move to twenty-five percent.
3. **Twenty-five percent of the patient's body weight is generally recommended when the goal of treatment is to decrease muscle spasm or stretch soft tissue in the lumbar spine.**
4. Fifty percent of the patient's body weight is required for mechanical separation of the lumbar spine, however, this amount of force would be excessive to diminish muscle spasm.

System Specific: Non-Systems
Content Outline: Equipment & Devices; Therapeutic Modalities

A physical therapist reviews a physician referral form that includes only the patient's name and the referring physician's signature. During the examination the patient indicates that she had knee surgery two weeks ago, however, is unable to provide more specific information. The therapist attempts to call the physician's office, but is unable to reach anyone. The MOST appropriate therapist action is:

1. initiate treatment based on the results of the examination
2. initiate treatment based on an established protocol following knee surgery
3. initiate treatment, however, avoid resistive exercises and high-level functional activities
4. **delay treatment until orders are received from the referring physician**

Correct Answer: 4 (Criteria for Standards of Practice)

Physical therapists should not initiate treatment for patients following surgery until they have adequate medical information to develop an effective plan of care. Presently, the therapist only knows that the patient had knee surgery two weeks ago and was referred to physical therapy by their surgeon.

1. Initiating treatment without specific knowledge of the surgical procedure could be considered a negligent act and may unnecessarily jeopardize the integrity of the surgical procedure.
2. Initiating treatment based on an established protocol following knee surgery is too generic of an approach since there are a multitude of different protocols for each of the various types of commonly performed knee surgeries. It is critical that the physical therapist receives additional information on the surgical procedure directly from the referring physician or an appropriate intermediary (i.e., the referring physician's office).
3. Initiating treatment while avoiding resistive exercises and high-level functional activities limits the scope of the physical therapy session, however, it does not ensure that the chosen interventions are appropriate based on the patient's current status.
4. **Delaying treatment until orders are received from the referring physician ensures that the physical therapist has all of the relevant information prior to developing a plan of care. This action allows the therapist to be fully informed about relevant contraindications and precautions and allows the therapist to develop a plan of care based on the anticipated outcomes.**

System Specific: Non-Systems
Content Outline: Safety & Professional Roles; Teaching/Learning; Research

Exam One: Question 23

A physical therapist employed in an acute care hospital reviews the results of recent laboratory testing for one of his patients. A note in the medical record indicates that the patient was dehydrated at the time the blood sample was taken. Which finding would be MOST likely based on the patient's hydration status?

1. increased coagulation time
2. decreased hematocrit level
3. **increased blood urea nitrogen level**
4. decreased hemoglobin level

> **Correct Answer: 3** (Goodman - Pathology p. 1640)

A blood urea nitrogen (BUN) test measures the amount of nitrogen in the blood that comes from the waste product urea. Urea is made when protein is broken down in the body.

1. Prothrombin time and partial thromboplastin time measure the coagulation of the blood. Increased coagulation time indicates an increased time to form a clot. Neither test is affected by hydration status.
2. Hematocrit measures the percentage of red blood cells in a volume of blood. Hematocrit may be increased when the body's water content is decreased from dehydration, diarrhea, vomiting, excessive sweating, severe burns, and the use of diuretics.
3. **A blood urea nitrogen test is performed to assess kidney function. An increased blood urea nitrogen level can be indicative of dehydration, renal failure or heart failure. Normal blood urea nitrogen levels for adults are 10-20 mg/dL.**
4. Hemoglobin is the iron-containing molecule of red blood cells that binds with oxygen. A low hemoglobin level is indicative of anemia and suggests the oxygen-carrying capacity of the blood is decreased. Hemoglobin may be increased when the body's water content is decreased from dehydration, diarrhea, vomiting, excessive sweating, severe burns, and the use of diuretics.

System Specific: Other Systems
Content Outline: Foundations for Evaluation, Differential Diagnosis, & Prognosis

Exam One: Question 24

A patient four days status post transtibial amputation is transported to physical therapy for a scheduled treatment session. Assuming an uncomplicated recovery, the MOST appropriate patient transfer to utilize from a wheelchair to a mat table is:

1. two-person lift
2. hydraulic lift
3. **stand pivot**
4. sliding board

> **Correct Answer: 3** (Seymour p. 160)

Physical therapists should select transfers for patients based on their unique abilities and limitations. A patient status post transtibial amputation should be able to utilize their uninvolved lower extremity during the transfer and as a result, the therapist would not need to utilize a dependent transfer.

1. A two-person lift is used to transfer a patient between two surfaces of different heights or when transferring a patient to the floor.
2. A hydraulic lift is a device required for dependent transfers when a patient is obese, when there is only one therapist available to assist with the transfer or when the patient is totally dependent.
3. **A stand pivot transfer is used when a patient is able to stand and bear weight through one or both of the lower extremities. The patient must possess functional balance and the ability to pivot.**
4. A sliding board transfer is used for a patient who has sitting balance, some upper extremity strength, and can adequately follow directions.

System Specific: Non-Systems
Content Outline: Equipment & Devices; Therapeutic Modalities

Exam One: Question 25

A physical therapist positions a patient in supine prior to performing a manual muscle test of the supinator. To isolate the supinator and minimize the action of the biceps the therapist should position the patient's elbow in:

1. 30 degrees of elbow flexion
2. 60 degrees of elbow flexion
3. 90 degrees of elbow flexion
4. **terminal elbow flexion**

Correct Answer: 4 (Kendall p. 289)

The supinator is innervated by the radial nerve (C5, C6, C7) and acts to supinate the forearm. The biceps is innervated by the musculocutaneous nerve (C5-C6) and acts to flex the elbow and supinate the forearm. A therapist can isolate one muscle from another muscle with a similar action by placing the deemphasized muscle in a shortened position during the testing procedure. This finding is based on the length-tension relationship which specifies that a muscle can generate the greatest tension at its resting length.

1. The biceps is significantly lengthened in this position, however, 30 degree of elbow flexion allows the biceps to generate a reasonable amount of force.
2. The biceps is slightly lengthened in 60 degrees of elbow flexion, however, the muscle is able to generate a significant amount of force since the position is relatively close to the muscle's resting length.
3. The biceps is typically tested with the elbow in 90 degrees of flexion and therefore this is an undesirable position to minimize the action of the muscle.
4. **Placing the biceps in a maximally shortened position significantly limits the muscle's ability to function as a supinator. Physical therapists should avoid maximum pressure in this position since the shortened position of the biceps can result in significant cramping.**

System Specific: Musculoskeletal System
Content Outline: Examination

Exam One: Question 26

During an examination a physical therapist attempts to determine a patient's general willingness to use an affected body part. What objective information would be the MOST useful for the therapist?

1. bony palpation
2. **active movement**
3. passive movement
4. sensory testing

Correct Answer: 2 (Magee p. 28)

There are a multitude of tests and measures commonly utilized in physical therapy. Physical therapists must be familiar with these tests and measures and understand the relevance and type of information gathered.

1. Bony palpation is a passive technique that would not require the patient to actively participate.
2. **Active movement requires the patient to perform unassisted voluntary range of motion. The activity provides the therapist with information on the patient's willingness to use the affected body part, available range of motion, strength, and coordination.**
3. Passive movement refers to the arc of motion attained by a therapist without assistance from the patient. Passive range of motion is generally slightly greater than active range of motion. The activity provides the therapist with information on the integrity of the articular surfaces, extensibility of the joint capsule, ligaments, muscles, fascia, and skin.
4. Sensory testing is an umbrella term that includes the examination of superficial sensations, deep sensations, and combined cortical sensations. The vast majority of sensory tests would require the patient to verbalize and would not require the active use an affected body part.

System Specific: Musculoskeletal System
Content Outline: Examination

Exam One: Question 27

A patient with right hemiplegia is observed during gait training. The patient performs sidestepping towards the hemiplegic side. The physical therapist may expect the patient to compensate for weakened abductors by:

1. hip hiking of the unaffected side
2. lateral trunk flexion towards the affected side
3. **lateral trunk flexion towards the unaffected side**
4. hip extension of the affected side

> **Correct Answer: 3** (O'Sullivan p. 734)

Gait deviations result from many factors including potential weakness of the affected muscle groups, diminished proprioception, impaired trunk control, decreased awareness of the affected side, and contractures.

1. Hip hiking of the unaffected (left) side would not serve any purpose when side stepping to the right. The left lower extremity can step towards the right without the need to hip hike since motor function on the left is unaffected.
2. Lateral trunk flexion towards the affected (right) side while attempting to side step to the right will only further load the right lower extremity making it more difficult to step toward the right.
3. **Lateral trunk flexion towards the unaffected (left) side can compensate for weak hip abductors while sidestepping. This action unweights the right lower extremity and utilizes momentum along with the abductors to perform sidestepping.**
4. Hip extension of the affected (right) lower extremity would be important if the person was attempting to step backwards, but would not be a component of sidestepping.

System Specific: Neuromuscular & Nervous Systems
Content Outline: Interventions

Exam One: Question 28

A patient reports to a scheduled physical therapy session 25 minutes late. The patient has not been seen previously in physical therapy and was scheduled in a 45 minute block of time. The patient referral indicates the patient is 10 days status post arthroscopic medial meniscectomy. The MOST appropriate therapist action is:

1. **begin the examination**
2. design a home exercise program
3. consult with the patient's physician
4. ask the patient to reschedule

> **Correct Answer: 1** (Criteria for Standards of Practice)

Physical therapists have to possess effective time management skills and adapt their schedule as necessary when warranted. It is important for therapists to attempt to accommodate patients when they happen to be early or late for scheduled appointments, however, they must also be careful that the accommodations do not disadvantage other patients.

1. **The physical therapist should have ample time (i.e., 20 minutes) to begin the examination. This may be particularly important in the described scenario because the patient is 10 days status post arthroscopic surgery.**
2. Although the patient may benefit from a home exercise program, it would be inappropriate to design a home exercise program without first completing a thorough examination.
3. The physician is responsible for the medical management of the patient, however, it is not necessary for a physical therapist to provide the physician with information related to timeliness.
4. Asking the patient to reschedule is a viable option, however, since there is still 20 minutes remaining in the session it is likely that the therapist can effectively use the time.

System Specific: Non-Systems
Content Outline: Safety & Professional Roles; Teaching/Learning; Research

Exam One: Question 29

A physical therapist identifies that an infant is unable to roll from prone to supine. Which reflex could interfere with the infant's ability to roll?

1.   **asymmetrical tonic neck reflex**
2.   Moro reflex
3.   positive support reflex
4.   symmetrical tonic neck reflex

Correct Answer: 1 (Ratliffe p. 25)

The asymmetrical tonic neck reflex interferes with rolling secondary to the tonal influence that is stimulated by turning of the head towards the side when preparing to roll.

1.   **The onset of the asymmetrical tonic neck reflex is at birth. When the infant turns its head to one side, the upper and lower extremities on the face-side will extend while the upper and lower extremities on the skull-side flex. Without integration, the child will be unable to roll.**
2.   The Moro reflex is stimulated by a sudden change in position of the head (i.e., when the head drops into extension). There is immediate abduction, extension, and splaying of the fingers followed by adduction of the upper extremities across the chest. This will normally cause an infant to cry.
3.   The positive support reflex is stimulated as weight is placed on the balls of the feet when the infant is upright. This produces an extension response within the lower extremities and trunk.
4.   The symmetrical tonic neck reflex is stimulated by movement of the head. With flexion, the upper extremities flex and lower extremities extend; with extension, the upper extremities extend and lower extremities flex.

System Specific: Neuromuscular & Nervous Systems
Content Outline: Interventions

Exam One: Question 30

A physical therapist reviews a laboratory report for a 41-year-old male diagnosed with chronic obstructive pulmonary disease. Which of the following would be considered a normal hemoglobin value?

1.   10 gm/dL
2.   **15 gm/dL**
3.   20 gm/dL
4.   25 gm/dL

Correct Answer: 2 (Paz p. 230)

Hemoglobin is the protein in red blood cells that carries oxygen. A blood test can determine how much hemoglobin is in the blood. The range of normal values for adult men is approximately 14 – 18 gm/dL.

1.   10 gm/dL is well below the normal range for adult men. Lower than normal hemoglobin levels can be due to anemia, acute blood loss, lead poisoning, nutritional deficiencies of iron, folate, and vitamins B_{12} and B_6.
2.   **Although the exact lower and upper values of normal may vary slightly depending on the source, 15 gm/dL is well within the range of normal.**
3.   20 gm/dL is well above the normal range for adult males. Higher than normal hemoglobin levels may be due to cor pulmonale, pulmonary fibrosis, and polycythemia vera (i.e., abnormal increase in blood cells).
4.   25 gm/dL is well above the normal range for adult males.

System Specific: Other Systems
Content Outline: Foundations for Evaluation, Differential Diagnosis, & Prognosis

Exam One: Question 31

A patient diagnosed with an incomplete spinal cord lesion presents with muscle paralysis on the ipsilateral side of the lesion and a loss of pain, temperature, and sensitivity on the contralateral side of the lesion. This presentation BEST describes:

1. posterior cord syndrome
2. central cord syndrome
3. anterior cord syndrome
4. **Brown-Sequard's syndrome**

Correct Answer: 4 (Umphred p. 607)

Brown-Sequard's syndrome is an incomplete spinal cord lesion resulting in hemisection of the spinal cord. There is paralysis and loss of vibration and position sense on the same side as the lesion (corticospinal tract and dorsal columns) and loss of pain and temperature sense on the opposite side of the lesion (lateral spinothalamic tract).

1. Posterior cord syndrome is a rare incomplete lesion that results from compression of the posterior spinal artery with subsequent loss of pain perception, stereognosis, proprioception, and two-point discrimination below the level of the lesion. Motor function remains intact.

2. Central cord syndrome is an incomplete lesion resulting from hyperextension. Damage to the spinothalamic tract, corticospinal tract, and dorsal columns produce greater upper extremity involvement than lower extremity; greater motor deficits exist as compared to sensory deficits.

3. Anterior cord syndrome is an incomplete lesion that results from compression to the anterior part of the spinal cord and anterior spinal artery. Presentation consists of a bilateral loss of motor function and pain and temperature sense below the level of the lesion (corticospinal and spinothalamic tracts).

4. **Brown-Sequard's syndrome most commonly occurs from a stab or bullet wound. True hemisection of the cord is rare; most injuries are irregular in nature with a mixture of symptoms.**

System Specific: Neuromuscular & Nervous Systems
Content Outline: Foundations for Evaluation, Differential Diagnosis, & Prognosis

Exam One: Question 32

A physical therapist reviews a physician's examination of a patient scheduled for physical therapy. The examination identifies excessive medial displacement of the elbow during ligamentous testing. Which ligament is typically involved with medial instability of the elbow?

1. annular
2. radial collateral
3. **ulnar collateral**
4. volar radioulnar

Correct Answer: 3 (Hertling p. 360)

The medial collateral ligament, also termed the ulnar collateral ligament, is a fan shaped ligament that serves to restrict medial angulation of the ulna on the humerus.

1. The annular ligament is a strong, well-defined band that attaches to the anterior and posterior margins of the radial notch of the ulna. It acts as a restraining ligament preventing the downward displacement of the radial head.

2. The radial collateral ligament is a strong, triangular band attaching to a depression below the lateral epicondyle of the humerus and the lateral margin of the ulna. The ligament is assessed for potential instability by applying a varus force to the distal forearm.

3. **The ulnar collateral ligament extends from the medial epicondyle to the medial margin of the ulna's trochlear notch and is assessed for potential instability by applying valgus force to the distal forearm.**

4. The volar radioulnar ligament is located at the wrist joint and would not be implicated in an unstable elbow.

System Specific: Musculoskeletal System
Content Outline: Clinical Application of Foundational Sciences

Exam One: Question 33

A patient is unable to take in an adequate supply of nutrients by mouth due to the side effects of radiation therapy. As a result, the patient's physician orders the implementation of tube feeding. What type of tube is MOST commonly used for short-term feeding?

1. endobronchial
2. **nasogastric**
3. endotracheal
4. tracheostomy

> **Correct Answer: 2** (Pierson p. 288)

Patients in an acute care environment often utilize a variety of lines, tubes, and equipment. It is important for physical therapists to possess a basic understanding of these devices and be aware of signs and symptoms that may indicate the need for formal intervention.

1. An endobronchial tube, also called Carlen's catheter, is a flexible catheter for bronchospirometry and for isolation of a portion of the lung to control secretions into the remainder of the tracheobronchial tree during general anesthesia.
2. **A nasogastric tube is a plastic tube inserted through a nostril that extends into the stomach. The device is commonly used for liquid feeding, medication administration or to remove gas from the stomach. A gastric tube is inserted directly into the stomach for long-term feeding.**
3. An endotracheal tube is an airway catheter inserted in the trachea for endotracheal intubation.
4. A tracheostomy refers to an opening made in the trachea in order to insert a catheter or tube, most often to facilitate breathing.

System Specific: Non-Systems
Content Outline: Equipment & Devices; Therapeutic Modalities

Exam One: Question 34

A physical therapist employed in an acute care hospital prepares to work on standing balance with a patient rehabilitating from abdominal surgery. The patient has been on extended bed rest following the surgical procedure and has only been out of bed a few times with the assistance of the nursing staff. The MOST important objective measure to assess after assisting the patient from supine to sitting is:

1. **systolic blood pressure**
2. diastolic blood pressure
3. perceived exertion
4. oxygen saturation rate

> **Correct Answer: 1** (Pierson p. 337)

Orthostatic hypotension results from an inability to compensate quickly for changes in blood pressure. When a person stands up suddenly, gravity tends to cause blood to pool in the veins of the legs and lower body. As a result, the amount of blood returned to the heart is reduced and blood pressure falls. Dizziness or light-headedness is the most common symptom. Normally, the body quickly responds to a decrease in blood pressure, however, compensatory mechanisms may malfunction or function too slowly in patients who have been on extended bed rest.

1. **During bed rest, when the leg muscles are not used regularly, blood pools in the leg veins and is not pumped back to the heart. This results in diminished blood volume which serves to reduce blood pressure. Systolic blood pressure is the maximum arterial pressure during systole or contraction of the left ventricle. It is the most important measure to assess in a patient moving from supine to sitting after prolonged bed rest because of the risk of orthostatic hypotension. A decrease in systolic blood pressure of 20 mm Hg or greater is indicative of orthostatic hypotension.**
2. Diastolic blood pressure refers to the arterial pressure during diastole (between ventricular contractions), therefore, it is not as useful a measure to assess the patient's response to sitting up.
3. Rating of perceived exertion is a subjective measure of how hard the body is working. It is based on the sensations experienced during physical activity including increased heart rate, respiration rate, sweating, and muscle fatigue. It is not a useful measure to assess the patient's response to sitting up.
4. Oxygen saturation measures the percentage of hemoglobin binding sites in the blood bound to oxygen. It is not affected by changing positions.

System Specific: Other Systems
Content Outline: Interventions

Exam One: Question 35

A physical therapist inspects a burn obtained as a result of iontophoresis. The therapist describes the burn as an acidic reaction. If the therapist is correct, the pH of the skin would MOST likely be:

1. **2**
2. 4
3. 6
4. 8

> ### Correct Answer: 1 (Prentice - Therapeutic Modalities p. 175)

Iontophoresis utilizes a continuous direct current which moves ions through the body's tissues. The direct current alters the normal pH of the skin and makes the patient susceptible to a chemical burn. The pH is a measure of the degree to which a solution is acidic or alkaline. Usually a pH of 7.0 indicates neutrality, a pH of less than 7.0 indicates acidity, and a pH of more than 7.0 indicates alkalinity. In this particular case, the acidic or alkaline reaction would be based on the relative change from the skin's normal pH of 3-4. Decreasing current density by increasing the size of the cathode relative to the anode can reduce the risk of a chemical burn.

1. **A pH of 2 would be considered an acidic reaction since it is below the typical pH of the skin.**
2. The normal pH of the skin is 3-4 and therefore a pH of 4 would fall at the upper limit of the normal range.
3. A pH of 6 would be considered an alkaline reaction since it is above the typical pH of the skin.
4. The pH of the skin would not typically reach a level approaching 8. This level exceeds the pH of the blood which is between 7.35-7.45.

System Specific: Integumentary System
Content Outline: Clinical Application of Foundational Sciences

Exam One: Question 36

A physical therapist attempts to palpate the lunate by moving his finger immediately distal to Lister's tubercle. Which wrist motion will allow the therapist to facilitate palpation of the lunate?

1. extension
2. **flexion**
3. radial deviation
4. ulnar deviation

> ### Correct Answer: 2 (Hoppenfeld p. 69)

The lunate is located in the center of the proximal row of carpals between the scaphoid and the triquetrum. The lunate is distinguished by its crescent-like outline and is just proximal to the capitate.

1. Extension and flexion of the wrist can be helpful to identify the lunate and capitate articulation, however, extension in isolation would not facilitate palpation of the lunate.
2. **The lunate is palpable just distal to the radial tubercle. Flexion of the wrist facilitates palpation of the lunate.**
3. Radial deviation would not be helpful to facilitate palpation of the lunate because the carpal bone is a midline structure.
4. Ulnar deviation would not be helpful to facilitate palpation of the lunate. Ulnar deviation can be used to facilitate palpation of the navicular since the motion causes the navicular to slide out from under the radial styloid process.

System Specific: Musculoskeletal System
Content Outline: Clinical Application of Foundational Sciences

Exam One: Question 37

A physician indicates that a patient rehabilitating from a cerebrovascular accident has significant perceptual deficits. Which anatomical region would MOST likely be affected by the stroke?

1. primary motor cortex
2. **somatosensory cortex**
3. basal ganglia
4. cerebellum

Correct Answer: 2 (DeMyer p. 54)

A lesion affecting the somatosensory cortex often results in numerous impairments including loss of sensation, perception, proprioception, and diminished motor control.

1. The primary motor cortex is located in the precentral gyrus within the frontal lobe and contains the largest concentration of corticospinal neurons. This area lies directly in front of the central sulcus and primarily controls contralateral voluntary movements.
2. **The somatosensory cortex occupies the postcentral gyrus which is directly behind the central sulcus. The structure is responsible for complex processing of sensory information and damage can cause severely impaired perception. The somatosensory cortex receives information regarding touch, temperature, pain, and discriminative senses including stereognosis and position sense.**
3. The basal ganglia are a group of nuclei (putamen, caudate nucleus, globus pallidus) that are located at the base of the cerebral cortex. The basal ganglia influences movement and postural control.
4. The cerebellum regulates movement, muscle tone, and postural control. Symptoms of a cerebellar lesion include ataxia, tremor, hypotonia, and asthenia.

System Specific: Neuromuscular & Nervous Systems
Content Outline: Clinical Application of Foundational Sciences

Exam One: Question 38

A physical therapist treats a patient referred to physical therapy with incontinence. The patient describes her difficulty beginning after the birth of her son. After completing an examination the therapist concludes that the patient has extremely weak pelvic floor muscles. When instructing the patient in a pelvic floor muscle strengthening program, the MOST appropriate position to initiate treatment is:

1. sidelying
2. sitting
3. standing
4. **supine**

Correct Answer: 4 (Hall p. 413)

A patient with weak pelvic floor muscles should be instructed in strengthening exercises in a position that minimizes the influence of gravity on the pelvic floor. As the patient's strength improves more challenging positions will be utilized for strengthening.

1. Although sidelying would be an acceptable position, it is more awkward than the supine position for most patients when initiating a pelvic floor muscle strengthening program.
2. Sitting requires the pelvic floor to contract against the resistance of gravity which would be too challenging for the initiation of pelvic floor exercises.
3. Standing requires the pelvic floor to contract against the resistance of gravity which would be too challenging for the initiation of pelvic floor exercises.
4. **Patients with extremely weak pelvic floor muscles should initiate strengthening exercises in a horizontal plane in order to avoid gravity exerting a downward force on the pelvic floor.**

System Specific: Other Systems
Content Outline: Interventions

Exam One: Question 39

A physical therapist prepares to administer the Berg Balance Scale to a patient rehabilitating from a cerebrovascular accident. Which of the following tools is considered a necessary piece of equipment when administering this outcome measure?

1. reflex hammer
2. goniometer
3. **stopwatch**
4. stethoscope

Correct Answer: 3 (Physical Therapist's Clinical Companion p. 105)

The Berg Balance Scale is used for assessing a patient's risk of falling. The Berg consists of 14 tasks of everyday life that are scored according to a 0-4 scale. The maximum total score is 56, with a score of less than 45 indicating the patient is at an increased risk for falls. Observation and scoring should take approximately 15-20 minutes.

1. A reflex hammer may be used when examining a patient who has sustained a cerebrovascular accident, however, it is not a tool utilized for the Berg Balance Scale. A reflex hammer is most commonly used to assess deep tendon reflexes.
2. A goniometer may be used to quantify range of motion in a patient who has sustained a cerebrovascular accident, however, it is not a tool utilized for the Berg Balance Scale.
3. **Necessary equipment to administer the Berg includes a stopwatch, two chairs, a ruler, and a step stool.**
4. A stethoscope is used to assess respiratory rate, breath sounds, heart rate, and Korotkoff's (heart) sounds.

System Specific: Non-Systems
Content Outline: Safety & Professional Roles; Teaching/Learning; Research

Exam One: Question 40

A physical therapist employed in a school setting observes a 10-year-old boy attempt to move from the floor to a standing position. During the activity, the boy has to push on his legs with his hands in order to attain an upright position. This type of finding is MOST commonly associated with:

1. cystic fibrosis
2. Down syndrome
3. **Duchenne muscular dystrophy**
4. spinal muscular atrophy

Correct Answer: 3 (Campbell p. 427)

Duchenne muscular dystrophy is a sex-linked disorder characterized by progressive muscular weakness beginning between the ages of two and five. Life expectancy with Duchenne muscular dystrophy is late teens to early twenties due to respiratory or cardiac failure. The described method of standing upright is termed Gowers' sign.

1. Cystic fibrosis is a progressive autosomal recessive genetic disorder of the exocrine glands. The primary findings include pancreatic insufficiency, excessive pulmonary secretions within the lungs, and excessive electrolyte secretion of the sweat glands. Life expectancy has increased to 35 years of age.
2. Down syndrome (trisomy 21) is a chromosomal disorder that has an increased incidence in children of older parents. A moderate to severe decrease in cognition is typical, however, the mean life expectancy is 50-60 years of age.
3. **Gowers' sign is a descriptive term used to describe a specific method patient's with muscular dystrophy often use to assume an upright position. The disease causes mechanical weakening and cell destruction. Pseudohypertrophy of the calf muscles is often the first observed finding, however, all muscles are eventually affected including respiratory and cardiac muscles.**
4. Spinal muscular atrophy is a progressive autosomal recessive genetic disorder characterized by anterior horn cell degeneration, paralysis, and intact cognition. Spinal muscular atrophy - type 1 has a life expectancy of less than three years while type 2 has a slower progression and type 3 has a normal life expectancy.

System Specific: Other Systems
Content Outline: Foundations for Evaluation, Differential Diagnosis, & Prognosis

Exam One: Question 41

A physical therapist uses repeated contractions to strengthen the quadriceps of a patient that fails to exhibit the desired muscular response throughout a portion of the range of motion. This proprioceptive neuromuscular facilitation technique should be applied:

1. with the extremity placed into a shortened range within the pattern
2. **at the point where the desired muscular response begins to diminish**
3. at the end of the available range of motion
4. with a maximal contraction of the antagonistic muscle group

> **Correct Answer: 2** (Sullivan p. 71)

Repeated contractions should be applied at the point where the contraction begins to diminish. The technique utilizes an isometric contraction followed by subsequent manual stretching and resisted isotonic movement. Repeated contractions assist with enhancing motor neuron recruitment and strengthening of a muscle or group of muscles.

1. Hold-relax active movement is a technique to improve initiation of movement to muscles tested at 1/5 or less. An isometric contraction is performed once the extremity is passively placed into a shortened range within the pattern. Overflow and facilitation may be used to assist with the contraction. Upon relaxation, the extremity is moved into a lengthened position with a quick stretch. The patient then returns the extremity to the shortened position through an isotonic contraction.
2. **Repeated contractions, alternating isometrics, resisted progression, and timing for emphasis are all PNF techniques that are applied with the goal and purpose of increasing strength.**
3. Hold-relax is a technique that applies an isometric contraction at the end of available range to increase range of motion. The contraction is facilitated for all muscle groups at the limiting point in the range. Relaxation occurs and the extremity moves through the newly acquired range to the next point of limitation until there are no further gains in range of motion.
4. Contract-relax is a technique that applies a maximal contraction of the antagonistic muscle group as the extremity reaches the point of limitation. The therapist resists movement for eight to ten seconds with relaxation to follow. The technique is repeated until there are no further gains in range of motion.

System Specific: Neuromuscular & Nervous Systems
Content Outline: Interventions

Exam One: Question 42

A patient rehabilitating from extensive burns to the right upper extremity often complains of severe pain in the arm during physical therapy treatment sessions. The present plan of care emphasizes range of motion, stretching, and positioning. The MOST appropriate action to address the patient's complaint is to:

1. reduce the frequency and duration of the treatment sessions
2. **schedule treatment sessions when the patient's pain medication is most effective**
3. avoid treatment activities that are uncomfortable for the patient
4. request that the referring physician increase the dosage of the patient's pain medication

> **Correct Answer: 2** (Paz p. 277)

Rehabilitation following a burn is extremely painful. Scheduling therapy to coincide with the maximum benefit from pain medication is a high priority. The reduction of pain level will allow for progression with the established plan of care.

1. Reducing the frequency and duration of treatment will not allow for adequate intervention and burn care. Patient participation may decrease as well secondary to pain if they are not treated in coordination with the pain medication schedule.
2. **A patient should receive the optimal benefit of pain medication during their scheduled therapy session. Greater tolerance may allow the patient to make more rapid progress in therapy.**
3. Patients with burns will likely have discomfort with all activities and treatments. Avoiding certain treatments (e.g., stretching) would be negligent.
4. The physician is responsible for prescribing the correct amount of medication. Increasing the dosage of the pain medication may not benefit the patient if physical therapy is not performed at an appropriate time.

System Specific: Integumentary System
Content Outline: Interventions

Exam One: Question 43

A patient in the intensive care unit rehabilitating from a serious infection is connected to a series of lines and tubes. Which lower extremity intravenous infusion site would be the MOST appropriate to administer an intravenous line?

1. median cubital vein
2. basilic vein
3. cephalic vein
4. **saphenous vein**

> **Correct Answer: 4** (Pierson p. 289)

The majority of intravenous insertions are made into superficial veins. Appropriate veins exist in the upper extremity, lower extremity, and scalp.

1. The median cubital vein is the communication between the basilic and cephalic veins in the cubital fossa.
2. The basilic vein is a large and superficial vein of the upper limb that assists with drainage of the hand and forearm.
3. The cephalic vein is located along the anterolateral surface of the biceps and is often visible through the skin.
4. **The saphenous vein is a superficial vein that extends from the foot to the saphenous opening. The vein is the only listed option that is located in the lower extremity.**

System Specific: Cardiac, Vascular, & Pulmonary Systems
Content Outline: Foundations for Evaluation, Differential Diagnosis, & Prognosis

Test Taking Tip: On occasion, examination questions appear to be considerably more difficult than they actually are. In this particular item, candidates do not have to possess specific knowledge related to each of the options, rather they need to recognize that only one of the options is located in the lower extremity. Candidates must be sure they interpret each question correctly and attempt to make the question as simple as possible. Candidates who can do this consistently on the examination often score higher than other candidates with similar academic knowledge.

Exam One: Question 44

A physical therapist reviews a medical chart to determine when a patient was last medicated. The chart indicates the patient received medication at 2300 hours. Assuming it is now 8:00 a.m., how long ago did the patient receive the medication?

1. 5 hours
2. **9 hours**
3. 15 hours
4. 18 hours

> **Correct Answer: 2** (Nosse p. 217)

Military time counts the hours per day from 0100 hours (1 a.m.) through 2400 hours (12 a.m.).

1. Five hours prior to 8 a.m. would be 0300 hours military time or 3 a.m.
2. **Nine hours is the time that has elapsed from 2300 hours (11 p.m.) through 0800 hours (8 a.m.).**
3. Fifteen hours prior to 8 a.m. would be 1700 hours military time or 5 p.m.
4. Eighteen hours prior to 8 a.m. would be 1400 hours military time or 2 p.m.

System Specific: Non-Systems
Content Outline: Safety & Professional Roles; Teaching/Learning; Research

Exam One: Question 45

A physical therapist examines the foot of a 17-year-old female referred to physical therapy with lower leg pain. After placing the foot in subtalar neutral, the therapist determines that the medial border of the foot along the first metatarsal is higher than the lateral border of the foot along the fifth metatarsal. This position would MOST appropriately be documented as:

1. **forefoot varus**
2. forefoot valgus
3. rearfoot varus
4. rearfoot valgus

> **Correct Answer: 1** (Brotzman p. 354)

Malalignment of the foot and ankle can alter the normal biomechanics of gait and distribute abnormal forces to other joints in the kinematic chain. Physical therapists must carefully assess the individual and collective functioning of the rearfoot, midfoot, and forefoot when assessing the foot and ankle.

1. **Forefoot varus refers to an inverted position of the forefoot in relationship to the rearfoot with the subtalar joint in a neutral position. Patients with low arches in weight bearing often exhibit forefoot varus with the subtalar joint in a neutral position.**
2. Forefoot valgus refers to an everted position of the forefoot in relation to the rearfoot with the subtalar joint in a neutral position. Forefoot valgus is often associated with high arches or cavus feet.
3. Rearfoot varus refers to the calcaneus assuming a position of inversion (calcaneus varus) with the subtalar joint in a neutral position. Three to four degrees of inversion is considered to be within normal limits.
4. Rearfoot valgus refers to the calcaneus assuming a position of eversion (calcaneus valgus) with the subtalar joint in a neutral position. Rearfoot valgus is often a result of compensation for forefoot varus.

System Specific: Musculoskeletal System
Content Outline: Examination

Exam One: Question 46

A physical therapist reviews the medical record of a patient recently admitted to an inpatient rehabilitation hospital. The patient sustained a traumatic head injury in a motor vehicle accident five weeks ago. The medical record indicates that the patient is often disoriented and can frequently become agitated with little provocation. The MOST appropriate location for the therapist to make initial contact with the patient is:

1. **in the patient's room**
2. in the physical therapy gym
3. in a private treatment room
4. in the physical therapy waiting room

> **Correct Answer: 1** (Umphred p. 550)

A patient with a head injury that is confused and can become agitated is likely functioning at level IV on the Rancho Los Amigos Scale.

1. **The patient's room is the most appropriate first meeting place since the patient will be familiar with the surroundings and may therefore be less distractible. The patient may tend to become agitated in the gym due to overstimulation from other patients and the overall level of activity.**
2. The physical therapy gym is a good option for the treatment of the general population, but becomes more difficult following brain injury due to the patient's decreased attention, lack of focus, and potential agitation.
3. A private treatment room may be too isolated if assistance is needed. Since the patient has a poor attention span, it will be helpful to use familiar surroundings, pictures, and personal effects.
4. The physical therapy waiting room is not an appropriate place to treat a patient. This patient would likely have a difficult time adjusting to the various distractions in the waiting room.

System Specific: Neuromuscular & Nervous Systems
Content Outline: Interventions

Exam One: Question 47

A physical therapist instructs a patient positioned in supine to bring her left leg toward her chest and maintain the position using her left arm. Assuming the therapist observes the reaction shown in the picture, what muscle would MOST likely have insufficient length?

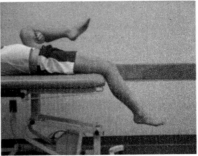

1. iliopsoas
2. quadratus lumborum
3. **rectus femoris**
4. sartorius

Correct Answer: 3 (Magee p. 692)

The left hip and knee are flexed to the chest to flatten the lumbar spine and stabilize the pelvis. A hip flexion contracture would be denoted by the right leg rising off the table. The length of the rectus femoris can be assessed by examining the relative position of the knee (i.e., amount of knee flexion).

1. The iliopsoas acts to flex the hip. Tightness in the muscle could be identified using the Thomas test, however, the patient's right leg remains on the table which would be an indication of sufficient length in the one-joint hip flexors.
2. The quadratus lumborum originates on the iliolumbar ligament and the iliac crest. The muscle inserts on the inferior border of the last rib and the transverse processes of the upper four lumbar vertebrae. As a result, the muscle does not act on the hip.
3. **Extension of the right knee is an indication that the patient has tightness in the two-joint rectus femoris muscle. A patient without tightness in the rectus femoris would typically present with the knee in 90 degrees of flexion while maintaining the position.**
4. The sartorius is a two-joint muscle that crosses both the hip and knee. The muscle acts to flex, laterally rotate, and abduct the hip joint. The Thomas test is not specific enough to address tightness in the sartorius due to the diversity of the muscle's action. To specifically identify sartorius tightness the physical therapist would need to identify hip flexion, lateral rotation, and abduction of the hip during the Thomas Test.

System Specific: Musculoskeletal System
Content Outline: Examination

Exam One: Question 48

A physical therapist employed in a rehabilitation hospital treats a patient status post traumatic brain injury. During the treatment session the therapist notices that the patient's toes are discolored below a bivalved lower extremity cast. The cast was applied approximately five hours ago in an attempt to reduce a plantar flexion contracture. The MOST appropriate therapist action is to:

1. discontinue use of the anterior portion of the cast
2. contact the staff nurse and request that the cast is removed
3. refer the patient to an orthotist
4. **remove the cast**

Correct Answer: 4 (O'Sullivan p. 920)

Discoloration of the patient's toes is an indication that the cast may be too tight and is impeding the patient's circulation. This would serve as a red flag to remove the cast for further inspection. The bivalved cast design allows for easy removal.

1. A bivalved cast consists of anterior and posterior portions secured with Velcro straps for total contact. Both portions are necessary to provide proper positioning and therapeutic stretch.
2. The therapist would not need to request a staff nurse to remove the cast. The therapist would remove the bivalved cast in order to further assess skin integrity and circulation.
3. Referral to an orthotist occurs when there is a need for an orthotic device. If the orthotist applied the serial cast, the therapist would still immediately remove the cast due to the discoloration of the foot. The therapist would then call the orthotist with an update on the patient's status.
4. **A therapist is qualified to monitor a patient's lower extremity circulation when using a cast and if necessary is capable of removing a bivalved cast.**

System Specific: Non-Systems
Content Outline: Equipment & Devices; Therapeutic Modalities

Exam One: Question 49

A physical therapist attempts to obtain information on the ability of noncontractile tissue to allow motion at a specific joint. Which selective tissue tension assessment would provide the therapist with the MOST valuable information?

1. active range of motion
2. active-assistive range of motion
3. **passive range of motion**
4. resisted isometrics

> **Correct Answer: 3** (Norkin p. 7)

Passive range of motion provides the physical therapist with information regarding the integrity of noncontractile tissues.

1. Active range of motion requires active contraction of muscles, which are composed of contractile tissue. Performing active range of motion will not allow an assessment of the noncontractile elements of a joint.
2. Active-assistive range of motion requires active contraction of muscles, which are composed of contractile tissue. While the therapist is assisting the patient in the movement, it is impossible to assess only the noncontractile elements of the joint since the musculature is actively contracting.
3. **Passive range of motion provides the therapist with information on the integrity of the articular surfaces and the extensibility of the joint capsule and associated ligaments. Passive range of motion is independent of a patient's strength.**
4. Resisted isometrics requires active contraction of the surrounding musculature. As a result, there is no ability to assess the noncontractile tissues of the joint.

System Specific: Musculoskeletal System
Content Outline: Examination

Exam One: Question 50

A physical therapist attempts to transfer a dependent patient from a wheelchair to a bed. The therapist is concerned about the size of the patient, but is unable to secure another staff member to assist with the transfer. Which type of transfer would allow the therapist to move the patient with the GREATEST ease?

1. dependent standing pivot
2. **hydraulic lift**
3. sliding board
4. assisted standing pivot

> **Correct Answer: 2** (Pierson p. 201)

The hydraulic lift can be used as a safe and efficient method to transfer large and/or dependent patients with little physical exertion. The transfer can be performed by one therapist under most circumstances.

1. A dependent standing pivot transfer would not be appropriate for a therapist that is concerned about the patient's size. This transfer requires the therapist to perform 100% of the activity.
2. **The hydraulic lift transfer allows the therapist to transfer the patient independently from the wheelchair to the bed without jeopardizing patient or staff safety.**
3. A sliding board transfer requires the patient to possess adequate sitting balance and actively participate in the transfer. This type of transfer would not be appropriate for a dependent patient.
4. An assisted standing pivot transfer requires the patient to stand and participate in the transfer.

System Specific: Non-Systems
Content Outline: Equipment & Devices; Therapeutic Modalities

Exam One: Question 51

A physically active 19-year-old male receives pre-operative instruction prior to anterior cruciate ligament reconstruction. The patient's past medical history includes a medial meniscectomy of the contralateral knee eight months ago. The MOST likely functional level of the patient following rehabilitation is:

1. able to participate in light recreational activities
2. able to participate in all recreational activities
3. able to return to recreational and competitive athletic activities with a derotation brace
4. **able to return to previous functional level**

> **Correct Answer: 4** (Kisner p. 734)

Anterior cruciate ligament (ACL) reconstruction refers to the use of a graft to replace a damaged anterior cruciate ligament. The graft is placed through drilled holes in the femoral and tibial tunnels and then anchored with a fixation device.

1. The patient's anticipated functional level following anterior cruciate ligament reconstruction would allow the patient to participate in activities that are higher level than "light recreational activities."
2. "Recreational activities" would not typically include vigorous activities such as competitive sports. The patient should be able to return to his previous functional level which likely includes a combination of recreational activities and more physically challenging pursuits.
3. Derotation bracing can be an effective method to limit instability in patients with an anterior cruciate ligament deficient knee, however, research associated with the use of derotation bracing following anterior cruciate ligament reconstruction has shown little evidence to support enhanced knee function or reduced reinjury rates.
4. **A physically active, young patient should return to his previous functional level within 4-6 months following anterior cruciate ligament reconstruction.**

System Specific: Musculoskeletal System
Content Outline: Foundations for Evaluation, Differential Diagnosis, & Prognosis

Exam One: Question 52

A patient rehabilitating from an upper extremity injury uses a latissimus pull-down machine. The therapist specifically instructs the patient to pull the bar down behind her head. This action emphasizes strengthening of the:

1. **rhomboids and middle trapezius**
2. biceps brachii and pectoralis major
3. teres minor and middle trapezius
4. pectoralis major and rhomboids

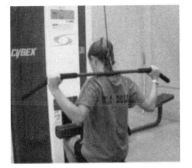

> **Correct Answer: 1** (Kendall p. 326)

Knowledge of functional anatomy allows physical therapists to analyze various resistive exercises and identify the primary muscles involved.

1. **The rhomboids and middle trapezius both function as strong adductors of the scapula. Adduction of the scapula (retraction) is required in order to complete the latissimus pull-down exercise with the bar positioned behind the patient's head. Physical therapists should use caution when using this exercise since without proper instruction, patients may have a tendency to significantly flex their neck.**
2. The biceps brachii acts to flex the elbow joint, supinate the forearm, and assists with shoulder flexion. The pectoralis major acts to adduct and medially rotate the humerus. The muscles primary actions are not consistent with the exercise.
3. The teres minor acts to laterally rotate the shoulder joint and stabilize the head of the humerus in the glenoid cavity. The middle trapezius acts to adduct the scapula. The teres minor would not be emphasized in the exercise.
4. The pectoralis major acts to adduct and medially rotate the humerus. The rhomboids act to adduct and elevate the scapula. The pectoralis major would not be emphasized in the exercise.

System Specific: Musculoskeletal System
Content Outline: Interventions

Exam One: Question 53

A physical therapist adjusts the on:off time on an electrical stimulation unit prior to beginning treatment. When using the unit for muscle re-education the MOST appropriate on:off ratio is:

1. 5:1
2. 15:1
3. **1:5**
4. 1:15

Correct Answer: 3 (Prentice - Therapeutic Modalities p. 131)

The on:off ratio should be determined based on the established therapeutic objectives. The on:off ratio for muscle strengthening is most often expressed as 1:5 while a ratio of 1:1 may be more appropriate for a therapeutic objective such as relieving muscle spasm.

1. On time should be less than off time in order to prevent muscle fatigue. The ratio is expressed in the same order that the words appear in the ratio statement "on:off" and therefore a ratio of 5:1 would result in five times greater on time than off time.
2. A ratio of 15:1 would result in severe muscle fatigue due not only to the excessive period of on time, but also to the inadequate period of off time.
3. **The initial on:off ratio should be 1:5 in order to minimize muscle fatigue. As the patient gets stronger, the on:off ratio may be altered to 1:4 or 1:3.**
4. A ratio of 1:15 would provide excessive periods of rest following each contraction and would result in extremely long treatment sessions.

System Specific: Non-Systems
Content Outline: Equipment & Devices; Therapeutic Modalities

Exam One: Question 54

A physical therapist is scheduled to administer a whirlpool treatment to a patient that is HIV positive. The therapist is concerned about her ability to complete the treatment since she sustained a small paper cut on her fourth digit approximately three hours ago. The MOST appropriate therapist action is:

1. refuse to treat the patient and document the rationale in the medical record
2. **treat the patient using appropriate medical asepsis**
3. ask the patient to reschedule their appointment
4. select another appropriate treatment procedure

Correct Answer: 2 (Pierson p. 30)

Standard precautions are designed for the care of all patients in hospitals regardless of the medical diagnosis. Health care professionals that follow established standard precautions do not place themselves or the patient at any significant risk for being contaminated or infected by pathogenic microorganisms.

1. A physical therapist cannot refuse to treat patients based on the presence of HIV or any other potentially infectious condition.
2. **A physical therapist should treat a patient that is HIV positive using established medical asepsis techniques to prevent the possible transmission of blood or body fluids.**
3. The physical therapist has an obligation to treat the patient despite their HIV status. Rescheduling the patient without adequate cause would be a violation of the patient's right to receive necessary health care services.
4. The question does not provide any evidence that the current treatment procedure is inappropriate for the patient. As a result, it would be unnecessary to select another treatment procedure.

System Specific: Integumentary System
Content Outline: Interventions

Exam One: Question 55

A physical therapist examines a patient referred to physical therapy diagnosed with anterior compartment syndrome. The patient presents with an inability to dorsiflex the foot and a mild sensory disturbance between the first and second toes. The nerve MOST likely involved is the:

1. **deep peroneal nerve**
2. medial plantar nerve
3. tibial nerve
4. lateral plantar nerve

Correct Answer: 1 (Magee p. 900)

Anterior compartment syndrome often affects the deep peroneal nerve as it passes under the extensor retinaculum. The result of nerve compression ranges from a mild sensory disturbance to an inability to dorsiflex the foot.

1. **The deep peroneal nerve innervates the tibialis anterior, extensor hallucis longus and brevis, lumbricales, interossei, extensor digitorum brevis, and peroneus tertius muscles.**
2. The medial plantar nerve is the larger of the two branches of the tibial nerve. The nerve supplies cutaneous branches to the medial three and a half digits, and motor branches to the abductor hallucis, flexor digitorum brevis, flexor hallucis brevis, and the most medial lumbrical muscles.
3. The tibial nerve innervates the tibialis posterior, abductor and adductor hallucis, flexor hallucis longus and brevis, flexor digitorum longus and brevis, quadratus plantae, soleus, gastrocnemius, plantaris, and popliteus muscles.
4. The lateral plantar nerve is the smaller of the two branches of the tibial nerve. The nerve supplies cutaneous branches to the lateral one and a half toes and motor branches to muscles of the sole of the foot that are not supplied by the medial plantar nerve.

System Specific: Neuromuscular & Nervous Systems
Content Outline: Clinical Application of Foundational Sciences

Exam One: Question 56

A 35-year-old female is admitted to the hospital following a recent illness. Laboratory testing reveals a markedly high platelet count. This finding is typical with:

1. emphysema
2. metabolic acidosis
3. renal failure
4. **malignancy**

Correct Answer: 4 (Goodman - Differential Diagnosis p. 558)

Thrombocytosis refers to an increased number of blood platelets. This condition is usually temporary and can occur as a compensatory measure after severe hemorrhage, surgery, iron deficiency, and as a manifestation of certain cancers.

1. Emphysema is defined as an abnormal permanent enlargement of air spaces distal to the terminal bronchioles. Blood values will include an increase in red blood cells to carry the oxygen and abnormal carbon dioxide and carbon monoxide. Pulmonary function tests will show an increase in total lung capacity, functional residual capacity, and residual volume. The vital capacity is decreased.
2. Metabolic acidosis is an acid-base disorder defined as an accumulation of acids or a deficit of bases within the blood. Causes may include renal failure, starvation, diabetic or alcoholic ketoacidosis. Blood values will show a decrease in serum pH due to a decrease in HCO_3 or an increase in H+ ions. An arterial pH < 7.35 in the absence of an elevated $PaCO_2$ is considered metabolic acidosis.
3. Renal failure is defined as an abrupt or rapid decline in renal filtration and function. There are three categories: prerenal, intrinsic, and post renal failure. Typical causes include hypovolemia, congestive heart failure, dehydration, sepsis, and autoimmune diseases. Blood values include hypocalcemia, hyperkalemia, elevated blood urea nitrogen, creatinine, magnesium, and uric acid.
4. **Malignancy is defined as cells that have the ability to spread, invade, and destroy tissue. A tumor that is malignant may or may not respond to treatment or may return after removal. Blood values vary based on type, degree, and location of the malignancy, however, are often increased as a manifestation of an occult neoplasm such as lung cancer.**

System Specific: Other Systems
Content Outline: Foundations for Evaluation, Differential Diagnosis, & Prognosis

Exam One: Question 57

A physical therapist interviews a patient referred to physical therapy with a diagnosis of chronic bronchitis. What finding obtained during the patient interview is MOST closely associated with the patient's medical diagnosis?

1. **patient is a smoker**
2. patient has a sedentary lifestyle
3. patient has numerous allergies
4. patient has severe scoliosis

Correct Answer: 1 (Hillegass p. 274)

Smoking is a large risk factor for the development of chronic bronchitis. Over time, smokers will experience decreased alveolar ventilation and potentially hypoxia and acidosis. Persistent cough and sputum production create a cycle of impaired perfusion, oxygenation, and recurrent infection. Untreated, hypoxia can lead to cor pulmonale.

1. **Cigarette smoke irritates the bronchial lining and causes hypersecretion and hypertrophy of mucus producing cells of the larger bronchi. The excess secretion of mucus begins to obstruct the airways causing wheezing and coughing. The cilia begin to decrease in function and infection results from reduced clearance.**
2. A sedentary life style is a risk factor for cardiovascular disease. Regular, moderate physical activity helps prevent heart and blood vessel disease. Physical activity can assist in controlling cholesterol, diabetes, obesity, and blood pressure.
3. Allergies can enhance the effects of chronic bronchitis, but are not normally a causative factor in the development of the condition.
4. Scoliosis is classified as a restrictive lung disorder with more severe curves (>60) that produce reduced lung capacity and overall pulmonary insufficiency. Scoliosis, however, is not closely associated with the diagnosis of chronic bronchitis.

System Specific: Cardiac, Vascular, & Pulmonary Systems
Content Outline: Foundations for Evaluation, Differential Diagnosis, & Prognosis

Exam One: Question 58

A physical therapist reviews the medical record of a 46-year-old female diagnosed with myasthenia gravis. A recent physician entry indicates that the patient is currently taking immunosuppressive medication. Which laboratory test should be the MOST frequently monitored based on the patient's medication?

1. hematocrit
2. hemoglobin
3. platelet count
4. **white blood cell count**

Correct Answer: 4 (Ciccone p. 593)

Immunosuppressive medications are commonly used to prevent the rejection of organ transplant or to treat specific diseases caused by an autoimmune response. The medications lower a patient's resistance to infection.

1. Hematocrit measures the percentage of red blood cells in a volume of blood. Hematocrit may be decreased with anemia, nutritional deficiency, and leukemia. Hematocrit may be increased with dehydration, polycythemia, and burns.
2. Hemoglobin is the iron containing pigment in red blood cells that functions to carry oxygen in the blood. Low hemoglobin may indicate anemia or blood loss; elevated hemoglobin suggests polycythemia or dehydration.
3. Platelet count identifies the number of platelets present in whole blood. Platelets are small blood cells that are necessary for clotting. If the platelet level is high, it indicates increased risk of thrombosis and if the level is low, it indicates increased risk of bruising and bleeding.
4. **The majority of immunosuppressive medications act non-selectively and as a result the immune system is less able to resist infections and the spread of malignant cells. Leukopenia refers to a reduction in the number of leukocytes in the blood. The white blood cell count provides valuable information related to the degree of immunosuppression. It is essential for physical therapists to be aware of the patient's most recent white blood cell count prior to initiating treatment.**

System Specific: Other Systems
Content Outline: Foundations for Evaluation, Differential Diagnosis, & Prognosis

Exam One: Question 59

A physical therapist makes a conscious effort to demonstrate particular kinds of behavior that are significant and attainable for an eight-year-old patient. This type of behavior therapy is termed:

1. flooding
2. operant conditioning
3. role playing
4. **modeling**

> **Correct Answer: 4** (Wallace p. 364)

Physical therapists often employ a number of strategies to influence patient behavior or to promote learning. Knowledge of a wide variety of techniques and their relative utility can assist therapists to achieve better outcomes with their patients.

1. Flooding is a technique to help patients heal their traumatic memories. The goal is to expose patients to their traumatic memories with the goal of reintegrating their repressed emotions with their current awareness. Flooding is commonly used to treat people to handle specific phobias.
2. Operant conditioning is a process where learning occurs when an individual engages in specific behaviors in order to receive certain consequences. Examples of specific operant conditioning techniques include positive reinforcement, negative reinforcement, extinction, and punishment.
3. Role playing requires participants to take the place of someone else by acting the part of that person in a particular situation. The rationale associated with the technique is that people can learn more from acting out a particular situation than from purely discussing it.
4. **Modeling refers to the process of learning by watching others. Learning often occurs through observation alone without any specific verbal direction from the therapist.**

System Specific: Non-Systems
Content Outline: Safety & Professional Roles; Teaching/Learning; Research

Exam One: Question 60

A patient rehabilitating from knee surgery exhibits significant weakness in the involved extremity. During the most recent therapy session the patient was able to complete an independent straight leg raise as shown. What muscle is emphasized in the exercise?

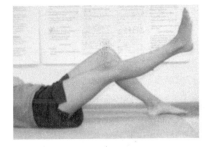

1. vastus medialis
2. **rectus femoris**
3. vastus lateralis
4. sartorius

> **Correct Answer: 2** (Kisner p. 745)

A straight leg raise is a commonly utilized lower extremity resistive exercise. The exercise requires dynamic hip flexion and an isometric contraction of the quadriceps. The resistance of gravity decreases gradually as the lower extremity is elevated.

1. A straight leg raise requires activation of muscles that cross both the hip and knee joints. The vastus medialis acts to extend the knee, but does not act on the hip. The muscle is innervated by the femoral nerve.
2. **The rectus femoris is the prime mover during a straight leg raise exercise. The muscle is a component of the quadriceps femoris muscle group and is innervated by the femoral nerve. The muscle is able to act on the hip as well as the knee due to the muscle originating on the anteroinferior iliac spine and the groove above the rim of the acetabulum.**
3. A straight leg raise requires activation of muscles that cross both the hip and knee joints. The vastus lateralis acts to extend the knee, but does not act on the hip. The muscle is innervated by the femoral nerve.
4. The sartorius is a two-joint muscle that crosses both the hip and knee. The muscle acts to flex, laterally rotate, and abduct the hip joint and is innervated by the femoral nerve. The muscle would likely be active during a straight leg raise, but would not be the prime mover.

System Specific: Musculoskeletal System
Content Outline: Interventions

Exam One: Question 61

A physical therapist reviews a laboratory report for a patient recently admitted to the hospital. The patient sustained burns over 25 percent of her body in a fire. Assuming the patient exhibits hypovolemia, which of the following laboratory values would be the MOST significantly affected?

1. **hematocrit**
2. erythrocyte sedimentation rate
3. oxygen saturation rate
4. prothrombin time

Correct Answer: 1 (Paz p. 266)

Hypovolemia refers to a state of decreased blood volume, most often related to a decrease in blood plasma. The reduction of blood volume often occurs following a burn due to the shift in fluid to the interstitium, which reduces plasma and intravascular fluid volume. This results in a variety of hemodynamic and circulatory changes, however, hematocrit would likely be the laboratory value most affected.

1. **Hematocrit is the volume percentage of red blood cells in whole blood. The hematocrit rises immediately after a severe burn and gradually decreases with fluid replacement.**
2. Erythrocyte sedimentation rate is a non-specific test for inflammatory disorders often associated with conditions such as cancer, autoimmune diseases, and infection. The test is based on how quickly red blood cells sink to the bottom of a test solution containing anticoagulated blood.
3. Oxygen saturation indicates the saturation of hemoglobin with oxygen. Normal oxygen saturation is 95-98 percent. Oxygen saturation is not related to total blood volume.
4. Prothrombin time is most commonly used to monitor oral anticoagulant therapy or to screen for selected bleeding disorders.

System Specific: Other Systems
Content Outline: Foundations for Evaluation, Differential Diagnosis, & Prognosis

Exam One: Question 62

A physical therapist performs autolytic debridement in an attempt to remove nonviable tissue from a stage IV pressure ulcer. Autolytic debridement removes necrotic tissue by using:

1. a sharp instrument
2. an externally applied force
3. **the body's own mechanisms**
4. a commercially prepared enzyme

Correct Answer: 3 (Sussman p. 204)

Autolytic debridement is typically performed using a moisture-retentive dressing. The dressing maintains a moist wound environment which promotes rehydration of viable tissue and allows the body's enzymes to digest necrotic tissue.

1. Sharp debridement requires the use of scalpel, scissors, and/or forceps to selectively remove nonviable tissue, foreign material or debris from a wound.
2. Wound irrigation removes nonviable tissue from the wound bed using pressurized fluid which serves as an externally applied force. Pulsatile lavage is an example of a specific wound irrigation technique.
3. **Autolytic debridement refers to using the body's own mechanisms to remove nonviable tissue. Common methods of autolytic debridement include transparent films, hydrocolloids, hydrogels, and alginates.**
4. Enzymatic debridement requires the application of a commercially prepared enzyme to the surface of nonviable tissue. The applied enzyme attempts to degrade the nonviable tissue through gradual digestion.

System Specific: Integumentary System
Content Outline: Interventions

Exam One: Question 63

A physical therapist is responsible for supervising a physical therapist assistant at an off site location. Which of the following would not necessitate a supervisory visit by the physical therapist?

1. a change in the patient's medical status
2. a modification in the patient's plan of care
3. a request by the physical therapist assistant
4. **an alteration in the patient's level of motivation**

> **Correct Answer: 4** (Guide to Physical Therapist Practice)

When a physical therapist delegates patient care responsibilities to physical therapist assistants or other supportive personnel, the physical therapist remains responsible for overseeing the physical therapy program.

1. A change in the patient's medical status requires reassessment and possibly a change in the established plan of care.
2. A physical therapist is solely responsible for modifying an established plan of care. A physical therapist assistant may be able to modify a parameter of an existing intervention within an established plan of care (i.e., changing the weight of a progressive resistive exercise).
3. The physical therapist is required to provide patient-related consultation at the request of another practitioner.
4. **Physical therapist assistants often deal with changes in patients' level of motivation. This observation in isolation would not warrant a supervisory visit by the physical therapist.**

System Specific: Non-Systems
Content Outline: Safety & Professional Roles; Teaching/Learning; Research

Exam One: Question 64

A physician instructs a 26-year-old male to utilize a knee derotation brace for all athletic activities. Which condition would MOST warrant the use of the derotation brace?

1. medial meniscus repair
2. anterior cruciate ligament reconstruction
3. **anterior cruciate ligament insufficiency**
4. posterior cruciate ligament reconstruction

> **Correct Answer: 3** (Kisner p. 723)

Derotation braces are most effective in patients with ligamentous instability, usually involving the anterior and posterior cruciate ligaments. The literature is inconclusive on the efficacy of functional bracing following reconstruction.

1. A patient with a medial meniscus repair would not tend to experience functional instability unless there were other structures involved such as the anterior cruciate ligament. Meniscal repairs are most often performed when the lesion is in the vascular outer third of the medial or lateral meniscus.
2. Anterior cruciate ligament reconstruction is typically performed due to disabling instability or frequent episodes of the knee giving way. The purpose of the surgical procedure is to reduce functional instability. Full return to vigorous activities following ACL reconstruction often takes four to six months.
3. **A patient with anterior cruciate ligament insufficiency would be far more likely to experience functional instability than a patient who had anterior cruciate ligament reconstruction. As a result, the patient with the insufficiency would be a better candidate for the derotation brace.**
4. Posterior cruciate ligament reconstruction is considerably less common than anterior cruciate ligament reconstruction. The purpose of the surgical procedure is to reduce functional instability. Full return to vigorous activities following PCL reconstruction often takes nine months to one year.

System Specific: Musculoskeletal System
Content Outline: Foundations for Evaluation, Differential Diagnosis, & Prognosis

Exam One: Question 65

A physical therapist obtains a gross measurement of hamstrings length by passively extending the lower extremity of a patient in short sitting. The MOST common substitution to exaggerate hamstrings length is:

1. weight shift to the contralateral side
2. anterior rotation of the pelvis
3. **posterior rotation of the pelvis**
4. hiking of the contralateral hip

Correct Answer: 3 (Magee p. 643)

The hamstrings muscles consist of the semitendinosus, semimembranosus, and biceps femoris. The semitendinosus and semimembranosus are considered the medial hamstrings since they insert on the medial surface of the tibia. The biceps femoris is considered the lateral hamstrings since the muscle inserts on the lateral surface of the tibia and the lateral surface of the head of the fibula.

1. Weight shifting to the contralateral side in short sitting without other compensatory movement would have minimal impact on measured hamstrings length.
2. Anterior rotation of the pelvis would tend to make the apparent hamstrings length shorter than the actual length due to the hamstrings origin on the tuberosity of the ischium.
3. **Posterior rotation of the pelvis would tend to make the apparent hamstrings length longer than the actual length due to the hamstrings origin on the tuberosity of the ischium. Patients often attempt to posteriorly rotate the pelvis in short sitting by leaning backwards.**
4. Hip hiking of the contralateral limb may cause the patient to weight shift toward the involved side. This adaptation would have minimal impact on measured hamstrings length.

System Specific: Musculoskeletal System
Content Outline: Examination

Exam One: Question 66

A physical therapist conducts an upper quarter screening examination on a patient diagnosed with rotator cuff tendonitis. With the patient in sitting, the MOST appropriate action to facilitate palpation of the rotator cuff is:

1. passive abduction of the humerus
2. active medial and lateral rotation of the humerus
3. **passive extension of the humerus**
4. active extension and flexion of the elbow

Correct Answer: 3 (Hoppenfeld p. 13)

The rotator cuff is composed of the supraspinatus, infraspinatus, teres minor, and subscapularis. The rotator cuff muscles are important in shoulder movement and in maintaining glenohumeral joint stability. Tenderness elicited during palpation may be due to localized inflammation, a tear or detachment of a tendon.

1. Passive abduction of the humerus would tend to keep the rotator cuff obscured beneath the acromion which would make palpation extremely difficult.
2. The therapist should make sure that the area being palpated is as relaxed as possible. As a result, active movement would be less desirable than passive movement.
3. **The rotator cuff lies directly beneath the acromion and therefore must be rotated out from underneath the acromion before it can be palpated. Passive extension of the humerus makes it possible for a therapist to palpate a portion of the rotator cuff although the individual muscles cannot be easily distinguished from each other.**
4. The rotator cuff acts on the shoulder and not the elbow. As a result, elbow flexion and extension would not influence palpation of the rotator cuff.

System Specific: Musculoskeletal System
Content Outline: Examination

Exam One: Question 67

A physical therapist prepares to formally assess the balance of a patient with a neurological disorder. The MOST appropriate method to assess the vestibular component of balance would be:

1. assess cutaneous sensation
2. **apply a perturbation to alter the body's center of gravity**
3. examine proprioception in a weight bearing posture
4. quantify visual acuity and depth perception

Correct Answer: 2 (Goodman - Pathology p. 1566)

Balance requires complex integration of the vestibular, visual, and somatosensory systems. Each system is responsive to specific stimuli and therefore can be assessed individually or collectively.

1. Cutaneous sensation is commonly assessed as part of a neurological examination, however, would not be directly associated with the vestibular system. Cutaneous sensory receptors include free nerve endings, Ruffini endings, hair follicle endings, and Meissner's corpuscles.
2. **The vestibular system reports information to the brain regarding the position and movement of the head with respect to gravity and movement. Assessment of the vestibular system often includes perturbations that require the body to make automatic adjustments that restore normal alignment.**
3. The somatosensory system provides information about the relative orientation and movement of the body in relation to the support surface. Examining proprioception in a weight bearing posture would be a common method used for assessment of the somatosensory system.
4. The visual system allows individuals to perceive movement and detect the relative orientation of the body in space. Visual receptors allow for perceptual acuity regarding verticality, motion of objects and self, environmental orientation, postural sway, and movements of the head and neck. Visual acuity and depth perception contribute to the feedback gathered by the visual system.

System Specific: Neuromuscular & Nervous Systems
Content Outline: Examination

Exam One: Question 68

A physical therapist inspects the skin of a child recently admitted to the hospital after sustaining a scald burn from hot water on his torso. The burn is moist and red with several areas of blister formation. The burn covers an area approximately four inches by three inches and blanches with direct pressure. The MOST likely burn classification is:

1. superficial
2. **superficial partial-thickness**
3. deep partial-thickness
4. full-thickness

Correct Answer: 2 (Goodman - Pathology p. 436)

The extent and severity of a burn is dependent on a variety of factors including age, duration of burn, type of burn, and affected area. Burns are most appropriately classified according to the depth of tissue destruction.

1. A superficial burn involves only the outer epidermis. The involved area may be red with slight edema. Healing occurs without evidence of scarring.
2. **A superficial partial-thickness burn involves the epidermis and the upper portion of the dermis. The involved area may be extremely painful and exhibit blisters. Healing occurs with minimal to no scarring in approximately two weeks. A superficial partial-thickness burn is relatively common since many scalding water burns and intense sunburns fall into this category. The primary difference in appearance between superficial and superficial partial-thickness burns is the presence of blistering. This category of burn is the most painful since all nerve endings remain intact.**
3. A deep partial-thickness burn involves complete destruction of the epidermis and the majority of the dermis. The involved area may appear discolored with broken blisters and edema. Damage to nerve endings may result in only moderate levels of pain. Healing occurs with hypertrophic scars and keloids.
4. A full-thickness burn involves complete destruction of the epidermis and dermis along with partial damage of the subcutaneous fat layer. The involved area often presents with eschar formation and minimal pain. Patients with full-thickness burns require grafts and may be susceptible to infection.

System Specific: Integumentary System
Content Outline: Foundations for Evaluation, Differential Diagnosis, & Prognosis

Exam One: Question 69

A physical therapist prepares to examine a patient's triceps using a reflex hammer. The MOST appropriate positioning of the patient's arm during the testing procedure is:

1. **shoulder extension and elbow flexion**
2. shoulder flexion and elbow extension
3. shoulder extension and elbow extension
4. shoulder flexion and elbow flexion

Correct Answer: 1 (Bickley p. 698)

Deep tendon reflexes are performed to test the integrity of the spinal reflex. A physical therapist should assess a deep tendon reflex by placing the tendon on slight stretch. A reflex hammer is used to sharply tap over the tendon. Reflexes can be graded as normal, exaggerated (hyper) or depressed (hypo) or can be graded on a scale of 0-4.

1. **Shoulder extension and elbow flexion would be the most appropriate position to test the triceps reflex. The reflex is best elicited with the patient in sitting or standing with the arm supported by the physical therapist. The therapist strikes the triceps tendon with a reflex hammer where it crosses the olecranon fossa. Stimulation of the triceps reflex elicits involuntary contraction of the triceps. An acceptable alternate position to test the triceps reflex would be shoulder abduction and elbow flexion.**
2. Shoulder flexion and elbow extension would not place the triceps tendon on adequate stretch to elicit the triceps reflex.
3. Shoulder extension and elbow extension would result in an ineffective position to elicit the triceps reflex since the triceps is already in a maximally shortened position.
4. Shoulder flexion and elbow flexion place the triceps on total stretch secondary to the origin and insertion of the triceps muscle. A deep tendon reflex should be tested with the tendon on slight stretch.

System Specific: Neuromuscular & Nervous Systems
Content Outline: Examination

Exam One: Question 70

If the forced expiratory volume in one second (FEV_1) test is negative for airway obstruction in 99% of individuals without lung disease, then the measurement of FEV_1 is:

1. sensitive
2. **specific**
3. reliable
4. valid

Correct Answer: 2 (Portney p. 620)

The validity of a diagnostic test, such as the FEV_1 test, is evaluated by its accuracy in assessing the presence or absence of a target condition such as airway obstruction. A test is considered to be specific when the test is negative in persons who do not have the disease. A highly specific test will rarely be positive when a person does not have the disease.

1. Sensitivity is the probability of obtaining a positive test among individuals who have the disease. In this example, neither condition was met: the test result was negative for airway obstruction and the individuals tested did not have lung disease.
2. **Specificity is the probability of obtaining a negative test among individuals without the disease (who should test negative). Because 99 of 100 individuals without lung disease had a negative FEV_1 test for airway obstruction, the test is highly specific.**
3. Reliability refers to the extent to which a test or measurement is consistent or yields the same result on repeated trials. In this example, there is no indication that the FEV_1 was administered more than once, therefore no estimate of reliability is possible.
4. Validity refers to the degree to which a test or measurement accurately reflects or assesses the specific concept the clinician is attempting to measure. Validity is concerned with the success at measuring what was set out to be measured. In this example, the data does not provide useful information for assessing the extent to which FEV_1 is a valid way to identify airway obstruction.

System Specific: Non-Systems
Content Outline: Safety & Professional Roles; Teaching/Learning; Research

Exam One: Question 71

A physician examines a 36-year-old male with shoulder pain. As part of the examination the physician orders x-rays. Which medical condition could be confirmed using this type of diagnostic imaging?

1. bicipital tendonitis
2. **calcific tendonitis**
3. supraspinatus impingement
4. subacromial bursitis

Correct Answer: 2 (Hertling p. 304)

The greater the density of the tissue, the more visible it will appear on x-ray. The majority of inflammatory conditions of the shoulder would be formally diagnosed using magnetic resonance imaging.

1. Bicipital tendonitis is an inflammatory process of the tendon of the long head of the biceps. The condition is characterized by subjective reports of a deep ache directly in front and on top of the shoulder made worse with overhead activities or lifting. Repeated full abduction and lateral rotation of the humeral head can lead to irritation that produces inflammation, edema, microscopic tears within the tendon, and degeneration of the tendon itself.

2. **Calcific tendonitis is often visible on x-ray due to the relative density of calcium. The greater the density of the tissue, the more visible it will appear on x-ray. The supraspinatus and infraspinatus tendons are common sites for calcific tendonitis.**

3. Supraspinatus impingement is caused by an inability of a weak supraspinatus muscle to adequately depress the head of the humerus in the glenoid fossa during elevation of the arm. The patient may experience a feeling of weakness and identify the presence of a painful arc of motion most commonly occurring between 60 and 120 degrees of active abduction.

4. Subacromial bursitis refers to inflammation of the subacromial bursa which lies between the deltoid muscle, supraspinatus tendon, and the fibrous capsule of the shoulder joint. The bursa facilitates movement of the deltoid muscle over the fibrous capsule of the shoulder joint and the supraspinatus tendon. The clinical presentation of the condition is very similar to the clinical presentation of supraspinatus impingement.

System Specific: Musculoskeletal System
Content Outline: Foundations for Evaluation, Differential Diagnosis, & Prognosis

Exam One: Question 72

A physical therapist designs a research study that will examine the effect of high voltage galvanic electrical stimulation on edema following arthroscopic knee surgery. The MOST appropriate method to collect data is:

1. anthropometric measurements
2. **circumferential measurements**
3. goniometric measurements
4. volumetric measurements

Correct Answer: 2 (Hertling p. 501)

Physical therapists must utilize appropriate tests and measures to quantify the relative effectiveness of selected interventions. Therapists should carefully consider the reliability and validity of selected tests and measures when analyzing the collected data.

1. Common anthropometric measurements used for adults include height, weight, body mass index (BMI), waist-to-hip ratio, and percentage of body fat. These measures are then compared to reference standards to assess items such as weight status and the risk for various diseases.

2. **Circumferential measurements using a flexible tape measure allow physical therapists to obtain a gross estimate of edema in the knee. Pre-test and post-test measurements provide information on the effect of the electrical stimulation on the edema.**

3. Goniometric measurements are obtained with a goniometer and are designed to quantify available range of motion. If electrical stimulation is effective in reducing the edema, the patient may have improved range of motion, however, this would still not directly quantify the relative change in edema.

4. Volumetric measurements are often used to quantify the presence of edema in the wrist and hand by examining the amount of water displaced following immersion. Comparison with the uninvolved extremity provides a baseline measure. It would be impractical to attempt this type of measurement at the knee joint.

System Specific: Non-Systems
Content Outline: Safety & Professional Roles; Teaching/Learning; Research

Exam One: Question 73

A physical therapist employed in an outpatient orthopedic clinic examines a patient diagnosed with cerebral palsy. The therapist has limited experience with cerebral palsy and is concerned about his ability to provide appropriate treatment. The MOST appropriate therapist action is:

1. inform the patient of your area of expertise
2. **co-treat the patient with another more experienced therapist**
3. treat the patient
4. refuse to treat the patient

> **Correct Answer: 2** (Guide for Professional Conduct)

Physical therapists must make decisions that are consistent with their professional training. Since the therapist is concerned about his ability to provide appropriate treatment, he is in need of some form of external assistance.

1. Informing the patient of their area of expertise would likely make the patient question the therapist's competence.
2. **By co-treating the patient, the therapist receives external assistance and at the same time improves his skills with a particular patient population.**
3. The question states that the therapist is concerned about his ability to treat the patient. This type of admission makes it inappropriate to simply treat the patient without utilizing available resources.
4. Refusing to treat the patient would not be necessary since the therapist has available resources to offer assistance.

System Specific: Non-Systems
Content Outline: Safety & Professional Roles; Teaching/Learning; Research

Exam One: Question 74

A patient status post Achilles tendon repair is examined in physical therapy. The physician referral includes a very specific post-operative protocol. If the therapist plans on deviating from the established protocol, the MOST appropriate action is to:

1. secure the patient's surgical report
2. complete a thorough examination
3. carefully document any modification
4. **contact the referring physician**

> **Correct Answer: 4** (Guide for Professional Conduct)

A protocol traditionally outlines a detailed plan or sequence to be followed when treating a patient with a selected medical condition.

1. Familiarity with the surgical report would be helpful for the therapist, however, would not provide adequate justification for deviating from the established protocol.
2. A thorough examination must be completed regardless of whether the referral includes a very specific protocol or simply an order to "evaluate and treat."
3. When possible the therapist should contact the referring physician prior to making any modifications to a protocol, however, when a modification does occur it is necessary to document the change.
4. **Protocols are often established by physicians to ensure that health care providers progress patients in a predictable manner without jeopardizing the patients' post surgical status. As a result, it is necessary to contact the referring physician when deviating from the established protocol.**

System Specific: Non-Systems
Content Outline: Safety & Professional Roles; Teaching/Learning; Research

Exam One: Question 75

A physical therapist examines the gait of a 62-year-old male with peripheral neuropathy. The therapist observes that the patient's right foot has a tendency to slap the ground during the loading response. The observation can BEST be explained by weakness of the:

1. iliopsoas
2. **tibialis anterior**
3. tibialis posterior
4. gastrocnemius

Correct Answer: 2 (Kendall p. 410)

Peripheral neuropathy is a broad term that describes a lesion to a peripheral nerve. The condition can be caused by a multitude of factors including diabetes, compression, trauma or nutritional deficiencies. Patients with peripheral neuropathy may exhibit motor, sensory, and autonomic changes including extreme sensitivity to touch, loss of sensation, muscle weakness, and loss of vasomotor tone.

1. The iliopsoas is formed by the iliacus and psoas major muscles and acts to flex the hip and assists in lateral rotation and abduction. The iliacus is innervated by the femoral nerve and the psoas major is innervated by the lumbar plexus.
2. **The tibialis anterior acts to dorsiflex the ankle joint and assists in inversion of the foot. The muscle is innervated by the deep peroneal nerve. Injury to the deep peroneal nerve (L4, L5, S1) may produce dramatic weakness in dorsiflexion and resultant foot drop at initial foot contact. The patient will likely try to compensate for this by excessive hip and knee flexion in an attempt to avoid dragging the toe.**
3. The tibialis posterior acts to invert the foot and assists in plantar flexion of the ankle joint. The muscle is innervated by the tibial nerve.
4. The gastrocnemius acts to plantar flex the ankle joint and assists in flexion of the knee joint. The muscle is innervated by the tibial nerve.

System Specific: Neuromuscular & Nervous Systems
Content Outline: Clinical Application of Foundational Sciences

Exam One: Question 76

A physical therapist compiles a table which identifies joint position at the hip, knee, ankle, and metatarsophalangeal joints for each subunit of the stance phase of gait. Which of the following is NOT accurate in describing normal joint position at the end of terminal stance?

1. 15 degrees of hip hyperextension
2. 0 degrees of knee extension
3. 0 degrees of ankle dorsiflexion
4. **10 degrees of metatarsophalangeal hyperextension**

Correct Answer: 4 (Levangie p. 461)

Rancho Los Amigos stages of gait include initial contact, loading response, midstance, terminal stance, pre-swing, initial swing, midswing, and terminal swing. Each stage requires a specific amount of available range of motion at each of the lower extremity joints. Terminal stance begins when the stance limb's heel rises and ends when the other foot touches the ground.

1. The hip is in 10-20 degrees of hyperextension at the end of terminal stance.
2. The knee is in neutral (i.e., 0 degrees) at the end of terminal stance.
3. The ankle is in neutral (i.e., 0 degrees) at the end of terminal stance.
4. **The metatarsophalangeal joints are in 30 degrees of hyperextension at the end of terminal stance.**

System Specific: Musculoskeletal System
Content Outline: Examination

Exam One: Question 77

A physical therapist positions a patient as shown in order to assess their claim of complete paresis of the right lower extremity. The therapist instructs the patient to perform a rapid straight leg raise with their left lower extremity. Which finding would BEST dispute the patient's claim?

1. The patient is unable to lift their left heel from the therapist's hand.
2. The patient experiences radiating pain into the right lower extremity.
3. **The patient exerts a downward force into the therapist's hand with their right heel.**
4. The patient reports severe pain while performing the straight leg raise.

Correct Answer: 3 (Magee p. 577)

The Hoover test is often employed as a gross test for malingering. The physical therapist places one hand underneath each calcaneus with the patient lying in supine. The patient is then asked to perform a straight leg raise on the uninvolved extremity while the therapist simultaneously assesses motor output on the involved side.

1. The Hoover test relies on assessing the reaction of the contralateral limb rather than the quality of the straight leg raise.
2. The Hoover test is designed to provide insight on potential malingering rather than serving as a provocative test intended to create radiating pain or other signs or symptoms.
3. **A rapid straight leg raise of the left (uninvolved) lower extremity should result in the patient exerting a downward force into the therapist's hand with the right (involved) heel. This action would be considered a normal response due to the effort associated with performing the straight leg raise, therefore disputing the patient's claim of complete paresis of the right lower extremity.**
4. The Hoover test is not influenced by the presence or absence of pain.

System Specific: Neuromuscular & Nervous Systems
Content Outline: Examination

Exam One: Question 78

A patient rehabilitating from a lower extremity injury has been non-weight bearing for three weeks. A recent physician entry in the medical record indicates the patient is cleared for weight bearing up to 25 pounds. The MOST appropriate device to use when instructing the patient on the new weight bearing status is:

1. an inclinometer
2. **a scale**
3. an anthropometer
4. a tape measure

Correct Answer: 2 (Pierson p. 225)

There are a variety of surgical procedures and medical conditions that require patients to limit the amount of weight being borne through a lower extremity. Failure to comply with prescribed weight bearing restrictions can jeopardize or significantly delay a patient's recovery. It is therefore critical for therapists to educate patients on their prescribed weight bearing status.

1. Inclinometers, also termed gravity-dependent goniometers, use gravity's effect on pointers and fluid levels to measure joint position and motion.
2. **A scale can be a valuable tool for a patient to use to better understand what a selected amount of weight bearing feels like since it offers immediate feedback in the form of pounds.**
3. An anthropometer is a device used to gather data on the measurements and proportions of the human body. Common uses include measuring long bone length, skin folds or use in motion analysis studies.
4. Tape measures are designed to quantify distance. A common use in physical therapy would be to assess leg length or conduct girth measurements.

System Specific: Musculoskeletal System
Content Outline: Interventions

Exam One: Question 79

A physical therapist observes a patient complete hip abduction and adduction exercises in standing. Which axis of movement is utilized with these particular motions?

1. frontal
2. vertical
3. **anterior-posterior**
4. longitudinal

> ### Correct Answer: 3 (Levangie p. 7)

Motions are described as occurring around three cardinal planes of the body (frontal, sagittal, transverse). Movement in the cardinal planes occur around three corresponding axes (anterior-posterior, medial-lateral, vertical). The axis of any cardinal plane movement is always found perpendicular to its corresponding plane.

1. The frontal (coronal) plane divides the body into anterior and posterior sections. Motions in the frontal plane occur around an anterior-posterior axis. Although the described motions, hip abduction and adduction, occur in the frontal (coronal) plane, the question specifically asks about the axis of movement.
2. The term vertical or longitudinal axis of motion is used when the axis of motion passes through the length of a long bone. Motions in the transverse plane such as medial and lateral rotation occur around a vertical axis. The transverse plane divides the body into upper and lower sections.
3. **Motions in the frontal (coronal) plane such as abduction and adduction occur around an anterior-posterior axis. The frontal plane divides the body into anterior and posterior sections.**
4. The term longitudinal and vertical are synonyms and therefore respond to the same axis of movement.

System Specific: Musculoskeletal System
Content Outline: Clinical Application of Foundational Sciences

Exam One: Question 80

A patient is treated using pulsed wave ultrasound at 1.2 W/cm^2 for seven minutes. The specific parameters of the pulsed wave are 2 msec on time and 8 msec off time for one pulse period. The duty cycle should be recorded as:

1. 10%
2. **20%**
3. 25%
4. 50%

> ### Correct Answer: 2 (Cameron p. 192)

Duty cycle is defined as the ratio of the on time to the total time. When ultrasound is used in a pulsed mode with a 20% or lower duty cycle, the heat produced during the on time of the cycle is dispersed during the off time and as a result, there is no measurable net increase in temperature. Ultrasound using a 20% or lower duty cycle would typically be used for nonthermal effects.

1. A 10% duty cycle would result if the parameters of the pulsed wave were 1 msec on time and 9 msec off time. Duty cycle = 1 msec / (1 msec + 9 msec) = .10 (100) = 10%.
2. **The question indicates that the parameters of the pulsed wave are 2 msec on time and 8 msec off time for one pulse period. As a result, duty cycle = 2 msec / (2 msec + 8 msec) = .20 (100) = 20%.**
3. This option may have been a common response for candidates who incorrectly answered the question since it is intuitive to take the on time and divide it by the off time. This calculation would be as follows: 2 msec / 8 msec = .25 (100) = 25%. Although the math is correct, the option remains incorrect since by definition duty cycle is defined as the ratio of the on time to the total time (not only the off time).
4. A 50% duty cycle would result any time the on time was the same as the off time. For example, if the parameters of the pulsed wave were 2 msec on time and 2 msec off time. Duty cycle = 2 msec / (2 msec + 2 msec) = .50 (100) = 50%.

System Specific: Non-Systems
Content Outline: Equipment & Devices; Therapeutic Modalities

Test Taking Tip: It is important for candidates to remove extraneous information from the question since this action allows candidates to focus more intently on the important aspects of the question. In this particular question, the fact that the therapist is using pulsed wave ultrasound at 1.2 W/cm^2 for seven minutes is irrelevant since answering the question correctly is based solely on determining the duty cycle from the given on and off time (total time).

Exam One: Question 81

A physical therapist examines the output from a single lead electrocardiogram of a patient with first degree atrioventricular heart block. The defining characteristic of this condition is:

1. inverted T wave
2. **prolonged PR interval**
3. bizarre QRS complex
4. ST segment depression

Correct Answer: 2 (Brannon p. 212)

The PR interval is the time required to conduct the cardiac impulse from the sinoatrial node to the atrioventricular node. This is normally 0.12 to 0.20 seconds. Heart blocks, also known as conduction blocks, are characterized as 1st, 2nd or 3rd degree according to the severity of the disturbance in the conduction of the cardiac impulse through the electrical conduction system. A first-degree heart block is relatively benign. The defining feature is a prolonged PR interval (> 0.20 sec.).

1. A normal T wave is rounded, symmetric, and upright. An inverted T wave is commonly associated with myocardial ischemia.
2. **The normal duration of the PR interval is 0.12 to 0.20 second. A prolonged PR interval (> 0.20 sec) is the defining feature of first-degree atrioventricular block.**
3. A bizarre QRS complex refers to the characteristic shape and configuration of a premature ventricular contraction (PVC) arising from an ectopic focus in the ventricle that occurs before the expected time of normal ventricular depolarization.
4. ST segment depression is a classic sign of myocardial ischemia.

System Specific: Cardiac, Vascular, & Pulmonary Systems
Content Outline: Foundations for Evaluation, Differential Diagnosis, & Prognosis

Exam One: Question 82

The first step a physical therapist should take to incorporate current best evidence into the practice of physical therapy is to:

1. **pose an answerable clinical question**
2. locate the most current best evidence from the literature
3. critically appraise the evidence for its validity, impact, and applicability
4. integrate the evidence into clinical decision making

Correct Answer: 1 (Sackett p. 3)

The first step in evidence-based practice is to pose an answerable clinical question. This action is considered the starting point for searching the literature for information related to the question. A well built, answerable clinical question usually has four components: 1) patient/problem of interest; 2) intervention; 3) comparison intervention(s), if relevant; 4) the clinical outcomes of interest. These components form the acronym P-I-C-O.

1. **The first step in evidence-based practice is to ask an answerable clinical question.**
2. The second step in evidence-based practice is to locate the best evidence to answer the question.
3. The third step in evidence-based practice is to critically appraise the evidence you find.
4. The fourth step in evidence-based practice is integrating the evidence, along with clinical experience and the patient's unique values and circumstances, to make clinical decisions.

System Specific: Non-Systems
Content Outline: Safety & Professional Roles; Teaching/Learning; Research

Exam One: Question 83

A patient diagnosed with ankylosing spondylitis exhibits a forward stooped posture. As part of the patient's care plan the physical therapist selects a number of active exercises that promote improved posture. Which proprioceptive neuromuscular facilitation pattern would be the MOST appropriate to achieve the therapist's objective?

1. D1 extension
2. D1 flexion
3. D2 extension
4. **D2 flexion**

> **Correct Answer: 4** (Sullivan p. 300)

A proprioceptive neuromuscular facilitation approach utilizes methods that promote or hasten the response of the neuromuscular mechanism through stimulation of the proprioceptors. The two diagonal patterns are commonly referred to as D1 and D2 where "D" stands for diagonal and "1" and "2" refer to specific patterns of movement. To improve the patient's standing posture the therapist should use a pattern that requires the patient to move the arms upward and away from the body (D2 flexion).

1. The command for D1 extension would be to open your hand and push down and away from your body.
2. The command for D1 flexion would be to close your hand and pull up and across your body.
3. The command for D2 extension would be to close your hand and pull down and across your body.
4. **The command for D2 flexion would be to open your hand and pull up and away from your body. The pattern emphasizes shoulder flexion, abduction, and lateral rotation which would facilitate improved standing posture.**

System Specific: Neuromuscular & Nervous Systems
Content Outline: Interventions

Exam One: Question 84

A physical therapist completing a balance assessment positions a patient in standing prior to administering the Romberg test. When administering the Romberg test it would be MOST important for the therapist to determine:

1. the width of the base of support necessary in order to maintain standing
2. the amount of time the patient is able to maintain the test position
3. **the amount of sway present during the testing period**
4. the complexity of tasks the patient is able to perform with eyes open and eyes closed

> **Correct Answer: 3** (Montgomery p. 191)

A positive Romberg test is indicative of a loss of proprioception often associated with a posterior column lesion in the spinal cord or a peripheral neuropathy.

1. The Romberg test is performed with the patient in standing with the feet together. The width of the base of support is not altered by the therapist during the test.
2. The Romberg test is most commonly administered during 30 second observational periods. The test does not attempt to quantify the amount of time a patient is able to maintain a static posture, rather the amount of sway present during the testing period.
3. **The amount of sway present during the testing period determines whether the Romberg test is positive or negative. A positive test is characterized by a patient being able to stand with no more than minimal sway with the eyes open, but presents with increased instability or falls with the eyes closed.**
4. The Romberg test is a static standing test where the variable being manipulated is whether the eyes are open or closed and not the complexity of the tasks.

System Specific: Neuromuscular & Nervous Systems
Content Outline: Examination

Exam One: Question 85

A physical therapist reviews the medical record of a patient diagnosed with peripheral arterial disease prior to initiating treatment. Which objective finding would MOST severely limit the patient's ability to participate in an ambulation exercise program?

1. **signs of resting claudication**
2. decreased peripheral pulses
3. cool skin
4. blood pressure of 165/90 mm Hg

> **Correct Answer: 1** (Kisner p. 830)

Peripheral arterial disease refers to a condition involving the arterial system that results in compromised circulation to the extremities. Resting claudication is typically considered a contraindication to active exercise in patients with peripheral arterial disease.

1. **Claudication pain is a symptom of ischemia of the lower extremity muscles caused by peripheral arterial disease. Resting claudication pain is typically considered a contraindication to exercise with peripheral arterial disease and may be an indication that the disease process is more advanced.**
2. Decreased peripheral pulses are a common sign associated with peripheral arterial disease, but would only severely limit ambulation if blood flow was markedly diminished or absent. Decreased peripheral pulses are a result of plaque buildup in the arteries which decreases blood flow and subsequently oxygen to the extremities.
3. Cool skin may be a sign of peripheral arterial disease, but would only severely limit ambulation if blood flow was markedly diminished or absent. Cool skin results from the diminished circulation, particularly in the extremities.
4. A blood pressure of 165/90 mm Hg is common during exercise and does not severely limit ambulation.

System Specific: Cardiac, Vascular, & Pulmonary Systems
Content Outline: Interventions

Exam One: Question 86

A patient with limited elbow and forearm range of motion is referred to physical therapy. When mobilizing the humeroradial articulation, the treatment plane is considered to be:

1. in the concave radial head, parallel to the long axis of the radius
2. **in the concave radial head, perpendicular to the long axis of the radius**
3. in the convex radial head, parallel to the long axis of the radius
4. in the convex radial head, perpendicular to the long axis of the radius

> **Correct Answer: 2** (Kisner p. 128)

The humeroradial joint is a uniaxial hinge joint between the capitulum of the humerus and the head of the radius. The humerus is convex and the radius is concave and therefore osteokinematic motion and arthrokinematic glide are in the same direction. The treatment plane is considered the plane perpendicular to a line running from the axis of rotation to the middle of the concave articular surface. The plane itself is located in the concave partner and is therefore determined by the position of the concave bone.

1. The radial head is the concave partner, however, the treatment plane is perpendicular and not parallel to the long axis of the radius.
2. **The radial head is the concave partner and the treatment plane is perpendicular to the long axis of the radius.**
3. The radial head is the concave partner and not the convex partner. The treatment plane is perpendicular and not parallel to the long axis of the radius.
4. The radial head is the concave partner and not the convex partner, however, the treatment plane is perpendicular to the long axis of the radius.

System Specific: Musculoskeletal System
Content Outline: Interventions

Exam One: Question 87

A physical therapist conducts an inservice on exercise guidelines for a group of senior citizens. As part of the inservice the therapist discusses the benefits of improving cardiovascular status through a low intensity activity such as a walking program. What frequency of exercise would be the MOST desirable to achieve the stated objective?

1. twice per day
2. one time per week
3. three times per week
4. **five times per week**

> **Correct Answer: 4** (American College of Sports Medicine p. 452)

To minimize medical problems and promote long-term compliance with this population, exercise intensity should start low and progress gradually according to individual tolerance and preference. Exercise performed at a moderate intensity should be performed for 30 minutes on most days of the week. If exercise is at a vigorous level, it should be performed at least three times per week. Since the cited exercise is low intensity, five times per week is the most appropriate option.

1. The therapist can recommend that individuals who have difficulty sustaining exercise for 30 minutes continuously, or who prefer shorter bouts of exercise, should exercise for shorter periods (e.g., 10 minutes) several times each day. This is not the most desirable combination of exercise intensity and frequency, however, to improve cardiovascular status.
2. One time per week is an inadequate frequency to improve cardiovascular fitness when exercising at low intensity.
3. Three times per week is an appropriate frequency if the exercise is at a vigorous level. It would not be the most desirable frequency for low intensity exercise.
4. **Since walking is a low intensity activity, more frequent exercise sessions are needed to improve cardiovascular status. Five times per week is the most desirable option.**

System Specific: Cardiac, Vascular, & Pulmonary Systems
Content Outline: Interventions

Exam One: Question 88

A physical therapist identifies the pisiform after palpating along the proximal row of carpals. Which carpal bone articulates with the pisiform?

1. trapezium
2. trapezoid
3. lunate
4. **triquetrum**

> **Correct Answer: 4** (Hoppenfeld p. 70)

The proximal row of carpal bones from lateral to medial consists of the scaphoid, lunate, triquetrum, and pisiform. The distal row of carpal bones from lateral to medial consists of the trapezium, trapezoid, capitate, and hamate. The carpal bones articulate with each other at synovial joints and are connected via ligaments to form a compact mass.

1. The trapezium is located on the lateral side of the carpus between the scaphoid and the first metacarpal. It is distinguished by a deep groove on its palmar surface.
2. The trapezoid is the smallest carpal bone in the distal row and is noted for its wedge shaped form. The inferior surface of the bone articulates with the proximal end of the second metacarpal bone and the superior surface articulates with the scaphoid.
3. The lunate is located in the center of the proximal row between the scaphoid and the triquetrum. The lunate is distinguished by its crescent-like outline.
4. **The triquetrum is located on the medial side of the proximal row of carpals between the lunate and pisiform. The triquetrum is the third most often fractured carpal bone. The pisiform is located within the flexor carpi ulnaris tendon and lies immediately superior to the triquetrum.**

System Specific: Musculoskeletal System
Content Outline: Clinical Application of Foundational Sciences

Exam One: Question 89

A physical therapist employed in an acute care hospital reviews the medical record of a patient diagnosed with congestive heart failure. The therapist would like to implement a formal exercise program, but is concerned about the patient's exercise tolerance. Which condition is MOST responsible for the patient's limited exercise tolerance?

1.   diminished lung volumes
2.   arterial oxygen desaturation
3.   **insufficient stroke volume during ventricular systole**
4.   excessive rise in blood pressure

> **Correct Answer: 3** (Hillegass p. 134)

Congestive heart failure refers to the heart's inability to maintain a cardiac output that is adequate to meet the demands of the tissues due to an abnormality in the pumping ability of the heart muscle.

1.   Diminished lung volumes are more commonly associated with obstructive or restrictive lung conditions and are not typically associated with congestive heart failure.
2.   The level of arterial oxygenation is not significantly impacted with congestive heart failure, rather the primary issue is that a smaller volume of blood is pumped with each contraction of the ventricles.
3.   **Congestive heart failure may be due to a diminished pumping ability of the ventricles due to muscle weakening (systolic dysfunction) or to stiffening of the heart muscle that impairs the ventricles' capacity to relax and fill (diastolic dysfunction). With systolic dysfunction, the weak heart pumps a smaller volume of blood for each contraction of the ventricles (stroke volume), reducing cardiac output. The resultant decrease in the delivery of oxygenated blood to the active tissues limits the patient's ability to exercise.**
4.   Most patients with congestive heart failure take multiple medications including diuretics, vasodilators, ACE inhibitors, and beta blockers. The medications serve to reduce the hemodynamic response to exercise. An excessive increase in blood pressure is therefore unlikely.

System Specific: Cardiac, Vascular, & Pulmonary Systems
Content Outline: Foundations for Evaluation, Differential Diagnosis, & Prognosis

Exam One: Question 90

A physical therapist measures a patient for a wheelchair. When measuring back height, which method is MOST accurate?

1.   measure from the seat of the chair to the base of the axilla and subtract two inches
2.   **measure from the seat of the chair to the base of the axilla and subtract four inches**
3.   measure from the seat of the chair to the acromion process and subtract two inches
4.   measure from the seat of the chair to the acromion process and subtract four inches

> **Correct Answer: 2** (Pierson p. 135)

There are a variety of specific measurements that must be performed when fitting a patient for a wheelchair. Failure to obtain accurate measurements can result in a wheelchair that is not appropriately sized. Ramifications include increased difficulty with mobility and potential complications such as pressure sores or skin breakdown.

1.   Measuring from the seat of the chair to the base of the axilla and subtracting two inches would result in the back height being at the mid-scapular level. This back height would be too high to allow for optimal mobility.
2.   **Back height should be determined by measuring from the seat of the chair to the base of the axilla and subtracting four inches. This method will allow the back height to fall below the inferior angle of the scapula. The height of the seat cushion used, if applicable, must be added to the obtained measurement.**
3.   Measuring from the seat of the chair to the acromion process and subtracting two inches would result in a back height that is excessive and would significantly restrict the patient's movement.
4.   Measuring from the seat of the chair to the acromion process and subtracting four inches is more desirable than option 3, but would still not allow the back height to fall below the inferior angle of the scapula.

System Specific: Non-Systems
Content Outline: Equipment & Devices; Therapeutic Modalities

Exam One: Question 91

A patient diagnosed with infrapatellar tendonitis completes a series of functional activities. After completing the activities the physical therapist instructs the patient to use ice massage over the anterior surface of the knee. The MOST appropriate treatment time is:

1. 3-5 minutes
2. **5-10 minutes**
3. 10-15 minutes
4. 15-20 minutes

Correct Answer: 2 (Cameron p. 145)

Ice massage is typically performed by freezing water in paper cups and applying the ice directly to the treatment area. Ice massage tends to create a more intense cooling since the ice is applied directly to a localized target area.

1. Sufficient cooling with ice massage would not occur with a 3-5 minute treatment time.
2. **Ice massage requires a treatment time of 5-10 minutes due to the intensity of the cooling.**
3. A treatment time of 10-15 minutes would be excessive with ice massage and could result in signs and symptoms of cold intolerance.
4. A treatment time of 15-20 minutes would be within the established range for an ice pack, but would not be acceptable for ice massage.

System Specific: Non-Systems
Content Outline: Equipment & Devices; Therapeutic Modalities

Exam One: Question 92

A physical therapist uses functional electrical stimulation as part of a treatment regimen designed to improve quadriceps strength. Which on:off time ratio would result in the MOST rapid onset of muscle fatigue?

1. 3:1
2. 1:4
3. **5:1**
4. 1:6

Correct Answer: 3 (Prentice - Therapeutic Modalities p. 128)

The on:off time ratio is simply a method to show the relative duration of the on time versus the off time. The muscle contracts during the on time and relaxes during the off time. The greater the on time in relation to the off time, the more rapid the onset of muscle fatigue.

1. An on:off time ratio of 3:1 indicates that there is three seconds of on time for every one second of off time. This ratio would promote fatigue, however, it is not the best answer.
2. An on:off time ratio of 1:4 indicates that there is one second of on time for every four seconds of off time. This ratio has significantly greater rest periods and therefore fatigue would not tend to be a large factor.
3. **An on:off time ratio of 5:1 indicates that there is five seconds of on time for every one second of off time. This ratio would promote rapid fatigue given the extremely large on time in relation to the short off time.**
4. An on:off time ratio of 1:6 indicates that there is one second of on time for every six seconds of off time. This ratio has the greatest rest period and therefore fatigue would not tend to be a factor.

System Specific: Non-Systems
Content Outline: Equipment & Devices; Therapeutic Modalities

Test Taking Tip: Candidates must be extremely careful to answer examination questions in a precise manner. In this particular question, candidates need to identify the on:off time ratio that would result in the most rapid onset of fatigue. The best answer would have the greatest amount of on time in relation to the amount of off time. The correct option must be expressed in the same manner that the ratio is presented, meaning that the on time represents the first number and the off time represents the second number. By reversing these numbers the physical therapist could possess the requisite academic knowledge to answer the question, but still fail to answer the question correctly.

Exam One: Question 93

According to proponents of evidence-based medicine, the BEST source of information upon which to make clinical decisions about therapy for an individual patient is:

1. cohort study
2. randomized controlled trial
3. **systematic review**
4. case report

> **Correct Answer: 3** (Sackett p. 133)

The hierarchy of evidence ranks the strength of the different types of clinical evidence, studies or clinical trials from those with the least amount of bias to those with the potential for the greatest amount of bias.

1. Cohort studies are observation studies in which subjects are classified according to the presence or absence of a particular risk factor or exposure and followed over time to determine disease outcomes. Cohort studies do not evaluate the effect of therapy.
2. In a randomized controlled trial, patients are randomized into an experimental and a control group. Both groups are followed up for the variables or outcomes of interest. Randomized-control trials provide strong evidence for or against a therapy, but are not considered to be the highest level of evidence.
3. **Systematic reviews are summaries of the medical literature that use explicit methods to perform a thorough literature search, a critical appraisal of individual studies, and statistical techniques to combine results. Systematic reviews are considered to provide the highest level of evidence for or against a therapy.**
4. A case report is an in-depth description of an interesting condition or response to treatment. A case report is the least rigorous form of research because of its inherent lack of control and limited generalizability.

System Specific: Non-Systems
Content Outline: Safety & Professional Roles; Teaching/Learning; Research

Exam One: Question 94

A physical therapist employed in an outpatient clinic observes a patient complete a series of exercises. During the treatment session the patient mentions to the therapist that he is experiencing angina. After resting for 20 minutes the patient's condition is unchanged, however, he insists it is something that he can work through. The MOST appropriate therapist action is:

1. allow the patient to resume exercise and continue to monitor the patient's condition
2. reduce the intensity of the exercise and continue to monitor the patient's condition
3. discontinue the treatment session and encourage the patient to make an appointment with his physician
4. **discontinue the treatment session and call an ambulance**

> **Correct Answer: 4** (Hillegass p. 642)

Changes in anginal symptoms may reflect a change in coronary status. Any increase or change in anginal symptoms should be recorded and receive immediate medical attention.

1. Continued angina after 20 minutes of rest is cause for concern as it may indicate a serious change in the patients' coronary status. The patient should not be allowed to exercise, even if he says he can work through it.
2. Reducing the intensity of exercise does not negate the fact that the patient has continued angina after 20 minutes of rest.
3. Discontinuing the treatment session is necessary, however, encouraging the patient to make an appointment with his physician does not ensure that the patient will receive immediate medical attention.
4. **If anginal symptoms are not relieved by stopping exercise, or the use of three sublingual nitroglycerin tablets (one taken every five minutes), the patient should be transported to the nearest hospital emergency center.**

System Specific: Cardiac, Vascular, & Pulmonary Systems
Content Outline: Foundations for Evaluation, Differential Diagnosis, & Prognosis

Exam One: Question 95

A 55-year-old male status post myocardial infarction is referred to physical therapy. The patient has a history of cardiac disease and is moderately obese. The patient's age-predicted maximal heart rate should be recorded as:

1. 190
2. 185
3. **165**
4. 155

Correct Answer: 3 (Brannon p. 254)

Heart rate is used as a guide to set exercise intensity because of the relatively linear relationship between heart rate and oxygen consumption. Although it is best to measure maximal heart rate during a progressive maximal exercise test, maximal heart rate is inversely related to age and may be estimated by the formula: 220 – age.

1. A patient with an age-predicted maximal heart of 190 would be 30 years old. $220 - 55 \neq 190$
2. A patient with an age-predicted maximal heart of 185 would be 35 years old. $220 - 55 \neq 185$
3. **A patient with an age-predicted maximal heart of 165 would be 55 years old. $220 - 55 = 165$**
4. A patient with an age-predicted maximal heart of 155 would be 65 years old. $220 - 55 \neq 155$

System Specific: Cardiac, Vascular, & Pulmonary Systems
Content Outline: Interventions

Exam One: Question 96

A physical therapist transports a patient in a wheelchair to the parallel bars in preparation for ambulation activities. The patient is status post abdominal surgery and has not ambulated in over two weeks. The MOST appropriate action to facilitate ambulation is:

1. assist the patient to standing
2. monitor the patient's vital signs
3. **demonstrate ambulation in the parallel bars**
4. secure an additional staff member to offer assistance

Correct Answer: 3 (Minor p. 266)

The physical therapist must provide clear and concise directions to the patient in order to minimize the risk associated with the activity. This may be particularly important in the described scenario since the patient has not ambulated in over two weeks and using the parallel bars is likely to be a novel activity.

1. Assisting the patient to standing will likely be necessary, however, this action without previously demonstrating the activity will place the patient at greater risk.
2. Monitoring a patient's vital signs (i.e., heart rate, blood pressure, respiration rate) may be necessary depending on the patient's response to the activity, however, it would not be considered the most appropriate action to facilitate ambulation.
3. **Demonstration allows the physical therapist to model the appropriate technique for the patient in a controlled learning environment.**
4. The stability provided by the parallel bars makes it unlikely the physical therapist would need to secure an additional staff member to offer assistance. Although this would be an acceptable option, it would not be as effective as demonstration.

System Specific: Non-Systems
Content Outline: Equipment & Devices; Therapeutic Modalities

Exam One: Question 97

A physical therapist prepares to transfer a patient from a wheelchair to a treatment table. The patient cannot stand independently, but is able to bear some weight through the lower extremities. The MOST appropriate transfer technique is:

1. sliding board transfer
2. hydraulic lift
3. **dependent squat pivot**
4. two-person lift

> **Correct Answer: 3** (Minor p. 221)

Physical therapists should select transfers that allow patients to participate in the transfer to the greatest extent possible. Although the patient cannot stand independently, they can bear some weight through the lower extremities.

1. A sliding board transfer is used for a patient who has some sitting balance, some upper extremity strength, and can adequately follow directions.
2. A hydraulic lift is a device required for dependent transfers when a patient is obese, when there is only one therapist available to assist with the transfer or when the patient is totally dependent.
3. **A dependent squat pivot transfer is used when a patient can bear some weight through the lower extremities, however, cannot transfer independently.**
4. A two-person lift is used to transfer a patient between two surfaces of different heights or when transferring a patient to the floor.

System Specific: Non-Systems
Content Outline: Safety & Professional Roles; Teaching/Learning; Research

Exam One: Question 98

A risk management committee composed of various members of the rehabilitation team is charged with identifying methods to prevent employee exposure to blood and body fluids. The MOST appropriate INITIAL action is:

1. provide follow-up to employees if exposed to blood and body fluids
2. provide free hepatitis B immunizations to staff
3. **develop an infection control policy that conforms to Occupational Safety and Health Administration guidelines**
4. educate staff about the policies

> **Correct Answer: 3** (Pierson p. 31)

The Occupational Safety and Health Administration (O.S.H.A.) requires that health care facilities provide employees with information and instruction in techniques to protect them from infectious diseases (e.g., blood borne diseases).

1. Health care facilities are required to provide follow up to employees exposed to blood and body fluids. This is an important action, however, the committee was charged with identifying methods to prevent employee exposure to blood and body fluids.
2. Health care facilities are required to offer the hepatitis B vaccine to employees who are at substantial risk of occupational exposure to hepatitis B. The vaccine does not have to be free, but usually is offered without charge or with a substantial discount.
3. **Health care facilities are required to have a formal infection control policy that is consistent with O.S.H.A. requirements. It is important for all health care facilities to establish a committee who develops an infection control policy and then closely monitors the policy to ensure that it remains consistent with current O.S.H.A. guidelines.**
4. Staff is required to be educated on established policies, however, the initial action needs to focus on developing a policy consistent with current O.S.H.A. guidelines.

System Specific: Non-Systems
Content Outline: Safety & Professional Roles; Teaching/Learning; Research

Exam One: Question 99

A physical therapist attempts to classify the amount of assistance a patient requires to complete a sit to stand transfer. After completing the transfer, the therapist estimates that he was required to exert approximately 20% of the physical work in order to ensure the transfer was completed safely. The MOST appropriate classification of the level of assistance would be:

1. independent
2. supervision
3. **minimal assistance**
4. moderate assistance

> **Correct Answer: 3** (Pierson p. 174)

Classifying transfer status allows health care providers to communicate information regarding the level of assistance necessary during a transfer to other health care providers. Categories range from independent to maximum assistance.

1. Independent transfers require a patient to perform all aspects of the transfer, including the set-up, without assistance from others.
2. Supervision is used when it is necessary for a therapist to observe throughout the completion of the task.
3. **Minimal assistance is used for patients who can perform at least 75% of the activity.**
4. Moderate assistance is used for patients who can perform at least 50% of the activity.

System Specific: Non-Systems
Content Outline: Safety & Professional Roles; Teaching/Learning; Research

Test Taking Tip: It is critical that candidates read each question carefully since even small lapses in concentration can lead to unnecessary test taking mistakes. In this particular question, it states clearly that the therapist estimates that he was required to exert approximately 20% of the physical work in order to ensure the transfer was completed safely. It would be very easy for a candidate to misinterpret this and believe that the patient was exerting 20% of the physical work instead of the physical therapist. Mistakes like this on the actual examination are particularly problematic since they result in candidates missing questions that they may have been academically prepared to answer correctly.

Exam One: Question 100

A patient explains to her therapist that she was instructed to bear up to five pounds of weight on her involved extremity. The patient's weight bearing status would be BEST described as:

1. non-weight bearing
2. toe touch weight bearing
3. **partial weight bearing**
4. weight bearing as tolerated

> **Correct Answer: 3** (Pierson p. 225)

Physical therapists often classify a patient's weight bearing status using specific terminology ranging from non-weight bearing to full weight bearing. It is important for therapists to fully understand these terms since failure to follow the prescribed weight bearing status can jeopardize the safety of the patient and result in professional negligence.

1. Non-weight bearing occurs when a patient is unable to place any weight through the involved extremity and is not permitted to touch the ground or any surface.
2. Toe touch weight bearing occurs when a patient is unable to place any weight through the involved extremity, however, may place the toes on the ground to assist with balance.
3. **Partial weight bearing occurs when a patient is allowed to put a particular amount of weight through the involved extremity. The amount of weight bearing is expressed as allowable pounds of pressure or as a percentage of total weight. Partial weight bearing requires an assistive device.**
4. Weight bearing as tolerated occurs when a patient determines the proper amount of weight bearing based on comfort. The amount of weight bearing can range from minimal to full.

System Specific: Non-Systems
Content Outline: Safety & Professional Roles; Teaching/Learning; Research

Exam One: Question 101

A physical therapist reviews the surgical report of a patient that sustained extensive burns in a fire. The report indicates that at the time of primary excision, cadaver skin was utilized to close the wound. This type of graft is termed:

1. **allograft**
2. autograft
3. heterograft
4. xenograft

Correct Answer: 1 (Paz p. 274)

Cadaver skin is removed from donors shortly after their deaths, then processed and distributed by skin and tissue banks. Cadaver skin is often used on patients with severe burns as a substitute until a graft of their own skin can be applied.

1. **An allograft is a temporary skin graft taken from another human, usually a cadaver, in order to cover a large burned area. A homograft is synonymous with the term allograft.**
2. An autograft is a permanent skin graft taken from a donor site on the patient's own body.
3. A heterograft is a temporary skin graft taken from another species.
4. A xenograft is synonymous with the term heterograft.

System Specific: Integumentary System
Content Outline: Foundations for Evaluation, Differential Diagnosis, & Prognosis

Exam One: Question 102

A physician completes a physical examination on a 16-year-old male who injured his knee while playing in a soccer contest yesterday. The physician's preliminary diagnosis is a grade II anterior cruciate ligament injury. Which of the following diagnostic tools would be the MOST appropriate in the IMMEDIATE medical management of the patient?

1. bone scan
2. computed tomography
3. magnetic resonance imaging
4. **x-ray**

Correct Answer: 4 (Magee p. 40)

A grade II anterior cruciate ligament injury most often presents with moderate pain and swelling, minimal instability of the joint, and decreased range of motion. The physician would make the diagnosis based on the patient's clinical presentation and the results of ligamentous testing such as the Lachman test, lateral pivot shift maneuver or anterior drawer test.

1. A bone scan is a diagnostic test that utilizes radioactive isotopes to identify areas of bone that are hypervascular or have an increased rate of bone mineral turnover. Bone scans are most commonly used to detect bone disease or stress fractures.
2. Computed tomography produces cross-sectional images based on x-ray attenuation. A computerized analysis of the changes in absorption produces a detailed reconstructed image. The test is commonly used to diagnose spinal lesions and in diagnostic studies of the brain.
3. Magnetic resonance imaging is a non-invasive diagnostic test that utilizes magnetic fields to produce an image of bone and soft tissue. The test is valuable in providing images of soft tissue structures such as muscles, menisci, ligaments, tumors, and internal organs. The test would be the most beneficial to confirm the presence of an anterior cruciate ligament injury, however, due to the cost of the diagnostic test and the availability of the testing units it is unlikely that the test would be used in the immediate medical management.
4. **X-ray is a radiographic photograph commonly used to assist with the diagnosis of musculoskeletal pathology such as fractures, dislocations, and bone loss. An x-ray is a relatively cost effective diagnostic test often utilized in the immediate medical management to rule out the possibility of an associated fracture.**

System Specific: Musculoskeletal System
Content Outline: Foundations for Evaluation, Differential Diagnosis, & Prognosis

Exam One: Question 103

A physical therapist performs goniometric measurements on a 38-year-old female rehabilitating from an acromioplasty. The therapist attempts to stabilize the scapula while measuring glenohumeral abduction. Failure to stabilize the scapula will lead to:

1. downward rotation and elevation of the scapula
2. downward rotation and depression of the scapula
3. **upward rotation and elevation of the scapula**
4. upward rotation and depression of the scapula

> **Correct Answer: 3** (Norkin p. 78)

Normal glenohumeral abduction is 0-120 degrees. When measuring glenohumeral abduction, the axis of the goniometer should be placed over the anterior aspect of the acromial process. The stationary arm should be positioned parallel to the midline of the anterior aspect of the sternum and the moveable arm should be positioned on the medial midline of the humerus. Failure to stabilize the scapula will result in the obtained range of motion value being greater than the actual amount of glenohumeral abduction available.

1. Glenohumeral abduction requires upward rotation of the scapula and not downward rotation.
2. Glenohumeral abduction requires upward rotation and elevation of the scapula and not downward rotation and depression.
3. **Failure to stabilize the scapula when measuring glenohumeral abduction will result in upward rotation and elevation of the scapula. When measuring shoulder complex abduction, the thorax should be stabilized to prevent lateral flexion of the trunk.**
4. Glenohumeral abduction requires elevation of the scapula and not depression.

System Specific: Musculoskeletal System
Content Outline: Examination

Exam One: Question 104

A physical therapist performs an examination on a 46-year-old male patient diagnosed with piriformis syndrome. The patient indicates he has experienced pain in his low back and buttock region for the last three weeks. Which motions would you expect to be weak and painful during muscle testing based on the patient's diagnosis?

1. **abduction and lateral rotation of the thigh**
2. abduction and medial rotation of the thigh
3. adduction and lateral rotation of the thigh
4. adduction and medial rotation of the thigh

> **Correct Answer: 1** (Magee p. 696)

Piriformis syndrome refers to a condition in which the piriformis muscle irritates the sciatic nerve causing pain in the buttocks and referred pain along the course of the sciatic nerve. The piriformis muscle originates on the anterior surface of the sacrum and the sacrotuberous ligament and inserts on the greater trochanter of the femur. The muscle is innervated by the sacral plexus.

1. **The patient would likely present with pain and weakness with resisted abduction and lateral rotation of the thigh since the motions are consistent with the action of the piriformis muscle.**
2. The patient would likely present with pain and weakness with resisted abduction of the thigh, however, would not with resisted medial rotation.
3. The patient would not likely experience pain and weakness with resisted adduction, however, may with lateral rotation.
4. The patient would not likely experience pain and weakness with resisted adduction or medial rotation of the thigh since the motions are the exact opposite of the piriformis muscle's action.

System Specific: Other Systems
Content Outline: Examination

Exam One: Question 105

A physical therapist examines a patient with a dorsal scapular nerve injury. Which muscles would you expect to be MOST affected by this condition?

1. serratus anterior, pectoralis minor
2. **levator scapulae, rhomboids**
3. latissimus dorsi, teres major
4. supraspinatus, infraspinatus

Correct Answer: 2 (Kendall p. 348)

Damage to a peripheral nerve can significantly impair muscle function. The severity of the impact ranges from a mild disturbance to denervation.

1. The serratus anterior is innervated by the long thoracic nerve and the pectoralis minor is innervated by the medial pectoral nerve.
2. **The levator scapulae and rhomboids are innervated by the dorsal scapular nerve.**
3. The latissimus dorsi is innervated by the thoracodorsal nerve and the teres major is innervated by the lower subscapular nerve.
4. The supraspinatus and infraspinatus are innervated by the suprascapular nerve.

System Specific: Other Systems
Content Outline: Clinical Application of Foundational Sciences

Test Taking Tip: In some cases, a physical therapist may not have a full complement of academic information available to answer a given question, however, may still be able to identify the correct option or at least eliminate one or more of the incorrect options. For example, in option 1 the therapist may know that the serratus anterior is innervated by the long thoracic nerve, but may not know the innervation of the pectoralis minor. By recognizing that at least one of the muscles listed in option 1 is not associated with the dorsal scapular nerve, the therapist can safely eliminate this option. Candidates should not become anxious or unsettled when they identify information that they are not familiar with on the National Physical Therapy Examination and instead attempt to answer the question based on their existing academic knowledge. Candidates can use this strategy to enhance their examination score.

Exam One: Question 106

A 13-year-old female diagnosed with cerebral palsy is referred to physical therapy. The patient exhibits slow, involuntary, continuous writhing movements of the upper and lower extremities. This type of motor disturbance is MOST representative of:

1. spasticity
2. ataxia
3. hypotonia
4. **athetosis**

Correct Answer: 4 (Tecklin p. 183)

Cerebral palsy is an umbrella term used to describe a group of non-progressive movement disorders that result from brain damage. Athetoid cerebral palsy involves damage to the cerebellum, cerebellar pathways or both.

1. Spasticity refers to an increased resistance to passive stretch. Spasticity is commonly observed with patients diagnosed with cerebral palsy due to upper motor neuron damage.
2. Ataxia is a generalized term used to describe motor impairments of cerebellar origin. It is characterized by the inability to perform coordinated movement and may affect gait, posture, and patterns of movements.
3. Hypotonia refers to decreased or absent tone where resistance to passive movement is decreased, stretch reflexes are diminished, and limbs are easily moved. Hypotonicity in children is often associated with motor delays.
4. **Athetosis refers to involuntary movements characterized as slow, irregular, and twisting. Peripheral movements occur without central stability. This type of motor disturbance makes it extremely difficult to maintain a static body position.**

System Specific: Neuromuscular & Nervous Systems
Content Outline: Clinical Application of Foundational Sciences

Exam One: Question 107

A physician refers a patient rehabilitating from a fractured femur to physical therapy for gait training. Which of the following would NOT be the responsibility of the physical therapist?

1. assessing balance
2. **determining weight bearing status**
3. selecting an assistive device
4. assessing endurance

Correct Answer: 2 (Guide for Professional Conduct)

Physical therapists have a high degree of autonomy, however, remain dependent on the physician for items such as determining weight bearing status.

1. Physical therapists assess balance using a variety of measures including the Berg Balance Scale, Functional Reach Test, Romberg Test, and the Tinetti Performance Oriented Mobility Assessment.
2. **Determining weight bearing status would be the responsibility of the physician. This decision is likely influenced by the amount of time since the fracture and the degree of healing observed through radiographs.**
3. Physical therapists would typically select an appropriate assistive device for a patient after considering a number of variables such as the prescribed weight bearing status, cognition, upper and lower extremity strength, balance, and coordination.
4. Physical therapists routinely assess endurance using measures such as Borg's Rating of Perceived Exertion Scale.

System Specific: Non-Systems
Content Outline: Safety & Professional Roles; Teaching/Learning; Research

Exam One: Question 108

A physical therapist instructs a 55-year-old patient with significant bilateral lower extremity paresis to transfer from a wheelchair to a mat table. The patient has normal upper extremity strength and has no other known medical problems. The MOST appropriate transfer technique is a:

1. dependent squat pivot transfer
2. **sliding board transfer**
3. two-person lift
4. hydraulic lift

Correct Answer: 2 (Pierson p. 177)

Physical therapists should select transfers for patients based on their unique abilities and limitations. Once a specific type of transfer is selected, the therapist should have the patient assist with the transfer to the greatest extent possible.

1. A dependent squat pivot transfer is used to transfer a patient who cannot stand independently, but can bear some weight through the trunk and lower extremities.
2. **A sliding board transfer is used for a patient who possesses sitting balance, good upper extremity strength, and can adequately follow directions. The use of the sliding board and the extent of upper extremity strength available make it possible for the patient to complete the transfer despite the presence of bilateral lower extremity paresis.**
3. A two-person lift is used to transfer a patient between two surfaces of different heights or when transferring a patient to the floor.
4. A hydraulic lift is a device required for dependent transfers when a patient is obese, when there is only one therapist available to assist with the transfer or when the patient is totally dependent.

System Specific: Non-Systems
Content Outline: Equipment & Devices; Therapeutic Modalities

Exam One: Question 109

A physical therapist instructs a patient to make a fist. The patient can make a fist, but is unable to flex the distal phalanx of the ring finger. This clinical finding can BEST be explained by:

1. a ruptured flexor carpi radialis tendon
2. a ruptured flexor digitorum superficialis tendon
3. **a ruptured flexor digitorum profundus tendon**
4. a ruptured extensor digitorum communis tendon

Correct Answer: 3 (Hoppenfeld p. 101)

The flexor digitorum profundus muscle originates on the anterior and medial surfaces of the proximal portion of the ulna, interosseous membrane, and deep antebrachial fascia. The muscle inserts via four tendons into the anterior surface of the bases of the distal phalanges.

1. The flexor carpi radialis muscle acts to flex and abduct the wrist and may assist in pronation of the forearm and in flexion of the elbow.
2. The flexor digitorum superficialis muscle acts to flex the proximal interphalangeal joints of the second through fifth digits, and assists in flexion of the metacarpophalangeal joints and flexion of the wrist.
3. **The flexor digitorum profundus muscle acts to flex the distal interphalangeal joints of the index, middle, ring, and little finger, and assists in flexion of the proximal interphalangeal and metacarpophalangeal joints. A ruptured flexor digitorum profundus tendon would therefore make it impossible to flex the distal phalanx.**
4. The extensor digitorum communis muscle acts to extend the metacarpophalangeal joints and in conjunction with the lumbricales and interossei, extends the interphalangeal joints of the second through fifth digits. The muscle assists in abduction of the index, ring, and little finger and in extension and abduction of the wrist.

System Specific: Musculoskeletal System
Content Outline: Foundations for Evaluation, Differential Diagnosis, & Prognosis

Test Taking Tip: Candidates will often benefit from attempting to narrow down the possible options to a given examination question by eliminating options that they know are incorrect. In this particular question, a candidate should recognize that the answer cannot be option 4 since a rupture to an extensor tendon would result in an inability to extend and not to flex. Candidates who can use this type of pragmatic approach often achieve higher scores on the examination.

Exam One: Question 110

A physical therapist implements an aquatic program for a patient rehabilitating from a lower extremity injury. The program requires the patient to run in place using a flotation device while tethered to the side of the pool using an elastic cord. Which action would be the MOST appropriate to increase resistance?

1. increase the water temperature
2. **increase the speed of movement**
3. increase the depth of the water
4. remove the flotation device

Correct Answer: 2 (Ruoti p. 20)

The therapeutic effects of immersion in water relate to the principles of hydrodynamics and thermodynamics. Some of the more relevant concepts associated with these principles include density, specific gravity, hydrostatic pressure, buoyancy, and viscosity.

1. Changes in the water temperature can influence variables such as oxygen uptake, but would not significantly influence resistance.
2. **The viscosity of water provides resistance to a body in motion. Viscosity refers to the thickness or resistance to the flow of a liquid. The faster the relative speed of the body, the greater the magnitude of resistance.**
3. Increasing the depth of the water would not result in a significant change in resistance since the patient is using a flotation device and therefore their level of immersion would remain relatively constant.
4. Removal of the flotation device would likely increase resistance since the patient may tend to move faster without the flotation device, however, it remains less desirable than simply continuing to use the belt and increasing the speed of movement.

System Specific: Other Systems
Content Outline: Clinical Application of Foundational Sciences

Exam One: Question 111

A physical therapist measures passive forearm pronation and concludes that the results are within normal limits. Which measurement would be classified as within normal limits?

1. 60 degrees
2. **80 degrees**
3. 100 degrees
4. 120 degrees

> **Correct Answer: 2** (Norkin p. 375)

Physical therapists should possess a thorough understanding of normal range of motion at different joints in the body. When measuring forearm pronation the axis of the goniometer is placed lateral to the ulnar styloid process. The proximal arm of the goniometer should be aligned parallel to the anterior midline of the humerus and the distal arm should be on the dorsal aspect of the forearm, just proximal to the styloid processes of the radius and ulna.

1. A value of 60 degrees of forearm pronation would be considered hypomobile.
2. **According to the American Academy of Orthopedic Surgeons and the American Medical Association normal forearm pronation is 0-80 degrees.**
3. A value of 100 degrees of forearm pronation would be considered hypermobile.
4. A value of 120 degrees of forearm pronation would be considered extremely hypermobile and would be unlikely given the joint structure of the superior and inferior radioulnar joints.

System Specific: Musculoskeletal System
Content Outline: Examination

Test Taking Tip: There are sometimes small differences in reported ranges when using different academic sources. In the case of range of motion, acceptable academic sources may include groups such as the American Academy of Orthopedic Surgeons and the American Medical Association. Candidates must resist the urge to become too obsessive when reviewing this type of content and be confident that a scored examination question on the National Physical Therapy Examination would not require a candidate to differentiate between two acceptable sources.

Exam One: Question 112

A physical therapist discusses the importance of proper posture with a patient rehabilitating from back surgery at the L3-L4 spinal level. Which body position would place the MOST pressure on the lumbar spine?

1. standing in the anatomical position
2. standing with 45 degrees of hip flexion
3. **sitting in a chair slouching forward**
4. sitting in a chair with reduced lumbar lordosis

> **Correct Answer: 3** (Hertling p. 880)

A study by Nachemson examined intradiskal pressures in the lumbar spine (L3 disc) as they relate to specific body positions. The order of body positions from the lowest total load to the greatest total load is as follows: lying in supine, sidelying, standing in the anatomical position, standing with 45 degrees of hip flexion, sitting in a chair with reduced lumbar lordosis, and sitting in a chair slouching forward.

1. Standing in the anatomical position resulted in the total load being greater than the load associated with lying in supine or sidelying.
2. Standing with 45 degrees of hip flexion resulted in the total load being greater than the load associated with lying in supine, sidelying, and standing in the anatomical position.
3. **Sitting in a chair slouching forward resulted in the total load being greater than any of the other five body positions measured.**
4. Sitting in a chair with reduced lumbar lordosis had the greatest total load of the positions measured with the only exception being sitting in a chair slouching forward.

System Specific: Musculoskeletal System
Content Outline: Interventions

Exam One: Question 113

A physical therapist works on transfer activities with a patient diagnosed with a complete C5 spinal cord injury. Which of the following muscles would the patient be able to utilize during the training session?

1. **brachioradialis**
2. pronator teres
3. extensor carpi radialis brevis
4. latissimus dorsi

Correct Answer: 1 (Kendall p. 294)

A patient with C5 tetraplegia would be able to utilize muscles innervated at or above the C5 spinal level.

1. **The brachioradialis is innervated by the radial nerve (C5-C6) and acts to flex the elbow joint and assists in pronating and supinating the forearm when these movements are resisted.**
2. The pronator teres is innervated by the median nerve (C6-C7) and acts to pronate the forearm and assists in flexion of the elbow joint.
3. The extensor carpi radialis brevis is innervated by the radial nerve (C6, C7, C8) and acts to extend the wrist and assists in wrist abduction.
4. The latissimus dorsi is innervated by the thoracodorsal nerve (C6, C7, C8) and with the origin fixed acts to medially rotate, adduct, and extend the shoulder joint.

System Specific: Neuromuscular & Nervous Systems
Content Outline: Clinical Application of Foundational Sciences

Exam One: Question 114

A physical therapist treats a 32-year-old female diagnosed with thoracic outlet syndrome. While exercising the patient begins to complain of feeling lightheaded and dizzy. The therapist immediately ushers the patient to a nearby chair and begins to monitor her vital signs. The therapist measures the patient's respiration rate as 10 breaths per minute, pulse rate as 45 beats per minute, and blood pressure as 115/85 mm Hg. Which of the following statements is MOST accurate?

1. **pulse rate and respiration rate are below normal levels**
2. pulse rate and blood pressure are above normal levels
3. blood pressure and respiration rate are above normal levels
4. the patient's vital signs are within normal limits

Correct Answer: 1 (Pierson p. 61)

Normal range for pulse rate is 60-100 beats per minute for an adult, while respiration rate is 12-18 breaths per minute. Normal blood pressures are 100-140 mm Hg systolic and 60-90 mm Hg diastolic.

1. **A pulse of 45 beats per minute and a respiratory rate of 10 breaths per minute are below the normal range and can contribute to the patient's complaints.**
2. A pulse of 45 beats per minute is below the normal range and a blood pressure of 115/85 mm Hg is within the normal range.
3. A blood pressure of 115/85 mm Hg is within the normal range and a respiration rate of 10 breaths per minute is below the normal range.
4. Blood pressure is the only vital sign that is within normal limits. Pulse rate and respiration rate are below normal.

System Specific: Cardiac, Vascular, & Pulmonary Systems
Content Outline: Clinical Application of Foundational Sciences

Exam One: Question 115

A physical therapist works with a patient diagnosed with anterior cruciate ligament insufficiency. The physician referral specifies closed kinematic chain rehabilitation. Which exercise would NOT be appropriate based on the physician order?

1. exercise on a stair machine
2. limited squats to 45 degrees
3. walking backwards on a treadmill
4. **isokinetic knee extension and flexion**

> **Correct Answer: 4** (Dutton p. 956)

Closed-chain activities involve the body moving over a fixed distal segment. Closed-chain activities are often integrated into lower extremity strengthening programs. Open-chain activities involve the distal segment, usually the hand or foot, moving freely in space.

1. Exercising on a stair machine requires the patient to maintain contact with the stair mechanism with their feet which would maintain the lower extremity in a fixed position.
2. Limited squats to 45 degrees require the feet to stay in contact with the ground while the hips and knees are gradually flexed and the trunk remains erect.
3. Walking backwards on a treadmill, or retro-walking, requires the lower extremity to be in contact with the treadmill for the majority of the activity. As a result, the activity would be considered a form of closed-chain exercise.
4. **Isokinetic knee extension and flexion requires the distal segment to move freely in space, as a result the exercise is considered to be a form of open-chain exercise. Isokinetic contractions occur when a muscle is contracting at the same speed throughout the entire available range.**

System Specific: Musculoskeletal System
Content Outline: Interventions

Exam One: Question 116

A patient paralyzed from the waist down discusses accessibility issues with an employer in preparation for her return to work. The patient is concerned about her ability to navigate a wheelchair in certain areas of the building. What is the MINIMUM space required to turn 180 degrees in a standard wheelchair?

1. 32 inches
2. 48 inches
3. **60 inches**
4. 72 inches

> **Correct Answer: 3** (Physical Therapist's Clinical Companion p. 330)

The Americans with Disabilities Act was designed to provide a clear and comprehensive national mandate for the elimination of discrimination. Title III provides information on public accommodations including minimum accessibility standards.

1. Thirty-two inches is the minimum required width of a doorway for wheelchair clearance, however, this space would not be adequate to turn 180 degrees in a standard wheelchair.
2. Forty-eight inches would be 12 inches less than the minimum required space to turn 180 degrees in a standard wheelchair.
3. **Sixty inches is the minimum required width to turn 180 degrees in a standard wheelchair according to the Americans with Disabilities Act.**
4. Seventy-two inches would be adequate to turn 180 degrees in a standard wheelchair, however, this value exceeds the minimum required space by 12 inches.

System Specific: Non-Systems
Content Outline: Safety & Professional Roles; Teaching/Learning; Research

Exam One: Question 117

A patient is referred to physical therapy following surgery to repair a torn rotator cuff. The physician referral does not include post-operative guidelines and also does not classify the extent or size of the tear. The physical therapist's MOST appropriate action is to:

1. consult various medical resources that discuss physical therapy management of rotator cuff repairs
2. consult various protocols of other surgeons in the area
3. **contact the referring physician and discuss the patient's care**
4. discuss the patient's care with other staff members who are more experienced in treating rotator cuff repairs

Correct Answer: 3 (Criteria for Standards of Practice)

Physical therapists should consult with the referring physician when there is inadequate information available to direct the patient's plan of care. This is particularly important in surgical cases since there can be large variability in the post-operative management of even similar conditions.

1. Medical resources can serve to educate the therapist in regard to the specific injury and the typical management, however, would not offer specific insight on the patient's unique needs.
2. There are a variety of surgical approaches that can be used to repair a rotator cuff tear and in addition each tear is unique in terms of its location and magnitude. As a result, the protocols of other physicians may have little relevance to the rehabilitation needs of the patient.
3. **The physician would be the only individual who could provide the necessary level of specificity related to the surgical procedure and the associated rehabilitation parameters.**
4. Consulting with staff members may be helpful to draw on their expertise, however, does not provide the necessary clarification related to the patient's situation.

System Specific: Non-Systems
Content Outline: Safety & Professional Roles; Teaching/Learning; Research

Exam One: Question 118

A 52-year-old, self-referred male is examined in physical therapy. The patient states that over the last three months he has experienced increasing neck stiffness and pain at night. He also communicates that he recently had several episodes of dizziness. The patient has a family history of cancer and has smoked two packs of cigarettes a day for over twenty years. The date of his last medical examination was ten years ago. The physical therapist's MOST appropriate action is to:

1. treat the patient conservatively and document any changes in the patient's status
2. inform the patient that he is not a candidate for physical therapy
3. refer the patient to an oncologist
4. **refer the patient to his primary care physician**

Correct Answer: 4 (Magee p. 2)

Physical therapists must carefully screen patients for any potential signs or symptoms (i.e., "red flags") that indicate the need for physician referral.

1. Failure to recognize the need to refer a patient to a physician despite the presence of "red flags" can jeopardize patient safety and may be considered professional negligence.
2. There is ample evidence provided that indicates the patient is not presently a candidate for physical therapy. Although this is important to convey to the patient, the need to refer the patient to a physician based on the presence of "red flags" is a greater priority since it addresses a potential underlying pathology.
3. The physical therapist should not attempt to make a medical diagnosis and would therefore be better served to refer the patient to the primary care physician. The physician would likely examine the patient and order a variety of laboratory and diagnostic testing and if necessary refer the patient to other medical personnel.
4. **The self-referred patient offers a medical history that reveals several significant issues including episodes of dizziness, neck stiffness with pain at night, and a family history of cancer. Based on the history and the date of the last medical examination, the patient should be referred to a physician.**

System Specific: Other Systems
Content Outline: Foundations for Evaluation, Differential Diagnosis, & Prognosis

Exam One: Question 119

A physical therapist wearing sterile protective clothing establishes a sterile field prior to changing a dressing on a wound. Which area of the protective clothing would NOT be considered sterile even before coming in contact with a non-sterile object?

1. gloves
2. sleeves of the gown
3. front of the gown above waist level
4. **front of the gown below waist level**

> **Correct Answer: 4** (Pierson p. 299)

Once a sterile field has been established a physical therapist must be careful to maintain the sterile field and minimize any chance of contamination. The four rules of asepsis that a therapist should follow are: 1.) know which items are sterile, 2.) know which items are not sterile, 3.) separate sterile items from non-sterile items, 4.) if a sterile item becomes contaminated, the situation must be remedied immediately.

1. Gloves offer protection to the therapist's hands to reduce the likelihood of becoming infected with microorganisms and decrease the risk of the patient receiving microorganisms from the physical therapist. Sterile gloves are considered to be sterile after they are applied.
2. A gown is used to protect the therapist's clothing from being contaminated or soiled by a contaminant. The gown also reduces the probability of the physical therapist transmitting a microorganism from their clothing to the patient. The sleeves of a sterile gown are considered to be sterile after they are applied.
3. The front of the gown above the waist level is considered to be sterile after the gown is applied.
4. **The front of the gown below the waist level is not considered to be sterile after the gown is applied since there is an increased chance of incidental contact with a non-sterile object without the physical therapist's knowledge.**

System Specific: Non-Systems
Content Outline: Safety & Professional Roles; Teaching/Learning; Research

Exam One: Question 120

A physical therapist transports a patient with multiple sclerosis to the gym for her treatment session. The patient is wheelchair dependent and uses a urinary catheter. When transporting the patient, the MOST appropriate location to secure the collection bag is:

1. in the patient's lap
2. on the patient's lower abdomen
3. on the wheelchair armrest
4. **on the wheelchair cross brace beneath the seat**

> **Correct Answer: 4** (Pierson p. 290)

Urine drains into a collection bag as a result of the effect of gravity; therefore the collection bag from a urinary catheter must be positioned below the level of the bladder.

1. Securing the collection bag in the patient's lap would result in the collection bag being at a similar level as the patient's bladder. The position would interfere with virtually any activity that required movement.
2. The lower abdomen is above the level of the bladder and would also interfere with any movement. Additionally, the patient may be embarrassed or bothered by having the collection bag in such a visible location.
3. The wheelchair armrest is above the level of the bladder and therefore would impede the flow of urine into the collection bag.
4. **Positioning the collection bag on the cross brace beneath the seat will allow it to be below the level of the bladder and will minimize the possibility that the bag or tubing will be pulled or snagged.**

System Specific: Non-Systems
Content Outline: Equipment & Devices; Therapeutic Modalities

Exam One: Question 121

A physical therapist employed by a home health agency visits a patient status post total knee arthroplasty. The patient was discharged from the hospital yesterday and according to the medical record had an unremarkable recovery. The physician orders include the use of a continuous passive motion machine. The MOST appropriate rate of motion would be:

1. **2 cycles per minute**
2. 4 cycles per minute
3. 6 cycles per minute
4. 8 cycles per minute

Correct Answer: 1 (Kisner p. 61)

A continuous passive motion (CPM) machine is a mechanical device designed to provide continuous motion for a particular joint using a predetermined range and speed. The primary indication for CPM use is to improve range of motion that may have been impaired secondary to a surgical procedure. CPM can be used to prevent motion loss by inhibiting the formation of adhesions and contractures. CPM has been shown to accelerate healing, improve the orientation of collagen fibers, and inhibit edema formation. Any joint may be indicated for CPM use, however, the knee is the most common joint treated with CPM.

1. **A rate of two cycles per minute (one cycle = 30 seconds) typically allows the patient to tolerate the CPM without difficulty.**
2. A rate of four cycles per minute (one cycle = 15 seconds) represents a faster rate than is typically recommended. Faster rates are not usually tolerated as well primarily due to a patient's post-surgical status.
3. A rate of six cycles per minute (one cycle = 10 seconds) would not typically allow the patient to sufficiently relax and may result in protective muscle guarding.
4. A rate of eight cycles per minute (one cycle = 7.5 seconds) would be excessive and would likely result in the patient activating the stop button.

System Specific: Non-Systems
Content Outline: Equipment & Devices; Therapeutic Modalities

Exam One: Question 122

A physical therapist attempts to examine the extent of ataxia in a patient's upper extremities. The preferred method to examine and document ataxia is:

1. manual muscle test
2. sensory test for light touch
3. functional assessment of rolling in bed
4. **finger to nose**

Correct Answer: 4 (DeMyer p. 380)

Ataxia refers to the inability to perform coordinated movements usually as a result of cerebellar pathology. Ataxia can affect gait, patterns of movement, and posture. The condition increases the incidence of errors in the rate, rhythm, and timing of responses.

1. Manual muscle tests are utilized to assess the strength of a muscle or muscle group. Ataxia is not necessarily due to weakness, rather the loss of muscular coordination.
2. A sensory test for light touch determines perception of tactile touch input. The test area is lightly touched or stroked using a brush, cotton ball or tissue. Sensory testing assesses the ascending pathways of the spinal cord.
3. Functional assessment of rolling in bed tests the overall mobility and strength of a patient, but is not a specific test for ataxia.
4. **A finger to nose test requires the patient to perform coordinated and controlled voluntary movement. A patient with ataxia may have difficulty completing the activity in an accurate and fluid manner.**

System Specific: Neuromuscular & Nervous Systems
Content Outline: Examination

Exam One: Question 123

An eleven-month-old child with cerebral palsy attempts to maintain a quadruped position. Which reflex would interfere with this activity if it was NOT integrated?

1. Galant reflex
2. **symmetrical tonic neck reflex**
3. plantar grasp reflex
4. positive support reflex

Correct Answer: 2 (Ratliffe p. 26)

Primitive reflexes are reflexes which begin in utero or in early infancy. Most of these reflexes become integrated as the infant ages. Integration denotes that the reflex is no longer present when the stimulus is provided. Failure to integrate primitive reflexes can lead to impaired movement.

1. The Galant reflex is stimulated by stroking lateral to the spine. The response is lateral sidebending to the same side as the side of the stimulus. An infant would typically be able to maintain the quadruped position if this reflex was stimulated.

2. **Head positioning is the stimulus for the symmetrical tonic neck reflex. When the head is flexed, the upper extremities flex and the lower extremities extend. When the head extends the upper extremities extend and the lower extremities flex. The reaction of the extremities would not allow the infant to maintain a quadruped position.**

3. The plantar grasp reflex is stimulated by placing pressure on the ball of the foot, generally in standing. The response is for the toes to curl or flex. The reflex will have no impact on an infant's ability to maintain quadruped since the balls of the feet are not in contact with the floor.

4. The positive support reflex is stimulated by bearing weight through the feet. The response is for the lower extremities to extend, thereby allowing the infant to bear weight through the lower extremities. The reflex will have no impact on an infant's ability to maintain quadruped since they are not bearing weight through the feet.

System Specific: Neuromuscular & Nervous Systems
Content Outline: Interventions

Exam One: Question 124

A physical therapist attempts to schedule a patient for an additional therapy session after completing the examination. The physician referral indicates the patient is to be seen two times a week. The therapist suggests several possible times to the patient, but the patient insists she can only come in on Wednesday at 4:30. The therapist would like to accommodate the patient, but already has two patients scheduled at that time. The MOST appropriate action is to:

1. schedule the patient on Wednesday at 4:30
2. attempt to move one of the patients scheduled on Wednesday at 4:30 to a different time
3. **schedule the patient with another physical therapist on Wednesday at 4:30**
4. inform the referring physician the patient will only be seen once this week in therapy

Correct Answer: 3 (Guide for Professional Conduct)

The *Guide for Professional Conduct* published by the American Physical Therapy Association states that physical therapists shall respect the rights and dignity of all individuals. It is therefore necessary for the physical therapist to consider not only what is best for the patient in question, but also what is best for all of the patients being treated by the physical therapist.

1. Scheduling the patient on Wednesday at 4:30 will result in the physical therapist having three patients scheduled at the same time. It is unlikely that the physical therapist will be able to provide the requisite level of care for each patient given the number of patients.

2. Attempting to move a patient who is already scheduled to another appointment is not considerate of the patient's particular needs. It is the physical therapist's responsibility to ensure that each patient in their care is treated with the utmost respect.

3. **Scheduling with another physical therapist will allow the patient to be seen two times per week as indicated on the referral and will accommodate the patient's schedule.**

4. Informing the physician that the patient cannot be seen two times per week in physical therapy is not usually considered necessary information to communicate to the physician. When possible physical therapists should attempt to provide patients with the necessary frequency of physical therapy visits.

System Specific: Non-Systems
Content Outline: Safety & Professional Roles; Teaching/Learning; Research

Exam One: Question 125

While reading the Methods section of a research report, a physical therapist notes the investigators used a repeated measures design. This form of experimental design:

1. **controls for differences between subjects**
2. keeps the subjects "blind" to the identity of the treatment group
3. ensures that subjects with similar characteristics are assigned to different treatment groups
4. selects a homogenous group of subjects

Correct Answer: 1 (Portney p. 172)

Researchers may employ a number of design strategies to manipulate and control variables and measurements to strengthen the validity of their experiment and demonstrate a cause-and-effect relationship between the independent and dependent variables.

1. **In a repeated measures design all subjects experience all levels of the independent variable. This provides an efficient method for controlling differences between subjects because characteristics that may affect the outcomes, such as gender, age, physical characteristics, remain constant for each subject. Differences in outcomes can be attributed to the treatment. Since each subject acts as his own control, a repeated measures design is also called a within-subjects design.**
2. In its most complete form, blinding involves hiding the identity of group assignments from the subjects, from those who provide treatment, from those who measure the outcome variables, and from those who analyze the data. A repeated measures design may or may not include "blinding."
3. The design strategy that ensures that subjects with similar characteristics are assigned to different treatment groups is called matching. A repeated measures design may or may not include matching.
4. By selecting subjects who are homogeneous with respect to a specific trait, the researcher eliminates these traits as variables that may interfere with the dependent variable. A repeated measures design may or may not use homogeneous subjects.

System Specific: Non-Systems
Content Outline: Safety & Professional Roles; Teaching/Learning; Research

Exam One: Question 126

A physical therapist reviews the parameters of several pain modulation theories using transcutaneous electrical nerve stimulation (TENS). When comparing sensory stimulation to motor stimulation, sensory stimulation requires:

1. greater phase duration
2. **greater frequency**
3. stronger amplitude
4. shorter treatment time

Correct Answer: 2 (Cameron p. 218)

Motor stimulation requires sufficient phase charge to elicit a muscle contraction. This is accomplished by using a low frequency and long phase duration. Sensory stimulation, also called conventional TENS, requires a sufficient phase charge to achieve a sensory response, but is below the motor threshold. This is accomplished by using a high frequency and short phase duration.

1. Phase duration is shorter with sensory level stimulation compared to motor level stimulation.
2. **Frequency is significantly greater with sensory level stimulation compared to motor level stimulation.**
3. Sensory level stimulation requires lower amplitude than motor level stimulation.
4. Treatment time is highly variable with sensory and motor stimulation TENS.

System Specific: Non-Systems
Content Outline: Equipment & Devices; Therapeutic Modalities

Exam One: Question 127

A physical therapist performs an examination on a 27-year-old male diagnosed with iliotibial band syndrome. The patient is an avid distance runner who routinely ran between 45-60 miles per week before experiencing pain in his knee. Standing posture reveals a varus position at the knee and a cavus foot. When palpating the lateral portion of the lower extremity, which area would MOST likely exhibit marked tenderness?

1. **lateral femoral condyle**
2. lateral joint line
3. lateral tibial condyle
4. fibular head

> **Correct Answer: 1** (Hertling p. 535)

Iliotibial band syndrome is characterized by localized pain approximately two centimeters above the knee joint line over the lateral femoral condyle. The syndrome can be caused by activities requiring frequent flexion of the knee such as running or cycling which produce an inflammatory reaction.

1. **The iliotibial band is a thickened strip of fascia that extends from the iliac crest to the tibial tubercle. In iliotibial band syndrome there is excessive contact between the iliotibial band and the lateral femoral condyle usually when the knee is in approximately 30 degrees of flexion.**
2. Tenderness along the lateral joint line is more commonly associated with a meniscal injury.
3. The lateral tibial condyle is not typically painful since the irritation tends to be superior in the area of the lateral femoral condyle.
4. The fibular head is located on the lateral side of the knee at the approximate level of the tibial tubercle. The bony structure serves as the insertion for the biceps femoris muscle, but would not typically be involved with iliotibial band syndrome.

System Specific: Musculoskeletal System
Content Outline: Foundations for Evaluation, Differential Diagnosis, & Prognosis

Exam One: Question 128

The measurement of blood pressure with an aneroid sphygmomanometer is said to have concurrent validity if the pressures measured by the sphygmomanometer are equal to the pressures measured at the same time by:

1. an electrocardiogram
2. **a pressure transducer inserted in the artery**
3. a physician using a mercury sphygmomanometer
4. a pulse oximeter

> **Correct Answer: 2** (Portney p. 103)

Concurrent validity is demonstrated when the measurement to be validated and a "gold standard" are measured at relatively the same time so that they both reflect the same incident or behavior.

1. Since the electrocardiogram does not measure blood pressure, it could not provide evidence of the concurrent validity of a measurement of blood pressure.
2. **For blood pressure measured by an aneroid sphygmomanometer to have concurrent validity, the systolic and diastolic pressures would have to be similar to the pressures measured simultaneously by another instrument considered to be the "gold standard." A pressure transducer inserted in the patient's artery provides a direct and precise measurement of blood pressure.**
3. Like the aneroid sphygmomanometer, a mercury sphygmomanometer provides an indirect measure of blood pressure. The device would not be nearly as accurate as a pressure transducer inserted directly in the artery.
4. Since a pulse oximeter does not measure blood pressure, it could not provide evidence of the concurrent validity of a measurement of blood pressure.

System Specific: Non-Systems
Content Outline: Safety & Professional Roles; Teaching/Learning; Research

Exam One: Question 129

A physical therapist transfers a patient in a wheelchair down a curb with a forward approach. Which of the following actions would be the MOST appropriate?

1. have the patient lean forward
2. have the wheelchair brakes locked
3. **tilt the wheelchair backwards**
4. position yourself in front of the patient

Correct Answer: 3 (Pierson p. 158)

When descending a curb using a forward approach, the wheelchair must remain tipped backward until the rear wheels are in contact with the surface below the curb.

1. The patient would likely fall forward out of the wheelchair if the patient leans forward as the wheelchair's front casters are lowered down a curb. The patient must keep their center of mass back so that the wheelchair can descend without forward momentum.
2. The wheelchair brakes need to remain off so that the wheelchair can roll down the curb under the direction of the physical therapist. If the brakes are locked, the wheelchair will not be able to move forward down the curb.
3. **The physical therapist must be competent in tilting the wheelchair back as it descends so that the activity does not create an unnecessary safety risk. The physical therapist must provide caregivers with consistent instructions on how to safely ascend and descend a curb.**
4. If the physical therapist is positioned in front of the patient then they will not be able to tilt the wheelchair backwards or effectively manage the wheelchair as it rolls down the curb. The patient may also come forward towards the therapist since the front casters will touch the ground first and allow for forward momentum.

System Specific: Non-Systems
Content Outline: Equipment & Devices; Therapeutic Modalities

Exam One: Question 130

A physical therapist working on an oncology unit reviews the medical chart of a male patient prior to initiating airway clearance techniques. The patient's cell counts are as follows: hematocrit 44%, white blood cells 8,500/mm^3, platelets 30,000/μl, hemoglobin levels 15 gm/dL. Which blood test value suggests that chest percussion for airway clearance is contraindicated?

1. hematocrit
2. white blood cells
3. **platelets**
4. hemoglobin

Correct Answer: 3 (Paz p. 736)

Certain blood values may influence the physical therapist's choice of interventions and goals for the treatment session. The platelet value is significantly below the normal value and would therefore result in percussion being contraindicated.

1. The hematocrit is within the normal range of 39-49% in males.
2. White blood cell count is within the normal range of 4,500 – 11,000/mm^3.
3. **The platelet count is well below the normal range of 150,000 – 450,00/μl. With a platelet count of 50,000/μl or less, the patient is thrombocytopenic and would be placed on thrombocytopenic precautions until the platelet count returns to normal. These precautions include restricting chest percussion due to the increased risk of bleeding. Alternative chest physical therapy techniques may include coughing, deep breathing exercises, and using an incentive spirometer.**
4. The hemoglobin is within the normal range for males (14-18 gm/dL).

System Specific: Other Systems
Content Outline: Interventions

Exam One: Question 131

A physical therapist treats a patient with a fractured left hip. The patient is weight bearing as tolerated and uses a large base quad cane for gait activities. Correct use of the quad cane would include:

1. using the quad cane on the left with the longer legs positioned away from the patient
2. **using the quad cane on the right with the longer legs positioned away from the patient**
3. using the quad cane on the left with the longer legs positioned toward the patient
4. using the quad cane on the right with the longer legs positioned toward the patient

> **Correct Answer: 2** (Minor p. 352)

A quad cane should be utilized in the upper extremity that is opposite from the affected lower extremity. The device is designed so that the longer legs are positioned away from the patient.

1. The quad cane should be used in the hand opposite the affected lower extremity.
2. **The quad cane, positioned in the right hand with the longer legs pointing away from the patient, will allow for proper distribution of the weight during gait and as a result, the patient will be less likely to trip over the longer legs of the cane.**
3. The quad cane should be used in the hand opposite the affected lower extremity with the longer legs of the quad cane positioned away from the patient.
4. The quad cane should be used with the longer legs positioned away from the patient so that the patient does not trip over them.

System Specific: Non-Systems
Content Outline: Equipment & Devices; Therapeutic Modalities

Exam One: Question 132

A 66-year-old female is referred to physical therapy with rheumatoid arthritis. During the examination the physical therapist notes increased flexion at the proximal interphalangeal joints and hyperextension at the metacarpophalangeal and distal interphalangeal joints. This deformity is MOST representative of:

1. **Boutonniere deformity**
2. mallet finger
3. swan neck deformity
4. ulnar drift

> **Correct Answer: 1** (Magee p. 404)

There are a number of common hand and finger deformities that are often associated with specific medical diagnoses. Physical therapists should be familiar with the clinical presentation of these deformities. Boutonniere deformity, swan neck deformity, and ulnar drift are commonly observed in patients with rheumatoid arthritis.

1. **Boutonniere deformity is characterized by extension of the metacarpophalangeal and distal interphalangeal joints and flexion of the proximal interphalangeal joint. The deformity is caused by a rupture of the central tendinous slip of the extensor hood.**
2. Mallet finger is characterized by the distal phalanx of the finger resting in a flexed position. The deformity is caused by a rupture or avulsion of the extensor tendon.
3. Swan neck deformity is characterized by flexion at the distal interphalangeal joints and hyperextension of the proximal interphalangeal joints. The deformity is caused by a contraction of the intrinsic muscles or tearing of the volar plate.
4. Ulnar drift is characterized by ulnar deviation of the digits due to weakening of the capsuloligamentous structures of the metacarpophalangeal joints and the accompanying effect on the extensor communis tendons.

System Specific: Musculoskeletal System
Content Outline: Foundations for Evaluation, Differential Diagnosis, & Prognosis

Exam One: Question 133

A patient diagnosed with piriformis syndrome is referred to physical therapy for one visit for instruction in a home exercise program. After examining the patient, the physical therapist feels the patient's rehabilitation potential is excellent, but is concerned that one visit will not be sufficient to meet the patient's needs. The MOST appropriate action is to:

1. schedule the patient for treatment sessions as warranted by the results of the examination
2. explain to the patient that recent health care reforms have drastically reduced the frequency of physical therapy visits covered by third party payers
3. explain to the patient that she can continue with physical therapy beyond the initial session, but will be liable for all expenses not covered by her insurance
4. **contact the referring physician and request approval for additional physical therapy visits**

Correct Answer: 4 (Criteria for Standards of Practice)

A physical therapist has an ethical and legal obligation to act in the patient's best interest.

1. Scheduling the patient for treatment sessions based on the results of the examination is appropriate, however, the physical therapist should contact the referring physician and attempt to have the visits approved.
2. Health care reforms have, in many cases, limited the frequency of physical therapy visits covered by third party payers, however, there is no indication that the patient would not have coverage for the additional visits.
3. Patients should understand that they may be responsible for the cost of unreimbursed physical therapy services, however, the physical therapist should take the necessary steps to insure that the services are both necessary and authorized by the referring physician.
4. **The physical therapist will need to seek physician approval for the additional visits in order to be working under a physician referral. Although this does not guarantee that the visits will be approved by the physician or that the visits will be covered by the third party payer, it provides the therapist with the opportunity to act in the patient's best interest.**

System Specific: Non-Systems
Content Outline: Safety & Professional Roles; Teaching/Learning; Research

Exam One: Question 134

A physical therapist completes lower extremity range of motion activities with a patient status post spinal cord injury. While performing passive range of motion, the therapist notices that the patient's urine is extremely dark and has a distinctive foul smelling odor. Which of the following is the MOST appropriate action?

1. verbally report the observation to the patient's physician
2. verbally report the observation to the patient's nurse
3. **document and verbally report the observation to the patient's nurse**
4. document and verbally report the observation to the director of rehabilitation

Correct Answer: 3 (Pierson p. 290)

Physical therapists should report any abnormality in a patient's urine to the appropriate member of the health care team since this may indicate a change in the patient's medical status. Documentation of urine may include comments related to appearance (i.e., color, smell, quantity).

1. Verbally reporting the observation to a physician without also documenting the finding would be an incomplete response.
2. The nurse would be the most logical health care professional to initially receive this information, however, the option does not include documentation.
3. **The nurse is an appropriate member of the health care team to receive this information and it is necessary to document the findings.**
4. The director of rehabilitation is an administrative position within the health care organization and therefore would not typically be directly involved in the patient's care.

System Specific: Other Systems
Content Outline: Foundations for Evaluation, Differential Diagnosis, & Prognosis

Exam One: Question 135

A rehabilitation manager designs a system to monitor the productivity of the physical therapists. Which piece of data would be the LEAST beneficial to accomplish the manager's objective?

1. number of generated timed treatment units
2. **results of patient satisfaction survey data**
3. total hours of direct patient treatment time
4. number of regular payroll hours

> **Correct Answer: 2** (Nosse p. 421)

Productivity is a term used to describe the efficiency of a given worker or group of workers. Productivity standards are used as performance targets to help direct management and staff. The established standards should be based on a measurable unit of output (e.g., billable units), objectively measured, understandable, and achievable.

1. The number of generated timed treatment units is most often expressed in 15 minute intervals and is necessary in order to determine the productivity of physical therapists.
2. **The results of patient satisfaction data would be considered a qualitative measure describing the general satisfaction of patients with selected aspects of the physical therapy services. Items commonly explored in this type of survey include direct patient care activities, staffing, environment, scheduling, hours of operation, and parking. Although measures of quality are often examined concurrently with productivity, they are not used to determine productivity.**
3. The total hours of direct patient treatment time is often compared to the number of generated timed treatment units.
4. The number of regular payroll hours is necessary to determine full-time equivalents. This measure is most often used to examine staffing patterns or staffing needs.

System Specific: Non-Systems
Content Outline: Safety & Professional Roles; Teaching/Learning; Research

Exam One: Question 136

A physical therapist observing a patient complete a leg curl exercise notices two prominent tendons visible on the posterior surface of the patient's left knee. The visible tendons are MOST likely associated with the:

1. semimembranosus and semitendinosus muscles
2. **semitendinosus and biceps femoris muscles**
3. popliteus and semitendinosus muscles
4. semimembranosus and biceps femoris muscles

> **Correct Answer: 2** (Kendall p. 418)

The hamstrings muscles include the semitendinosus, semimembranosus, and biceps femoris. The muscles primary action is to flex the knee. As a result, the tendons of each of the hamstrings muscles become more prominent with resisted knee flexion.

1. The semimembranosus and semitendinosus are hamstrings muscles that act to flex the knee joint, however, they are both located on the medial aspect of the posterior knee joint. The image shows two tendons, one that is located on the medial aspect of the posterior surface of the knee joint and the other on the lateral aspect.
2. **The semitendinosus and biceps femoris are hamstrings muscles whose tendons become prominent when performing a leg curl. The biceps femoris is the lateral tendon, while the semitendinosus is the medial tendon.**
3. The popliteus muscle is located deep within the posterior surface of the knee joint and would not appear as a tendinous cord-like structure. The semitendinosus is a medial hamstrings muscle that would be prominent on the medial aspect of the posterior surface of the knee joint.
4. The semimembranosus muscle is a medial hamstrings muscle, however, the muscle's tendon is not nearly as prominent as the semitendinosus. The biceps femoris is a lateral hamstrings muscle that would be prominent on the lateral aspect of the posterior surface of the knee joint.

System Specific: Musculoskeletal System
Content Outline: Clinical Application of Foundational Sciences

Exam One: Question 137

A physical therapist prepares to apply a hot pack to the low back of a patient diagnosed with degenerative disk disease. When examining the patient the therapist identifies several blisters on the patient's right side. The patient indicates they were caused by heat from a hot pack applied during the previous treatment session. The patient indicates he was hesitant to tell the therapist that the heat was too intense. The MOST appropriate therapist action is to:

1. **complete an incident report**
2. contact the referring physician
3. modify the documentation from the previous treatment session
4. avoid documenting the event since it occurred during the previous treatment session

Correct Answer: 1 (Scott - Promoting Legal and Ethical Awareness p. 81)

An incident report is a factual written summary of an adverse event designed to memorialize specific details of the event and to limit future liability of the organization. Information obtained from the incident report is often used to guide risk management initiatives.

1. **The physical therapist must complete the incident report since they directly observed the blistered skin and heard the patient relate the cause of the burn to the hot pack.**
2. The referring physician may be informed of the event, however, the need to complete the incident report would be a higher priority given the described scenario.
3. Modifying documentation from a previous treatment session is not acceptable and would be considered a fraudulent act.
4. The patient's revelation to the therapist is important information to document despite the fact that the activity in question occurred during the previous treatment session. The therapist should document the objective findings (i.e., blisters) and the patient's claim that the blisters were caused by heat from the hot pack.

System Specific: Non-Systems
Content Outline: Safety & Professional Roles; Teaching/Learning; Research

Exam One: Question 138

A physical therapist attempts to calculate the target heart rate range for a 32-year-old female with no significant past medical history. The patient's resting heart rate is recorded as 60 beats per minute and the maximal heart rate is 180 beats per minute. Using the heart rate reserve method (Karvonen formula) the patient's target heart rate range should be recorded as:

1. 96 - 120 beats per minute
2. **132 - 156 beats per minute**
3. 144 - 174 beats per minute
4. 164 - 185 beats per minute

Correct Answer: 2 (American College of Sports Medicine p. 455)

There are a number of formulas used to prescribe exercise intensity based on heart rate. The HR reserve method, also known as the Karvonen method, uses resting heart rate subtracted from the maximal heart rate to obtain the heart rate reserve. Adding 60% and 80% of the heart rate reserve to resting heart rate results in the target heart rate range.

Target heart rate range = $[(HR_{max} - HR_{rest}) *0.60$ and $0.80] + HR_{rest}$

1. 96 - 120 beats per minute is less than the target heart rate range calculated using the Karvonen formula and the patient's maximal and resting heart rates.
2. **Target heart rate range = [(180 – 60) * 0.60 and 0.80] + 60**
   = [120*0.60 and 120*0.80] + 60
   = (72 + 60) and (96 + 60)
   = 132 - 156 beats per minute
3. 144 - 174 beats per minute overlaps with a portion of the target heart rate range calculated from the Karvonen formula and the patient's maximal and resting heart rates, but is too high at the lower and upper ends.
4. 164 - 185 beats per minute is more than the target heart rate range calculated using the Karvonen formula and the patient's maximal and resting heart rates.

System Specific: Cardiac, Vascular, & Pulmonary Systems
Content Outline: Interventions

Exam One: Question 139

A 47-year-old patient with a diagnosis of CVA with left hemiplegia is referred for orthotic examination. Significant results of manual muscle testing include: hip flexion 3+/5, hip extension 3/5, knee flexion 3+/5, knee extension 3+/5, ankle dorsiflexion 2/5, and ankle inversion and eversion 1/5. Sensation is intact and no abnormal tone is noted. The MOST appropriate orthosis for this patient is a:

1. knee-ankle-foot orthosis with a locked knee
2. **plastic articulating ankle-foot orthosis**
3. metal upright ankle-foot orthosis locked in neutral
4. prefabricated posterior leaf spring orthosis

> **Correct Answer: 2** (Seymour p. 381)

The goal of an orthotic is to correct abnormal movement patterns and improve function using the least amount of intervention. A plastic ankle-foot orthosis (AFO) with an articulating ankle joint is the most appropriate orthotic based on the patient's strength, sensation and tone.

1. A knee-ankle-foot orthosis (KAFO) with a locked knee would be most appropriate for a patient that had no voluntary knee control. The locked knee ensures that the knee joint remains in an extended position and avoids genu recurvatum or collapsing of the knee during stance phase.
2. **The patient's strength at the hip and knee allows for an ankle-foot orthosis (AFO) to be used. A plastic AFO is appropriate since there is intact sensation and an articulating ankle joint is recommended to improve biomechanics during gait since there is an absence of tonal abnormalities.**
3. A metal upright AFO is normally prescribed for a patient that has fluctuating tone and/or a sensory deficit. An AFO may be locked in neutral at the ankle joint if an increase in tone exists or in the absence of voluntary motion.
4. A posterior leaf spring orthosis provides a dorsiflexion assist during gait. This type of AFO provides a spring-like dorsiflexion assist during terminal stance. Since the trim lines are posterior to the malleoli, dorsiflexion and plantar flexion can still occur during gait. The posterior leaf spring orthosis would not offer enough stability for the patient.

System Specific: Non-Systems
Content Outline: Equipment & Devices; Therapeutic Modalities

Exam One: Question 140

A physical therapist treats a patient diagnosed with Parkinson's disease. When working on controlled mobility, which of the following would BEST describe the physical therapist's objective?

1. facilitate postural muscle control
2. **promote weight shifting and rotational trunk control**
3. emphasize reciprocal extremity movement
4. facilitate tone and rigidity

> **Correct Answer: 2** (O'Sullivan p. 246)

Controlled mobility activities should emphasize weight shifting and trunk control with rotation. This type of activity may serve to decrease rigidity and improve the fluidity of gait in a patient with Parkinson's disease. Controlled mobility training is beneficial to all patient populations.

1. When a therapist facilitates postural muscle control through approximation, tapping or other facilitation techniques, the goal is to improve the overall postural stability of the patient.
2. **Controlled mobility is the ability to move within a weight bearing position or rotate around a long axis. Activities that promote weight shifting and rotational trunk control are examples of controlled mobility.**
3. Coordination training will often focus on reciprocal extremity movement in order to enhance the ability of a patient to reverse movement between opposing muscle groups.
4. A therapist may facilitate tone in a patient with hypotonia, but would not facilitate tone in a patient that presents with hypertonia or rigidity.

System Specific: Neuromuscular & Nervous Systems
Content Outline: Interventions

Exam One: Question 141

A physical therapist reviews the medical chart of a patient with a history of recurrent dysrhythmias. The therapist is concerned about the patient's past medical history and would like to monitor the patient during selected formal exercise activities. Which of the following monitoring devices would be the MOST beneficial?

1. pulmonary artery catheter
2. **electrocardiogram**
3. intracranial pressure monitor
4. pulse oximeter

Correct Answer: 2 (Hillegass p. 380)

An electrocardiogram (ECG) is a recording of the electrical activity of the heart over time produced by an electrocardiograph, usually via skin electrodes. It is a common monitoring device for patients with known or suspected cardiac abnormalities.

1. A pulmonary artery catheter monitors cardiovascular pressures in the pulmonary artery.
2. **The electrocardiogram provides a graphic record of the electrical activity of the heart at rest or during exercise. Dysrhythmia is a general term used to denote disturbances in the heart's rhythm, which are best monitored by an electrocardiogram.**
3. An intracranial pressure monitor consists of a small plastic tube usually inserted in the left or right anterior portion of the brain. The monitor is often used to assess the pressure surrounding the brain of patients in the intensive care unit who have sustained head trauma, brain hemorrhage, brain surgery or conditions in which the brain may swell.
4. A pulse oximeter is an instrument that uses a light-emitting diode, a photodiode signal detector, and a microprocessor to determine the percentage of oxygen saturation of arterial blood.

System Specific: Cardiac, Vascular, & Pulmonary Systems
Content Outline: Foundations for Evaluation, Differential Diagnosis, & Prognosis

Exam One: Question 142

A physical therapist observes a change in the muscle tone of an infant's extremities as a result of head rotation. Which developmental reflex would facilitate this type of response?

1. **asymmetrical tonic neck reflex**
2. symmetrical tonic neck reflex
3. symmetrical tonic labyrinthine reflex
4. crossed extension reflex

Correct Answer: 1 (Ratliffe p. 26)

Primitive and tonic reflexes are normally present during infancy and gradually are integrated throughout early development by the central nervous system. Physical therapists should be familiar with the stimulus, response, and age of integration of common pediatric reflexes.

1. **The asymmetrical tonic neck reflex normally occurs in infants from birth to 6 months of age when the head is rotated to one side. This reflex causes extension of the extremity toward the side of rotation.**
2. The symmetrical tonic neck reflex normally occurs in infants from 6 to 8 months of age and is fully integrated by 8 to 12 months of age. It is stimulated by placing the head in either flexion or extension. When the head is in flexion, the upper extremities will flex while the lower extremities extend. When the head is extended, the upper extremities will extend while the lower extremities flex.
3. The symmetrical tonic labyrinthine reflex normally occurs at birth and is fully integrated by 6 months of age. It is stimulated by placing the infant in either prone or supine. When in the prone position, the body and extremities exhibit increased flexor tone and are held in flexion; in supine, the body and extremities exhibit increased extensor tone and are held in extension.
4. The crossed extension reflex normally occurs at 28 weeks gestation and is fully integrated by 1-2 months of age. The reflex is stimulated by a noxious stimulus to the ball of the foot, while the lower extremity is fixed in extension. This will elicit a response of the opposite lower extremity in which it will flex, then adduct and extend.

System Specific: Neuromuscular & Nervous Systems
Content Outline: Interventions

Exam One: Question 143

A physical therapy program designs a study that uses performance on the Scholastic Aptitude Test as a predictor of grade point average in a physical therapy academic program. The results of the study identify that the overall correlation between the variables is r =.87. Which statement is MOST accurate based on the results of the study?

1. A high grade point average in a physical therapy program is caused by a high score on the Scholastic Aptitude Test.
2. **Students in a physical therapy program with high scores on the Scholastic Aptitude Test tend to have high grade point averages.**
3. There is no relationship between grade point average in a physical therapy program and performance on the Scholastic Aptitude Test.
4. There is an inverse relationship between grade point average in a physical therapy program and performance on the Scholastic Aptitude Test.

Correct Answer: 2 (Portney p. 525)

Correlation coefficients quantitatively describe the strength and magnitude of the relationship between two variables. The symbol "r" denotes the Pearson product-moment correlation coefficient, which is used to evaluate the strength and direction of the linear relationship between two continuous variables on the interval or ratio scales. The Pearson "r" can take values ranging from -1.00 (a perfect negative relationship) to 1.00 (a perfect positive relationship).

1. Correlation does not imply a causal relationship between two variables. A strong relationship between X and Y does not suggest that X causes Y or that Y causes X. Therefore, it cannot be said that the r = 0.87 suggests that a high score on the Scholastic Aptitude Test causes a high grade point average.
2. **A r = 0.87 indicates a good to excellent relationship between the Scholastic Aptitude Test (SAT) and grade point average (GPA). That is, low scores on the SAT tend to be associated with low GPAs and high scores on the SAT tend to be associated with high GPAs.**
3. No relationship between grade point average and performance on the Scholastic Aptitude Test would be indicated by an r = 0.0.
4. A r = 0.87 indicates a positive or direct relationship between grade point average in a physical therapy program and performance on the Scholastic Aptitude Test. A negative correlation coefficient would indicate an inverse relationship.

System Specific: Non-Systems
Content Outline: Safety & Professional Roles; Teaching/Learning; Research

Exam One: Question 144

A patient is referred to physical therapy with a C6 nerve root injury. Which of the following clinical findings would NOT be expected with this type of injury?

1. diminished sensation on the anterior arm and the index finger
2. weakness in the biceps and supinator
3. diminished brachioradialis reflex
4. **paresthesias of the long and ring fingers**

Correct Answer: 4 (Magee p. 22)

Involvement of a specific nerve root often results in predictable impairments including diminished sensation, muscle weakness, impaired reflexes, and paresthesias.

1. Diminished sensation on the anterior arm and index finger is characteristic of a C6 nerve root injury and is assessed using light touch from a cotton ball.
2. Weakness in the biceps and supinator muscles is characteristic of a C6 nerve root injury and is assessed through resistive testing as part of an upper quarter screening examination and/or specific manual muscle testing.
3. A diminished brachioradialis reflex is characteristic of a C6 nerve root injury and is assessed by striking the blunt end of a reflex hammer at the distal end of the radius with the patient's elbow flexed to 90 degrees and the upper extremity supported by the therapist.
4. **Paresthesias of the long and ring fingers are commonly associated with the C7 nerve root. Other findings of a C7 nerve root injury include weakness of the triceps and wrist flexors, and a diminished triceps reflex.**

System Specific: Neuromuscular & Nervous Systems
Content Outline: Clinical Application of Foundational Sciences

Exam One: Question 145

A 22-year-old male status post traumatic brain injury receives physical therapy services in a rehabilitation hospital. The patient is presently functioning at Rancho Los Amigos level VI. The patient has progressed well in therapy, however, has been bothered by diplopia. Which treatment strategy would be the MOST appropriate to address diplopia?

1. provide non-verbal instructions within the patient's direct line of sight
2. **place a patch over one of the patient's eyes**
3. ask the patient to turn his head to one side when he experiences diplopia
4. instruct the patient to carefully focus on a single object

Correct Answer: 2 (O'Sullivan p. 1159)

Diplopia refers to double vision resulting from defective function of the extraocular muscles that is typically caused by damage to the brain. A patient with diplopia is often instructed to wear a patch alternately over one of their eyes. Specific strengthening exercises of the extraocular muscles can serve to improve the patient's vision.

1. Verbal instruction is often more desirable than non-verbal instruction since double vision would tend to minimize the effectiveness of non-verbal instruction.
2. **A patient with diplopia will actually see two sets of the environment. If wearing the patch over the alternate eye does not resolve the problem, the patient may require prism glasses.**
3. The patient will not alleviate diplopia through positioning of the head. Double vision can result from damage to the brain and requires strengthening and the use of an eye patch.
4. A patient with diplopia can use the extraocular muscles of each eye, but they are not in focus. Verbal cueing to "focus" on a single object will not alleviate diplopia since strengthening is required.

System Specific: Neuromuscular & Nervous Systems
Content Outline: Interventions

Exam One: Question 146

A physical therapist completes an upper extremity manual muscle test on a patient diagnosed with rotator cuff tendonitis. Assuming the patient has the ability to move the upper extremities against gravity, which of the following muscles would NOT be tested with the patient in a supine position?

1. pronator teres
2. pectoralis major
3. biceps brachii
4. **middle trapezius**

Correct Answer: 4 (Kendall p. 329)

The middle fibers of the trapezius originate on the spinous processes of the first through fifth thoracic vertebrae and insert on the medial margin of the acromion and superior lip of the spine of the scapula. The muscle is innervated by the spinal accessory nerve and ventral ramus C2, C3, C4.

1. The pronator teres is tested in a supine position. The test arm is positioned with forearm pronation and partial elbow flexion. The therapist provides pressure at the lower forearm in the direction of forearm supination.
2. The pectoralis major is tested with the patient in a supine position. The test arm is flexed to 90 degrees at the shoulder with slight medial rotation and elbow extension. Pressure is applied against the forearm in the direction of horizontal abduction.
3. The biceps brachii is tested with the patient in a supine position. The test arm is flexed at the elbow to 90 degrees with supination of the forearm. The therapist provides pressure at the distal end of the forearm in the direction of forearm pronation.
4. **The middle trapezius is tested with the patient in a prone position. The test arm is abducted at the shoulder to 90 degrees with lateral rotation and elbow extension. The therapist provides pressure against the forearm in a downward direction.**

System Specific: Musculoskeletal System
Content Outline: Examination

Exam One: Question 147

A physical therapist prepares a patient education program for an individual with chronic venous insufficiency. Which of the following would NOT be appropriate to include in the patient education program?

1. wear shoes that accommodate to the size and shape of your feet
2. observe your skin daily for breakdown
3. **wear your compression stockings only at night**
4. keep your feet elevated as much as possible throughout the day

> **Correct Answer: 3** (Kisner p. 833)

Chronic venous insufficiency is a common disorder of the lower extremity veins in which the veins do not work properly and blood pools in the lower extremities, leading to increased pressure within the veins. If uncontrolled, fluid may leak into the surrounding tissues in the ankles and feet and may eventually cause skin breakdown and ulceration.

1. Wearing shoes that accommodate to the size and shape of the foot is an important component of an education program for a patient with venous insufficiency. Successful implementation of the program reduces the risk of skin abrasions, ulcerations, and wound infections.
2. Swelling, cellulitis, and chronic lower extremity ulcers are common complications of venous insufficiency. Daily observation of the skin is a necessary component of an education program for a patient with venous insufficiency.
3. **Patients with chronic venous insufficiency often wear graduated compression stockings which attempt to improve circulation by preventing backward flow through the veins of the lower extremities. It is recommended that compression stockings are applied in the morning, since swelling is usually minimal in the morning and left on during the day for activity such as ambulation, to promote blood flow to the heart and avoid venous stasis.**
4. Elevating the feet throughout the day reduces pressure in the lower extremity veins and helps to improve blood flow. Positioning guidelines would be part of an education program for a patient with venous insufficiency.

System Specific: Cardiac, Vascular, & Pulmonary Systems
Content Outline: Interventions

Exam One: Question 148

A physical therapist determines that a patient rehabilitating from ankle surgery has consistent difficulty with functional activities that emphasize the frontal plane. Which of the following would be the MOST difficult for the patient?

1. anterior lunge
2. **six-inch lateral step down**
3. six-inch posterior step up
4. eight-inch posterior step down

> **Correct Answer: 2** (Norkin p. 4)

The frontal plane divides the body into front and back halves. Movements in the frontal plane occur as side to side movements such as abduction or adduction. Rotary motion in the frontal plane occurs around an anterior-posterior axis.

1. An anterior lunge would require the patient to perform hip flexion and extension (returning from the lunged position) which are sagittal plane motions.
2. **A lateral step-down would require the patient to perform hip abduction and adduction which are frontal plane motions.**
3. A posterior step up would require the patient to perform hip flexion and extension which are sagittal plane motions.
4. The posterior step down, regardless of the height of the step, would require the patient to perform hip flexion and extension which are sagittal plane motions.

System Specific: Musculoskeletal System
Content Outline: Interventions

Test Taking Tip: On occasion a candidate has the ability to identify the correct answer to an examination question without possessing the requisite academic knowledge. In this question, the candidate may have noticed that options 1, 3, and 4 are motions that would occur in the same plane. The candidate may be unsure of the actual plane, however, recognizes that since the plane of movement would be the same in each instance, the options mutually exclude each other from being the correct answer. This is an example of using deductive reasoning strategies to eliminate one or more options. It is important to emphasize that deductive reasoning strategies should only be utilized when a candidate does not possess the necessary academic knowledge to answer the question.

Exam One: Question 149

A patient rehabilitating from a radial head fracture is examined in physical therapy. During the examination, the physical therapist notes that the patient appears to have an elbow flexion contracture. Which of the following would NOT serve as an appropriate active exercise technique to increase range of motion?

1. contract-relax
2. hold-relax
3. **maintained pressure**
4. rhythmic stabilization

> **Correct Answer: 3** (Sullivan p. 64)

Maintained pressure is an effective technique that can be used to increase range of motion by facilitating local muscle relaxation, however, it is a passive technique.

1. Contract-relax is a technique used to increase range of motion. As the extremity reaches the point of limitation, the patient performs a maximal contraction of the antagonistic muscle group. The therapist resists movement for eight to ten seconds with relaxation to follow. The technique should be repeated until no further gains in range of motion are noted.
2. Hold-relax is an isometric contraction used to increase range of motion. The contraction is facilitated at the limiting point in the range of motion. Relaxation occurs and the extremity moves through the newly acquired range to the next point of limitation until no further increases in range of motion occur.
3. **Maintained pressure over the belly or tendon of a muscle can produce a calming effect and create relaxation of the musculotendinous unit. The effects of pressure are immediate, with little evidence of long-term effects.**
4. Rhythmic stabilization is a technique used to increase range of motion and coordinate isometric contractions. The technique requires isometric contractions of all muscles around a joint against progressive resistance. The patient should relax and move into the newly acquired range and repeat the technique.

System Specific: Musculoskeletal System
Content Outline: Interventions

Exam One: Question 150

A patient with a lengthy medical history of cardiac pathology is referred to a phase II cardiac rehabilitation program. During the first session the physical therapist prepares to measure the patient's blood pressure by inflating the cuff 20 mm Hg above the patient's estimated systolic value. Which of the following values describes the MOST appropriate rate to release the pressure when obtaining the blood pressure measurement?

1. **2-3 mm Hg per second**
2. 3-5 mm Hg per second
3. 5-7 mm Hg per second
4. 8-10 mm Hg per second

> **Correct Answer: 1** (Pierson p. 63)

Deflating the cuff at a rate of 2-3 mm Hg per second is recommended to enable the physical therapist to identify normal Korotkoff's sounds and obtain a valid measure of the patient's blood pressure. Rates faster than 2-3 mm Hg will tend to increase the measurement error.

1. **After inflating the cuff to 20 mm Hg above the estimated systolic pressure, the therapist should carefully unscrew (open) the valve and deflate the bladder no more than 2-3 mm per second while listening for the Korotkoff's sounds.**
2. 3-5 mm Hg per second is faster than the recommended rate of 2-3 mm Hg per second.
3. 5-7 mm Hg per second is more than twice as fast as the recommended rate of 2-3 mm Hg per second.
4. 8-10 mm Hg per second is more than three times as fast as the recommended rate of 2-3 mm Hg per second.

System Specific: Cardiac, Vascular, & Pulmonary Systems
Content Outline: Examination

Exam One: Question 151

A physical therapist examines a patient who complains of occasional difficulty maintaining her balance when walking and frequent episodes of vertigo. The MOST likely cause of the patient's difficulty is a disorder of the:

1. visual system
2. somatosensory system
3. auditory system
4. **vestibular system**

> **Correct Answer: 4** (Goodman - Pathology p. 1566)

Vestibular disorders are extremely common in clinical practice and it is estimated that up to five percent of the population in the United States experience some type of dizziness.

1. The visual system allows individuals to perceive movement and detect the relative orientation of the body in space.
2. The somatosensory system provides information about the relative orientation and movement of the body in relation to a supporting surface.
3. The auditory system is the sensory system associated with hearing. The auditory system is highly involved in vestibular functions and as a result, anything that disrupts auditory information can also affect vestibular functioning.
4. **The vestibular system reports information to the brain regarding the position and movement of the head with respect to gravity and inertia. Abnormalities of the vestibular system result in dizziness and impaired balance.**

System Specific: Neuromuscular & Nervous Systems
Content Outline: Clinical Application of Foundational Sciences

Exam One: Question 152

As a component of a cognitive assessment, a physical therapist asks a patient to count from one to twenty-five by increments of three. Which cognitive function does this task MOST accurately assess?

1. **attention**
2. constructional ability
3. abstract ability
4. orientation

> **Correct Answer: 1** (O'Sullivan p. 230)

Attention is defined as the capacity of the brain to process information from the environment or from long-term memory. The complexity and familiarity of the task determines the degree of attention required to complete the task.

1. **Attention can be assessed by asking a patient to count from one to twenty-five by increments of three. The task should be relatively easy for most individuals, however, it requires the person to exert a sustained, consistent effort. Attention deficits are common with many neurological disorders including brain injury, stroke, and dementia.**
2. Constructional ability can be assessed by asking a person to copy figures consisting of varying sizes and shapes or to draw a known item such as a clock.
3. Abstract ability can be assessed by asking a person to interpret a common proverb or to describe similarities or differences between two objects.
4. Orientation can be assessed by asking a person to identify time (e.g., day, month, season), person (e.g., name), and place (e.g., city, state).

System Specific: Neuromuscular & Nervous Systems
Content Outline: Examination

Exam One: Question 153

An 86-year-old female is partial weight bearing on the left lower extremity after a total hip arthroplasty. Her upper extremity strength is 3+/5 and she resides alone. Which assistive device would be the MOST appropriate for the patient?

1. Lofstrand crutches
2. axillary crutches
3. large base quad cane
4. **walker**

Correct Answer: 4 (Pierson p. 219)

A physical therapist must select an assistive device based on the patient's weight bearing status and their abilities and limitations. The patient's post-operative status, age, and limited upper extremity strength make it important that the selected device offer adequate stability without relying too heavily on upper extremity strength.

1. Lofstrand crutches or forearm crutches allow altered levels of weight bearing. The patient, however, would not have the upper extremity strength and stability necessary to use the device.
2. Axillary crutches can be used with all levels of weight bearing, however, offer limited stability and require significantly more coordination than a walker.
3. A large base quad cane is a type of straight cane that has a broad base positioned on four short posts. The device provides a larger base of stability than a straight cane, however, does not allow for partial weight bearing.
4. **A walker provides the patient with the necessary stability without relying on significant upper extremity strength. The walker allows for varying degrees of weight bearing on the involved lower extremity.**

System Specific: Non-Systems
Content Outline: Equipment & Devices; Therapeutic Modalities

Exam One: Question 154

A patient with a suspected scaphoid fracture is referred to physical therapy. Which clinical sign is MOST indicative of a scaphoid fracture?

1. localized edema along the dorsum of the hand
2. crepitus with active range of motion
3. **localized bony tenderness in the anatomic snuff box**
4. pain with resisted wrist extension

Correct Answer: 3 (Hertling p. 425)

The scaphoid links the proximal and distal carpal rows and helps provide stability to the wrist. A scaphoid fracture can occur as a result of a fall on an outstretched hand. This injury can be serious due to the potential for avascular necrosis. The fracture is usually treated with prolonged immobilization of the wrist and thumb.

1. Localized edema would be commonly associated with a scaphoid fracture, however, since edema is associated with a multitude of injuries to the wrist and hand it does not necessarily provide direct evidence of a scaphoid fracture. Small amounts of edema in this area may minimize the concavity of the anatomic snuffbox.
2. Crepitus refers to a grinding, crackling or popping noise often associated with cartilage loss or degeneration. Crepitus with active range of motion cannot easily be localized to a specific bony structure in the wrist and hand.
3. **The anatomic snuff box is located between the tendons of the extensor pollicis longus and extensor pollicis brevis. The scaphoid bone can be palpated inside the snuff box. Tenderness of the scaphoid bone upon palpation is often associated with a fracture.**
4. The primary muscles that extend the wrist do not insert on the scaphoid and as a result, pain with resisted wrist extension is not typically associated with a scaphoid fracture.

System Specific: Musculoskeletal System
Content Outline: Foundations for Evaluation, Differential Diagnosis, & Prognosis

Exam One: Question 155

A patient on prolonged bed rest attempts to get out of bed. Upon attaining a standing position the patient complains of lightheadedness and blurred vision. The MOST appropriate explanation is:

1. **decrease in blood pressure**
2. decrease in respiratory rate
3. increase in pulse rate
4. adverse reaction to medication

> **Correct Answer: 1** (Pierson p. 337)

Lightheadedness and blurred vision are signs of decreased cerebral blood flow due to a drop in blood pressure. This often occurs when patients who have been on prolonged bed rest assume an upright position.

1. **Orthostatic hypotension refers to a decrease in blood pressure that often occurs in patients on prolonged bed rest when attempting to achieve an upright position.**
2. A decrease in respiratory rate is not associated with changes in position or symptoms of lightheadedness and blurred vision.
3. Although pulse rate may increase slightly when a patient on bed rest attempts to get out of bed, the relative magnitude of the change would not typically cause symptoms of lightheadedness and blurred vision.
4. There are a variety of medications that can cause lightheadedness or blurred vision, however, the described patient scenario (i.e., patient on extended bed rest, attaining a standing position) provides a more compelling case for the presented symptoms being caused by the decrease in blood pressure.

System Specific: Cardiac, Vascular, & Pulmonary Systems
Content Outline: Interventions

Exam One: Question 156

A patient's job requires him to move boxes weighing 35 pounds from a transport cart to an elevated conveyor belt. The patient can complete the activity, however, is unable to prevent hyperextension of the spine. The MOST appropriate physical therapist action is:

1. implement a pelvic stabilization program
2. design an abdominal strengthening program
3. review proper body mechanics
4. **use an elevated platform when placing boxes on the belt**

> **Correct Answer: 4** (Kisner p. 476)

Physical therapists often perform work site evaluations and make recommendations to modify existing work activities.

1. A pelvic stabilization program may be helpful to improve core stability, however, the question provides ample evidence that the problem is more likely related to the height of the elevated conveyor belt.
2. An abdominal strengthening program would also improve core stability, but would not accommodate for the height of the elevated conveyor belt.
3. Reviewing proper body mechanics may be desirable, however, the question states that the patient is unable to prevent hyperextension of the spine. Failure to prevent hyperextension of the spine is more likely to occur because of the height of the conveyor belt than lack of knowledge of proper body mechanics.
4. **In order to eliminate hyperextension of the spine it may be necessary to modify the workstation. The most reasonable modification would be to utilize an elevated platform in order to minimize the height of the conveyor belt. In many instances, it is possible to modify a work site without utilizing large amounts of resources (e.g., time, money).**

System Specific: Musculoskeletal System
Content Outline: Interventions

Exam One: Question 157

A 21-year-old male patient informs a physical therapist that additional therapy visits will not be covered by his medical insurance provider. The patient is 12 weeks status post anterior cruciate ligament reconstruction and has had an unremarkable post-operative progression. The MOST appropriate therapist action is:

1. offer to treat the patient pro bono
2. devise an affordable payment plan
3. request additional visits from the third party payer
4. **discharge the patient with a home exercise program**

> **Correct Answer: 4** (Kisner p. 734)

Physical therapists should discharge patients from physical therapy when the anticipated goals or expected outcomes have been achieved or the patient is no longer benefitting from physical therapy services.

1. Physical therapists are not permitted to offer pro bono services to selected patients based on factors such as reimbursement or the ability to pay. Therapists should strive to treat all patients equitably.
2. A payment plan permits a patient to pay for incurred physical therapy services in a gradual manner. This may be a more desirable option when a patient requires ongoing physical therapy services, but does not have adequate financial resources.
3. Requesting additional physical therapy visits from the third party payer is a possible option, however, based on the patient's diagnosis and post-operative progression additional visits may not be warranted.
4. **A patient 12 weeks status post anterior cruciate ligament reconstruction that has experienced an unremarkable recovery should be able to function independently using a well designed home exercise program. The program should incorporate activities such as jogging, strengthening, and agility drills.**

System Specific: Non-Systems
Content Outline: Safety & Professional Roles; Teaching/Learning; Research

Exam One: Question 158

A physical therapist monitors the blood pressure response to exercise of a 52-year-old male on a stationary bicycle. The therapist notes a relatively linear increase in systolic blood pressure with increasing exercise intensity. The change in the patient's systolic blood pressure with exercise is BEST explained by:

1. **increased cardiac output**
2. decreased peripheral resistance
3. increased oxygen saturation
4. decreased myocardial oxygen consumption

> **Correct Answer: 1** (Brannon p. 73)

Cardiac output is the volume of blood pumped into the systemic circulation per minute and is equal to the product of heart rate and stroke volume.

1. **The trend toward lower blood pressure during exercise brought about by a decrease in peripheral resistance is negated by an increase in cardiac output. The increased heart rate and force of contraction of the myocardium (stroke volume) has the net effect of increasing systolic blood pressure in a normal population.**
2. A decrease in peripheral resistance to blood flow tends to cause a decrease in blood pressure due to dilatation of blood vessels in the exercising muscles.
3. Oxygen saturation is not affected by exercise in individuals with healthy lungs. Oxygen saturation may decrease during exercise in patients with chronic lung disease.
4. An increase in heart rate while cycling will increase myocardial oxygen consumption as the heart muscle utilizes more oxygen. Cardiac output increases to supply oxygenated blood to the exercising muscles.

System Specific: Cardiac, Vascular, & Pulmonary Systems
Content Outline: Clinical Application of Foundational Sciences

Exam One: Question 159

A 64-year-old female patient is admitted to the hospital with a stage III decubitus ulcer over her right ischial tuberosity. The patient's past medical history includes severe chronic obstructive pulmonary disease. The MOST appropriate position for the patient is:

1. supine with pillows under the knees
2. prone with pillows under the knees
3. **left sidelying with pillows between the knees**
4. right sidelying with pillows between the knees

Correct Answer: 3 (Frownfelter p. 547)

Left sidelying would be the position of choice in order to relieve pressure on the ulcer and maximize the patient's respiration. Recognizing contraindications for chronic obstructive pulmonary disease as well as positioning for pressure relief will allow for safe and effective positioning to enhance recovery.

1. Although the supine position with pillows under the knees is a comfortable position that reduces lumbar lordosis and strain, there would be pressure directly over the right ischial tuberosity and this would hinder progress or worsen the decubitus ulcer.
2. A prone position would allow for pressure relief over the right ischial tuberosity, however, the patient has severe chronic obstructive pulmonary disease and should not lie in prone as breathing would be very difficult. Pillows are also not typically placed under the knees when a patient is in prone.
3. **Left sidelying does not compromise respiration and avoids placing stress on the right ischial tuberosity.**
4. A right sidelying position would assist the patient with breathing and would not compromise overall respiration, however, there would be significant pressure over the right ischial tuberosity.

System Specific: Integumentary System
Content Outline: Interventions

Exam One: Question 160

A physical therapist performs a manual muscle test on a patient's shoulder medial rotators. Which muscle would NOT be involved in this specific test?

1. pectoralis major
2. teres major
3. latissimus dorsi
4. **teres minor**

Correct Answer: 4 (Kendall p. 321)

The primary muscles being assessed while testing the shoulder medial rotators include the pectoralis major, latissimus dorsi, subscapularis, and teres major. The test is performed with the patient in supine and resistance is applied to the forearm in the direction of laterally rotating the humerus. The test can alternately be performed with the patient in prone.

1. The pectoralis major – upper fibers act to flex and medially rotate the shoulder joint, and horizontally adduct the humerus. The upper fibers are innervated by the lateral pectoral nerve. The pectoralis major – lower fibers act to depress the shoulder girdle and obliquely adduct the humerus. The lower fibers are innervated by the lateral and medial pectoral nerves.
2. The teres major acts to medially rotate, adduct, and extend the shoulder joint. The muscle is innervated by the lower subscapular nerve (C5, C6, C7).
3. The latissimus dorsi with the origin fixed acts to medially rotate, adduct, and extend the shoulder joint. The muscle is innervated by the thoracodorsal nerve (C6, C7, C8).
4. **The teres minor acts to laterally rotate the shoulder joint and stabilize the head of the humerus in the glenoid cavity. The muscle is innervated by the axillary nerve (C5, C6).**

System Specific: Musculoskeletal System
Content Outline: Clinical Application of Foundational Sciences

Exam One: Question 161

A patient in an acute care hospital has a catheter inserted into the internal jugular vein. The catheter travels through the superior vena cava and into the right atrium. The device permits removal of blood samples, administration of medication, and monitoring of central venous pressure. The device is BEST termed:

1. arterial line
2. central venous pressure catheter
3. **Hickman catheter**
4. Swan-Ganz catheter

Correct Answer: 3 (Pierson p. 286)

Patients in a medically compromised state often use a variety of lines, tubes, and special equipment. Physical therapists should be familiar with the handling and management of these devices and be aware of any precautions or contraindications.

1. An arterial line is a monitoring device consisting of a catheter that is inserted into an artery and attached to an electronic monitoring system. An arterial line is used to measure blood pressure or to obtain blood samples. The device is considered to be more accurate than traditional measures of blood pressure and does not require repeated needle punctures.

2. A central venous pressure catheter is a plastic intravenous tube used to measure pressure in the right atrium or the superior vena cava. Specifically, the device measures pressure associated with the filling of the right ventricle (i.e., diastolic pressure).

3. **A Hickman catheter (indwelling right atrial catheter) inserts into the right atrium of the heart. The catheter permits removal of blood samples, administration of medication, and monitoring of central venous pressure. Potential complications associated with the use of a Hickman catheter include sepsis and blood clots.**

4. A Swan-Ganz catheter is a soft, flexible catheter that is inserted through a vein and eventually into the pulmonary artery. The device is used to provide continuous measurements of pulmonary artery pressure. Patients must attempt to avoid activities that increase pressure on the catheter's insertion site.

System Specific: Cardiac, Vascular, & Pulmonary Systems
Content Outline: Foundations for Evaluation, Differential Diagnosis, & Prognosis

Exam One: Question 162

A patient informs her physical therapist that she noticed a small lump on her right breast while dressing. The patient was referred to physical therapy with lateral epicondylitis and has no significant past medical history. The MOST appropriate therapist action is:

1. inspect the lump
2. **instruct the patient to make an immediate appointment with her physician**
3. inform the patient she may have cancer
4. document the patient's comment in the medical record

Correct Answer: 2 (Goodman - Pathology p. 1022)

Ninety percent of breast cancer is discovered through self-identification. Research has demonstrated that in the United States one in nine women may be affected by breast cancer over the course of their life. As a result, it is imperative that the physical therapist impress upon the patient the importance of consulting with her physician.

1. Inspecting the lump would be inappropriate, especially when considering the patient's medical diagnosis. Physical therapists must refer patients to appropriate medical personnel when warranted based on the results of subjective and objective data.

2. **The patient's statement makes immediate contact with the physician imperative. The physical therapist should be careful not to alarm the patient, however, must stress the importance of an appointment with the physician.**

3. It would be inappropriate for the physical therapist to suggest that the patient may have cancer. Physical therapists cannot medically diagnose and should avoid suggestive comments related to a given diagnosis.

4. It is acceptable to document the patient's comments in the medical record, however, the priority needs to be related to follow-up with the physician.

System Specific: Other Systems
Content Outline: Examination

Exam One: Question 163

A physical therapist attempts to confirm the fit of a wheelchair for a patient recently admitted to a skilled nursing facility. After completing the assessment, the therapist determines the wheelchair has excessive seat width. Which adverse effect results from excessive seat width?

1. difficulty changing position within the wheelchair
2. insufficient trunk support
3. **difficulty propelling the wheelchair**
4. increased pressure to the distal posterior thighs

Correct Answer: 3 (O'Sullivan p. 1302)

Seat width is determined by measuring the widest aspect of the user's buttocks, hips or thighs and adding approximately two inches. This provides space for bulky clothing, orthoses or clearance of the trochanters from the armrest side panel. The standard seat width for an adult wheelchair is 18 inches.

1. Difficulty changing position within the wheelchair may be due to a wheelchair that is too small and constricts movement. A seat with excess width would not prohibit the patient from moving within the wheelchair.
2. Insufficient trunk support may be due to a wheelchair that has less back support than is recommended. Back support is measured from the seat of the chair to the floor of the axilla with the patient's shoulder flexed to 90 degrees and then subtract approximately four inches. This will allow the back height to be below the inferior angles of the scapulae. The standard back height is 16 - 16.5 inches.
3. **Difficulty propelling a wheelchair may be due to excessive seat width. This will require the patient to stabilize at the shoulders and excessively abduct the upper extremities to reach the wheels. This produces a less functional push and increases the difficulty maneuvering through tight spaces.**
4. Increased pressure to the distal posterior thighs typically results from excessive seat depth. Seat depth is measured from the patient's posterior buttocks, along the lateral thigh to the popliteal fold; then subtract approximately two inches to avoid pressure from the front edge of the seat against the popliteal space. The standard seat depth for an adult wheelchair is 16 inches.

System Specific: Non-Systems
Content Outline: Equipment & Devices; Therapeutic Modalities

Exam One: Question 164

A patient uses a self-administered assessment tool as a method to record daily progress. What type of reliability would be the MOST essential using this tool?

1. reliability of parallel forms
2. internal consistency
3. **intratester**
4. intertester

Correct Answer: 3 (Portney p. 87)

Since the assessment tool is used to record daily progress, it will be administered repeatedly. If changes in the scores are to be attributed to real progress made in physical therapy, and not to inconsistency or unreliable measurement, the tool should be evaluated for reliability.

1. Reliability of parallel forms refers to the consistency between results of two tests constructed in the same way from the same content domain. Parallel forms reliability is not an issue in this example because there is only one form of the assessment tool.
2. Internal consistency reliability refers to the consistency of results across items within a test. The reliability of the instrument is evaluated by estimating how well the different items within the test, which are supposed to reflect the same construct, do yield similar results. This is not of concern in the example.
3. **Intratester reliability refers to the extent to which scores on the tool obtained by the same tester are consistent. The tool should have intratester reliability so that any changes recorded can be attributed to progress in therapy and not to unreliable measurement.**
4. Intertester reliability refers to the extent of agreement of the scores recorded by two or more individuals. Interrater reliability addresses the consistency of the implementation of a rating system.

System Specific: Non-Systems
Content Outline: Safety & Professional Roles; Teaching/Learning; Research

Exam One: Question 165

A physical therapist administers the Mini-Mental State Examination to a patient recently admitted to an acute care medical facility. The MINIMUM patient score necessary in order to avoid being classified as possessing a cognitive impairment would be:

1. 18
2. **24**
3. 30
4. 34

> **Correct Answer: 2** (Physical Therapist's Clinical Companion p. 113)

The Mini-Mental State Examination can be used to screen for cognitive dysfunction or dementia. The 11 question measure assesses five areas of cognitive function: orientation, registration, attention/calculation, recall, and language. The measure takes approximately 5-10 minutes to complete. Possible scores obtained on the Mini-Mental State Examination range from 0-30.

1. A score less than 20 may be associated with dementia, delirium, schizophrenia or an affective disorder.
2. **A score of 24 is the minimum score to avoid being classified as having a cognitive impairment.**
3. A score of 30 is a perfect score and would indicate that the patient is cognitively within normal limits.
4. A score of 34 exceeds the maximum score that can be attained on the Mini-Mental State Examination.

System Specific: Neuromuscular & Nervous Systems
Content Outline: Examination

Exam One: Question 166

A physical therapist receives a referral to instruct a patient in stair training using axillary crutches. The patient is rehabilitating from a tibial fracture and is currently partial weight bearing on the involved extremity. The MOST important action prior to initiating the training session is:

1. apply a gait belt
2. maintain proper body mechanics
3. assess vital signs
4. **examine the patient's limitations and capabilities**

> **Correct Answer: 4** (Pierson p. 217)

It is essential to determine the patient's limitations and capabilities prior to initiating an activity such as stair training. Failure of the physical therapist to accurately assess the patient's current status may unnecessarily jeopardize patient safety.

1. Applying a gait belt is a useful strategy to promote safety, however, therapists can effectively guard patients without the use of a gait belt. This fact makes it more important for the therapist to assess the patient's limitations and capabilities.
2. Maintaining proper body mechanics while guarding a patient is extremely important, however, the question asks specifically about the most important action prior to initiating the training session.
3. Vital signs should be assessed during the examination, however, given the patient's diagnosis and the proposed activity, it would not be as critical as some of the other presented options.
4. **Critical areas to assess prior to initiating the training session include uninvolved lower extremity strength, upper extremity strength, and ability to follow instructions.**

System Specific: Non-Systems
Content Outline: Safety & Professional Roles; Teaching/Learning; Research

Exam One: Question 167

A physical therapist employed in an inpatient rehabilitation center works with a patient rehabilitating from a total knee arthroplasty. Which treatment activity would be the MOST appropriate to delegate to a physical therapy aide?

1. monitoring vital signs
2. measuring knee range of motion with a goniometer
3. **observing a patient complete a mat exercise program**
4. recording modality parameters in the medical record

Correct Answer: 3 (Guide to Physical Therapist Practice)

The physical therapy aide is a non-licensed worker who is specifically trained under the direction and supervision of a physical therapist. Activities performed by the physical therapy aide are limited to those tasks that do not require clinical decision making by the physical therapist.

1. Monitoring vital signs is a skilled activity and therefore would be inappropriate for a physical therapy aide. Failure to accurately monitor vital signs can jeopardize patient safety.
2. Performing goniometric measurements is a skilled activity taught to physical therapists and physical therapist assistants as part of their academic training. A physical therapy aide would therefore not be permitted to perform this type of activity.
3. **Observing a patient complete a mat exercise program could be considered an unskilled activity and therefore appropriate for the physical therapy aide. It would be inappropriate for the physical therapy aide to expand their duties beyond an observational role (i.e., modify, interpret, progress) since this would require clinical decision making.**
4. Physical therapy aides should not make entries in the medical record. Recording parameters associated with a specific intervention should be completed by the physical therapist or in some cases the physical therapist assistant who performed the intervention.

System Specific: Non-Systems
Content Outline: Safety & Professional Roles; Teaching/Learning; Research

Exam One: Question 168

A physical therapist discusses common cognitive and behavioral changes associated with stroke with family members of a patient with right hemisphere damage and resultant left hemiplegia. Which term does NOT accurately describe the MOST typical patient presentation?

1. poor judgment
2. impulsive
3. quick
4. **overly cautious**

Correct Answer: 4 (Umphred p. 870)

Physical therapists should be aware of commonly encountered behavioral differences in patients status post stroke with left hemisphere versus right hemisphere damage.

1. Patients with right hemisphere damage often have difficulty in grasping the whole idea of a task or activity and therefore may have difficulty with reasoning and judgment.
2. Patients with right hemisphere damage are often impulsive and tend to overestimate their abilities and underestimate their limitations. This combination makes the patient a greater safety risk compared to a patient with left hemisphere damage.
3. Patients with right hemisphere damage often are quick when performing mobility or tasks. Feedback must be given to encourage the patient to slow down and focus on each of the sequential steps of the activity.
4. **Patients with left hemisphere damage often are described as cautious, anxious, and disorganized. They often have difficulties communicating and in processing information in a sequential manner.**

System Specific: Neuromuscular & Nervous Systems
Content Outline: Foundations for Evaluation, Differential Diagnosis, & Prognosis

Test Taking Tip: A candidate may have considered eliminating options 2 and 3 simply because the terms impulsive and quick are so similar. There are obvious hemispheric differences following stroke, however, they are most often described in general terms which would make it extremely unlikely that impulsive and quick would be used to describe opposing hemispheres. As a result, a candidate may be willing to eliminate both options from consideration even without the requisite academic knowledge.

Exam One: Question 169

A physical therapist gathers a variety of equipment prior to administering a series of sensory tests. Which form of sensation would be examined by utilizing a tuning fork?

1. joint position
2. **vibration**
3. stereognosis
4. barognosis

Correct Answer: 2 (Bickley p. 692)

A tuning fork is a small two pronged metal device that provides a fixed tone when struck. The base of the device is placed on a bony prominence after being struck and the patient attempts to perceive the vibratory stimulus. If vibration sense is intact, the patient will perceive the vibration. If there is impairment, the patient will be unable to distinguish between vibration and nonvibration.

1. Joint position sense and the awareness of joints at rest is termed proprioceptive awareness. This can be assessed by the therapist holding a joint in a static position followed by the patient verbally describing the position or duplicating the position with the contralateral extremity.

2. **Vibration sense can be assessed by placing a tuning fork vibrating at 128 Hz over a bony prominence. Vibration sense is often the first sensation to be compromised in the presence of a peripheral neuropathy.**

3. Stereognosis refers to the ability of a patient to identify objects placed in the hand without visual assistance. The objects are typically small and familiar such as a coin, key, comb, and pen.

4. Barognosis refers to the recognition of weight. The patient is asked to identify the comparative weights of similar sized objects presented in a series.

System Specific: Neuromuscular & Nervous Systems
Content Outline: Examination

Exam One: Question 170

A physical therapist discusses the process of learning to drive an adapted van with a patient rehabilitating from a spinal cord injury. What is the highest spinal cord injury level where this activity would be a realistic independent functional outcome?

1. C4
2. **C6**
3. T1
4. T3

Correct Answer: 2 (Umphred p. 632)

A patient with a spinal cord injury would need to have adequate upper extremity active movement to manipulate the hand controls. Prior to driving, an individual would have several unique tests that determine range of motion, strength, vision, and reaction time. The test is usually performed by a physical therapist, occupational therapist or a certified driving instructor.

1. A patient with a C4 spinal cord injury would not have adequate upper extremity movement to independently manipulate hand controls. The diaphragm and trapezius would be innervated.

2. **A patient with a C6 spinal cord injury would possess the requisite upper extremity movement to drive an adapted van with hand controls and use a lift to get the wheelchair in and out of the vehicle. The extensor carpi radialis, infraspinatus, latissimus dorsi, pectoralis major, pronator teres, serratus anterior, and teres minor would be innervated.**

3. A patient with a T1 spinal cord injury would be able to drive an adapted van. The patient would have full upper extremity innervation including a strong grasp. The option is not the correct response since the question asks the highest spinal cord injury level where driving is a realistic functional outcome.

4. A patient with a T3 spinal cord injury would also be able to drive an adapted van. The patient's clinical presentation would be consistent with the patient at the T1 level.

System Specific: Neuromuscular & Nervous Systems
Content Outline: Foundations for Evaluation, Differential Diagnosis, & Prognosis

Exam One: Question 171

A physical therapist searches the literature to find an appropriate cardiovascular screening test to identify individuals with known cardiovascular disease who should have a medical examination before starting an exercise program. The physical therapist should choose a screening test with:

1. **high positive predictive value**
2. low positive predictive value
3. high discriminant validity
4. high internal consistency

> **Correct Answer: 1** (Portney p. 622)

To be clinically useful, a screening test should be efficient to use and yield accurate responses. The accuracy of the screening test is assessed by its predictive value.

1. **A positive predictive value estimates the probability that a person who tests positive on the screening test actually has the condition the screening test is intended to detect. A test with a high positive predictive value provides a strong estimate of the actual number of patients who have the condition.**
2. A screening test with a low positive predictive value would not be clinically useful as it would not accurately identify individuals with the condition or disease.
3. Discriminant validity is a way to assess the construct validity of a measurement. When measurements that are believed to assess different characteristics are shown to be different, or have a low correlation, then one measurement is said to have discriminant validity with respect to the second measurement. This is not the most important attribute for a screening test.
4. Internal consistency is a form of reliability of a measurement, assessing the degree to which a set of items in an instrument all measure the same trait. This is not the most important attribute for a screening test.

System Specific: Non-Systems
Content Outline: Safety & Professional Roles; Teaching/Learning; Research

Exam One: Question 172

A patient classifies the intensity of exercise as a 16 using Borg's (20-point) Rating of Perceived Exertion Scale. This classification BEST corresponds to:

1. 40 percent of the maximum heart rate range
2. 60 percent of the maximum heart rate range
3. 70 percent of the maximum heart rate range
4. **85 percent of the maximum heart rate range**

> **Correct Answer: 4** (Brannon p. 316)

Borg's Rating of Perceived Exertion Scale (RPE) may be used as an alternative means to monitor the intensity of exercise once the patient becomes familiar with the feeling of exertion associated with exercise at the appropriate target level. The 20-point RPE scale ranges from a minimum value of 6 to a maximum value of 20.

1. A rating of 16 is relatively close to the maximum value and would therefore not correspond to a heart rate percent that is less than 50% of heart rate range.
2. 60% of the heart rate range corresponds to an RPE of 12 to 13 (somewhat hard).
3. 70% of the heart rate range corresponds to an RPE of 14 or 15 (between somewhat hard and hard).
4. **A rating of 16 (hard+) on the 20-point RPE scale corresponds to 85% of the heart rate range.**

System Specific: Cardiac, Vascular, & Pulmonary Systems
Content Outline: Interventions

Exam One: Question 173

A male patient rehabilitating from a lower extremity injury is referred to physical therapy for gait analysis. The physical therapist begins the session by observing the patient at free speed walking. The normal degree of toe-out at this speed is:

1. 3 degrees
2. **7 degrees**
3. 14 degrees
4. 21 degrees

Correct Answer: 2 (Levangie p. 524)

The degree of toe-out is measured by determining the angle formed by each foot's line of progression and a line intersecting the center of the heel and the second toe.

1. A measurement of 3 degrees of toe-out may be associated with walking at a relative fast rate of speed since the normal degree of toe-out decreases as the speed of walking increases.
2. **The degree of toe-out during free speed walking is approximately 7 degrees.**
3. A measurement of 14 degrees is greater than normal and may be associated with a wide range of orthopedic or neurologic abnormalities.
4. A measurement of 21 degrees is excessive and may be associated with more severe orthopedic or neurologic abnormalities.

System Specific: Musculoskeletal System
Content Outline: Clinical Application of Foundational Sciences

Exam One: Question 174

A patient with Alzheimer's disease is referred to physical therapy for instruction in an exercise program. The MOST appropriate INITIAL step is:

1. provide verbal and written instructions
2. frequently repeat multiple step directions
3. **assess the patient's cognitive status**
4. avoid using medical terminology

Correct Answer: 3 (Bickley p. 151)

Physical therapists should attempt to provide exercise instructions that are consistent with the abilities and limitations of the target audience. This is particularly important with Alzheimer's disease since cognitive status can vary greatly from patient to patient.

1. Providing verbal and written instructions is an effective method to improve patient understanding and can be particularly important in the case of a home exercise program. The breadth and depth of the instructions would be heavily influenced by the patient's cognitive status.
2. Repetition is an effective technique to enhance learning and memory. The appropriate amount of repetition will be dictated in part by the patient's cognitive status.
3. **It is essential for the physical therapist to determine the patient's cognitive status prior to providing formal exercise instruction. The patient's cognitive status will have a significant impact on a variety of factors including the ability to interpret instructions, the ability to perform exercises correctly, and the ability to recall elements of the exercise program.**
4. Physical therapists should avoid using medical terminology whenever possible. Although this is good advice, it would not be as important as assessing the patient's cognitive status.

System Specific: Neuromuscular & Nervous Systems
Content Outline: Foundations for Evaluation, Differential Diagnosis, & Prognosis

Exam One: Question 175

A physician provides a group of physical therapists with an overview of diagnostic imaging techniques commonly used in clinical practice. Which imaging technique would NOT be considered invasive?

1. arthrography
2. myelography
3. discography
4. **computed tomography**

> **Correct Answer: 4** (Magee p. 62)

Diagnostic imaging techniques are often used to confirm a clinical opinion. Familiarity with these techniques will allow the physical therapist to play a more active role in the medical management of their patients and assist them to comprehend and perhaps interpret the results of diagnostic imaging.

1. Arthrography is an invasive test utilizing a contrast medium to provide visualization of joint structures through radiographs. Soft tissue disruption can be identified by leakage from the joint cavity and capsule. The test is commonly used at peripheral joints such as the hip, knee, ankle, elbow, and wrist.
2. Myelography is an invasive test that combines fluoroscopy and radiography to evaluate the spinal subarachnoid space. The test utilizes a contrast medium that is injected into the epidural space by spinal puncture. Myelography is used to identify bone displacement, disk herniation, spinal cord compression or tumors.
3. Discography is an invasive test that involves injecting a radiopaque dye into the nucleus pulposus of an intervertebral disc using radiographic guidance. The technique can be used to identify disruptions of the nucleus pulposus or the annulus fibrosus.
4. **Computed tomography is a non-invasive imaging technique that uses cross-sectional images based on x-ray attenuation. Computer enhancement allows the imaging to have significantly better contrast resolution when compared to conventional x-rays.**

System Specific: Musculoskeletal System
Content Outline: Foundations for Evaluation, Differential Diagnosis, & Prognosis

Exam One: Question 176

A physical therapist completing a lower quarter screening examination attempts to palpate the tendon of the tibialis anterior. The MOST appropriate therapist action to facilitate palpation is:

1. ask the patient to actively move the foot into dorsiflexion and eversion
2. **ask the patient to actively move the foot into dorsiflexion and inversion**
3. passively move the patient's foot into dorsiflexion and eversion
4. passively move the patient's foot into dorsiflexion and inversion

> **Correct Answer: 2** (Kendall p. 410)

The tibialis anterior acts to dorsiflex the ankle joint and assists in inversion of the foot. The muscle is innervated by the deep peroneal nerve.

1. Active movement would be helpful to facilitate palpation of the tendon, however, the tibialis anterior assists to invert the foot and not evert.
2. **The action of the tibialis anterior is to dorsiflex the ankle and invert the foot. To facilitate palpation of the tendon the patient must actively move in the direction of the muscle's action.**
3. Passive movement would not be as useful as active movement to assist with facilitation of a contractile structure.
4. Dorsiflexion of the ankle and inversion of the foot is consistent with the action of the tibialis anterior, however, passive movement would not be as desirable as active movement to facilitate palpation of the tendon.

System Specific: Musculoskeletal System
Content Outline: Clinical Application of Foundational Sciences

Exam One: Question 177

A physical therapist transports a patient with a brain injury to the physical therapy gym. Each day after arriving in the gym, the patient asks the therapist, "Where am I?" Recognizing the patient has short-term memory loss, the therapist's MOST appropriate response should be:

1. You know where you are.
2. You are in the same place you were yesterday at this time.
3. **You are in the physical therapy gym for your treatment session.**
4. You are in the hospital because of your injury.

Correct Answer: 3 (O'Sullivan p. 914)

A patient's question should be answered in a direct and forthcoming manner whenever possible.

1. The statement implies that the patient knows where they are and is simply withholding information. The more likely reality is that the patient's short-term memory loss is responsible for the difficulty with orientation.
2. The statement provides information for the patient by informing them that they were in the same location that they were yesterday, however, because of the short-term memory loss this may still be of little value.
3. **The statement provides a specific and informative response to the question asked by the patient. Frequent repetition is a component of any treatment plan for patients with short-term memory loss.**
4. The statement provides some useful information for the patient, but lacks the specificity of option 3 given that the patient has been transported to the physical therapy gym.

System Specific: Neuromuscular & Nervous Systems
Content Outline: Interventions

Exam One: Question 178

A physical therapist completes a balance assessment on a patient recently admitted to a skilled nursing facility. The therapist concludes that the patient is able to maintain their balance without support in standing, however, cannot maintain balance during weight shifting or with any form of external perturbation. The MOST appropriate balance grade would be:

1. normal
2. good
3. **fair**
4. poor

Correct Answer: 3 (O'Sullivan p. 254)

The patient's ability to maintain balance in standing and inability to maintain balance with weight shifting or outside challenges is typical of a patient with fair standing balance.

1. A balance grade of normal indicates that the patient would weight shift in all directions and accept maximal perturbation while maintaining their balance.
2. A balance grade of good indicates that the patient would maintain balance without support and accept moderate perturbation while maintaining their balance.
3. **A balance grade of fair indicates that the patient would maintain balance without support, but cannot weight shift without losing their balance.**
4. A balance grade of poor indicates that the patient would require some assistance in order to maintain balance in standing and cannot weight shift or accept any perturbation.

System Specific: Neuromuscular & Nervous Systems
Content Outline: Examination

Exam One: Question 179

A physical therapist completes a respiratory assessment on a patient with T2 paraplegia. As a component of the assessment, the therapist measures the amount of chest excursion during inspiration. The MOST appropriate patient position to conduct the measurement is:

1. sitting
2. **supine**
3. prone
4. sidelying

> **Correct Answer: 2** (Umphred p. 626)

The primary muscles of inspiration are the diaphragm and external intercostals. The primary muscles of expiration are the abdominals and internal intercostals. Normal mechanics of inspiration allow for an increase in the diameter of the thorax. Normal mechanics of resting expiration is through recoil of the lungs, however, the abdominals and internal intercostals contribute in several ways. The loss of these muscles significantly decreases the overall respiratory efficiency. Supine is the most appropriate position to assess chest excursion and initially strengthen.

1. The sitting position is a higher level activity for patients with any form of respiratory weakness and compromise. Patients should be assessed and initiate strengthening in the supine position with the goal of progressing to a sitting position. Abdominal binders assist the patient with respiration in sitting by maintaining pressure that is normally lost in patients with lesions at T12 or above.

2. **The supine position creates support and resistance to the diaphragm. There is a direct correlation between the amount of chest expansion and intercostal strength.**

3. The prone position would not be recommended for a patient with a spinal cord injury due to the patient's body weight and force of gravity upon the weakened muscles of respiration.

4. The sidelying position would not be indicated for measurement of chest excursion during inspiration since one portion of the thorax would be supported by the surface that the patient is sidelying on.

System Specific: Cardiac, Vascular, & Pulmonary Systems
Content Outline: Examination

Exam One: Question 180

A physical therapist working in an outpatient physical therapy clinic guards a patient descending a curb with axillary crutches. Based on the photograph, the MOST likely patient scenario is:

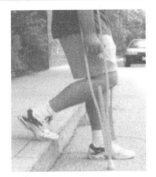

1. **partial weight bearing secondary to a left lateral ankle sprain**
2. partial weight bearing secondary to a right lateral ankle sprain
3. toe touch weight bearing secondary to a left lateral ankle sprain
4. toe touch weight bearing secondary to a right lateral ankle sprain

> **Correct Answer: 1** (Pierson p. 260)

When descending a curb with axillary crutches the involved lower extremity and crutches are moved from the curb to the ground, while the upper extremities and the uninvolved lower extremity are used to slowly lower the body.

1. **The patient should use the upper extremities and the uninvolved lower extremity to slowly lower the body when descending a curb. As a result, the patient's left ankle would be the involved ankle. Partial weight bearing occurs when a patient is allowed to put a particular amount of weight through the involved extremity.**

2. If the right ankle was the involved ankle, the patient would use the upper extremities and the left lower extremity to slowly lower the body when descending a curb.

3. The patient's left ankle is the involved ankle, however, the picture does not depict toe touch weight bearing. Toe touch weight bearing occurs when a patient is unable to place any weight through the involved extremity, however, can place the toes on the ground to assist with balance.

4. The right ankle is not the involved ankle and the depicted weight bearing status is better described as partial weight bearing.

System Specific: Non-Systems
Content Outline: Equipment & Devices; Therapeutic Modalities

Exam One: Question 181

A physical therapist prepares a patient recovering from a total hip arthroplasty using a posterolateral surgical approach for discharge from the hospital. The patient is a 65 year old and resides alone. Assuming an uncomplicated recovery, which of the following pieces of adaptive equipment would NOT be necessary for home use?

1. long handled shoehorn
2. raised toilet seat
3. **sliding board**
4. tub bench

Correct Answer: 3 (Kisner p. 657)

Contraindications following total hip arthroplasty using a posterolateral surgical approach include hip flexion greater than 90 degrees, adduction, and medial rotation beyond neutral. Adaptive equipment allows the patient to perform necessary activities of daily living without compromising the integrity of the total hip arthroplasty.

1. A long handled shoehorn allows the patient to put on shoes without flexing the affected hip greater than 90 degrees.
2. A raised toilet seat allows the patient to use the toilet without flexing the hips greater than 90 degrees. A normal toilet seat requires greater than 90 degrees of hip flexion.
3. **A patient scheduled for discharge from the hospital following total hip arthroplasty surgery should be able to perform transfers independently without using a sliding board.**
4. A tub bench provides a stable base for the patient to use when showering. The stability offered by the tub bench allows the patient to safely shower without concerns or fear of falling.

System Specific: Non-Systems
Content Outline: Equipment & Devices; Therapeutic Modalities

Exam One: Question 182

A physical therapist records the end-feel associated with forearm supination as firm in the medical record. Which of the following is NOT consistent with an end-feel categorized as firm?

1. muscular stretch
2. capsular stretch
3. **soft tissue approximation**
4. ligamentous stretch

Correct Answer: 3 (Norkin p. 8)

Supination occurs in the transverse plane around a longitudinal axis with the patient in the anatomical position. Normal supination is 0-80 degrees. The end-feel is typically classified as firm due to tension in the palmar radioulnar ligament of the inferior radioulnar joint, interosseous membrane, pronator teres, and pronator quadratus muscles.

1. Muscular stretch is a type of firm end-feel described as a "rubbery" feel resembling what would be felt at the extremes of a straight leg raise due to tension in the hamstrings muscles.
2. Capsular stretch is a type of firm end-feel with a "leathery" feeling with slight creep. An example is extension of the metacarpophalangeal joints of the fingers resulting from tension in the anterior capsule.
3. **Soft tissue approximation is a type of soft end-feel. This type of end-feel could occur with knee flexion resulting from contact between the soft tissue of the posterior leg and the posterior thigh.**
4. Ligamentous stretch is a type of firm end-feel with no give or creep. This type of end-feel could occur with forearm supination resulting from tension in the palmar radioulnar ligament of the inferior radioulnar joint and interosseous membrane.

System Specific: Musculoskeletal System
Content Outline: Clinical Application of Foundational Sciences

Exam One: Question 183

A physical therapist examines several superficial reflexes on a patient diagnosed with an upper motor neuron lesion. When assessing the cremasteric reflex the MOST appropriate stimulus is:

1. stroke the skin beneath the costal margins and above the inguinal ligament
2. **stroke the skin of the superior and medial thigh**
3. prick the skin of the perianal region
4. prick the skin of the glans penis

> **Correct Answer: 2** (DeMyer p. 333)

The physical therapist should stroke the skin in the area of the superior and medial thigh in order to elicit the cremasteric reflex. The anticipated response is elevation of the testicle on the same side as the stimulus.

1. Stroking the skin beneath the costal margins and above the inguinal ligament assesses the abdominal reflex. A normal response will produce a contraction of the abdominal muscles in the stimulated quadrant.
2. **Stroking of the skin of the superior and medial thigh will elicit the cremasteric reflex. Upper and lower motor neuron disorders as well as a spinal injury at the L1-L2 level can cause the reflex to be absent.**
3. Pricking the skin of the perianal region assesses the superficial anal reflex. A normal response will produce a contraction of the rectal sphincter.
4. Pricking the skin of the glans penis assesses the bulbocavernosus reflex. A normal response will produce a contraction of the bulbous urethra.

System Specific: Neuromuscular & Nervous Systems
Content Outline: Examination

Exam One: Question 184

A 35-year-old male diagnosed with ankylosing spondylitis is referred to physical therapy for instruction in a home exercise program. Which general treatment objective would be the MOST beneficial for the patient?

1. strengthening of the rectus abdominus
2. strengthening of the internal and external obliques
3. strengthening of the quadratus lumborum
4. **strengthening of the back extensors**

> **Correct Answer: 4** (Dutton p. 237)

Ankylosing spondylitis is a form of systemic rheumatic arthritis that results in inflammation of the axial skeleton with subsequent back pain. The condition is associated with an increase in thoracic kyphosis and loss of the lumbar curve. The patient often develops a forward stooped posture observed in standing.

1. Strengthening of the rectus abdominus will produce a flexion moment in the trunk. This will further accentuate the thoracic kyphosis and decrease the lumbar lordosis.
2. Strengthening of the internal and external obliques when contracting bilaterally will produce a flexion moment of the trunk and when contracting unilaterally will produce a rotary moment of the trunk. General core strengthening is desirable, however, the emphasis would be on strengthening the back extensors.
3. Strengthening of the quadratus lumborum will produce a lateral bending of the trunk when performed in a closed-chain activity and a hip hiking movement when performed in an open-chain activity. These motions would not be the emphasis of a strengthening program for a patient with ankylosing spondylitis. The quadratus lumborum also assists with extension, however, the muscle is just one of many muscles that serve this function.
4. **Extension exercises are often an important component of a comprehensive plan of care to assist patients with ankylosing spondylitis to maintain the normal curves of the spine while at the same time limiting the forward bending nature of the disease.**

System Specific: Musculoskeletal System
Content Outline: Interventions

Exam One: Question 185

A 73-year-old male patient receiving outpatient physical therapy begins to experience acute angina. The patient indicates he uses nitroglycerin to alleviate the angina. The MOST appropriate mode of administration is:

1. oral
2. buccal
3. **sublingual**
4. topical

Correct Answer: 3 (Ciccone p. 309)

Drugs can be administered through the alimentary canal or through nonalimentary routes. Each route has distinct advantages and disadvantages.

1. Oral administration is the most common method of administration. It is considered the easiest form of taking medication when self-medication is required and is relatively safe since drugs enter the system in a fairly controlled manner.
2. Buccal administration occurs when the drug is placed between the cheeks and gums. Drugs administered in this manner are absorbed through the oral mucosa.
3. **Sublingual administration occurs when placing drugs under the tongue. Sublingual administration of nitroglycerin is the most appropriate mode of administration with acute angina due to the rapid absorption into the systemic circulation.**
4. Topical administration refers to the application of drugs topically to the surface of the skin or mucous membranes. Topical administration is used most often to treat the outer layer of the skin and not other areas since most medications are absorbed poorly through the epidermis and into the systemic circulation.

System Specific: Cardiac, Vascular, & Pulmonary Systems
Content Outline: Clinical Application of Foundational Sciences

Exam One: Question 186

A physical therapist prepares to conduct a manual muscle test of the hip flexors. Assuming a grade of poor, the MOST appropriate testing position is:

1. prone
2. **sidelying**
3. supine
4. standing

Correct Answer: 2 (Kendall p. 422)

A grade of poor indicates that the hip flexors can produce movement with gravity-eliminated, but cannot function against gravity. Muscles acting to flex the hip include the iliopsoas, sartorius, rectus femoris, and pectineus.

1. A prone position would place the hip flexors in an elongated position and make it impossible for the therapist to offer resistance in a direction opposite of the muscle's action.
2. **The hip flexors would need to be tested in sidelying due to the grade of "poor." If the hip flexors were given a grade of "good" or "normal" the recommended testing position would be sitting upright with the knees bent over the side of the table.**
3. A supine position would not be considered gravity-eliminated and therefore would not be appropriate given the muscle's current grade. A supine position is sometimes employed as a substitute for sitting upright, most often in situations where the muscle's strength is "good" or "normal."
4. Testing the hip flexors in standing would be problematic since the muscles would need to work against gravity and it would be impossible to adequately stabilize the patient during the testing.

System Specific: Musculoskeletal System
Content Outline: Examination

Exam One: Question 187

A physical therapist administers the Functional Reach Test to a patient rehabilitating from a neurological disorder. Which bony landmark would be the MOST appropriate to utilize when formally measuring the distance the patient reached during each trial?

1. distal tip of the third digit
2. **third metacarpal**
3. radial styloid process
4. ulnar styloid process

> **Correct Answer: 2** (Montgomery p. 192)

The Functional Reach Test was developed to assess standing balance and the risk for falls. The test is reliable, however, the standard error of measurement may be relatively high and the test measures sway only in a forward direction. A person is required to stand upright against a wall with a static base of support. The patient is then asked to make a fist and raise the arm nearest the wall to 90 degrees of shoulder flexion. The therapist records the beginning position on a yardstick. The patient is then asked to lean forward as far as possible and the ending position is recorded. The beginning position is then subtracted from the ending position to obtain the final value.

1. The distal tip of the third digit is in the midline of the hand, but is not the identified landmark used on the Functional Reach Test.
2. **The Functional Reach Test requires the therapist to measure the position of the patient's third metacarpal on the yardstick after making a fist.**
3. The radial styloid process is located on the lateral side of the distal radius with the hand in the anatomic position. The most prominent part of the radial styloid process is just proximal to the carpal joint.
4. The ulnar styloid process is located on the medial side of the ulna with the hand in the anatomic position. The ulna articulates with the distal radius, but does not articulate with the carpals.

System Specific: Non-Systems
Content Outline: Safety & Professional Roles; Teaching/Learning; Research

Exam One: Question 188

A physical therapist measures elbow flexion while a patient grasps the handgrip of a walker in standing. The therapist records elbow flexion as 35 degrees. Which statement BEST describes the height of the walker?

1. the walker height is too low for the patient
2. **the walker height is too high for the patient**
3. the walker height is appropriate for the patient
4. not enough information is given to assess walker height

> **Correct Answer: 2** (Pierson p. 225)

A patient using a properly fitting walker should exhibit 20–25 degrees of elbow flexion. This position of the elbow would allow the patient to most effectively use the upper extremities during ambulation. A walker can be used with all levels of weight bearing and offers a large base of support which promotes stability.

1. A walker height that is too low for the patient would result in elbow flexion less than the recommended 20-25 degrees. Any deviation from the recommended fit would decrease the efficiency of using the walker and increase the potential safety risk.
2. **A walker height that is too high for the patient would result in elbow flexion greater than the recommended 20-25 degrees.**
3. Elbow flexion of 35 degrees exceeds the upper limit of the acceptable range of elbow flexion (i.e., 20-25 degrees) when using a walker. As the height of the walker increases, the amount of elbow flexion will also increase.
4. The amount of elbow flexion is the primary indicator of the relative height of the walker. As a result, there is ample information provided to assess the height of the walker.

System Specific: Non-Systems
Content Outline: Equipment & Devices; Therapeutic Modalities

Exam One: Question 189

A physical therapist often makes errors when completing daily documentation. Which of the following statements would be the MOST appropriate advice to the therapist when an error occurs?

1. use correction fluid as needed on your documentation
2. **place a single line through the error, write "error", date, and initial it**
3. use pencil when completing your documentation
4. use erasable ink when completing your documentation

Correct Answer: 2 (Shamus-Effective Documentation p. 10)

Physical therapists often make mistakes when writing entries in the medical record. It is critical that when this occurs, therapists correct the mistake in a manner that makes the medical record accurate and also makes it clear how the record was altered.

1. Correction fluid provides a mechanism to correct mistakes, however, obscures the original entry.
2. **Place a single line through the error, write "error", date, and initial it provides the physical therapist with a valid method to correct the mistake while preserving the integrity of the original entry.**
3. Pencil is not acceptable to utilize when completing documentation since it is not permanent.
4. Erasable ink is not acceptable since by virtue of being "erasable" it lacks permanence.

System Specific: Non-Systems
Content Outline: Safety & Professional Roles; Teaching/Learning; Research

Exam One: Question 190

A 22-year-old male rehabilitating from a motor vehicle accident is referred to physical therapy for gait training. The patient sustained multiple injuries including a fractured tibia and a traction injury to the brachial plexus. The patient is partial weight bearing and has good upper extremity strength. The MOST appropriate assistive device is:

1. axillary crutches
2. **Lofstrand crutches**
3. walker with platform attachment
4. cane

Correct Answer: 2 (Pierson p. 222)

Physical therapists often have to consider a variety of factors when determining an appropriate assistive device for a patient. In this particular question, the therapist has to consider the patient's brachial plexus injury and the present weight bearing status.

1. Axillary crutches would accommodate the patient's weight bearing status, however, have the potential to transmit pressure through the axillary region which could exacerbate the brachial plexus injury.
2. **Lofstrand or forearm crutches avoid transmitting pressure to the brachial plexus area and accommodate for the weight bearing status of the involved lower extremity. The patient's age and upper extremity strength make Lofstrand crutches the most appropriate device.**
3. A walker with a platform attachment would be an appropriate option for the patient, however, given the patient's age and upper extremity strength the device may offer more stability than the patient requires.
4. A cane or bilateral canes do not permit partial weight bearing and instead are used to promote balance.

System Specific: Non-Systems
Content Outline: Equipment & Devices; Therapeutic Modalities

Exam One: Question 191

A physical therapist asks a patient to complete a visual analogue scale designed to assess pain intensity. The scale consists of a 10 centimeter line with descriptive labels at each end. Which terminology would be the MOST appropriate for the FIRST label?

1. **no pain**
2. mild pain
3. weak pain
4. faint pain

> ### Correct Answer: 1 (Magee p. 9)

A visual analogue scale is a tool used to assess pain intensity using a 10-15 cm line with the left anchor indicating "no pain" and the right anchor indicating "the worst pain you can have." The level of perceived pain is indicated on the line and is reassessed frequently over the course of physical therapy to qualify changes in the pain level and to assess progress.

1. **The left anchor of a visual analogue pain scale is often described as no pain, pain free or the absence of pain.**
2. Mild pain is defined as not acute or serious. The term mild pain would be more appropriately used on a verbal descriptor scale where a patient may be asked to point to a term that best matches their pain (e.g., slight pain, mild pain, moderate pain, severe pain).
3. Weak pain is characterized as not strong or lacking force. This would correspond to a rating on the lower portion of the visual analogue scale, but would not be used as an anchor definition.
4. Faint pain is characterized as lacking strength or vividness. This would correspond to a rating slightly above the visual analogue scale's left anchor.

System Specific: Other Systems
Content Outline: Examination

Exam One: Question 192

The MOST important contribution case reports make to evidence-based practice in physical therapy is:

1. A case report demonstrates a causal relationship between treatment and outcome in a single patient.
2. **A case report provides information that can be used to generate inductive hypotheses for future studies.**
3. A case report provides data on the natural history of disease states.
4. A case report uses triangulation to test a hypothesis with more than one source of data.

> ### Correct Answer: 2 (Portney p. 316)

Describing interesting, new and unique cases is one means of building a foundation for clinical science.
The case report is a practical approach to research in the clinical sciences because it is directly applicable to patient care, but it is also the least rigorous because of its lack of control and limited generalizability.

1. Due to the lack of control and the number of different interventions the patient may receive (medical, surgical, nursing, social, recreational, etc.), it is not reasonable to try to suggest a direct causal relationship between one treatment and the outcome in a single patient.
2. **Case reports are important for generating and testing theory and for providing information that may be used to generate inductive hypotheses that can be tested by exploratory or experimental methods.**
3. Longitudinal studies of many patients followed for a long period of time are the preferred means of studying the natural history of a disease.
4. Case reports do not triangulate data from multiple sources to test hypotheses. In most case reports, the data comes from a single patient.

System Specific: Non-Systems
Content Outline: Safety & Professional Roles; Teaching/Learning; Research

Exam One: Question 193

A physical therapist treats an infant diagnosed with torticollis with marked lateral flexion of the neck to the right. As part of the infant's plan of care the therapist performs passive stretching activities to improve the patient's range of motion. The MOST appropriate stretch for the patient is:

1. lateral flexion to the right and rotation to the right
2. lateral flexion to the left and rotation to the left
3. lateral flexion to the right and rotation to the left
4. **lateral flexion to the left and rotation to the right**

Correct Answer: 4 (Long p. 190)

Torticollis is characterized by lateral flexion of the head toward the affected side and rotation toward the unaffected side. The condition is caused by a contracture of the sternocleidomastoid muscle.

1. Stretching in lateral flexion to the right would be inappropriate since the question indicates that the patient presents with marked lateral flexion of the neck to the right. The direction of the stretch for the rotation component is accurate.
2. Stretching in lateral flexion to the left would be beneficial, however, patients with torticollis present with rotation to the opposite side. As a result, the rotation component should be stretched to the right and not the left.
3. This option more accurately characterizes the clinical presentation of the patient than it does the necessary stretch. The question indicates that the patient presents with marked lateral flexion of the neck to the right and therefore it would not make sense to stretch to the right. The direction of stretch for the rotation component is also inaccurate.
4. **Stretching the patient in lateral flexion to the left and rotation to the right is the correct answer since it is opposite of the patient's current contracture (i.e., marked lateral flexion of the neck to the right and rotation to the left).**

System Specific: Musculoskeletal System
Content Outline: Foundations for Evaluation, Differential Diagnosis, & Prognosis

Test Taking Tip: It is possible for a candidate to eliminate two of the presented options without having any specific knowledge related to torticollis. The question indicates that the patient presents with marked lateral flexion of the neck to the right. Based on the that particular clinical finding it becomes apparent that the stretch would need to be in the opposite direction (i.e., to the left). Often when presented with information that is unfamiliar, candidates fail to recognize that they can still narrow down the presented options. It is critically important for candidates to use this valuable skill since it can significantly increase the probability of identifying the correct response.

Exam One: Question 194

A physical therapist instructs a patient to close her eyes and hold out her hand. The therapist places a series of different weights in the patient's hand one at a time. The patient is then asked to identify the comparative weight of the objects. This method of sensory testing is used to examine:

1. **barognosis**
2. graphesthesia
3. recognition of texture
4. stereognosis

Correct Answer: 1 (O'Sullivan p. 147)

Barognosis, graphesthesia, recognition of texture, and stereognosis are considered combined cortical sensations.

1. **Barognosis refers to the ability of a patient to identify the comparative weight of objects in a series. This can be done by placing a series of different weights in the same hand or by placing different weights in each hand simultaneously.**
2. Graphesthesia refers to the ability of a patient to verbally identify letters or numbers traced on the palm of the hand typically with a fingertip or the eraser of a pencil.
3. Recognition of texture refers to the ability to differentiate among various textures such as cotton, wool or silk. Items may be identified by name or texture such as rough or smooth.
4. Stereognosis refers to the ability to identify an object without sight. Objects used are typically easily obtainable and familiar objects such as a coin, key or comb. Patients are asked to verbally identify the object by name.

System Specific: Neuromuscular & Nervous Systems
Content Outline: Examination

Exam One: Question 195

A physical therapist assesses the pulse rate of a patient exercising on a treadmill. The therapist notes that the rhythm of the pulse is often irregular. The MOST appropriate action to ensure an accurate measurement of pulse rate is:

1. select a different pulse site
2. **measure the pulse rate for 60 seconds**
3. use a different stethoscope
4. document the irregular pulse rate in the patient's medical record

> **Correct Answer: 2** (Pierson p. 58)

An irregular pulse rate is characterized by beats occurring at varying intervals. The lack of predictability will increase measurement error particularly when the time used to assess the pulse is relatively small (e.g., 15 seconds).

1. Pulse site will not have an impact on the regularity or irregularity of the pulse.
2. **The longer the duration of the measurement, the closer the obtained measure will be to the patient's actual pulse rate. Although 60 seconds may seem excessive to assess the pulse in a patient with a regular heart rhythm, it is often necessary in the presence of an irregular rhythm in order to ensure a valid measure of pulse rate.**
3. The question does not provide any evidence to suggest that the stethoscope used is defective. In addition, the type of stethoscope used would primarily influence the quality of audible sound and not other items such as rhythm.
4. Documenting the irregular rhythm is necessary, however, the question specifically asks for the most appropriate method to ensure an accurate measurement of pulse rate.

System Specific: Cardiac, Vascular, & Pulmonary Systems
Content Outline: Examination

Exam One: Question 196

A physical therapist participates in a community fitness program by conducting anthropometric measurements designed to determine percent body fat. Which site is NOT typically utilized when measuring skinfolds?

1. suprailiac
2. subscapular
3. triceps
4. **lateral calf**

> **Correct Answer: 4** (American College of Sports Medicine p. 269)

Measuring body composition by determining skinfold measurements is based on the principle that the amount of subcutaneous fat is proportional to the total amount of body fat. The technique provides a better estimate of body fat than height, weight, and circumference; however, is not as accurate as hydrostatic weighing.

1. The suprailiac site is taken by obtaining a diagonal fold; in line with the natural angle of the iliac crest taken in the anterior axillary line immediately superior to the iliac crest.
2. The subscapular site is taken by obtaining a diagonal fold; 1-2 cm below the inferior angle of the scapula.
3. The triceps site is taken by obtaining a vertical fold; on the posterior midline of the upper arm, halfway between the acromion and olecranon process, with the arm held freely to the side of the body.
4. **The lateral calf is not a site used for obtaining skinfold measurements, rather the medial calf is used. The medial calf site is taken by obtaining a vertical fold; at the maximum circumference of the calf on the midline of its medial border.**

System Specific: Other Systems
Content Outline: Examination

Exam One: Question 197

A physical therapist prepares to administer ultrasound to a patient with lateral epicondylitis. When applying ultrasound the amount of heat absorbed is LEAST dependent upon:

1. the intensity
2. the duration of exposure
3. **the choice of the coupling agent**
4. the size of the area sonated

Correct Answer: 3 (Prentice – Therapeutic Modalities p. 378)

A number of factors play a significant role in determining the amount of heat absorbed using ultrasound. Physical therapists must ensure that the selected parameters are consistent with the desired physiologic effect.

1. Intensity refers to the power per unit area of the sound head, most often expressed in W/cm^2. The amount of heat absorbed will increase as the intensity increases assuming that other parameters remain constant.
2. The amount of heat absorbed will increase as the duration of exposure increases assuming that the other parameters remain constant. The duration of exposure is measured in minutes.
3. **A coupling agent is used to transmit ultrasound energy between the transducer and the target area since ultrasound waves do not travel well through air. Examples of coupling agents include gels, lotions, bladders or water. The choice of coupling agent has a relatively small impact when compared to the other presented options.**
4. The amount of heat absorbed will increase as the size of the area sonated decreases assuming that other parameters remain constant. Surface area is most often measured in cm^2. Surface area two to three times the size of the transducer typically requires a duration of five minutes of treatment.

System Specific: Non-Systems
Content Outline: Equipment & Devices; Therapeutic Modalities

Exam One: Question 198

A physical therapist employed in a rehabilitation hospital utilizes the services of a physical therapy aide. Which variable BEST determines the extent to which physical therapy aides are involved in patient care activities?

1. the number of years of experience
2. the scope of formal training
3. **the discretion of the physical therapist**
4. the quantity of continuing education courses

Correct Answer: 3 (Guide to Physical Therapist Practice)

The physical therapy aide is a non-licensed worker who is specifically trained under the direction and supervision of a physical therapist. Activities performed by the aide are limited to those tasks that do not require clinical decision making by the physical therapist.

1. Regardless of the number of years of training the aide remains a non-licensed health care provider.
2. The scope of the formal training of the physical therapy aide may influence how the aide is utilized, however, to what extent this factor is considered will depend on the judgment of the physical therapist.
3. **The determination of what tasks are appropriately directed to the aide must be made by the physical therapist or, where allowable by law or regulations, the physical therapist assistant.**
4. The quantity of continuing education courses may provide the physical therapy aide with specialized knowledge in selected areas of clinical practice, however, how this influences the aides' role in patient care activities remains the responsibility of the physical therapist.

System Specific: Non-Systems
Content Outline: Safety & Professional Roles; Teaching/Learning; Research

Exam One: Question 199

A physical therapist prepares to treat a patient with cystic fibrosis using postural drainage. The MOST appropriate patient position when treating the superior segments of the lower lobes is:

1. sitting, leaning over a folded pillow at a 30 degree angle
2. head down on left side, 1/4 turn backward
3. supine with two pillows under the knees
4. **prone with two pillows under the hips**

Correct Answer: 4 (Rothstein p. 445)

Postural drainage for the superior segments of the lower lobes requires the physical therapist to clap over the middle of the back at the tip of the scapula on either side of the spine.

1. Sitting, leaning over a folded pillow at a 30 degree angle describes the postural drainage position for the posterior segments of the upper lobes.
2. Head down on left side, 1/4 turn backward describes the postural drainage position for the right middle lobe.
3. Supine with two pillows under the knees describes the postural drainage position for the anterior segments of the left and right upper lobes.
4. **Prone with two pillows under the hips describes the postural drainage position for the superior segments of the left and right lower lobes.**

System Specific: Cardiac, Vascular, & Pulmonary Systems
Content Outline: Interventions

Exam One: Question 200

A patient rehabilitating from a knee injury completes an isokinetic examination. The patient produces 88 ft/lbs of torque with the hamstrings at 120 degrees per second. Assuming normal quadriceps/hamstrings ratio, which of the following MOST accurately reflects the predicted quadriceps value?

1. 67 ft/lbs
2. 109 ft/lbs
3. **136 ft/lbs**
4. 183 ft/lbs

Correct Answer: 3 (Hamill p. 236)

The most commonly accepted ratio of quadriceps to hamstrings strength is 3:2. As the speed of movement increases above 200 degrees per second the ratio approaches 1:1.

1. A quadriceps value of 67 ft/lbs would indicate that the quadriceps are not as strong as the recorded hamstrings value (i.e., 0.8:1.0).
2. A quadriceps value of 109 ft/lbs would result in a quadriceps/hamstrings ratio of slightly greater than 1:1 (i.e., 1.2:1.0).
3. **A quadriceps value of 136 ft/lbs would result in a quadriceps/hamstrings ratio of approximately 3:2 (i.e., 1.5:1.0).**
4. A quadriceps value of 183 ft/lbs would result in a quadriceps/hamstrings ratio of over 2:1 (i.e., 2.1:1.0).

System Specific: Musculoskeletal System
Content Outline: Examination

Notes

Physical Therapy Exam Two

DIRECTION

"If you don't know where you are going you could wind up some place else." - Yogi Berra

Candidates must be proactive throughout the study process and avoid relying on their past accomplishments. Candidates that assess their progress throughout the study plan and make appropriate modifications often outperform candidates that prepare for the National Physical Therapy Examination in a more random fashion.

Exam Two: Question 1

A physical therapist using an electrical stimulation device attempts to quantify several characteristics of a monophasic waveform. When measuring phase charge, the standard unit of measure is the:

1. **coulomb**
2. ampere
3. ohm
4. second

Correct Answer: 1 (Prentice - Therapeutic Modalities p. 84)

Physical therapists should possess an understanding of the basic principles associated with electricity. As part of this knowledge, therapists should be aware of the standard units associated with commonly utilized electrical terminology.

1. **A coulomb is a term used to describe electrical charge. One coulomb equals 6.25×10^{18} electrons per second.**
2. An ampere is a unit of measure used to describe the rate of current. One ampere equals the delivery of one coulomb of electrical charge per second.
3. An ohm is a unit used to describe resistance or electrical impedance. An electrical circuit with high resistance (ohms) will have less flow (amperes) than a circuit with less resistance and the same voltage.
4. A second is a unit used to measure time. There are 60 seconds in a minute. Common terms used with electrical current include microseconds and milliseconds.

System Specific: Non-Systems
Content Outline: Equipment & Devices; Therapeutic Modalities

Exam Two: Question 2

A physical therapist assesses the functional strength of a patient's hip extensors while observing the patient move from standing to sitting. What type of contraction occurs in the hip extensors during this activity?

1. concentric
2. **eccentric**
3. isometric
4. isokinetic

Correct Answer: 2 (Levangie p. 376)

The gluteus maximus and the hamstrings muscles function as primary hip extensors. These muscles contract in an eccentric fashion when moving from standing to sitting.

1. Concentric contractions require a shortening of the involved muscle. The hip extensors would lengthen when moving from standing to sitting and therefore the contraction would not be labeled concentric.
2. **Eccentric contractions require a lengthening of the involved muscle. The contraction generally occurs when there is a need to decelerate a body part. The hip extensors would lengthen when moving from standing to sitting.**
3. Isometric contractions do not change the length of a muscle or produce movement. As a result, the hip extensors cannot contract isometrically when moving from standing to sitting.
4. Isokinetic contractions occur when a muscle contracts and shortens at a constant speed. This can occur only when a muscle's maximal force of contraction exceeds the total load on the muscle. The hip extensors would not lengthen at a constant speed when moving from standing to sitting.

System Specific: Musculoskeletal System
Content Outline: Clinical Application of Foundational Sciences

Exam Two: Question 3

A patient referred to physical therapy with chronic low back pain has failed to make any progress toward meeting established goals in over three weeks of treatment. The physical therapist has employed a variety of treatment techniques, but has yet to observe any sign of subjective or objective improvement in the patient's condition. The MOST appropriate action would be to:

1. transfer the patient to another therapist's schedule
2. re-examine the patient and establish new goals
3. continue to modify the patient's treatment plan
4. **alert the referring physician to the patient's status**

Correct Answer: 4 (Criteria for Standards of Practice)

Physical therapists must be willing to consult with a referring physician when there is ample evidence suggesting that the patient is not benefitting from physical therapy services.

1. There is no supporting evidence to suggest that the patient's failure to make progress is influenced by the patient-therapist relationship or the therapist's level of competence.
2. Re-examining the patient and establishing new goals is a viable option, however, failing to make progress during a relatively long period of time (i.e., three weeks) necessitates formal communication with the physician.
3. Modifying an established treatment plan is desirable when progress has not been made or the rate of progress is not satisfactory. Although a desirable option, the length of time the patient has failed to make progress would necessitate formal communication with the physician.
4. **Formal communication should occur with the referring physician when a patient fails to make progress in physical therapy. This is particularly relevant in the described scenario since the physical therapist has employed a variety of treatment techniques and has not observed any sign of subjective or objective improvement.**

System Specific: Non-Systems
Content Outline: Safety & Professional Roles; Teaching/Learning; Research

Exam Two: Question 4

A patient recently admitted to an acute care hospital is referred to physical therapy. The physical therapist documents the following clinical signs: pallor, cyanosis, and cool skin. These clinical signs are MOST consistent with:

1. cor pulmonale
2. **anemia**
3. hypertension
4. diaphoresis

Correct Answer: 2 (Paz p. 405)

Anemia refers to a reduction in the number of circulating red blood cells or a reduction in hemoglobin. Anemia is the most common disorder of the blood. The three main categories of anemia include excessive blood loss (i.e., hemorrhage), excessive blood cell destruction (i.e., hemolysis), and deficient red blood cell production (i.e., hematopoiesis).

1. Cor pulmonale is right-sided heart failure arising from disease of the lungs. Signs of right ventricular failure are elevated central venous pressure with distension of the neck veins. Ascites (accumulation of fluid in the peritoneal cavity) and peripheral edema of the feet and ankles are common. Individuals with heart failure often experience fatigue and exercise intolerance.
2. **A decrease in the number of red blood cells that carry oxygen in the blood results in a variety of symptoms including pallor, cyanosis, cool skin, vertigo, weakness, headache, and malaise.**
3. Hypertension, or increased blood pressure, is diagnosed when diastolic blood pressure equals or exceeds 90 mm Hg or when systolic blood pressure equals or exceeds 140 mm Hg. Hypertension often goes unrecognized as mild to moderate elevations in blood pressure usually are not symptomatic.
4. Diaphoresis refers to profuse perspiration and is often associated with shock or other emergent medical conditions.

System Specific: Cardiac, Vascular, & Pulmonary Systems
Content Outline: Foundations for Evaluation, Differential Diagnosis, & Prognosis

Exam Two: Question 5

A physical therapist employed by a home health care agency knocks on the door of a patient that has a scheduled therapy session. After waiting several minutes, the therapist concludes the patient is not at home. The MOST appropriate therapist action is:

1. **contact the patient and reschedule**
2. notify the patient's insurance provider
3. notify the referring physician
4. discharge the patient from physical therapy

Correct Answer: 1 (Criteria for Standards of Practice)

Physical therapists must decide how to handle missed appointments based on the relative frequency of occurrence and the rationale presented by the patient. There is not any information provided that indicates the patient has missed previous appointments and therefore the situation should be treated as an isolated incident.

1. **There are a number of possible reasons why the patient may have missed the appointment such as an unexpected emergency or neglecting to write down the scheduled appointment. As a result, the therapist should focus on rescheduling the patient's session.**
2. The insurance provider would receive information on therapy sessions attended, however, it would be unnecessary to notify the provider about a single missed appointment.
3. Physicians need to be updated on patient progress and relevant changes in medical status, however, missing a scheduled appointment would not meet this type of criteria.
4. A single missed appointment would not be sufficient grounds to discharge the patient from physical therapy. If missing scheduled appointments was a recurring theme, this option would be more plausible.

System Specific: Non-Systems
Content Outline: Safety & Professional Roles; Teaching/Learning; Research

Exam Two: Question 6

A physical therapist receives a referral for a two-month-old infant diagnosed with osteogenesis imperfecta. After completing the examination, the therapist discusses the physical therapy plan of care with the infant's parents. The PRIMARY goal of therapy should be:

1. improve muscle strength and diminish tone
2. facilitate protected weight bearing
3. **promote safe handling and positioning**
4. diminish pulmonary secretions

Correct Answer: 3 (Ratliffe p. 254)

Osteogenesis imperfecta is an autosomal disorder of collagen synthesis that affects bone metabolism. Children with osteogenesis imperfecta often have delayed developmental milestones secondary to ongoing fractures with immobilization, hypermobility of joints, and poorly developed muscles. The disorder is classified into four types with diverse clinical presentations ranging from normal appearance with mild symptoms to severe involvement that can be fatal during infancy.

1. The patient would likely have diminished muscle strength due to atrophy, hypermobility of joints, and multiple fractures. Improving strength is therefore desirable, however, would not be the primary goal of therapy for the patient. In addition, tone is not typically altered with osteogenesis imperfecta.
2. Protected weight bearing is desirable in order to reduce the risks associated with fracture and prevent disuse atrophy. Given the patient's age this goal would not be the primary focus of therapy.
3. **A patient with osteogenesis imperfecta is extremely susceptible to fractures during even basic activities such as being carried or bathing. As a result, safe handling and positioning would be the primary goal. This information would be critical to convey to all caregivers, perhaps most notably, the infant's parents.**
4. Osteogenesis imperfecta is a disorder of collagen synthesis that affects bone metabolism. The disorder would not directly influence pulmonary secretions.

System Specific: Musculoskeletal System
Content Outline: Foundations for Evaluation, Differential Diagnosis, & Prognosis

Exam Two: Question 7

A physical therapist elects to utilize the Six-Minute Walk Test as a means of quantifying endurance for a patient rehabilitating from a lengthy illness. Which variable would be the MOST appropriate to measure when determining the patient's endurance level with this objective test?

1. perceived exertion
2. heart rate response
3. elapsed time
4. **distance walked**

> **Correct Answer: 4** (Paz p. 915)

The Six-Minute Walk Test is used to determine a patient's functional exercise capacity. The test is commonly used upon admission, discharge, and to monitor progress or decline throughout physical therapy. This tool is administered to various populations including those with cardiac impairments, pulmonary disease, chronic conditions, and patients recovering from orthopedic surgical procedures.

1. The patient is instructed to walk as quickly as they can and attempt to cover as much ground as possible within the six minute period. The therapist does not attempt to record the patient's perceived exertion, however, the patient must let the therapist know if they experience chest pain or dizziness.
2. The heart rate response will likely increase as the intensity and duration of the test increases, however, the test is not designed to examine the heart rate response. Heart rate, blood pressure, oxygen saturation, and a dyspnea score are typically assessed prior to and after the administration of the test.
3. The elapsed time for the Six-Minute Walk Test is six minutes, as the name implies, and therefore does not vary during the administration of the test.
4. **The test requires the therapist to measure the distance the patient walks within a six minute period with rest periods permitted as necessary.**

System Specific: Cardiac, Vascular, & Pulmonary Systems
Content Outline: Examination

Exam Two: Question 8

A physician orders an electrocardiogram (ECG) for a patient diagnosed with congestive heart failure. The medical record indicates the patient is currently taking digitalis. What effect would you expect digitalis to have on the patient's ECG?

1. sinus tachycardia
2. **lengthened PR interval**
3. lengthened QT interval
4. elevated ST segment

> **Correct Answer: 2** (Brannon p. 227)

Digitalis is a medication given to increase the force of myocontractility and is often prescribed for patients with heart failure. Increased contractility increases cardiac output and decreases preload, cardiac workload, and myocardial oxygen demand, thus reducing the clinical effects of congestive heart failure.

1. Sinus tachycardia is a fast heart rate (greater than 100 bpm) that has its origin in the SA node.
2. **By increasing conduction time through the AV node, digitalis prolongs the PR interval on the ECG.**
3. The QT interval measures the depolarization and repolarization time of the ventricles and extends from the beginning of the QRS complex to the end of the T wave. Digitalis may produce shortening of the QT interval.
4. The ST segment represents the beginning of ventricular repolarization and is generally isoelectric. In healthy African American men it can be elevated as much as 2 mm. The ST segment is also elevated in an acute myocardial infarction. Digitalis may produce sagging in the ST segment.

System Specific: Cardiac, Vascular, & Pulmonary Systems
Content Outline: Foundations for Evaluation, Differential Diagnosis, & Prognosis

Exam Two: Question 9

A physical therapist completes an examination on a five-year-old boy diagnosed with Duchenne muscular dystrophy. The referral indicates that the boy was diagnosed with the disease less than one year ago. Assuming a normal progression, which of the following findings would be the FIRST to occur?

1. distal muscle weakness
2. **proximal muscle weakness**
3. impaired respiratory function
4. inability to perform activities of daily living

> **Correct Answer: 2** (Ratliffe p. 241)

Duchenne muscular dystrophy is an inherited disorder, characterized by rapidly worsening muscle weakness that starts in the proximal muscles of the lower extremities and pelvis, and later affects all voluntary muscles.

1. Distal muscles are affected later in the course of the disease process.
2. **Muscle weakness and atrophy begin in the proximal muscles of the lower extremities and pelvis, then progresses to the muscles of the shoulders and neck, followed by loss of upper extremity muscles and respiratory muscles.**
3. The muscles of respiration are not initially affected in patients with Duchenne muscular dystrophy.
4. As the condition progresses, weakness begins to interfere with activities of daily living.

System Specific: Other Systems
Content Outline: Foundations for Evaluation, Differential Diagnosis, & Prognosis

Exam Two: Question 10

A physical therapist obtains an x-ray of a 14-year-old female recently referred to physical therapy after experiencing an increase in back pain following activity. The patient previously participated in competitive gymnastics, however, states that her back was unable to tolerate the intensity of training. Based on the presented x-ray, the therapist would expect the patient's medical diagnosis to be:

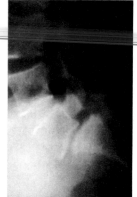

1. spondylitis
2. spondylolysis
3. **spondylolisthesis**
4. spondyloptosis

> **Correct Answer: 3** (Magee p. 515)

There are a variety of commonly encountered medical conditions that significantly impact the lumbar spine. Physical therapists should be familiar with the clinical presentation and management of these medical conditions.

1. Spondylitis refers to inflammation of a vertebra.
2. Spondylolysis refers to a defect in the pars interarticularis or the arch of the vertebra. This is most common in the L5 vertebra, but can also occur in other lumbar or thoracic vertebra.
3. **Spondylolisthesis refers to the forward displacement of one vertebra over another. The x-ray involves spondylolisthesis at the L5-S1 level. Individuals involved in physical activities such as weight lifting, gymnastics or football are particularly susceptible to this condition. The severity of the spondylolisthesis is classified on a scale of 1-5 based on how much a given vertebral body has slipped forward over the vertebral body beneath it.**
4. Spondyloptosis refers to the condition where a vertebral body is completely off of the adjacent vertebral body (grade 5).

System Specific: Musculoskeletal System
Content Outline: Foundations for Evaluation, Differential Diagnosis, & Prognosis

Exam Two: Question 11

A physical therapist completes a developmental assessment on a five-month-old infant. If the therapist elects to examine the infant's palmar grasp reflex, which of the following stimuli is the MOST appropriate?

1. contact to the ball of the foot in upright standing
2. **maintained pressure to the palm of the hand**
3. noxious stimulus to the palm of the hand
4. sudden change in the position of the head

> **Correct Answer: 2** (O'Sullivan p. 240)

Primitive reflexes are reflexes which begin during gestation or in early infancy. Most of these reflexes become integrated as the infant ages. Integration indicates that the reflex is no longer present when the stimulus is provided. Failure to integrate primitive reflexes can lead to impaired movement and function.

1. Contact to the ball of the foot in an upright position will elicit the plantar grasp reflex, resulting in curling of the toes. The reflex begins at 28 weeks of gestation and is fully integrated by 9 months of age.
2. **The palmar grasp reflex is elicited through maintained pressure to the palm of the hand resulting in finger flexion. The reflex begins at birth and is integrated at approximately four to six months of age.**
3. The palmar grasp reflex is stimulated by maintained pressure to the palm of the hand and not via noxious stimuli.
4. A sudden change in the position of the head will stimulate the Moro reflex and will cause extension, abduction of the upper extremities, hand opening and crying; followed by flexion and adduction of the upper extremities across the chest. The reflex begins at 28 weeks of gestation and is fully integrated by 5-6 months of age.

System Specific: Neuromuscular & Nervous Systems
Content Outline: Examination

Exam Two: Question 12

A physical therapist treats a nine-year-old child diagnosed with cystic fibrosis. As part of the treatment session the therapist attempts to improve the efficiency of the patient's breathing. The MOST appropriate technique to encourage full expansion at the base of the lungs is:

1. manual percussion over the posterior portion of the ribs with the patient in prone
2. **manual contacts with pressure over the lateral borders of the ribs with the patient in supine**
3. manual vibration over the lateral portion of the ribs with the patient in sidelying
4. manual cues over the epigastric area with the patient in supine

> **Correct Answer: 2** (Frownfelter p. 553)

Applying direct pressure with the hands on the lateral borders of the ribs with the patient in supine can promote a more efficient breathing pattern. Physical therapy management for a child with cystic fibrosis may include bronchial drainage techniques, chest percussion, vibration, and suctioning.

1. Manual percussion over the posterior ribs with the patient in prone describes the postural drainage position and technique used for airway clearance, not lung expansion, of the posterior basal lung segments
2. **Direct pressure of the hands over the lateral ribs can facilitate expansion of the basal lobes of the lungs.**
3. Manual vibration over the lateral portion of the ribs in sidelying describes the postural drainage position and technique used for airway clearance, not expansion, of the lateral basal lung segments.
4. The epigastric area refers to the upper central region of the abdomen. Manual cues on this area would not encourage expansion at the base of the lungs.

System Specific: Cardiac, Vascular, & Pulmonary Systems
Content Outline: Interventions

Exam Two: Question 13

A physician discusses a patient's plan of care with a physical therapist. The patient is a 29-year-old male that sustained deep partial-thickness burns to the anterior surface of his lower extremities. The physician discusses the possibility of discontinuing use of the topical antibiotic silver sulfadiazine after identifying an irregularity in the patient's laboratory results. Which finding could be MOST related to the use of silver sulfadiazine?

1. **leukopenia**
2. peripheral edema
3. hypokalemia
4. altered pH balance

Correct Answer: 1 (Paz p. 357)

Silver sulfadiazine is a topical antibiotic that works by interfering with bacterial nucleic acid production by disrupting folic acid synthesis in susceptible bacteria. The antibiotic is a broad spectrum agent that can be applied directly to the skin. Additional problems encountered with sulfa drugs include gastrointestinal distress and allergic reactions.

1. **Silver sulfadiazine is a sulfa drug that can produce a decrease in the number of circulating white blood cells (leukopenia), usually below 5,000 mm^3.**
2. Peripheral edema refers to the swelling of tissues in the lower limbs due to the accumulation of fluid. Peripheral edema frequently is associated with heart failure, venous insufficiency, pregnancy, kidney disease, and selected pharmacological agents.
3. Hypokalemia refers to an abnormally low potassium concentration in the blood. The condition can be caused by vomiting, diarrhea, burns, uncontrolled diabetes mellitus, diuretic therapy, and steroid therapy.
4. The pH is a measure of the degree to which a solution is acidic or alkaline. A pH of 7.0 indicates neutrality, a pH of less than 7.0 indicates acidity, a pH of more than 7.0 indicates alkalinity. The body's fluids are usually between 7.35-7.45. Topical agents such as mafenide acetate would be more likely to alter pH.

System Specific: Integumentary System
Content Outline: Interventions

Exam Two: Question 14

A patient recently admitted to the hospital with an acute illness is referred to physical therapy. During a scheduled treatment session the patient asks what effect anemia will have on his ability to complete a formal exercise program. The MOST appropriate therapist response is:

1. you may feel as though your muscles are weak
2. you may experience frequent nausea
3. your aerobic capacity may be reduced
4. **you may have a tendency to become fatigued**

Correct Answer: 4 (Goodman - Pathology p. 685)

Anemia refers to a reduction in the number of circulating red blood cells or reduction in hemoglobin. Symptoms of anemia include pallor of the skin, vertigo, and general malaise.

1. Although a patient may sense that their muscles are weak, fatigue will have a greater impact on the patient's ability to complete a formal exercise program.
2. Nausea refers to the sensation of unease and discomfort in the stomach with an urge to vomit. Nausea is a common side effect of many medications and is commonly associated with chemotherapy, pregnancy, and general anesthesia. Nausea is not typically associated with anemia.
3. Anemia may adversely affect aerobic capacity. However, this is not a term that most patients would readily understand.
4. **Anemia is a common cause of fatigue. Fatigue often results since there are an inadequate number of red blood cells available to transport oxygen to the tissues of the body.**

System Specific: Other Systems
Content Outline: Clinical Application of Foundational Sciences

Exam Two: Question 15

When performing range of motion exercises with a patient that sustained a head injury, a physical therapist notes that the patient lacks full elbow extension and classifies the end-feel as hard. The MOST likely cause is:

1. **heterotopic ossification**
2. spasticity of the biceps
3. anterior capsular tightness
4. triceps weakness

> **Correct Answer: 1** (Goodman - Pathology p. 1237)

Heterotopic ossification refers to abnormal bone growth in tissue and is relatively common in patients following head injury. Signs and symptoms include decreased range of motion, local swelling, and warmth.

1. **The presence of abnormal bone growth in tissue (i.e., heterotopic ossification) could result in an end-feel that is classified as hard due to the bony contact.**
2. Spasticity of the biceps would tend to produce a firm end-feel due to the presence of increased muscle tone.
3. Anterior capsular tightness would tend to produce a firm end-feel. Other common examples of a firm end-feel include muscular, ligamentous, and fascial shortening.
4. Muscle weakness would not be associated with an end-feel of any type since by definition end-feel is a passive assessment.

System Specific: Other Systems
Content Outline: Foundations for Evaluation, Differential Diagnosis, & Prognosis

Exam Two: Question 16

A physical therapist develops a problem list after examining a patient with a transtibial amputation. Which of the following would be the MOST appropriate entry in the patient problem list?

1. donning and doffing prosthesis requires verbal cues
2. donning and doffing prosthesis requires verbal cues and minimal assist of one
3. **dependence with donning and doffing prosthesis**
4. independent donning and doffing prosthesis in one week

> **Correct Answer: 3** (Quinn p. 34)

The problem list, located in the assessment portion of a S.O.A.P. note, should summarize the significant findings from the examination. Since the problem list relates back to the subjective and objective portion of the note, each entry should be described in broad terms. Items in the problem list should be capable of being influenced or changed by physical therapy intervention.

1. The entry describes the patient's current difficulty, but should be expressed in a more general manner without qualifiers (i.e., requires verbal cues).
2. The entry is similar to option 1 with an additional qualifier (i.e., minimal assist of one).
3. **The entry summarizes the patient's problem without providing unnecessary specificity which would already be included in the objective section of the S.O.A.P. note.**
4. The entry more closely approximates a goal since it describes a hypothesized future level of performance.

System Specific: Non-Systems
Content Outline: Safety & Professional Roles; Teaching/Learning; Research

Exam Two: Question 17

A physical therapist monitors a 6 foot 3 inch, 275 pound male's blood pressure using the brachial artery. Which of the following is MOST important when selecting an appropriate size blood pressure cuff for the patient?

1. patient age
2. percent body fat
3. somatotype
4. **extremity circumference**

Correct Answer: 4 (Pierson p. 62)

If the bladder of the blood pressure cuff is too narrow in relation to the circumference of the patient's arm, the reading will be erroneously high. Conversely, if the bladder is too wide, the reading will be erroneously low.

1. The patient's age is relevant to differentiate whether the patient is an infant, child or adult, however, age becomes a poor predictor of extremity circumference once an individual becomes an adult.
2. A patient with a high percent body fat may need a larger cuff, however, the measure is not nearly as sensitive as extremity circumference.
3. Somatotype is a term used to classify a system of body typing. The most common classifications of somatotype include endomorph, mesomorph, and ectomorph. This information may be useful, however, would not be nearly as specific as a more direct measure such as extremity circumference.
4. **The width of a bladder should be approximately 40% of the circumference of the midpoint of the limb. Bladder width for an average size adult is 5-6 inches.**

System Specific: Cardiac, Vascular, & Pulmonary Systems
Content Outline: Examination

Exam Two: Question 18

A patient informs a physical therapist that he has to use the bathroom immediately after being transported outside the hospital to practice car transfers. The physical therapist's MOST appropriate response to meet the patient's physical need is to:

1. ask the patient if it is an emergency
2. complete the transfer training as quickly as possible and allow the patient to use the bathroom
3. **transport the patient back into the hospital to use the bathroom**
4. instruct the patient that in the future he should use the bathroom before beginning physical therapy

Correct Answer: 3 (Code of Ethics)

The *Code of Ethics* published by the American Physical Therapy Association states that "A physical therapist shall respect the rights and dignity of all individuals and shall provide compassionate care."

1. Asking the patient if it is an emergency places the patient in an awkward situation since they may not have a clear idea of how long they can wait to use the bathroom or how long the transfer training will take. The response could also be interpreted by the patient as insensitive since they have already requested to use the bathroom.
2. The fact that the patient has to use the bathroom would likely impact their ability to fully engage in the transfer training. In addition, the patient may not be able to delay their need to use the bathroom until the training session has been completed.
3. **Transporting the patient back into the hospital shows respect for the patient's request and addresses the physical need in a timely manner.**
4. The response does not address the immediate patient need to use the bathroom. The action would be more compelling if the patient had made the same request on several different occasions, however, it still would not be the immediate response.

System Specific: Non-Systems
Content Outline: Safety & Professional Roles; Teaching/Learning; Research

Exam Two: Question 19

A physical therapist works with a patient status post stroke on a mat program. The therapist assists the patient in lateral weight shifting activities while positioned in prone on elbows. Which therapeutic exercise technique would allow the patient to improve dynamic stability with this activity?

1. alternating isometrics
2. **approximation**
3. rhythmic initiation
4. timing for emphasis

Correct Answer: 2 (Sullivan p. 27)

Facilitation techniques are designed to reduce the effects of impairments and disabilities while promoting motor recovery and improved function. It is important to select a facilitation technique whose purpose is consistent with the established therapeutic objectives.

1. Alternating isometrics are designed to facilitate isometric holding first in agonists acting on one side of the joint, followed by holding of the antagonist muscle groups. This technique is indicated when there is instability in weight bearing, poor static postural control, and/or weakness.
2. **Approximation is a therapeutic exercise technique designed to facilitate contraction and stability through joint compression. The compression force is most often applied to joints through gravity acting on body weight, manual contacts or weight belts.**
3. Rhythmic initiation is a facilitation technique that begins with voluntary relaxation followed by passive movement through increments in range. This is followed by active-assistive movements progressing to resisted movements. The technique is indicated when there is a need to relax, hypertonicity, inability to initiate movement, motor learning deficits, and communication deficits.
4. Timing for emphasis is a facilitation technique that uses maximum resistance to elicit a sequence of contractions from major muscle components of a pattern of motion. This technique allows overflow to occur from strong to weak muscles. The technique is indicated when there is weakness and/or incoordination and is commonly used in conjunction with repeated contractions.

System Specific: Neuromuscular & Nervous Systems
Content Outline: Interventions

Exam Two: Question 20

A patient informs a physical therapist how frustrated she feels after being examined by her physician. The patient explains that she becomes so nervous, she cannot ask any questions during scheduled office visits. The therapist's MOST appropriate response is to:

1. offer to go with the patient to her next scheduled physician visit
2. offer to call the physician and ask any relevant questions
3. **suggest that the patient write down questions for the physician and bring them with her to the next scheduled visit**
4. tell the patient it is a very normal response to be nervous in the presence of a physician

Correct Answer: 3 (Davis p. 95)

The physical therapist should attempt to identify a strategy or strategies that the patient can use to take a more active role during visits with the physician.

1. It is probably not realistic for the physical therapist to go with the patient to her next scheduled visit. In addition, the action places the burden on the therapist and does not promote a long-term change in the patient's current behavior.
2. Offering to call the physician and ask any relevant questions is similar to the previous option, however, may be slightly more practical. The action, however, does not require the patient to take a more active role and instead uses the physical therapist as an intermediary.
3. **Writing down questions allows the patient to reflect on the information she would like to gather in advance and provides the structure necessary to reduce the influence of the patient's anxiety during office visits.**
4. Acknowledging that many people are nervous in the presence of a physician may make the patient momentarily feel better, however, it does not provide the patient with a viable method to change her current behavior.

System Specific: Non-Systems
Content Outline: Safety & Professional Roles; Teaching/Learning; Research

Exam Two: Question 21

A physical therapist observes an electrocardiogram of a patient on beta-blockers. Which of the following electrocardiogram changes could be facilitated by beta-blockers?

1. **sinus bradycardia**
2. sinus tachycardia
3. premature ventricular contractions
4. ST segment sagging

> **Correct Answer: 1** (Brannon p. 134)

Beta-adrenergic blocking agents (beta-blockers) decrease heart rate, blood pressure, and myocardial contractility.

1. **Sinus bradycardia is a slow sinus rhythm of less than 60 beats per minute. It may occur from beta-blocker medication, during sleep, in physically fit individuals, acute myocardial infarction, carotid sinus pressure, and in response to increased vagal tone due to pain.**
2. Sinus tachycardia is a rapid sinus rhythm of greater than 100 beats per minute. It is usually caused by something that increases sympathetic activity, such as excitement, pain, fever, hypoxia, exercise, and stimulants. Beta-blockers have the opposite effect on heart rate.
3. A premature ventricular contraction (PVC) is a premature beat arising from an ectopic focus in the ventricle. PVCs may be precipitated by anxiety, tobacco, alcohol, caffeine, and any condition causing myocardial ischemia. PVCs are not caused by beta-blockers.
4. ST segment sagging or depression is indicative of myocardial ischemia and is not caused by beta-blockers.

System Specific: Cardiac, Vascular, & Pulmonary Systems
Content Outline: Clinical Application of Foundational Sciences

Exam Two: Question 22

An athlete is forced to contemplate knee surgery after spraining the anterior cruciate ligament (ACL) while playing soccer. Which situation would provide the MOST direct support for an anterior cruciate ligament reconstruction?

1. grade III ACL sprain with a grade I posterior cruciate ligament (PCL) sprain
2. grade III ACL sprain with a lateral meniscus tear
3. grade II ACL sprain with a medial meniscus tear
4. **functional instability**

> **Correct Answer: 4** (Kisner p. 726)

Surgical intervention is based on the amount of functional instability, however, is also influenced by a number of other variables including skeletal maturity, previous ligament injury, activity level, and age.

1. A grade III ACL sprain refers to a complete tear of the ACL. A grade I PCL sprain refers to a mild injury to the PCL without discernable laxity.
2. A grade III ACL sprain refers to a complete tear of the ACL. The addition of a lateral meniscus tear would likely enhance the instability already caused by the complete tear of the ACL.
3. A grade II ACL sprain refers to a moderate tear of the ACL with discernable laxity with the presence of an endpoint. The amount of laxity would be compounded by the presence of the medial meniscus tear. Meniscal tears contribute to knee instability since the meniscus, when healthy, contribute to the stability of the knee.
4. **Many individuals are able to continue to function at high levels despite a variety of ligamentous and meniscal injuries, therefore functional instability provides the most direct support for an anterior cruciate ligament reconstruction.**

System Specific: Musculoskeletal System
Content Outline: Foundations for Evaluation, Differential Diagnosis, & Prognosis

Exam Two: Question 23

A physical therapist employed in a long-term care setting attempts to identify a screening tool that examines a patient's ability to perform a variety of activities of daily living independently. The therapist would like to readminister the tool to assess patient progress. The MOST appropriate screening tool is the:

1. **Barthel Index**
2. Berg Balance Scale
3. Functional Reach Test
4. Tinetti Performance Oriented Mobility Assessment

> **Correct Answer: 1** (Physical Therapist's Clinical Companion p. 104)

There are a vast number of available screening tools utilized in physical therapy. A selected screening tool must be both valid and reliable and the individuals administering the tool must be qualified and capable in order to obtain meaningful results.

1. **The Barthel Index consists of ten activities of daily living and is often used as a screening tool in rehabilitation, long-term care settings, and home care. Scoring ranges from 0-100 in increments of 5. A score of 100 indicates that the patient is independent.**
2. The Berg Balance Scale consists of 14 tasks of everyday life activities that are scored according to a 0-4 scale. The maximum total score possible is 56, with a score of less than 45 indicating the patient is at risk for multiple falls.
3. The Functional Reach Test was developed to assess standing balance and the risk for falls. A person is required to stand upright against a wall with a static base of support. The patient is asked to make a fist and raise the arm nearest the wall to 90 degrees of shoulder flexion. The patient is then asked to lean forward as far as possible. The beginning position is subtracted from the ending position in order to obtain the final value.
4. The Tinetti Performance Oriented Mobility Assessment measures balance and gait using an ordinal scale of 0-2. The test has a total possible score of 28. Patients scoring less than 19 are considered to be at high risk for falling.

System Specific: Non-Systems
Content Outline: Safety & Professional Roles; Teaching/Learning; Research

Exam Two: Question 24

A patient rehabilitating from a lower extremity injury is referred to physical therapy for hydrotherapy treatments. The physical therapist would like the patient to fully extend the involved lower extremity while sitting in the hydrotherapy tank. Which type of whirlpool would NOT allow the patient to extend the involved lower extremity?

1. Hubbard tank
2. **highboy tank**
3. lowboy tank
4. walk tank

> **Correct Answer: 2** (Michlovitz p. 127)

Whirlpools consist of a tank that holds water and a turbine that produces movement of the water. Whirlpools are available in a variety of shapes and sizes. The type of whirlpool selected is primarily influenced by the size and shape of the body part to be treated and the established therapeutic objectives.

1. A Hubbard tank is used for full-body immersion. Approximate dimensions for the Hubbard tank are a depth of four feet, a length of eight feet, and a width of six feet.
2. **A highboy tank is designed for immersion of larger body parts. The length of a highboy tank does not permit a patient to fully extend the lower extremities in sitting, however, its depth permits immersion to the midthoracic region.**
3. A lowboy tank is also designed for immersion of larger body parts. The length of a lowboy tank permits a patient to fully extend the lower extremities in sitting, however, its depth is significantly less than the highboy.
4. A walk tank would allow for near full body immersion with the patient in an upright posture. The patient would have the ability to bear weight through the lower extremities and simulate selected functional activities.

System Specific: Non-Systems
Content Outline: Equipment & Devices; Therapeutic Modalities

Exam Two: Question 25

While examining a patient diagnosed with Achilles tendonitis, a physical therapist notes that the foot and ankle appear to be pronated. Which motions combine to create pronation in a non-weight bearing foot?

1. **abduction, dorsiflexion, eversion**
2. adduction, dorsiflexion, inversion
3. abduction, plantar flexion, eversion
4. adduction, plantar flexion, inversion

Correct Answer: 1 (Magee p. 854)

Pronation and supination are triplanar multi-joint motions that occur between the hindfoot, the midfoot, and the forefoot. A non-weight bearing foot is synonymous with the term open-chain.

1. **Pronation of the foot consists of abduction of the forefoot, dorsiflexion of the subtalar and midtarsal joints, and eversion and inward rotation of the heel.**
2. Pronation requires abduction of the forefoot and eversion of the heel, instead of adduction of the forefoot and inversion of the heel.
3. Pronation requires dorsiflexion and not plantar flexion of the subtalar and midtarsal joints.
4. Supination of the foot consists of adduction of the forefoot, plantar flexion of the subtalar and midtarsal joints, and inversion and outward rotation of the heel.

System Specific: Musculoskeletal System
Content Outline: Clinical Application of Foundational Sciences

Exam Two: Question 26

A physical therapist performs goniometric measurements on a patient rehabilitating from injuries sustained in a motor vehicle accident. When measuring rotation of the cervical spine, which of the following landmarks would be the MOST appropriate for the axis of the goniometer?

1. centered over the external auditory meatus
2. **centered over the center of the cranial aspect of the head**
3. centered over the C7 spinous process
4. centered over the midline of the occiput

Correct Answer: 2 (Norkin p. 324)

Cervical rotation occurs in the transverse plane around a vertical axis. The patient should be positioned sitting in a chair with back support. The cervical spine should be positioned in neutral.

1. Centering the axis of the goniometer over the external auditory meatus would be appropriate when measuring the range of motion for cervical flexion and extension. The stationary arm should be either perpendicular or parallel to the ground, while the moving arm should be aligned with the base of the nares.
2. **The axis of the goniometer should be positioned over the center of the cranial aspect of the head when measuring rotation of the cervical spine. The stationary arm should be parallel to an imaginary line between the two acromial processes, while the moving arm should be aligned with the tip of the nose.**
3. Centering the axis of the goniometer over the C7 spinous process would be appropriate when measuring the range of motion for cervical sidebending. The stationary arm should be aligned with the spinous processes of the thoracic vertebrae (perpendicular to the ground), while the moving arm is aligned with the dorsal midline of the head, using the occipital protuberance for reference.
4. Centering the axis of the goniometer over the midline of the occiput is not a commonly used landmark for cervical spine range of motion.

System Specific: Musculoskeletal System
Content Outline: Examination

Exam Two: Question 27

A physical therapist performs girth measurements on a patient rehabilitating from knee surgery. The therapist takes the measurements 5 cm and 10 cm above the superior pole of the patella with the patient in supine. The girth measurements are recorded as 32 cm and 37 cm on the right and 34 cm and 40 cm on the left. Which of the following conclusions can be made regarding the strength of the patient's quadriceps?

1. The right quadriceps will be capable of producing a greater force than the left.
2. The left quadriceps will be capable of producing a greater force than the right.
3. The right and left quadriceps will be capable of producing equal force.
4. **Not enough information is given to form a conclusion.**

> **Correct Answer: 4** (Magee p. 805)

Girth (circumferential) measurements using a flexible tape measure are commonly used to obtain a gross estimate of muscle atrophy or edema.

1. The circumference of the right quadriceps at the two identified measurement sites is less than the circumference of the equivalent sites on the left quadriceps. The obtained measurements would not likely support the statement that the right quadriceps are stronger than the left.
2. The circumference of the left quadriceps at the two identified measurement sites is greater than the circumference of the equivalent sites on the right quadriceps. The therapist may therefore hypothesize that the right quadriceps are stronger than the left, however, girth measurements are not used to determine strength.
3. The right and left quadriceps could be capable of producing equal force despite different circumferences, however, this is impossible to prove or disprove using girth measurements.
4. **The physical therapist cannot rely on girth measurements to determine strength and would instead need to utilize a formal test and measure for strength such as manual muscle testing or isokinetic testing.**

System Specific: Musculoskeletal System
Content Outline: Foundations for Evaluation, Differential Diagnosis, & Prognosis

Exam Two: Question 28

A physical therapist instructs a patient to expire maximally after taking a maximal inspiration. The therapist can use these instructions to measure the patient's:

1. expiratory reserve volume
2. inspiratory reserve volume
3. total lung capacity
4. **vital capacity**

> **Correct Answer: 4** (Brannon p. 293)

Vital capacity is the maximum volume of gas that can be exhaled after a maximum inhalation.

1. Expiratory reserve volume (ERV) is the additional volume of air that can be exhaled beyond the normal tidal exhalation. ERV is one component of vital capacity.
2. Inspiratory reserve volume (IRV) is the additional volume of air that can be inhaled beyond the normal tidal inhalation. IRV is one component of vital capacity.
3. Total lung capacity is the maximum volume to which the lungs can be expanded. It is the sum of vital capacity and residual volume: TLC = VC + RV.
4. **Vital capacity is the maximum volume of gas that can be exhaled after a maximum inhalation. It is equal to the sum of inspiratory reserve volume, tidal volume, and expiratory reserve volume: VC = IRV + TV + ERV.**

System Specific: Cardiac, Vascular, & Pulmonary Systems
Content Outline: Examination

Exam Two: Question 29

A physical therapist participating in a research project decides it will be necessary to utilize a relatively large sample. By including a large number of subjects, the researcher hopes to increase:

1. the effect size
2. **the likelihood of rejecting the null hypothesis**
3. the validity of the outcome measurements
4. the reliability of the outcome measurements

> **Correct Answer: 2** (Portney p. 423)

Sample size is critical to the probability that a statistical test will lead to rejection of the null hypothesis (i.e., statistical power). Besides sample size, statistical power is a function of the significance criterion (alpha), the variance in the data, and the effect size.

1. Effect size is a statistical expression of the magnitude of the difference between different treatments or the magnitude of the relationship between variables. Sample size has no specific effect on the effect size.
2. **The larger the sample, the greater the probability that a statistical test will lead to rejection of the null hypothesis. Small samples are less likely to represent the population of interest. Therefore, true differences or relationships (whatever is being tested) are more likely to be detected in large samples.**
3. Validity of measurement refers to the degree to which an instrument measures what it is intended to measure. Sample size has no specific effect on the validity of measurements.
4. Reliability of measurement refers to the consistency with which an instrument or rater measures a variable. Sample size has no specific effect on the reliability of measurements.

System Specific: Non-Systems
Content Outline: Safety & Professional Roles; Teaching/Learning; Research

Exam Two: Question 30

A physical therapist monitors a patient's vital signs while exercising in a phase I cardiac rehabilitation program. The patient is status post myocardial infarction and has progressed without difficulty while involved in the program. Which of the following vital sign recordings would exceed the typical limits of a phase I program?

1. heart rate elevated 18 beats per minute above resting level
2. respiration rate of 18 breaths per minute
3. **systolic blood pressure decreased by 25 mm Hg from resting level**
4. diastolic blood pressure less than 100 mm Hg

> **Correct Answer: 3** (Brannon p. 4)

Physical therapists should closely monitor the response to exercise of patients in a phase I cardiac rehabilitation program. A drop in the systolic blood pressure of 20 mm Hg or greater is indicative of exercise hypotension and is an indication to stop exercise.

1. An increase in heart rate of 18 beats per minute above resting heart rate is acceptable. Most guidelines for phase I cardiac rehabilitation recommend that heart rate not exceed 120 beats per minute or a heart rate more than 20 beats above resting for post myocardial infarction patients or a heart rate more than 30 beats above resting for post-surgical patients.
2. Dyspnea is a reason to terminate exercise during phase I exercise. However, a respiration rate of 18 breaths per minute is at the upper limit of the normal range and would not typically cause a patient to report a sense of dyspnea.
3. **A decrease in systolic pressure of 25 mm Hg exceeds the 20 mm Hg limit allowed during exercise in a phase I cardiac rehabilitation program.**
4. A diastolic blood pressure of 110 mm Hg is considered the upper limit for exercise in phase I cardiac rehabilitation. A diastolic pressure less than 110 mm Hg is acceptable.

System Specific: Cardiac, Vascular, & Pulmonary Systems
Content Outline: Interventions

Exam Two: Question 31

A physical therapist establishes the following short-term goal for a patient rehabilitating from total knee arthroplasty surgery: Patient will ambulate with a walker 50% weight bearing and moderate assist of 1 for 20 feet within one week. Three days later, the patient successfully achieves the established goal. Which of the following would be the MOST appropriate revision of the short-term goal?

1. ambulate with walker 75% weight bearing and moderate assist of 1 for 30 feet within one week
2. ambulate with walker 50% weight bearing and moderate assist of 2 for 30 feet within one week
3. **ambulate with walker 50% weight bearing and minimal assist of 1 for 30 feet within one week**
4. ambulate with walker 75% weight bearing and minimal assist of 1 for 10 feet within one week

Correct Answer: 3 (Guide for Professional Conduct)

Physical therapists must frequently revise short-term goals to facilitate the achievement of an established long-term goal.

1. The physician would be the health care professional responsible for modifying the patient's weight bearing status. The physical therapist would typically modify parameters associated with level of assistance, frequency, and duration.
2. The goal maintains the patient's present weight bearing status while it increases the assistance from 1 to 2 and increases the ambulation distance by 10 feet. The item does not provide adequate justification to increase the level of assistance based solely on an increase in ambulation distance of 10 feet.
3. **The goal maintains the patient's present weight bearing status while it decreases the level of assistance from moderate to minimal and increases the ambulation distance by 10 feet. This would appear to be a reasonable modification based on the previously achieved goal and the surgical procedure.**
4. Increasing the patient's weight bearing status from 50% to 75% would be inappropriate without physician approval.

System Specific: Non-Systems
Content Outline: Safety & Professional Roles; Teaching/Learning; Research

Exam Two: Question 32

A physician orders a nasogastric tube for a patient on an acute rehabilitation unit. Which of the following does NOT accurately describe a potential use of the nasogastric tube?

1. administer medications directly into the gastrointestinal tract
2. obtain gastric specimens
3. remove fluid or gas from the stomach
4. **obtain venous blood samples from the stomach**

Correct Answer: 4 (Pierson p. 288)

A nasogastric tube is a plastic tube that enters the body through a nostril and terminates in a patient's stomach. As a result, the tube is not used for obtaining venous samples.

1. A nasogastric tube can administer medications directly into the gastrointestinal tract. The patient can also be fed nutrients directly through the nasogastric tube if they are unable to take in adequate nutrition orally. Oral feeding or drinking is contraindicated when the nasogastric tube is in place, but exercise is permitted with caution. Head and neck movements should be closely monitored.
2. A nasogastric tube can be used to obtain gastric specimens. The tube is best taped to the patient's face so that it does not easily become dislodged.
3. A nasogastric tube can be used to remove fluid or gas from the stomach and may be utilized to keep the stomach empty after surgery. This would also allow the bowels to rest if needed.
4. **An intravenous line can be used to obtain venous blood samples (but not from the stomach). Intravenous lines also infuse fluids, nutrients, medications, and electrolytes. A nasogastric tube does not obtain venous samples.**

System Specific: Other Systems
Content Outline: Foundations for Evaluation, Differential Diagnosis, & Prognosis

Exam Two: Question 33

When observing a patient ambulating, a physical therapist notes that the patient's gait has the following characteristics: narrow base of support, short bilateral step length, and decreased trunk rotation. This gait pattern is often observed in patients with a diagnosis of:

1. CVA
2. **Parkinson's disease**
3. post-polio syndrome
4. multiple sclerosis

Correct Answer: 2 (Paz p. 190)

Patients with Parkinson's disease often exhibit gait abnormalities due to difficulty initiating movement, rigidity, absence of equilibrium responses, and diminished associated reactions.

1. A patient that has experienced a CVA may present with a wide range of diverse impairments, however, a common finding is hemiplegia or hemiparesis. Other characteristics may include gait deviations secondary to weakness and tonal influence. Patients often present with foot drop and decreased stability at the ankle, knee, and hip.
2. **The gait of a patient with Parkinson's disease is characterized by a decrease in stride length and velocity. As the disease progresses, the patient appears to be attempting to catch up with their center of gravity as the step length becomes smaller; this is termed festination. Festination places the patient at higher risk for a fall.**
3. The gait of a patient with post-polio syndrome is characterized by asymmetrical gait patterns secondary to weakness, fatigue, and pain.
4. The gait of a patient with multiple sclerosis is characterized by impaired trunk control and balance. There is often circumduction to assist with foot clearance and ataxia due to weakness and tonal influence.

System Specific: Neuromuscular & Nervous Systems
Content Outline: Foundations for Evaluation, Differential Diagnosis, & Prognosis

Exam Two: Question 34

A physical therapist prepares to complete an assisted standing pivot transfer with a patient that requires moderate assistance. In order to increase a patient's independence with the transfer, which of the following instructions would be the MOST appropriate?

1. I want you to help me perform the transfer.
2. **Try to utilize your own strength to complete the transfer.**
3. Only grab onto me if it is absolutely necessary.
4. Pretend you were home alone and needed to complete the transfer.

Correct Answer: 2 (Purtilo p. 168)

When treating a patient there must be clear and specific instructions given prior to the initiation of any task. Failure to offer clear and specific instructions increases the probability of an unwanted action. Requesting that the patient utilize their own strength to complete the transfer is the most appropriate instruction for the patient.

1. The statement, "I want you to help me perform the transfer," states that the therapist wants the patient to assist, but does not give the patient exact expectations on how to perform during the transfer.
2. **The statement, "Try to utilize your own strength to complete the transfer," is a direct statement that explains the exact expectations of the patient during the transfer.**
3. The statement, "Only grab onto me if it is absolutely necessary," does not encourage any kind of active participation on the patient's behalf and allows for a "high risk" behavior of grabbing onto the therapist at the patient's discretion.
4. The statement, "Pretend you were home alone and needed to complete the transfer," would not be appropriate since the patient currently requires moderate assistance and if they were "pretending to be alone" they would not follow the correct and safe method for transferring independently.

System Specific: Non-Systems
Content Outline: Safety & Professional Roles; Teaching/Learning; Research

Exam Two: Question 35

A physical therapist instructs a patient with a lower extremity amputation to wrap her residual limb. The patient has mildly impaired sensation on several localized areas of the residual limb. Which of the following would be the LEAST acceptable method of securing the bandage?

1. **clips**
2. safety pins
3. tape
4. Velcro

> **Correct Answer: 1** (Seymour p. 132)

Bandaging of the residual limb is an important aspect of care in rehabilitation following amputation. Goals include shaping, stabilizing the volume, and desensitization of the residual limb. Patients should avoid the use of clips for securing the bandage due to the potential risk for damage to the skin of the residual limb.

1. **Clips should not be used to secure bandages, especially for patients that exhibit impaired sensation. Failure of the patient to recognize that a clip is causing damage to the residual limb could lead to a wound that would significantly delay rehabilitation progress.**
2. Safety pins should not be used on a patient with impaired sensation. If the pin opens, there is risk for damage to the patient's residual limb. Although safety pins are not desirable, they are not as dangerous as clips.
3. Tape would be one of the most acceptable methods for securing the bandage since the tape does not pose any risk to the residual limb.
4. Velcro is an acceptable method to secure the bandage, however, it is not as feasible and affordable as tape.

System Specific: Integumentary System
Content Outline: Interventions

Exam Two: Question 36

A physical therapist attempts to identify a patient's risk factors for coronary artery disease as part of a health screening. The patient's heart rate is recorded as 78 beats per minute and blood pressure as 110/70 mm Hg. A recent laboratory report indicates a total cholesterol level of 170 mg/dL with high-density lipoproteins reported as 20 mg/dL and low-density lipoproteins as 110 mg/dL. Which of the following values would be considered atypical?

1. heart rate
2. blood pressure
3. **high-density lipoproteins (HDL)**
4. low-density lipoproteins (LDL)

> **Correct Answer: 3** (American Heart Association)

A value less than 40 mg/dL is considered low for HDL cholesterol. Values of 60 mg/dL or greater are considered high. A low HDL value is strongly associated with an increased risk for coronary artery disease.

1. 78 beats per minute is a normal resting heart rate. The range of normal is 60–100 beats per minute.
2. A systolic blood pressure of 110 mm Hg and a diastolic blood pressure of 70 mm Hg are considered within normal limits for blood pressures.
3. **A HDL cholesterol level of 20 mg/dL is very low and is associated with an increased risk of coronary artery disease. The patient would likely be treated by their physician with pharmacological and non-pharmacological therapies to raise the HDL cholesterol level.**
4. The optimal level of low-density lipoprotein cholesterol is less than 100. A value of 110 mg/dL is considered near optimal. High levels of LDL cholesterol increase the risk of coronary artery disease.

System Specific: Other Systems
Content Outline: Foundations for Evaluation, Differential Diagnosis, & Prognosis

Exam Two: Question 37

A physical therapist performs palpation with a patient positioned in standing as part of a respiratory assessment. Which structure would be the MOST appropriate to assess with the therapist positioned behind the patient?

1. mediastinum
2. upper chest wall motion
3. middle chest wall motion
4. **lower chest wall motion**

> **Correct Answer: 4** (Frownfelter p. 223)

Palpation of chest wall motion is performed segmentally to compare the motion over the upper, middle, and lower lobes while the patient is breathing quietly and while breathing deeply.

1. The physical therapist palpates the mediastinum to evaluate for deviation of the trachea by inserting the tip of the index finger in the suprasternal notch. This is done facing the patient.
2. The physical therapist evaluates upper chest wall expansion by placing the palms of the hands anteriorly over the chest wall from the fourth rib upward. The therapist's fingers are stretched over the trapezius and the thumbs placed together along the midline of the chest. The therapist faces the patient.
3. The physical therapist evaluates middle chest wall expansion by placing the fingers laterally over the posterior axillary folds with the thumbs together along the midline of the chest. The therapist faces the patient.
4. **The lower chest wall expansion is evaluated with the patient's back to the therapist and the therapist's fingers wrapped around the anterior axillary folds with the tips of the thumbs together at the vertebral spines.**

System Specific: Cardiac, Vascular, & Pulmonary Systems
Content Outline: Examination

Exam Two: Question 38

A physical therapist prepares a whirlpool treatment for a scheduled patient. Which treatment area would place the patient at the GREATEST risk for hyperthermia?

1. wrist and hand
2. **thigh**
3. elbow
4. foot and ankle

> **Correct Answer: 2** (Cameron p. 264)

Whirlpool treatments stress the body's ability to dissipate heat and therefore can result in hyperthermia or other forms of heat illness. The larger the portion of the body immersed in the whirlpool the greater the level of heat stress.

1. Whirlpool treatment to the wrist and hand would require only a small portion of the upper extremity to be immersed.
2. **Whirlpool treatment to the thigh would require the patient to be immersed up to the waist, possibly including a portion of the torso, depending on the configuration of the whirlpool tank. This level of immersion would place the patient at the greatest risk for hyperthermia.**
3. Whirlpool treatment to the elbow would require the majority of the upper extremity to be immersed. This is greater than the level of immersion for the wrist and hand, but it still represents a relatively small percentage of the total body surface.
4. Whirlpool treatment to the foot and ankle would require the lower extremity to be immersed only to the midcalf.

System Specific: Non-Systems
Content Outline: Equipment & Devices; Therapeutic Modalities

Exam Two: Question 39

A group of physical therapists conducts scoliosis screenings on adolescents as part of physical therapy week. The MOST appropriate action after identifying an adolescent with a moderate scoliotic curve is to:

1. **refer the adolescent for further orthopedic assessment**
2. educate the adolescent as to the cause of the scoliosis
3. devise an exercise program for the adolescent
4. instruct the adolescent in the importance of proper posture

Correct Answer: 1 (Goodman - Pathology p. 1113)

A patient with moderate scoliosis should be referred to an orthopedic physician since treatment for moderate curves (measured between 25 and 40 degrees) requires a spinal orthosis and physical therapy intervention for posture, flexibility, strengthening, respiratory function, and proper utilization of the spinal orthosis.

1. **Scoliosis is a condition that will respond to treatment best when detected early. Common postural findings with scoliosis include increased spacing between the elbow and trunk during standing, leg length discrepancy, uneven shoulder and hip heights, and prominence on one side of the pelvis or breast (due to rotation of the curve).**
2. Although education regarding scoliosis is important, the most appropriate action when identifying a moderate curve is to refer the patient to a physician for further assessment and treatment. The physician will educate the patient based on their findings regarding the scoliosis.
3. A physician should always evaluate a patient with moderate scoliosis prior to the development and implementation of an exercise program.
4. Postural training will not rectify or maintain a moderate scoliotic curve. Moderate curves require multifaceted treatment and physician involvement.

System Specific: Non-Systems
Content Outline: Safety & Professional Roles; Teaching/Learning; Research

Exam Two: Question 40

A physical therapist checks the water temperature of the hot pack machine after several patients report the heat being very strong. Which of the following temperatures would be acceptable?

1. 64 degrees Celsius (147 degrees Fahrenheit)
2. **71 degrees Celsius (160 degrees Fahrenheit)**
3. 83 degrees Celsius (181 degrees Fahrenheit)
4. 94 degrees Celsius (201 degrees Fahrenheit)

Correct Answer: 2 (Cameron p. 161)

A hot pack must be stored in hot water between 158 to 167 degrees Fahrenheit (70 to 75 degrees Celsius). Six to eight towel layers should be applied between the hot pack and the treatment surface. The size and shape of the hot pack varies depending on the size and contour of the treatment area.

1. 64 degrees Celsius (147 degrees Fahrenheit) would be less than the recommend water temperature in the hot pack unit. As a result, the hot pack would not possess the necessary thermal energy with the traditional number of towel layers.
2. **71 degrees Celsius (160 degrees Fahrenheit) is consistent with the recommended range of water temperature and therefore the hot pack will possess the requisite amount of thermal energy.**
3. 83 degrees Celsius (181 degrees Fahrenheit) would be greater than the recommended water temperature and therefore may create a potential safety risk for the patient without adding additional towel layers.
4. 94 degrees Celsius (201 degrees Fahrenheit) would be significantly greater than the recommended water temperature and would place the patient at significant risk for a superficial burn.

System Specific: Non-Systems
Content Outline: Equipment & Devices; Therapeutic Modalities

Exam Two: Question 41

A physical therapist employed in an outpatient physical therapy clinic attempts to obtain informed consent from a 17-year-old male prior to initiating a formal exercise test. The patient signs the informed consent form, however, the patient's parents dropped him off at the clinic and are now unavailable to sign the form. The MOST appropriate therapist action is:

1. complete the exercise test
2. secure another physical therapist to witness the exercise test
3. contact the referring physician and request approval to complete the exercise test
4. **reschedule the exercise test**

> **Correct Answer: 4** (Scott - Promoting Legal and Ethical Awareness p. 222)

Obtaining informed consent from patients before exercise testing is an important ethical and legal consideration. Physical therapists have an obligation to obtain informed consent from patients prior to initiating intervention activities. If a patient is under the age of 18 the therapist is required to obtain informed consent from the patient and a parent or legal guardian.

1. The physical therapist should have a valid consent form before performing the exercise test.
2. Having another physical therapist witness the test is not a substitute for legal informed consent.
3. Having the physician approve the test is not a substitute for legal informed consent.
4. **A patient's status as a minor makes it necessary that a parent or legal guardian sign the consent form. The physical therapist should reschedule the test to a time when a parent can sign the consent form.**

System Specific: Non-Systems
Content Outline: Safety & Professional Roles; Teaching/Learning; Research

Exam Two: Question 42

A physical therapist attempts to obtain a general assessment of a patient's cognitive status. The patient is a 62-year-old female three days status post total hip arthroplasty. The MOST appropriate action is:

1. review the patient's medical record
2. **conduct a patient interview**
3. conduct a physical examination
4. consult with family members

> **Correct Answer: 2** (Bickley p. 55)

A patient interview provides a physical therapist with an opportunity to assess patient cognition. This approach is often more appropriate than relying on a previous entry in the medical record, particularly with a patient status post surgery.

1. It is important to review a patient's medical record prior to the initial examination so that the therapist has an understanding of past medical history, current medical status, physician orders, and any precautions or contraindications, however, this is not the optimal choice for assessment of the patient's cognitive status.
2. **Conducting a patient interview allows the therapist to evaluate the patient's cognitive status through a routine screening of person, place, and time or through more extensive testing such as the Mini Mental State Examination.**
3. A physical examination would focus on a patient's physical attributes and impairments. Items such as muscle strength, range of motion, and anthropometric measurements are examples of common components of a physical examination.
4. Consultation with family members may assist in certain scenarios, however, cannot replace direct screening of the patient when assessing cognition.

System Specific: Other Systems
Content Outline: Examination

Exam Two: Question 43

A physical therapist attempts to secure a wheelchair for a patient with an incomplete spinal cord injury. The patient is a 28-year-old female that is very active and relies on a wheelchair as her primary mode of transportation. Which type of wheelchair design would be the MOST appropriate for the patient?

1. standard chair with a rigid frame
2. **lightweight chair with a rigid frame**
3. standard chair with a folding frame
4. lightweight chair with a folding frame

> **Correct Answer: 2** (Physical Therapist's Clinical Companion p. 324)

A lightweight wheelchair will be significantly easier for the patient to propel and maneuver, while a rigid frame provides the necessary durability and strength required for an active individual.

1. A standard chair would not be optimal secondary to the increased weight of the chair and the patient's decreased strength due to the incomplete spinal cord injury.
2. **A lightweight wheelchair is easier to propel and maneuver. The chair is made from stainless steel or aluminum which also enhances durability. The rigid frame allows for strength and a smoother ride for the patient.**
3. A standard wheelchair with a folding frame would not be optimal secondary to the increased weight of the chair which would necessitate greater effort for mobility and transportation. The folding frame would not possess the durability required for an active individual.
4. The lightweight wheelchair is a better choice for the patient, however, the folding frame is not an optimal choice based on the patient's activity level.

System Specific: Non-Systems
Content Outline: Equipment & Devices; Therapeutic Modalities

Exam Two: Question 44

A physical therapist attempts to select an assistive device for a patient rehabilitating from a traumatic brain injury. The patient is occasionally impulsive, however, has fair standing balance and good upper and lower extremity strength. Which of the following would be the MOST appropriate assistive device?

1. cane
2. axillary crutches
3. Lofstrand crutches
4. **walker**

> **Correct Answer: 4** (Pierson p. 219)

A walker would be the most appropriate assistive device to use since the patient can stand without support, however, has only fair standing balance and is impulsive at times. A walker does not require a great deal of coordination.

1. A cane is appropriate to assist with balance and stability, however, it does not provide a large amount of assistance due to the small base of support. A cane would not be appropriate for a patient that presents with impulsivity and only fair standing balance.
2. Axillary crutches are appropriate for patients of all weight bearing levels, however, require a higher level of coordination. Injury can occur to axillary vessels and nerves if used improperly. The device would not be appropriate for the patient based on their present balance and the medical diagnosis.
3. Lofstrand crutches are an option for patients that need more support than a cane. The crutches provide minimal stability and require functional standing balance and coordination for use. Lofstrand crutches would not be appropriate for a patient with fair balance and impulsivity.
4. **A walker is appropriate for patients of varying weight bearing levels. The device offers the greatest amount of stability due to its large base of support. The stability offered by the walker is necessary due to the patient's fair standing balance and impulsivity. Proper supervision would be necessary based on the patient's diagnosis.**

System Specific: Non-Systems
Content Outline: Equipment & Devices; Therapeutic Modalities

Exam Two: Question 45

A physical therapist examines a 16-year-old male diagnosed with left knee anterior cruciate ligament insufficiency. During the examination a Lachman test is performed. Ideally, the therapist should perform the test with the knee in:

1. **20-30 degrees flexion**
2. 30-40 degrees flexion
3. 40-50 degrees flexion
4. 80-90 degrees flexion

Correct Answer: 1 (Magee p. 767)

The Lachman test is perhaps the most common ligamentous instability test designed to assess the integrity of the anterior cruciate ligament. It is typically performed with the patient in a supine position and the knee flexed 20-30 degrees. The therapist applies an anterior directed force to the tibia on the femur. A positive test is indicated by excessive anterior translation of the tibia on the femur with a diminished or absent end-point and may be indicative of an anterior cruciate ligament injury.

1. **20-30 degrees of knee flexion is generally accepted as the amount of knee flexion used for the Lachman test. The position approximates a functional position and all parts of the anterior cruciate ligament are relatively taut.**
2. 30-40 degree of knee flexion is slightly greater than the recommended amount of knee flexion for the Lachman test.
3. 40-50 degrees is significantly greater than the recommended amount of knee flexion for the Lachman test.
4. 80-90 degrees of knee flexion more closely approximates the position of the knee when performing the anterior drawer test.

System Specific: Musculoskeletal System
Content Outline: Examination

Exam Two: Question 46

A patient with cerebellar dysfunction exhibits signs of dysmetria. Which of the following activities would be the MOST difficult for the patient?

1. rapid alternating pronation and supination of the forearms
2. **placing feet on floor markers while walking**
3. walking at varying speeds
4. marching in place

Correct Answer: 2 (Umphred p. 840)

Dysmetria refers to an inability to modulate movement where patients will either overestimate or underestimate their targets. The cerebellum is normally responsible for the timing, force, extent, and direction of the limb movement in order to correctly reach a target.

1. Dysdiadochokinesia refers to the inability to perform rapid alternating movements such as pronation and supination of the forearms. As speed increases there is typically a rapid loss of range of movement and rhythm of movement. This condition is a result of damage to the cerebellum.
2. **Dysmetria occurs with cerebellar lesions and is defined as the inability to appropriately reach a target. An example of dysmetria would be the inability of a patient to place their feet on floor markers successfully while walking.**
3. Difficulty walking at varying speeds is common with cerebellar pathology, however, the activity is not associated with dysmetria.
4. Patients with cerebellar lesions often have difficulty modulating movement. As a result, irregular stepping patterns and poor upright stance make activities such as marching in place difficult.

System Specific: Neuromuscular & Nervous Systems
Content Outline: Interventions

Exam Two: Question 47

A physical therapist examines a patient referred to physical therapy diagnosed with a medial collateral ligament sprain. During the examination the patient appears to be relaxed and comfortable, however, is extremely withdrawn. Which of the following questions would be the MOST appropriate to further engage the patient?

1. Is this the first time you have injured your knee?
2. Have you ever been to physical therapy before?
3. How long after your injury did you see a physician?
4. **What do you hope to achieve in physical therapy?**

> **Correct Answer: 4** (Goodman – Differential Diagnosis p. 38)

Physical therapists often use a variety of strategies to increase the level of patient participation in treatment sessions. Open-ended questions allow patients to answer with a myriad of responses, while closed-ended questions can often be answered with a yes or no response.

1. The question can be answered with a simple "yes or no" and therefore would be unlikely to increase patient participation.
2. The question would also require a simple "yes or no" response.
3. The question requires the patient to respond with an amount of time. The response, although not a "yes or no," would be equally unlikely to further engage the patient.
4. **The question requires the patient to provide some level of insight towards their physical therapy goals and may provide a foundation for a meaningful exchange between the patient and therapist. The information obtained by the therapist can be valuable when designing an appropriate plan of care.**

System Specific: Non-Systems
Content Outline: Safety & Professional Roles; Teaching/Learning; Research

Exam Two: Question 48

A physical therapist conducts a pre-operative training session for a patient scheduled for surgery to repair a large rotator cuff tear. The patient is a 54-year-old male who is employed as an insurance agent. During the pre-operative training session the patient inquires as to the amount of time before he is able to return to recreational activities such as tennis and golf. The MOST appropriate time frame is typically:

1. 6-8 weeks
2. 12-14 weeks
3. **24-28 weeks**
4. 36-40 weeks

> **Correct Answer: 3** (Brotzman p. 99)

The majority of rotator cuff tears occur in individuals greater than 40 years of age with a history of recurrent shoulder symptoms. A large tear is most often considered to be between 3-5 centimeters in diameter.

1. At 6-8 weeks following surgery the patient may be ready to begin to focus on strength, endurance, and neuromuscular control while continuing to attain or maintain range of motion. Since the tear was classified as "large" in some cases the patient may not be permitted to perform strengthening exercises until 10-12 weeks.
2. At 12-14 weeks following surgery the patient focuses on task specific strengthening activities. The activities occur in a controlled environment and the patient is closely monitored.
3. **At 24-28 weeks the patient is typically allowed to return to recreational activities such as tennis and golf. Strengthening activities may continue during this period since studies have shown that on average patients regain approximately 80% of their strength in the involved shoulder compared to the uninvolved shoulder in the first six months following surgery. The actual rate of recovery is influenced significantly by the size of the tear.**
4. At 36-40 weeks the patient typically has returned to their previous lifestyle and continues to gain strength in the involved shoulder. Studies have shown that even after one year only 90% of the strength in the shoulder has been achieved compared to the uninvolved shoulder.

System Specific: Musculoskeletal System
Content Outline: Foundations for Evaluation, Differential Diagnosis, & Prognosis

Exam Two: Question 49

A physical therapist determines a patient's heart rate by counting the number of QRS complexes in a six second electrocardiogram strip. Assuming the therapist identifies eight QRS complexes in the strip, the patient's heart rate should be recorded as:

1. 40 beats per minute
2. 60 beats per minute
3. **80 beats per minute**
4. 100 beats per minute

Correct Answer: 3 (Brannon p. 193)

The QRS complex reflects the depolarization of the ventricles during the cardiac cycle. If the heart rhythm is regular, the minute heart rate can be determined by counting the number of QRS complexes in 6 seconds on the electrocardiogram paper, then multiply this number by 10 to get the heart rate for one minute.

1. For a heart rate of 40 beats per minute, there would be four QRS complexes in six seconds.
2. For a heart rate of 60 beats per minute, there would be six QRS complexes in six seconds.
3. **Eight QRS complexes per six second interval x 10 (six second intervals per minute) = 80 QRS complexes per minute.**
4. For a heart rate of 100 beats per minute, there would be 10 QRS complexes in six seconds.

System Specific: Cardiac, Vascular, & Pulmonary Systems
Content Outline: Examination

Exam Two: Question 50

A physical therapist prepares to apply a sterile dressing to a wound after debridement. The therapist begins the process by drying the wound using a towel. The therapist applies medication to the wound using a gauze pad and then applies a series of dressings that are secured using a bandage. Which step would NOT warrant the use of sterile technique?

1. **bandage**
2. dressings
3. medication
4. towel

Correct Answer: 1 (Pierson p. 307)

Application of a bandage does not require sterile technique since the bandage does not come in direct contact with the wound. All other aspects of the scenario require sterile technique to protect the wound and surrounding area, the patient, and the caregiver from contamination.

1. **A bandage is applied over a dressing. The function of a bandage is to keep the dressing in position, provide a barrier between the dressing and the environment, provide pressure, and protect the wound. Since the bandage does not come in direct contact with the area surrounding the wound, sterile technique is not required.**
2. A dressing for a wound is usually comprised of several layers. The function of a dressing is to prevent contamination to the wound, keep microorganisms within the wound from infecting other areas, assist with healing, apply pressure, absorb drainage, and prevent further injury to the wound. Application of all layers of a dressing requires sterile technique.
3. The application of medication is part of the dressing in this scenario and should be applied using sterile technique.
4. If the patient is using the towel directly on the area of the wound, the towel must be sterile and the therapist must use sterile technique to avoid contamination.

System Specific: Integumentary System
Content Outline: Interventions

Exam Two: Question 51

A physical therapist develops a chart detailing expected functional outcomes for a variety of spinal cord injuries. Which is the highest spinal cord injury level at which independent transfers with a sliding board would be feasible?

1. C4
2. **C6**
3. T1
4. T3

Correct Answer: 2 (Rothstein p. 404)

The ability to independently transfer with a sliding board following a spinal cord injury is primarily dependent on the patient's available motor and sensory innervation. In addition to performing independent sliding board transfers, a patient with a C6 spinal cord injury should be able to perform independent bed mobility, coughing, skin inspection, and pressure relief with equipment and adaptations.

1. A patient with a C4 spinal cord injury would not have adequate upper extremity movement to be capable of completing the transfer. Primary muscles innervated include the diaphragm and trapezius.
2. **A patient with a C6 spinal cord injury would possess the requisite upper extremity strength to make the transfer feasible. Primary muscles innervated include the extensor carpi radialis, infraspinatus, latissimus dorsi, pectoralis major, pronator teres, serratus anterior, and teres minor.**
3. A patient with a T1 spinal cord injury would possess full upper extremity innervation and should be able to complete the transfer. The option is not the correct response since the item asks the highest spinal cord injury level where the transfer is feasible.
4. A patient with a T3 spinal cord injury should also be able to complete the transfer. The patient's clinical presentation would be consistent with the patient at the T1 level.

System Specific: Neuromuscular & Nervous Systems
Content Outline: Foundations for Evaluation, Differential Diagnosis, & Prognosis

Exam Two: Question 52

A patient rehabilitating from a spinal cord injury has significant lower extremity spasticity which often results in the patient's feet becoming dislodged from the wheelchair footrests. The MOST appropriate modification to address this problem is:

1. hydraulic reclining unit
2. elevating legrests
3. **heel loops and/or toe loops**
4. detachable swing-away legrests

Correct Answer: 3 (O'Sullivan p. 976)

There are a variety of wheelchair components that can assist patients to achieve maximum function, comfort, stability, and protection. The specific components selected are based on the unique needs of each patient.

1. A hydraulic reclining unit would allow the patient to recline in the actual chair. Semireclining chairs recline to approximately 30 degrees from the vertical and fully reclining chairs recline to a horizontal position.
2. Elevating legrests allow the entire front rigging to be elevated and maintained at varying heights. Patients with inadequate knee flexion, a long leg cast or circulatory compromise may use this type of adaptation.
3. **Heel loops and/or toe loops can maintain the foot on the footrest. This is often necessary in the presence of spasticity.**
4. Detachable swing-away legrests allow the front rigging to be pivoted outward away from the wheelchair frame. This adaptation allows the wheelchair to be positioned closer to objects and provides more unobstructed space to transfer.

System Specific: Non-Systems
Content Outline: Equipment & Devices; Therapeutic Modalities

Exam Two: Question 53

A physical therapist utilizes a manual assisted cough technique on a patient with a midthoracic spinal cord injury. When completing this technique with the patient in supine, the MOST appropriate location for the therapist's hand placement is:

1. manubrium
2. **epigastric area**
3. xiphoid process
4. umbilical region

Correct Answer: 2 (O'Sullivan p. 959)

The degree of respiratory impairment is related to the level of the spinal cord injury, residual muscle function, trauma at the time of injury, and premorbid respiratory status. Weakness or paralysis of the external oblique muscles compromises the patient's ability to cough and expel secretions.

1. The manubrium is the broad, quadrangular shaped upper part of the sternum. This region is too high to provide effective pressure support for coughing.
2. **The epigastric area is the upper central region of the abdomen, located between the costal margins and the subcostal plane. Applying manual hand pressure inwards and upwards over the epigastric area can assist the patient to cough and promote airway clearance.**
3. The xiphoid process is a small cartilaginous extension to the lower part of the sternum that is usually ossified in the adult. Pressure over this region should be avoided.
4. The umbilical region is the area surrounding the umbilicus (i.e., belly button). This region is too low to provide effective pressure support for coughing.

System Specific: Cardiac, Vascular, & Pulmonary Systems
Content Outline: Interventions

Exam Two: Question 54

A patient 72 hours status post stroke is referred to physical therapy. As part of the patient care program, the physical therapist makes positioning recommendations to the nursing staff. How often should turning occur?

1. every thirty minutes
2. **every two hours**
3. every four hours
4. every six hours

Correct Answer: 2 (Pierson p. 90)

During the initial stages of rehabilitation a patient status post stroke should be repositioned in bed on a regular basis. Failure to reposition could result in contractures or excessive pressure to the skin and associated structures. The greatest pressure typically occurs to tissues that cover bony prominences.

1. Turning a patient on a 30 minute interval would be desirable to reduce the risk of tissue damage, however, the time frame would place an unrealistic burden on the nursing staff without adequate clinical justification.
2. **Turning a patient on a two hour interval is the most widely accepted positioning rule. This interval is sufficient to reduce the risk of tissue damage and is realistic for the nursing staff.**
3. Turning a patient every four hours is inadequate and would place the patient at significant risk for tissue damage.
4. Turning a patient every six hours is also inadequate. The greater the interval beyond two hours, the greater the probability that the patient will experience tissue damage.

System Specific: Integumentary System
Content Outline: Interventions

Exam Two: Question 55

A physical therapist prepares to use soft tissue massage as part of a treatment plan for a patient with an adductor strain. The MOST appropriate therapist action prior to initiating treatment is:

1. utilize proper draping
2. **explain the treatment procedure and obtain patient consent**
3. ask another therapist to be present during the treatment session
4. describe the benefits of soft tissue massage on muscle strains

> **Correct Answer: 2** (Scott - Promoting Legal and Ethical Awareness p. 224)

The *Criteria for Standards of Practice for Physical Therapy* published by the American Physical Therapy Association state that "Within the patient/client management process, the physical therapist and the patient/client establish and maintain an ongoing collaborative process of decision making that exists throughout the provision of services."

1. Proper draping is essential given the location of the adductors, however, explaining the treatment procedure and obtaining consent would be the prerequisite activity.
2. **Explaining the treatment procedure and obtaining patient consent provides the patient with a broad understanding of the intervention and permits them with the opportunity to refuse. Failure to take this action may result in the therapist assuming unnecessary legal risk.**
3. Asking another physical therapist to be present provides the therapist with a witness who could verify that the intervention was applied in a professional manner. Although this is a commonly used risk management strategy, it ignores the patient's right to be involved in decision making.
4. A patient should be aware of the benefits associated with a specific intervention, however, this would likely be a component of explaining the treatment procedure and obtaining patient consent.

System Specific: Non-Systems
Content Outline: Safety & Professional Roles; Teaching/Learning; Research

Exam Two: Question 56

A physical therapist moves a patient from sidelying to supine after the patient was unable to maintain the manual muscle test position for the hip abductors. Assuming the patient is able to complete full range of motion in the horizontal plane, the MOST appropriate muscle grade is:

1. fair
2. fair minus
3. **poor**
4. poor minus

> **Correct Answer: 3** (Kendall p. 20)

Physical therapists are required to modify the traditional manual muscle testing position when a patient is unable to complete range of motion against gravity. The primary hip abductors are the gluteus minimus and gluteus medius.

1. A grade of fair is characterized by the patient completing range of motion against gravity without manual resistance.
2. A grade of fair minus is characterized by the patient being unable to complete the range of motion against gravity, but does complete more than half of the range.
3. **A grade of poor is characterized by the patient completing range of motion with gravity eliminated.**
4. A grade of poor minus is characterized by the patient being unable to complete range of motion in a gravity eliminated position.

System Specific: Musculoskeletal System
Content Outline: Examination

Exam Two: Question 57

A physical therapist completes a lower quarter screening examination on a patient diagnosed with trochanteric bursitis. Assuming a normal end-feel, which of the following classifications would be MOST consistent with hip extension?

1. soft
2. **firm**
3. hard
4. empty

Correct Answer: 2 (Norkin p. 196)

End-feel is the type of resistance that is felt when passively moving a joint through the end range of motion.

1. A soft end-feel results in a yielding compression that halts further movement. An example of a soft end-feel would be associated with knee flexion secondary to compression of soft tissue.
2. **The end-feel most often associated with hip extension is firm due to tension in the anterior joint capsule and the iliofemoral ligament.**
3. A hard or bony end-feel results in an unyielding sensation most often caused by bone to bone contact. An example of a hard or bony end-feel would be elbow extension.
4. An empty end-feel results when pain prevents reaching the end of range of motion. Resistance is not felt, although protective muscle splinting or muscle spasm may be detected. An empty end-feel is always considered abnormal.

System Specific: Musculoskeletal System
Content Outline: Clinical Application of Foundational Sciences

Exam Two: Question 58

A physician utilizes diagnostic imaging to show motion within a joint through x-ray. This type of imaging is BEST termed:

1. computed tomography
2. **fluoroscopy**
3. discography
4. radionuclide scanning

Correct Answer: 2 (Magee p. 64)

Knowledge of diagnostic imaging techniques allows therapists to better understand the rationale associated with physician orders for imaging and the interpretation of the obtained results.

1. Computed tomography is a non-invasive imaging technique that uses cross-sectional images based on x-ray attenuation. Computer enhancement allows the imaging to have significantly better contrast resolution when compared to conventional x-rays.
2. **Fluoroscopy refers to examination by means of the fluoroscope. A fluoroscope allows an examiner to observe the actions of joints, organs or entire systems of the body. The instrument requires a specific body segment to be placed between a fluorescent screen and an x-ray tube. X-rays from the tube pass through the body and project images on the screen.**
3. Discography is an invasive imaging technique that involves injecting a radiopaque dye into the nucleus pulposus of an intervertebral disc using radiographic guidance. The technique can be used to identify disruptions of the nucleus pulposus or the annulus fibrosus.
4. Radionuclide scanning is an invasive imaging technique that can be used in conjunction with bone scans to identify areas where there is a high level of bone turnover relative to the rest of the bone. The technique requires the intravenous injection of chemicals labeled with isotopes.

System Specific: Musculoskeletal System
Content Outline: Foundations for Evaluation, Differential Diagnosis, & Prognosis

Exam Two: Question 59

A physical therapist reviews the medical record of a patient recently admitted to the intensive care unit. A note from the patient's physician indicates an order for arterial blood gas analysis six times daily. Which type of indwelling line would be used to collect the necessary samples?

1. intravenous line
2. **arterial line**
3. central venous line
4. pulmonary artery line

Correct Answer: 2 (Pierson p. 286)

Samples for blood gas analysis may be obtained from different regions of the vascular bed. Arterial samples are taken from either a needle puncture or indwelling catheter in a peripheral artery.

1. An intravenous line consists of a short catheter inserted through the skin into a peripheral vein. Intravenous lines are used as a route to administer medications or fluids.
2. **An arterial line consists of a catheter inserted through the skin into an artery connected to pressure tubing, a transducer, and a monitor. The device can be used for continuous direct blood pressure readings and to sample arterial blood for arterial blood gas analysis. The radial and brachial arteries are the most common sites for an arterial line.**
3. A central venous line consists of a catheter inserted through the skin into a large vein, usually the superior vena cava or inferior vena cava, or within the right atrium of the heart to measure right atrial pressure. The catheter also may be used as a route for medication or fluid administration, blood sampling, and emergency placement of a pacemaker.
4. A pulmonary artery line is a balloon-tipped catheter introduced via the internal jugular vein or subclavian vein passing through the right atrium, tricuspid valve, right ventricle, pulmonary valve, and into the pulmonary artery. It is used to monitor cardiovascular pressures and to sample mixed venous blood for gas analysis.

System Specific: Other Systems
Content Outline: Foundations for Evaluation, Differential Diagnosis, & Prognosis

Exam Two: Question 60

A physical therapist completes a family training session with a patient rehabilitating from a spinal cord injury. During the training the patient asks a question regarding their functional ability following rehabilitation. The MOST appropriate therapist response is to:

1. explain that it is difficult to predict since all patients progress differently
2. **provide information on the expected prognosis based on the nature and severity of the injury**
3. refer the patient to the director of rehabilitation
4. refer the patient to the physiatrist

Correct Answer: 2 (Purtilo p. 33)

Patients often ask physical therapists questions about their functional abilities following rehabilitation. It is reasonable for the therapist to provide the patient with information on this topic given the patient's level of motor and sensory innervation.

1. The statement, although accurate, does not directly address the patient's question. Physical therapists should attempt to answer questions posed by patients in a direct and forthcoming manner whenever possible.
2. **Physical therapists can share information with patients related to projected functional outcomes following rehabilitation. Physical therapists should be careful to make sure that the topics addressed fall within their scope of practice.**
3. The director of rehabilitation is typically responsible for oversight of the therapy services provided by the various health care disciplines. The position is primarily administrative and therefore the director would not typically be well suited to respond to questions regarding expected patient outcome.
4. Referring the patient to the physiatrist, although appropriate, would be a more attractive option if the question posed by the patient was directly related to their medical management or another similar topic that would fall under the scope of practice of the physiatrist.

System Specific: Neuromuscular & Nervous Systems
Content Outline: Foundations for Evaluation, Differential Diagnosis, & Prognosis

Exam Two: Question 61

A patient positioned in standing with their arm positioned at their side with 90 degrees of elbow flexion completes shoulder medial and lateral rotation exercises using a piece of elastic tubing. Which plane of the body is utilized with this activity?

1. coronal
2. frontal
3. sagittal
4. **transverse**

> ### Correct Answer: 4 (Levangie p. 7)

Medial and lateral rotation with the arm positioned at the side with 90 degrees of elbow flexion occurs in a transverse plane.

1. The coronal plane divides the body into anterior and posterior sections. Motions in the coronal plane occur around an anterior-posterior axis.
2. The terms frontal and coronal are synonyms and describe the same plane of movement.
3. The sagittal plane divides the body into left and right halves. Motions in the sagittal plane occur around a medial-lateral axis.
4. **The transverse plane divides the body into upper and lower sections. Motions in the transverse plane occur around a vertical axis.**

System Specific: Musculoskeletal System
Content Outline: Clinical Application of Foundational Sciences

Test Taking Tip: A candidate should recognize that the frontal plane and the coronal plane are synonyms and as a result refer to the same plane of movement. Therefore, 1 and 2 can be eliminated as potential answers to the question since they mutually exclude each other.

Exam Two: Question 62

A physical therapist uses a self-care assessment to examine change over time in rehabilitation programs. The assessment uses a seven-point scale to examine 18 items. The collected information is based on observations of patient performance. This type of assessment MOST closely describes:

1. **Functional Independence Measure**
2. Functional Status Index
3. Physical Self-Maintenance Scale
4. Katz Index of Activities of Daily Living

> ### Correct Answer: 1 (Van Deusen p. 425)

There are a variety of outcome measures which examine self-care and activities of daily living. Physical therapists should have general knowledge of the more commonly used measures and consider the conceptual and measurement model, reliability, validity, responsiveness, and interpretability inherent to each measure.

1. **The Functional Independence Measure (FIM) tests a subject in multiple areas to determine the overall degree of disability experienced by an adult rehabilitation patient. The tool is part of the Uniform Data System for Medical Rehabilitation. A seven-point scale is utilized to examine 18 areas, which include self-care, sphincter control, transfers, locomotion, communication, and social cognitive activities. The FIM is commonly used to examine changes in disability status that occur over time.**
2. The Functional Status Index was developed as a comprehensive ADL assessment for adults living in the community. The 18 items include the following domains: gross mobility, personal care, social/role activities, hand activities and home chores. Scores are generated in three areas: dependence, difficulty, and pain.
3. The Physical Self-Maintenance Scale (PSMS) is a Guttman scale containing six items of self-care. The PSMS was designed as a disability measure for use in planning and evaluating treatment in elderly people living in the community or within institutions. The scale is based on the theory that human behavior can be ordered in a hierarchy of complexity. The hierarchy runs from physical health through self-maintenance ADL and IADL, cognition, time use (hobbies), and social interaction.
4. The Katz Index of Activities of Daily Living uses a nominal scale index to identify self-care problems and the level of assistance required within six areas: bathing, dressing, toileting, transfers, continence, and feeding. It is a simple and quick assessment tool used to efficiently gather self-care information and predict outcome and the need for ongoing assistance.

System Specific: Non-Systems
Content Outline: Safety & Professional Roles; Teaching/Learning; Research

Exam Two: Question 63

A physical therapist working on a pulmonary rehabilitation unit works with a patient on therapeutic positioning. The patient has experienced a lengthy inpatient hospitalization and was only recently referred to physical therapy. The patient has significant weakness of the diaphragm and is hypertensive. The MOST appropriate patient position to initiate treatment is:

1. prone
2. supine
3. Trendelenburg
4. **reverse Trendelenburg**

Correct Answer: 4 (Hillegass p. 658)

The reverse Trendelenburg position refers to a position in which the patient's head is elevated on an inclined plane in relation to the feet.

1. The prone position would be a difficult position in which to teach the patient diaphragmatic breathing since the weight of the abdominal contents on the diaphragm makes it more difficult for a weakened diaphragm to contract.

2. In supine, the weight of the abdominal contents on the diaphragm makes it more difficult for a weakened diaphragm to contract. Also, the supine position can reduce the functional residual volume of the lungs by as much as fifty percent.

3. In the Trendelenburg position the patient's head is lower than their feet. The position is used to facilitate drainage from the lower lobes of the lungs and to increase blood pressure in hypotensive patients. The position would tend to increase the blood pressure of a patient that is already hypertensive.

4. **The reverse Trendelenburg position is recommended to reduce hypertension and facilitate movement of the diaphragm by using gravity to reduce the weight of the abdominal contents on the diaphragm.**

System Specific: Other Systems
Content Outline: Interventions

Exam Two: Question 64

A physical therapist performs rescue breathing on a patient that collapsed in the physical therapy gym. Which of the following is NOT accurate when performing rescue breathing on an adult?

1. maintain open airway with head tilt-chin lift
2. give one breath every five to six seconds
3. pinch nose shut
4. **continue for 30 seconds; approximately twelve breaths**

Correct Answer: 4 (American Heart Association)

Rescue breathing is a cardiopulmonary resuscitation technique designed for a patient that exhibits a pulse, but is not breathing.

1. A physical therapist should use the head tilt-chin lift maneuver to open the airway of an adult victim without evidence of head or neck trauma. If a cervical spine injury is suspected, the airway should be opened using a jaw thrust without head extension.

2. Rescue breathing is performed on an adult with a pulse for a full cycle of 60 seconds with breaths occurring every five to six seconds. Each breath should be given over one second regardless of whether an advanced airway is in place. Each breath should cause a visible rise in the chest. The pulse should be checked after two minutes.

3. To perform mouth-to-mouth rescue breaths, open the victim's airway, pinch the victim's nose, and create an airtight mouth-to-mouth seal providing 10-12 breaths per minute.

4. **Twelve breaths in 30 seconds is approximately twice the recommended breathing rate. Rescue breaths are performed at a rate of 10-12 breaths per minute for adult victims with a pulse that requires ventilatory support.**

System Specific: Non-Systems
Content Outline: Safety & Professional Roles; Teaching/Learning; Research

Exam Two: Question 65

A physical therapist observes an intravenous line that is tangled around a patient's bed rail. What type of medical asepsis is indicated prior to coming in contact with the intravenous line?

1. gloves
2. gloves, gown
3. gloves, gown, mask
4. **none**

Correct Answer: 4 (Pierson p. 289)

An intravenous (I.V.) system can be used to infuse fluids, electrolytes, nutrients, and medication. The I.V. line most commonly consists of plastic tubing and is considered a non-sterile object.

1. Gloves offer protection to the physical therapist's hands to reduce the likelihood of becoming infected with microorganisms from a patient and reduce the risk of the patient receiving microorganisms from the physical therapist. Gloves would not be necessary when handling an I.V. line.
2. A gown is used to protect the physical therapist's clothing from being contaminated or soiled by a contaminant. The gown also reduces the probability of the physical therapist transmitting a microorganism from their clothing to the patient. Gloves and gown would not be necessary when handling an I.V. line.
3. A mask is designed to reduce the spread of microorganisms that are transmitted through the air. The mask protects the physical therapist from inhalation of particles or droplets that may contain pathogens and also reduces the transmission of pathogens from the physical therapist to the patient. Gloves, gown, and mask would not be necessary when handling an I.V. line.
4. **The tubing is a non-sterile object that would not require the use of protective clothing. The physical therapist can reposition the I.V. line through direct hand contact.**

System Specific: Non-Systems
Content Outline: Safety & Professional Roles; Teaching/Learning; Research

Exam Two: Question 66

A physical therapist presents an inservice to the rehabilitation staff that compares traditional gait terminology with Rancho Los Amigos terminology. Which pair of descriptive terms describes the same general point in the gait cycle?

1. midstance to heel off and initial swing
2. **heel strike and initial contact**
3. foot flat to midstance and loading response
4. toe off and midswing

Correct Answer: 2 (Rothstein p. 678)

Traditional gait terminology and Rancho Los Amigos terminology can be used to describe the various components of gait. There are a fair number of similarities between the two classification systems, however, there are also a number of differences. Rancho Los Amigos terminology tends to be more descriptive since it describes intervals of gait, usually with a well defined beginning and end point.

1. Midstance to heel off occurs during stance phase. Initial swing begins when the stance foot lifts from the floor and ends with maximal knee flexion during swing (i.e., swing phase).
2. **Heel strike and initial contact are both terms that describe the moment that the heel contacts the ground and stance phase begins.**
3. The loading response corresponds to the amount of time between initial contact and the beginning of the swing phase for the other leg. This is not the same point in the gait cycle as foot flat to midstance since the loading response does not include the period of time when the other foot is off the floor until the body is directly over the stance limb (i.e., midstance).
4. Toe off is the point in which only the toe of the stance limb remains on the ground, however, midswing occurs during swing phase.

System Specific: Musculoskeletal System
Content Outline: Examination

Exam Two: Question 67

A physical therapist selects a therapeutic ultrasound generator with a frequency of 3.0 MHz. Which condition would MOST warrant the use of this frequency?

1. lumbar paravertebral muscle spasm
2. hip flexion contracture
3. quadriceps strain
4. **anterior talofibular ligament sprain**

Correct Answer: 4 (Cameron p. 192)

A higher frequency results in greater attenuation of energy in superficial structures. As a result, an ultrasound generator with a frequency of 3.0 MHz may be more desirable than a generator with a frequency of 1.0 MHz when treating a superficial structure.

1. The lumbar paravertebral muscles refer to a relatively diverse group of muscles next to the spine. The muscles collectively support the spine and produce movement. The relative depth of the muscles would make it necessary to utilize a frequency of 1.0 MHz to reach the target area.
2. A hip flexion contracture typically results from shortening of the iliopsoas muscle. The iliopsoas is formed by the iliacus and psoas major muscles and is considered to be the most powerful flexor of the hip. Ultrasound in this area would require a frequency of 1.0 MHz due to the depth of the muscle.
3. The quadriceps muscles are a large muscle group consisting of the rectus femoris, vastus lateralis, vastus medialis, and vastus intermedius. A strain in this area would require a frequency of 1.0 MHz due to the depth of the structures.
4. **The anterior talofibular ligament is a thickening of the anterior joint capsule that extends from the anterior surface of the lateral malleolus to the lateral facet of the talus and the lateral surface of the talar neck. The ligament is only two to five millimeters thick and therefore a frequency of 3.0 MHz would be adequate.**

System Specific: Non-Systems
Content Outline: Equipment & Devices; Therapeutic Modalities

Exam Two: Question 68

A physical therapist employed in a rehabilitation hospital utilizes a variety of transfer techniques to move patients of various functional abilities. Which type of transfer would NOT be classified as dependent?

1. sliding transfer
2. hydraulic lift
3. **sliding board transfer**
4. two-person lift

Correct Answer: 3 (Minor p. 224)

Physical therapists should select transfers for patients based on their unique abilities and limitations. Types of transfers range from completely dependent to independent.

1. The sliding transfer is considered a dependent transfer most often used when transferring a patient in supine from a treatment table or bed to a similar surface. When performing the transfer therapists often use a "draw" sheet to move the patient from one surface to the other.
2. The hydraulic lift is a device required for dependent transfers when a patient is obese, there is only one therapist available to assist with the transfer or the patient is totally dependent.
3. **The sliding board transfer is used for a patient that possesses sitting balance, upper extremity strength, and can adequately follow directions. The transfer is used when patients can assist or are independent.**
4. The two-person lift is considered a dependent transfer used to transfer a patient between two surfaces of different heights or when transferring a patient to the floor.

System Specific: Non-Systems
Content Outline: Equipment & Devices; Therapeutic Modalities

Exam Two: Question 69

A 28-year-old male referred to physical therapy by his primary physician complains of recurrent ankle pain. As part of the treatment program, the therapist uses ultrasound over the peroneus longus and brevis tendons. The MOST appropriate location for ultrasound application is:

1. inferior to the sustentaculum tali
2. over the sinus tarsi
3. **posterior to the lateral malleolus**
4. anterior to the lateral malleolus

Correct Answer: 3 (Kendall p. 412)

The peroneus longus and brevis are innervated by the superficial peroneal nerve (L4, L5, S1) and act to evert the foot and assist in plantar flexion of the ankle joint. The peroneus longus also acts to depress the head of the first metatarsal.

1. The sustentaculum tali is a horizontal eminence arising from the medial surface of the calcaneus. The bony prominence serves as the attachment for several ligaments including the plantar calcaneonavicular ligament, also known as the spring ligament.
2. The sinus tarsi is a small osseous canal which runs into the ankle under the talus bone. The structure is at the same approximate level as the lateral malleolus.
3. **The peroneus longus and brevis tendons pass posterior to the lateral malleolus. The peroneus longus inserts on the lateral side of the base of the first metatarsal and first cuneiform, while the peroneus brevis inserts on the tuberosity of the fifth metatarsal.**
4. The tendon of the extensor digitorum longus can be palpated slightly anterior to the lateral malleolus.

System Specific: Non-Systems
Content Outline: Equipment & Devices; Therapeutic Modalities

Exam Two: Question 70

A physical therapist treats a patient rehabilitating from an Achilles tendon repair using cryotherapy. Which cryotherapeutic agent would provide the GREATEST magnitude of tissue cooling?

1. frozen gel packs
2. **ice massage**
3. Fluori-Methane spray
4. cold water bath

Correct Answer: 2 (Cameron p. 145)

Cryotherapy is a commonly used therapeutic intervention in rehabilitation. Primary uses of cryotherapy include reducing inflammation, pain control, and spasticity management. Physical therapists must be aware of contraindications and precautions of cryotherapy as well as signs or symptoms of cold intolerance.

1. Frozen gel packs contain silica gel and are available in a variety of shapes and sizes. The packs are stored in a refrigeration unit and are usually applied with a moist towel. Cold packs may not maintain uniform contact with the treatment surface and require a treatment time of 15-30 minutes.
2. **Ice massage is typically performed by freezing water in paper cups and applying the ice directly to the treatment area. Ice massage tends to create a more intense cooling since the ice is applied directly to a localized target area. The treatment time is 5-10 minutes using ice massage due to the intensity of the cooling.**
3. Fluori-Methane is a commonly used vapocoolant spray. Vapocoolant sprays allow for a brief cooling to a very localized area of application. The vapocoolant spray is applied in parallel strokes along the skin in the area of trigger points. Stretching immediately follows the application of the vapocoolant spray.
4. A cold water bath is commonly used for immersion of the distal extremities. A basin or whirlpool is most often used to hold the cold water. A cold bath requires water temperature ranging from 55 to 64 degrees Fahrenheit (13 to 18 degrees Celsius). The body part typically requires a treatment time of 5 to 15 minutes to attain the desired therapeutic effects.

System Specific: Non-Systems
Content Outline: Equipment & Devices; Therapeutic Modalities

Exam Two: Question 71

A physical therapist treats a 32-year-old female rehabilitating from a closed head injury presently functioning at Rancho Los Amigos level IV. The therapist treats the patient in her home for 60 minute sessions, three times per week. Recently the therapist has noticed that the patient becomes increasingly combative as the session progresses and believes the deterioration in behavior is linked to the patient becoming fatigued. The MOST appropriate treatment modification is:

1. reduce the treatment sessions to 30 minutes, three times per week
2. reduce the frequency of the treatment sessions to two times per week
3. **increase the rest periods during existing treatment sessions**
4. increase the treatment sessions to 90 minutes, two times per week

> **Correct Answer: 3** (O' Sullivan p. 913)

The Rancho Los Amigos Levels of Cognitive Functioning Scale is used to describe cognitive and behavioral recovery in individuals following traumatic brain injury. A patient at level IV is labeled "Confused-Agitated."

1. Reducing the treatment sessions to 30 minutes in length would result in a fifty percent decrease in therapy time. It is possible that this may be necessary, however, the therapist should attempt to modify other parameters of treatment prior to implementing such a drastic reduction in therapy time.
2. Reducing the frequency of the sessions to two times per week would likely have minimal impact on the patient's behavior without reducing the length of the sessions or incorporating more frequent rest periods.
3. **A patient functioning at level IV may be particularly susceptible to changes in behavior based on fatigue. Ideally, the physical therapist should attempt to maintain the integrity of the current treatment regimen, however, if increased rest periods do not produce an observable change in the patient's behavior it may be appropriate to modify other parameters such as the frequency or length of treatment.**
4. It is likely that the length of the session, currently 60 minutes, may be more challenging for the patient than the frequency of the sessions. As a result, increasing the duration of the treatment sessions to 90 minutes would likely exacerbate the current situation.

System Specific: Neuromuscular & Nervous Systems
Content Outline: Interventions

Exam Two: Question 72

A physical therapist positions a patient in supine in preparation for goniometric measurements. When measuring medial rotation of the shoulder, the therapist should position the fulcrum:

1. on the lateral midline of the humerus using the lateral epicondyle as a reference
2. perpendicular to the floor
3. along the midaxillary line of the thorax
4. **over the olecranon process**

> **Correct Answer: 4** (Norkin p. 84)

According to the American Academy of Orthopaedic Surgeons normal shoulder medial rotation is 0-70 degrees.

1. The lateral midline of the humerus using the lateral epicondyle as a reference should be used to align the moveable arm of the goniometer when measuring shoulder flexion and extension.
2. The stationary arm of the goniometer should be aligned parallel or perpendicular to the floor when measuring medial rotation of the shoulder.
3. The midaxillary line of the thorax should be used to align the stationary arm of the goniometer when measuring shoulder flexion and extension.
4. **The fulcrum of the goniometer should be aligned over the olecranon process. The moveable arm of the goniometer should be aligned with the ulna, using the olecranon and ulnar styloid as a reference when measuring medial rotation of the shoulder.**

System Specific: Musculoskeletal System
Content Outline: Examination

Exam Two: Question 73

A physical therapist examines a patient diagnosed with left-sided heart failure. Which finding is NOT typically associated with this condition?

1. pulmonary edema
2. persistent cough
3. **dependent edema**
4. muscular weakness

> **Correct Answer: 3** (Hillegass p. 107)

Heart failure refers to the heart's inability to maintain a cardiac output that is adequate to meet the demands of the tissues due to an abnormality in the pumping ability of the heart muscle. Left-sided heart failure means it is the left side of the heart that is failing which causes fluid to build up behind the left ventricle. Left-sided failure is frequently caused by myocardial infarction, hypertension or aortic valve disease.

1. Pulmonary edema is the abnormal accumulation of fluid in the alveolar spaces of the lungs. This is the "congestion" of congestive heart failure. It is often caused by increased pulmonary hydrostatic pressure from left-sided heart failure.

2. Patients with left-sided failure may be in respiratory distress and have a cough that produces pink, frothy (blood-tinged) sputum.

3. **Dependent edema is associated with right-sided heart failure. Fluid backs up behind the right ventricle and produces the accumulation of fluid in the liver, abdomen, and ankles.**

4. Muscle weakness, fatigue, and decreased exercise tolerance are universal among patients with left-sided heart failure due to the decreased blood flow to the extremities.

System Specific: Cardiac, Vascular, & Pulmonary Systems
Content Outline: Foundations for Evaluation, Differential Diagnosis, & Prognosis

Exam Two: Question 74

A physical therapist monitors a patient with a single lead electrocardiogram. After carefully examining the obtained data, the therapist classifies the rhythm as sinus bradycardia. Which description is MOST indicative of this condition?

1. R-R interval is irregular with a rate between 100 and 200 beats per minute
2. R-R interval is irregular with a rate between 40 and 100 beats per minute
3. R-R interval is regular with a rate greater than 100 beats per minute
4. **R-R interval is regular with a rate less than 60 beats per minute**

> **Correct Answer: 4** (Brannon p. 195)

The electrocardiogram is composed of a number of different waves – P, R, T, sometimes U – and the terms "irregular" and "regular" usually refer to the rhythm of the heart rate (i.e., the distance between similar waves). A sinus rhythm indicates that the cardiac impulse originates in the sinoatrial node. Sinus bradycardia is a sinus rhythm with a heart rate of less than 60 beats per minute.

1. Irregular R-R intervals with a heart rate between 100 and 200 beats per minute is characteristic of atrial tachycardia. Atrial tachycardia is defined as three or more consecutive premature atrial complexes, where an ectopic focus in either atria initiates an impulse before the SA node.

2. Irregular R-R intervals with a heart rate between 40 and 100 beats per minute is characteristic of sinus arrhythmia. Sinus arrhythmia is an irregularity in rhythm where the cardiac impulse is initiated at the SA node, but with a variable quickening and slowing of the impulse formation.

3. Regular R-R intervals with a heart rate greater than 100 beats per minute is sinus tachycardia.

4. **Regular R-R intervals with a heart rate of less than 60 beats per minute is sinus bradycardia.**

System Specific: Cardiac, Vascular, & Pulmonary Systems
Content Outline: Clinical Application of Foundational Sciences

Exam Two: Question 75

A physical therapist washes his hands thoroughly after treating a patient with a suspected infection. Which statement regarding hand washing is NOT accurate?

1. **wash all hand and wrist jewelry**
2. wash your hands, wrists, and two to three inches of your distal forearms
3. wash for at least 30 seconds
4. select warm water to allow soap to lather easily

Correct Answer: 1 (Pierson p. 33)

Hand washing is one of the most effective methods to reduce and prevent the spread of microorganisms.

1. **All hand and wrist jewelry should be removed prior to hand washing. Washing the hands without removing jewelry will increase the likelihood of microorganism transmission.**
2. Hand washing should include the wrist and a portion of the distal forearm. Washing of the wrist and the distal forearm should include both friction and rotary motions.
3. Hand washing should occur for a minimum of 30 seconds and longer in instances where a physical therapist has treated a patient known to have an infection.
4. Warm water allows the soap to lather more easily and causes minimum irritation to the skin.

System Specific: Non-Systems
Content Outline: Safety & Professional Roles; Teaching/Learning; Research

Exam Two: Question 76

A physical therapist uses a 3.0 MHz ultrasound beam at 1.5 W/cm² to treat a patient diagnosed with carpal tunnel syndrome. The MAJORITY of ultrasound energy will be absorbed within a depth of:

1. **1-2 centimeters**
2. 2-3 centimeters
3. 4-5 centimeters
4. 5-6 centimeters

Correct Answer: 1 (Cameron p. 192)

Frequency should be selected according to the depth of tissues to be treated. The most common frequency settings are 1 MHz and 3 MHz. A frequency setting of 1 MHz is used for heating of deeper tissues (up to five centimeters) where a setting of 3 MHz is used for heating superficial tissues with a depth of penetration of less than two centimeters.

1. **Tissues 1-2 centimeters in depth can be effectively treated with ultrasound using a frequency of 3 MHz.**
2. Tissues 2-3 centimeters in depth require ultrasound using a frequency of 1 MHz since a frequency of 3 MHz would not provide sufficient depth.
3. Tissues up to 5 centimeters in depth can be treated with ultrasound using a frequency of 1 MHz.
4. Tissues greater than 5 centimeters in depth are not effectively treated with ultrasound.

System Specific: Non-Systems
Content Outline: Equipment & Devices; Therapeutic Modalities

Exam Two: Question 77

A physical therapist serves as an accessibility consultant for a local retail store. What is the MINIMUM width required for a patient using a wheelchair to safely traverse through a doorway?

1. 24 inches
2. 30 inches
3. **32 inches**
4. 36 inches

Correct Answer: 3 (Minor p. 401)

The Americans with Disabilities Act was designed to provide a clear and comprehensive national mandate for the elimination of discrimination. Title III provides information on public accommodations including minimum accessibility standards.

1. The seat width in an average adult size wheelchair is 18 inches. As a result, 24 inches would not be nearly sufficient to accommodate the remainder of the wheelchair and still have adequate space available to propel the wheelchair through the doorway.
2. A wheelchair would likely be able to traverse through a doorway that was 30 inches wide, however, it would not meet the minimum width required by the Americans with Disabilities Act.
3. **The Americans with Disabilities Act requires that the minimum width of a doorway is 32 inches.**
4. The Americans with Disabilities Act requires that the minimum width of a corridor (hallway) is 36 inches. This width allows the patient to change the direction of the wheelchair within the corridor.

System Specific: Non-Systems
Content Outline: Safety & Professional Roles; Teaching/Learning; Research

Exam Two: Question 78

A physical therapist reviews the medical record of a 52-year-old male status post myocardial infarction. The patient is currently in the coronary care unit and is scheduled to begin cardiac rehabilitation tomorrow. Which potential complication of a myocardial infarction is the patient MOST susceptible to:

1. heart failure
2. **arrhythmias**
3. thrombus formation
4. heart structural damage

Correct Answer: 2 (Brannon p. 102)

Myocardial infarction has four major complications: arrhythmias, heart failure, thrombolytic complications, and damage to the heart structures.

1. Heart failure is a syndrome that reflects an inability of the heart to maintain a cardiac output sufficient to meet the oxygen and nutritional needs of the tissues. Heart failure is not as common as arrhythmias.
2. **Arrhythmias are caused by abnormalities in cardiac impulse generation, conduction, or both and occur in 90% of individuals who have experienced a myocardial infarction.**
3. Venous or mural thrombi can occur due to venous stasis after myocardial infarction. Thrombus formation is not as common as arrhythmias.
4. Damage to the papillary muscle, ventricle wall, and intraventricular septum can occur after a myocardial infarction. Heart structural damage is not as common as arrhythmias.

System Specific: Cardiac, Vascular, & Pulmonary Systems
Content Outline: Foundations for Evaluation, Differential Diagnosis, & Prognosis

Exam Two: Question 79

A physical therapist positions a patient in prone on a treatment plinth in preparation for a hot pack. When preparing the hot pack for the low back, the therapist should utilize:

1. 2-4 towel layers
2. 4-6 towel layers
3. **6-8 towel layers**
4. 8-10 towel layers

Correct Answer: 3 (Cameron p. 162)

A hot pack must be stored in hot water between 158 to 167 degrees Fahrenheit (70 to 75 degrees Celsius). As a result, it is necessary to use a barrier between the hot packs' canvas or nylon covered case and the body part to be treated. Most often towels or hot pack covers are used. Hot pack covers count for two towel layers because of their thickness.

1. Two to four towel layers would be inadequate and would result in the patient being at risk for excessive heat.
2. Four to six towel layers may be inadequate to properly protect the patient from excessive heat. It is possible to use only four to six towel layers in instances where the patient complains of not feeling enough heat or the therapist is aware that the hot pack may not possess its typical amount of heat. Therapist's must be cautious, however, to avoid removing towels during the session since increased skin temperature may diminish the patient's thermal sensitivity and their ability to accurately assess heat tolerance.
3. **Six to eight towel layers placed between a hot pack and the treatment surface is generally adequate to allow for the necessary transmission of heat without jeopardizing patient safety.**
4. Eight to ten towel layers may be excessive and as a result would significantly diminish the transmission of heat.

System Specific: Non-Systems
Content Outline: Equipment & Devices; Therapeutic Modalities

Test Taking Tip: When an option provides a range of answers, it is essential that candidates are satisfied with both the lower and upper limit of the range. For example, in option 2 a candidate may be satisfied with six towel layers, however, may feel that four towel layers would be inadequate. As a result, a candidate should not select option 2.

Exam Two: Question 80

A physical therapist attempts to determine if a wheelchair is the appropriate size for a patient recently admitted to a rehabilitation program. As part of the assessment, the therapist examines the distance from the front edge of the seat to the posterior aspect of the lower leg. If the seat depth is appropriate, how much space should exist between these two landmarks?

1. 1 inch
2. **2 inches**
3. 4 inches
4. 6 inches

Correct Answer: 2 (Pierson p. 137)

Seat depth is determined by measuring from the patient's posterior buttock, along the lateral thigh to the popliteal fold; then subtracting approximately 2 inches to avoid pressure from the front edge of the seat against the popliteal space. Normal seat depth in an adult size wheelchair is 16 inches.

1. One inch of space may result in the patient experiencing increased pressure in the popliteal area or even potentially compromised circulation since the amount of space between the front edge of the seat and the popliteal space is less than the recommended amount of two inches.
2. **Two inches of space between the front edge of the seat and the popliteal space is the recommended amount of space. This distance corresponds to the width of three or four fingers.**
3. Four inches of space may result in the patient experiencing decreased trunk stability, increased weight bearing on the ischial tuberosities due to the body weight being shifted posteriorly secondary to the lack of support to the thighs, and poor balance since the base of support has been reduced.
4. Six inches of space would serve to exacerbate the difficulties discussed in option 3.

System Specific: Non-Systems
Content Outline: Equipment & Devices; Therapeutic Modalities

Exam Two: Question 81

A patient using a wheelchair arranges for a local contractor to build a ramp that will allow entry into the patient's house. What is the MAXIMUM recommended grade for the ramp?

1. 6.2%
2. **8.3%**
3. 9.5%
4. 10.4%

Correct Answer: 2 (O'Sullivan p. 409)

Percent grade reflects the angle of inclination. The percent grade is determined by taking the rise and dividing the value by the run and then multiplying the number by 100 to convert the value to a percentage. A percent grade of 100% would be completely vertical and a percent grade of 0% would be completely horizontal.

1. A grade of 6.2% would be acceptable for the ramp, however, the item asks for the maximum recommended grade.
2. **A grade of 8.3% would result from a ramp that had one inch of rise for every 12 inches of run. This value represents the maximum percent grade of a ramp according to the Americans with Disabilities Act.**
3. A grade of 9.5% exceeds the maximum percent grade of a ramp allowable according to the Americans with Disabilities act by 1.2%.
4. A grade of 10.4% exceeds the maximum percent grade of a ramp allowable according to the Americans with Disabilities act by 2.1%.

System Specific: Non-Systems
Content Outline: Safety & Professional Roles; Teaching/Learning; Research

Exam Two: Question 82

A 16-year-old female accompanied by her mother receives exercise instructions. During the treatment session the mother makes several comments to her daughter that appear to be extremely upsetting and result in the daughter losing concentration. The MOST appropriate physical therapist action is:

1. document the mother's comments in the medical record
2. ask the patient if her mother is verbally abusive
3. **ask the mother to return to the waiting area**
4. discontinue the treatment session

Correct Answer: 3 (Purtilo p. 344)

The physical therapist's primary concern should be to establish an environment that is conducive to instructing the patient in the exercise program. Failure to address the negative interaction between the mother and daughter may limit the effectiveness of the session.

1. Documentation may be an appropriate option, however, it does not address the primary objective which is to allow the patient to receive exercise instructions in an appropriate learning environment.
2. It would be inappropriate to ask the child a question about this topic, particularly in the presence of the mother.
3. **The therapist increases the likelihood that the child will be able to concentrate on the exercise instructions by asking the mother to return to the waiting area. The question provides ample information to hypothesize that the mother's actions may be the reason the child is upset.**
4. The child appears to be upset and is losing concentration, however, there is no indication that the session is hopeless and therefore the decision to discontinue the treatment session would be premature without first trying to modify the current learning environment.

System Specific: Non-Systems
Content Outline: Safety & Professional Roles; Teaching/Learning; Research

Exam Two: Question 83

A physical therapist working on a medical/surgical rotation returns from a morning inservice and finds a number of items that require her attention. Which of the following items should be given the highest priority?

1. **a patient requiring pre-operative instruction**
2. an incomplete exercise flow sheet
3. an unfinished wheelchair order form
4. a written note from a staff dietician

> **Correct Answer: 1** (Code of Ethics)

Physical therapists routinely have to multi-task, however, as part of this process therapists need to be able to prioritize the importance of selected activities.

1. **Pre-operative instruction most often occurs in close proximity to a scheduled surgical procedure. As a result, delaying the pre-operative instruction may result in the patient not receiving the necessary instruction or the surgery being delayed or cancelled.**
2. It is important to document exercise activities using a flow sheet or other suitable tracking form, however, the activity can be deferred without immediate consequence.
3. It is important to submit all order forms for equipment or other devices in a timely manner. This need is particularly important in today's health care environment due to the reduced length of stay. Despite the importance this would not supersede the need to complete the pre-operative instruction.
4. The physical therapist should read and, if necessary, respond to the note from the staff dietician, however, this would not supersede the need for the direct patient care activity.

System Specific: Non-Systems
Content Outline: Safety & Professional Roles; Teaching/Learning; Research

Exam Two: Question 84

A physical therapist employed in a busy outpatient orthopedic clinic attempts to determine a schedule for calibration and maintenance of an ultrasound unit. The MOST important factor for the therapist to consider when determining an appropriate schedule is:

1. beam nonuniformity ratio
2. **frequency of use**
3. cost associated with calibration and maintenance
4. availability of qualified personnel to inspect the unit

> **Correct Answer: 2** (Belanger p. 237)

Electrical equipment must be calibrated and maintained by qualified personnel on a regular schedule consistent with the manufacturer's recommendations. The regular schedule, once established, can be modified based on variables such as increased frequency of use or reports of faulty performance.

1. Beam nonuniformity ratio (BNR) refers to the ratio of intensity of the highest peak to the average intensity of all peaks. The BNR is determined by the intrinsic biophysical properties of the piezoelectric transducer. The BNR of an ultrasound device would not be a factor in determining a calibration and maintenance schedule.
2. **The frequency of use of an ultrasound device is extremely important when determining a schedule for calibration and maintenance. Ultrasound units used frequently may be calibrated several times a year, while a unit used sparingly would likely warrant a longer interval.**
3. The cost associated with calibration and maintenance of the ultrasound unit should not be a factor in establishing a calibration and maintenance schedule. Relying on a variable such as cost implies that when there are ample resources available calibration and maintenance take place and when resources are not available calibration and maintenance can be deferred.
4. The availability of qualified personnel to inspect the ultrasound unit would not be a factor in determining a calibration and maintenance schedule. If appropriate personnel are not available within the health care organization, there are a variety of external companies who can provide the necessary service.

System Specific: Non-Systems
Content Outline: Equipment & Devices; Therapeutic Modalities

Exam Two: Question 85

A patient rehabilitating from a fractured acetabulum is referred to physical therapy for ambulation activities. The patient has been on bed rest for three weeks and appears to be somewhat apprehensive about weight bearing. The MOST appropriate device to use when initiating ambulation activities is:

1. **parallel bars**
2. walker
3. axillary crutches
4. straight cane

> **Correct Answer: 1** (Pierson p. 219)

A physical therapist must carefully assess a patient's needs prior to initiating ambulation activities. The question provides ample evidence that the patient will need a secure and stable environment to initiate ambulation.

1. **The magnitude of the injury (i.e., fractured acetabulum), the length of time the patient has been on bed rest, and the degree of patient apprehension make it imperative that the therapist initiate ambulation in a controlled and stable environment (i.e., parallel bars).**
2. A walker is a relatively stable assistive device, however, the parallel bars provide a safer environment to initiate ambulation. It is likely that the patient will quickly transition to the walker in subsequent sessions.
3. Axillary crutches allow altered weight bearing levels, but would not likely provide the level of stability required given the presented information.
4. A straight cane does not permit partial weight bearing, if desired, and offers significantly less stability than any of the other presented options.

System Specific: Non-Systems
Content Outline: Equipment & Devices; Therapeutic Modalities

Exam Two: Question 86

A seven-year-old boy sitting in the physical therapy waiting area suddenly grasps his throat and appears to be in distress. The boy slowly stands, but is obviously unable to breathe. The physical therapist recognizing the signs of an airway obstruction should administer:

1. **abdominal thrusts**
2. chest thrusts
3. back blows
4. finger sweep

> **Correct Answer: 1** (American Heart Association)

An airway obstruction in a child or an adult is best treated by using abdominal thrusts.

1. **Abdominal thrusts (Heimlich maneuver) can be used on a child until the object is expelled or the victim becomes unresponsive. Abdominal thrusts are not recommended for infants (less than one year of age) because of an increased risk of injury.**
2. If abdominal thrusts are ineffective, the health care provider may consider using chest thrusts. Research has demonstrated that approximately 50% of the episodes of airway obstruction were not relieved by a single technique. As a result, the likelihood of success may be increased when using combinations of back blows, abdominal thrusts, and chest thrusts.
3. Back blows combined with chest thrusts are the recommended procedures for attempting to expel a foreign body airway obstruction in infants. Deliver five back blows (slaps) followed by five chest thrusts repeatedly until the object is expelled or the victim becomes unresponsive.
4. A finger sweep is recommended if the health care provider can see solid material obstructing the airway of an unresponsive patient. In the question, the boy is conscious.

System Specific: Non-Systems
Content Outline: Safety & Professional Roles; Teaching/Learning; Research

Exam Two: Question 87

A physical therapist assesses a patient's upper extremity deep tendon reflexes as part of a screening examination. The MOST appropriate location to elicit the brachioradialis reflex is the:

1. radial tuberosity
2. antecubital fossa
3. biceps tendon
4. **styloid process of the radius**

> **Correct Answer: 4** (Dutton p. 659)

The brachioradialis muscle is innervated by the radial nerve via the C5-C6 nerve root, however, the reflex is largely a function of C6. The brachioradialis muscle is the only muscle in the body that extends from the distal end of one bone to the distal end of another.

1. The radial tuberosity is an oval projection from the medial surface of the radius, immediately distal to the neck. The biceps brachii tendon inserts on the radial tuberosity.
2. The antecubital fossa is a triangular cavity of the elbow that contains the tendon of the biceps, the median nerve, and the brachial artery.
3. The biceps reflex (C5-C6) is tested by tapping over the biceps tendon or the thumb of the therapist placed directly over the biceps tendon in the antecubital fossa.
4. **The brachioradialis reflex is tested by tapping the brachioradialis tendon at the distal end of the radius with the flat edge of the reflex hammer.**

System Specific: Neuromuscular & Nervous Systems
Content Outline: Clinical Application of Foundational Sciences

Exam Two: Question 88

A physical therapist prepares to assist a patient with a sliding board transfer from a wheelchair to a mat table. Which of the following would be the MOST appropriate INITIAL instruction to the patient?

1. place the sliding board under your buttocks
2. move your buttocks onto the mat table
3. complete a series of push-ups
4. **secure the wheelchair brakes**

> **Correct Answer: 4** (Minor p. 224)

Securing the wheelchair brakes is the most appropriate action when initiating a transfer from a wheelchair.

1. Placing the sliding board under the buttocks occurs after the wheelchair is positioned, after the wheelchair brakes are secure, and after the armrests are removed.
2. Moving the buttocks onto the mat table is performed after the patient has actually slid out of the wheelchair, onto and across the sliding board, and is ready to complete the transfer.
3. Completing a series of push ups is performed after the sliding board is placed under the buttocks in order to move across the sliding board.
4. **Securing the wheelchair brakes is always the most appropriate action when initiating a transfer from a wheelchair. It is a safety concern that must be addressed in order for the patient to safely complete the transfer.**

System Specific: Non-Systems
Content Outline: Equipment & Devices; Therapeutic Modalities

Exam Two: Question 89

A physical therapist completes a respiratory assessment on a patient in an acute care hospital. The examination reveals decreased breath sounds and decreased fremitus. This finding is MOST indicative of:

1. **pleural effusion**
2. pulmonary edema
3. consolidation
4. atelectasis

> **Correct Answer: 1** (Hillegass p. 213)

Decreased breath sounds and decreased fremitus are most likely caused by pleural effusion or pneumothorax. Pulmonary edema, consolidation, and atelectasis are often associated with decreased breath sounds and increased fremitus.

1. **Pleural effusion is an accumulation of fluid between the layers of the membrane that lines the lungs and chest cavity. Abnormal lung pressures secondary to congestive heart failure often cause transudative pleural effusion. Exudative effusion results from inflammation of the pleura caused by lung disease.**
2. Pulmonary edema is an accumulation of fluid in the alveolar spaces. The condition is most often associated with decreased breath sounds and increased fremitus.
3. Consolidation refers to an area of the lung that is filled with fluid. The fluid may be edema, inflammatory exudate, pus, water or blood. The condition is most often associated with decreased breath sounds and increased fremitus on the side of the consolidation.
4. Atelectasis is the absence of gas in part or all of a lung due to a collapse of the lung tissue. The condition is most often associated with decreased breath sounds and increased fremitus.

System Specific: Cardiac, Vascular, & Pulmonary Systems
Content Outline: Foundations for Evaluation, Differential Diagnosis, & Prognosis

Exam Two: Question 90

A physical therapist records the parameters of an electrical stimulation treatment in a patient's medical record. The standard unit of measure when recording alternating current frequency is:

1. volt
2. **hertz**
3. coulomb
4. pulses per second

> **Correct Answer: 2** (Cameron p. 236)

Frequency controls, often labeled rate, determine the type of response or muscle contraction that electrical stimulation will produce. As the frequency of any waveform is increased, the amplitude tends to increase and decrease more rapidly.

1. Voltage refers to the electrical force capable of moving charged particles through a conductor between two regions or points.
2. **Hertz is a unit of measure which describes the number of cycles per second when using alternating current.**
3. A coulomb is the amount of electrical charge transported in one second by a steady current of one ampere.
4. Pulses per second is utilized to describe the frequency of pulsed current.

System Specific: Non-Systems
Content Outline: Equipment & Devices; Therapeutic Modalities

Exam Two: Question 91

A physical therapist working in cardiac rehabilitation progresses a patient involved in a phase II program through an established exercise protocol. The patient weighs 70 kg and has progressed without difficulty through the rehabilitation program. The protocol indicates the patient should be performing activities requiring 3-4 METs. An example of an appropriate activity would be:

1. level walking at 1 mph
2. jogging at 5 mph
3. cycling at 10 mph
4. **walking on a treadmill at 3 mph**

> **Correct Answer: 4** (Brannon p. 317)

One metabolic equivalent is the amount of oxygen consumed at rest and is equal to approximately 3.5 milliliters of oxygen per kilogram of body weight per minute. Other recreational activities requiring 3-4 METs include cycling at 6 mph and golfing while pulling a bag cart.

1. Level walking at 1 mph is approximately 1.5 to 2 METs.
2. Jogging at 5 mph is approximately 6 to 7 METs.
3. Cycling at 10 mph is approximately 5 to 6 METs.
4. **Walking on a treadmill at 3 mph is approximately 3 to 4 METs.**

System Specific: Cardiac, Vascular, & Pulmonary Systems
Content Outline: Interventions

Exam Two: Question 92

A physical therapist utilizes continuous ultrasound to supply thermal effects to a patient rehabilitating from a lower extremity injury. During the treatment session, the patient suddenly becomes startled and reports feeling an electrical shock from the ultrasound machine. The MOST appropriate therapist action is to:

1. decrease the intensity of the ultrasound
2. modify the duty cycle
3. discontinue ultrasound treatment
4. **unplug the machine and label – "defective, do not use"**

> **Correct Answer: 4** (Prentice – Therapeutic Modalities p. 48)

Any equipment that is potentially defective should be formally inspected prior to being used to treat patients.

1. Decreasing the intensity of the ultrasound will diminish the total amount of sound energy delivered to tissues, however, it does not significantly protect the patient from the potential harm of a malfunctioning ultrasound unit.
2. Modifying the duty cycle would be used to increase or decrease the amount of sound energy delivered to tissues or to emphasize to a greater or lesser extent the thermal or non-thermal effects, however, the option does not offer adequate protection for the patient.
3. Discontinuing ultrasound treatment, although appropriate, places other patients at risk by exposing them to potential harm from a malfunctioning ultrasound unit. It is an appropriate therapist response to discontinue any physical agent when the patient reports an abnormal response to treatment such as "feeling an electrical shock."
4. **By unplugging the machine and labeling it – "defective, do not use," the therapist not only guarantees that the current treatment is stopped, but also eliminates any potential risk from using the ultrasound unit with other patients. The unit requires a formal inspection from a qualified individual prior to being used again.**

System Specific: Non-Systems
Content Outline: Equipment & Devices; Therapeutic Modalities

Exam Two: Question 93

A physical therapy department embarks on a quality improvement program. Results from a random sample of patient charts reveal that 40% of the charts do not include a discharge summary. A logical next step to the quality improvement program would be:

1. dismiss the findings because discharge summaries are not directly related to the quality of patient care
2. discipline the staff members who did not complete the discharge summaries and continue to monitor the situation
3. dismiss the findings because a random sample does not provide accurate information
4. **notify the staff that discharge summaries are to be completed on all patients and continue to monitor the situation**

Correct Answer: 4 (Nosse p. 295)

Quality improvement refers to activities or programs designed to achieve a desired degree or grade of care. Findings from quality improvement initiatives should be communicated directly to staff in a manner that is constructive, instead of punitive.

1. Discharge summaries are an essential component of physical therapy documentation and offer important information that can be used as part of a quality improvement program.
2. Disciplining staff members based on the identification of a significant finding from a quality improvement program would be considered a punitive action, especially given the fact that the problem had not been previously addressed.
3. A random sample of patient charts is a commonly used form of sampling that allows individuals to draw inferences without having to examine every patient chart. Given the significance of the findings (i.e., 40% of patient charts did not include a discharge summary), it would be inappropriate to dismiss the findings.
4. **The identified finding is unacceptable and therefore compels the therapist to act. By notifying staff of the findings the therapist has emphasized the importance of completing discharge summaries. Continued monitoring is necessary to determine if the staffs' performance improves. Failure to improve may warrant disciplinary action.**

System Specific: Non-Systems
Content Outline: Safety & Professional Roles; Teaching/Learning; Research

Exam Two: Question 94

A physical therapist employed in a rehabilitation hospital examines a patient that exhibits several signs and symptoms of anemia. Which question would be the MOST useful to gather additional information related to anemia?

1. Does it hurt to take a deep breath?
2. **Do you experience heart palpitations or shortness of breath at rest or with mild exertion?**
3. Do you frequently experience dizziness, headaches or blurred vision?
4. Are you susceptible to bruising?

Correct Answer: 2 (Goodman - Differential Diagnosis p. 263)

Anemia is a condition in which the number of red blood cells is reduced. Due to the reduction of red blood cells, delivery of oxygen to the tissues is impaired. Symptoms of anemia include pallor, cyanosis, cool skin, weakness, and malaise.

1. Pain with deep breathing may be from pleurisy, pneumothorax or from an injury to the muscles, ribs, cartilage or nerves of the chest.
2. **Heart palpitations and shortness of breath are symptoms of anemia.**
3. Dizziness, headaches or blurred vision are signs and symptoms commonly associated with hypertension.
4. Susceptibility to bruising is a sign of a coagulation disorder, possibly from recent use of thrombolytic agents after a myocardial infarction or hemophilia.

System Specific: Other Systems
Content Outline: Foundations for Evaluation, Differential Diagnosis, & Prognosis

Exam Two: Question 95

A physical therapist performs postural drainage to the anterior basal segments of the lower lobes. During the treatment session the patient suddenly complains of dizziness and mild dyspnea. The MOST appropriate therapist action is:

1. reassure the patient that the response is normal
2. assess the patient's vital signs
3. **elevate the patient's head**
4. call for assistance

> **Correct Answer: 3** (Hillegass p. 650)

Postural drainage is the assumption of one or more body positions that allow gravity to drain secretions from each of the patient's lung segments. In each position, the segmental bronchus of the area to be drained is positioned perpendicular to the floor. Postural drainage to the anterior basal segment of the lower lobes would require the bottom of the bed to be elevated 18-20 inches.

1. A subjective complaint of dizziness and mild dyspnea would exceed a "normal" patient response. The physical therapist must act based on the patient's comment even though it would not be entirely unexpected given the necessary patient position for postural drainage of the anterior basal segment of the lower lobes.
2. Assessing the patient's vital signs is a desirable option, however, only after the patient is repositioned with the head elevated.
3. **Dizziness and dyspnea are signs of intolerance to the head down postural drainage position required to drain the anterior basal segments of the lower lobes. Elevating the patient's head will likely relieve the symptoms.**
4. Calling for assistance is not necessary since the patient's symptoms should subside once the head is elevated.

System Specific: Other Systems
Content Outline: Interventions

Exam Two: Question 96

A terminally ill patient completes a formal document that names his daughter as the individual to make health care decisions in the event that he is unable. This type of advanced directive is termed:

1. living will
2. physician's directive
3. **durable power of attorney**
4. euthanasia

> **Correct Answer: 3** (Scott – Promoting Legal and Ethical Awareness p. 194)

Durable power of attorney for health care decisions refers to a legal document that delegates decision making to a specified individual in the event another individual is found to be incompetent to make a medical decision.

1. A living will is a legal document that a person uses to make known his or her wishes regarding life prolonging medical treatments. It can also be referred to as an advance directive, health care directive or a physician's directive.
2. The term "physician's directive" is synonymous with a living will.
3. **The power associated with the durable power of attorney becomes operative when and if the patient becomes legally incompetent to make decisions. The patient often designates a spouse, relative, friend or attorney to act on their behalf.**
4. Euthanasia is the act of ending a person's life and usually pertains to patients in either vegetative states or that are terminally ill. Passive euthanasia is the practice of withholding or withdrawing life sustaining devices and measures. Active euthanasia involves the deliberate intervention in order to facilitate a person's death.

System Specific: Non-Systems
Content Outline: Safety & Professional Roles; Teaching/Learning; Research

Exam Two: Question 97

A patient recently diagnosed with a deep venous thrombophlebitis is placed on heparin. The PRIMARY side effect associated with heparin is:

1. hypotension
2. depression
3. **excessive anticoagulation**
4. thrombocytopenia

Correct Answer: 3 (Ciccone p. 352)

Anticoagulant agents delay or prevent blood coagulation (clotting). Heparin is an anticoagulant used to prevent and treat disorders such as pulmonary embolism, which result from vascular thrombosis. Heparin inhibits coagulation by preventing the conversion of prothrombin to thrombin and by preventing the release of thromboplastin from platelets.

1. Hypotension, a lower than normal systolic or diastolic blood pressure, is not a side effect of heparin.
2. Depression, a mood disorder characterized by loss of interest or pleasure in living, is not a side effect associated with heparin.
3. **The most common side effect of heparin is abnormal bleeding. A physical therapist should be careful to avoid excessive contact or bumping of the limbs of a patient on heparin since this may cause bruising or bleeding.**
4. Thrombocytopenia, or an abnormal decrease in the number of blood platelets, has been associated with heparin use, but is not the primary side effect.

System Specific: Cardiac, Vascular, & Pulmonary Systems
Content Outline: Clinical Application of Foundational Sciences

Exam Two: Question 98

A patient is asked to complete a pain questionnaire. The patient selects words such as cramping, dull, and aching to describe the pain. What related structure is MOST consistent with the pain description?

1. nerve root
2. **muscle**
3. bone
4. vascular

Correct Answer: 2 (Magee p. 7)

The patient interview provides a physical therapist with an opportunity to identify specific characteristics of pain. Subjective pain descriptors can provide valuable information related to a patient's condition. Characteristics to explore may include location, intensity, description, duration, and pattern.

1. Nerve root pain is often characterized as sharp, shooting, and burning. The pain tends to travel in the distribution of the specific nerve root.
2. **Muscle pain is often characterized as cramping, dull, and aching. The pain tends to worsen when the involved muscle contracts or is lengthened.**
3. Bone pain is often characterized as deep, intolerable, boring, and highly localized.
4. Vascular pain is often characterized as diffuse, throbbing, aching, and poorly localized. The pain is often referred to other parts of the body.

System Specific: Other Systems
Content Outline: Foundations for Evaluation, Differential Diagnosis, & Prognosis

Exam Two: Question 99

A physical therapist examines a patient with suspected vascular compression in the shoulder region. Which special test would be LEAST beneficial to confirm the therapist's suspicions?

1. Adson maneuver
2. Halstead maneuver
3. **Froment's sign**
4. Wright Test

> **Correct Answer: 3** (Magee p. 442)

There are a variety of special tests designed to identify vascular compression in the shoulder. When performing the tests, a positive sign is often indicated by diminution or disappearance of a pulse or reproduction of neurological signs or symptoms.

1. Adson maneuver is performed with the patient in sitting or standing. The therapist monitors the radial pulse and asks the patient to rotate their head to face the test shoulder. The patient is then asked to extend their head while the therapist laterally rotates and extends the patient's shoulder. A positive test is indicated by an absent or diminished radial pulse.

2. The Halstead maneuver is performed with the patient sitting over the edge of a table. The therapist palpates the radial pulse and applies a downward traction on the symptomatic side. The patient is then asked to extend the head and turn away from the tested side. A positive test is indicated by an absent or diminished pulse.

3. **Froment's sign requires a patient to grasp a piece of paper between the thumb and index finger. A positive test is indicated by flexion of the terminal phalanx of the thumb caused by paralysis of the adductor pollicis longus. The test is used to assess the integrity of the ulnar nerve.**

4. The Wright test or hyperabduction test is performed with the patient in sitting or supine. The therapist moves the patient's arm overhead in the frontal plane while monitoring the patient's radial pulse. A positive test is indicated by an absent or diminished radial pulse and may be indicative of compression in the costoclavicular space.

System Specific: Neuromuscular & Nervous Systems
Content Outline: Examination

Exam Two: Question 100

A 29-year-old female status post Colles' fracture is referred to physical therapy. The patient has moderate edema in her fingers and the dorsum of her hand and complains of pain during active range of motion. The MOST appropriate method to quantify the patient's edema is:

1. **volumetric measurements**
2. circumferential measurements
3. girth measurements
4. anthropometric measurements

> **Correct Answer: 1** (Magee p. 446)

Volumetric measurements are often used to quantify the presence of edema in the wrist and hand by examining the amount of water displaced following immersion.

1. **A patient with moderate edema in the fingers and dorsum of the hand would displace more water than the contralateral extremity due to the involved limb's increased volume. Although the contralateral extremity serves as an effective baseline measure, it is important to recognize that there may normally be a small difference between the dominant and non-dominant hand.**

2. Circumferential measurements using a flexible tape measure are most commonly used to obtain a gross estimate of edema or muscle atrophy. The test would not commonly be used for the hand due to the difficulty associated with obtaining an accurate measurement because of the relative nonuniformity of the hand.

3. Girth measurements are synonymous with circumferential measurements.

4. Common anthropometric measurements used for adults include height, weight, body mass index (BMI), waist-to-hip ratio, and percentage of body fat. These measures are then compared to reference standards to assess items such as weight status and the risk for various diseases.

System Specific: Other Systems
Content Outline: Examination

Exam Two: Question 101

A physical therapist inspects a wound over the sacrum of a 58-year-old female. The therapist would MOST accurately classify the presented wound as:

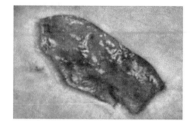

1. stage I
2. stage II
3. **stage III**
4. stage IV

> **Correct Answer: 3** (Sussman p. 89)

The National Pressure Ulcer Advisory Panel pressure ulcer staging criteria was developed for use with pressure ulcers. The staging criteria range from I - IV.

1. A stage I ulcer is characterized by an observable pressure related alteration of intact skin whose indicators, as compared to an adjacent or opposite area on the body, may include changes in skin color, skin temperature, skin stiffness or sensation.
2. A stage II ulcer is characterized by partial-thickness skin loss that involves the epidermis and/or dermis. The ulcer is superficial and presents clinically as an abrasion, a blister or a shallow crater.
3. **A stage III ulcer is characterized by full-thickness skin loss that involves damage or necrosis of subcutaneous tissue that may extend down to, but not through, underlying fascia. The ulcer presents clinically as a deep crater with or without undermining adjacent tissue.**
4. A stage IV ulcer is characterized by full-thickness skin loss with extensive destruction, tissue necrosis or damage to muscle, bone or supporting structures (e.g., tendon, joint capsule).

System Specific: Integumentary System
Content Outline: Examination

Exam Two: Question 102

A physical therapist observes a patient's breathing as part of a respiratory assessment. Which muscle of respiration is MOST active during forced expiration?

1. diaphragm
2. external intercostals
3. **internal intercostals**
4. upper trapezius

> **Correct Answer: 3** (Frownfelter p. 59)

Unlike quiet expiration, which is mainly a passive process primarily dependent on the elastic properties of lung tissue, forced expiration is an active process. In addition to the rectus abdominis, external and internal obliques, and transverse abdominis contracting to compress the abdominal viscera, the ribs are pulled downward by action of the internal intercostals and quadratus lumborum.

1. The diaphragm is the principal inspiratory muscle.
2. The external intercostals act to lift the ribs during deep inspiration.
3. **The internal intercostals assist to pull the ribs downward during forced expiration.**
4. The upper trapezius acts as an accessory muscle of inspiration by assisting to elevate and stabilize the scapulae.

System Specific: Cardiac, Vascular, & Pulmonary Systems
Content Outline: Clinical Application of Foundational Sciences

Exam Two: Question 103

A physical therapist treats a patient who sustained a right lateral ankle sprain less than six hours ago. The therapist contemplates the use of cold water immersion as a cryotherapeutic agent. What would be the primary limitation of this type of intervention?

1. decreased cell metabolism
2. excessive vasoconstriction of blood vessels
3. **the involved extremity cannot be elevated**
4. decreased nerve conduction velocity

> **Correct Answer: 3** (Cameron p. 267)

There are a wide range of cryotherapeutic agents commonly used in physical therapy including cold whirlpool, ice packs, ice massage, cold sprays, and contrast baths. Physical therapists should be aware of the advantages and limitations of each of the identified cryotherapeutic agents.

1. Cryotherapy decreases metabolic reactions including those involved in the inflammatory process.
2. Cryotherapy initially causes local vasoconstriction of smooth muscles in an attempt to conserve heat. Vasoconstriction is responsible for decreasing the formation and accumulation of edema.
3. **Cold water immersion is an acceptable form of cryotherapy, however, is not ideal when treating an acute lower extremity injury since the injured limb cannot be elevated. Inflammation is most effectively controlled if the cryotherapeutic agent is applied in conjunction with elevation and compression. Several other cryotherapeutic agents such as ice packs or cryocuff may be more desirable interventions.**
4. Cryotherapy decreases the nerve conduction velocity of both sensory and motor nerves. Cryotherapy has the greatest effect on the conduction velocity of myelinated and small fibers, and the least effect on the conduction velocity of unmyelinated and large fibers.

System Specific: Non-Systems
Content Outline: Equipment & Devices; Therapeutic Modalities

Exam Two: Question 104

A physical therapist reviews the results of a pulmonary function test for a 58-year-old male patient recently admitted to the hospital. The therapist notes that the patient's total lung capacity is significantly increased when compared to established norms. Which medical condition would MOST likely produce this type of result?

1. chronic bronchitis
2. **emphysema**
3. spinal cord injury
4. pulmonary fibrosis

> **Correct Answer: 2** (Frownfelter p. 87)

Emphysema is a chronic obstructive pulmonary disease characterized by an abnormal and permanent enlargement of the air spaces distal to the terminal bronchiole, accompanied by destructive changes in their walls. Changes in lung tissue resulting from these anatomic changes include loss of elastic recoil, collapse of airways during exhalation, and airflow obstruction.

1. In chronic bronchitis there is hypertrophy of the submucosal glands in the large and small bronchi and trachea with hypersecretion of mucus sufficient to cause a productive cough. Pulmonary function tests demonstrate a forced expiratory volume in one second (FEV_1) of < 65% of the predicted value. Total lung capacity is not increased in true chronic bronchitis.
2. **As a result of the pathologic changes to the lung tissue in emphysema, the lungs become hyperinflated. Due to the loss of elastic recoil, obstruction to airflow is seen as an increase in total lung capacity, residual volume, and functional residual capacity.**
3. Spinal cord injury is a neuromuscular cause of restrictive lung dysfunction. Characteristic changes in pulmonary function tests may include decreases in total lung capacity, vital capacity, and inspiratory capacity.
4. Pulmonary fibrosis is an inflammatory process affecting the alveoli that grossly distorts the architecture of the lung. These changes cause a decrease in lung compliance and a decrease in lung volumes including total lung capacity, vital capacity, functional residual capacity, and residual volume.

System Specific: Cardiac, Vascular, & Pulmonary Systems
Content Outline: Foundations for Evaluation, Differential Diagnosis, & Prognosis

Exam Two: Question 105

A physical therapist observes a patient's skin shortly after applying moist heat to the low back. The therapist identifies several signs of heat intolerance including uneven blotching and a surface rash. The MOST appropriate action is to:

1. continue with the present treatment
2. select an alternate superficial heating agent
3. limit moist heat exposure to five minutes
4. **discontinue the moist heat and document the findings**

> **Correct Answer: 4** (Cameron p. 162)

Physical therapists should frequently monitor a patient's response when using a hot pack. The patient should feel only a mild to moderate sensation of heat and formal inspection of the skin should occur intermittently. Therapists should avoid having the patient lie directly on the hot pack since body weight will tend to squeeze water from the pack and accelerate the rate of heat transfer to the tissues. In addition, local circulation could be reduced through compression of vessels which would serve to reduce the dissipation of heat.

1. Continuing with treatment after identifying signs of heat intolerance would unnecessarily jeopardize patient safety.
2. Heat intolerance can be associated with a variety of superficial heating agents and not solely moist heat. As a result, it would be inappropriate to simply select an alternate superficial heating agent.
3. Limiting the exposure to moist heat may be useful to minimize the severity of the reaction, however, since the question provides ample evidence of heat intolerance it is necessary to discontinue the intervention.
4. **Treatment should be discontinued when there is any sign of heat intolerance. It is important to document the observation in order to alert other possible providers to the patient's reaction and to make the incident part of the patient's permanent medical record.**

System Specific: Non-Systems
Content Outline: Equipment & Devices; Therapeutic Modalities

Exam Two: Question 106

A physical therapist prepares a patient status post CVA with global aphasia for discharge from a rehabilitation hospital. The patient will be returning home with her husband and daughter. The MOST appropriate form of education to facilitate a safe discharge is to:

1. **perform hands-on training sessions with the patient and family members**
2. videotape the patient performing transfers and activities of daily living
3. provide written instructions on all activities of daily living and functional tasks
4. meet with family members to discuss the patient's present status and abilities

> **Correct Answer: 1** (O'Sullivan p. 761)

In order to facilitate a safe discharge, it is imperative that the physical therapist is certain that the patient and family are aware of and can perform the necessary activities of daily living (ADLs) and functional tasks that will be required. The most effective manner in which to ascertain the family's readiness is to have them perform the required tasks and observe their competence.

1. **Hands-on training sessions provide unique opportunities for the therapist to assess the competence of family members in a structured environment.**
2. Videotaping the necessary transfers and ADLs will provide the family with a visual aid, however, it does not ensure that they are able to safely perform the tasks with the patient.
3. Providing written instructions on all ADLs and functional tasks is an important part of a home exercise program and should be included in all discharge plans. This action, however, does not ensure that family members are able to perform the tasks safely with the patient.
4. Meeting with the family member to discuss the patient's present status and abilities is an important part of any discharge planning, however, it will not provide the therapist with enough information on the family's competence with the required tasks.

System Specific: Other Systems
Content Outline: Interventions

Exam Two: Question 107

A physical therapist treats a 36-year-old male status post knee surgery. The therapist performs goniometric measurements to quantify the extent of the patient's extension lag. Which of the following would NOT provide a plausible rationale for the extension lag?

1. muscle weakness
2. **bony obstruction**
3. inhibition by pain
4. patient apprehension

> **Correct Answer: 2** (Kisner p. 891)

Patients that demonstrate an extension lag have greater passive extension than active extension. The difference in the passive and active extension range of motion is used to quantify the amount of the lag.

1. Muscle weakness would provide a plausible rationale for an extension lag since force production is necessary to produce active motion. Inability to produce adequate force to move the tibia on the femur while performing active extension would produce the lag.

2. **A bony obstruction would not produce an extension lag since passive range of motion and active range of motion would be equal. In essence, the obstruction would interfere with the ability to perform both passive and active knee extension.**

3. Inhibition by pain would provide a plausible rationale for an extension lag. The amount of pain produced during an active muscle contraction may make it impossible for the muscle to generate the required amount of force to actively extend the tibia on the femur. The difference in the passive extension versus the active extension would determine the amount of the extension lag.

4. Patient apprehension would provide a plausible rationale for an extension lag since the patient may be unwilling to actively move the knee through the available active range of motion due to fear or anxiety.

System Specific: Musculoskeletal System
Content Outline: Clinical Application of Foundational Sciences

Exam Two: Question 108

A patient successfully completes ten anterior lunges. The physical therapist would like to modify the activity to maximally challenge the patient in the sagittal plane. Which of the following modifications would be the MOST appropriate?

1. anterior lunge with concurrent bilateral elbow flexion to 45 degrees with five pound weights
2. **anterior lunge with concurrent bilateral shoulder flexion to 90 degrees with five pound weights**
3. anterior lunge with concurrent unilateral shoulder flexion to 90 degrees with a five pound weight
4. anterior lunge with concurrent bilateral shoulder abduction to 45 degrees with five pound weights

> **Correct Answer: 2** (Norkin p. 4)

The sagittal plane divides the body into left and right halves. Motions in the sagittal plane include flexion and extension. In order to maximally challenge the patient in this plane, candidates should choose the option that moves the patient's center of gravity furthest outside the base of support in the sagittal plane.

1. Bilateral elbow flexion would challenge the patient in the sagittal plane, however, the movement would not significantly change the center of gravity since the upper extremities would be held close to the body.

2. **Bilateral shoulder flexion would create the largest forward movement and would therefore provide the greatest challenge for the patient due to the center of gravity moving forward outside the base of support.**

3. Unilateral shoulder flexion would challenge the patient in the sagittal plane, however, it would not provide as much of a challenge as the bilateral shoulder flexion due to the decreased amount of mass moving outside the base of support (one upper extremity versus two upper extremities).

4. Bilateral shoulder abduction would challenge the patient in the frontal plane.

System Specific: Musculoskeletal System
Content Outline: Interventions

Exam Two: Question 109

A physical therapist teaches a patient positioned in supine to posteriorly rotate her pelvis. The patient has full active and passive range of motion in the upper extremities, but is unable to achieve full shoulder flexion while maintaining a posterior pelvic tilt. Which of the following could BEST explain these findings?

1. capsular tightness
2. **latissimus dorsi tightness**
3. pectoralis minor tightness
4. quadratus lumborum tightness

Correct Answer: 2 (Kendall p. 325)

A posterior pelvic tilt results in the posterior superior iliac spines of the pelvis moving posteriorly and inferiorly. This motion results in hip extension and lumbar spine flexion.

1. The capsular pattern at the glenohumeral joint is lateral rotation, abduction, and medial rotation. A capsular pattern of restriction at the glenohumeral joint would limit range of motion, however, would not be influenced by the position of the pelvis.
2. **Shortening of the latissimus dorsi often results in a limitation of shoulder flexion or abduction due to the muscle's origin on the external lip of the iliac crest and its insertion on the intertubercular groove of the humerus.**
3. Pectoralis minor tightness may have a direct effect on shoulder range of motion, however, would not be influenced by the position of the pelvis. Pectoralis minor tightness is often best identified by positioning a patient in supine with the arms at their side and the palms facing upward. The relative tightness of the muscle is determined by the extent to which the shoulder is raised from the table and the amount of resistance felt to downward pressure on the shoulder.
4. Quadratus lumborum tightness may affect the ability of the pelvis to achieve the posterior pelvic tilt position required in the question, however, would not affect shoulder range of motion since the muscle does not directly attach to the shoulder joint.

System Specific: Musculoskeletal System
Content Outline: Interventions

Exam Two: Question 110

A physical therapist observes a burn on the dorsal surface of a patient's arm. The wound area is mottled red with a number of blisters. The therapist informs the patient that healing should take place in less than three weeks. This description is MOST indicative of a:

1. superficial burn
2. **superficial partial-thickness burn**
3. deep partial-thickness burn
4. full-thickness burn

Correct Answer: 2 (Goodman - Pathology p. 436)

The burn classification system most commonly utilized uses the terms superficial, partial-thickness (superficial and deep), and full-thickness. The system provides a general description of the most common clinical findings associated with each type of burn.

1. A superficial burn involves only the outer epidermis. The involved area may be red with slight edema. Healing occurs without evidence of scarring in 3-7 days.
2. **A superficial partial-thickness burn involves the epidermis and the upper portion of the dermis. The involved area may be extremely painful and exhibit blisters. Healing occurs with minimal to no scarring in 14-21 days.**
3. A deep partial-thickness burn involves complete destruction of the epidermis and the majority of the dermis. The involved area may appear to be discolored with broken blisters and edema. Damage to nerve endings may result in only moderate levels of pain. Healing occurs with the potential for hypertrophic scars and keloids in 21-28 days.
4. A full-thickness burn involves complete destruction of the epidermis and dermis along with partial damage of the subcutaneous fat layer. The involved area often presents with eschar formation and minimal to no pain. Patients with full-thickness burns require grafts and may be susceptible to infection.

System Specific: Integumentary System
Content Outline: Foundations for Evaluation, Differential Diagnosis, & Prognosis

Exam Two: Question 111

A group of physical therapists develops a research project that examines the effect of increased abdominal muscle strength on forced vital capacity and forced expiratory volume. In order to conduct the study, the therapists are required to have the approval of the hospital Institutional Review Board. The PRIMARY purpose of the committee is to:

1. protect the hospital from unnecessary litigation
2. **ensure the rights of research subjects are protected**
3. examine the design of the research project
4. assess the financial ramifications of the research project

Correct Answer: 2 (Portney p. 52)

Federal regulations require an Institutional Review Board (IRB) review all research proposals prior to implementation to ensure that the rights of research subjects are protected.

1. By ensuring the rights of research subjects, the IRB may protect the hospital from litigation, however, protection from litigation is not the primary purpose of the committee.
2. **Ensuring the rights of research subjects is the primary purpose of the IRB. To do this, the IRB evaluates the scientific merit of the project, the competence of the investigators, the risk to subjects, and the feasibility of the project based on available resources.**
3. In evaluating the scientific merit of the project, the IRB will examine the research design. This is done to ensure that the rights of research subjects are protected since if the project is not scientifically sound, there can be no benefit.
4. In evaluating the research proposal, the IRB will consider the feasibility of the project based on the identified resources.

System Specific: Non-Systems
Content Outline: Safety & Professional Roles; Teaching/Learning; Research

Exam Two: Question 112

Members of a community health task force evaluate a proposal for a new adolescent screening program. Several members of the task force raise questions as to the validity of the screening instrument. Which measure of validity examines the instrument's ability to identify diseased persons by comparing true positives?

1. adaptability
2. selectivity
3. **sensitivity**
4. specificity

Correct Answer: 3 (Portney p. 620)

The validity of a diagnostic test is evaluated by its ability to accurately assess the presence or absence of the target condition. A diagnostic test can have four possible outcomes: true positive, true negative, false positive, and false negative.

1. Adaptability is not a measure of the accuracy or validity of a diagnostic or screening test.
2. Selectivity is not a measure of the accuracy or validity of a diagnostic or screening test.
3. **Sensitivity is a measure of the validity of a screening test, based on the probability that the screening test will be positive in someone with the disease or target condition (i.e., true positive).**
4. Specificity is a measure of the validity of a screening test, based on the probability that the screening test will be negative in someone who does not have the disease or target condition (i.e., true negative).

System Specific: Non-Systems
Content Outline: Safety & Professional Roles; Teaching/Learning; Research

Exam Two: Question 113

A physical therapist attempts to quantify a patient's endurance level by administering a maximal exercise test. What is the PRIMARY limitation of a maximal exercise test?

1. **Maximal exercise testing requires participants to exercise to the point of volitional fatigue.**
2. Maximal exercise testing does not typically allow a steady state heart rate at each work rate.
3. Maximal exercise testing is not useful in diagnosing coronary artery disease.
4. Maximal exercise testing requires progressive stages of increasing work intensities without rest intervals.

Correct Answer: 1 (American College of Sports Medicine p. 352)

The decision to use a maximal or submaximal exercise test depends largely on the reasons for the test and the availability of the appropriate equipment and personnel. Maximal exercise testing offers increased sensitivity for diagnosing coronary artery disease in asymptomatic individuals and provides a better estimate of maximum oxygen uptake than a submaximal test.

1. **The primary limitation of a maximal exercise test is that it requires the individual to exercise to the point of volitional fatigue. Some subjects terminate the exercise test due to fatigue or exercise intolerance before reaching their physiological maximum. This reduces the sensitivity of the estimate of maximum oxygen uptake.**
2. Most standardized exercise test protocols have the individual exercise at two or three minute intervals before increasing to a higher workload. This type of design allows the subject to come to a steady state heart rate for each workload before increasing the workload.
3. Maximal exercise testing is used to help diagnose coronary artery disease and offers better sensitivity than submaximal exercise testing.
4. Most standard exercise test protocols are continuous and do not allow formal rest intervals, however, this is not considered the primary limitation of the test.

System Specific: Cardiac, Vascular, & Pulmonary Systems
Content Outline: Examination

Exam Two: Question 114

A physical therapist prepares to complete a sensory examination on a patient rehabilitating from a lower extremity burn. Which of the following would serve as the BEST predictor of altered sensation?

1. presence of a skin graft
2. **depth of burn injury**
3. percentage of body surface affected
4. extent of hypertrophic scarring

Correct Answer: 2 (Rothstein p. 960)

Patients with burns often experience a number of sensory changes. These changes can include impaired sensation or increased sensitivity. Although many factors contribute to sensory alteration, the depth of the burn appears to be the best predictor.

1. Skin grafts are typically used with full-thickness burns and although there is a predictable pattern of sensory alteration with full-thickness burns, the absence of a skin graft would not be useful to predict sensory changes in less severe burns (i.e., superficial and partial-thickness).
2. **It is possible to predict the relative extent of sensory alteration based on the depth of the burn. For example, a superficial partial-thickness burn is characterized by extreme pain and significant sensitivity to temperature change, while a full-thickness burn is characterized by an absence of pain and inability to identify temperature change.**
3. The percentage of body surface affected provides information on the size or extent of the burn, but does not provide information on other important variables such as the depth or severity of the burn.
4. Hypertrophic scarring refers to an overgrowth of dermal constituents that remain within the boundaries of the wound. This occurs as a result of scar formation when the burn extends into the dermis. Hypertrophic scarring results in poor cosmesis and the development of contractures that may limit function. The presence of hypertrophic scarring provides only limited information regarding the extent of altered sensation.

System Specific: Integumentary System
Content Outline: Foundations for Evaluation, Differential Diagnosis, & Prognosis

Exam Two: Question 115

In a randomized control trial, the best way for a researcher to protect against the biases associated with the patient's and investigator's knowledge of the treatment the patient is receiving is to:

1. randomly assign patients to the intervention group
2. perform an intent-to-treat analysis of the data
3. **use a double-blind research design**
4. use a single-blind research design

Correct Answer: 3 (Portney p. 170)

Blinding is a form of experimental control implemented to protect against bias since both the patients' knowledge of their treatment and the investigator's expectations can influence performance or the recording and reporting of the outcomes under study.

1. Random assignment of patients to groups is recommended to ensure that each individual has an equal chance of being assigned to any group so that no systematic bias exists with respect to the attributes that might differentially affect the outcomes. Random assignment does not protect against the biases associated with the patient's and investigator's knowledge of the treatment the patient is receiving.

2. In an intent-to-treat analysis, the data is analyzed according to the original random assignments, according to the way subjects were intended to be treated, regardless of the treatment they actually received. An intent-to-treat analysis does not protect against the biases associated with the patient's and investigator's knowledge of the treatment the patient is receiving.

3. **Protection against bias associated with the patient's and investigator's knowledge of the treatment is best achieved by a double-blind research design. In a double-blind study, neither the subject nor the investigator is aware of the identity of the treatment group to which the subject was assigned until after the data is collected and the subject has completed the study.**

4. In a single-blind study, only the investigator is kept unaware of the identity of the treatment group to which the subject was assigned. The potential for bias from the patient remains uncontrolled.

System Specific: Non-Systems
Content Outline: Safety & Professional Roles; Teaching/Learning; Research

Exam Two: Question 116

A physician orders compression garments for an ambulatory patient who has significant difficulty with lower extremity edema. How much pressure would typically be necessary to control lower extremity edema?

1. 10 mm Hg
2. 18 mm Hg
3. 25 mm Hg
4. **35 mm Hg**

Correct Answer: 4 (Cameron p. 331)

Compression garments are available in different thicknesses and different levels of pretension. The garments offer varying levels of pressure ranging from 10 mm Hg to 50 mm Hg. The amount of pressure selected must be determined based on the intended goals of the therapeutic intervention.

1. A pressure of 10 mm Hg would not be adequate to control lower extremity edema in an ambulatory patient.

2. A pressure of 16-18 mm Hg is characteristic of off the shelf stockings used to prevent deep vein thrombosis in patients who are in bed.

3. A pressure of 20-30 mm Hg is used to control scar tissue formation.

4. **A pressure of 30-40 mm Hg is used to control edema in ambulatory patients.**

System Specific: Non-Systems
Content Outline: Equipment & Devices; Therapeutic Modalities

Exam Two: Question 117

A physical therapist monitors the vital signs of a 52-year-old male during a graded exercise test. The patient was prompted to seek medical assistance two weeks ago after becoming short of breath on two separate occasions. When interpreting the data collected during the exercise test, which finding would serve as the BEST indicator that the patient had exerted a maximal effort?

1. **failure of the heart rate to increase with further increases in intensity**
2. rise in systolic blood pressure of 50 mm Hg when compared to the resting value
3. rating of 12 on a perceived exertion scale
4. rating of 2/4 on the dyspnea scale

Correct Answer: 1 (American College of Sports Medicine p. 352)

Failure of the heart rate to increase with further increases in intensity occurs when the patient can no longer meet the demands imposed by the exercise, signifying the patient has produced a maximal effort.

1. **Failure of the heart rate to increase with further increases in exercise intensity is an objective indicator that the patient made a maximal effort during graded exercise testing.**
2. The normal response to exercise is a progressive increase in systolic blood pressure, typically 10 mm Hg per MET, with a possible plateau at peak exercise. A rise in systolic blood pressure of 50 mm Hg over the resting rate is common during graded exercise testing, however, is not necessarily an indication of a maximal effort.
3. A rating of 12 on the 6-20 perceived exertion scale corresponds only to a perception of "fairly light" to "somewhat hard." A rating of > 17 ("very hard") is an indicator of a maximal effort.
4. A rating of 2 out of 4 on the dyspnea scale corresponds to a perception of "moderate, bothersome" degree of breathlessness. This level does not indicate a maximal effort.

System Specific: Cardiac, Vascular, & Pulmonary Systems
Content Outline: Interventions

Exam Two: Question 118

A physical therapist performs an examination on a patient with hip-knee-ankle-foot orthoses. The patient can ambulate independently with the orthoses and Lofstrand crutches, however, due to the high energy expenditure often becomes fatigued very rapidly. Which disorder would be MOST consistent with this scenario?

1. amyotrophic lateral sclerosis
2. peripheral neuritis
3. neurogenic arthropathy
4. **spina bifida**

Correct Answer: 4 (Physical Therapist's Clinical Companion p. 314)

A hip-knee-ankle foot orthosis (HKAFO) consists of bilateral knee-ankle-foot orthoses with an extension to the hip joints with use of a pelvic band. The orthosis can control rotation at the hip and abduction/adduction. The orthosis is heavy and restricts patients to a swing-to or swing-through gait pattern. The HKAFO is indicated for patients with hip, foot, knee, and ankle weakness.

1. Amyotrophic lateral sclerosis is a chronic degenerative disease that produces both upper and lower motor neuron impairments. Motor weakness typically presents in a distal to proximal progression. The weakness combined with fatigue make it unlikely the patient would be able to ambulate with HKAFOs.
2. Peripheral neuritis refers to the inflammation of the nerves and is synonymous with the term peripheral neuropathy. Since every peripheral nerve has a highly specialized function, a wide array of symptoms can occur when nerves are damaged. Symptoms may include numbness, tingling, paresthesia, sensitivity to touch, and muscle weakness. As a result, it is difficult to determine the type of orthoses that would be appropriate based on the diagnosis alone.
3. Neurogenic arthropathy is a rapidly destructive arthropathy due to impaired pain perception and position sense, which can result from various underlying disorders, most commonly diabetes and stroke. Symptoms may include joint swelling, effusion, deformity, and instability. Treatment most often consists of joint immobilization which slows the disease progression.
4. **Spina bifida is a neural tube defect characterized by defective closure of the vertebral column. Although the exact clinical presentation of spina bifida can vary considerably, HKAFOs are often employed to assist pediatric patients with ambulation activities. The high energy cost of ambulating with the orthosis often makes community ambulation difficult.**

System Specific: Neuromuscular & Nervous Systems
Content Outline: Foundations for Evaluation, Differential Diagnosis, & Prognosis

Exam Two: Question 119

A physician orders electromyography for a patient with a brachial plexus injury to objectively determine the extent of pathology. Which of the following responses is MOST indicative of a normal muscle at rest?

1. **electrical silence**
2. spontaneous potentials
3. polyphasic potentials
4. occasional motor unit potentials

Correct Answer: 1 (Cameron p. 81)

Electromyography is a test that assesses the health of the muscles and the nerves controlling the muscles. A needle electrode is inserted through the skin into the muscle. The electrical activity detected by this electrode is displayed on an oscilloscope, and may be heard through a speaker. The presence, size, and shape of the wave form (i.e., the action potential) produced on the oscilloscope provides information about the ability of the muscle to respond when the nerves are stimulated.

1. **A normally innervated muscle is electrically silent at rest. Once the insertion activity (caused by the trauma of needle insertion) resolves, there should be no action potential on the oscilloscope.**
2. Spontaneous electrical potentials, like fibrillations and positive sharp waves, are seen in an acutely denervated muscle. Fibrillation and positive sharp waves are the result of spontaneous discharge of a single muscle fiber.
3. Polyphasic potentials are the electrical potentials from a denervated motor unit. A motor unit that exhibits five or more phases is referred to as polyphasic.
4. Occasional motor unit potentials occurring during minimal effort muscle contractions two to three weeks after injury suggest neurapraxia (a temporary failure of nerve conduction in the absence of structural nerve changes due to blunt injury, compression or ischemia).

System Specific: Other Systems
Content Outline: Foundations for Evaluation, Differential Diagnosis, & Prognosis

Exam Two: Question 120

A physical therapist completes a quantitative gait analysis on a patient rehabilitating from a lower extremity injury. As part of the examination the therapist measures the number of steps taken by the patient in a 30 second period. This measurement technique can be used to measure:

1. acceleration
2. **cadence**
3. velocity
4. speed

Correct Answer: 2 (Levangie p. 523)

Time and distance parameters are often used to provide a basic description of gait. Commonly used temporal variables include stance time, single limb and double support time, cadence, and speed. Commonly used distance variables include stride length, step length, width of base of support, and degrees of toe-out.

1. Acceleration is the rate of change of velocity with respect to time.
2. **Cadence is defined as the number of steps taken by a person per unit of time. Walking with increased cadence decreases the duration of double support time. A cadence of 110 steps per minute is typical in a male, while 116 steps per minute is typical in a female.**
3. Velocity is the rate of linear forward motion of the body which is measured most often in centimeters per second, meters per second or miles per hour. Walking velocity equals distance walked divided by time.
4. Speed is usually classified as slow, free or fast. Free speed of gait refers to a person's normal walking speed.

System Specific: Musculoskeletal System
Content Outline: Examination

Exam Two: Question 121

Members of a health promotion task force design a program that annually will screen individuals in selected retirement communities for osteoporosis. Which screening tool would be the MOST cost effective and reliable to incorporate as part of the program?

1. physical activity survey
2. dietary analysis
3. **measuring height**
4. urinalysis screening

Correct Answer: 3 (Goodman – Differential Diagnosis p. 502)

Osteoporosis is a metabolic bone disorder where the rate of bone resorption accelerates while the rate of bone formation slows down. This reduction of bone mass decreases the overall bone density and strength. The disease is more common in women and in particular postmenopausal women who are not taking hormone replacement therapy.

1. Physical activity is critical throughout the lifespan to maintain and possibly increase peak bone mass. The effect of exercise on slowing the decline of bone mineral density later in life has been found to be only modest. Regular activity has been found to decrease the incidence of hip fractures in individuals greater than 65 years of age.
2. A dietary analysis is an important component of a comprehensive plan of care for a patient with osteoporosis. This is important at all ages and in particular with postmenopausal women who require more than 1,500 mg of calcium daily. Adequate levels of Vitamin D are also necessary to assist in the absorption of dietary calcium. A dietary analysis would be expensive to implement and analyze and would be heavily influenced by a variety of other factors other than the presence or absence of osteoporosis.
3. **Measuring a person's height is an inexpensive and relatively reliable method to screen for osteoporosis. Patients with osteoporosis often lose height due to a reduction in bone mass, postural changes (e.g., kyphosis, Dowager's hump), and vertebral compression fractures.**
4. A urinalysis screening would be of minimal benefit since osteoporosis is a metabolic bone disorder and the primary affect of the condition is on the musculoskeletal system.

System Specific: Other Systems
Content Outline: Examination

Exam Two: Question 122

A physical therapist treats a patient diagnosed with lateral epicondylitis using iontophoresis. The therapist uses dexamethasone with a current intensity of 3 mA for 20 minutes. How often during the treatment session should the therapist check the skin?

1. every minute
2. **every three to five minutes**
3. every ten minutes
4. at the conclusion of the treatment session

Correct Answer: 2 (Prentice - Therapeutic Modalities p. 175)

Iontophoresis is the process by which medications are induced through the skin into the body by means of continuous direct current electrical stimulation. Sensitivity reactions most often occur due to the use of direct current, and in some cases, due to a particular therapeutic ion. A physical therapist should frequently check the patient's skin for a sensitivity reaction during iontophoresis treatment.

1. Checking the skin every minute would be both impractical and unnecessary since the time period is too short.
2. **An interval of three to five minutes provides the necessary frequency to detect an adverse reaction and take the necessary corrective action.**
3. An interval of ten minutes would be too long especially given the duration of the iontophoresis treatment (i.e., 20 minutes). Checking the skin at ten minute intervals would make it difficult for the physical therapist to detect a sensitivity reaction in a timely manner.
4. Checking the skin at the conclusion of treatment is common, however, additional skin checks need to occur at regular intervals throughout the duration of the 20 minute session.

System Specific: Non-Systems
Content Outline: Equipment & Devices; Therapeutic Modalities

Exam Two: Question 123

A physical therapist strongly suspects a patient is intoxicated after arriving for his treatment session. When asked if he has been drinking, the patient indicates he consumed six or seven alcoholic beverages before driving to therapy. The therapist's MOST appropriate action is to:

1. continue to treat the patient, assuming he can remain inoffensive to other patients
2. modify the patient's present treatment program to minimize the effects of alcohol
3. **contact a member of the patient's family to take the patient home**
4. instruct the patient to leave the clinic

> **Correct Answer: 3** (Guide for Professional Conduct)

A physical therapist should never treat a patient under the influence of alcohol. Therapists should be aware of signs and symptoms associated with intoxication and be willing to take necessary action to avoid harm to the patient and others when this situation is identified.

1. The amount of alcohol consumed would make it unsafe for the patient to participate in physical therapy. Effects of alcohol include impaired judgment, delayed reactions, impaired memory, and poor coordination.
2. Modifying the program to minimize the effects of alcohol condones the patient's behavior and makes it likely the same behavior would occur in the future.
3. **Contacting a member of the patient's family allows the physical therapist to discontinue the session and at the same time provides the patient with a safe method to return home.**
4. Instructing the patient to leave the clinic could create a safety issue for the patient and possibly others, particularly if the patient is driving a motor vehicle.

System Specific: Non-Systems
Content Outline: Safety & Professional Roles; Teaching/Learning; Research

Exam Two: Question 124

A physical therapist orders a wheelchair with a reclining back for a patient in a rehabilitation hospital. Which type of legrests would be the MOST appropriate for the wheelchair?

1. swing-away
2. detachable
3. **elevating**
4. fixed

> **Correct Answer: 3** (Pierson p. 146)

The specific features of a wheelchair depend on the patient's needs, abilities, and established goals. A wheelchair with a reclining back allows the back to be adjusted to various positions from vertical to fully horizontal. The wheelchair would require a removable headrest to support the head when the wheelchair is reclined and elevating legrests to promote patient comfort and maintain stability of the wheelchair.

1. Swing-away legrests allow the patient to position the wheelchair closer to objects and provide greater space at the front of the chair for the feet during transfers.
2. Detachable legrests provide similar benefits to those described for swing-away legrests.
3. **Elevating legrests promote patient comfort and stability when the wheelchair is in a reclined position. This feature may be necessary when a patient is unable to fully flex the knees or when knee flexion should be avoided. The legrests include a calf panel which provides necessary support for the lower leg.**
4. Fixed legrests are relatively common on wheelchairs used primarily for transport within a health care facility. The legrests have hinged footrests or footplates that allow for slightly more room when the patient rises or places the feet on the floor.

System Specific: Non-Systems
Content Outline: Equipment & Devices; Therapeutic Modalities

Exam Two: Question 125

A patient rehabilitating from cardiac surgery is monitored using an arterial line. The PRIMARY purpose of an arterial line is to:

1. measure right atrial pressure
2. measure heart rate and oxygen saturation
3. measure pulmonary artery pressure
4. **measure blood pressure**

Correct Answer: 4 (Pierson p. 286)

An arterial line is inserted directly into an artery and is used to continuously monitor blood pressure or to obtain blood samples.

1. Right atrial pressure, (i.e., blood pressure in the right atrium) is measured by a balloon tipped catheter which is advanced from the femoral, brachial or internal jugular vein into the pulmonary artery. A common version is the Swan-Ganz catheter.
2. In addition to the primary purpose of measuring blood pressure, an arterial line can be used as an access point for sampling arterial blood. Oxygen saturation can be determined by the analysis of blood gases, however, an arterial line does not monitor heart rate.
3. Like right atrial pressure, pulmonary artery pressure is measured by a Swan-Ganz catheter or another form of pulmonary artery catheter.
4. **An arterial line is a monitoring device consisting of a catheter that is inserted into an artery and attached to an electronic monitoring system. The device is considered to be more accurate than traditional measures of blood pressure and does not require repeated needle punctures.**

System Specific: Cardiac, Vascular, & Pulmonary Systems
Content Outline: Foundations for Evaluation, Differential Diagnosis, & Prognosis

Exam Two: Question 126

A physical therapist listens to the lung sounds of a 56-year-old male with chronic bronchitis. The patient was admitted to the hospital two days ago after complaining of shortness of breath and difficulty breathing. While performing auscultation the therapist identifies distinct lung sounds with a high constant pitch during exhalation. This type of sound is MOST consistent with:

1. crackles
2. rales
3. rhonchi
4. **wheezes**

Correct Answer: 4 (Frownfelter p. 219)

Wheezes are described as high-pitched, musical sounds made by air passing through narrowed tracheobronchial airways.

1. Crackles are discontinuous, adventitious breath sounds heard during auscultation of the lungs due to fluid accumulation in the distal airways or when collapsed alveoli reopen during inspiration.
2. Rales are synonymous with crackles.
3. Rhonchi are lower-pitched, continuous, adventitious breath sounds occurring during inspiration or expiration and are caused by the turbulence of air passing through secretions in large and mid-sized bronchi.
4. **Wheezes are continuous, high-pitched, adventitious breath sounds that are most frequently heard on exhalation and are associated with airway obstruction or bronchospasm. There can also be inspiratory wheezing caused by movement of air through secretions. Wheezes are commonly associated with asthma and bronchitis.**

System Specific: Cardiac, Vascular, & Pulmonary Systems
Content Outline: Examination

Exam Two: Question 127

A physical therapist administers iontophoresis to a patient with a lower extremity ulceration in an attempt to promote tissue healing. Which ion would BEST meet the stated objective?

1. acetate
2. magnesium
3. lidocaine
4. **zinc**

> **Correct Answer: 4** (Prentice - Therapeutic Modalities p. 172)

Iontophoresis refers to the transcutaneous delivery of ions into the body for therapeutic purposes using an electrical current. Physical therapists must possess an in-depth awareness of the most appropriate ions to treat specific conditions.

1. Acetate, from acetic acid, is a negatively charged ion used to treat calcific deposits.
2. Magnesium, from magnesium sulfate, is a positively charged ion used as a muscle relaxant and vasodilator.
3. Lidocaine, from xylocaine, is a positively charged ion used to treat pain and inflammation associated with acute inflammatory conditions.
4. **Zinc, from zinc oxide, is a positively charged ion used to promote healing, most often with open lesions and ulcerations.**

System Specific: Non-Systems
Content Outline: Equipment & Devices; Therapeutic Modalities

Exam Two: Question 128

A twelve-month-old child with cerebral palsy demonstrates an abnormal persistence of the positive support reflex. During therapy this would MOST likely interfere with:

1. sitting activities
2. **standing activities**
3. prone on elbows activities
4. supine activities

> **Correct Answer: 2** (Ratliffe p. 27)

The positive support reflex promotes extension of the lower extremities and trunk with weight bearing through the balls of the feet. If this reflex persists, it can interfere with standing, ambulation, balance reactions and weight shifting in standing, and can lead to plantar flexion contractures.

1. Sitting activities would not be influenced by the positive support reflex since there would not be stimulation to the ball of the foot. An infant is usually able to sit unsupported at six to seven months.
2. **The positive support reflex is elicited by contact of the ball of the foot with the floor surface when placed into a standing position. The reflex causes rigid extension of the lower extremities and trunk with weight bearing. This reflex is typically integrated at two to four months of age.**
3. Prone on elbows activities would not be influenced by the positive support reflex since there would not be stimulation to the ball of the foot. An infant is usually able to maintain the prone on elbows position at three to four months.
4. Supine activities would not be influenced by the positive support reflex since there would not be stimulation to the ball of the foot while in supine.

System Specific: Neuromuscular & Nervous Systems
Content Outline: Interventions

Exam Two: Question 129

A physical therapist treats a patient with limited shoulder range of motion. The therapist hypothesizes that the patient's range of motion limitation is due to pain and not a specific tissue restriction. Which graded oscillation techniques would be the MOST appropriate to treat this patient?

1. **grades I, II**
2. grades II, III
3. grades III, IV
4. grades IV, V

Correct Answer: 1 (Kisner p. 116)

Graded oscillation techniques include grade I, II, III, IV, and V. The type of grade selected is dependent on the intended treatment objective.

1. **Grade I refers to small amplitude oscillations at the beginning of the range. Grade II refers to large amplitude oscillations performed within the range, but not reaching the limit of range. Grade I and II are primarily used to treat pain by stimulating mechanoreceptors.**
2. Grade II was previously defined. Grade III refers to large amplitude oscillations performed to the limit of available range and stressed into tissue resistance.
3. Grade III was previously defined. Grade IV refers to small amplitude oscillations performed at the limit of available range and stressed into the tissue resistance. Grade III and IV are primarily used as stretching maneuvers.
4. Grade IV was previously defined. Grade V refers to small amplitude, high velocity thrust techniques used to break up adhesions.

System Specific: Musculoskeletal System
Content Outline: Interventions

Exam Two: Question 130

A patient diagnosed with lateral epicondylitis is referred to physical therapy. The therapist elects to use iontophoresis over the lateral epicondyle. Which type of current would the physical therapist use to administer the treatment?

1. **direct**
2. alternating
3. pulsatile
4. interferential

Correct Answer: 1 (Cameron p. 223)

Iontophoresis refers to the transcutaneous delivery of ions into the body for therapeutic purposes using an electrical current.

1. **Direct current is characterized by an uninterrupted flow of electrons toward the positive pole. This type of current is necessary to move the charged ions across the dermal barrier. Polarity remains constant and is determined by the physical therapist based on treatment goals and the polarity of the chosen ion.**
2. Alternating current is characterized by the bidirectional (constantly changing) continuous flow of electrons. Electrons flowing in an alternating current move from the negative to positive pole, reversing direction when the polarity is reversed.
3. Pulsatile current is characterized by three or more pulses grouped together and may be unidirectional or bidirectional. A series of unidirectional pulses is known as monophasic pulsed current and a series of bidirectional pulses is known as biphasic pulsed current.
4. Interferential current combines two high frequency alternating waveforms that are biphasic. The two waveforms are delivered through two sets of electrodes through separate channels in the same simulator.

System Specific: Non-Systems
Content Outline: Equipment & Devices; Therapeutic Modalities

Exam Two: Question 131

A physical therapist sets up a patient for mechanical traction to the lumbar spine. The therapist's objective is to provide soft tissue stretch to surrounding muscles. Assuming the therapist uses a force equivalent to 25% of the patient's body weight and the patient has tolerated treatment without difficulty on several other occasions, the MOST appropriate duration of treatment is:

1. 5 minutes
2. 10 minutes
3. **25 minutes**
4. 40 minutes

Correct Answer: 3 (Cameron p. 299)

Physical therapists must carefully select the parameters associated with mechanical traction (i.e., force, hold/relax times, duration) based on the desired outcomes.

1. A duration of five minutes would be appropriate for a brief trial of traction. This may be warranted if the patient's initial symptoms are severe. Shorter treatment times are generally recommended for the initial session or in the acute phase of rehabilitation.

2. A duration of 10 minutes would be appropriate for an initial session if the patient's symptoms are mild or moderate.

3. **A duration of 25 minutes would be appropriate when attempting to stretch soft tissue in a patient who has previously tolerated traction without difficulty. A duration of 20-30 minutes is most often recommended for stretching soft tissue or reducing muscle spasm. This amount of time allows for a prolonged stretch without compromising the integrity of other structures.**

4. A duration of 40 minutes or more using spinal traction is not necessary since the literature has shown that treatment of this duration generally provides no additional benefit.

System Specific: Non-Systems
Content Outline: Equipment & Devices; Therapeutic Modalities

Exam Two: Question 132

A physical therapist designs an exercise program for a patient rehabilitating from cardiac surgery. During the treatment session the therapist monitors the patient's oxygen saturation rate. Which of the following would be MOST representative of a normal oxygen saturation rate?

1. 82%
2. 87%
3. 92%
4. **97%**

Correct Answer: 4 (Brannon p. 296)

Oxygen saturation (SaO_2) measures the percentage of hemoglobin saturated with oxygen. The normal range for oxygen saturation is between 95-98% in healthy individuals.

1. A value of 82% SaO_2 demonstrates significant hypoxemia resulting in the patient requiring continuous use of supplemental oxygen. Exercise would be contraindicated at this level.

2. A value of 87% SaO_2 is below the range for acceptable oxygen saturation. The patient would likely use supplemental oxygen at rest and with exercise. The patient should maintain 90% SaO_2 or better with supplemental oxygen use.

3. A value of 92% SaO_2 is not within normal limits for oxygen saturation. In most cases, the patient would be monitored to ensure that SaO_2 does not fall below 90% during exertion or exercise.

4. **A value of 97% SaO_2 is within the specified range of 95-98% for normal arterial oxygen saturation.**

System Specific: Cardiac, Vascular, & Pulmonary Systems
Content Outline: Examination

Exam Two: Question 133

A physical therapist attempts to assess the integrity of the L4 spinal level. Which deep tendon reflex would provide the therapist with the MOST useful information?

1. lateral hamstrings
2. medial hamstrings
3. **patellar reflex**
4. Achilles reflex

Correct Answer: 3 (Magee p. 805)

Deep tendon reflexes are assessed to examine the integrity of the afferent and efferent peripheral nervous systems and the ability of the central nervous system to inhibit the reflex. The physical therapist should attempt to assess the reflex by striking the tendon with the reflex hammer after placing the tendon on slight stretch.

1. The lateral hamstrings reflex is innervated at the S1-S2 spinal level.
2. The medial hamstrings reflex is innervated at the L5-S1 spinal level.
3. **The patellar reflex is innervated at the L3-L4 spinal level.**
4. The Achilles reflex is innervated at the S1-S2 spinal level.

System Specific: Neuromuscular & Nervous Systems
Content Outline: Clinical Application of Foundational Sciences

Exam Two: Question 134

A physical therapist examines a patient diagnosed with rotator cuff tendonitis in physical therapy. The physician referral indicates the patient should be seen three times a week, however, after examining the patient the therapist feels once a week is adequate. The MOST appropriate therapist action is to:

1. **schedule the patient once a week and notify the referring physician of your rationale**
2. schedule the patient as indicated on the physician referral
3. ask the patient how often they would like to be seen in physical therapy
4. attempt to determine if the patient's insurance will cover physical therapy visits three times a week

Correct Answer: 1 (Guide for Professional Conduct)

The *Guide for Professional Conduct* published by the American Physical Therapy states that a physical therapist shall avoid overutilization of physical therapy services.

1. **The physical therapist should determine the frequency of physical therapy sessions based solely on the needs of the patient. The therapist should communicate the rationale for the change in the frequency of the physical therapy sessions to the physician.**
2. Scheduling the patient three times a week when it is not necessary would result in overutilization of physical therapy services. The *Code of Ethics* published by the American Physical Therapy Association states that a physical therapist shall seek only such remuneration as is deserved and reasonable for physical therapy services.
3. The patient's wishes should always be considered, however, only the physical therapist can determine the actual frequency of physical therapy visits necessary.
4. If the additional visits are not necessary it does not matter if the services will be reimbursed by the patient's insurance.

System Specific: Non-Systems
Content Outline: Safety & Professional Roles; Teaching/Learning; Research

Exam Two: Question 135

A patient receiving physical therapy services in an outpatient clinic explains that he has felt nauseous since having his methotrexate medication level altered. The MOST appropriate physical therapist action is to:

1. explain to the patient that nausea is very common when altering medication levels
2. ask the patient to stop taking the prescribed medication
3. request that the patient make an appointment with the physician
4. **request that the patient contact the physician's office**

> **Correct Answer: 4** (Ciccone p. 226)

Methotrexate is used as a disease-modifying agent in the treatment of rheumatoid arthritis. Adverse effects include nausea, gastrointestinal distress, hemorrhage, cough, shortness of breath, and lower extremity edema. Nausea refers to the sensation of unease and discomfort in the stomach with an urge to vomit. Although nausea is not a medical emergency, it is appropriate for the patient to inform the physician of any persistent side effects as soon as possible.

1. A physical therapist may inform a patient about common side effects of medications, however, the patient's acknowledgement of feeling nauseous after having their medication level altered would still require contact with the physician.
2. A physical therapist is not able to ask a patient to discontinue the use of a prescribed medication. This action is the sole responsibility of the physician.
3. A recommendation to make an appointment with the physician is appropriate, however, would not typically be as timely as contacting the physician's office. Given the patient's present status (i.e., feeling nauseous), it is necessary to advocate for an immediate resolution to the problem.
4. **A patient should contact the physician's office whenever they experience side effects that may be associated with prescribed medication. Direct contact with the physician is an immediate response which makes the physician aware of the patient's present status and allows them to potentially modify or discontinue medication.**

System Specific: Other Systems
Content Outline: Clinical Application of Foundational Sciences

Exam Two: Question 136

A physical therapist completes a fitness screening on a 34-year-old male prior to prescribing an aerobic exercise program. Which value is MOST representative of the patient's age-predicted maximal heart rate?

1. 168
2. 174
3. **186**
4. 196

> **Correct Answer: 3** (Minor p. 83)

Age-predicted maximal heart rate can be determined as follows: 220-age.

1. Based on the formula of 220 - age, the rate of 168 is too low for this patient's age-predicted maximal heart rate.
2. Based on the formula of 220 - age, the rate of 174 is too low for this patient's age-predicted maximal heart rate.
3. **Based on the formula of 220 - age, the rate of 186 is equal to this patient's age-predicted maximal heart rate.**
4. Based on the formula of 220 - age, the rate of 196 is too high for this patient's age-predicted maximal heart rate. This would be an unsafe rate for exercise.

System Specific: Cardiac, Vascular, & Pulmonary Systems
Content Outline: Examination

Exam Two: Question 137

A physical therapist observes a patient ambulating in the clinic. The therapist notes that the patient's pelvis drops on the left during left swing phase. This deviation is usually caused by weakness of the:

1. left gluteus medius
2. **right gluteus medius**
3. left gluteus minimus
4. right gluteus minimus

> **Correct Answer: 2** (Magee p. 966)

A Trendelenburg gait pattern is characterized by excessive lateral trunk flexion and weight shifting over the stance leg. The gait pattern is often seen with lesions of the superior gluteal nerve, L5 radiculopathy, and poliomyelitis.

1. The gluteus medius acts to abduct the hip joint. The anterior fibers medially rotate and may assist in flexion of the hip joint. The posterior fibers laterally rotate and may assist in extension. Weakness of the left gluteus medius would be characterized by the pelvis dropping on the right during right swing phase.
2. **Weakness of the right gluteus medius would be characterized by the pelvis dropping on the left during left swing phase.**
3. The gluteus minimus acts to abduct and medially rotate the hip and may assist in hip flexion. Weakness of the left gluteus minimus would be identified by diminished strength in medial rotation and abduction of the left hip.
4. Weakness of the right gluteus minimus would be identified by diminished strength in medial rotation and abduction of the right hip.

System Specific: Musculoskeletal System
Content Outline: Foundations for Evaluation, Differential Diagnosis, & Prognosis

Exam Two: Question 138

A physical therapist examines a patient diagnosed with cerebellar degeneration. Which of the following clinical findings is NOT typically associated with this condition?

1. **athetosis**
2. dysmetria
3. nystagmus
4. dysdiadochokinesia

> **Correct Answer: 1** (O'Sullivan p. 201)

Athetosis is a term used to describe slow, writhing, and involuntary movements that may occur with damage to the basal ganglia.

1. **Athetosis is characterized by extraneous and involuntary movements, slowness of movement, and alterations in muscle tone. Athetoid movements may look "wormlike" with a rotatory component evident.**
2. Dysmetria occurs with cerebellar lesions and is defined as the inability to appropriately reach a target. The cerebellum is normally responsible for the timing, force, extent, and direction of the limb movement in order to correctly reach the target.
3. Nystagmus can occur with cerebellar lesions and is usually classified as gaze-evoked nystagmus. The patient will attempt to look toward an object in the periphery, but the eyes will drift involuntarily back to neutral. This may occur unilaterally or bilaterally depending on the cause of cerebellar dysfunction.
4. Dysdiadochokinesia occurs with cerebellar lesions and is defined as the inability to perform rapid alternating movements.

System Specific: Neuromuscular & Nervous Systems
Content Outline: Foundations for Evaluation, Differential Diagnosis, & Prognosis

Exam Two: Question 139

A physical therapist examines a 36-year-old female referred to physical therapy after experiencing back pain two weeks ago. The patient identifies the majority of pain in the buttock and lateral thigh and denies any referred pain down the posterior leg. Presently she rates the pain as a "3" on a 0-10 scale, however, indicates that the pain is a "6" or a "7" during activity or at night. This description MOST closely resembles:

1. sacroilitis
2. iliolumbar syndrome
3. piriformis syndrome
4. **trochanteric bursitis**

> **Correct Answer: 4** (Goodman – Differential Diagnosis p. 751)

There are a multitude of medical diagnoses that are associated with low back pain. Physical therapists should be familiar with the typical clinical presentation of these diagnoses and be able to identify a given diagnosis after completing a thorough examination.

1. Sacroilitis refers to inflammation of one or both of the sacroiliac joints. The patient is typically tender to palpation directly over the sacroiliac joint.

2. Iliolumbar syndrome, also known as iliac crest pain syndrome, is caused by inflammation or a tear of the iliolumbar ligament. The condition often leads to referred pain in the pelvis or groin. The patient is often tender to palpation over the iliac crest and pain tends to be exacerbated with sidebending.

3. Piriformis syndrome refers to a condition in which the piriformis muscle irritates the sciatic nerve causing pain in the buttocks and referred pain along the course of the sciatic nerve. The primary patient complaint is buttock pain that is made worse by sitting, stair climbing or squatting.

4. **Trochanteric bursitis refers to inflammation of the trochanteric bursa, which is a pad-like sac that protects the soft tissue structures that cross the posterior portion of the greater trochanter. The patient is often extremely sensitive to palpation over the bursa and may experience lateral thigh pain that is exacerbated by activity or periods of prolonged rest.**

System Specific: Musculoskeletal System
Content Outline: Foundations for Evaluation, Differential Diagnosis, & Prognosis

Exam Two: Question 140

A physical therapist completes a sensory assessment on a 61-year-old female diagnosed with multiple sclerosis. As part of the assessment the therapist examines stereognosis, vibration, and two-point discrimination. What type of receptor is primarily responsible for generating the necessary information?

1. deep sensory receptors
2. **mechanoreceptors**
3. nociceptors
4. thermoreceptors

> **Correct Answer: 2** (O'Sullivan p. 134)

Mechanoreceptors generate information related to discriminative sensations. The information is then mediated through the dorsal column-medial lemniscal system. Examples of mechanoreceptors include free nerve endings, Merkel's disks, Ruffini endings, hair follicle endings, Meissner's corpuscles, and Pacinian corpuscles.

1. Deep sensory receptors are sensory receptors that are located in the muscles, tendons, and joints. Muscle and joint receptors are both classified as deep sensory receptors and include Golgi tendon organs, Pacinian corpuscles, muscle spindle, Ruffini endings, free nerve endings, and joint receptors. They evaluate position sense, proprioception, muscle tone, and movement.

2. **Mechanoreceptors are sensory receptors that respond to mechanical deformation of the area surrounding a receptor. They are responsible for sensations of touch, pressure, itch, tickle, vibration, and discriminative touch.**

3. Nociceptors are specialized peripheral free nerve endings that are found throughout different tissues within the body that respond to noxious stimuli and result in the perception of pain. A painful stimulus will ascend through the spinal cord via the lateral spinothalamic tract. Several areas of the brain provide specific responses to the painful stimulus.

4. Thermoreceptors are sensory receptors that respond to changes in temperature. Stimulation of the cold or warm receptors will ascend through the spinal cord via the lateral spinothalamic tract.

System Specific: Neuromuscular & Nervous Systems
Content Outline: Clinical Application of Foundational Sciences

Exam Two: Question 141

A physical therapist is employed at a physician owned physical therapy clinic that charges by the modality. One of the physicians, who is an owner of the practice, requests that all of his patients receive a minimum of heat, ultrasound, and electrical stimulation during each session. The therapist feels that the majority of patients receive little benefit from the treatment regimen. The MOST appropriate IMMEDIATE action is:

1. ignore the physician's request and treat each patient as you feel is indicated
2. **discuss with the physician the rationale for requesting modalities on each patient**
3. report the physician's conduct to the American Medical Association
4. inform the physician that he is abusing the health care system

> **Correct Answer: 2** (Guide for Professional Conduct)

The *Guide for Professional Conduct* states that physical therapists seek remuneration for their services that is deserved and reasonable.

1. The physical therapist must treat each patient as they feel is indicated, however, it would be inappropriate to ignore the physician's request without addressing the issue directly.
2. **The physical therapist should have a candid conversation with the physician and attempt to understand the rationale for the physician's current approach. The physical therapist can use the opportunity to educate the physician on appropriate utilization of physical therapy services.**
3. The physical therapist should address the issue directly with the physician prior to considering a formal complaint with an external licensing agency.
4. Informing a physician that he is abusing the health care system would likely place the physician in a defensive posture and negate any opportunity to have a meaningful conversation. In addition, the action could be considered slanderous.

System Specific: Non-Systems
Content Outline: Safety & Professional Roles; Teaching/Learning; Research

Exam Two: Question 142

A physical therapist completes a developmental assessment on an infant. At what age should an infant begin to sit with hand support for an extended period of time?

1. **6-7 months**
2. 8-9 months
3. 10-11 months
4. 12-15 months

> **Correct Answer: 1** (Ratliffe p. 46)

Infants typically develop the stability to sit with hand support in the sixth to seventh month.

1. **Sitting for a prolonged period of time with upper extremity support usually occurs at 6-7 months of age. The infant will also bring objects to midline, hold a bottle with two hands, and roll to prone.**
2. When an infant is 8-9 months of age, they will typically manipulate toys in sitting, raise themselves from supine to sit, pull to stand with support, and transfer objects with a controlled release.
3. When an infant is 10-11 months of age, they will typically stand briefly without support, transition from supine to sitting or quadruped, pull to stand through half kneel, and use a pincer grasp.
4. When an infant is 12 months of age, they will typically stand up through quadruped, use a wide array of sitting positions, walk without support, creep up stairs, throw a ball in sitting, and mark paper with crayons.

System Specific: Other Systems
Content Outline: Clinical Application of Foundational Sciences

Exam Two: Question 143

A physical therapist collects data as part of a preseason athletic screening program designed to identify individuals susceptible to heat illness. Which of the following measures would be the MOST valuable to collect?

1. height
2. weight
3. **percent body fat**
4. vital capacity

> **Correct Answer: 3** (American College of Sports Medicine p. 551)

A variety of factors can increase a patient's susceptibility to heat illness. Some of the more common risk factors include age extremes (i.e., children, elderly), excessive muscle mass or obese individuals, previous history of heat illness, salt or water depletion, and acute or chronic illness.

1. Height without additional information such as weight would provide little benefit to identify individuals susceptible to heat illness.
2. Weight without additional information such as height would provide little benefit to identify individuals susceptible to heat illness.
3. **Patients with a higher percent body fat are more susceptible to heat illness since the larger the person is, the more difficult it will be to dissipate excess heat since the body's cooling system cannot work quickly enough. In addition, research has revealed that overweight individuals may generate up to 18% greater heat production than underweight individuals.**
4. Vital capacity is defined as the maximal volume forcefully expired after a maximal inspiration. The pulmonary function test measure would not be useful in isolation to identify individuals susceptible to heat illness.

System Specific: Other Systems
Content Outline: Foundations for Evaluation, Differential Diagnosis, & Prognosis

Exam Two: Question 144

A physical therapist employed in an acute care hospital works with a patient on bed mobility activities. The therapist would like to incorporate a strengthening activity for the hip extensors that will improve the patient's ability to independently reposition in bed, however, the patient does not have adequate strength to perform bridging. The MOST appropriate exercise activity is:

1. anterior pelvic tilts
2. heel slides
3. straight leg raises
4. **isometric gluteal sets**

> **Correct Answer: 4** (O'Sullivan p. 525)

Bridging occurs when a patient positioned in hooklying lifts their buttocks and low back from a fixed surface. The activity can be used to facilitate pelvic motion and for strengthening the hip extensors.

1. An anterior pelvic tilt requires the anterior superior iliac spines of the pelvis to move anteriorly and inferiorly. Anterior pelvic tilts result in hip flexion and increased lumbar spine extension. The hip flexors and back extensors are the primary muscles active during the exercise.
2. Heel slides require the patient to lie on their back with the hips and knees flexed and the feet flat on the floor. The patient attempts to straighten the leg by sliding the heel on the floor while maintaining the low back in a flattened position. The patient then returns the leg to the upright starting position. The exercise is most often used as an active stretching technique to promote knee flexion.
3. Straight leg raises combine dynamic hip flexion with an isometric contraction of the quadriceps. The rectus femoris is the primary muscle active during the exercise.
4. **Isometric gluteal sets are an appropriate precursor to bridging since the activity incorporates the hip extensors.**

System Specific: Musculoskeletal System
Content Outline: Interventions

Exam Two: Question 145

A patient on supplemental oxygen participates in a series of active exercises. During the exercise session the patient's oxygen saturation falls to the lower limit of her established acceptable range of 92-95%. When asked by the physical therapist how she is feeling the patient reports that she feels fine. The MOST appropriate therapist action is:

1. **continue the exercise session**
2. increase the amount of oxygen
3. discontinue the exercise session
4. contact the patient's physician

> **Correct Answer: 1** (Paz p. 441)

Supplemental oxygen is most commonly administered by a nasal cannula at flow rates between one and six liters per minute.

1. **Since the oxygen saturation rate has not fallen below the patient's established acceptable range and the patient reports feeling fine it is reasonable to continue with the exercise session.**
2. Physical therapists should not routinely increase the amount of oxygen even if the patient's oxygen saturation level falls below their acceptable range as the increased levels of oxygen may depress the hypoxic drive in patients with chronically high $PaCO_2$ (partial pressure of carbon dioxide).
3. Since the oxygen saturation level did not fall below the acceptable range, it is not necessary to discontinue the exercise session.
4. The acceptable oxygen saturation level for exercise should be established by the patient's physician. Since the oxygen saturation level did not fall below the acceptable range, contacting the physician is not necessary.

System Specific: Cardiac, Vascular, & Pulmonary Systems
Content Outline: Interventions

Exam Two: Question 146

A physical therapist performs segmental breathing exercises with a patient following atelectasis. Which manual contact would be the MOST appropriate to emphasize lingula expansion?

1. **place the hands on the left side of the chest below the axilla**
2. place the hands below the clavicle on the anterior chest wall
3. place the hands over the posterior aspect of the lower ribs
4. place the hands on the right side of the chest below the axilla

> **Correct Answer: 1** (Tan p. 735)

Segmental breathing, also known as localized breathing or thoracic expansion exercise, is intended to improve regional ventilation in patients with pulmonary disease and to prevent and treat pulmonary complications after surgery. The technique combines positioning with tactile and verbal cueing and resistance to enhance expansion of a specific lung segment to facilitate chest wall motion and increase ventilation.

1. **The lingula is a segment of the left upper lobe. Placing the hands on the left side of the chest below the axilla would provide tactile stimulation to facilitate expansion of the chest wall to improve ventilation of the left upper lobe.**
2. Placing the hands below the clavicle on the anterior chest wall would provide tactile stimulation to the anterior segments of the upper lobes, but not the lingula.
3. Placing the hands over the posterior aspect of the lower ribs would provide tactile stimulus over the lateral basal segments of the right and left lower lobes, not the lingula.
4. Placing the hands on the right side of the chest below the axilla would be overlying the right middle lobe, not the lingula.

System Specific: Cardiac, Vascular, & Pulmonary Systems
Content Outline: Interventions

Exam Two: Question 147

A patient with C5 tetraplegia exercises on a mat table. Suddenly, the patient begins to demonstrate signs and symptoms of autonomic dysreflexia including headache and sweating above the level of the lesion. The MOST appropriate assessment to validate the presence of autonomic dysreflexia is:

1. pulse rate
2. **blood pressure**
3. respiratory rate
4. oxygen saturation

> **Correct Answer: 2** (Umphred p. 622)

Autonomic dysreflexia occurs when a noxious stimulus below the level of the lesion triggers the autonomic nervous system causing a sudden elevation in blood pressure. The condition is common in patients with spinal cord lesions above the T6 level. Symptoms include profuse sweating, goose bumps below the level of the lesion, and vasodilation (flushing) above the level of injury. This condition should be treated as a medical emergency.

1. Pulse rate can be somewhat variable with autonomic dysreflexia and therefore it is not particularly useful when attempting to validate the presence of the condition.
2. **A significant increase in the patient's blood pressure is associated with autonomic dysreflexia. As a result, the measure should be assessed when attempting to confirm the presence of the condition. Management of autonomic dysreflexia includes placing the patient in an upright position in an attempt to control the rising blood pressure.**
3. Respiration rate may increase slightly with autonomic dysreflexia, but the measurement would not be useful to validate the presence of the condition.
4. Oxygen saturation rate measures the oxygen saturation of blood. This measure would not be immediately impacted by the presence of autonomic dysreflexia.

System Specific: Neuromuscular & Nervous Systems
Content Outline: Foundations for Evaluation, Differential Diagnosis, & Prognosis

Exam Two: Question 148

A patient rehabilitating from a spinal cord injury informs a therapist that he will walk again. Which type of injury would make functional ambulation the MOST unrealistic?

1. **complete T9 paraplegia**
2. posterior cord syndrome
3. Brown-Sequard's syndrome
4. cauda equina injury

> **Correct Answer: 1** (Umphred p. 647)

The ability to functionally ambulate following a spinal cord injury is primarily dependent on the patient's available motor and sensory innervation and the associated energy requirements.

1. **A patient with complete T9 paraplegia would possess full upper extremity innervation and would be able to utilize the lower abdominals and intercostals. The patient would not possess any lower extremity innervation and therefore, functional ambulation would be unrealistic.**
2. Posterior cord syndrome refers to a relatively rare incomplete lesion caused by compression of the posterior spinal artery. The condition is characterized by loss of pain perception, proprioception, two-point discrimination, and stereognosis. Motor function is preserved.
3. Brown-Sequard's syndrome refers to an incomplete lesion usually caused by a stab wound, which produces hemisection of the spinal cord. The condition is characterized by paralysis and loss of vibratory and position sense on the same side as the lesion and loss of pain and temperature sense on the opposite side of the lesion.
4. Cauda equina injury occurs below the L1 spinal level where the long nerve roots transcend. Cauda equina injuries can be complete, however, are frequently incomplete due to the large number of nerve roots in the area. The condition is characterized by flaccidity, areflexia, and impairment of bowel and bladder function. Full recovery is not typical due to the distance needed for axonal regeneration.

System Specific: Neuromuscular & Nervous Systems
Content Outline: Foundations for Evaluation, Differential Diagnosis, & Prognosis

Exam Two: Question 149

A physical therapist monitors a 29-year-old male with a C6 spinal cord injury positioned on a tilt table. After elevating the tilt table to 30 degrees, the patient begins to complain of nausea and dizziness. The patient's blood pressure is measured as 70/35 mm Hg. The patient's signs and symptoms are MOST indicative of:

1. spinal shock
2. postural hypertension
3. autonomic dysreflexia
4. **orthostatic hypotension**

> **Correct Answer: 4** (Umphred p. 621)

Patients status post spinal cord injury are particularly susceptible to several potentially emergent conditions. Physical therapists must closely monitor patients for signs and symptoms associated with these conditions and, if necessary, provide appropriate and immediate medical management.

1. Spinal shock refers to a physiologic response that occurs between 30 and 60 minutes after trauma to the spinal cord and can last up to several weeks. The patient presents with total flaccid paralysis and loss of all reflexes below the level of injury.

2. Postural hypertension is a term used to describe dizziness caused by a change in position in the presence of high blood pressure (systolic blood pressure greater than 140 mm Hg and diastolic greater than 90 mm Hg). A far more common term is postural hypotension which is synonymous with orthostatic hypotension.

3. Autonomic dysreflexia occurs when a noxious stimulus below the level of the lesion triggers the autonomic nervous system causing a sudden elevation in blood pressure. If not treated, this condition can lead to convulsions, hemorrhage, and death. The condition frequently occurs in patients with lesions above T6.

4. **Orthostatic hypotension or postural hypotension occurs due to a loss of sympathetic control of vasoconstriction in combination with absent or severely reduced muscle tone. A decrease in systolic blood pressure greater than 20 mm Hg after moving from supine to sitting is typically indicative of orthostatic hypotension.**

System Specific: Other Systems
Content Outline: Foundations for Evaluation, Differential Diagnosis, & Prognosis

Exam Two: Question 150

A physical therapist attempts to examine the relationship between scores on a functional balance measure and another measurement whose validity is known. This type of example BEST describes:

1. face validity
2. predictive validity
3. **concurrent validity**
4. content validity

> **Correct Answer: 3** (Portney p. 103)

Concurrent validity refers to the relationship between test scores and either criterion states or measurements whose validity is known.

1. Face validity refers to whether the test "looks valid" to those who take and administer it. It refers, not to what the test actually measures, but to what it appears superficially to measure.

2. Predictive validity is a form of validity that is demonstrated when a score is helpful in predicting a specific future outcome. Examples of tests with predictive validity are career or aptitude tests, which are helpful in determining who is likely to succeed or fail in certain subjects or occupations.

3. **Concurrent validity is demonstrated when a test score correlates well with a measure that has previously been validated. This is the circumstance in the example, where the functional balance measure would have concurrent validity if a strong relationship can be shown between its scores and scores on a previously validated measurement.**

4. Content validity refers to the extent to which a measure represents all facets of a given concept or construct.

System Specific: Non-Systems
Content Outline: Safety & Professional Roles; Teaching/Learning; Research

Exam Two: Question 151

A physical therapist prepares to treat a patient with continuous ultrasound. Which general rule BEST determines the length of treatment when using ultrasound?

1. two minutes for an area that is two times the size of the transducer face
2. **five minutes for an area that is two times the size of the transducer face**
3. five minutes is the maximum treatment time regardless of the treatment area
4. ten minutes is the maximum treatment time regardless of the treatment area

> **Correct Answer: 2** (Prentice - Therapeutic Modalities p. 377)

The duration of ultrasound treatment is based on a number of variables including the treatment goal, the size of the area to be treated, and the effective radiating area of the transducer face.

1. Two minutes would not be enough time to use ultrasound in an area that was two times the size of the transducer face.
2. **An accepted recommendation is that ultrasound can be administered to an area two to three times the size of the effective radiating area of the transducer face in a five minute period. This recommendation equates to roughly twice the size of the transducer face.**
3. There is not a specified maximum amount of time when using ultrasound. Most often ultrasound is used for periods ranging from five to eight minutes in duration.
4. Ten minutes is a relatively long duration for treatment with ultrasound, however, this could be plausible in situations where the size of the area to be treated is large.

System Specific: Non-Systems
Content Outline: Equipment & Devices; Therapeutic Modalities

Exam Two: Question 152

A physical therapist attempts to prevent alveolar collapse in a patient following thoracic surgery. Which breathing technique would be the MOST beneficial to achieve the established goal?

1. inspiratory muscle trainer
2. mechanical percussors
3. **incentive spirometer**
4. flutter valve

> **Correct Answer: 3** (Hillegass p. 529)

An incentive spirometer provides visual or in some cases auditory feedback as the patient takes a maximum inspiration. Incentive spirometry increases the amount of air that is inspired and as a result, can be used as a treatment to prevent alveolar collapse after thoracic surgery.

1. Inspiratory muscle trainers are handheld breathing training devices used primarily to increase the strength and endurance of the muscles of inspiration. They are not used to prevent alveolar collapse after thoracic surgery.
2. Mechanical percussors are electronically or pneumatically powered devices employed as a substitute for manual percussion with the hands. They can be used to help mobilize bronchial secretions after thoracic surgery, but only if the patient was retaining secretions.
3. **Incentive spirometers are devices that provide visual or other feedback while the patient performs sustained maximal inspirations. The device is most often used following upper abdominal or thoracic surgery. Indications may include chest wall pain, loss of mobility, weakness of the muscles of inspiration, and to prevent or treat atelectasis.**
4. Flutter valves are mucus clearance devices that combine positive expiratory pressure with high frequency oscillations at the airway opening during exhalation.

System Specific: Cardiac, Vascular, & Pulmonary Systems
Content Outline: Interventions

Exam Two: Question 153

A physical therapist reviews the surface anatomy of the hand in preparation for a patient status post wrist arthrodesis. Which bony structure does NOT articulate with the lunate?

1. **trapezium**
2. radius
3. capitate
4. scaphoid

> **Correct Answer: 1** (Hoppenfeld p. 66)

The lunate is located in the center of the proximal row between the scaphoid and the triquetrum. The lunate is distinguished by its crescent-like outline. The proximal row of carpal bones from lateral to medial consists of the scaphoid, lunate, triquetrum, and pisiform. The distal row of carpal bones from lateral to medial consists of the trapezium, trapezoid, capitate, and hamate.

1. **The trapezium is located on the lateral side of the carpus between the scaphoid and the first metacarpal. It is distinguished by a deep groove on its palmar surface. The proximal portion of the trapezium articulates with the scaphoid. The distal portion articulates with the base of the second metacarpal.**

2. The radius articulates with the wrist at the radiocarpal joint. The concave surface of the distal end of the radius articulates with the scaphoid and lunate of the proximal row of carpals.

3. The capitate is the most central and largest of the carpal bones. The proximal portion of the capitate articulates with the lunate and scaphoid. The distal portion articulates with the base of the third metacarpal.

4. The scaphoid links the proximal and distal carpal rows and helps provide stability to the wrist. Patients who fracture the proximal aspect of the scaphoid are susceptible to avascular necrosis due to disrupted blood supply. The proximal portion of the scaphoid articulates with the radius. The distal portion articulates with the trapezium and trapezoid. The medial surface articulates with the lunate and capitate.

System Specific: Musculoskeletal System
Content Outline: Clinical Application of Foundational Sciences

Exam Two: Question 154

A physical therapist conducts a sensory assessment on numerous areas of a patient's face. The cranial nerve MOST likely assessed using this type of testing procedure is:

1. facial nerve
2. oculomotor nerve
3. **trigeminal nerve**
4. trochlear nerve

> **Correct Answer: 3** (Magee p. 74)

The cranial nerves refer to twelve pairs of nerves that have their origin in the brain. The majority of cranial nerves contain both sensory and motor fibers, however, there are several exceptions including the oculomotor and trochlear nerves.

1. The afferent component of the facial nerve (cranial nerve VII) can be assessed by examining a patient's ability to accurately identify sweet and salty substances. The efferent component is tested by performing a manual muscle test of selected muscles involved in facial expression.

2. The efferent component of the oculomotor nerve (cranial nerve III) can be assessed by asking a patient positioned in sitting to follow an object such as a writing utensil with their eyes as it is moved vertically, horizontally, and diagonally. The therapist should make sure the patient does not rotate their head during the testing and should inspect the patient's eyes for asymmetry or ptosis.

3. **The afferent component of the trigeminal nerve (cranial nerve V) can be assessed by examining sensation of the face and jaw. The efferent component is assessed by examining the muscles of mastication.**

4. The efferent component of the trochlear nerve (cranial nerve IV) can be assessed by asking a patient positioned in sitting to follow an object such as a writing utensil with their eyes as it is moved in an inferior direction. The therapist should make sure the patient does not move their head downward.

System Specific: Neuromuscular & Nervous Systems
Content Outline: Examination

Exam Two: Question 155

A physical therapist treats a patient in a medical intensive care unit. The therapist notices that intravenous solution appears to be infusing into the tissues surrounding the dorsum of the patient's hand. The MOST appropriate therapist action is:

1. **contact nursing**
2. reposition the intravenous line
3. remove the intravenous line
4. document the incident in the medical record

> **Correct Answer: 1** (Pierson p. 289)

An intravenous system consists of a sterile fluid source, a pump, a clamp, and a catheter to insert into a vein. An intravenous system can be used to infuse fluids, electrolytes, nutrients, and medication. The described scenario suggests that the catheter has become dislodged from the superficial vein. Nursing should be immediately alerted to any problems with the intravenous system.

1. **Nurses have the requisite training necessary to adjust, modify or discontinue the use of an intravenous system. In some instances, other health care providers are permitted to make selected modifications, however, only after being adequately instructed and trained.**
2. Repositioning the intravenous line for the purpose of straightening the tubing or removing an object that is occluding the tubing is an appropriate activity for a physical therapist. The action would not be useful to address the primary issue which is the intravenous solution infusing into the tissues of the hand.
3. Removing the intravenous line is a skilled activity that should be performed by a nurse.
4. Documenting the incident is appropriate, however, addressing the patient care issue would remain the priority.

System Specific: Non-Systems
Content Outline: Safety & Professional Roles; Teaching/Learning; Research

Exam Two: Question 156

A physical therapist completes a cognitive function test on a patient status post stroke. As part of the test, the therapist examines the patient's abstract ability. Which of the following tasks would be the MOST appropriate?

1. orientation to time, person, and place
2. copy drawn figures of varying size and shape
3. **discuss how two objects are similar**
4. identify letters or numbers traced on the skin

> **Correct Answer: 3** (O'Sullivan p. 232)

A patient with impaired abstract thinking may have involvement of the frontal lobe, diffuse encephalopathy or psychiatric illness.

1. Orientation can be assessed by asking a person to identify time (e.g., day, month, season), person (e.g., name), and place (e.g., city, state). Disorientation is most commonly associated with traumatic brain injury, delirium, and advanced dementia.
2. Copying drawn figures of varying size and shape assesses constructional ability. Impairments in constructional ability are often associated with damage to the parietal lobe or stroke.
3. **Abstract ability is commonly tested using two specific methods. The first method is by asking a patient to describe how two items such as a cat and a mouse are similar. The other method is by asking a patient to interpret the meaning of a proverb such as "a rolling stone gathers no moss." Patients with difficulty in abstract thinking may provide answers that tend to be literal or concrete.**
4. The ability to recognize symbols, letters or numbers traced on the skin refers to graphesthesia. Patients with language or speech disorders secondary to stroke can identify the correct figure by pointing at an image located in a table instead of through verbal identification.

System Specific: Neuromuscular & Nervous Systems
Content Outline: Examination

Exam Two: Question 157

A patient fails to attain established physical therapy goals within the number of visits approved by the patient's third party payer. The patient has made progress in therapy, however, has been slowed somewhat by an adverse reaction to medication. The MOST appropriate physical therapist action is:

1. request additional visits from the referring physician
2. **request additional visits from the third party payer**
3. inform the patient that physical therapy services may not be fully covered by the third party payer
4. discharge the patient from physical therapy with a home exercise program

> **Correct Answer: 2** (Criteria for Standards of Practice)

According to the *Criteria for Standards of Practice for Physical Therapy* published by the American Physical Therapy Association, "The physical therapist discharges the patient/client from physical therapy when the anticipated goals or expected outcomes for the patient/client have been achieved. The physical therapist discontinues intervention when the patient/client is unable to continue to progress toward goals or when the physical therapist determines that the patient/client will no longer benefit from physical therapy."

1. The question does not provide any evidence suggesting that the physician has limited the patient's number of physical therapy visits or that an established limit has been reached.
2. **A physical therapist should attempt to secure approval for additional physical therapy visits when there is ample evidence that the patient is progressing towards the established goals.**
3. It is reasonable for the physical therapist to provide information to the patient regarding reimbursement when possible, however, the greater priority would be to have the additional visits approved by the third party payer.
4. It would not be in the best interest of the patient to be discharged from physical therapy since they have made progress, however, have yet to attain the established goals.

System Specific: Non-Systems
Content Outline: Safety & Professional Roles; Teaching/Learning; Research

Exam Two: Question 158

A physical therapist documents in the medical record that a patient has moved from stage 5 to stage 6 of Brunnstrom's Stages of Recovery. This type of transition is characterized by:

1. absence of associated reactions
2. **disappearance of spasticity**
3. voluntary movement begins outside of synergy patterns
4. normal motor function

> **Correct Answer: 2** (Brunnstrom p. 47)

Brunnstrom separates neurological recovery into seven separate stages based on progression through abnormal tone and spasticity. The seven stages of recovery describe tone, reflex activity, and volitional movement.

1. In stage 2, movement occurs primarily in the form of associated reactions and spasticity begins to develop. In stage 3 voluntary movement begins within basic limb synergies.
2. **In stage 5, spasticity is still present although it continues to decrease. Stage 6 is characterized by the disappearance of spasticity and the ability to complete isolated joint movements in a coordinated fashion.**
3. In stage 4, movement patterns are not dictated solely by limb synergies and voluntary movement patterns begin outside of limb synergies.
4. In stage 7, normal motor function is restored.

System Specific: Neuromuscular & Nervous Systems
Content Outline: Examination

Exam Two: Question 159

A physical therapist preparing a hot pack notices the water in the hot pack unit is cloudy. The MOST probable explanation is:

1. power failure
2. **seepage from a hot pack**
3. ineffective heating element
4. thermostat set too low

> **Correct Answer: 2** (Cameron p. 161)

A hot pack consists of a canvas or nylon covered pack filled with hydrophilic silicate gel that provides a moist heat. The size and shape of the hot pack varies depending on the size and contour of the treatment area.

1. A power failure would result in the water temperature being low. As a result, the hot packs would not possess the necessary amount of heat to transfer to the target area.
2. **A disruption in the canvas case may cause small quantities of the silicate to be released into the water which often results in the water appearing cloudy.**
3. An ineffective heating element would fail to heat the water or would heat it to less than the desired temperature. A change in water temperature would not significantly influence the clarity of the water.
4. A thermostat that is set too low would not heat the water within the hot pack unit to the desired temperature.

System Specific: Non-Systems
Content Outline: Equipment & Devices; Therapeutic Modalities

Test Taking Tip: A power failure, ineffective heating element, and a thermostat set too low would all result in insufficient heating. Since the options would result in the same objective finding it would be unlikely that one of the options would be correct and the others would be incorrect. In essence, the options mutually exclude each other from being correct.

Exam Two: Question 160

A physical therapist designs a home exercise program for a patient rehabilitating from a lower extremity injury. Which step would be the MOST appropriate to maximize patient compliance?

1. limit the exercise program to 10 minutes
2. select a maximum of five different exercises
3. **select exercises consistent with the patient's rehabilitation goals**
4. avoid physically demanding exercises

> **Correct Answer: 3** (Kisner p. 20)

Many factors can influence patient compliance with a home exercise program, however, regardless of the construction of the program it is essential that the program is designed to be consistent with the patient's rehabilitation goals.

1. An exercise program that can be completed in a relatively short period of time is more likely to be completed since patients have a better opportunity to fit the program into their existing schedule.
2. Limiting the number of exercises tends to promote compliance since it is easier for the patient to focus and complete each exercise.
3. **Patients are typically highly motivated to complete home exercise programs when they believe the exercises will help them to achieve their personal rehabilitation goals. Options such as limiting the length of the exercise program and limiting the number of exercises are helpful strategies to promote compliance, however, they would not be as critical as aligning the exercises with the patient's rehabilitation goals.**
4. There is no information presented which implies the patient is averse to physically demanding activities.

System Specific: Non-Systems
Content Outline: Safety & Professional Roles; Teaching/Learning; Research

Test Taking Tip: Many items on the National Physical Therapy Examination require candidates to differentiate between good, better, and best options. Candidates must therefore carefully assess the relative value of each of the presented options. In this particular item, candidates must differentiate between several options that are plausible and attractive. Candidates must remain open minded when examining each of the options and avoid the tendency to select the first viable option that they encounter since in many cases there is an additional option that may be better.

Exam Two: Question 161

A physical therapist performs gait training activities with an eight-year-old child who utilizes a reciprocating gait orthosis. Which medical diagnosis is MOST often associated with the use of this type of orthotic device?

1. cerebral palsy
2. Down syndrome
3. Legg-Calve-Perthes disease
4. **spina bifida**

> **Correct Answer: 4** (Tecklin p. 256)

A reciprocating gait orthosis is a type of hip-knee-ankle-foot orthosis that incorporates a cable connecting the two hip joint mechanisms. The device assists the child to advance the lower extremities during ambulation.

1. Cerebral palsy is an umbrella term used to describe a group of non-progressive movement disorders that result from brain damage. Clinical presentation includes motor delays, abnormal muscle tone and motor control, reflex abnormalities, poor postural control, and balance impairments.

2. Down syndrome (trisomy 21) occurs when there is an error in cell division. Clinical manifestations include hypotonia, flattened nasal bridge, Simian line (palmar crease), epicanthal folds, enlargement of the tongue, and developmental delay.

3. Legg-Calve-Perthes disease is the name given to idiopathic osteonecrosis of the capital femoral epiphysis of the femoral head. Clinical presentation includes short limb, high greater trochanter, quadriceps atrophy, and adductor spasm. Bracing using a Scottish-Rite brace may be used in an attempt to contain the femoral head in the acetabulum.

4. **Spina bifida is a congenital neural tube defect that generally occurs in the lumbar spine, but can also occur at the sacral, thoracic, and cervical levels. Classifications include occulta, meningocele, and myelomeningocele. Since the impairments associated with some of the classifications of spina bifida can include motor and sensory loss below the vertebral defect a reciprocating gait orthosis is often used.**

System Specific: Non-Systems
Content Outline: Equipment & Devices; Therapeutic Modalities

Exam Two: Question 162

A physical therapist instructs a patient rehabilitating from thoracic surgery how to produce an effective cough. Which patient position would be the MOST appropriate to initiate treatment?

1. standing
2. **sitting**
3. sidelying
4. hooklying

> **Correct Answer: 2** (Kisner p. 868)

An effective cough requires an inspiration greater than tidal volume, followed by closure of the glottis, abdominal muscle contraction, and sudden opening of the glottis for the forceful expulsion of the inspired air.

1. Although it is possible to perform a maximal inhalation needed for an effective cough, the standing position would not be the MOST appropriate position to initiate treatment after thoracic surgery.

2. **Sitting upright will maximize all of the steps needed to produce an effective cough.**

3. The sidelying position does not promote the maximal inhalation needed for an effective cough.

4. The hooklying position does not promote the maximal inhalation needed for an effective cough. Hooklying refers to a position where the patient is lying in supine with their hips and knees bent and the feet flat on the floor with the arms positioned at the their side.

System Specific: Cardiac, Vascular, & Pulmonary Systems
Content Outline: Interventions

Exam Two: Question 163

A physical therapist provides pre-operative instructions for a patient scheduled for hip arthroplasty surgery. As part of the session, the therapist discusses the importance of preventing deep vein thrombosis following surgery. Which finding is the BEST indicator that the patient is at minimal risk of acquiring a deep vein thrombosis?

1. ability to perform ankle pumps and muscle setting exercises
2. **ability to ambulate on a frequent schedule**
3. ability to achieve full hip range of motion within the allowable limits
4. ability to utilize pneumatic compression devices and elastic stockings

Correct Answer: 2 (Kisner p. 833)

Deep vein thrombosis results from the formation of a blood clot that becomes dislodged and is termed an embolus. This is a serious medical condition since the embolus may obstruct a selected artery. Patients are often at risk for acquiring a deep vein thrombosis after surgery. Other risk factors include advanced age, obesity, infection, tobacco, and air travel.

1. Ankle pumps and muscle setting exercises are beneficial, but would not produce the magnitude of muscle pumping action compared to an activity such as ambulation since the exercises tend to involve muscles working in relative isolation.
2. **The ability to ambulate on a frequent schedule requires a significant amount of muscle pumping action generated from contraction of the lower extremity muscles. The initiation of this activity signifies that the patient is progressing toward a more dynamic state which significantly decreases the risk of acquiring deep vein thrombosis.**
3. Range of motion is a desirable activity following surgery since it requires muscle activity and promotes circulation, however, the intensity of the activity is relatively low when compared to ambulation.
4. Pneumatic compression devices and elastic stockings are often utilized following surgery since they can help to prevent coagulation and the formation of a thrombus. The interventions are less desirable than an activity like ambulation, however, can be successfully integrated into a comprehensive program to prevent deep vein thrombosis.

System Specific: Other Systems
Content Outline: Interventions

Exam Two: Question 164

A physical therapist performs an examination on an 84-year-old female in the physical therapy gym. The patient answers the therapist's questions in a very soft voice and appears to be intimidated by the bustling environment. The MOST appropriate therapist action is:

1. ask the patient if she understands why she was referred to physical therapy
2. tell the patient to relax and speak louder
3. **complete the examination in a private treatment room**
4. ask the patient about her rehabilitation goals

Correct Answer: 3 (Purtilo p. 344)

A physical therapist should make every attempt to ensure that the patient is comfortable with the environment. The fact that the patient is speaking with a very soft voice and appears to be intimidated by the bustling environment provides adequate justification that the environment is less than ideal.

1. Asking the patient if she understands why she was referred to physical therapy may provide insight toward the patient's awareness of her current abilities and limitations, however, it ignores the fact that the patient appears to be uncomfortable with the existing environment.
2. Telling the patient to relax and speak louder forces the patient to adapt to the existing environment without attempting to modify it.
3. **Completing the examination in a private treatment room attempts to create a more desirable environment for the initial session. A private treatment room offers a secure, quiet location that can be much less intimidating than a physical therapy gym.**
4. Asking the patient about her rehabilitation goals may provide the therapist with important information on how to design an appropriate plan of care, however, it does not address the immediate need which is to modify the existing environment.

System Specific: Non-Systems
Content Outline: Safety & Professional Roles; Teaching/Learning; Research

Exam Two: Question 165

A group of physical therapists design a research study which examines the reliability of the Functional Independence Measure. To measure reliability the therapists utilize a test-retest design. What is the MOST significant source of error with this type of research design?

1. sampling error
2. tendency to rate too strictly or leniently
3. change in test forms due to sampling of items
4. **change in subject situation over time**

> **Correct Answer: 4** (Portney p. 85)

The repeatability of scores on the Functional Independence Measure (FIM) from one test administration to another provides evidence of test-retest reliability.

1. Sampling error refers to the differences between samples drawn from the same population due to chance. This is not an issue in test-retest design for reliability because the same individuals are tested each time.
2. In a test-retest design for reliability, the therapists rating the patients use the same scoring rules on each occasion.
3. In a test-retest design for reliability, the FIM would be administered both times, therefore the form of the test would not change.
4. **Because test-retest design necessitates an interval of time between test administrations, a real change in the patient's function during this time would adversely affect the reliability score.**

System Specific: Non-Systems
Content Outline: Safety & Professional Roles; Teaching/Learning; Research

Exam Two: Question 166

A patient status post knee surgery receives instructions on the use of a continuous passive motion machine. Which of the following would be the MOST essential to ensure patient safety?

1. instructions on progression of range of motion
2. utilization of proximal and distal stabilization straps
3. recommendations for cryotherapy following treatment sessions
4. **orientation to remote on/off switch**

> **Correct Answer: 4** (Kisner p. 62)

The continuous passive motion machine (CPM) is a mechanical device designed to provide continuous motion at a particular joint using a predetermined range and speed. The primary indication for CPM use is to improve range of motion that may have been impaired secondary to a surgical procedure.

1. The physical therapist would likely provide the patient with a description of the anticipated range of motion progression, however, this does not ensure patient safety.
2. The CPM includes proximal and distal stabilization straps which serve to stabilize the upper and lower leg and ensure the knee joint is aligned with the axis of the CPM. Utilization of the straps is a standard procedure when using the CPM.
3. Cryotherapy could be used following the treatment session with the CPM, however, this action would do little to protect the patient while using the CPM.
4. **Physical therapists must orient patients to the CPM's remote on/off switch since the device allows patients to terminate the treatment immediately without direct assistance from a health care provider.**

System Specific: Non-Systems
Content Outline: Equipment & Devices; Therapeutic Modalities

Exam Two: Question 167

A physical therapist instructs a patient rehabilitating from a rotator cuff repair in a home exercise program. The patient is a 27-year-old male who is illiterate. The MOST appropriate action to promote compliance with the exercise program is:

1. ask the patient to memorize the exercises
2. use short sentences consisting of simple words
3. **draw pictures to describe the exercises**
4. do not utilize a home exercise program

> **Correct Answer: 3** (Kisner p. 22)

Illiterate refers to the inability to read or write simple sentences. Functional illiteracy refers to the inability of an individual to use reading, writing, and computational skills efficiently in everyday life situations. It is estimated that seven million individuals in the United States are illiterate and 27 million individuals are unable to read well enough to complete a job application.

1. Memorizing the exercises would be a formidable challenge for many patients. The absence of a handout for the patient to refer to would likely decrease compliance and may increase the probability of the exercises being performed incorrectly.
2. Physical therapists should try to keep exercise instructions as simple as possible, however, given the patient's illiteracy this modification may still be inadequate to meet the patient's needs.
3. **Pictures provide the patient with an image of the exercises without relying solely on formal written instructions or memorization.**
4. Home exercise programs are a critical component of almost any patient care plan and can be effective with patients that are illiterate. Physical therapists should use alternate forms of educational media (e.g., pictures) whenever possible since it is an erroneous assumption to believe that the vast majority of patients possess basic reading and writing skills.

System Specific: Non-Systems
Content Outline: Safety & Professional Roles; Teaching/Learning; Research

Exam Two: Question 168

A physical therapist treats a patient status post femur fracture with external fixation. While monitoring the patient during an exercise session, the therapist observes clear drainage from a distal pin site. The MOST appropriate therapist action is:

1. discontinue the exercise session and contact the referring physician
2. use a gauze pad to absorb the drainage and notify nursing
3. **use a gauze pad to absorb the drainage and continue with the exercise session**
4. document the finding and discontinue the exercise session

> **Correct Answer: 3** (Pierson p. 294)

External fixation devices provide stabilization to fracture sites through the use of pins that are inserted into bone fragments. Clear drainage from a pin site is not uncommon and should not be viewed as a sign of infection or any other serious medical complication.

1. Clear drainage from a distal pin site would not warrant discontinuing the exercise session or contacting the referring physician. If the scenario offered compelling data suggestive of infection, it would be appropriate to notify the referring physician and/or the nurse.
2. The gauze pad is an acceptable method to absorb the drainage. The observation of clear drainage from a distal pin site is relatively common and therefore would not require consultation with nursing.
3. **The exercise session can continue after the drainage has been absorbed.**
4. Documenting the observation would be acceptable, however, the presented scenario does not provide adequate justification for discontinuing the exercise session.

System Specific: Integumentary System
Content Outline: Interventions

Exam Two: Question 169

A physical therapist reviews the medical record of a patient with a suspected head injury. During testing using the Glasgow Coma Scale, the patient exhibited spontaneous eye opening, was able to follow selected motor commands, and was considered to be "oriented" based on verbal responses. The MOST likely score assigned to the patient would be:

1. 6
2. 12
3. **15**
4. 18

Correct Answer: 3 (O'Sullivan p. 900)

The Glasgow Coma Scale is a neurological assessment tool used initially after injury to determine arousal and cerebral cortex function. The assessment tool utilizes an ordinal scale ranging from 3-15 with a higher score representing a greater level of consciousness. The Glasgow Coma Scale examines eye opening, motor response, and verbal response. The scale was initially used to assess level of consciousness after head injury and is often used on selected patients in acute care or following trauma.

1. A score of 8 or less is indicative of a severe head injury.
2. A score of 9-12 is indicative of a moderate head injury.
3. **A score of 15 is the highest attainable score on the Glasgow Coma Scale. A score of 13-15 is indicative of a mild head injury.**
4. A score of 18 is not possible on the Glasgow Coma Scale since the maximum score is 15.

System Specific: Neuromuscular & Nervous Systems
Content Outline: Examination

Exam Two: Question 170

A physical therapist uses a subjective pain scale to assess pain intensity in a patient with multiple sclerosis. The pain scale consists of a 10 cm line with each end anchored by one extreme of perceived pain intensity. The patient is asked to mark on the line the point that best describes their present pain level. This type of scale is BEST termed:

1. Descriptor Differential Scale
2. Verbal Rating Scale
3. **Visual Analogue Scale**
4. Numerical Rating Scale

Correct Answer: 3 (Van Deusen p. 127)

There are a variety of commonly used pain scales in physical therapy. Physical therapists should have familiarity with the various scales and be able to select an appropriate scale based on the breadth and depth of information they are hoping to collect.

1. The Descriptor Differential Scale consists of 12 descriptor items each centered over 21 horizontal dashes. At the extreme left dash is a minus sign and at the extreme right dash is a plus sign. Patients are asked to rate the magnitude of their pain in terms of each descriptor.
2. A Verbal Rating Scale is most often used to assess pain affect. The scale typically consists of a series of adjectives describing increasing levels of unpleasantness such as "distracting," "oppressive" or "agonizing."
3. **A Visual Analogue Scale is a tool used to assess pain intensity using a 10-15 centimeter line with the left anchor indicating "no pain" and the right anchor indicating "the worst pain you can have." The level of perceived pain is indicated on the line and is reassessed frequently over the course of physical therapy to qualify changes in the pain level and to assess progress.**
4. A Numerical Rating Scale asks patients to rate their perceived level of pain intensity on a numerical scale from 0-10 or 0 - 100. The 0 represents "no pain" and the 10 or 100 represents "pain as bad as it could be."

System Specific: Other Systems
Content Outline: Examination

Exam Two: Question 171

A physical therapist assesses end-feel while completing passive plantar flexion range of motion. The therapist classifies the end-feel as firm. Which of the following structures does NOT contribute to the firm end-feel?

1. tension in the anterior joint capsule
2. tension in the tibialis anterior
3. tension in the anterior talofibular ligament
4. **tension in the calcaneofibular ligament**

> **Correct Answer: 4** (Norkin p. 260)

End-feel refers to the type of resistance that is felt when passively moving a joint through the end range of motion.

1. The anterior joint capsule experiences increased tension with passive plantar flexion range of motion which contributes to a firm end-feel.
2. The tibialis anterior acts to dorsiflex the ankle joint and invert the foot. As a result, the muscle would experience increased tension while lengthening during passive plantar flexion range of motion.
3. The anterior talofibular ligament resists movement into plantar flexion and inversion. The ligament would therefore experience increased tension during passive plantar flexion range of motion.
4. **Tension in the calcaneofibular ligament is often associated with the normal end-feel of dorsiflexion (i.e., firm). Other structures contributing to an end-feel associated with dorsiflexion include the posterior joint capsule, soleus, Achilles tendon, posterior portion of the deltoid ligament, and the posterior talofibular ligament.**

System Specific: Musculoskeletal System
Content Outline: Clinical Application of Foundational Sciences

Exam Two: Question 172

A physical therapist prepares to use phonophoresis as a component of a patient's plan of care, but is concerned about the potential of the ultrasound to exacerbate the patient's current inflammation. The MOST effective method to address the therapist's concern is:

1. utilize ultrasound with a frequency of 1 MHz
2. limit treatment time to five minutes
3. **incorporate a pulsed 20% duty cycle**
4. select an ultrasound intensity less than 1.5 W/cm²

> **Correct Answer: 3** (Cameron p. 192)

Physical therapists must select ultrasound treatment parameters that are consistent with the desired therapeutic outcome. Failure to select appropriate parameters can lead to poor outcomes and potentially jeopardize patient safety.

1. The frequency of ultrasound selected primarily determines the depth of penetration. A frequency setting of 1 MHz is used for heating of deeper tissues (up to five centimeters).
2. Limiting the treatment time to five minutes does effectively control the duration of ultrasound, but it does not address several other critical factors that significantly influence changes in tissue temperature (e.g., duty cycle, intensity).
3. **When ultrasound is used in a pulsed mode with a 20% or lower duty cycle, the heat produced during the on time of the cycle is dispersed during the off time and as a result there is no measurable net increase in temperature. Ultrasound using a 20% or lower duty cycle would typically be used for nonthermal effects.**
4. Limiting the intensity of ultrasound to less than 1.5 W/cm² is helpful to avoid exacerbating the patient's current inflammation, however, the patient's condition could still be exacerbated at many intensity levels below 1.5 W/cm².

System Specific: Non-Systems
Content Outline: Equipment & Devices; Therapeutic Modalities

Exam Two: Question 173

A physical therapist attempts to assess the integrity of the first cranial nerve. Which test would provide the therapist with the desired information?

1. the patient protrudes the tongue while an examiner checks lateral deviation
2. the patient completes a vision examination
3. the patient performs a shoulder shrug against resistance
4. **the patient is asked to identify familiar odors with the eyes closed**

Correct Answer: 4 (Tan p. 14)

Lesions affecting the cranial nerves often produce specific and predictable alterations. As a result, it is often desirable to perform cranial nerve testing.

1. The hypoglossal nerve (cranial nerve XII) is assessed by asking the patient to protrude the tongue. A positive test may be indicated by an inability to fully protrude the tongue or the tongue deviating to one side during protrusion.
2. The optic nerve (cranial nerve II) is assessed by asking the patient to identify objects or read selected items from a chart or diagram. A positive test may be indicated by an inability to identify objects at a reasonable distance.
3. The accessory nerve (cranial nerve XI) is assessed by asking a patient, positioned in sitting with the arms at their side, to shrug their shoulders and maintain the position while the therapist applies resistance through the shoulders in the direction of shoulder depression. A positive test may be indicated by an inability to maintain the test position against resistance.
4. **The olfactory nerve (cranial nerve I) is assessed by placing an item with a familiar odor under the patient's nostril and the patient is then asked to identify the odor. A positive test may be indicated by an inability to identify familiar odors.**

System Specific: Neuromuscular & Nervous Systems
Content Outline: Examination

Exam Two: Question 174

A patient eight days status post anterior cruciate ligament reconstruction using a patellar tendon autograft is examined in physical therapy. Which of the following exercises would be the MOST appropriate based on the patient's post-operative status?

1. limited range isokinetics at 30 degrees per second
2. unilateral leg press
3. **mini-squats in standing**
4. active knee extension in short sitting

Correct Answer: 3 (Kisner p. 732)

Anterior cruciate ligament reconstruction refers to the use of a graft to replace a damaged anterior cruciate ligament. The graft is placed through drilled holes in the femoral and tibial tunnels and then anchored with a fixation device. The focus of the early post-operative period is to protect the healing graft and donor site, and at the same time avoid post-operative complications such as adhesions, contractures, and articular degeneration.

1. Performing isokinetics at 30 degrees per second on a patient eight days status post anterior cruciate ligament reconstruction could potentially jeopardize the integrity of the graft.
2. A unilateral leg press is similar to a squat, however, it is usually performed in a supine position. The exercise is not as desirable as the mini-squat given the patient's post-operative status since the leg press activity is unilateral and therefore the patient would not have the benefit of using the uninvolved lower extremity to assist, if necessary. In addition, the mini-squat implies limited range where the unilateral leg press does not.
3. **A mini-squat is a closed chain exercise typically performed in standing that enables the patient to vary the force through the involved extremity by simply shifting their weight. This exercise significantly limits the amount of knee flexion and as a result does not place a great deal of stress through the reconstructed knee. When completing mini-squats in standing it is important that the knees do not move anterior to the toes as the hips descend since this will increase the shear forces of the tibia and could unnecessarily stress the graft.**
4. Active knee extension in short sitting is an open kinetic chain activity that places a significant amount of force on the anterior surface of the knee and in particular, the patellar tendon donor area.

System Specific: Musculoskeletal System
Content Outline: Interventions

Exam Two: Question 175

A physical therapy department in an acute care hospital utilizes physical therapy aides to perform a variety of patient care services. What health care professional is directly responsible for the actions of the physical therapy aide?

1. **the physical therapist of record**
2. the physical therapist assistant of record
3. the director of physical therapy
4. the director of rehabilitation

> **Correct Answer: 1** (Guide to Physical Therapist Practice)

The physical therapy aide is a non-licensed worker who is specifically trained under the direction and supervision of a physical therapist. Activities performed by the aide are limited to those tasks that do not require clinical decision making by the physical therapist.

1. **The determination of what tasks are appropriately directed to the aide must be made by the physical therapist. As a result, the physical therapist would be responsible for the actions of the aide.**
2. The physical therapist assistant can direct and supervise the aide in selected jurisdictions, however, the physical therapist is able to function in this capacity in all jurisdictions. The availability of an option that includes the physical therapist makes the physical therapist assistant option less desirable.
3. The director of physical therapy is an administrative position that would typically be responsible for the daily operations of the physical therapy department.
4. The director of rehabilitation is an administrative position within the health care organization. The position would typically be responsible for the oversight of a number of different departments including physical therapy, occupational therapy, and speech-language pathology.

System Specific: Non-Systems
Content Outline: Safety & Professional Roles; Teaching/Learning; Research

Exam Two: Question 176

A physical therapist is scheduled to treat a patient requiring droplet precautions. What type of protective equipment would be necessary prior to entering the patient's room?

1. gloves
2. **mask**
3. gloves and mask
4. gloves, gown, and mask

> **Correct Answer: 2** (Pierson p. 38)

Droplet precautions are designed to prevent transmission of infectious agents through close respiratory or mucous membrane contact. Droplets are most often deposited on the host's nasal mucosa, conjunctivae or mouth. Examples of diseases requiring droplet precautions include pertussis, influenza, and diphtheria.

1. Gloves would be required for contact precautions, but would not be required for droplet precautions.
2. **Droplet precautions require individuals coming within three feet of the patient to wear a mask, however, it is prudent to wear the mask upon entering the room of a patient on droplet precautions to avoid any inadvertent exposure.**
3. A mask is required when working with a patient with droplet precautions, however, gloves are not.
4. Only a mask is required when treating a patient with droplet precautions. Gloves, gown, and mask are typically required with direct contact with a patient with contact precautions.

System Specific: Non-Systems
Content Outline: Safety & Professional Roles; Teaching/Learning; Research

Exam Two: Question 177

A physical therapist collects data as part of a research project that requires direct observation of children performing selected gross motor activities. The therapist is concerned about the influence of an observer on the children's performance. The MOST effective strategy to control for this source of error is to:

1. provide initial and refresher observer training
2. increase observer awareness of the influence of their background
3. **have an observer spend time with the children before direct observation**
4. ask the children to ignore the presence of the observer

Correct Answer: 3 (Portney p. 310)

A research project should be designed to eliminate as many extraneous variables as possible. Failure to eliminate or at least reduce the potential impact of an observer on the children's performance would be a significant limitation of the study.

1. Observer training would be beneficial in order to provide the observers with a better sense of their purpose, role, and actions. This action would be desirable, but would not address the nuance of the observer for the children.
2. An individual's background can influence their observations particularly when the data collected is open for interpretation. This option also focuses on the observer and not the children.
3. **Spending time with the children prior to direct observation will allow the children to feel more at ease and as a result their performance may be more reflective of their current abilities.**
4. Asking the children to ignore the presence of the observer would likely serve to bring additional attention to the observer and therefore influence behavior.

System Specific: Non-Systems
Content Outline: Safety & Professional Roles; Teaching/Learning; Research

Exam Two: Question 178

A patient reports to a physical therapist that she completely tore one of the ligaments in her ankle. If the patient's comment is accurate, the injury to the ligament is MOST likely classified as a:

1. grade I sprain
2. **grade III sprain**
3. grade I strain
4. grade III strain

Correct Answer: 2 (Dutton p. 1128)

Ligamentous injuries are termed sprains and are graded based on the amount of tissue damage that the ligament has sustained. A strain refers specifically to an injury involving a muscle or tendon.

1. A first degree sprain involves a stretch of the ligament where there is no discontinuity of the ligament. The injury usually results in minimal if any joint hypermobility.
2. **A third degree sprain involves a complete rupture or break in the continuity of a ligament. The injury usually results in gross instability and laxity.**
3. A first degree strain involves minimal disruption in the continuity of a muscle or tendon. The question asks specifically about a ligament tear or sprain.
4. A third degree strain involves a complete rupture or break in the continuity of a muscle or tendon. The question is asking about a ligament tear or a sprain.

System Specific: Musculoskeletal System
Content Outline: Clinical Application of Foundational Sciences

Exam Two: Question 179

A physical therapist prepares to treat a patient diagnosed with impingement syndrome with iontophoresis directly over the insertion of the supraspinatus muscle. What bony landmark BEST corresponds to this site?

1. lesser tubercle of the humerus
2. **greater tubercle of the humerus**
3. supraspinous fossa of the scapula
4. deltoid tuberosity of the humerus

Correct Answer: 2 (Kendall p. 314)

Impingement syndrome is a commonly used term describing mechanical impingement of the rotator cuff tendon beneath the anteroinferior portion of the acromion. Symptoms of impingement syndrome include difficulty reaching up behind the back, pain with overhead use of the arm, and weakness of the shoulder muscles.

1. The subscapularis muscle originates on the subscapular fossa of the scapula and inserts on the lesser tubercle of the humerus. The muscle is innervated by the subscapular nerve.
2. **The supraspinatus muscle inserts on the greater tubercle of the humerus. The muscle is innervated by the suprascapular nerve.**
3. The supraspinatus muscle originates on the supraspinous fossa of the scapula. The question asks about the insertion of the muscle.
4. The deltoid tuberosity is the insertion point for the three heads of the deltoid. The anterior deltoid originates on the lateral third of the clavicle, the middle deltoid originates on the acromion process, and the posterior deltoid originates on the spine of the scapula. The deltoid is innervated by the axillary nerve.

System Specific: Musculoskeletal System
Content Outline: Clinical Application of Foundational Sciences

Exam Two: Question 180

A patient status post motor vehicle accident is referred to physical therapy. The patient has multiple injury sites including the hand, wrist, elbow, and knee. As part of the patient care plan, the physical therapist attempts to increase tissue temperature at each of the involved sites. The MOST appropriate thermal agent is:

1. diathermy
2. ultrasound
3. **hydrotherapy**
4. hot packs

Correct Answer: 3 (Michlovitz p. 128)

There are a large number of thermal agents that are used in physical therapy. When selecting the most appropriate thermal agent, physical therapists must consider a number of variables including the location and size of the area or areas to be treated.

1. Diathermy refers to the application of shortwave or microwave electromagnetic energy to produce heat within tissues. Diathermy relies on inductive coil applicators or capacitive plates which provide energy to a localized area.
2. Ultrasound uses inaudible acoustic mechanical vibrations of high frequency to produce thermal and nonthermal effects. Ultrasound is most often performed by placing a transducer in direct contact with a body surface or through a medium such as water. The size of the ultrasound transducer would significantly limit the surface area treated with ultrasound.
3. **Hydrotherapy transfers heat through conduction or convection and is administered in tanks of varying size ranging from extremity whirlpools to Olympic size pools. The ability to select the size of the tank makes hydrotherapy an attractive option considering the multiple injury sites.**
4. A hot pack consists of a canvas or nylon covered pack filled with a hydrophilic silicate gel that provides a moist heat. The size and shape of the hot pack varies depending on the size and contour of the treatment area, however, the number of different injury sites makes the use of hot packs impractical.

System Specific: Non-Systems
Content Outline: Equipment & Devices; Therapeutic Modalities

Exam Two: Question 181

A physical therapist presents an inservice on graded oscillation techniques. Which grades of oscillation are the MOST appropriate for stretching maneuvers?

1. I, II
2. I, III
3. II, III
4. **III, IV**

Correct Answer: 4 (Kisner p. 116)

Physical therapists must select the appropriate rate, rhythm, and intensity of mobilization techniques. Graded oscillation techniques range from grades I-V. Grades I and II oscillations are used primarily to treat joints limited by pain, while grades III and IV oscillations are used as stretching maneuvers. Grade V oscillations are thrust techniques used to snap adhesions at the limit of available motion.

1. Grade I oscillations refer to small amplitude rhythmic oscillations performed at the beginning of the range. Grade II oscillations refer to large amplitude rhythmic oscillations performed within the range, but not reaching the limit of the range and not returning to the beginning of the range. Grade I and II oscillations are used to treat joints limited by pain. The oscillations inhibit pain by stimulating mechanoreceptors that block nociceptive pathways at the spinal cord or brain stem.
2. Grade I oscillations were previously defined. Grade III oscillations refer to large amplitude rhythmic oscillations performed up to the limit of the available motion and are stressed into the tissue resistance. Grade I oscillations are used primarily to treat joints limited by pain, while grade III oscillations are used as stretching maneuvers.
3. Grade II and III oscillations were previously defined. Grade II oscillations are used primarily to treat joints limited by pain, while grade III oscillations are used as stretching maneuvers.
4. **Grades III oscillations were previously defined. Grade IV oscillations refer to small amplitude rhythmic oscillations performed at the limit of the available motion and are stressed into the tissue resistance. Grades III and IV oscillations are used as stretching maneuvers.**

System Specific: Musculoskeletal System
Content Outline: Interventions

Exam Two: Question 182

A physical therapist examines the breath sounds of a 55-year-old male diagnosed with pulmonary disease. The therapist identifies rales during both inspiration and expiration. This finding is MOST representative of:

1. pleural effusion
2. pulmonary fibrosis
3. **impaired secretion clearance**
4. localized stenosis

Correct Answer: 3 (Hillegass p. 627)

Auscultation of the lungs with a stethoscope is an examination procedure physical therapists use to identify abnormalities in lung sounds. Abnormal lung sounds may suggest problems with ventilation or airway clearance.

1. Pleural effusion is the accumulation of fluid in the pleural space. Lung sounds are usually decreased, but a pleural friction rub may be heard if the pleural surfaces are inflammed.
2. Pulmonary fibrosis is a type of restrictive lung dysfunction characterized by changes to the alveoli and lung architecture from an inflammatory process. The inflammatory changes cause scarring and fibrotic lesions in the lungs which result in decreased lung compliance, lung volumes, diffusing capacity, increased pulmonary arterial pressure, and work of breathing. Auscultation often reveals decreased breath sounds.
3. **Crackles or rales are abnormal breath sounds heard during auscultation of the lungs with a stethoscope. Crackles are extra sounds caused by the "popping open" of small airways blocked by secretions or fluid and may be heard during both the inspiratory and expiratory phases of the breathing cycle.**
4. Localized stenosis is not a term associated with breath sounds.

System Specific: Cardiac, Vascular, & Pulmonary Systems
Content Outline: Foundations for Evaluation, Differential Diagnosis, & Prognosis

Exam Two: Question 183

The components of a clinical question posed in order to search the literature for information about the effectiveness of a therapy include:

1. subjective, objective, assessment, plan (S.O.A.P.)
2. **patient or problem, intervention, comparison, outcome (P-I-C-O)**
3. validity, reliability, applicability
4. diagnosis, prognosis, intervention

> **Correct Answer: 2** (Portney p. 10)

Asking a patient-centered clinical question is the first step in searching the literature for information about the effectiveness of a therapy.

1. Subjective, objective, assessment, and plan (S.O.A.P.) refer to the elements commonly used for recording daily notes of a patient's physical therapy sessions.
2. **The acronym P-I-C-O helps to focus on the appropriate pieces of information needed to search the literature for information about the effectiveness of a therapy. The P refers to the target population or characteristics of the patient or problem of interest. The I refers to the intervention being considered. The C refers to the comparison or control condition that may be considered along with the intervention and is most appropriate when the need is to compare the effectiveness of two or more interventions. The O refers to the outcomes or measurements that will be relevant to understanding the effect of the interventions.**
3. Validity, reliability, and applicability are properties of measurements.
4. Diagnosis, prognosis, and intervention are elements of the patient/client management model as described in the *Guide to Physical Therapist Practice*, along with examination, and evaluation.

System Specific: Non-Systems
Content Outline: Safety & Professional Roles; Teaching/Learning; Research

Exam Two: Question 184

A physical therapist completes a study which examines the effect of goniometer size on the reliability of passive shoulder joint measurements. The therapist concludes that goniometric measurements of passive shoulder range of motion can be highly reliable when taken by a single therapist, regardless of the size of the goniometer. This study demonstrates the use of:

1. interrater reliability
2. **intrarater reliability**
3. internal validity
4. external validity

> **Correct Answer: 2** (Norkin p. 41)

Reliability, or the extent to which a measurement is consistent and free from error, is a prerequisite of any measurement. There are a number of types of reliability that may be estimated: test-retest, rater (intrarater and interrater), alternate forms, and internal consistency.

1. Interrater reliability refers to the reproducibility of measurements made by two or more raters who measure the same group of subjects.
2. **Intrarater reliability refers to the reproducibility of measurements made by one individual across two or more trials.**
3. Internal validity focuses on cause and effect relationships. Specifically, is there evidence that, given a statistical relationship between the independent variable and dependent variable in an experiment, one causes the other.
4. External validity refers to the extent to which the results of a study can be generalized beyond the study sample to persons, settings, and times that are different from those employed in the experimental situation. External validity is concerned with the usefulness of the information outside the experimental situation.

System Specific: Non-Systems
Content Outline: Safety & Professional Roles; Teaching/Learning; Research

Exam Two: Question 185

A physical therapist employed in an acute care hospital examines a patient rehabilitating from surgery. The patient has diabetes, however, has no other significant past medical history. Which of the following situations would MOST warrant IMMEDIATE medical attention?

1. **signs of confusion and lethargy**
2. systolic blood pressure increase of 20 mm Hg during exercise
3. lack of significant clinical findings following the examination
4. discovery of significant past medical history unknown to the physician

> **Correct Answer: 1** (Goodman - Differential Diagnosis p. 493)

Confusion and lethargy in a patient with diabetes are signs of hypoglycemia or low blood glucose. If untreated, hypoglycemia can rapidly progress towards a life-threatening situation.

1. **It is important to treat hypoglycemia immediately using glucose tablets or sugar in order to raise blood glucose levels.**
2. An increase in systolic blood pressure of 20 mm Hg is a normal response to exercise.
3. The lack of significant findings in the examination does not warrant immediate medical attention.
4. Discovery of significant unknown medical history warrants referral to the physician for possible future examination and follow-up, but does not warrant immediate medical attention.

System Specific: Other Systems
Content Outline: Interventions

Exam Two: Question 186

A patient with a peripheral nerve injury is examined in physical therapy. The patient's primary symptoms result from an injury to the superficial peroneal nerve. The MOST likely area of sensory alteration is:

1. sole of the foot
2. plantar surface of the toes
3. **lateral aspect of the leg and dorsum of the foot**
4. triangular area between the first and second toes

> **Correct Answer: 3** (Kendall p. 369)

The superficial peroneal nerve innervates the peroneus longus and brevis. It is a branch of the sciatic nerve.

1. The sole of the foot receives cutaneous innervation from the medial and lateral plantar nerves, which are branches of the tibial nerve. The tibial nerve is a branch of the sciatic nerve.
2. The plantar surface of the toes are innervated by the medial and lateral plantar nerves, which are branches of the tibial nerve. The tibial nerve is a branch of the sciatic nerve.
3. **A peripheral nerve injury affecting the superficial peroneal nerve often results in sensory alterations along the lateral aspect of the leg and dorsum of the foot.**
4. The triangular area between the first and second toes is innervated by the deep peroneal nerve. It is a branch of the sciatic nerve.

System Specific: Neuromuscular & Nervous Systems
Content Outline: Clinical Application of Foundational Sciences

Exam Two: Question 187

A physical therapist reviews a physician examination which indicates diminished sensation in the L3 dermatome. The MOST appropriate location to confirm the physician's findings is:

1. dorsum of the foot
2. **anterior thigh**
3. groin
4. lateral calf

> **Correct Answer: 2** (Magee p. 22)

A dermatome refers to an area of skin supplied by a dorsal root of a spinal nerve.

1. Sensation in the dorsum of the foot is supplied by the L5 and S1 spinal nerves. The L5 dermatome corresponds to the medial portion of the dorsum of the foot and the S1 dermatome corresponds to the lateral portion of the dorsum of the foot.
2. **Sensation in the anterior thigh is supplied by the L2 and L3 spinal nerves.**
3. Sensation in the groin is supplied by the S3 and S4 spinal nerves. The S3 dermatome corresponds to the groin and medial thigh and the S4 dermatome corresponds to the perineum, genitals, and lower sacrum.
4. Sensation in the lateral calf is supplied by the L5 spinal nerve.

System Specific: Neuromuscular & Nervous Systems
Content Outline: Clinical Application of Foundational Sciences

Exam Two: Question 188

A physical therapist attempts to obtain a history from a patient that recently immigrated to the United States. The patient does not speak English and seems to be intimidated by the hospital environment. The MOST appropriate action is to:

1. ask the patient to communicate in writing
2. ask another physical therapist to complete the examination
3. move the patient to a private treatment room
4. **request an interpreter**

> **Correct Answer: 4** (Haggard p. 39)

A physical therapist must utilize available resources to ensure that all patients receive quality health care. Title VI, of the Civil Rights Act of 1964 prohibits exclusion from services and discrimination on grounds of race, color or national origin. This extends to people with non-English or limited English proficiency. Failure to request an interpreter given the patient's obvious need would be a violation of the patient's rights.

1. Communicating in writing is not desirable in this situation since it is unlikely that the patient would be able to communicate in a written form that would be understood by the physical therapist. In addition, writing alone does not provide the patient with an effective method of communication especially in the hospital environment.
2. This option may be more desirable if it was clear that the other physical therapist possessed the necessary language skills to communicate effectively with the patient.
3. Moving the patient to a private treatment room may address the patient's intimidation with the hospital environment, however, it does not address the more critical communication element.
4. **An interpreter would provide the patient and physical therapist with an effective method to communicate with each other. This action would ensure that the patient can actively participate in their care and that the physical therapist can appropriately direct future sessions.**

System Specific: Non-Systems
Content Outline: Safety & Professional Roles; Teaching/Learning; Research

Exam Two: Question 189

A physical therapist prepares to perform volumetric measurements as a means of quantifying edema. Which patient would appear to be the MOST appropriate candidate for this type of objective measure?

1. **a 38-year-old female with a Colles' fracture**
2. a 27-year-old male with bicipital tendonitis
3. a 48-year-old male with a rotator cuff tear
4. a 57-year-old male with pulmonary edema

Correct Answer: 1 (Magee p. 446)

Volumetric measurements are commonly used to measure edema in the distal extremities. The measurement is typically performed by examining the amount of water displaced from a cylinder following immersion of an affected body part. It would be impractical to use this type of measurement in an area other than a distal extremity.

1. **A Colles' fracture refers to a fracture of the distal end of the radius. The injury would likely result in swelling in the wrist and hand which could be quantified with volumetric measurements.**
2. The location of the biceps tendon would require immersion of the upper extremity or the entire shoulder complex. The size of the upper extremity would make this unrealistic.
3. The location of the rotator cuff would require immersion of the entire shoulder complex which would also be unrealistic due to the size of the area.
4. Pulmonary edema refers to swelling or fluid accumulation in the lungs. This condition would be impossible to assess using volumetric measurements.

System Specific: Cardiac, Vascular, & Pulmonary Systems
Content Outline: Foundations for Evaluation, Differential Diagnosis, & Prognosis

Exam Two: Question 190

A three-year-old child throws frequent temper tantrums, usually contrived to gain attention. The physical therapist, recognizing the child's objective, refuses to acknowledge the action. This type of behavior therapy is BEST termed:

1. aversive conditioning
2. **extinction**
3. operant conditioning
4. rational emotive imagery

Correct Answer: 2 (Wortman p. 136)

By refusing to acknowledge the child's tantrums the physical therapist avoids reinforcing the behavior. As a result, the tantrums may decrease in frequency and eventually disappear.

1. Aversive conditioning is a behavioral therapy technique which reduces the appeal of a behavior by associating the behavior with physical or psychological discomfort. In aversive conditioning, the individual is exposed to an unpleasant stimulus while engaging in the targeted behavior. The goal would be to create an aversion to the targeted behavior.
2. **Extinction is the withholding of reinforcement for a previously reinforced behavior which decreases the future probability of that behavior. The goal of extinction is a reduction or a loss in the strength of a conditioned response when the unconditioned stimulus or reinforcement is withheld.**
3. Operant conditioning is learning that takes place when the learner recognizes the connection between the behavior and its consequences.
4. Rational emotive imagery is a form of intense mental practice for learning new emotional and physical habits. The behavioral technique focuses on uncovering irrational beliefs which may lead to unhealthy negative emotions and replacing them with more productive rational alternatives.

System Specific: Non-Systems
Content Outline: Safety & Professional Roles; Teaching/Learning; Research

Exam Two: Question 191

A 61-year-old male referred to physical therapy complains of an excessive cough, sputum production, and shortness of breath. The patient indicates that he has been bothered by some combination of these symptoms for over 10 years. The patient's present condition is MOST indicative of:

1. idiopathic hypoventilation
2. chronic hypoxemia
3. Parkinson's disease
4. **chronic bronchitis**

> **Correct Answer: 4** (Paz p. 70)

Excessive cough, sputum production, and shortness of breath are common symptoms of chronic obstructive pulmonary disease. Chronic bronchitis is defined as hypersecretion of mucus sufficient to cause a productive cough on most days for three months during two consecutive years.

1. Hypoventilation is a state in which a reduced amount of air enters the alveoli, resulting in decreased levels of oxygen and increased levels of carbon dioxide in the blood. It can be caused by shallow breathing, slow breathing or diminished lung function.
2. Chronic hypoxemia is a condition in which the arterial oxygenation is habitually below normal (PaO_2 of less than 80 mm Hg).
3. Parkinson's disease is a primary degenerative disorder of the nervous system characterized by a decrease in the production of dopamine in the basal ganglia.
4. **Chronic bronchitis is a form of obstructive pulmonary disease that is characterized by increased mucus secretions from the bronchioles and structural changes to the bronchi. Persistent cough, wheezing, shortness of breath, and cyanosis are common symptoms.**

System Specific: Cardiac, Vascular, & Pulmonary Systems
Content Outline: Foundations for Evaluation, Differential Diagnosis, & Prognosis

Exam Two: Question 192

A patient appears to be somewhat anxious after learning her treatment will include soft tissue massage. The MOST appropriate massage stroke to begin treatment is:

1. **effleurage**
2. vibration
3. petrissage
4. tapotement

> **Correct Answer: 1** (De Domenico p. 14)

Massage is a manual therapeutic modality that produces physiologic effects through different types of stroking, rubbing, and pressure. The specific massage technique to utilize depends on the established goals and the desired physiologic effects.

1. **Effleurage is a massage technique that is usually light in stroke and produces a reflexive response. The technique is often performed at the beginning and at the end of a massage to allow the patient to relax and should be directed towards the heart. Effleurage is also often used as a transitional stroke between different massage strokes.**
2. Vibration is a massage technique that places the therapist's hands or fingers firmly over an area and utilizes a rapid shaking motion that causes vibration to the treatment area. The therapist initiates this motion from the forearm while maintaining firm contact with the treatment area.
3. Petrissage is a massage technique described as kneading where the muscle is squeezed and rolled under the therapist's hands. Petrissage can be performed with two hands over larger muscle groups or with as few as two fingers over smaller muscles.
4. Tapotement is a massage technique that provides stimulation through rapid and alternating movements such as tapping, hacking, cupping, and slapping. The primary purpose of tapotement is to enhance circulation and stimulate peripheral nerve endings.

System Specific: Other Systems
Content Outline: Interventions

Exam Two: Question 193

A patient two days status post arthrotomy of the knee completes a quadriceps setting exercise while lying supine on a mat table. During the exercise the patient begins to experience severe pain. The MOST appropriate physical therapist action is:

1. have the patient perform the exercise in sidelying
2. have the patient flex the knee prior to initiating the exercise
3. place a pillow under the ankle
4. **discontinue the exercise**

> **Correct Answer: 4** (Kisner p. 745)

A quadriceps setting exercise requires the patient to perform an isometric contraction of the quadriceps muscle. The resistive activity places minimal stress on the knee compared to many other resistive activities and as a result is often utilized early in a post-operative program.

1. Sidelying is often used to diminish the influence of gravity, however, in the described scenario the patient is performing an isometric activity with the lower extremity supported. As a result, it is possible that the patient would have more difficulty and associated pain completing the activity in sidelying.
2. Flexing the knee prior to initiating the exercise may decrease the patient's discomfort, however, the severity of the pain makes it critical that the exercise is discontinued.
3. Placing a pillow under the ankle would result in further extension of the knee. Given the patient's relative acuity secondary to their post-operative status, this position would likely increase the patient's pain.
4. **Severe pain in a patient rehabilitating from a surgical procedure is an acceptable reason to immediately discontinue an exercise. It is reasonable to attempt to modify an activity in the presence of pain, however, given the severity of the pain and the absence of information on the cause of the pain, discontinuing the exercise is a more desirable option.**

System Specific: Musculoskeletal System
Content Outline: Interventions

Exam Two: Question 194

A physical therapist enters a private treatment area and observes a patient collapsed on the floor. The patient appears to be moving slightly, however, seems to be in need of medical assistance. The MOST IMMEDIATE therapist action is:

1. **check for unresponsiveness**
2. monitor airway, breathing, and circulation
3. position the patient
4. phone emergency medical services

> **Correct Answer: 1** (American Heart Association)

The first step in performing a primary survey is to determine responsiveness.

1. **To check for responsiveness, tap the victim on the shoulder and ask, "Are you all right?" If the patient is unresponsive (i.e., no movement or response to stimulation), the therapist should phone 911, get an automatic external defibrillator, provide cardiopulmonary resuscitation, and use the AED, if necessary.**
2. Monitoring airway, breathing, and circulation describes all of the elements of cardiopulmonary resuscitation.
3. Positioning the patient is only necessary if the patient is unresponsive and needs cardiopulmonary resuscitation. If an unresponsive victim is face down, the therapist should roll the victim to a face up position to open the airway.
4. The therapist should phone emergency medical services only after determining the patient is unresponsive.

System Specific: Non-Systems
Content Outline: Safety & Professional Roles; Teaching/Learning; Research

Exam Two: Question 195

A 48-year-old female rehabilitating from a fractured femur asks questions about her expected functional level following rehabilitation. Assuming an uncomplicated recovery, the MOST accurate prediction of functional level would be based on the patient's:

1. frequency of physical therapy visits
2. previous medical history
3. **previous functional level**
4. compliance with a home exercise program

> **Correct Answer: 3** (Hertling p. 101)

A variety of factors can be useful when attempting to predict a patient's future functional level. Which variable is the most important is often determined by the unique characteristic of the patient's current disease or medical condition.

1. The frequency of physical therapy visits may be associated with the patient's rate of progress, however, it is not as strong of a predictor of functional level as the other options.
2. The previous medical history of a patient is often valuable information when predicting a patient's functional level, however, the option is more limited in scope than the patient's previous functional level. If the patient's previous medical history was significant there is a reasonable chance that it would already be reflected in the patient's previous functional level.
3. **A relatively young patient rehabilitating from a fractured femur should have a near complete recovery. As a result, the patient's previous functional level would serve as the best predictor of the patient's future functional level.**
4. A patient that is compliant with a home exercise program may have fewer complications than a patient who is less compliant, however, this variable alone remains a poor predictor of functional level.

System Specific: Musculoskeletal System
Content Outline: Foundations for Evaluation, Differential Diagnosis, & Prognosis

Exam Two: Question 196

A physical therapist attempts to strengthen the lumbricales on a patient with a low metatarsal arch. Which exercise would be the MOST appropriate?

1. resisted extension of the metatarsophalangeal joint
2. **resisted flexion of the metatarsophalangeal joint**
3. resisted abduction of the metatarsophalangeal joint
4. resisted adduction of the metatarsophalangeal joint

> **Correct Answer: 2** (Kendall p. 404)

The lumbricales act to flex the metatarsophalangeal joints and assist in extending the interphalangeal joints of the second through fifth digits. The lumbricales are innervated by the tibial nerve.

1. The extensor digitorum longus extends the metatarsophalangeal joints of the second through fifth digits. The extensor digitorum brevis extends the metatarsophalangeal joints of the first through fourth digits.
2. **Resisted flexion of the metatarsophalangeal joint can be used to strengthen the lumbricales. This can be performed with manual resistance or by gathering a towel or another similar object placed on the floor.**
3. The dorsal interossei abduct the second through fourth digits from the axial line through the second digit and assist in flexion of the metatarsophalangeal joints.
4. The plantar interossei adduct the third, fourth, and fifth digits toward the axial line through the second digit and assist in flexion of the metatarsophalangeal joints.

System Specific: Musculoskeletal System
Content Outline: Interventions

Exam Two: Question 197

A 46-year-old male rehabilitating from a radial head fracture misses his third consecutive physical therapy treatment session. The therapist called the patient after the second missed appointment, but did not receive a return phone call. The MOST appropriate physical therapist action is:

1. contact the patient's insurance provider
2. design a home exercise program for the patient
3. schedule the patient with another physical therapist
4. **discharge the patient from physical therapy**

> **Correct Answer: 4** (Shamus – Effective Documentation p. 219)

Patients receiving physical therapy services should demonstrate a commitment to attaining established goals. Failure to attend scheduled therapy sessions, particularly without providing advanced notice, is a strong indication that the patient is not currently exhibiting an appropriate level of commitment.

1. The situation should be formally addressed in the physical therapy clinic prior to contemplating the need to inform the insurance provider.
2. Designing a home exercise program for the patient could be a viable alternative, however, for this to be the correct response there would need to be evidence that suggests the patient has difficulty attending physical therapy sessions due to time constraints or other life activities.
3. The question does not provide any evidence to suggest that there is a conflict between the patient and the therapist or that the patient-therapist relationship is associated with the missed physical therapy sessions.
4. **Multiple missed appointments without a response to a phone call warrants discharging the patient from physical therapy. Failure to act in this manner limits the availability of physical therapy services for other patients.**

System Specific: Non-Systems
Content Outline: Safety & Professional Roles; Teaching/Learning; Research

Exam Two: Question 198

A physical therapist treats a patient with a decubitus ulcer using whirlpool. After treating the wound for 10 treatment sessions, the wound still shows little evidence of granulation. The MOST appropriate action is:

1. begin aggressive debridement
2. recommend a wound culture
3. apply aseptic ointment to the wound
4. **discontinue whirlpool treatments**

> **Correct Answer: 4** (Sussman p. 199)

The *Criteria for Standards of Practice for Physical Therapy* published by the American Physical Therapy Association specifies the following: "The physical therapist re-examines the patient/client as necessary during an episode of care to evaluate progress or change in patient/client status and modifies the plan of care accordingly or discontinues physical therapy services."

1. Debridement is typically warranted when there is nonviable tissue present. Debridement can be selective debridement (e.g., sharp, enzymatic, and autolytic) or non-selective debridement (e.g., wet-to-dry dressings, wound irrigation, and hydrotherapy). The question indicates that the wound has not shown evidence of healing after hydrotherapy, however, it does not specify that the wound needs to be debrided.
2. A wound culture is a test in which microorganisms from a wound are grown in a special growth medium. It is performed to identify the microorganism causing an infection in a wound or an abscess. The described scenario does not offer direct evidence suggesting the need for a wound culture and in addition it would be a higher priority to discontinue the ineffective intervention.
3. Aseptic ointment is often used on contaminated or high risk wounds and can be applied to non-contaminated wounds that demonstrate early signs of infection. The question does not provide direct evidence to support aseptic ointment and in addition it would be a higher priority to discontinue the ineffective intervention.
4. **Physical therapists have an obligation to discontinue ineffective interventions. If the selected intervention was beneficial it is likely that 10 treatment sessions would have been adequate to generate supporting evidence such as signs of healing (e.g., presence of granulation tissue).**

System Specific: Integumentary System
Content Outline: Interventions

Exam Two: Question 199

A physical therapist instructs a patient rehabilitating from a low back injury in a series of five pelvic stabilization exercises. The patient indicates he understands the exercises, however, frequently becomes confused and is unable to perform them correctly. The MOST appropriate therapist action is:

1. repeat the exercise instructions
2. **reduce the number of exercises in the series**
3. select a different treatment option
4. conclude the patient is not a candidate for physical therapy

> **Correct Answer: 2** (Haggard p. 107)

A physical therapist should attempt to simplify the exercise session in order to reduce the patient's confusion.

1. Repeating the exercise instructions can be valuable, however, given that the patient "frequently becomes confused" this action is unlikely to resolve the patient's problem.
2. **Reducing the number of exercises in the series serves to simplify the program. Five pelvic stabilization exercises is a significant number for the patient to learn, and as a result, it is reasonable to hypothesize that the number of exercises may be the primary reason for the patient's difficulty.**
3. There is not enough evidence available to suggest that the patient is unable to learn the exercises or that the exercises, if performed appropriately, are not of value. As a result, selecting a different treatment option is not justified.
4. A therapist should attempt to alter the learning environment or the method of providing patient instruction prior to concluding that a patient is not a candidate for physical therapy.

System Specific: Non-Systems
Content Outline: Safety & Professional Roles; Teaching/Learning; Research

Exam Two: Question 200

A physical therapist employed in a rehabilitation hospital prepares to perform a stand pivot transfer with a 42-year-old male rehabilitating from a motor vehicle accident. Prior to initiating the transfer, the therapist notices that the patient is wearing only a pair of hospital issued non-skid socks on his feet. The MOST appropriate therapist action is to:

1. ask another therapist for assistance and complete a dependent transfer
2. have the patient complete a sliding board transfer
3. perform the stand pivot transfer without socks
4. **perform the stand pivot transfer with the patient wearing the hospital-issued socks**

> **Correct Answer: 4** (Pierson p. 176)

Physical therapists should not permit patients to perform transfer activities with standard socks since this action unnecessarily jeopardizes patient safety.

1. The physical therapist should have the patient actively participate in the transfer whenever possible. The use of non-skid socks is acceptable and would not impact the patient's ability to participate in the stand pivot transfer.
2. The question does not provide evidence to suggest that the stand pivot transfer is not appropriate for the patient. As a result, there is no reason to select an alternate type of transfer.
3. Patients should not complete transfers in bare feet. This action would create an unnecessary safety risk since the patient may slip if their feet are sweaty or if they fail to provide adequate traction. In addition, the patient increases their risk of acquiring or transmitting microorganisms.
4. **The hospital-issued socks are appropriate for transfers since the non-skid surface incorporates rubberized material that significantly improves traction when compared to traditional socks.**

System Specific: Non-Systems
Content Outline: Safety & Professional Roles; Teaching/Learning; Research

Notes

Physical Therapy
Exam Three

EXCELLENCE

"Aiming for perfection is always a goal in progress." - Thomas J. Watson Jr.

Candidates do not have to be perfect to pass the National Physical Therapy Examination, however, should attempt to strive for perfection. The relative importance of the examination makes it imperative that candidates become intolerant of any risk of failure.

Exam Three: Question 1

A physical therapist would like to minimize the likelihood of a burn when using iontophoresis. Which action would be the MOST consistent with the therapist's objective?

1.   **increase the size of the cathode relative to the anode**
2.   decrease the space between the electrodes
3.   increase the current intensity
4.   decrease the moisture of the electrodes

> ### Correct Answer: **1** (Prentice - Therapeutic Modalities p. 167)

Current density (mA/cm^2) is calculated by taking the current amplitude (mA) and dividing by the surface area (cm^2). Greater current density will result in an increased risk of an electrochemical burn.

1.   **Increasing the size of the cathode relative to the anode serves to decrease current density and therefore reduces the probability of a burn when using iontophoresis. The cathode refers to the negatively charged electrode in a direct current system and the anode refers to the positively charged electrode. The accumulation of positively charged ions in a small area creates an alkaline reaction that is more likely to create tissue damage. As a result, it is desirable to increase the size of the cathode.**
2.   Decreasing the space between the electrodes decreases the surface area and therefore increases current density resulting in an increased risk of an electrochemical burn.
3.   Increasing the current intensity will increase the force and speed of propulsion of the ions and increase ion uptake. The result of this is increased current density and an increased risk of an electrochemical burn.
4.   Commercially produced electrodes most commonly used with iontophoresis have a small chamber covered by a semipermeable membrane which houses the ionized solution. This type of electrode eliminates the need to soak a more traditional electrode in water or saline and instead, is simply self-adherent.

System Specific: Non-Systems
Content Outline: Equipment & Devices; Therapeutic Modalities

Exam Three: Question 2

A physical therapist reviews a patient coverage form that lists the parameters used during a recent ultrasound treatment to the right anterior shoulder: 1.5 W/cm^2, pulsed 20%, 1 MHz, 6 minutes. Assuming the objective of the ultrasound was to increase tissue temperature, which parameter would be the MOST critical for the therapist to alter?

1.   time
2.   **duty cycle**
3.   frequency
4.   intensity

> ### Correct Answer: **2** (Cameron p. 192)

Physical therapists must select specific parameters when using ultrasound based on the desired physiological effect. Failure to select the correct parameters will minimize the effectiveness of the session and could potentially jeopardize patient safety in extreme cases.

1.   The duration of the ultrasound is an important parameter, however, it is typically determined based on the size of the area to be treated and not by the desired increase in tissue temperature.
2.   **Duty cycle is defined as the ratio of the on time to the total time. When ultrasound is used in a pulsed mode with a 20% or lower duty cycle, the heat produced during the on time of the cycle is dispersed during the off time and as a result there is no measurable net increase in temperature. To increase tissue temperature it would be necessary to significantly increase the duty cycle or use a continuous mode.**
3.   The frequency of ultrasound selected primarily determines the depth of penetration. A frequency setting of 1 MHz is used for heating of deeper tissues (up to five centimeters). A frequency setting of 3 MHz produces a more rapid heating with a depth of penetration of less than two centimeters.
4.   Intensity for continuous ultrasound is normally set between .5 to 2.0 W/cm^2 for thermal effects. Pulsed ultrasound is normally set between .5 to .75 W/cm^2 with a 20% duty cycle for nonthermal effects.

System Specific: Non-Systems
Content Outline: Equipment & Devices; Therapeutic Modalities

Exam Three: Question 3

A physical therapist examines a patient with a C6 spinal cord injury. Which muscle would NOT be innervated based on the patient's level of injury?

1. biceps
2. deltoid
3. **triceps**
4. diaphragm

> **Correct Answer: 3** (Magee p. 22)

A patient with a C6 spinal cord injury would not possess motor, sensory or reflex function below the C6 level. As a result, any muscle or structure innervated below this level would not be active.

1. The biceps muscle is innervated by the musculocutaneous nerve (C5-C6).
2. The deltoid muscle is innervated by the axillary nerve (C5-C6).
3. **The triceps muscle is innervated by the radial nerve (C7-C8).**
4. The diaphragm is innervated by the phrenic nerve (C3, C4, C5).

System Specific: Neuromuscular & Nervous Systems
Content Outline: Clinical Application of Foundational Sciences

Exam Three: Question 4

A physical therapist attempts to assess the integrity of the vestibulocochlear nerve by administering the Rinne test on a patient with a suspected upper motor neuron lesion. After striking the tine of the tuning fork to begin vibration, which bony prominence should the therapist utilize to position the stem of the tuning fork?

1. midline of the skull
2. occipital protuberance
3. inion
4. **mastoid process**

> **Correct Answer: 4** (Magee p. 115)

The Rinne test is designed to compare bone conduction hearing with air conduction hearing. A therapist uses a vibrating tuning fork placed on the mastoid process and then placed next to the ear. Air conducted sound should be approximately twice as long as bone conducted sound.

1. The Weber test is another commonly used hearing test that requires placing a tuning fork on the midline of the skull on the patient's forehead.
2. The occipital protuberance refers to a prominence on the outer surface of the occipital bone.
3. The inion refers to the most prominent projecting point of the occipital bone at the midline of the base of the skull. The inion marks the center of the superior nuchal line.
4. **The mastoid process refers to a protruding bony area in the lower part of the skull situated behind the ear.**

System Specific: Neuromuscular & Nervous Systems
Content Outline: Examination

Exam Three: Question 5

A physical therapist prepares to apply a topical antibiotic to a small portion of the upper arm of a patient with a deep partial-thickness burn. When applying the topical antibiotic the therapist should utilize which form of medical asepsis?

1. gloves
2. **sterile gloves**
3. sterile gloves, gown
4. sterile gloves, gown, mask

> **Correct Answer: 2** (Paz p. 290)

Topical antibiotics are often utilized in the treatment of burns. They serve to reduce bacterial count, provide a covering for the wound, reduce stiffness, and reduce evaporative loss. Since topical antibiotics are applied directly to the affected area, sterile gloves should be worn.

1. Gloves offer protection to the physical therapist's hands to reduce the likelihood of becoming infected with microorganisms from a patient and reduce the risk of the patient receiving microorganisms from the physical therapist. Non-sterile gloves are typically used with intact skin.
2. **Topical antibiotics are applied directly to the burn and therefore require the use of sterile gloves. Failure to use sterile technique increases the probability of contamination.**
3. A gown is used to protect the physical therapist's clothing from being contaminated or soiled by a contaminant. The gown also reduces the probability of the physical therapist transmitting a microorganism from their clothing to the patient. The size and the location of the burn make it unnecessary to use a gown.
4. A mask is designed to reduce the spread of microorganisms that are transmitted through the air. The mask protects the physical therapist from inhalation of particles or droplets that may contain pathogens and also reduces the transmission of pathogens from the physical therapist to the patient. The mask would not be necessary since there is minimal risk of microorganisms being transmitted through the air in the described scenario.

System Specific: Integumentary System
Content Outline: Interventions

Exam Three: Question 6

A patient involved in a motor vehicle accident sustains a proximal fibula fracture. The fracture damaged the motor component of the common peroneal nerve. Ankle dorsiflexion and eversion are tested as 2/5. The MOST appropriate intervention to assist the patient with activities of daily living would be:

1. electrical stimulation
2. **orthosis**
3. exercise program
4. aquatic program

> **Correct Answer: 2** (Seymour p. 31)

There are a variety of interventions that can assist patients to perform activities of daily living following a peripheral nerve injury. Physical therapists must select the most appropriate interventions to accomplish each of the established goals. In this particular question, the candidate is asked to identify the most appropriate intervention to assist the patient with activities of daily living.

1. Electrical stimulation can be used to facilitate motor activity within the affected muscle, however, the effectiveness of this intervention may be limited depending on the severity of the damage to the nerve. In addition, the intervention would not immediately assist the patient with activities of daily living.
2. **The use of an orthosis would ensure adequate foot clearance and stability during activities of daily living. This form of intervention would have an immediate impact on the patient's ability to perform activities of daily living.**
3. An exercise program would be beneficial for the patient for a variety of reasons. The patient will need to perform selected movements in a different manner since the lower extremity musculature has been affected. Exercise will also be necessary to strengthen the surrounding musculature to provide additional stability. Despite the stated benefits, the intervention would not provide the same magnitude of benefit as the orthosis when performing activities of daily living.
4. An aquatic program allows the patient to exercise in a decreased weight bearing environment, however, the intervention is unlikely to have an immediate impact on the patient's ability to perform activities of daily living.

System Specific: Other Systems
Content Outline: Interventions

Exam Three: Question 7

A physical therapist discusses the importance of a proper diet with a patient diagnosed with congestive heart failure. Which of the following substances would MOST likely be restricted in the patient's diet?

1. high-density lipoproteins
2. low-density lipoproteins
3. **sodium**
4. triglycerides

> **Correct Answer: 3** (Goodman - Pathology p. 572)

Patients with congestive heart failure tend to have excessive fluid retention in the pulmonary and systemic circulation. As a result, a diet high in potassium is prescribed, while items high in sodium are restricted.

1. High-density lipoproteins (HDL) are the smallest particles in the classes of lipoproteins. They are composed of proteins, cholesterol, and a small amount of triglyceride. HDL plays an important role in lipid metabolism by transporting cholesterol back to the liver from the cells. High levels of HDL reduce the incidence of coronary artery disease. There is no association between HDL and congestive heart failure.

2. Low-density lipoproteins (LDL) are the major carriers of cholesterol in plasma. Elevated LDL is a cause of coronary artery disease. There is no association between LDL and congestive heart failure.

3. **Due to poor cardiac output in congestive heart failure, renal and extrarenal sensors initiate a process to retain fluid to increase arterial blood flow. Retention of sodium is part of that process. By controlling sodium intake and water retention, congestive heart failure can be more effectively controlled.**

4. Triglycerides are combinations of glycerol and fatty acids. Elevated triglycerides are not independently predictive of coronary artery disease, but are associated with known risk factors for atherosclerosis, including low HDL cholesterol level and uncontrolled diabetes. There is no association between triglycerides and congestive heart failure.

System Specific: Cardiac, Vascular, & Pulmonary Systems
Content Outline: Interventions

Exam Three: Question 8

A physical therapist instructs a patient with a pulmonary disease in energy conservation techniques. Which of the following techniques would be the MOST effective when assisting a patient to complete a selected activity without dyspnea?

1. diaphragmatic breathing
2. **pacing**
3. pursed-lip breathing
4. ventilatory muscle training

> **Correct Answer: 2** (Kisner p. 865)

Pacing is a technique that can allow patients to complete functional activities without shortness of breath or dyspnea.

1. Diaphragmatic breathing is a breathing technique that can decrease the work of breathing by lowering respiratory rate, increasing tidal volume, and decreasing the use of accessory muscles of respiration by facilitating use of the diaphragm. Diaphragmatic breathing can be used with pacing when necessary.

2. **Pacing is an integral component of energy-saving techniques used by patients who present with dyspnea during activity. Pacing refers to dividing an activity into component parts so that the patient does not exceed the limits of their breathing capacity throughout each portion of the task. For example, climbing up stairs is performed only on exhalation and by taking only one or two steps at a time.**

3. Pursed-lip breathing is a breathing technique performed by inhaling through the nose and exhaling through pursed lips. Patients with chronic obstructive pulmonary disease have been shown to benefit from pursed lip breathing by decreasing respiratory rate, increasing tidal volume, and decreasing the sense of dyspnea. When used in isolation the technique would not be as effective as pacing to assist the patient to complete the activity without dyspnea.

4. Ventilatory muscle training is accomplished by devices called inspiratory muscle trainers, which strengthen the inspiratory muscles by providing resistance to inspiration.

System Specific: Cardiac, Vascular, & Pulmonary Systems
Content Outline: Interventions

Exam Three: Question 9

A physical therapist reviews the medical record of a patient 24 hours status post total hip arthroplasty. A recent entry in the medical record indicates that the patient was placed on anticoagulant medication. Which of the following laboratory values would be MOST affected based on the patient's current medication?

1. hematocrit
2. hemoglobin
3. **prothrombin time**
4. white blood cell count

> **Correct Answer: 3** (Physical Therapist's Clinical Companion p. 145)

Anticoagulant drugs are often prescribed post-operatively for patients at risk for acquiring deep vein thrombosis.

1. Hematocrit is used in the identification of abnormal states of hydration, polycythemia, and anemia. A low hematocrit may result in a feeling of weakness, chills or dyspnea. A high hematocrit may result in an increased risk of thrombus.
2. Hemoglobin is used to assess blood loss, anemia, and bone marrow suppression. Low hemoglobin may indicate anemia or recent hemorrhage, while elevated hemoglobin suggests hemoconcentration caused by polycythemia or dehydration.
3. **Prothrombin time is often used as a screening procedure to examine extrinsic coagulation factors (V, VII, X, prothrombin, and fibrinogen) and to determine the effectiveness of oral anticoagulant therapy. An abnormal prothrombin time is most often caused by liver disease, injury or by treatment with blood thinners. Abnormal values can place patients at risk for side effects ranging from a high likelihood of bleeding to a high likelihood of developing a clot.**
4. White blood cell count is commonly used to identify the presence of infection, allergens, bone marrow integrity or the degree of immunosuppression. An increase in white blood cell count can occur after hemorrhage, surgery, coronary occlusion or malignant growth.

System Specific: Other Systems
Content Outline: Foundations for Evaluation, Differential Diagnosis, & Prognosis

Exam Three: Question 10

A physical therapist discusses the plan of care for a 61-year-old male diagnosed with spinal stenosis with the referring physician. During the discussion the physician shows the therapist a picture of the patient's spine obtained through computed tomography. What color would vertebrae appear when using this imaging technique?

1. black
2. light gray
3. dark gray
4. **white**

> **Correct Answer: 4** (Magee p. 62)

Computed tomography produces cross-sectional images based on x-ray attenuation. The test is commonly used to diagnose spinal lesions and in diagnostic studies of the brain. The relative color of each item using computed tomography is dependent on the relative density. The greater the density, the less penetration of x-rays and the whiter the image will appear. Specific structures listed in descending degree of density are metal, bone, soft tissue, water, fat, and air.

1. Cerebrospinal fluid would appear as black using computed tomography since it is radiolucent.
2. Soft tissue structures would appear as various shades of gray depending on their relative density.
3. A structure that is darker gray has less relative density than a structure that appears as a lighter shade of gray.
4. **Vertebrae are composed of extremely dense bone and therefore appear to be white.**

System Specific: Musculoskeletal Systems
Content Outline: Foundations for Evaluation, Differential Diagnosis, & Prognosis

Exam Three: Question 11

A physical therapist identifies a number of substances that influence circulation. Which of the following substances is stimulated by decreased arterial pressure and acts as a vasoconstrictor?

1. **angiotensin**
2. histamine
3. epinephrine
4. norepinephrine

> **Correct Answer: 1** (Ciccone p. 297)

Physical therapists should possess a general sense of the role of different substances and their influence on normal body processes such as circulation.

1. **Angiotensin is a polypeptide in the blood that causes vasoconstriction, increased blood pressure, and the release of aldosterone from the adrenal cortex. Release of angiotensin is stimulated by decreased arterial pressure.**
2. Histamine is an endogenous chemical that is involved in the normal regulation of a variety of physiologic functions such as gastric secretion as well as various hypersensitivity or allergic reactions.
3. Epinephrine is a naturally occurring hormone released by the adrenal glands. The hormone is released in the fight or flight response. The hormone boosts the supply of oxygen and glucose to the brain and muscles while suppressing other non-emergency body processes such as digestion.
4. Norepinephrine serves dual roles as a hormone and neurotransmitter. Norepinephrine affects parts of the brain where attention and responding actions are controlled and in conjunction with epinephrine underlies the fight or flight response by increasing heart rate, releasing glucose from energy stores, and increasing blood flow to skeletal muscles.

System Specific: Cardiac, Vascular, & Pulmonary Systems
Content Outline: Clinical Application of Foundational Sciences

Exam Three: Question 12

A patient diagnosed with C5 tetraplegia receives physical therapy services in a rehabilitation hospital. The patient has made good progress in therapy and is scheduled for discharge in one week. During a treatment session, the patient informs the physical therapist that one day in the future he will walk again. The MOST appropriate therapist response is:

1. Your level of injury makes walking unrealistic.
2. **Future advances in spinal cord research may make your goal a reality.**
3. You can have a rewarding life even if confined to a wheelchair.
4. Completing your exercises on a regular basis will help you to walk.

> **Correct Answer: 2** (Umphred p. 639)

Physical therapists should encourage patients to reach for their goals even in cases where presently it may be unrealistic. In this scenario, the patient is not asking the therapist directly about their future functional level, rather the patient is simply sharing their optimism about the possibility of one day being able to walk. It would, therefore, be inappropriate for the therapist to do anything to diminish this optimism.

1. The response is accurate, however, it would serve to significantly dampen the patient's current enthusiasm and is not warranted given the described scenario.
2. **Responding in this manner leaves open the possibility that the patient may one day walk, without providing the patient with a sense of false hope.**
3. The response would likely be construed as negative given the patient's proclamation and is made worse by the terminology selected (i.e., "confined to a wheelchair").
4. The response implies that compliance with an exercise program can facilitate walking. This is not accurate based on the patient's level of injury and therefore may provide the patient with a sense of false hope.

System Specific: Neuromuscular & Nervous Systems
Content Outline: Foundations for Evaluation, Differential Diagnosis, & Prognosis

Exam Three: Question 13

A physical therapist performs several surface palpations on a patient diagnosed with an acromioclavicular injury. Which anatomical landmark is MOST consistent with the location of the therapist's finger?

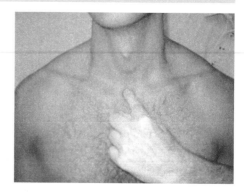

1. manubrium
2. sternoclavicular joint
3. **suprasternal notch**
4. xiphoid process

> **Correct Answer: 3** (Hoppenfeld p. 6)

Physical therapists must possess knowledge of surface anatomy and be able to identify anatomical structures through observation or palpation. It is often important to inspect the integrity of selected structures within a reasonable proximity of the primary injury.

1. The manubrium refers to the broad upper portion of the sternum. The manubrium has a quadrangular shape and articulates with the clavicles and the first two ribs.

2. The sternoclavicular joint consists of the clavicle articulating with the manubrium of the sternum.

3. **The anatomical landmark consistent with the therapist's finger is the suprasternal notch. The suprasternal notch refers to the "V" shaped notch at the top of the sternum.**

4. The xiphoid process refers to the small extension of the lower portion of the sternum. The xiphoid process is cartilaginous at birth and usually ossifies and unites with the body of the sternum by 40 years of age.

System Specific: Musculoskeletal System
Content Outline: Clinical Application of Foundational Sciences

Exam Three: Question 14

A physical therapist discusses the plan of care for a patient rehabilitating from total hip arthroplasty surgery (posterolateral approach) with the patient's surgeon. During the discussion the surgeon indicates that he would like the patient to continue to wear a knee immobilizer in order to help prevent hip dislocation. The PRIMARY rationale for this action is:

1. The knee immobilizer serves as a constant reminder to the patient that the hip is susceptible to injury.
2. **The knee immobilizer reduces hip flexion by maintaining knee extension.**
3. The knee immobilizer facilitates quadriceps contraction during weight bearing activities.
4. The knee immobilizer limits post-operative edema and as a result, promotes lower extremity stability.

> **Correct Answer: 2** (Paz p. 105)

Hip flexion greater than 90 degrees is often considered a contraindication following total hip arthroplasty surgery using a posterolateral surgical approach. Other contraindications in the early post-operative phase include restricting adduction and medial rotation beyond neutral.

1. A knee immobilizer can serve as an external feedback mechanism to remind the patient that the hip is vulnerable to injury, however, this would not be the primary rationale to use the device.

2. **A knee immobilizer limits hip flexion by maintaining the knee in an extended position. The immobilizer can be particularly helpful in patients who are unable to maintain posterior hip precautions independently.**

3. A knee immobilizer is commonly used following knee surgery to provide stability to the lower extremity. The immobilizer is most often prescribed in the presence of quadriceps weakness to prevent "buckling" or "giving way" of the knee. The knee immobilizer would, however, offer limited stability to a patient following total hip arthroplasty surgery.

4. The knee immobilizer offers some compression to the knee, however, would have little impact on the patient's post-operative edema particularly since the surgery involved the hip. In addition, limiting post-operative edema would play a relatively minor role in promoting lower extremity stability.

System Specific: Non-Systems
Content Outline: Equipment & Devices; Therapeutic Modalities

Exam Three: Question 15

A physical therapist administers a submaximal exercise test to a patient in a cardiac rehabilitation program. The protocol requires the patient to ride a cycle ergometer for a predetermined amount of time using progressive workloads. In order to predict the patient's maximum oxygen uptake it is necessary to determine the relationship between:

1. heart rate and rate of perceived exertion
2. **heart rate and workload**
3. blood pressure and rate of perceived exertion
4. blood pressure and workload

> **Correct Answer: 2** (American College of Sports Medicine p. 308)

Because maximal exercise testing is not always feasible, practitioners often rely on submaximal exercise tests to assess cardiorespiratory fitness. In addition to the heart rate response, it is recommended that the individual's functional response to exercise is examined.

1. Rate of perceived exertion (RPE) is one of the indices commonly measured as a response to exercise. However, oxygen uptake cannot be determined from heart rate and RPE.
2. **The physical therapist can use the heart rate response to one or more submaximal workloads to predict maximum oxygen uptake.**
3. Rate of perceived exertion (RPE) and blood pressure are commonly measured as a response to exercise. However, oxygen uptake cannot be determined from blood pressure and RPE.
4. Blood pressure is one of the indices commonly measured as a response to exercise. However, oxygen uptake cannot be determined from blood pressure and workload.

System Specific: Cardiac, Vascular, & Pulmonary Systems
Content Outline: Interventions

Exam Three: Question 16

A physical therapist employed in a large medical center reviews the chart of a 63-year-old male referred to physical therapy for pulmonary rehabilitation. The chart indicates the patient has smoked one to two packs of cigarettes a day since the age of 25. The admitting physician documented that the patient's thorax was enlarged with flaring of the costal margins and widening of the costochondral angle. Which pulmonary disease does the chart MOST accurately describe?

1. asthma
2. bronchiectasis
3. chronic bronchitis
4. **emphysema**

> **Correct Answer: 4** (Hillegass p. 277)

Due to the pathologic changes in alveoli, patients with emphysema often have increased total lung capacity from "air trapping." Over time, many patients develop a barrel-shaped configuration of the thorax. The anteroposterior diameter enlarges to approximate the transverse diameter. The diaphragm is depressed and the sternum pushed forward with the ribs attached in a horizontal, not angular, fashion. As a result, the chest appears continuously in the inspiratory position.

1. Asthma is a chronic inflammatory disease of the airways. Clinical features include cough, dyspnea, and wheezing, but not an enlarged thorax.
2. Bronchiectasis is a permanent, abnormal dilatation of one or more bronchi caused by destruction of the elastic and muscular components of the bronchial walls. Common clinical features include recurrent pulmonary infections with cough and copious mucopurulent sputum, but not an enlarged thorax.
3. Chronic bronchitis is defined as hypersecretion of mucus sufficient to cause a productive cough on most days for three months during two consecutive years, but not an enlarged thorax.
4. **Emphysema is an obstructive pulmonary disease characterized by destruction of alveoli leading to hyperinflation of the lungs. A barrel-shaped configuration of the thorax is a common clinical feature of the disease.**

System Specific: Cardiac, Vascular, & Pulmonary Systems
Content Outline: Foundations for Evaluation, Differential Diagnosis, & Prognosis

Exam Three: Question 17

A physical therapist reviews the results of pulmonary function testing on a 44-year-old female diagnosed with emphysema. Assuming the patient's testing was classified as unremarkable, which of the following lung volumes would MOST likely approximate 10% of the patient's total lung capacity?

1. **tidal volume**
2. inspiratory reserve volume
3. residual volume
4. functional residual capacity

> **Correct Answer: 1** (Frownfelter p. 153)

Tidal volume is the total volume of air inhaled or exhaled during quiet breathing. Total lung capacity is the maximum volume of air to which the lungs can be expanded. Normal tidal volume is approximately 10% of total lung capacity.

1. **While there is wide variability in tidal volume in the normal population, the average for a healthy adult is around 500 mL (± 100 mL). Total lung capacity is the maximum volume of air to which the lungs can be expanded, typically 4,000 – 6,000 mL. Thus, normal tidal volume is approximately 10% of total lung capacity.**

2. Inspiratory reserve volume is the additional volume of air that can be inhaled beyond the normal tidal inhalation. The inspiratory reserve volume varies, however, should represent approximately 55% to 60% of the total lung capacity.

3. Residual volume is the volume of air remaining in the lungs after a forced expiratory effort. This volume is usually 1,000 mL, and approximates 25% of total lung capacity.

4. Functional residual capacity is the amount of air remaining in the lungs at the end of a normal tidal exhalation. This volume approximates 40% of total lung capacity.

System Specific: Cardiac, Vascular, & Pulmonary Systems
Content Outline: Examination

Exam Three: Question 18

A physical therapist measures a patient's shoulder complex medial rotation with the patient positioned in supine, the glenohumeral joint in 90 degrees of abduction, and the elbow in 90 degrees of flexion. The therapist records the patient's shoulder medial rotation as 0 - 70 degrees and classifies the end-feel as firm. Which portion of the joint capsule is primarily responsible for the firm end-feel?

1. anterior joint capsule
2. **posterior joint capsule**
3. inferior joint capsule
4. superior joint capsule

> **Correct Answer: 2** (Norkin p. 84)

The glenohumeral joint is a synovial ball and socket joint, in which the round head of the humerus (convex) articulates with the shallow glenoid cavity (concave) of the scapula. The glenohumeral joint has three degrees of freedom. The capsule of the glenohumeral joint is reinforced by the superior glenohumeral ligament, middle glenohumeral ligament, inferior glenohumeral ligament, and the coracohumeral ligament.

1. A firm end-feel caused by the anterior joint capsule would most often be associated with lateral rotation of the glenohumeral joint as the humeral head slides anteriorly on the glenoid fossa.

2. **A firm end-feel caused by the posterior joint capsule would most often be associated with medial rotation of the glenohumeral joint as the humeral head slides posteriorly on the glenoid fossa.**

3. A firm end-feel caused by the inferior joint capsule would most often be associated with flexion and abduction of the glenohumeral joint. In flexion, the humeral head moves posteriorly and inferiorly, and in abduction the humeral head moves inferiorly.

4. A firm end-feel caused by the superior joint capsule would most often be associated with extension and adduction of the glenohumeral joint. In extension, the humeral head moves anteriorly and superiorly, and in adduction the humeral head moves superiorly.

System Specific: Musculoskeletal System
Content Outline: Clinical Application of Foundational Sciences

Exam Three: Question 19

A physician suspects a stress fracture in a 16-year-old distance runner after completing an examination. Assuming the physician's preliminary diagnosis is correct, which of the following diagnostic tests would be the MOST appropriate to identify the stress fracture?

1. **bone scan**
2. magnetic resonance imaging
3. telethermography
4. ultrasound scan

> **Correct Answer: 1** (Magee p. 63)

Physical therapists should be familiar with commonly employed diagnostic tests since the results of these tests are frequently encountered in the medical record. Awareness of the purpose of the diagnostic tests may also assist the physical therapist to make specific recommendations to the referring physician when appropriate.

1. **A bone scan is a diagnostic test that utilizes radioactive isotopes to identify areas of bone that are hypervascular or have an increased rate of bone mineral turnover. Bone scans can demonstrate bone disease or stress fractures with as little as 4-7% bone loss.**
2. Magnetic resonance imaging is a non-invasive diagnostic test that utilizes magnetic fields to produce an image of bone and soft tissue. The test is valuable in providing images of soft tissue structures such as muscles, menisci, ligaments, tumors, and internal organs.
3. Telethermography is a diagnostic test that demonstrates thermal alterations in the body. For example, a hyperthermic image may be observed in the presence of an inflammatory reaction or a hypothermic image may be observed in the presence of compression or a degenerative process.
4. Ultrasound can be used as a diagnostic test by administering high frequency sound waves into the tissues. The depth of each structure is determined based on the amount of time it takes for an echo to return to the transducer. Ultrasound provides good image detail and cross-sectional multi-planar images.

System Specific: Musculoskeletal System
Content Outline: Foundations for Evaluation, Differential Diagnosis, & Prognosis

Exam Three: Question 20

A physical therapist positions a patient in prone to measure passive knee flexion. Range of motion may be limited in this position due to:

1. active insufficiency of the knee extensors
2. active insufficiency of the knee flexors
3. **passive insufficiency of the knee extensors**
4. passive insufficiency of the knee flexors

> **Correct Answer: 3** (Kisner p. 44)

Passive insufficiency occurs when a two-joint muscle is passively stretched across two joints at the same time resulting in an inability to permit normal elongation simultaneously over both joints. When the muscle is in a lengthened position, the actin filaments are pulled away from the myosin heads so that they cannot create as many cross-bridges. Active insufficiency occurs when a two-joint muscle is incapable of shortening to the extent necessary to produce full range of motion at all joints crossed simultaneously. When the muscle is in a shortened position the overlap of actin and myosin reduces the number of sites available for cross-bridge formation.

1. Active insufficiency occurs with active movement and not passive movement. The question specifically asks about passive knee flexion.
2. Active insufficiency occurs with active movement and not passive movement.
3. **Passive insufficiency refers to a lack of muscle length. When performing passive knee flexion the two-joint knee extensors are placed on stretch and therefore in the presence of insufficient length, may contribute to a limitation in knee flexion.**
4. When performing passive knee flexion, the knee flexors would shorten and therefore would not limit knee flexion range of motion.

System Specific: Musculoskeletal System
Content Outline: Examination

Exam Three: Question 21

A physical therapist incorporates electrical stimulation as part of the plan of care for a patient rehabilitating from a lower extremity injury. Which of the following recommendations would be LEAST effective to minimize electrode resistance?

1. keep the sponge interface well moistened
2. **use small electrodes**
3. maintain even, firm contact with the skin
4. remove hair from the skin

Correct Answer: 2 (Prentice - Therapeutic Modalities p. 84)

Resistance refers to the opposition to electron flow in a conducting material.

1. Water serves as a conductive substance that reduces electrode resistance.
2. **Small electrodes increase electrode resistance, while large electrodes decrease electrode resistance.**
3. Uneven or inadequate contact or pressure from the electrodes increases electrode resistance and can severely limit the effectiveness of electrotherapy.
4. Hair can cause nonuniform conduction at the skin-electrode interface and therefore it is important that the skin be appropriately prepared by cleaning and potentially clipping if necessary.

System Specific: Non-Systems
Content Outline: Equipment & Devices; Therapeutic Modalities

Exam Three: Question 22

A physical therapist reviews the results of a pulmonary function test. Assuming normal values, which of the following measurements would you expect to be the GREATEST?

1. **vital capacity**
2. tidal volume
3. residual volume
4. inspiratory reserve volume

Correct Answer: 1 (Brannon p. 48)

Vital capacity is defined as the amount of air that can be exhaled following a maximal inspiratory effort.

1. **Vital capacity is comprised of inspiratory reserve volume (IRV), tidal volume (TV), and expiratory reserve volume (ERV). Vital capacity is approximately 4,000 - 5,000 mL, but varies directly with height and indirectly with age.**
2. Tidal volume is the amount of air inspired and expired during normal resting ventilation. This volume is approximately 500 mL.
3. The lungs are not emptied of air even after maximal exhalation. The residual volume is the amount of air remaining in the lungs after the expiratory reserve volume has been exhaled. This volume is approximately 900 - 1,200 mL.
4. Inspiratory reserve volume is the volume that can be inhaled in excess of tidal breathing. This volume is approximately 2,300 - 3,000 mL.

System Specific: Cardiac, Vascular, & Pulmonary Systems
Content Outline: Examination

Exam Three: Question 23

A patient involved in a motor vehicle accident sustains an injury to the posterior cord of the brachial plexus. Which muscle would NOT be affected by the injury?

1. **infraspinatus**
2. subscapularis
3. latissimus dorsi
4. teres major

> **Correct Answer: 1** (Kendall p. 248)

The brachial plexus extends from the neck to the axilla and arises from the ventral rami of the fifth through eighth cervical nerves and most of the first thoracic nerve. The brachial plexus innervates the entire upper extremity as well as the muscles of the scapula. Knowledge of its components is critical to proper identification and treatment of upper extremity impairments.

1. **The infraspinatus muscle is innervated by the suprascapular nerve (C4, C5, C6) that extends from the superior trunk of the brachial plexus.**
2. The subscapularis is innervated by the upper (C5, C6) and lower subscapular nerve (C5, C6, C7) which extends from the all three trunks of the brachial plexus, via the posterior cord.
3. The latissimus dorsi is innervated by the thoracodorsal nerve (C6, C7, C8) which extends from all three trunks of the brachial plexus, via the posterior cord.
4. The teres major is innervated by the lower subscapular nerve (C5, C6, C7) which extends from all three trunks of the brachial plexus, via the posterior cord.

System Specific: Neuromuscular & Nervous Systems
Content Outline: Clinical Application of Foundational Sciences

Exam Three: Question 24

A physical therapist designs a training program for a patient without cardiovascular pathology. The therapist calculates the patient's age-predicted maximal heart rate as 175 beats per minute. Which of the following would be an acceptable target heart rate for the patient during cardiovascular exercise?

1. 93 beats per minute
2. **135 beats per minute**
3. 169 beats per minute
4. 195 beats per minute

> **Correct Answer: 2** (American College of Sports Medicine p. 455)

The target heart rate for exercise can be approximated using a percentage of the maximum heart rate, which can be estimated as 220 − age. With this approach, 70-85% of maximum heart rate or 50-70% of maximum oxygen uptake (VO_{2max}) is the recommended exercise intensity according to the American College of Sports Medicine. If the maximal heart rate is 175 beats per minute, the target heart rate range is (70% x 175) to (85% x 175), or 123 to 149 beats per minute. Some sources recommend a more broadly defined target heart rate range of 60-90%. In either case, the correct answer would be option 2.

1. 93 beats per minute is below the recommended range for exercise intensity. 93 beats per minute corresponds to 53% of the maximum heart rate.
2. **135 beats per minute is within the recommended range for exercise intensity. 135 beats per minute corresponds to 77% of the maximum heart rate.**
3. 169 beats per minute is above the recommended range for exercise intensity. 169 beats per minute corresponds to 97% of the maximum heart rate.
4. 195 beats per minute is above the recommended range for exercise intensity. 195 beats per minute corresponds to 111% of the maximum heart rate.

System Specific: Cardiac, Vascular, & Pulmonary Systems
Content Outline: Interventions

Exam Three: Question 25

A patient with complete C5 tetraplegia works on a forward raise for pressure relief. The patient utilizes loops that are attached to the back of the wheelchair to assist with the forward raise. Which muscles need to be particularly strong in order for the patient to be successful with the forward raise?

1. brachioradialis, brachialis
2. rhomboids, levator scapulae
3. **biceps, deltoids**
4. triceps, flexor digitorum profundus

> **Correct Answer: 3** (Rothstein p. 404)

A patient with C5 tetraplegia would not have muscles innervated below the C5 level. Primary innervations and actions for each of the muscles are listed.

1. The brachioradialis (C5-C6) and brachialis (C5-C6) would both be innervated. The primary action of the brachioradialis and brachialis is to flex the elbow.
2. The rhomboids (C4-C5) and levator scapulae (C3-C5) would both be innervated. The rhomboids adduct and rotate the scapula downward. The levator scapulae elevate and rotate the scapula downward.
3. **The biceps (C5-C6) and deltoids (C5-C6) would both be innervated. The deltoids (anterior, middle, posterior) assist with all shoulder motions with the exception of adduction. The biceps act to flex the shoulder, flex the elbow, and supinate the forearm.**
4. The triceps (C7-C8) and flexor digitorum profundus (C8-T1) would not be innervated in a patient with C5 tetraplegia.

System Specific: Neuromuscular & Nervous Systems
Content Outline: Clinical Application of Foundational Sciences

Exam Three: Question 26

A patient sustained a fracture of the acetabulum that was treated with open reduction and internal fixation. The injury occurred in a motor vehicle accident approximately seven weeks ago. Which objective measure would be the MOST influential variable when determining the patient's weight bearing status?

1. visual analogue pain scale rating
2. **radiographic confirmation of bone healing**
3. lower extremity manual muscle testing
4. balance and coordination assessment

> **Correct Answer: 2** (Brotzman p. 147)

The primary determinant of weight bearing status following a fracture is based on the relative stability of the fracture. The amount of time since the injury (i.e., seven weeks) should allow for bone healing to be visible using diagnostic imaging.

1. The pain level following a fracture is not directly correlated with the relative stability of the acetabulum.
2. **An X-ray is a radiographic photograph commonly used to assist with the diagnosis of musculoskeletal problems such as fractures, dislocations, and bone loss. The diagnostic tool provides the physician with the best indicator of the relative stability of the fracture and therefore would be the most influential variable when determining weight bearing status.**
3. A manual muscle test would assess the relative strength of selected muscles, but would not provide information on the relative stability of the fracture.
4. A balance and coordination assessment may be useful when determining an appropriate assistive device or the level of assistance needed, however, this is not directly related to the relative stability of the fracture.

System Specific: Musculoskeletal System
Content Outline: Foundations for Evaluation, Differential Diagnosis, & Prognosis

Exam Three: Question 27

A patient two weeks status post transtibial amputation is instructed by his physician to remain at rest for two days after contracting bronchitis. The MOST appropriate position for the patient in bed is:

1. supine with a pillow under the patient's knees
2. supine with a pillow under the patient's thighs and knees
3. **supine with the legs extended**
4. sidelying in the fetal position

> **Correct Answer: 3** (Seymour p. 145)

It is important for a patient with a transtibial amputation to keep the knee extended in order to prevent shortening of the hamstrings muscles and avoid developing a flexion contracture at the knee.

1. Lying in supine with a pillow under the knees is a comfortable position for the patient after transtibial amputation. However, placing a pillow under the knee puts the knee in a partially flexed position. This promotes the development of hamstrings muscle tightness, which may lead to a flexion contracture at the knee.
2. Lying in supine with a pillow under the thighs puts the hip and knee in a flexed position. This promotes the development of hip flexor and hamstrings muscle tightness, which may lead to flexion contractures at the hip or knee.
3. **The supine position with the legs extended is the most appropriate position since it promotes lengthening of the hip flexors and hamstrings muscles and prevents the development of flexion contractures.**
4. Sidelying in the fetal position places the hips and knees in a flexed position. This promotes the development of hip flexor and hamstrings muscle tightness, which may lead to flexion contractures at the hip or knee.

System Specific: Other Systems
Content Outline: Interventions

Exam Three: Question 28

A physical therapist tests a small area of skin for hypersensitivity prior to using a cold immersion bath. The patient begins to demonstrate evidence of cold intolerance within 60 seconds after cold application. The MOST appropriate response is to:

1. limit cold exposure to ten minutes or less
2. select an alternate cryotherapeutic agent
3. continue with the cold immersion bath
4. **discontinue cold application and document the findings**

> **Correct Answer: 4** (Cameron p. 140)

Signs of cold intolerance include pain, cyanosis, wheals, mottling, increased pulse rate, and a significant drop in blood pressure.

1. Limiting cold exposure to ten minutes or less would still place the patient at significant risk for an adverse reaction to the cold since the patient exhibited evidence of cold intolerance in 60 seconds.
2. Selecting an alternate cryotherapeutic agent would minimally decrease the likelihood of cold intolerance since the magnitude of tissue cooling is relatively uniform across different cryotherapeutic agents.
3. Continuing with the cold immersion bath after observing evidence of cold intolerance would place the patient at significant risk for experiencing a more severe reaction to the cold.
4. **A physical therapist should immediately stop the application of cold when any sign of cold intolerance is observed.**

System Specific: Non-Systems
Content Outline: Equipment & Devices; Therapeutic Modalities

Exam Three: Question 29

A 27-year-old female diagnosed with anterior compartment syndrome reports to an outpatient clinic for physical therapy services. While reviewing the physician referral supplied by the patient, the physical therapist identifies that the referral form is over 90 days old. The MOST appropriate therapist action is:

1. continue with the session since the existing referral is acceptable
2. **attempt to contact the physician's office by telephone to receive verbal orders**
3. send the physician written correspondence requesting an updated referral
4. discontinue the session until the patient secures an updated referral

Correct Answer: 2 (Nosse p. 217)

Physical therapists should attempt to ensure that physician referrals are as current as possible. This action is a risk management strategy that increases the probability of patients being appropriate candidates for physical therapy services.

1. Ninety days is a significant amount of time and it is possible that the patient's health status or another relevant variable has changed during this period.
2. **Contacting the physician's office by telephone provides the fastest, most direct method to update the referral without further delaying treatment. Relying on a verbal order would not be problematic in this case since the physical therapist already has the original referral.**
3. Sending the physician written correspondence requesting an updated referral would unnecessarily delay physical therapy services.
4. Discontinuing the session until the patient secures an updated referral would delay physical therapy services. The option places the burden for retrieving the referral on the patient and although this is acceptable, the task could likely be handled without difficulty by the physical therapist or the office staff.

System Specific: Non-Systems
Content Outline: Safety & Professional Roles; Teaching/Learning; Research

Exam Three: Question 30

A physical therapist assesses the deep tendon reflexes of a patient as part of a lower quarter screening examination. The therapist determines that the right and left patellar tendon reflex and the left Achilles tendon reflex are 2+, while the right Achilles tendon reflex is absent. The clinical condition that could BEST explain this finding is:

1. cerebral palsy
2. multiple sclerosis
3. **peripheral neuropathy**
4. intermittent claudication

Correct Answer: 3 (Goodman – Differential Diagnosis p. 746)

A reflex is a motor response to a sensory stimulation that can be used to assess the integrity of the nervous system. Deep tendon reflexes (DTR) elicit a muscle contraction when the muscle's tendon is stimulated. A grade of 2+ would be considered a normal response.

1. Cerebral palsy is a neuromuscular disorder of posture and controlled movement, however, the clinical presentation is highly variable based on the area and extent of central nervous system damage. It is unlikely that a reflex would be absent in an upper motor neuron disorder like cerebral palsy.
2. Multiple sclerosis is a chronic autoimmune inflammatory disease of the central nervous system characterized by demyelination of the myelin sheaths that surround nerves within the brain and spinal cord. Symptoms can include visual problems, paresthesias and sensory changes, clumsiness, weakness, ataxia, balance dysfunction, and fatigue. Deep tendon reflexes would not typically be absent with multiple sclerosis since it is an upper motor neuron disorder.
3. **Peripheral neuropathy is a broad term that describes a lesion to a peripheral nerve. Patients with peripheral neuropathy may exhibit motor, sensory, and autonomic changes including extreme sensitivity to touch, loss of sensation, muscle weakness, and loss of vasomotor tone. Deep tendon reflexes may be asymmetrical based on the location of the involved peripheral nerve and usually present as diminished or absent.**
4. Intermittent claudication occurs as a result of insufficient blood supply and ischemia in active muscles. Symptoms most commonly include pain and cramping in muscles distal to the occluded vessel. Deep tendon reflexes would not typically be affected.

System Specific: Neuromuscular & Nervous Systems
Content Outline: Foundations for Evaluation, Differential Diagnosis, & Prognosis

Exam Three: Question 41

A physical therapist employed in a work hardening program performs an examination on a patient diagnosed with fibromyalgia. During the examination the therapist identifies an inconsistency between the measured lumbar range of motion and the amount of lumbar range of motion observed while lifting a milk crate from the floor to a table. The MOST appropriate therapist action is:

1. **avoid discussing the identified inconsistency with the patient**
2. confront the patient with the identified inconsistency
3. discuss the identified inconsistency with the referring physician
4. discharge the patient from physical therapy

> **Correct Answer: 1** (O'Sullivan p. 1127)

Symptom magnification is best identified by inconsistencies in the presentation of function. Physical therapists should be extremely cautious to avoid labeling patients as "symptom magnifiers" or "malingerers" without adequate evidence to support their hypothesis.

1. **There is not enough information presented to form a definitive conclusion and therefore the physical therapist should not address the observation with the patient. The therapist would be better served by continuing the examination and gathering additional information during future treatment sessions.**
2. The physical therapist has identified a given inconsistency, however, it would be inappropriate to immediately confront the patient based on a single observation.
3. There are a variety of legitimate reasons why a physical therapist could observe an inconsistency such as the described scenario. As a result, the finding does not warrant consultation with the physician.
4. There is not any presented information that would suggest the patient is not a candidate for physical therapy.

System Specific: Non-Systems
Content Outline: Safety & Professional Roles; Teaching/Learning; Research

Exam Three: Question 42

A former patient calls to ask for advice after injuring his low back in a work related accident. The patient explains that he cannot bend down and touch his toes without severe pain and has muscle spasms throughout the entire low back. The physical therapist works in a state without direct access, but would like to help the former patient. The MOST appropriate response would be:

1. explain to the patient that you would be happy to treat him, however, since you have not completed a formal examination it would be unfair to prescribe treatment
2. arrange a time for the patient to come into your clinic for immediate treatment
3. prescribe flexion exercises and ice every three hours
4. **refer the patient to a qualified physician**

> **Correct Answer: 4** (Guide for Professional Conduct)

The *Guide for Professional Conduct* published by the American Physical Therapy Association states: "A physical therapist shall make professional judgments that are in the patient/client's best interests."

1. The physical therapist correctly recognizes that the patient cannot be treated without a formal examination, however, needs to also consider that the patient was hurt in a work related accident and works in a state without direct access.
2. Arranging a time for treatment without first completing an examination is inappropriate.
3. Prescribing exercises of any type without adequate clinical justification can be considered a negligent act.
4. **Referring the patient to a physician will allow the patient to receive a thorough examination, and if indicated, a referral to physical therapy.**

System Specific: Non-Systems
Content Outline: Safety & Professional Roles; Teaching/Learning; Research

Exam Three: Question 39

A patient rehabilitating from congestive heart failure is examined in physical therapy. During the examination the patient begins to complain of pain. The MOST IMMEDIATE physical therapist action is to:

1. notify the nursing staff to administer pain medication
2. contact the referring physician
3. discontinue the treatment session
4. **ask the patient to describe the location and severity of the pain**

> **Correct Answer: 4** (Magee p. 5)

Congestive heart failure is characterized by the inability of the heart to maintain adequate cardiac output. Before the physical therapist can adequately respond to the patient's report of pain, it is essential to gather additional information.

1. Administering pain medication is premature until more information is known about the pain. Once additional information is collected, the nursing staff will be able to make a more informed decision.
2. Contacting the physician is premature until more information is known about the location and severity of the pain. This type of detailed information is necessary to provide the physician with a better sense of what the patient is currently experiencing.
3. Discontinuing the treatment session based on a subjective report of pain is a viable option particularly given the patient's diagnosis, however, the physical therapist would need to gather additional information about the pain prior to making a definitive decision.
4. **Having the patient describe the location and severity of the pain is the most immediate action the physical therapist should take. The information can be collected in a timely manner and may be useful to determine the relative seriousness of the patient's subjective report of pain.**

System Specific: Other Systems
Content Outline: Examination

Exam Three: Question 40

A physical therapist reviews the medical record of a patient diagnosed with chronic obstructive pulmonary disease. The medical record indicates that the patient's current condition is consistent with chronic respiratory acidosis. Which testing procedure was likely used to identify this condition?

1. **arterial blood gas analysis**
2. pulmonary function testing
3. graded exercise testing
4. pulse oximetry

> **Correct Answer: 1** (Paz p. 60)

Arterial blood gas analysis (ABG) provides information on the functioning of the lungs (i.e., oxygenation and elimination of carbon dioxide). Respiratory acidosis is characterized by elevated $PaCO_2$ and below normal pH due to hypoventilation.

1. **Abnormal acid-base balance will result in respiratory alkalosis, respiratory acidosis, metabolic alkalosis or metabolic acidosis depending on the cause. These conditions can become life threatening without intervention to normalize the pH within the body, which is typically 7.35-7.45. ABG analysis provides values for $PaCO_2$, PaO_2, O_2 saturation, and CO_2.**
2. Pulmonary function testing is a series of measurements that measure and evaluate how well the lungs take in and release air and how well they move oxygen into and remove carbon dioxide from the blood. There are reference values based on height, weight, sex, and age and results are considered abnormal if they are not within 80% of these reference values for a given test.
3. Graded exercise testing is used to measure the response of the heart to a graded increase in oxygen demand. Exercise occurs using a systematic protocol that can assess other variables such as evaluation of arrhythmias, functional capacity, and significance of coronary artery disease.
4. An oximeter is a photoelectric device used to determine the oxygen saturation of blood. The device is most commonly applied to the finger or the ear. Oximetry is often used by therapists to assess activity tolerance.

System Specific: Cardiac, Vascular, & Pulmonary Systems
Content Outline: Foundations for Evaluation, Differential Diagnosis, & Prognosis

Exam Three: Question 37

During a balance assessment of a patient with left hemiplegia, it is noted that in sitting the patient requires minimal assistance to maintain the position and cannot accept any additional challenge. The physical therapist would appropriately document the patient's sitting balance as:

1. normal
2. good
3. fair
4. **poor**

Correct Answer: 4 (O'Sullivan p. 254)

Sitting balance can be graded in an objective manner by using a scale that ranges from poor to normal. A patient that requires assistance to maintain a sitting position would be graded as having poor sitting balance.

1. A grade of normal is indicative of a person that is able to sit unsupported, move in and out of the base of support, and accept maximal challenge without loss of balance.
2. A grade of good is indicative of a person that is able to sit unsupported, move in and out of the base of support, and accept some challenge without loss of balance.
3. A grade of fair is indicative of a person that is able to maintain their balance in sitting unsupported, but cannot accept any challenge or go outside of their base of support without loss of balance.
4. **A grade of poor is indicative of a person that is unable to maintain their balance in sitting without external support or assistance.**

System Specific: Neuromuscular & Nervous Systems
Content Outline: Examination

Exam Three: Question 38

A physical therapist is treating a patient with a head injury who begins to perseverate. In order to refocus the patient and achieve the desired therapeutic outcome, the therapist should:

1. focus on the topic of perseveration for a short period of time in order to appease the patient
2. **guide the patient into an interesting new activity and reward successful completion of the task**
3. take the patient back to his room for quiet time and attempt to resume therapy once he has stopped perseverating
4. continue with repetitive verbal cues to cease perseveration

Correct Answer: 2 (O'Sullivan p. 723)

Perseveration is the continued repetition of a word, phrase or movement. Initiating a new activity during therapy may allow the patient to redirect attention and subsequently receive positive reinforcement for attending to the selected task.

1. It is not necessary to attempt to appease the patient since the patient cannot independently move beyond whatever they are perseverating on. Staying with the topic will not assist in moving forward.
2. **Patients with a lesion in the premotor or prefrontal cortex often exhibit perseveration. Since the patient typically continues the repetition of a word, phrase or movement after the cessation of the original stimulus, the best intervention would be to redirect the patient away from the current activity.**
3. The patient will not benefit from "quiet time" since the patient is not perseverating due to a behavioral issue. Redirecting the patient may successfully allow the patient to move forward and continue with therapy without interruption.
4. Verbal cueing is not an effective technique to cease perseveration. The patient typically requires a redirection of their attention to another activity or environment.

System Specific: Neuromuscular & Nervous Systems
Content Outline: Interventions

Exam Three: Question 35

The goals for a patient status post total knee arthroplasty include general conditioning and independent household mobility. Which component of the patient's treatment would be the MOST appropriate to delegate to a physical therapy aide?

1. stair training
2. progressive gait training with a straight cane
3. patient education regarding the surgical procedure
4. **ambulation with a walker for endurance**

Correct Answer: 4 (Guide to Physical Therapist Practice)

A physical therapy aide is a non-licensed worker, trained under the direction of a physical therapist, who requires continuous on-site supervision. A physical therapist is required, before delegating any component of a treatment plan, to have an understanding of the physical therapy aide's level of training as well as the patient's current abilities.

1. Stair training is a skilled activity that requires the constant supervision of a licensed physical therapist. The term "training" implies that the patient is being taught a new skill. Delegating this type of skilled activity to a physical therapy aide is inappropriate and would potentially jeopardize patient safety.

2. Progressive gait training implies that there will be some progression within the activity based on the patient's performance. The decision to progress a patient during an activity is the responsibility of the physical therapist and would be inappropriate for a physical therapy aide.

3. Patient education regarding the surgical procedure requires an individual to possess specific knowledge of the actual surgical procedure performed by the surgeon. A physical therapy aide does not possess the educational background to provide the patient with this information.

4. **A physical therapist, and in some jurisdictions a physical therapist assistant, may delegate ambulation activities to an aide if the physical therapist feels the aide's training is adequate to complete the activity. This decision would be heavily influenced by the patient's current status and competence with ambulation. Ambulation for endurance implies that the patient already possesses basic competence with the activity.**

System Specific: Non-Systems
Content Outline: Safety & Professional Roles; Teaching/Learning; Research

Exam Three: Question 36

A physical therapist examines the heart sounds of a 48-year-old female status post coronary artery bypass graft. When auscultating, the therapist identifies the heart sound associated with closing of the mitral and tricuspid valves. This heart sound BEST describes:

1. **S1**
2. S2
3. S3
4. S4

Correct Answer: 1 (Hillegass p. 122)

The heart sounds are the noises generated by the beating heart and the resultant flow of blood through it. The therapist uses a stethoscope to listen for these sounds, which provide important information about the condition of the heart.

1. **The first heart sound, S1 (the lub of the lub-dub), is associated with the closing of the mitral and tricuspid valves, corresponding to the onset of ventricular systole.**

2. The second heart sound, S2, (the dub of the lub-dub), is associated with the closing of the aortic and pulmonary valves, corresponding to the onset of ventricular diastole.

3. A third heart sound, S3, occurs early in diastole while the ventricle is rapidly filling. The sound occurs immediately after S2 (lub-dub-dub). The S3 sound may occur in healthy children and young adults, and is referred to as a physiologic third heart sound. It also indicates a loss of ventricular compliance in the presence of heart disease or heart failure. In this case, it is called a ventricular gallop.

4. A fourth heart sound, S4, occurs late in diastole just before S1 (la-lub-dub) and is associated with atrial contraction and an increased resistance to ventricular filling. The heart sound is referred to as an atrial gallop. The sound is common in patients with hypertension, a history of myocardial infarction or coronary bypass surgery.

System Specific: Cardiac, Vascular, & Pulmonary Systems
Content Outline: Clinical Application of Foundational Sciences

Exam Three: Question 33

A physical therapist attempts to palpate the tibialis posterior tendon. To facilitate palpation of this structure the therapist should:

1.   **ask the patient to invert and plantar flex the foot**
2.   ask the patient to evert and dorsifex the foot
3.   ask the patient to invert and dorsiflex the foot
4.   passively evert and plantar flex the foot

> ### Correct Answer: 1 (Kendall p. 411)

A tendon is a band of dense fibrous tissue forming the termination of a muscle which attaches the muscle to a bone. A tendon becomes more prominent when the associated muscle is active. The tendon of the tibialis posterior can be palpated posterior and inferior to the medial malleolus.

1.   **The tibialis posterior originates on the interosseous membrane, lateral portion of the posterior surface of the tibia, and proximal two thirds of the medial surface of the fibula. The muscle acts to invert the foot and assists with plantar flexion of the ankle joint. As a result, the tendon is more prominent with active inversion and plantar flexion.**
2.   Eversion and dorsiflexion are opposite of the action of the tibialis posterior. As a result, the active movement would not facilitate palpation of the muscle's tendon.
3.   The tibialis anterior acts to dorsiflex the ankle joint and assists with inversion of the foot. As a result, the tendon is more prominent with active dorsiflexion and inversion. The tendon of the muscle is easily palpated where it crosses the ankle joint to its insertion on the medial aspect of the base of the first metatarsal and the medial cuneiform bone.
4.   Passive movement would not be as desirable as active movement to facilitate palpation of the tendon since muscular activity is necessary to make the tendon prominent. In addition, the tibialis posterior inverts the foot and assists with plantar flexion of the ankle joint.

System Specific: Musculoskeletal System
Content Outline: Clinical Application of Foundational Sciences

Exam Three: Question 34

A physical therapist participating in a research project elects to use a simple random sample to draw a sample from the population. By selecting this type of sample, the researcher ensures:

1.   the data collected from the sample will be normally distributed
2.   the sample size will be large
3.   the sample will have proportional representation from all parts of the population
4.   **that every member of the population has an equal opportunity of being chosen**

> ### Correct Answer: 4 (Portney p. 148)

Probability samples are created through a process of random selection. Each selection is independent and every member of the population has an equal chance of being selected for the sample.

1.   Simple random sampling does not ensure that the data collected will be normally distributed. The shape of the distribution of the data collected from the sample is independent of the type of sample.
2.   Simple random sampling does not determine the size of the sample.
3.   To ensure that the sample will have proportional representation from all parts of the population, the therapist would create a proportional stratified sample.
4.   **A simple random sample is unbiased; each member of the population has an equal chance of being chosen.**

System Specific: Non-Systems
Content Outline: Safety & Professional Roles; Teaching/Learning; Research

Exam Three: Question 31

An employee with a disclosed disability informs her employer that she is unable to perform an essential function of her job unless her workstation is modified. Which of the following would provide the employer with a legitimate reason for NOT granting the employee's request?

1. the accommodation would cost hundreds of dollars
2. the accommodation would require an expansion of the employee's present workstation
3. **the accommodation would fundamentally alter the operation of the business**
4. the accommodation would not address the needs of other employees

Correct Answer: 3 (Pierson p. 349)

The Americans with Disabilities Act was designed to provide a clear and comprehensive national mandate for the elimination of discrimination. Employers are required to make reasonable accommodations for qualified individuals with a disability who satisfy the job-related requirements of a position held or desired.

1. An accommodation that costs hundreds of dollars does not necessarily indicate that the accommodation is unreasonable or creates an "undue hardship" for the employer.
2. Workstation modifications are common and are most often designed to allow a qualified employee or applicant to perform an essential job function.
3. **An accommodation that fundamentally alters the operation of a business would be considered an "undue hardship."**
4. The Americans with Disabilities Act applies primarily, but not exclusively, to "disabled" individuals. It is not necessary to ensure that an accommodation made for a qualified individual addresses the needs of other employees.

System Specific: Non-Systems
Content Outline: Safety & Professional Roles; Teaching/Learning; Research

Exam Three: Question 32

A group of health care professionals participates in a family conference for a patient with a spinal cord injury. During the conference one of the participants summarizes the patient's progress with bathing and dressing activities. This type of information is typically conveyed by a/an:

1. nurse
2. physical therapist
3. **occupational therapist**
4. case manager

Correct Answer: 3 (Van Deusen p. 303)

Physical therapists work closely with a large number of health care providers in a variety of settings. Roles and responsibilities may vary slightly in different practice settings and in different states due to established state practice acts.

1. Nurses work to promote health, prevent disease, and help patients cope with illness. Patient care activities are extremely diverse including tasks such as assisting physicians during treatments and examinations, administering medications, recording symptoms and reactions, and instructing patients and families.
2. Physical therapists provide services to help restore function, improve mobility, relieve pain, and prevent or limit permanent physical disabilities of patients suffering from injuries or disease. Physical therapists engage in examination, evaluation, diagnosis, prognosis, and intervention in an effort to maximize patient outcomes.
3. **Occupational therapists help people improve their ability to perform activities of daily living, work, and leisure skills. Occupational therapists most commonly work with individuals who have conditions that are mentally, physically, developmentally or emotionally disabling.**
4. Case managers coordinate health care services appropriate to achieve established rehabilitation goals. Work activities include implementing and coordinating a medical care plan with health care providers and the patient.

System Specific: Non-Systems
Content Outline: Safety & Professional Roles; Teaching/Learning; Research

Test Taking Tip: Candidates must remember that the National Physical Therapy Examination is a national examination that is not specifically influenced by the rules or regulations of a given state. When answering examination questions, candidates must carefully consider national standards which are often heavily influenced by positions of the American Physical Therapy Association or other professional associations. By remembering this important concept, candidates will be able to make informed decisions when answering questions related to this theme.

Exam Three: Question 43

A physical therapist treats a patient with superficial partial-thickness burns to the anterior surface of his lower legs. In an attempt to assist the patient to control the pain associated with the burns, the therapist rewards the patient with a lengthy rest period after successfully completing an exercise sequence. This type of psychological approach is MOST representative of:

1. distraction
2. extinction
3. classical conditioning
4. **operant conditioning**

Correct Answer: 4 (Richard p. 486)

Physical therapists often use specific teaching and learning strategies to influence or shape patient behavior. Many of the most common strategies employed are derived from the field of educational psychology. Physical therapists should be familiar with commonly used teaching and learning strategies and recognize opportunities to integrate them into patient care activities.

1. Distraction is a general term that refers to something that diverts attention.
2. Extinction refers to removing selected variables that reinforce a specific behavior. It can also refer to the lack of any consequence following a behavior. The theory is that when a behavior is inconsequential, producing neither favorable nor unfavorable consequences, it will occur with less frequency.
3. Classical conditioning is a process where learning occurs when an unconditioned stimulus is repeatedly preceded by a neutral stimulus. The neutral stimulus serves as a conditioned stimulus and the learned reaction that results is termed the conditioned response.
4. **Operant conditioning is learning that takes place when the learner recognizes the connection between the behavior (completing an exercise progression) and its consequences (lengthy rest period).**

System Specific: Non-Systems
Content Outline: Safety & Professional Roles; Teaching/Learning; Research

Exam Three: Question 44

A physical therapist reviews a research study that examines knee flexion range of motion two weeks following arthroscopic surgery. Assuming knee flexion range of motion two weeks after arthroscopic surgery is a normally distributed variable, what percentage of patients in the population would achieve a goniometric measurement value between the mean and one standard deviation above the mean?

1. 14%
2. **34%**
3. 48%
4. 68%

Correct Answer: 2 (Portney p. 399)

Because of the standard properties of the normal distribution, it is possible to determine the proportional areas under the curve represented by the standard deviation. 34.13% of the area under the curve of a normal distribution is bounded by the mean and 1 standard deviation above or below the mean.

1. 14% is the approximate area under the normal curve between 1 and 2 standard deviations above or below the mean.
2. **34% is the approximate area under the normal curve bounded by 1 standard deviation above or below the mean.**
3. 48% is the approximate area under the normal curve bounded by 2 standard deviations above or below the mean.
4. 68% is the approximate area under the normal curve bounded by 1 standard deviation below the mean and 1 standard deviation above the mean.

System Specific: Non-Systems
Content Outline: Safety & Professional Roles; Teaching/Learning; Research

Exam Three: Question 45

A physical therapist uses intermittent compression to treat a patient with an acute ankle sprain. The patient is positioned in supine with the leg elevated on a 40 degree wedge. The therapist uses an inflation pressure of 50 mm Hg with an on:off time of 40 seconds on and 20 seconds off. The treatment time is scheduled for 20 minutes. After five minutes of treatment the patient reports some discomfort in the ankle. The MOST appropriate modification to the current treatment parameters would be:

1. increase the inflation pressure
2. **increase the off time**
3. increase the total treatment time
4. increase the elevation of the leg

Correct Answer: 2 (Prentice - Therapeutic Modalities p. 489)

Intermittent compression is often used in combination with elevation to limit edema following an acute ankle sprain. The physical therapist should modify the parameters of the intervention based on relevant subjective data such as a report of discomfort.

1. Increasing the inflation pressure would likely serve to exacerbate the patient's pain level.
2. **Increasing the off time greater than the current 20 second interval would provide the patient with a greater rest period and may therefore decrease the patient's discomfort.**
3. Increasing the total treatment time without modifying other parameters (e.g., on:off time, inflation pressure) would likely result in the level of discomfort remaining the same or worsening as the session continues.
4. Increasing the elevation of the leg beyond 40 degrees would not likely decrease the patient's discomfort without concurrently decreasing another treatment parameter.

System Specific: Non-Systems
Content Outline: Equipment & Devices; Therapeutic Modalities

Exam Three: Question 46

A physical therapist examines the electrocardiogram of a patient during exercise. What change in the electrocardiogram would be most indicative of myocardial ischemia?

1. P wave changes
2. PR interval changes
3. QRS complex changes
4. **ST segment changes**

Correct Answer: 4 (Brannon p. 183)

ST segment depression is the most common manifestation of exercise-induced myocardial ischemia.

1. The P wave is normally the first wave of the ECG tracing and represents depolarization of the atria. Normally, the P wave is upright, rounded, and symmetric with only one P wave for each QRS complex. Abnormal configuration of P waves occurs in various conditions including wandering atrial pacemaker, premature atrial complexes, atrial tachycardia, atrial fibrillation, atrial flutter, and nodal or junctional arrhythmias.
2. The PR interval represents the time (in seconds) from the beginning of the P wave (onset of atrial depolarization) to the beginning of the QRS complex (onset of ventricular depolarization). The normal PR interval duration range is from 0.12 seconds - 0.20 seconds, measured from the initial deflection of the P wave to the initial deflection of the QRS complex. A prolonged PR interval can correspond to impaired AV node conduction and results in various types of heart block.
3. The QRS complex represents depolarization of the ventricles. Abnormal configuration of the QRS complex occurs in various conditions including premature ventricular contractions, ventricular tachycardia, and ventricular fibrillation.
4. **The ST segment is the portion of the ECG tracing from the end of the S wave to the beginning of the T wave. It represents the initiating of ventricular repolarization and is a sensitive indicator of ischemia of the ventricles. The standard criterion for a positive exercise test is greater than or equal to 1 mm of horizontal or downsloping ST segment depression.**

System Specific: Cardiac, Vascular, & Pulmonary Systems
Content Outline: Foundations for Evaluation, Differential Diagnosis, & Prognosis

Exam Three: Question 47

A physical therapist treats a patient diagnosed with chronic arterial disease. The patient exhibits cool skin, decreased sensitivity to temperature changes, and intermittent claudication with activity. The primary treatment goal is to increase the patient's ambulation distance. The MOST appropriate ambulation parameters to facilitate achievement of the goal are:

1. **short duration, frequent intervals**
2. short duration, infrequent intervals
3. long duration, frequent intervals
4. long duration, infrequent intervals

> **Correct Answer: 1** (Kisner p. 830)

Intermittent claudication occurs as a result of insufficient blood supply and ischemia in active muscles. The condition occurs with activity, subsides during periods of rest, and as a result can limit the duration of exercise activities. Symptoms most commonly include pain and cramping in muscles distal to the occluded vessel.

1. **Treadmill and track walking are the most effective modes of exercise to reduce claudication. The initial workloads are set to elicit claudication symptoms within three to five minutes. This is followed by a period of standing or sitting to allow symptoms to resolve. The exercise-rest-exercise pattern is repeated throughout the exercise session. Because of the short duration of each bout of exercise before the onset of symptoms, more frequent exercise bouts are indicated.**

2. Because the patient can only exercise for shorter durations before the onset of symptoms, exercising at infrequent intervals would not allow the patient to progress toward the goal of increasing ambulation distance.

3. Patients who experience claudication from chronic arterial disease usually can only walk for short periods before the onset of pain limits their ability to continue exercise. Therefore, long duration of exercise with frequent intervals is not a realistic plan to progress toward the goal of increasing ambulation distance.

4. Although the infrequent intervals may provide the patient with less total activity, the long duration of the exercise remains problematic.

System Specific: Other Systems
Content Outline: Interventions

Exam Three: Question 48

A patient rehabilitating from a bone marrow transplant is referred to physical therapy for instruction in an exercise program. The physical therapist plans to use oxygen saturation measurements to gain additional objective data related to the patient's exercise tolerance. Assuming the patient's oxygen saturation was measured as 95% at rest, which of the following guidelines would be the MOST appropriate?

1. discontinue exercise when the patient's oxygen saturation is below 95%
2. **discontinue exercise when the patient's oxygen saturation is below 90%**
3. discontinue exercise when the patient's oxygen saturation is below 85%
4. discontinue exercise when the patient's oxygen saturation is below 80%

> **Correct Answer: 2** (Paz p. 441)

An oxygen saturation at rest greater than 95% is considered to be within normal limits. A rate of 90% or less is often used as a guideline to discontinue exercise activities. Supplemental oxygen may be indicated if oxygen saturation is 90% or less.

1. An oxygen saturation of 95% is within normal limits.

2. **When oxygen saturation falls below 90% exercise should be discontinued and the patient should rest. This corresponds to a partial pressure of oxygen (PaO_2) of approximately 60 mm Hg, which represents a state of arterial hypoxemia. This is the most common indication for supplemental oxygen therapy.**

3. A patient with an oxygen saturation of 85% is in a state of hypoxemia. Exercise should have been terminated before this level of hypoxemia was reached.

4. A patient with an oxygen saturation of 80% is in a severe hypoxemic state. Exercise should have been terminated before this level of hypoxemia was reached.

System Specific: Other Systems
Content Outline: Interventions

Exam Three: Question 49

A physical therapist reviews a patient's medical history prior to administering intermittent compression. Which of the following conditions would be considered a contraindication to the use of this mechanical device?

1. venous stasis ulcer
2. **acute pulmonary edema**
3. intermittent claudication
4. lymphedema

Correct Answer: 2 (Prentice - Therapeutic Modalities p. 496)

Intermittent compression is effective in controlling edema since it increases the extravascular hydrostatic pressure and circulation. Intermittent compression is most commonly used to control edema due to venous insufficiency or lymphatic dysfunction.

1. Venous stasis ulcers occur secondary to inadequate functioning of the venous system resulting in inadequate circulation and eventual tissue damage and ulceration. Intermittent compression improves venous circulation and facilitates the healing of previously formed ulcers.
2. **Acute pulmonary edema should not be treated with intermittent compression since the shift of fluid from the peripheral to the central circulation may significantly increase stress on the heart.**
3. Intermittent claudication occurs when blood flow is not adequate to meet the demand of the peripheral tissue, most often during activity. The result is ischemia which produces symptoms such as muscle pain, numbness, tingling, and fatigue. Intermittent claudication would not be a contraindication for intermittent compression.
4. Lymphedema refers to an abnormal accumulation of tissue fluid in the interstitial spaces. Stagnation of the tissue fluid promotes the inflammatory response and increases the probability of infection. Intermittent compression is commonly used to treat lymphedema.

System Specific: Non-Systems
Content Outline: Equipment & Devices; Therapeutic Modalities

Exam Three: Question 50

A 62-year-old female is restricted from physical therapy for two days following surgical insertion of a urinary catheter. This type of procedure is MOST commonly performed with a:

1. condom catheter
2. Foley catheter
3. **suprapubic catheter**
4. Swan-Ganz catheter

Correct Answer: 3 (Pierson p. 290)

An internal or indwelling catheter is inserted through the urethra and into the bladder. Females can utilize internal catheters, while males can use internal or external catheters.

1. An external catheter is applied over the shaft of the penis and is held in place by a padded strap or adhesive tape. The catheter has no practical application for females.
2. A Foley catheter is an indwelling urinary tract catheter that has a balloon attachment at one end. The balloon, which is filled with air or sterile water, must be deflated before the catheter can be removed. The catheter does not require surgical insertion.
3. **A suprapubic catheter is an indwelling urinary catheter that is surgically inserted directly into the patient's bladder. Insertion of a suprapubic catheter is performed under general anesthesia.**
4. A Swan-Ganz catheter is a soft, flexible catheter that is inserted through a vein into the pulmonary artery. The device is used to provide continuous measurements of pulmonary artery pressure.

System Specific: Other Systems
Content Outline: Foundations for Evaluation, Differential Diagnosis, & Prognosis

Exam Three: Question 51

A physical therapist attempts to auscultate over the aortic valve. Which of the following areas is the MOST appropriate to isolate the desired valve?

1. second left intercostal space at the left sternal border
2. **second right intercostal space at the right sternal border**
3. fourth left intercostal space along the lower left sternal border
4. fifth left intercostal space at the midclavicular line

> **Correct Answer: 2** (Rothstein p. 504)

Auscultation of the heart requires selective listening for each component of the cardiac cycle over the main topographic areas for auscultation.

1. The second left intercostal space at the left sternal border denotes the pulmonary area and is best for auscultating the pulmonary valve.
2. **The second right intercostal space at the right sternal border denotes the aortic area and is best for auscultating the aortic valve.**
3. The fourth left intercostal space along the lower left sternal border denotes the tricuspid area and is best for auscultating the tricuspid valve.
4. The fifth left intercostal space at the midclavicular line denotes the mitral area or apex of the heart and is best for auscultating the mitral valve.

System Specific: Cardiac, Vascular, & Pulmonary Systems
Content Outline: Clinical Application of Foundational Sciences

Exam Three: Question 52

A physical therapist attempts to estimate the energy expenditure in calories for a patient performing a selected activity for 15 minutes. Assuming the therapist has a metabolic equivalent value for the activity, what other variables are necessary in order to obtain an estimate of the patient's energy expenditure?

1. patient's height
2. **patient's body weight**
3. patient's stroke volume
4. patient's residual volume

> **Correct Answer: 2** (Rothstein p. 540)

To estimate the energy expended (calories) of an activity, it is necessary to know the patient's body weight (kg) and the metabolic equivalent (MET) value of the activity.

1. Height is not needed to estimate the energy expenditure of an activity. Height and weight are needed to calculate body mass index.
2. **A metabolic equivalent (MET) is a measure of oxygen consumption, 1 MET = 3.5 mL O_2 per kg of body weight per minute. Therefore, the caloric expenditure of any activity can be estimated using the number of METs for the activity, the body weight (kg), and the duration of the activity.**
3. Stroke volume is the volume of blood ejected from the ventricles with each contraction. Stroke volume is not needed to estimate the energy expenditure of an activity. Stroke volume and heart rate are needed to calculate cardiac output.
4. Residual volume is the volume of air that remains in the lungs after a maximum forced exhalation. Residual volume is not needed to estimate the energy expenditure of an activity.

System Specific: Cardiac, Vascular, & Pulmonary Systems
Content Outline: Examination

Exam Three: Question 53

A patient in a work hardening program completes a training program consisting of ten different exercises requiring upper and lower extremity strength and endurance. The patient indicates that he is frustrated since he has been unable to increase the weight on a selected carrying activity in over two weeks. The MOST appropriate physical therapist action is:

1. provide the patient with verbal encouragement
2. attempt to substitute a different exercise for the carrying activity
3. **vary the order of the exercises**
4. decrease the number of repetitions

> **Correct Answer: 3** (Prentice – Techniques p. 379)

Physical therapists must be able to modify existing training programs based on the rate of patient progress and the stated therapeutic objectives.

1. Verbal encouragement is desirable, however, given the two week time frame it is likely that an attempt to modify the program would be more appropriate.

2. The described scenario does not provide enough evidence to indicate that the carrying activity should be discontinued. The question states only that the patient is frustrated since he has been unable to increase the weight. It would therefore be more valuable to modify the program in a manner that allows the patient to progress with the originally selected activity.

3. **Varying the order of the exercises in the program is a strategy often employed when a patient experiences a plateau. For example, by encountering the activity earlier in the program the patient may be less fatigued and able to progress.**

4. The question discusses the patient's inability to increase the weight on the carrying activity, however, it does not discuss the number of repetitions. If the therapist decreases the number of repetitions from the present level it may deemphasize the focus on endurance.

System Specific: Other Systems
Content Outline: Interventions

Exam Three: Question 54

A patient prepares for discharge from a rehabilitation hospital after completing three months of therapy. The patient has made significant progress in his rehabilitation, however, expresses concern that his previous employer may not want him to return to work due to his injury. The MOST appropriate action is to:

1. explain to the patient that to return to work after a serious injury is very difficult
2. **inform the patient of his rights according to the Americans with Disabilities Act**
3. request that the patient consider vocational retraining
4. refer the patient to a psychologist to assist with the transition back to work

> **Correct Answer: 2** (Minor p. 399)

The Americans with Disabilities Act (ADA) is federal legislation designed to eliminate discrimination against individuals with disabilities. Physical therapists have an ethical obligation to make patients aware of their rights according to the ADA.

1. A physical therapist should be empathetic and supportive about the patient's return to work, however, it is more critical to make the patient aware of their rights according to the ADA.

2. **The patient may have some of their expressed concern eliminated by learning that they have certain rights according to the ADA.**

3. The question does not provide any evidence to suggest that the patient is unable to complete their previous role at work. As a result, it would be premature to suggest vocational retraining.

4. The patient is worried that the employer may not want him to return to work, however, the question does not imply that the patient's concern has a psychological origin.

System Specific: Non-Systems
Content Outline: Safety & Professional Roles; Teaching/Learning; Research

Exam Three: Question 55

A physical therapist employed in an acute care hospital attempts to identify a standardized instrument that measures level of consciousness. The MOST appropriate standardized instrument is the:

1. **Glasgow Coma Scale**
2. Modified Rankin Scale
3. Barthel Index
4. Sickness Impact Profile

> **Correct Answer: 1** (Rothstein p. 360)

The Glasgow Coma Scale provides a practical method for assessing the degree of conscious impairment in the critically ill patient. The scale utilizes eye opening, verbal responses, and motor responses to determine the level of consciousness and degree of dysfunction.

1. **The Glasgow Coma Scale is a neurological assessment tool used initially after injury to determine arousal and cerebral cortex function. A score of eight or less correlates to a severe brain injury, a score of 9 to 12 indicates a moderate brain injury, and a score of 13 to 15 indicates a mild brain injury.**
2. The Modified Rankin Scale measures independence rather than the performance of specific tasks. The scale is a measure of disability or dependence in activities of daily living and is frequently used with patients with CVA.
3. The Barthel Index measures the patient's performance in 10 activities of daily living. It is considered a reliable disability scale for patients with CVA. Scored items relate to self-care (feeding, grooming, bathing, dressing, bowel and bladder care, and toileting) and mobility (ambulation, transfers, and stair climbing).
4. The Sickness Impact Profile is a generic measure used to evaluate the impact of disease on both physical and emotional functioning. Patients are asked to respond to the items based on their current status.

System Specific: Neuromuscular & Nervous Systems
Content Outline: Examination

Exam Three: Question 56

A physical therapist critically analyzes the methodology used in a published research study. Which type of sampling procedure would result in the GREATEST degree of sampling error?

1. simple random sample
2. systematic sample
3. **cluster sample**
4. stratified random sample

> **Correct Answer: 3** (Portney p. 152)

Cluster sampling involves successive random sampling of a series of units in the population. Cluster sampling is often utilized when a researcher is unable to know all elements in the population in advance.

1. A simple random sample is a type of probability sample where every element of the population has an equal chance of being selected for the sample.
2. A systematic sample is a type of probability sample where elements are chosen from lists of population members using specified intervals, such as every 4th element.
3. **A cluster sample is a probability sample in which large subgroups (clusters) are randomly selected first, and then smaller units are selected from the clusters. Because the technique requires two or more samples to be drawn, each sample is subject to sampling error, potentially compounding the accuracy of the final sample.**
4. A stratified random sample is a type of probability sample in which elements of the population are chosen at random from homogenous groups based on some characteristic. Organizing elements into homogenous groups before selection decreases the sampling error.

System Specific: Non-Systems
Content Outline: Safety & Professional Roles; Teaching/Learning; Research

Exam Three: Question 57

A physical therapist attempts to identify an appropriately sized wheelchair for a patient recently referred to a rehabilitation hospital. The physical therapist determines that the patient's hip width in sitting and the measurement from the back of the buttocks to the popliteal space are each 16 inches. Given these measurements, which of the following wheelchair specifications would BEST fit this patient?

1. seat width 16 inches, seat depth 14 inches
2. seat width 18 inches, seat depth 18 inches
3. seat width 16 inches, seat depth 18 inches
4. **seat width 18 inches, seat depth 14 inches**

Correct Answer: 4 (Pierson p. 135)

Seat width is determined by measuring the widest aspect of the user's buttocks, hips or thighs and adding two inches. Seat depth is measured from the user's posterior buttock, along the lateral thigh to the popliteal fold; then subtracting two inches. In the described scenario, seat width and depth should be calculated as follows: seat width = hip width (16 inches) + 2 inches = 18 inches; seat depth = posterior buttock to the popliteal space (16 inches) - 2 inches = 14 inches.

1. The described wheelchair would have inadequate seat width, however, the seat depth would be appropriate. Inadequate seat width could result in the development of a pressure sore.
2. The described wheelchair would have appropriate seat width, however, the seat depth would be excessive. Excessive seat depth could result in increased pressure in the popliteal area leading to discomfort or circulatory compromise.
3. The described wheelchair would have inadequate seat width and the seat depth would be excessive.
4. **A seat width of 18 inches and a seat depth of 14 inches are consistent with the presented formula based on the obtained measurements.**

System Specific: Non-Systems
Content Outline: Equipment & Devices; Therapeutic Modalities

Exam Three: Question 58

A physical therapist employed in an acute care hospital conducts an initial interview with a patient referred to physical therapy. During the interview, the therapist asks the patient if he feels dependent on coffee, tea or soft drinks. Which clinical scenario would MOST appropriately warrant this type of question?

1. a 27-year-old female status post arthroscopic medial meniscectomy
2. **a 42-year-old male with premature ventricular contractions**
3. a 37-year-old female with restrictive pulmonary disease
4. a 57-year-old male with respiratory alkalosis

Correct Answer: 2 (Brannon p. 206)

Premature ventricular contractions (PVCs) are premature beats arising from an ectopic focus in one of the ventricles of the heart. Coffee, tea, and soft drinks may contain caffeine, a stimulant that may precipitate premature ventricular contractions. Other causes of PVCs are nicotine, stress, alcohol, and certain electrolyte imbalances.

1. It would not be important to know if a patient who is post arthroscopic medial meniscectomy has a dependence on coffee, tea, and soft drinks, since these drinks would have no affect on their condition or course of physical therapy.
2. **It would be important to know if a patient known to have PVCs has a dependence on coffee, tea, and soft drinks since these drinks may contain caffeine, a stimulant that can precipitate PVCs. The physical therapist should inform the patient about the possible connection between these drinks and the occurrence of PVCs.**
3. It would not be important to know if a patient who has restrictive pulmonary disease has a dependence on coffee, tea, and soft drinks, since these drinks have no known affect on their condition or course of physical therapy.
4. It would not be important to know if a patient with respiratory alkalosis has a dependence on coffee, tea, and soft drinks, since these drinks would have no affect on their condition or course of physical therapy.

System Specific: Cardiac, Vascular, & Pulmonary Systems
Content Outline: Foundations for Evaluation, Differential Diagnosis, & Prognosis

Exam Three: Question 59

A physical therapist assigns a manual muscle test grade of 4 to patient A and a grade of 2 to patient B. Which of the following is the BEST interpretation of the strength of the patients?

1. patients A and B have equal strength
2. **patient A is stronger than patient B**
3. patient A is twice as strong as patient B
4. patient B is twice as strong as patient A

Correct Answer: 2 (Portney p. 68)

Manual muscle test grades are examples of ordinal measurements, which in essence represent labels specifying relative rank or position. Ordinal measurements are rank-ordered into categories that have a "greater than – less than" relationship. The intervals between ranks on an ordinal scale may not be consistent and may not be known.

1. The numerical scale used in manual muscle testing ranks the strength by strongest (equivalent to the grade of 5) and weakest (equivalent to the grade of 0). In this situation, the grades are not equal, 4 does not equal 2 therefore they cannot have equal strength.
2. **Based on the traditional 0 – 5 manual muscle grading scale, a grade of 4 represents more muscle strength than a grade of 2.**
3. The numerical scale does not provide an "absolute" value, therefore, it is impossible to say that a grade of 4 is two times stronger than a grade of 2. Furthermore, the testing positions of these grades are not the same and as a result they cannot be compared in this manner.
4. The numerical order of the manual muscle testing scale indicates that a grade of 5 is the strongest and a grade of 0 is the weakest. Therefore, a grade of 2 cannot indicate greater strength than a grade of 4.

System Specific: Non-Systems
Content Outline: Safety & Professional Roles; Teaching/Learning; Research

Exam Three: Question 60

A physical therapist inspects a patient's wound prior to applying a dressing. When documenting the findings in the medical record the therapist classifies the exudate from the wound as serous. Based on the documentation, the MOST likely color of the exudate is:

1. **clear**
2. pink
3. red
4. yellow

Correct Answer: 1 (Sussman p. 216)

It is normal during the stages of healing to observe exudate from a wound. The physical therapist should inspect the various types of exudate and determine whether it is a normal response to healing or an abnormal response that needs to be reported.

1. **Serous exudate is described as clear or light color fluid with a thin, watery consistency. This particular type of exudate is normal during the inflammatory and proliferative phases of healing.**
2. Serosanguinous (pink) exudate can be a normal exudate in a healthy healing wound.
3. Sanguinous (red) exudate indicates a bloody discharge which may be indicative of either new blood vessel growth (normal healing tissue) or a disruption of blood vessels (abnormal).
4. Purulent (yellow) exudate is generally indicative of infection.

System Specific: Integumentary System
Content Outline: Examination

Exam Three: Question 61

A patient coverage form indicates selective debridement is to be performed on a patient rehabilitating from a lower extremity burn. Based on the coverage form, the MOST likely intervention would be:

1. whirlpool
2. wet-to-dry dressings
3. **enzymatic debridement**
4. wound irrigation

Correct Answer: 3 (Sussman p. 201)

Selective debridement involves removing only nonviable tissues from a wound. Non-selective debridement involves removing both viable and nonviable tissues from a wound.

1. Whirlpool uses a turbine to produce agitation and aeration which creates movement of the water in the tank. The movement of the water results in the softening and loosening of adherent necrotic tissue. The inability to isolate necrotic tissue using whirlpool makes the intervention a form of non-selective debridement.

2. Wet-to-dry dressings refer to the application of a moistened gauze dressing placed in an area of necrotic tissue. The dressing is then allowed to dry completely and is later removed along with the necrotic tissue that has adhered to the gauze. This type of debridement should be used sparingly on wounds with both necrotic tissue and viable tissue since granulation tissue will be traumatized in the process. As a result, a wet-to-dry dressing is a form of non-selective debridement.

3. **Enzymatic debridement is considered to be selective since the topical preparation of the enzymes used (collagenolytic, proteolytic) will greatly influence the treatment outcome.**

4. Wound irrigation removes necrotic tissue from the wound bed using pressurized fluid. Most devices permit varying pressure settings and provide suction for removal of the exudate and debris. Wound irrigation is a form of non-selective debridement.

System Specific: Integumentary System
Content Outline: Interventions

Exam Three: Question 62

A physical therapist participates in a community-based screening program designed to identify individuals with osteoporosis. Which group would have the highest risk for developing osteoporosis?

1. **Caucasian females over the age of 60**
2. Black females over the age of 60
3. Caucasian females under the age of 40
4. Black females under the age of 40

Correct Answer: 1 (Goodman - Differential Diagnosis p. 504)

Osteoporosis is a metabolic bone disease characterized by increased bone resorption resulting in a reduction in bone mass. Osteoporosis is more prevalent in females than in males, in older than younger individuals, and in Caucasians than Blacks.

1. **Caucasian females experience an increased incidence of osteoporosis compared to black females. The relative risk of osteoporosis increases with age since there is decreased production of estrogen and a greater loss of bone density following menopause.**

2. Black females have an increased risk of osteoporosis with increasing age, however, this group is at less risk than Caucasian females because bone mass has a positive correlation to the color and pigmentation of the skin. Therefore, Black females generally have greater bone mass than the statistically equivalent Caucasian females.

3. Caucasian females under the age of 40 are typically not at high risk for osteoporosis. Bone mass will normally peak between 25 and 35 years of age, followed by a progressive increase in bone resorption compared to bone formation that may result, decades later, in osteopenia and osteoporosis.

4. Blacks under the age of 40 are typically not at high risk for osteoporosis. Bone mass will normally peak between 25 and 35 years of age. Bone resorption and bone formation occur in a similar manner as described in option 3.

System Specific: Other Systems
Content Outline: Foundations for Evaluation, Differential Diagnosis, & Prognosis

Exam Three: Question 63

A physical therapist positions a patient in sidelying in preparation for postural drainage activities. Which lung segment would be indicated based on the patient's position?

1. posterior basal segment of the lower lobes
2. anterior apical segment of the upper lobes
3. **lateral basal segment of the lower lobes**
4. anterior segment of the upper lobes

> **Correct Answer: 3** (Frownfelter p. 341)

When performing postural drainage, the physical therapist should position the patient so that the bronchus of the involved lung segment is perpendicular to the ground. Specific positioning for each lung segment allows gravity to assist in the drainage of the secretions.

1. Posterior basal segment of the lower lobes would require positioning in prone with a pillow under the hips with the foot of the bed elevated 18-20 inches from the floor.
2. The anterior apical segment of the upper lobes would require a seated position where the patient is leaning back at a 30 degree angle against the therapist.
3. **The lateral basal segment of the lower lobes requires positioning in sidelying with an inclination of 20 inches of the foot of the bed.**
4. The anterior segment of the upper lobes would require a supine position with a pillow under the knees.

System Specific: Cardiac, Vascular, & Pulmonary Systems
Content Outline: Interventions

Exam Three: Question 64

A patient with acute back pain is given a transcutaneous electrical nerve stimulation unit to use at home. The physical therapist provides detailed instructions on the care and use of the unit. Which of the following activities is NOT the responsibility of the patient?

1. modulate the current intensity
2. application of new electrodes
3. change the battery
4. **alter the pulse rate and width**

> **Correct Answer: 4** (Cameron p. 214)

Physical therapists routinely educate patients on how to use various portable electrical devices such as a transcutaneous electrical nerve stimulation (TENS) unit at home. Therapists must be sure that patients understand which parameters they are able to modify and which parameters should be modified by the patient.

1. Patients need to adjust the current intensity of the TENS with each use. Current intensity refers to the movement of charged particles and is most often measured in amperes.
2. Electrodes often need to be replaced during the course of treatment since they may no longer adequately adhere to the skin.
3. Changing the battery of a TENS unit is a relatively easy task that does not require changing any of the specified treatment parameters.
4. **Specific pulse rates and widths are selected by the therapist based on the TENS technique selected. Common techniques include sensory level stimulation, motor level stimulation, brief intense sensory level stimulation, and noxious level stimulation. Pulse rate and width should not be altered by the patient throughout the duration of treatment, unless specified by the therapist.**

System Specific: Non-Systems
Content Outline: Equipment & Devices; Therapeutic Modalities

Exam Three: Question 65

A patient with chronic pulmonary dysfunction is placed on a corticosteroid medication to reduce mucosal edema and inflammation. The MOST common cardiovascular side effect of corticosteroids is:

1. palpitations
2. arrhythmias
3. **increased blood pressure**
4. tachycardia

Correct Answer: 3 (Ciccone p. 378)

Increased blood pressure or hypertension is a side effect that is associated with heavy or prolonged use of corticosteroids (also known as glucocorticoids). Other side effects include osteoporosis, muscle wasting, skin breakdown, cataracts, adrenocorticosuppression, and hyperglycemia.

1. A palpitation is a sensation in which a person is aware of an irregular, hard or fast heartbeat that may skip or beat irregularly. The word palpitation is sometimes used synonymously with arrhythmia, however, a palpitation may or may not be caused by an arrhythmia. Many palpitations are benign, but the underlying cause is important to diagnose.
2. An arrhythmia is defined as a significant deviation from normal sinus rhythm. Many medications have potential side effects of arrhythmias including other cardiac medications, tricyclic antidepressants, and minerals such as calcium.
3. **Corticosteroid use can increase blood pressure secondary to the sodium and water retention properties of the corticosteroid. Long-term use of corticosteroids must be closely monitored due to the stated adverse effects.**
4. Tachycardia refers to a heart rate in excess of 100 beats per minute in an adult. It may occur normally in response to fever, exercise or excitement. Many substances have potential side effects of tachycardia including alcohol, caffeine, nicotine, and certain anti-anxiety and cardiac medications.

System Specific: Other Systems
Content Outline: Clinical Application of Foundational Sciences

Exam Three: Question 66

A physical therapist inspects a wound that has large quantities of exudate which requires frequent dressing changes. If the therapist applies a dressing that cannot handle the quantity of exudate present, the MOST likely outcome is:

1. **maceration**
2. granulation
3. epithelialization
4. infection

Correct Answer: 1 (Sussman p. 114)

Transparent film is an example of a type of dressing that would be unable to handle a significant amount of exudate. Conversely, an alginate dressing would be a better choice for a wound with a significant amount of exudate since the dressing is highly permeable and would therefore tend to absorb the exudate.

1. **Maceration refers to a softening of connective tissue fibers due to excessive moisture. The result is a loss of pigmentation and a wound that is highly susceptible to breakdown or enlargement.**
2. Granulation refers to perfused, fibrous connective tissue that replaces a fibrin clot in a healing wound. The tissue is highly vascular and fills the defects of full-thickness wounds.
3. Epithelialization refers to the process of epidermal resurfacing and appears as pink or red skin.
4. Signs and symptoms of infection include the production of pus, redness, pain, and swelling. More generalized symptoms of infection may include fever, chills, and an increased pulse rate. Laboratory values associated with infection include an increased erythrocyte sedimentation rate and white blood cell count.

System Specific: Integumentary System
Content Outline: Interventions

Exam Three: Question 67

A patient refuses physical therapy services after being transported to the gym. The physical therapist explains the potential consequences of refusing treatment, however, the patient does not reconsider. The MOST appropriate INITIAL therapist action is:

1. treat the patient
2. convince the patient to have therapy
3. contact the referring physician
4. **document the incident in the medical record**

> **Correct Answer: 4** (Scott - Promoting Legal and Ethical Awareness p. 231)

The *Guide for Professional Conduct* published by the American Physical Therapy Association states that "A physical therapist shall respect the patient's/client's right to make decisions regarding the recommended plan of care, including consent, modification or refusal."

1. A therapist does not have the right to treat a patient against their wishes.
2. The therapist is obligated to inform the patient of the potential consequences of refusing treatment, however, the purpose of this action is to allow the patient to make an informed decision and not to "convince" them to have therapy.
3. Contacting the referring physician when a patient refuses treatment is appropriate and necessary, however, it would not be the "initial" therapist action.
4. **The therapist must document that the patient refused treatment and was informed of the potential consequences associated with this decision. Failure to document this important information in a timely manner could place the therapist at unnecessary legal risk.**

System Specific: Non-Systems
Content Outline: Safety & Professional Roles; Teaching/Learning; Research

Exam Three: Question 68

A physical therapist completes an examination on a 36-year-old female diagnosed with multiple sclerosis. After completing the examination, the therapist should FIRST:

1. develop long-term goals
2. develop short-term goals
3. **develop a problem list**
4. justify the need for physical therapy services

> **Correct Answer: 3** (Quinn p. 34)

A physical therapist should generate a problem list after completing an examination. The problem list will assist the physical therapist to determine the patient's need for physical therapy services, the frequency of therapy sessions, and the short and long-term goals.

1. The development of long-term goals is vital to the plan of care. The physical therapist will generate long-term goals based on current patient status, typical expected outcome based on diagnosis, patient goals, and the expected time frame of physical therapy services.
2. Short-term goals are developed to assist in attaining a long-term goal in a step by step manner. The physical therapist will generate short-term goals with a predetermined time frame based on current patient status and the established long-term goal.
3. **Once an examination has been completed, the physical therapist reviews all of the data and generates a problem list. The problem list assists the therapist to determine if physical therapy services are warranted and to develop an effective and individualized plan of care.**
4. A physical therapist must justify the need for physical therapy services based on the results of the examination, however, the problem list would be developed first to assist the therapist to make an informed decision.

System Specific: Non-Systems
Content Outline: Safety & Professional Roles; Teaching/Learning; Research

Exam Three: Question 69

An electrical equipment safety committee develops a policy to limit electrical hazards arising from ground faults. Which action would be the MOST appropriate to meet the committee's objective?

1. report all equipment defects or failures
2. **manually test each ground fault circuit interrupter on a monthly basis**
3. follow manufacturer recommendations for electrical equipment care and service
4. mandate an introductory inservice on all new electrical equipment

> **Correct Answer: 2** (Prentice - Therapeutic Modalities p. 98)

Policies are used to guide or in some instances, standardize certain behaviors within an organization. It is important to recognize that the question asks specifically about a policy related to electrical hazards arising from ground faults.

1. The identification of defects or failures is essential for corrective action to be taken, however, the action is reactive rather than proactive.
2. **Ground fault circuit interrupters are designed to identify the presence of ground faults and quickly switch off power to that circuit. The automatic device provides personal protection from electrical shock. Manually testing each ground fault circuit interrupter on a fixed interval allows for proactive monitoring.**
3. Manufacturers' recommendations for electrical equipment care and service should be followed. This action, although desirable, does not specifically address the goal of limiting electrical hazards arising from ground faults.
4. Physical therapists should be oriented to all new electrical equipment and possess a thorough understanding of how to operate the equipment prior to clinical use. This action in isolation does not specifically address the prevention of ground faults.

System Specific: Non-Systems
Content Outline: Safety & Professional Roles; Teaching/Learning; Research

Exam Three: Question 70

A 21-year-old female is examined in physical therapy after sustaining a grade I ankle sprain two days ago in a marching band competition. The patient's description of the mechanism of injury is consistent with inversion and plantar flexion. Which of the following ligaments would MOST likely be affected?

1. **anterior talofibular ligament**
2. calcaneofibular ligament
3. anterior tibiofibular ligament
4. deltoid ligament

> **Correct Answer: 1** (Magee p. 859)

A grade I ankle sprain is a minor injury that involves stretching of the ligament or perhaps a small partial tear of the ligament. Treatment consists of rest, ice, compression, and elevation.

1. **The anterior talofibular ligament is a thickening of the anterior joint capsule that extends from the anterior surface of the lateral malleolus to the lateral facet of the talus and the lateral surface of the talar neck. The ligament functions to resist ankle inversion with the foot in plantar flexion. Regardless of the position of the foot, the anterior talofibular ligament is the most likely ligament torn with an inversion injury.**
2. The calcaneofibular ligament is a round cord that passes posteroinferiorly from the tip of the lateral malleolus to the lateral surface of the calcaneus. The ligament functions to resist ankle inversion and dorsiflexion.
3. The anterior tibiofibular ligament provides support to the distal tibiofibular joint. The ligament resists distal and posterior glide of the fibula.
4. The deltoid ligament refers to the collective medial ligaments of the ankle. The ligament as a whole attaches proximally to the medial aspect of the medial malleolus and fans out to the various distal attachments.

System Specific: Musculoskeletal System
Content Outline: Clinical Application of Foundational Sciences

Exam Three: Question 71

A physical therapist prepares to administer iontophoresis over the anterior surface of a patient's knee. The therapist would like to keep the current density low in order to avoid skin irritation. Which of the listed parameters would BEST accomplish the therapist's objective?

1. **current amplitude of 4 mA; electrode with an area of 12 cm²**
2. current amplitude of 4 mA; electrode with an area of 4 cm²
3. current amplitude of 3 mA; electrode with an area of 6 cm²
4. current amplitude of 3 mA; electrode with an area of 4 cm²

> **Correct Answer: 1** (Cameron p. 223)

The current density may be altered either by increasing or decreasing current intensity or by changing the size of the electrode. Current density with iontophoresis equals current amplitude (mA) divided by electrode size (cm²). Failure to select appropriate treatment or failure to monitor the patient's response to treatment creates an unnecessary safety risk.

1. **Current density = 4 mA / 12 cm² = .33 mA/cm²**
2. Current density = 4 mA / 4 cm² = 1.0 mA/cm²
3. Current density = 3 mA / 6 cm² = .50 mA/cm²
4. Current density = 3 mA / 4 cm² = .75 mA/cm²

System Specific: Non-Systems
Content Outline: Equipment & Devices; Therapeutic Modalities

Exam Three: Question 72

To practice physical therapy according to the tenets of evidence-based medicine, a physical therapist must:

1. use tests and measurements with known reliability and validity
2. use systematic reviews and randomized controlled trials as sources of research evidence
3. **integrate the best research evidence, clinical expertise, and patient values in clinical decision-making**
4. respect the rights and dignity of patients

> **Correct Answer: 3** (Sackett p. 1)

Evidence-based medicine is the integration of the best research evidence with clinical expertise and patient values. Best research evidence refers to clinically relevant research, especially patient-centered clinical research. Clinical expertise refers to the clinician's clinical skills and past experiences, but also may refer to published clinical practice guidelines. Patient values refer to the unique preferences, concerns, and expectations each patient brings to the clinical encounter.

1. Using tests and measurements with known reliability and validity is important to the practice of physical therapy, but is not specific to evidence-based practice.
2. Using systematic reviews and randomized controlled trials as sources of research evidence is important to the practice of physical therapy, but is not specific to evidence-based practice.
3. **Evidence-based medicine is the integration of the best research evidence with clinical expertise and patient values.**
4. Respecting the rights and dignity of patients is important to the practice of physical therapy, but is not specific to evidence-based practice.

System Specific: Non-Systems
Content Outline: Safety & Professional Roles; Teaching/Learning; Research

Exam Three: Question 73

A physical therapist completes a coordination assessment on a 67-year-old patient with central nervous system involvement. After reviewing the results of the assessment, the therapist concludes the clinical findings are indicative of cerebellar dysfunction. Which finding is NOT associated with cerebellar dysfunction?

1. dysmetria
2. **hypertonia**
3. ataxia
4. nystagmus

Correct Answer: 2 (O'Sullivan p. 198)

Cerebellar pathology is often characterized by incoordinated movement. Specific motor impairments associated with cerebellar pathology include ataxia, hypotonicity, dysmetria, dysdiadochokinesia, nystagmus, tremor, and scanning speech.

1. Dysmetria refers to the inability to control the range of a movement and the force of muscular activity. The result of this is often overshooting or undershooting.
2. **Cerebellar dysfunction would typically be associated with hypotonia and not hypertonia. Hypotonia causes the patient to have difficulty fixating the limb, leading to incoordination with movement.**
3. Ataxia refers to the inability to perform coordinated movements. Ataxia can affect gait, patterns of movement, and posture. The condition increases the incidence of errors in the rate, rhythm, and timing of responses.
4. Nystagmus refers to abnormal eye movement that entails nonvolitional, rhythmic oscillation of the eyes. The speed of movement is typically faster in one direction than the other direction.

System Specific: Neuromuscular & Nervous Systems
Content Outline: Foundations for Evaluation, Differential Diagnosis, & Prognosis

Exam Three: Question 74

A patient status post open knee meniscectomy is referred to physical therapy for neuromuscular electrical stimulation. The MOST beneficial frequency of treatment to promote strengthening is:

1. two times per day
2. one time per week
3. **three times per week**
4. once every two weeks

Correct Answer: 3 (Prentice - Therapeutic Modalities p. 131)

The question indicates that the focus of the intervention is to increase strength and therefore it is necessary for the intervention to be performed multiple times each week. Frequency is also influenced by variables such as intensity, repetitions, and sets.

1. One time per day would be excessive since the intensity of the strengthening activity would require more recovery time. Failure to have sufficient recovery time may lead to delayed-onset muscle soreness, excessive microtrauma, and possible injury.
2. One time per week is insufficient based on the stated goal of promoting muscle strength. This frequency may be more appropriate for a maintenance program.
3. **Three times per week is a general guideline for strengthening activities. The frequency allows for adequate intensity and sufficient rest time to minimize microtrauma and avoid delayed onset muscle soreness.**
4. Once every two weeks is insufficient for virtually any therapeutic purpose, most notably strengthening.

System Specific: Non-Systems
Content Outline: Equipment & Devices; Therapeutic Modalities

Exam Three: Question 75

A 67-year-old male with longstanding cardiac pathology is referred to physical therapy. The medical record indicates the patient is taking Nitrostat. The PRIMARY indication for this medication is:

1. to strengthen the heart's pumping force
2. **to produce a general vasodilation of vascular structures**
3. to increase excretion of sodium and water
4. to decrease electrical conduction

> **Correct Answer: 2** (Ciccone p. 309)

Nitrates are commonly used to treat angina pectoris. Potential adverse reactions when using nitrates includes headache, hypotension, dizziness, vertigo, weakness, and flushing. Nitrostat and NitroQuick are commonly used brand names of nitrates.

1. Cardiac glycosides are a category of drugs that increase the myocardial contraction force. Cardiac glycosides increase myocardial contractility by elevating intracellular calcium levels and facilitating actin-myosin interaction in cardiac cells.
2. **Nitrates are administered to produce a general vasodilation throughout the body. Nitrates decrease the amount of blood returning to the heart as well as the amount of work the heart must perform which decreases myocardial oxygen demand.**
3. Diuretics decrease the volume of water within the vascular system by increasing the renal excretion of sodium and water.
4. Antiarrythmics such as sodium channel blockers normalize the rate of sodium entry into cardiac tissues and thereby help control cardiac excitation and conduction.

System Specific: Cardiac, Vascular, & Pulmonary Systems
Content Outline: Clinical Application of Foundational Sciences

Exam Three: Question 76

A physical therapist interviews a patient recently involved in a motor vehicle accident. The patient sustained multiple lower extremity injuries as a result of the accident and appears to be very depressed. In an attempt to encourage active dialogue the therapist asks open-ended questions. Which of the following would NOT be considered an open-ended question?

1. How does your knee feel today?
2. What are your goals for physical therapy?
3. **Do you have trouble sleeping at night?**
4. Tell me about your present condition?

> **Correct Answer: 3** (Goodman - Differential Diagnosis p. 38)

Open-ended questions allow patients to answer with a myriad of responses, while closed-ended questions can often be answered with a yes or no response.

1. The question "How does your knee feel today?" provides the patient with a variety of potential answers and will likely result in the patient elaborating about the pain level today in relation to the baseline pain level.
2. The question "What are your goals for physical therapy?" provides the patient with the opportunity to elaborate on what they hope to achieve in physical therapy and is often extremely helpful for the therapist when designing an individualized program for the patient.
3. **The question "Do you have trouble sleeping at night?" would likely be answered by a simple "yes" or "no" and therefore is considered to be a closed-ended question.**
4. The question "Tell me about your present condition?" requires the patient to provide the therapist with a variety of information related to the history of their medical condition and current status.

System Specific: Non-Systems
Content Outline: Safety & Professional Roles; Teaching/Learning; Research

Exam Three: Question 77

A group of physical therapists employed in an acute care hospital is responsible for developing departmental guidelines for electrical equipment care and safety. What is the MINIMUM required testing interval for electrical equipment?

1. 3 months
2. 6 months
3. **12 months**
4. 24 months

> **Correct Answer: 3** (Belanger p. 237)

Electrical equipment should be inspected according to the specified intervals outlined by the manufacturer. The regular schedule, once established, can be modified based on variables such as increased frequency of use or reports of faulty performance.

1. Three months would be a reasonable testing interval for devices that are used more frequently or devices that tend to have greater difficulty remaining properly calibrated.
2. Six months would be a reasonable testing interval for some equipment, although the question asks for the minimum required testing interval.
3. **Testing intervals may often be more frequent than every twelve months, however, it is unacceptable for any electrical equipment to be uninspected for more than a twelve-month period.**
4. Twenty-four months would typically exceed all manufacturer's recommendations for equipment testing.

System Specific: Non-Systems
Content Outline: Equipment & Devices; Therapeutic Modalities

Test Taking Tip: Candidates must pay close attention to specific qualifiers used within the question. The question asks for "the MINIMUM required testing interval." In some cases, candidates fail to identify this type of qualifier and as a result select another option. In this particular question a candidate could easily select a three month or six month interval based on the premise that more frequent inspection would lead to better functioning electrical equipment with less risk to the patient. Although this is correct, the question is specifically asking the candidate to identify "the MINIMUM required testing interval."

Exam Three: Question 78

A physical therapist participates in a research study to determine the effect of noise level on the ability to perform a physical skill. In the study, noise is the:

1. **independent variable**
2. dependent variable
3. criterion variable
4. extraneous variable

> **Correct Answer: 1** (Portney p. 129)

The independent variable is also known as the experimental or predictor variable. It is the condition, intervention or characteristic that will predict or cause an outcome in an experimental study.

1. **Noise level is the independent variable because it is the condition or characteristic that the researcher will manipulate to see how it changes physical skill.**
2. The dependent variable is also known as the outcome variable, which is the response or effect that is presumed to vary with the independent variable. Physical skill is the dependent variable because it is presumed to vary depending on noise level.
3. The term criterion variable is a synonym for dependent variable.
4. An extraneous variable is also known as a nuisance or intervening variable. An extraneous variable is any factor that is not related to the purpose of the study, but that may affect the dependent variable.

System Specific: Non-Systems
Content Outline: Safety & Professional Roles; Teaching/Learning; Research

Exam Three: Question 79

A patient with a C6 spinal cord injury is examined in physical therapy. Which objective finding would be the strongest indication the spinal cord injury is NOT complete?

1. intact sensation on the lateral portion of the shoulder
2. absent triceps reflex
3. **diminished sensation over the hypothenar eminence**
4. weakness of the biceps muscle

> **Correct Answer: 3** (Goodman - Pathology p. 1502)

A patient with a complete C6 spinal cord injury would not possess motor, sensory or reflex function below the C6 level. As a result, any identified finding below this level could provide evidence that the injury is not complete.

1. The dermatome associated with the lateral portion of the shoulder is C5 and therefore sensation in this area would typically be intact in a complete spinal cord injury at the C6 level.
2. The triceps reflex is associated with the C7-C8 nerve root and therefore the reflex would be absent in a complete spinal cord injury at the C6 level.
3. **The dermatome that corresponds to the hypothenar eminence is at the C8 level. As a result, the finding of diminished sensation (not absent) at a level below the level of injury (i.e., C6) indicates that the injury is incomplete.**
4. The biceps muscle is innervated by C5-C6 and therefore weakness is often associated with a spinal cord injury at this level.

System Specific: Neuromuscular & Nervous Systems
Content Outline: Foundations for Evaluation, Differential Diagnosis, & Prognosis

Exam Three: Question 80

When is it considered acceptable for a clinical trial to include a non-treatment control group as a basis for comparison with a new experimental therapy?

1. **when there is no known effective form of therapy to treat the patient's condition**
2. when the experimental therapy has shown positive results in animal studies
3. when the study is approved by the facility's Institutional Review Board (IRB)
4. when subjects are randomly assigned to a group

> **Correct Answer: 1** (Portney p. 49)

According to the current Declaration of Helsinki, in research with human beings, a placebo control may be used in clinical conditions for which no treatments have been effective or when the purpose of the research is to determine if a particular treatment is not effective. In all cases, the researcher is obliged to inform the potential human subjects when the study includes a control group.

1. **A non-treatment control group may be used in clinical conditions for which no treatments have been effective.**
2. Positive results in animal studies do not make the use of a non-treatment control group acceptable in research on humans.
3. Federal regulations in the United States require that an Institutional Review Board (IRB) research proposals using human subjects prior to implementation to ensure that the rights of the subjects are protected. However, review by the IRB does not make the use of a non-treatment control group acceptable.
4. Random assignment to groups is the best way to control for confounding variables that could affect the outcomes of the study. However, it does not make the use of a non-treatment control group acceptable.

System Specific: Non-Systems
Content Outline: Safety & Professional Roles; Teaching/Learning; Research

Exam Three: Question 81

A physical therapist treats a patient diagnosed with spinal stenosis. As part of the treatment program the patient lies prone on a treatment plinth with a hot pack draped over the low back. The MOST effective method to monitor the patient while using the hot pack is:

1. check on the patient at least every ten minutes
2. **supply the patient with a bell to ring if the hot pack becomes too hot**
3. instruct the patient to remove the hot pack if it becomes too hot
4. select an alternate superficial heating modality

> **Correct Answer: 2** (Michlovitz p. 162)

A hot pack consists of a canvas or nylon covered pack filled with a hydrophilic silicate gel that provides a moist heat. A hot pack must be stored in hot water between 158 to 167 degrees Fahrenheit (70 to 75 degrees Celsius). Application requires six to eight layers of towels around the hot pack. Given the potential for burns, formal measures must be adopted to ensure safe use throughout the treatment session.

1. Checking on a patient on a frequent basis is desirable, however, 10 minutes is not frequent enough particularly when considering that the duration of treatment with a hot pack may only be 20 minutes.
2. **Supplying the patient with a bell to ring if the hot pack becomes too intense provides a form of instant communication with the therapist.**
3. It may be challenging for the patient to independently remove the hot pack based on the selected positioning. In addition, this option places the burden solely on the patient to make a definitive decision on whether or not to continue using the hot pack. This decision should be made by the therapist with feedback from the patient.
4. There is no need to discontinue a selected intervention in the absence of data to support this decision. Hot packs can be a safe and effective form of superficial heat when applied with the necessary precautions.

System Specific: Non-Systems
Content Outline: Equipment & Devices; Therapeutic Modalities

Exam Three: Question 82

A physical therapist asks a patient to complete a pain questionnaire. The questionnaire utilizes an ascending numeric scale ranging from "0" equaling no pain to "10" equaling excruciating pain. This type of measurement scale is BEST described as:

1. nominal
2. **ordinal**
3. interval
4. ratio

> **Correct Answer: 2** (Portney p. 68)

Four scales of measurement have been identified – nominal, ordinal, interval, ratio – each with its own set of rules for manipulating and interpreting numerical data.

1. The nominal scale of measurement is also known as the classificatory scale. Objects or things are classified in categories according to some criterion, e.g., name, letter, or symbol, which do not have any quantitative value. The nominal scale is the lowest scale of measurement.
2. **The ordinal scale of measurement requires that the categories be ranked or ordered according to some defined characteristic or property, so that the numbers on the scale have a greater than – less than relationship. The intervals between ranks need not be equal, and may not be known, as is the case with measurement of pain on a 0 to 10 scale. While an "8" indicates greater pain than a "4" it cannot be said to represent twice as much pain because the magnitude of pain associated with each number is unknown and may vary among patients. Also, the difference between an 8 and 4 does not indicate the same difference in pain as the difference between a 6 and 2.**
3. The interval scale has the rank-order characteristics of an ordinal scale, but also demonstrates known and equal distances or intervals between the units of measurement. This latter property permits relative difference and equivalence to be determined. Measures of temperature on the Fahrenheit and Celsius scales are at the interval level.
4. The ratio scale is the highest level of measurement because, in addition to the known and equal distances or intervals, the scale has an absolute zero point representing a total absence of the property being measured. Range of motion, height, weight, and force are examples of clinical measurements on the ratio scale.

System Specific: Non-Systems
Content Outline: Safety & Professional Roles; Teaching/Learning; Research

Exam Three: Question 83

An attorney contacts you by phone and requests specific information on a patient he claims to represent. Questions asked include the extent of the patient's disability and his willingness to return to work. The MOST appropriate response is:

1. answer the questions asked by the attorney
2. **request the attorney provide a completed release of patient medical information form**
3. tell the attorney not to bother you at work
4. send the attorney a copy of the patient's medical records

Correct Answer: 2 (Scott - Promoting Legal and Ethical Awareness p. 78)

Physical therapists have an ethical and legal obligation to appropriately secure protected health information. Releasing this type of information without written patient consent would be considered a negligent act.

1. Answering questions asked by the attorney without the appropriate release forms would violate the rights of the patient.
2. **The attorney should be reminded of the appropriate procedure to obtain medical records.**
3. It is inappropriate to be rude to the attorney despite the fact that the attorney should be aware of the appropriate procedure to obtain medical records.
4. Sending the attorney a copy of the patient's medical records violates the patient's rights since there is no indication that the attorney has followed the appropriate procedure to have the records released.

System Specific: Non-Systems
Content Outline: Safety & Professional Roles; Teaching/Learning; Research

Exam Three: Question 84

A patient four weeks status post anterior cruciate ligament reconstruction questions a physical therapist as to why he is still partial weight bearing. An acceptable rationale is:

1. **the patient does not have full active knee extension**
2. the patient has good quadriceps strength
3. the patient has fair hamstrings strength
4. the patient has diminished superficial cutaneous sensation

Correct Answer: 1 (Kisner p. 733)

The physician is responsible for determining a patient's weight bearing status following surgery. Physical therapists should possess an understanding of relevant factors associated with the prescribed weight bearing status and understand what is necessary for the patient to progress to full weight bearing.

1. **A patient status post anterior cruciate ligament reconstruction surgery may continue to use an assistive device for weight bearing if they do not possess full active knee extension. Ambulation on a flexed knee can result in excessive irritation of the patellofemoral joint.**
2. The quadriceps control the amount of knee flexion during initial contact (loading response) and then extend the knee toward midstance. The quadriceps also control the amount of knee flexion during pre-swing (heel off to toe off) and prevent excessive heel rise during initial swing. Good quadriceps strength would be adequate for full weight bearing on the involved lower extremity assuming the absence of other relevant clinical findings. A grade of good indicates that the patient completes range of motion against gravity with moderate resistance.
3. The hamstrings are responsible for controlling the forward swing of the leg during terminal swing. The hamstrings provide posterior support to the knee capsule when the knee is extended during stance. Fair hamstrings strength would be adequate for full weight bearing on the involved lower extremity assuming the absence of other relevant clinical findings. A grade of fair indicates that the patient completes range of motion against gravity without manual resistance.
4. Diminished superficial cutaneous sensation is common following surgery particularly in close proximity to an incision. The presence of diminished superficial cutaneous sensation would not influence a patient's weight bearing status.

System Specific: Musculoskeletal System
Content Outline: Interventions

Exam Three: Question 85

A physical therapist palpates medially along the spine of the scapula. Which spinous process is at the same level as the vertebral end of the spine?

1. T2
2. **T3**
3. T4
4. T5

Correct Answer: 2 (Hoppenfeld p. 11)

Physical therapists often use selected bony prominences to assist them to identify a specific vertebral level. For example, in the lumbar spine the top of the iliac crest is at the same level as the L4-L5 interspace and in the sacral spine the posterior superior iliac spine is at the same level as S2.

1. The scapula's medial border extends from the level of spinous processes T2-T7.
2. **The vertebral end of the spine of the scapula is at the same level as the spinous process of T3.**
3. The spinous process of T4 is slightly below the level of the vertebral end of the spine of the scapula. Like all thoracic vertebrae, T4 articulates with the ribs and possesses a spinous process that is easily identifiable, particularly when the spine is flexed.
4. The spinous process of T5 is significantly inferior to the level of the vertebral end of the spine of the scapula. The body of the middle four vertebrae in the thoracic spine (T5-T8) when viewed from the superior aspect are heart shaped and their vertebral foramina are circular.

System Specific: Musculoskeletal System
Content Outline: Clinical Application of Foundational Sciences

Exam Three: Question 86

A physical therapist observes a patient status post transfemoral amputation lying in supine with a pillow positioned under the residual limb. This position results in the patient being MOST susceptible to a:

1. knee extension contracture
2. knee flexion contracture
3. **hip flexion contracture**
4. hip extension contracture

Correct Answer: 3 (Seymour p. 145)

Proper positioning is required to avoid a contracture of the residual limb. A patient with a transfemoral amputation is particularly susceptible to a hip flexion contracture.

1. A patient with a transfemoral amputation would not possess a knee joint on the affected side. As a result, a contracture involving the affected lower extremity would only involve the hip.
2. A patient with a transtibial amputation lying in supine with a pillow under the residual limb would be more likely to develop a knee flexion contracture.
3. **A hip flexion contracture can occur if the patient lies supine with a pillow under the residual limb. The positioning into hip flexion along with the relative strength of the hip flexors places the patient at high risk for contracture. Intermittent prone lying is often a recommended activity following a transfemoral amputation.**
4. Lying in supine would not make the patient susceptible to a hip extension contracture since the hip remains in a neutral or a flexed position when in supine.

System Specific: Musculoskeletal System
Content Outline: Foundations for Evaluation, Differential Diagnosis, & Prognosis

Test Taking Tip: This question demonstrates how easy it can be to make a test taking mistake on the National Physical Therapy Examination. Some candidates may have selected option 2 knee flexion contracture after reading key words such as supine and pillow under the residual limb. If they selected option 2 it is likely that they were thinking about a transtibial amputation despite the fact that the question clearly indicates transfemoral amputation. Candidates must be careful to identify key words within the question and possess a clear understanding of what the question is asking prior to identifying the correct answer. Test taking mistakes result in a candidate's score not representing their true ability and as a result, make them more at risk for failing the National Physical Therapy Examination. Increased awareness of individual tendencies is one proactive approach to reduce the frequency of test taking mistakes.

Exam Three: Question 87

A physical therapist conducts an examination on a patient diagnosed with Parkinson's disease. Which of the following clinical findings would the therapist expect to identify?

1. aphasia
2. ballistic movements
3. severe muscle atrophy
4. **cogwheel rigidity**

Correct Answer: 4 (O'Sullivan p. 200)

Parkinson's disease is a degenerative disorder characterized by a decrease in production of dopamine (neurotransmitter) within the corpus striatum portion of the basal ganglia. Clinical presentation may include hypokinesia, difficulty initiating and stopping movement, festinating and shuffling gait, bradykinesia, poor posture, and "cogwheel" or "lead pipe" rigidity.

1. Aphasia is an acquired neurological communication impairment caused by damage to the brain. The condition is most commonly associated with brain injury, head trauma, CVA, tumor or infection.
2. Ballistic movements refer to large amplitude involuntary movements affecting the proximal limb musculature, manifested in jerking, flinging movements of the extremity. Ballismus usually results from a lesion in the subthalamic nucleus. Often only one side of the body is involved, resulting in hemiballismus.
3. Severe muscle atrophy is an expected clinical finding in diseases that affect the nerves that control muscles (e.g., poliomyelitis, amyotrophic lateral sclerosis, Guillain-Barre syndrome) and diseases affecting the muscles directly (e.g., muscular dystrophy, myotonia congenita).
4. **Cogwheel rigidity refers to a jerky, rachet-like resistance to passive movement as muscles sequentially tense and relax. The condition is most often associated with Parkinson's disease.**

System Specific: Neuromuscular & Nervous Systems
Content Outline: Foundations for Evaluation, Differential Diagnosis, & Prognosis

Exam Three: Question 88

A patient rehabilitating from a CVA requires an orthosis due to occasional dragging of the toe during swing phase. The patient presents with weakness of the dorsiflexors and has good medial/lateral stability at the ankle. The MOST appropriate option for the patient is:

1. solid ankle-foot orthosis
2. tone reducing foot orthosis
3. **posterior leaf spring orthosis**
4. custom articulating ankle-foot orthosis with anterior trim lines

Correct Answer: 3 (Seymour p. 383)

A posterior leaf spring (PLS) orthosis is a type of ankle-foot orthosis that provides a dorsiflexion assist during swing phase. The trim line is posterior to the malleoli and as a result the device offers minimal medial or lateral ankle support.

1. A solid ankle-foot orthosis (AFO) is typically indicated for diminished strength of the dorsiflexors, plantar flexors, evertors or invertors. The solid AFO will control the ankle and influence the knee joint during gait. The solid AFO maintains the ankle in a static position, however, may assist with tonal influence and lower extremity weakness. The AFO provides more stability than the patient requires.
2. A tone reducing foot orthosis is typically indicated to decrease hypertonicity and normalize tone. The foot orthosis provides total contact under the foot allowing for areas of pressure that function to decrease tone.
3. **The PLS orthosis is designed with flexibility so that both dorsiflexion and plantar flexion can occur during the gait cycle. The PLS allows for improved biomechanics during gait secondary to its flexibility and therefore would be the most appropriate type of orthosis for the patient given their level of medial/lateral stability.**
4. A custom articulating ankle-foot orthosis (AFO) with anterior trim lines typically provides total contact and a significant amount of stability. The articulating joint promotes improved biomechanics allowing the tibia to advance over the foot during stance phase. The patient, however, would not require the level of stability offered by this type of AFO.

System Specific: Non-Systems
Content Outline: Equipment & Devices; Therapeutic Modalities

Exam Three: Question 89

A physical therapist prescribes a wheelchair for a 34-year-old patient with bilateral lower extremity amputations. The MOST important feature of a wheelchair designed for the patient should be:

1. friction surface handrims
2. **the drive wheels are set behind the vertical back supports**
3. reclining back with elevating legrests
4. removable armrests

Correct Answer: 2 (Seymour p. 160)

A patient with bilateral lower extremity amputations requires offset rear wheels to accommodate for the change in the center of gravity. An anti-tipping device may also be used to prevent the wheelchair and patient from falling backwards.

1. Friction surface handrims are used when patients do not have a functional grip or strength to adequately propel a wheelchair. Patients with C6-C7 tetraplegia commonly rely on this feature.
2. **A wheelchair with offset rear wheels is an adaptation that moves the axis posterior to the center support and provides greater stability during propulsion over varying surfaces. An active patient will use all available options to enhance the stability of the chair.**
3. A wheelchair with a reclining back and elevating legrests would be appropriate for a patient that does not tolerate an upright posture or possess postural control. This would not be appropriate for a patient with bilateral amputations since it would move the center of gravity in a posterior direction as the chair reclines.
4. Removable armrests are appropriate for many patients including those with bilateral amputations to improve safety and ease of transfers, however, the most important adaptation should be the offset rear wheels to ensure safety within the wheelchair.

System Specific: Non-Systems
Content Outline: Equipment & Devices; Therapeutic Modalities

Exam Three: Question 90

A physical therapist assesses a patient's heart rate by measuring the time necessary for 30 beats. Assuming the therapist measures this value as 22 seconds, the patient's heart rate should be recorded as:

1. **82 beats per minute**
2. 86 beats per minute
3. 90 beats per minute
4. 95 beats per minute

Correct Answer: 1 (Pierson p. 60)

To determine the beats per minute, calculate the number of beats in one second, then multiply the obtained value by 60 seconds per minute.

1. **The number of beats in one second = 1.36 (30 beats / 22 seconds = 1.36 beats per second). Multiplying 1.36 beats per second by 60 seconds per minute yields heart rate in beats per minute: 1.36 beats per second x 60 seconds per minute = 81.6 beats per minute (rounded up to 82).**
2. 1.36 beats per second x 60 seconds per minute ≠86
3. 1.36 beats per second x 60 seconds per minute ≠90
4. 1.36 beats per second x 60 seconds per minute ≠95

System Specific: Cardiac, Vascular, & Pulmonary Systems
Content Outline: Examination

Exam Three: Question 91

A patient diagnosed with Guillain-Barre syndrome works on weight shifting activities while standing in the parallel bars. The PRIMARY objective of this activity is to improve:

1. mobility
2. stability
3. **controlled mobility**
4. skill

> **Correct Answer: 3** (Sullivan p. 77)

Functional training uses postures and activities to improve motor control. Physical therapists select activities for patients that are designed to progressively increase the effects of gravity and body weight.

1. Mobility, the first stage of motor control, refers to the ability to initiate movement through a functional range of motion.
2. Stability, the second stage of motor control, refers to the ability to maintain a position or posture through cocontraction and tonic holding around a joint.
3. **Controlled mobility, the third stage of motor control, refers to the ability to move within a weight bearing position or rotate around a long axis.**
4. Skill, the fourth stage of motor control, refers to the ability to consistently perform functional tasks and manipulate the environment with normal postural reflex mechanisms and balance reactions. Skill activities include ADLs and community locomotion.

System Specific: Neuromuscular & Nervous Systems
Content Outline: Interventions

Exam Three: Question 92

A physical therapist asks a physical therapist assistant to complete a lower extremity isokinetic test on a patient. The physical therapist assistant is willing to complete the test, however, indicates it has been quite some time since they have set up the isokinetic device. The MOST appropriate physical therapist action is:

1. provide verbal cueing for the physical therapist assistant prior to beginning the set up
2. instruct the physical therapist assistant to refer to the owner's manual
3. **observe the physical therapist assistant complete the set up**
4. ask another physical therapist assistant to complete the set up

> **Correct Answer: 3** (Nosse p. 217)

A physical therapist should establish and maintain an ongoing professional relationship with a physical therapist assistant. The physical therapist should delegate appropriate patient care duties to the physical therapist assistant that are within their established scope of practice. The physical therapist assistant must clearly communicate their needs to the physical therapist and work in a collaborative manner.

1. Verbal cueing allows the physical therapist to assist the physical therapist assistant to set up the isokinetic device through verbal input, however, it does not ensure that the device is set up correctly.
2. Referring the physical therapist assistant to the owner's manual provides the physical therapist assistant with a general reference to guide them through the set up, but like the previous option does not ensure that the device is set up correctly.
3. **Observing the physical therapist assistant complete the set up allows the physical therapist to assist the physical therapist assistant as needed and at the same time ensures the device is set up correctly. Direct involvement of the physical therapist is collaborative and may assist the physical therapist assistant to complete the set up independently in the future.**
4. The physical therapist assistant is capable of completing the set up with assistance. As a result, it is not necessary to secure another physical therapist assistant to complete the set up. In addition, the question does not provide direct evidence that another physical therapist assistant is available who possesses the requisite knowledge to complete the activity.

System Specific: Non-Systems
Content Outline: Safety & Professional Roles; Teaching/Learning; Research

Exam Three: Question 93

A physical therapist administers ultrasound over a patient's anterior thigh. After one minute of treatment, the patient reports feeling a slight burning sensation under the soundhead. The therapist's MOST appropriate action is to:

1. explain to the patient that what she feels is not out of the ordinary when using ultrasound
2. **temporarily discontinue treatment and examine the amount of coupling agent utilized**
3. discontinue treatment and contact the referring physician
4. continue with treatment utilizing the current parameters

Correct Answer: 2 (Michlovitz p. 89)

A patient report of a slight burning sensation under the soundhead can be due to inadequate coupling, loosening of the crystal or hot spots due to a high beam nonuniformity ratio.

1. A complaint of a slight burning sensation would be an abnormal response when using ultrasound. As a result, it would be inappropriate to inform the patient that what she feels is "not out of the ordinary." It may be normal to feel a dull warming, however, a slight burning sensation would require an immediate response.

2. **The complaint of a slight burning sensation may indicate improper coupling. By temporarily discontinuing the treatment and examining the amount of coupling agent used, the physical therapist may be able to continue with treatment. If the physical therapist adds coupling agent and the patient reports a similar sensation the intervention should be discontinued and the ultrasound unit should be formally inspected by a qualified technician.**

3. Discontinuing treatment would be an acceptable option, however, there is not presently a need to contact the referring physician. A physical therapist may elect to contact the physician in situations where the patient has been injured by a physical therapy intervention or if there has been a change in the patient's medical status.

4. Continuing with treatment utilizing the current parameters is not appropriate since the patient has already reported a slight burning sensation. Failure to respond specifically to the patient's subjective report creates an unnecessary safety risk.

System Specific: Non-Systems
Content Outline: Equipment & Devices; Therapeutic Modalities

Exam Three: Question 94

A patient ambulating in the physical therapy gym suddenly grabs the physical therapist's arm and indicates that he feels faint. The MOST appropriate IMMEDIATE action is:

1. assess the patient's pulse rate
2. ask the patient if he has ever previously fainted
3. loosen tight clothing
4. **assist the patient to a sitting position**

Correct Answer: 4 (Code of Ethics)

The physical therapist must take immediate action to ensure patient safety. By assisting the patient to a chair, the therapist can adequately assess the patient without compromising patient safety.

1. Assessing the patient's pulse rate may provide the physical therapist with additional information on the patient's current medical status, however, the more immediate concern would be to assist the patient to a stable and secure position to minimize the risk of a fall.

2. Gathering additional information on the patient's past medical history will eventually be warranted, however, the action does not specifically address the immediate safety concern.

3. Loosening tight clothing may assist the patient to be more comfortable, however, this action would not be appropriate until the patient is in a secure position.

4. **The physical therapist's primary responsibility is to preserve patient safety. Assisting the patient to a sitting position takes the patient out of immediate danger. Each of the remaining options is viable, however, only after patient safety has been preserved.**

System Specific: Cardiac, Vascular, & Pulmonary Systems
Content Outline: Interventions

Exam Three: Question 95

A physical therapist uses a manual wheelchair during a training session with a patient with C5 quadriplegia. Which wheelchair would be the most appropriate based on the patient's level of injury?

1. manual wheelchair with sip and puff controls
2. **manual wheelchair with handrim projections**
3. manual wheelchair with friction surface handrims
4. manual wheelchair with standard handrims

Correct Answer: 2 (O'Sullivan p. 962)

A patient with C5 tetraplegia would typically be able to utilize a manual wheelchair with handrim projections to assist with propulsion. The projections are typically angled at 30 degrees and may have friction surfaces for greater ease of movement.

1. Sip and puff controls are used only on power wheelchairs. These types of controls are most often used on patients with C4 tetraplegia. Innervation at the C4 level includes the diaphragm, trapezius, face, and neck muscles.
2. **A manual wheelchair with handrim projections would be appropriate to use during a training session for a patient with C5 quadriplegia, however, may not be used as the primary mode of mobility due to the limited upper extremity muscle innervation and the associated endurance issues.**
3. A manual wheelchair with friction surface handrims would be more appropriate for a patient with C6-C7 tetraplegia secondary to the motor innervation at the C6 and C7 levels.
4. A patient with paraplegia (full upper extremity innervation) can propel a wheelchair without adaptation of the wheelrims. Standard handrims are used for patients with injury at the C8 level and below.

System Specific: Non-Systems
Content Outline: Equipment & Devices; Therapeutic Modalities

Exam Three: Question 96

A physical therapist employed in a rehabilitation hospital creates a professional development plan as part of his annual performance appraisal. Which of the following would be the MOST appropriate plan to facilitate the therapist's development in his present practice setting?

1. attend continuing education courses approved by the Federation of State Boards of Physical Therapy
2. attend continuing education courses featuring nationally recognized experts
3. attend a minimum of two continuing education courses annually
4. **attend continuing education courses related to primary patient care responsibilities**

Correct Answer: 4 (Guide for Professional Conduct)

Facilitating the physical therapist's development in his present practice setting requires the physical therapist to attend continuing education courses related to his primary care responsibilities. Continuing education courses allow the physical therapist to refine existing skills and learn new skills. By taking courses related to primary patient care responsibilities the therapist will be able to immediately integrate selected skills into their daily practice.

1. The Federation of State Boards of Physical Therapy does not approve continuing education courses.
2. Attending continuing education courses featuring nationally recognized experts does not ensure that the courses will be more beneficial to the therapist than courses taught by less known speakers. The physical therapist should evaluate each course based on its relevant merit and the direct relevance to their patient care duties.
3. The quality of the continuing education courses a physical therapist attends is a more important variable to consider than the actual number of courses attended. For example, a physical therapist could attend several courses with little direct relevance to their present patient care duties and as a result receive little practical benefit.
4. **The physical therapist should attend continuing education courses that directly relate to their primary patient care responsibilities. Developing this particular skill set will allow the physical therapist to improve the quality of patient care within their current practice setting.**

System Specific: Non-Systems
Content Outline: Safety & Professional Roles; Teaching/Learning; Research

Exam Three: Question 97

A male physical therapist examines a female diagnosed with subacromial bursitis. After taking a thorough history, the therapist asks the patient to change into a gown. The patient seems very uneasy about this suggestion, but finally agrees to use the gown. The MOST appropriate course of action would be to:

1. continue with treatment as planned
2. attempt to treat the patient without using the gown
3. **bring a female staff member into the treatment room and continue with treatment**
4. offer to transfer the patient to a female physical therapist

Correct Answer: 3 (Nosse p. 217)

The physical therapist should be sensitive to the patient's apparent discomfort with the situation, however, must also take appropriate steps to manage their relative risk. Physical therapists must be willing to modify their approach with each patient encounter based on the unique presented circumstances.

1. The patient's original reluctance to wear the gown makes it prudent to have a witness present during treatment. The decision to continue with treatment without any formal action places the physical therapist at unnecessary risk.
2. Failure to wear the gown may make it more difficult for the physical therapist to treat the patient or depending on the chosen intervention could risk damaging or soiling the patient's clothes.
3. **The male physical therapist should bring a female staff member into the treatment room. The presence of a witness is a form of risk management that protects the physical therapist in the event of any alleged misconduct and may make the patient more comfortable.**
4. It would be impractical to transfer a patient to another physical therapist simply because the patient seemed to be uncomfortable when asked to change into the gown.

System Specific: Non-Systems
Content Outline: Safety & Professional Roles; Teaching/Learning; Research

Exam Three: Question 98

A physical therapist treats a patient status post CVA. Which action would be MOST likely to facilitate elbow extension in a patient with hemiplegia?

1. **turn the head to the affected side**
2. turn the head to the unaffected side
3. extend the lower extremities
4. flex the lower extremities

Correct Answer: 1 (Sullivan p. 19)

Patients status post CVA are likely to exhibit abnormal tonic reflexes. Eliciting the reflexes will produce sustained posturing and abnormal movement patterns.

1. **The asymmetrical tonic neck reflex produces extension of the affected upper extremity when the patient's head is turned toward the affected side. The upper extremity on the skull side will flex.**
2. If the patient's head is turned toward the unaffected side, the unaffected upper extremity will extend and the affected upper extremity will flex due to the influence of the asymmetrical tonic neck reflex (ATNR).
3. The symmetrical tonic labyrinthine reflex (STLR) promotes a tendency for extension when a patient is in supine and reduced extensor influence when the patient is in prone. STLR would not facilitate elbow extension in isolation as noted with ATNR.
4. Flexion of the lower extremities does not have a direct influence on upper extremity flexion or extension.

System Specific: Neuromuscular & Nervous Systems
Content Outline: Interventions

Exam Three: Question 99

A physical therapist examines a patient three days following shoulder surgery. The patient complains of general malaise and reports a slightly elevated body temperature during the last twenty-four hours. Physical examination reveals an edematous shoulder that is warm to the touch. A small amount of yellow fluid is observed seeping from the incision. The MOST appropriate therapist action is:

1. send the patient to the emergency room
2. **communicate the information to the referring physician**
3. document the findings in the medical record
4. ask the patient to make an appointment with the referring physician

Correct Answer: 2 (Anemaet p. 547)

Physical therapists must be aware of any signs or symptoms of infection, particularly in patients following surgery. Common signs of infection include elevated body temperature, purulent exudate, swelling, edema, and redness.

1. The patient's presentation requires the physical therapist to take formal action, but would not be indicative of an emergent condition that requires the patient to be seen in the emergency room.
2. **The possibility of infection in a patient three days status post surgery warrants immediate consultation with the referring physician.**
3. The subjective and objective information gathered by the physical therapist should be documented in the medical record, however, this action would not address the primary issue which is the possibility of an infection.
4. Asking the patient to make an appointment with the physician is not an appropriate action since it places the burden solely on the patient. The physical therapist is responsible for communicating any potential change in a patient's medical status to the physician in a timely manner.

System Specific: Other Systems
Content Outline: Interventions

Exam Three: Question 100

A physical therapist instructs a patient how to fall safely to the floor when using axillary crutches. Which of the following should be the FIRST to occur in the case of a forward fall?

1. reach towards the floor
2. turn your face towards one side
3. **release the crutches**
4. flex the trunk and head

Correct Answer: 3 (Pierson p. 271)

Physical therapists are responsible for instructing patients how to properly use various assistive devices. The instructions typically include training in fall prevention and strategies to minimize injury in the event of a fall.

1. Reaching forward toward the floor would be a desirable action in the event of a forward fall, however, the question specifically asks for the "first" action.
2. Turning the face towards one side would be a desirable action in the event of a forward fall to minimize the relative trauma to the face, however, this would not be the "first" action.
3. **A patient should release the crutches in the event of a forward fall in order to utilize the upper extremities to minimize the impact of the fall.**
4. Flexing the trunk and head are instructions that are necessary when teaching a patient to properly fall backward. The coupled motions are used to facilitate the patient to fall on their buttocks instead of directly landing on their head.

System Specific: Non-Systems
Content Outline: Safety & Professional Roles; Teaching/Learning; Research

Exam Three: Question 101

A physical therapist instructs a patient in residual limb wrapping. Which bandage would be the MOST appropriate to utilize for a patient with a transfemoral amputation?

1. two-inch
2. four-inch
3. **six-inch**
4. eight-inch

Correct Answer: 3 (Seymour p. 132)

A six-inch bandage is used to wrap the residual limb of a patient with a transfemoral amputation. The bandage should be applied in a figure-eight pattern using angular turns. The bandage provides a pressure gradient that is greatest distally with decreasing pressure proximally. The bandage should be applied well into the groin area to avoid an adductor roll and should be rewrapped approximately every four hours in order to maintain proper pressure and fit.

1. A two-inch bandage would not be appropriate for wrapping the residual limb of a patient following transfemoral amputation due to the large surface area. The limited width of the bandage may have a tendency to cause a tourniquet effect.
2. A four-inch bandage would be appropriate when wrapping the residual limb of a patient following a transtibial amputation, however, would not be the most appropriate for a transfemoral amputation.
3. **A patient with a transfemoral amputation should wrap the residual limb with two to three six-inch bandages and include a hip spica to assist with securing the bandage. The six-inch bandage is appropriately sized to cover the necessary surface area of the thigh and waist.**
4. An eight-inch bandage is too wide for use on a typical residual limb. The patient would be at an increased risk for multiple wrinkles and folds since the residual limb would not possess the necessary surface area to accommodate the eight-inch bandage.

System Specific: Integumentary System
Content Outline: Interventions

Exam Three: Question 102

A physical therapist measures body composition using skinfold measurements prior to initiating an exercise program. When measuring the abdominal skinfold the MOST appropriate method is:

1. **utilize a vertical fold approximately 2 cm to the right of the umbilicus**
2. utilize a horizontal fold approximately 2 cm to the right of the umbilicus
3. utilize a vertical fold approximately 2 cm to the left of the umbilicus
4. utilize a horizontal fold approximately 2 cm to the left of the umbilicus

Correct Answer: 1 (American College of Sports Medicine p. 269)

Anthropometry studies body dimensions and includes the use of skinfold measurements. The theory associated with skinfold measurements is that the amount of subcutaneous fat is proportional to the total amount of body fat. The exact proportion of subcutaneous to total fat varies with gender, age, and ethnicity. Acceptable skinfold sites include the biceps, triceps, abdominal, suprailiac, thigh, chest, midaxillary, medial calf, and subscapular areas. Each site has specific guidelines for attaining measurements in order to maximize consistency and decrease measurement error. A healthy range of body fat is 12-18% for males and 18-23% for females.

1. **The abdominal skinfold site utilizes a vertical fold approximately 2 cm to the right of the umbilicus.**
2. The abdominal skinfold requires the use of a vertical fold and not a horizontal fold.
3. All skinfold measurements are made using the right side of the body.
4. The abdominal skinfold requires the use of a vertical fold using the right side of the body.

System Specific: Musculoskeletal System
Content Outline: Examination

Exam Three: Question 103

A physical therapist observes that a patient has an exaggerated heel strike on the left during ambulation activities. Which term is MOST consistent with heel strike using Rancho Los Amigos nomenclature?

1. terminal swing
2. loading response
3. **initial contact**
4. midstance

Correct Answer: 3 (Levangie p. 520)

The phases of gait are classified based on either points in time (traditional terminology) or periods of time (Rancho Los Amigos terminology). It is important for physical therapists to be familiar with both sets of terminology. Standard terminology includes heel strike, foot flat, midstance, heel off, toe off, acceleration, midswing, and deceleration. Rancho Los Amigos terminology includes initial contact, loading response, midstance, terminal stance, pre-swing, initial swing, midswing, and terminal swing.

1. Terminal swing begins when the tibia is perpendicular to the floor and ends when the foot touches the ground.
2. Loading response corresponds to the amount of time between initial contact and the beginning of the swing phase for the other leg.
3. **Initial contact is the beginning of the stance phase that occurs when the foot touches the ground.**
4. Midstance corresponds to the point in stance phase when the other foot is off the floor until the body is directly over the stance limb.

System Specific: Musculoskeletal System
Content Outline: Examination

Exam Three: Question 104

A physical therapist obtains the past medical history of a patient recently referred to physical therapy after being diagnosed with adhesive capsulitis. Which medical condition is associated with an increased incidence of adhesive capsulitis?

1. **diabetes mellitus**
2. hemophilia
3. peripheral vascular disease
4. osteomalacia

Correct Answer: 1 (Goodman – Pathology p. 494)

Adhesive capsulitis refers to an inflammation and adherence of the articular capsule resulting in limited joint play and restricted active and passive movement. The condition is more common in women than in men and tends to appear in the fourth, fifth, and sixth decades of life.

1. **Diabetes mellitus is a group of metabolic diseases characterized by high blood sugar levels that result from defects in insulin secretion, the actions of insulin, or both. Patients with diabetes mellitus have an increased incidence of adhesive capsulitis and often experience a longer duration of symptoms and greater limitation of motion.**
2. Hemophilia is a bleeding disorder of genetic etiology. It is a sex-linked autosomal recessive trait. Patients with hemophilia are prone to hemarthrosis, intramuscular hemorrhage, and secondary complications from hematomas. The condition is not associated with an increased incidence of adhesive capsulitis.
3. Peripheral vascular disease refers to any disease or pathology of the circulatory system outside of the brain and heart. The disease is characterized by narrowing of the arteries, and reduced blood flow to the legs, arms, brain and other organs. The cause, in most cases, is atherosclerosis. The condition is not associated with an increased incidence of adhesive capsulitis.
4. Osteomalacia refers to softening of the bone without loss of bone matrix. There is insufficient mineralization of the bone matrix normally caused by insufficient calcium absorption and increased renal phosphorus losses. Symptoms include bone pain, aching, fatigue, and periarticular tenderness. The condition is not associated with an increased incidence of adhesive capsulitis.

System Specific: Other Systems
Content Outline: Foundations for Evaluation, Differential Diagnosis, & Prognosis

Exam Three: Question 105

A physical therapist notices that a patient with a transfemoral amputation consistently takes a longer step with the prosthetic limb than the contralateral limb. The MOST likely cause of the deviation is:

1. weak abdominal muscles
2. **hip flexion contracture**
3. weak residual limb
4. fear and insecurity

Correct Answer: 2 (Seymour p. 232)

A hip flexion contracture on the prosthetic side can result in an uneven step length. Hip flexion contractures are the most common type of contracture following a transfemoral amputation. Activities such as prone lying can decrease the incidence of developing the contracture.

1. A patient with weak abdominal muscles may have difficulty maintaining standard step length secondary to weakness of the trunk and inadequate stability. The physical therapist would not tend to observe an increased step length secondary to weakened abdominals.
2. **A hip flexion contracture would cause decreased hip extension during late stance on the prosthetic side allowing for a shorter step on the uninvolved side and a longer step with the prosthetic limb.**
3. A patient with a weak residual limb would not typically take a longer step with the prosthetic limb since the hip flexors would be weak and unable to create the necessary force. A weak limb would typically result in a shorter step on the prosthetic side or the use of compensatory techniques (vaulting or circumduction) to advance the prosthesis.
4. A patient that exhibits fear and insecurity would typically demonstrate an overall shorter step length bilaterally. The patient may exhibit a shuffling gait in order to minimize single stance phase on either lower extremity.

System Specific: Musculoskeletal System
Content Outline: Foundations for Evaluation, Differential Diagnosis, & Prognosis

Exam Three: Question 106

A physical therapist designs a research study that examines body composition as a function of aerobic exercise and diet. Which method of data collection would provide the therapist with the MOST valid measurement of body composition?

1. anthropometric measurements
2. bioelectrical impedance
3. **hydrostatic weighing**
4. skinfold measurements

Correct Answer: 3 (American College of Sports Medicine p. 268)

Body composition is defined as the relative percentage of body weight that is comprised of fat and fat-free tissue. There are multiple methods for testing the percentage of body fat including hydrostatic weighing, skinfold measurements, plethysmography, body mass index (BMI), and bioelectrical impedance analysis.

1. Common anthropometric measurements used for adults include height, weight, BMI, waist-to-hip ratio, and percentage of body fat. These measures are then compared to reference standards to assess items such as weight status and the risk for various diseases.
2. Bioelectric impedance measures body composition by using electrical current to determine the resistance or opposition to current flow. The technique is based on the principle that resistance to electrical current is inversely related to the composition of water within the body. Limitations include the requisite hydration status of the patient and the ability of the examiner to follow the established testing protocol.
3. **Hydrostatic weighing calculates the density of the body by immersing a person in water and measuring the amount of water that becomes displaced. The percentage of body fat is then determined by calculating the measured amount of water displaced in an equation based on Archimedes' principle. This measurement technique is considered the criterion or gold standard for determining body composition. Limitations include the relative availability and expense of the necessary equipment and the amount of time needed to administer the technique.**
4. Skinfold measurements can be used to determine the overall percentage of body fat through the measurement of nine standardized sites. The theory associated with skinfold measurements is that the amount of subcutaneous fat is proportional to the total amount of body fat. Limitations of this method include the availability of an experienced examiner as well as variance from the standards based on gender, age, and ethnicity.

System Specific: Other Systems
Content Outline: Examination

Exam Three: Question 107

A physical therapist examines a patient diagnosed with post-polio syndrome. Which of the following areas is the least likely to be affected based on the patient's diagnosis?

1. strength
2. **sensation**
3. endurance
4. functional mobility

Correct Answer: 2 (Goodman - Pathology p. 1624)

Post-polio syndrome is a term used to describe symptoms that occur years after the onset of poliomyelitis. The condition is characterized by a weakening of the muscles that were originally affected by polio. Symptoms include progressive muscle weakness, fatigue, and muscle atrophy.

1. Patients with post-polio syndrome experience a decrease in strength. This finding may be related to the degeneration of individual nerve terminals in the motor units that remain after the initial illness.
2. **The polio virus attacks specific neurons in the brainstem and anterior horn cells of the spinal cord. As a result, sensation is not typically affected.**
3. Endurance is compromised in patients with post-polio syndrome secondary to the loss of strength, vasomotor abnormalities, joint pain, and myalgias.
4. Functional mobility will decrease as a result of the patient's loss of strength and endurance. Pain will also often increase with physical activity which may result in the patient becoming less active.

System Specific: Neuromuscular & Nervous Systems
Content Outline: Foundations for Evaluation, Differential Diagnosis, & Prognosis

Exam Three: Question 108

A physical therapist prepares to perform manual vibration as a means of airway clearance with a patient diagnosed with chronic obstructive pulmonary disease. When performing vibration the MOST appropriate form of manual contact over the affected lung segment is:

1. contact with a cupped hand
2. **contact with the entire palmar surface of the hand**
3. contact with the ulnar border of the hand
4. contact with the distal phalanx of the middle finger

Correct Answer: 2 (Hillegass p. 651)

Vibration is administered by contracting the muscles of the upper extremities and intentionally causing a vibration to the chest wall with the hands. Vibration should produce a gentle, high frequency force and is a viable alternative to percussion in acutely ill patients with chest wall discomfort or pain.

1. Contact with a cupped hand would be indicated when performing percussion. Percussion refers to a rhythmical clapping applied over an affected lung segment. Percussion is used to loosen retained secretions.
2. **Vibration requires the palmar aspect of the physical therapist's hands to be in full contact with the affected lung segment. The therapist may elect to partially or fully overlap the hands during manual vibration. Vibration is applied at the end of a deep inspiration and is maintained through the end of expiration.**
3. Contact with the ulnar border of the hand can be used as a method to assess tactile fremitus. Tactile fremitus refers to the vibration of spoken words felt through the chest wall. The palmar surface of one or both hands can also be used. Tactile fremitus provides information about the density of the lungs and the thoracic cavity.
4. Mediate percussion is used to evaluate changes in lung density. The technique requires the physical therapist to place the middle finger of one hand flat on the chest wall along the intercostal space between two ribs while the other fingers are lifted off of the chest wall. The opposing hand acts as a fulcrum using the middle finger to strike the middle finger of the opposite hand positioned on the chest wall. The quality of the generated sound provides the therapist with information on lung density.

System Specific: Cardiac, Vascular, & Pulmonary Systems
Content Outline: Interventions

Exam Three: Question 109

A physical therapist completes an upper quarter screening examination on a patient with a suspected cervical spine lesion. Which objective finding is NOT consistent with C5 involvement?

1. **muscle weakness in the supinator and wrist extensors**
2. diminished sensation in the deltoid area
3. muscle weakness in the deltoid and biceps
4. diminished biceps and brachioradialis reflexes

Correct Answer: 1 (Magee p. 22)

Involvement of a specific nerve root often results in predictable impairments including diminished sensation, muscle weakness, impaired reflexes, and paresthesias.

1. **Muscle weakness of the supinator (C5, C6, C7) and the extensor digitorum (C6, C7, C8) is associated with C6 involvement.**
2. Diminished sensation in the deltoid area and the anterior aspect of the entire arm to the base of the thumb is associated with the C5 dermatome.
3. Muscle weakness of the deltoid (C5, C6) and the biceps (C5, C6) is associated with the C5 myotome.
4. Diminished biceps (C5, C6) and brachioradialis (C5, C6) reflexes are associated with C5 involvement.

System Specific: Neuromuscular & Nervous Systems
Content Outline: Foundations for Evaluation, Differential Diagnosis, & Prognosis

Exam Three: Question 110

A physical therapist employed in a rehabilitation hospital reviews the medical record of a 26-year-old patient recently admitted to the facility. The medical record indicates that the patient sustained a spinal cord injury four weeks ago in a diving accident. Which medical diagnosis would result in the patient being MOST susceptible to autonomic dysreflexia?

1. T4 paraplegia
2. T12 paraplegia
3. cauda equina injury
4. posterior cord syndrome

Correct Answer: 1 (O'Sullivan p. 943)

Autonomic dysreflexia is caused when a noxious stimulus below the level of the lesion triggers the autonomic nervous system causing a sudden elevation in blood pressure. Symptoms include profuse sweating, bradycardia, goose bumps, headache, and vasodilation (flushing) above the level of the injury. This condition should be treated as a medical emergency.

1. **Autonomic dysreflexia is common in patients with spinal cord lesions above the T6 level. The condition should be treated as a medical emergency. Immediate medical management includes assisting the patient to a sitting position in an attempt to reduce blood pressure and examining the urinary drainage system since this often serves as the noxious stimulus that triggers the autonomic response.**
2. A patient with T12 paraplegia would not typically be at risk for autonomic dysreflexia since the level of the lesion is below T6.
3. Cauda equina injury occurs below the L1 spinal level where the long nerve roots transcend. Characteristics include flaccidity, areflexia, and impairment of bowel and bladder function. Full recovery is not typical due to the distance needed for axonal regeneration.
4. Posterior cord syndrome refers to a relatively rare incomplete lesion caused by compression of the posterior spinal artery and is characterized by loss of pain perception, proprioception, two-point discrimination, and stereognosis. Motor function is preserved.

System Specific: Neuromuscular & Nervous Systems
Content Outline: Foundations for Evaluation, Differential Diagnosis, & Prognosis

Exam Three: Question 111

A physical therapist utilizes neuromuscular electrical stimulation by attaching an electrode over the motor point of the peroneus longus. The MOST appropriate location to attach the electrode is:

1. along the lateral border of the popliteal fossa
2. **on the anterolateral surface of the lower leg**
3. proximal to the first metatarsophalangeal joint
4. immediately inferior to the lateral malleolus

Correct Answer: 2 (Kendall p. 365)

A motor point refers to a point on the skin where the application of an electrical stimulus via an electrode will cause the contraction of an underlying muscle. A physical therapist can attempt to identify a motor point based on their knowledge of a muscle's origin and insertion.

1. The popliteal fossa refers to an area or shallow depression located on the posterior surface of the knee. The area is significantly superior to the origin and insertion of the peroneus longus and therefore could not serve as a motor point for the muscle.
2. **The peroneus longus originates on the head and upper two-thirds of the lateral surface of the fibula and inserts on the lateral side of the base of the first metatarsal and the medial cuneiform. The muscle acts to evert the foot and assists in plantar flexion of the ankle joint. The anterolateral surface of the lower leg is consistent with the muscle's motor point.**
3. A motor point proximal to the first metatarsophalangeal joint would likely be associated with one of the intrinsic muscles of the foot.
4. While the location immediately inferior to the lateral malleolus would correspond to an area that the peroneus longus passes over, by the time the muscle reaches this distal point, it is mostly tendon and therefore an electrical stimulus would not produce the desired motor response.

System Specific: Non-Systems
Content Outline: Equipment & Devices; Therapeutic Modalities

Exam Three: Question 112

A patient diagnosed with shoulder pain of unknown etiology is referred by his physician for magnetic resonance imaging. Results of the test reveal a partial tear of the infraspinatus muscle. Which muscle group would be the MOST seriously affected by the injury?

1. **shoulder lateral rotators**
2. shoulder medial rotators
3. shoulder abductors
4. shoulder adductors

Correct Answer: 1 (Kendall p. 321)

The infraspinatus muscle originates on the medial two-thirds of the infraspinous fossa of the scapula and inserts on the greater tubercle of the humerus. The muscle is innervated by the suprascapular nerve.

1. **The primary action of the infraspinatus is lateral rotation of the shoulder joint. The muscle also plays an important role in stabilizing the head of the humerus in the glenoid cavity. Other muscles that function as shoulder lateral rotators include the teres minor and posterior deltoid.**
2. The shoulder medial rotators include the subscapularis, teres major, pectoralis major, latissimus dorsi, and anterior deltoid muscles.
3. The shoulder abductors include the middle deltoid and supraspinatus muscles.
4. The shoulder adductors include the pectoralis major, latissimus dorsi, and teres major muscles.

System Specific: Musculoskeletal System
Content Outline: Clinical Application of Foundational Sciences

Exam Three: Question 113

A physical therapist reads in the medical record that a wound located near a patient's ischial tuberosity was classified as "Black" using the Red-Yellow-Black system. The MOST relevant finding associated with a "Black" classification would be the presence of:

1. granulation tissue
2. exudate
3. slough
4. **eschar**

Correct Answer: 4 (Sussman p. 91)

The Red-Yellow-Black Wound system uses a wound's surface color to direct treatment. A red wound is the most desirable, followed by yellow, and then black.

1. Granulation tissue is produced during the proliferative phase of wound healing and is rich with macrophages, fibroblasts, collagen, and blood vessels. Granulation tissue is classified as "Red" using the Red-Yellow-Black system.

2. Exudate is a fluid rich in protein and cellular debris that has escaped from blood vessels due to inflammation. The characteristics of exudate from a given wound assist physical therapists to diagnose wound infection, evaluate the effectiveness of selected interventions, and monitor wound healing. Exudate is not part of the Red-Yellow-Black system.

3. Slough is a form of necrotic tissue that is usually moist, stringy, and viscous and is most often yellow in color. Slough is classified as "Yellow" using the Red-Yellow-Black system.

4. **Eschar describes a particular type of necrosis, usually presenting as brown or black with a hard or soft appearance. Eschar is indicative of full-thickness tissue destruction. Eschar is classified as "Black" using the Red-Yellow-Black system.**

System Specific: Integumentary System
Content Outline: Foundations for Evaluation, Differential Diagnosis, & Prognosis

Exam Three: Question 114

A physical therapist instructs a patient with a unilateral amputation to ascend and descend stairs. Which amputation level would you expect to have the MOST difficulty performing the described task?

1. transmetatarsal
2. transtibial
3. **transfemoral**
4. Symes

Correct Answer: 3 (Tan p. 245)

As the level of amputation increases, the necessary energy expenditure, balance, and coordination required to complete functional activities also increases.

1. A transmetatarsal amputation will have very little effect on a patient's ability to ascend and descend stairs. A transmetatarsal amputation is an amputation that occurs through the midsection of the metatarsals.

2. A transtibial amputation will result in an increased energy expenditure of approximately twenty-five percent with mobility compared to a person with two healthy lower extremities. The amount is significantly less than the increased energy expenditure associated with a transfemoral amputation.

3. **A transfemoral amputation will have the largest impact on energy expenditure during functional activities. A patient ambulating with a transfemoral prosthesis has an increased energy expenditure of approximately two times that of a person with two healthy lower extremities. As a result, ascending and descending stairs will be the most difficult for a patient with a transfemoral amputation.**

4. A Syme's amputation occurs when the ankle is disarticulated and the heel pad is attached to the distal tibia. The amputation causes an increased energy expenditure during mobility, but due to the long length of the lever arm and distal point of amputation, the increase in energy expenditure is minimal.

System Specific: Musculoskeletal System
Content Outline: Foundations for Evaluation, Differential Diagnosis, & Prognosis

Exam Three: Question 115

A physical therapist receives a referral for a 48-year-old female diagnosed with lung cancer. The patient reports smoking three packs of cigarettes a day for the last 25 years. Assuming the patient was diagnosed with cancer two months ago, which of the following pieces of data would provide the therapist with the MOST valuable information when establishing the plan of care and the associated goals?

1. premorbid lifestyle
2. **staging of cancer**
3. past medical history
4. motivation level

Correct Answer: 2 (Goodman – Pathology p. 350)

Lung cancer is the most frequent form of cancer in the United States and refers to a malignancy of the epithelium of the respiratory tract. The majority of lung cancers are detected on routine chest x-ray in patients presenting with an unrelated medical condition. The staging of the cancer is used to estimate prognosis and to determine appropriate intervention strategies.

1. The patient's premorbid lifestyle is relevant, however, would not be the primary factor when establishing the plan of care and associated goals.

2. **The TNM Classification System (T=tumor, N=node, M=metastasis) is a commonly used cancer classification system that describes the extent of a particular malignant tumor. "T" refers to the extent of the primary tumor, "N" refers to the absence or presence and extent of regional lymph node metastasis, and "M" refers to the absence or presence of distant metastasis. This type of staging offers guidance to health care professionals when determining treatment options, life expectancy, and prognosis for complete resolution.**

3. Past medical history provides a basic snapshot of a patient's overall health status. This information would be considered when establishing the plan of care and associated goals, but it would not be as critical as other pieces of information (i.e., cancer staging).

4. Motivation level is particularly important once a plan of care is established, however, the patient's motivation level would be of only modest value when establishing the plan of care and associated goals.

System Specific: Other Systems
Content Outline: Foundations for Evaluation, Differential Diagnosis, & Prognosis

Exam Three: Question 116

A physical therapist treats a 54-year-old male rehabilitating from a tibial plateau fracture. While completing a resistive exercise the patient indicates that lifting weights often causes him to void small amounts of urine. The MOST appropriate therapist action is:

1. refer the patient to a support group
2. instruct the patient in pelvic floor muscle strengthening exercises
3. discontinue resistive exercises as part of the established plan of care
4. **educate the patient about incontinence**

Correct Answer: 4 (Kisner p. 581)

Incontinence refers to an inability to control the release of urine, feces or gas and is a common occurrence for many men and women. The causes of incontinence may include weak pelvic floor muscles or medical conditions such as an enlarged prostate, prostatitis, cancer, neurological disorders or obstruction. Proper diagnosis is necessary in order to effectively treat this condition.

1. The use of a support group would be a potential adjunct activity for the patient, however, at this time, education is the appropriate action.

2. It would be inappropriate to begin pelvic floor exercises without a referral from a physician since the cause of the incontinence is unknown.

3. The physical therapist should not discontinue resistive exercises since strengthening is a necessary component of a rehabilitation program for a patient following a tibial plateau fracture. This action also does not directly address the current issue of uncontrolled voiding of urine.

4. **The patient may significantly benefit from formal education about incontinence. The action would provide the patient with necessary information and make the patient more likely to see a physician about this issue. A vast majority of patients with incontinence can be successfully treated with non-invasive measures such as pelvic floor exercises.**

System Specific: Other Systems
Content Outline: Interventions

Exam Three: Question 117

A patient two days status post transfemoral amputation demonstrates decreased strength and generalized deconditioning. Which of the following positions should be utilized when instructing the patient to wrap their residual limb?

1. sidelying
2. standing
3. **supine**
4. prone

Correct Answer: 3 (Seymour p. 124)

A physical therapist should instruct a patient to wrap their residual limb in a manner that allows full access to the residual limb and provides a secure and stable environment that does not jeopardize patient safety.

1. A sidelying position would make it difficult for the patient to utilize the upper extremities to manipulate the bandage. Viewing the residual limb in sidelying would also be more difficult than in supine.
2. Standing on the uninvolved lower extremity would not provide an adequate base of support for wrapping the residual limb. Wrapping the residual limb in standing requires high levels of coordination and balance.
3. **A supine position would provide the patient with adequate access to the residual limb and provide a secure and stable environment to complete the wrapping.**
4. A prone position would make it extremely challenging for the patient to wrap the residual limb and would make it impossible for the patient to inspect the wrapping. A prone position may be contraindicated for patients with particular cardiac or respiratory pathologies.

System Specific: Integumentary
Content Outline: Interventions

Exam Three: Question 118

A physical therapist employed in an outpatient private practice receives a referral for a patient diagnosed with spondylolisthesis. Which of the following scenarios would be MOST consistent with the medical diagnosis?

1. **a 13-year-old female gymnast with no significant medical history**
2. a 17-year-old female tennis player with a 15 degree lateral curvature of the spine
3. a 28-year-old male machinist with a history of recurrent low back pain
4. a 67-year-old male with a previous diagnosis of ankylosing spondylitis

Correct Answer: 1 (Dutton p. 1565)

Spondylolisthesis refers to a condition where one vertebra slips forward on the one below it due to a bilateral fracture of the pars interarticularis. This condition most commonly occurs at L4-L5 or L5-S1.

1. **Children ages 10-15 who are involved in activities such as gymnastics, weight lifting, volleyball, and pole vaulting are particularly susceptible to spondylolisthesis.**
2. Lateral curvature of the spine is indicative of scoliosis and not spondylolisthesis. Scoliosis has many causes including changes in bony structure of the spine (i.e., wedging of a vertebral body), neuromuscular disorders (i.e., cerebral palsy, muscular dystrophy) or an impairment of an extremity (i.e., leg length discrepancy). Scoliosis can also have idiopathic etiology.
3. This patient's age and occupation are not typically consistent with the incidence of spondylolisthesis. The recurrence of the patient's low back pain is more suggestive of a muscular strain than a fracture.
4. Ankylosing spondylitis is a systemic condition that is characterized by inflammation of the spine and larger peripheral joints. The chronic inflammation causes destruction of the ligamentous-osseous junction with subsequent fibrosis and ossification of the area. Men are at a two to three time greater risk than women and onset is typically seen between twenty and forty years of age.

System Specific: Musculoskeletal System
Content Outline: Foundations for Evaluation, Differential Diagnosis, & Prognosis

Exam Three: Question 119

A patient diagnosed with Cushing's syndrome is referred to physical therapy. Which of the following signs and symptoms is NOT consistent with this syndrome?

1. distension of the abdomen
2. swelling in the facial area
3. **adrenal hypoplasia**
4. cardiac hypertrophy

Correct Answer: 3 (Goodman - Pathology p. 481)

Cushing's syndrome is produced by an excess of free circulating cortisol from the adrenal cortex. Physical therapists may be more likely to treat patients who have developed medication-induced Cushing's syndrome, usually after receiving large doses of cortisol or cortisol derivatives.

1. Distention of the abdomen and subsequent central obesity is consistent with Cushing's syndrome. Weakening of the muscles and elastic tissue in combination with abnormal fat distribution results in distention of the abdomen. Thinning of the skin with striae on the breasts, axillary areas, and abdomen are often observed.
2. Swelling in the facial area is a common characteristic of Cushing's syndrome. This condition is often referred to as "moon-shaped face."
3. **Cushing's syndrome is a condition characterized by hyperfunction of the adrenal cortex. Addison's disease is a condition characterized by hypoplasia of the adrenal cortex.**
4. Physiological manifestations of Cushing's syndrome include hypertension caused by potassium depletion, and sodium and water retention. Hypertension can result in left ventricular hypertrophy and increased risk of congestive heart failure or CVA.

System Specific: Other Systems
Content Outline: Foundations for Evaluation, Differential Diagnosis, & Prognosis

Exam Three: Question 120

A physical therapist completes an examination on a patient diagnosed with complete C7 tetraplegia. The patient problem list includes inability to complete an independent bed to wheelchair transfer, decreased passive lower extremity range of motion, tissue breakdown over the ischial tuberosities, and decreased upper extremity strength. Which of the following treatment activities should be given the highest priority?

1. **pressure relief activities**
2. transfer training using a sliding board
3. self-range of motion activities
4. upper extremity strengthening exercises

Correct Answer: 1 (O'Sullivan p. 465)

A physical therapist should give the highest priority to educating the patient on appropriate skin care including pressure relief activities. A patient with C7 tetraplegia can perform lateral and forward weight shifting in the wheelchair to assist with pressure relief.

1. **Education and instruction in pressure relief activities is the highest priority for a patient that has compromised sensation. The patient can perform independent relief through weight shifting each two-hour period to avoid further skin breakdown and infection.**
2. Transfer training using a sliding board will be a component of the treatment plan, but would not be the highest priority. Weight shifting is a precursor to performing a sliding board transfer.
3. Self-range of motion will be a component of the treatment plan. Patients must maintain an expected length in each muscle group in order to function at maximum potential. Pressure relief must be given the highest priority, however, so that the patient can progress through rehabilitation without skin breakdown.
4. Upper extremity strengthening will be a component of the treatment plan and focuses on maximizing strength in the available muscles. Although strengthening is desirable, failure to prevent tissue breakdown will place the patient at considerable risk for serious medical complications.

System Specific: Neuromuscular & Nervous Systems
Content Outline: Interventions

Exam Three: Question 121

A physical therapist treats a 56-year-old male status post transfemoral amputation with a hip flexion contracture. As part of the treatment regimen the therapist performs passive stretching exercises to the involved hip. The MOST appropriate form of passive stretching is:

1. **moderate tension over a prolonged period of time**
2. moderate tension over a brief period of time
3. maximal tension over a prolonged period of time
4. maximal tension over a brief period of time

Correct Answer: 1 (Kisner p. 79)

The effectiveness of a stretching program is influenced by a multitude of variables including intensity, duration, speed, frequency, and mode of stretch. Physical therapists must carefully select the parameters of a stretching program based on the established therapeutic goals.

1. **Moderate tension over a prolonged period of time would be the most appropriate form of stretching for the hip flexors. Moderate tension will minimize muscle guarding and the duration of the stretch will promote gradual gains in muscle length.**
2. Moderate tension over a brief period of time is an appropriate option, however, the time period would be less effective than a prolonged period of time to increase muscle length.
3. Maximal tension over a prolonged period of time would not likely be tolerated by the patient. The amount of tension would result in significant muscle guarding that would limit the effectiveness of the stretching activity.
4. Maximal tension over a brief period of time may be a slightly better option than the prolonged period of time, however, the intensity of the stretch would still likely result in muscle guarding that would limit the effectiveness of the stretching activity.

System Specific: Musculoskeletal System
Content Outline: Interventions

Exam Three: Question 122

A physical therapist treats a patient diagnosed with Parkinson's disease. When working on controlled mobility, which of the following would BEST describe the physical therapist's objective?

1. facilitate postural muscle control
2. **promote weight shifting and rotational trunk control**
3. emphasize reciprocal extremity movement
4. facilitate tone and rigidity

Correct Answer: 2 (Sullivan p. 77)

Controlled mobility refers to the ability to move within a weight bearing position or rotate around a long axis. Controlled mobility is one component of the Stages of Motor Control (mobility, stability, controlled mobility, and skill).

1. Stability refers to the ability to maintain a position or posture through cocontraction and tonic holding around a joint. Unsupported sitting with midline control is an example of stability.
2. **Controlled mobility activities should emphasize weight shifting and trunk control with rotation. This type of activity may serve to decrease rigidity and improve the fluidity of gait in a patient with Parkinson's disease.**
3. A patient must possess prerequisite stability and dynamic postural control in order to perform reciprocal extremity movement. Coordination training often focuses on reciprocal extremity movement.
4. Facilitation techniques are used to increase tone in patients with hypotonia. These techniques are not often used to treat Parkinson's disease since patients with this condition typically exhibit hypertonia or in more severe cases, rigidity.

System Specific: Neuromuscular & Nervous Systems
Content Outline: Interventions

Exam Three: Question 123

A physical therapist assesses the strength of selected lower extremity muscles on a patient rehabilitating from a knee injury. The pictured test would be MOST effective to examine the strength of the:

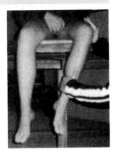

1. hip abductors
2. hip adductors
3. hip medial rotators
4. **hip lateral rotators**

Correct Answer: 4 (Kendall p. 430)

The hip lateral rotators include the gluteus maximus, obturator internus, obturator externus, piriformis, gemelli, and sartorius. Weakness of the lateral rotators usually results in medial rotation of the femur accompanied by pronation of the foot and a tendency toward a valgus position at the knee.

1. The strength of the hip abductors is assessed with the patient in sidelying with the test leg raised. The physical therapist should apply pressure to the distal aspect of the femur, pushing the leg downward in an attempt to adduct the thigh. The hip abductors include the gluteus minimus, gluteus medius, piriformis, and obturator internus.

2. The strength of the hip adductors is assessed with the patient in sidelying with the test leg closest to the surface adducted. The physical therapist should apply pressure to the distal aspect of the femur, pushing the leg downward in an attempt to abduct the thigh. The hip adductors include the adductor longus, adductor brevis, adductor magnus, and gracilis.

3. The strength of the hip medial rotators is assessed with the patient in sitting. The physical therapist should apply pressure to the lateral side of the leg above the ankle, pushing the leg inward in an attempt to rotate the thigh laterally. The hip medial rotators include the pectineus, adductor longus, tensor fasciae latae, gluteus minimus, and gluteus medius.

4. **The strength of the hip lateral rotators is assessed with the patient in sitting. The physical therapist should apply pressure to the medial side of the leg above the ankle, pushing the leg outward in an attempt to rotate the thigh medially.**

System Specific: Musculoskeletal System
Content Outline: Examination

Exam Three: Question 124

A physical therapist employed in a rehabilitation hospital treats a patient status post traumatic brain injury. During the treatment session the therapist notices that the patient's toes are discolored below a bivalved lower extremity cast. The cast was applied approximately five hours ago in an attempt to reduce a plantar flexion contracture. The MOST appropriate therapist action is to:

1. discontinue the use of the anterior portion of the cast
2. contact the staff nurse and request that the cast is removed
3. refer the patient to an orthotist
4. **remove the cast**

Correct Answer: 4 (Tan p. 501)

Discoloration of the patient's toes is an indication that the cast is too tight and is likely impeding the patient's circulation. This objective finding would make it necessary to remove the bivalved cast for further inspection.

1. The anterior and posterior portions of the bivalved cast would need to be removed in order to assess the patient's skin integrity and circulation. Removal of only the anterior portion of the cast would not be adequate to fully inspect the lower extremity.

2. The physical therapist would be able to remove the bivalved cast by simply unfastening the Velcro straps which secure the anterior and posterior portions. As a result, the physical therapist would not need to rely on the nurse.

3. Referral to an orthotist is not necessary since a bivalved cast is easily removed and the observed finding requires immediate attention.

4. **A physical therapist possesses the requisite skills and training to remove the bivalved cast.**

System Specific: Non-Systems
Content Outline: Equipment & Devices; Therapeutic Modalities

Exam Three: Question 125

A physical therapist treats a 26-year-old male with complete C6 tetraplegia. During treatment the patient makes a culturally insensitive remark that the therapist feels is offensive. The MOST appropriate therapist action is to:

1. document the incident in the medical record
2. transfer the patient to another physical therapist's schedule
3. discharge the patient from physical therapy
4. **inform the patient that the remark was offensive and continue with treatment**

> **Correct Answer: 4** (Purtilo p. 343)

A physical therapist must make a patient aware of behavior that is unacceptable. Failure to address the issue directly with the patient may serve to reinforce the behavior.

1. Documentation would be more appropriate in instances such as a patient's refusal of physical therapy services, a fall or injury or to provide a status update for various members of the health care team.
2. The patient should not be transferred to another physical therapist's schedule due to a culturally insensitive remark. A physical therapist must be able to provide direct feedback to patients regarding their status, progress, and behaviors when necessary.
3. Discharge from physical therapy should only occur when all attainable goals are met or when a patient makes a decision to cease physical therapy services. It would be inappropriate for a physical therapist to discharge a patient for making a culturally insensitive remark, particularly since there is no indication that a similar incident has occurred previously.
4. **The physical therapist should provide immediate feedback to the patient when an inappropriate behavior is witnessed. A culturally insensitive remark would not warrant the interruption or cessation of the existing plan of care.**

System Specific: Non-Systems
Content Outline: Safety & Professional Roles; Teaching/Learning; Research

Exam Three: Question 126

A physical therapist asks a patient who has been inconsistent with his attendance in physical therapy, why he is having difficulty keeping scheduled appointments. The patient responds that it is difficult to understand the scheduling card that lists the appointments. The therapist's MOST appropriate action would be to:

1. contact the referring physician to discuss the patient's poor attendance in therapy
2. make sure the patient is given a scheduling card at the conclusion of each session
3. **write down the patient's appointments on a piece of paper in a manner that the patient can understand**
4. discharge the patient from physical therapy

> **Correct Answer: 3** (Falvo p. 165)

In order to determine if the patient's poor attendance in therapy is due to difficulty understanding the scheduling card, the information must be presented in a manner the patient can understand.

1. Contacting the referring physician may eventually be warranted, however, the initial focus should be directed toward improving the patient's understanding of his scheduled appointments.
2. Since the patient has expressed that he has difficulty reading the scheduling card, it would not be helpful to provide the same card at more frequent intervals.
3. **The physical therapist can improve the patient's understanding of the scheduling card by writing the appointments in a more understandable format.**
4. A patient should not be discharged from physical therapy unless the physical therapist has already taken steps to improve the patient's compliance with scheduled appointments.

System Specific: Non-Systems
Content Outline: Safety & Professional Roles; Teaching/Learning; Research

Exam Three: Question 127

A physical therapist treats a patient status post right cerebrovascular accident with resultant left hemiplegia for a colleague on vacation. A note left by the primary therapist indicates that the patient exhibits "pusher syndrome." When examining the patient's sitting posture, which of the following findings would be MOST likely?

1. **sitting with increased lean to the left along with increased weight bearing through the left buttocks**
2. sitting with increased lean to the right along with increased weight bearing through the right buttocks
3. sitting with increased weight bearing through the right buttocks and the head rotated to the right; unresponsive to stimuli on the left
4. sitting with unequal weight bearing and the head rotated to the left; unresponsive to stimuli on the right

> **Correct Answer: 1** (O'Sullivan p. 750)

Pusher syndrome is characterized by a significant lateral deviation toward the hemiplegic side. Pusher syndrome more commonly occurs in patients that have sustained a right CVA. Therapeutic intervention for a patient that exhibits pusher syndrome may include the use of a mirror, a small wedge placed under the left lateral thigh, weight shifting across midline, and facilitation techniques for trunk control.

1. **A patient with right CVA (left hemiplegia) with pusher syndrome would typically exhibit a lateral lean to the left in sitting with increased weight bearing on the left buttocks.**
2. A patient with right CVA (left hemiplegia) without pusher syndrome would typically exhibit less weight bearing through the left side due to the existing sensory and motor deficits. Intervention would include midline orientation and weight shifting in sitting.
3. A patient with right CVA (left hemiplegia) who demonstrates the inability to interpret stimuli on the left side of the body is exhibiting unilateral neglect. Neglect is most often associated with a lesion of the right frontal lobe of the brain.
4. A patient with right CVA (left hemiplegia) would not typically rotate the head towards the affected (left) side, but rather away from it secondary to neglect. The patient would be more responsive to stimuli on the right.

System Specific: Neuromuscular & Nervous Systems
Content Outline: Foundations for Evaluation, Differential Diagnosis, & Prognosis

Exam Three: Question 128

A physical therapist working in a school system develops long-term goals as part of an Individualized Educational Plan for a child with Down syndrome. The MOST appropriate time frame to attain these goals is:

1. one month
2. four months
3. six months
4. **one year**

> **Correct Answer: 4** (Tecklin p. 659)

An Individualized Educational Plan (IEP) is designed for any school-aged child that requires therapy services. Long-term goals are based on a one-year plan. These services are provided through federal legislation through the Individuals with Disabilities Education Act (IDEA).

1. A goal with a one-month time frame is designed for a patient that requires therapeutic intervention for an injury or condition that will steadily progress and improve. This time frame is not within the framework of the IEP.
2. A four-month time frame may be an appropriate interval to informally reassess the child and quantify the actual progress towards the established goals, however, it is typically an insufficient amount of time to expect the established goals to be accomplished.
3. A six-month time frame may be an appropriate interval for review of established goals for the IEP since it is a midpoint in the year. This time frame, however, is not typically sufficient to accomplish the long-term goals.
4. **Federal legislation mandates the review of an IEP on a one-year basis. Goals relate to improving a child's educational experience. IDEA also provides for children 0-5 years of age through early intervention programs.**

System Specific: Non-Systems
Content Outline: Safety & Professional Roles; Teaching/Learning; Research

Exam Three: Question 129

A two-year-old with T10 spina bifida receives physical therapy for gait training. Initially, the preferred method to teach a child how to maintain standing is with the use of:

1. bilateral hip-knee-ankle-foot orthoses (HKAFO) and forearm crutches
2. **parapodium and the parallel bars**
3. bilateral knee-ankle-foot orthoses (KAFO) and the parallel bars
4. bilateral ankle-foot orthoses (AFO) and the parallel bars

Correct Answer: 2 (Tecklin p. 254)

The parapodium provides the necessary amount of support and is optimal to assist with standing activities for children with thoracic and high level lumbar lesions. The parallel bars are the most stable assistive device to initiate standing and gait training.

1. HKAFOs would require a swing-through or reciprocal gait pattern. Using HKAFOs with forearm crutches requires a high level of balance and energy expenditure and is not appropriate for initial standing activities.
2. **The parapodium is a HKAFO with a thoracolumbar orthosis that supports the trunk and lower extremities. It has a large base of support and is used with or without an assistive device. This would be ideal for a patient with T10 spina bifida to initiate standing within the parallel bars.**
3. A patient with T10 spina bifida would not initially use KAFOs in the parallel bars when working on standing activities due to the deficits in strength and sensation below the T10 level.
4. A patient with T10 spina bifida would not possess the necessary motor function to use bilateral AFOs.

System Specific: Neuromuscular & Nervous Systems
Content Outline: Interventions

Exam Three: Question 130

A physical therapist notices a small area of skin irritation under the chin of a patient wearing a Philadelphia collar. The patient expresses that the area is not painful, but is becoming increasingly itchy. The MOST appropriate therapist action is:

1. instruct the patient to apply 1% hydrocortisone cream to the area twice daily
2. apply powder to the area and instruct the patient to avoid scratching
3. **provide the patient with a liner to use as a barrier between the skin and the orthosis**
4. discontinue use of the orthosis until the skin has become less irritated

Correct Answer: 3 (Physical Therapist's Clinical Companion p. 316)

Patients can experience itching or skin irritation when using a cervical orthosis. Since an orthosis is applied directly over the skin, it is imperative to utilize a liner that maximizes comfort, promotes cleanliness, limits moisture, and reduces skin irritation. Failure to select an appropriate liner may result in skin breakdown.

1. Hydrocortisone may be used to treat an existing area of irritation, however, it does not address the primary cause of irritation.
2. Powder may assist to temporarily reduce friction over a particular area, but it does not address the primary cause of irritation.
3. **Liners made from lambs' wool are commonly utilized and prevent chafing and irritation of the patient's skin. This liner is easily donned and provides an adequate barrier between the skin and orthosis.**
4. Discontinuing the use of the cervical orthosis would be undesirable since it is prescribed based on medical necessity.

System Specific: Non-Systems
Content Outline: Equipment & Devices; Therapeutic Modalities

Exam Three: Question 131

A patient with muscle weakness and compromised balance uses a four-point gait pattern with two canes. The physical therapist would like to instruct the patient to ascend and descend the stairs according to the normal flow of traffic. When ascending stairs the MOST practical method is to:

1. **use the handrail with the right hand and place the two canes in the left hand**
2. use the handrail with the left hand and place the two canes in the right hand
3. place one cane in each hand and avoid using the handrail
4. place the two canes in the left hand and avoid using the handrail

> **Correct Answer: 1** (Minor p. 386)

Since the normal flow of traffic assumes ascending on the right and descending on the left, the patient should grasp the railing with the right hand and use the two canes in the left hand when ascending and descending the stairs.

1. **Since the patient does not have unilateral weakness, it is most appropriate to ascend the stairs on the right in order to utilize the handrail and remain consistent with the normal flow of traffic.**
2. Since the normal flow of traffic assumes ascending on the right and descending on the left, the patient would be going against the normal flow of traffic by grasping the handrail with the left hand and using the two canes in the right hand.
3. The patient should use a handrail when available in order to improve stability and balance.
4. Failure to use the handrail would significantly increase the patient's relative risk of falling.

System Specific: Non-Systems
Content Outline: Equipment & Devices; Therapeutic Modalities

Exam Three: Question 132

A patient rehabilitating from a total hip arthroplasty receives home physical therapy services. The patient is currently full weight bearing and is able to ascend and descend stairs independently. The patient expresses that her goal following rehabilitation is to walk one mile each day. The MOST appropriate plan to accomplish the patient's goal is to:

1. continue home physical therapy services until the patient's goal is attained
2. refer the patient to an outpatient orthopedic physical therapy clinic
3. **design a home exercise program that emphasizes progressive ambulation**
4. admit the patient to a rehabilitation hospital

> **Correct Answer: 3** (Guide for Professional Conduct)

The patient's goal of walking one mile each day does not warrant continued physical therapy services. The physical therapist should assist the patient to achieve their individual goals by implementing a home exercise program that includes progressive ambulation.

1. Home physical therapy is warranted for patients that are "homebound." This patient would not qualify for home physical therapy services secondary to her current functional status.
2. The patient's current functional status does not appear to warrant continued physical therapy services regardless of practice setting. Since the patient is now independent in the home and her goal includes ambulating one mile each day, the outpatient orthopedic clinic is not an appropriate setting. The patient can meet her goal independently by following a home program.
3. **The physical therapist can assist the patient with her long-term goal by designing a home exercise program that incorporates ongoing exercise and progressive ambulation activities. This patient would not typically qualify for further physical therapy services.**
4. A rehabilitation hospital is appropriate for patients with functional deficits and acute rehabilitation needs. The patient's current functional status makes the intensity of rehabilitation offered in this setting unnecessary.

System Specific: Musculoskeletal System
Content Outline: Interventions

Exam Three: Question 133

A physical therapist completes a work site analysis for a patient with T3 paraplegia. The patient is employed in the marketing department of an advertising agency and relies on a wheelchair for daily locomotion. Which of the following is likely to be the MOST significant architectural barrier for the patient?

1. hardwood floors
2. **an entrance ramp (one inch of vertical rise for every six inches of ramp length)**
3. one-quarter inch thresholds at each door
4. pedestal type sinks

Correct Answer: 2 (O'Sullivan p. 409)

An entrance ramp that has one inch of vertical rise for every six inches of ramp length would not satisfy the 1:12 (rise:run) minimum ratio identified in the Americans with Disabilities Act (ADA).

1. Hardwood floors allow for easier propulsion, turning, and function with the wheelchair. Floor surfaces must be firm, stable, and slip resistant. A patient would expect increased difficulty using a wheelchair on carpet or outside terrain.
2. **An entrance ramp designed with one inch of vertical rise for every six inches of ramp length would be twice as steep as the 1:12 (rise:run) minimum ratio. The 1:12 ratio allows for a maximum ramp grade of 8.3 percent.**
3. A threshold of one-quarter inch is an acceptable height as a transition surface. Thresholds with beveled edges up to one-half inch are permissible.
4. Pedestal type sinks would not serve as an architectural barrier since the underside of the sink is open and allows for close wheelchair access. A sink encased with a vanity style cabinet would be more restrictive.

System Specific: Non-Systems
Content Outline: Safety & Professional Roles; Teaching/Learning; Research

Exam Three: Question 134

A physical therapist selects an assistive device for a patient rehabilitating from a recent illness. Which assistive device provides the LEAST stability?

1. **Lofstrand crutches**
2. walker
3. parallel bars
4. axillary crutches

Correct Answer: 1 (Minor p. 296)

Lofstrand crutches have a full or half-cuff that fits over a patient's forearms. The patient holds the crutch by grasping the handgrip that extends from the vertical axis of the crutch. Lofstrand crutches allow for greater ease of movement, but provide less overall stability than axillary crutches.

1. **Lofstrand crutches can be used with all levels of weight bearing, however, require the highest level of coordination for proper use. The Lofstrand crutches can be used with two-point, three-point, four-point, swing-to, and swing-through gait patterns.**
2. A walker can be used with all levels of weight bearing. The walker has a significant base of support and offers good stability. A walker is used with a three-point gait pattern.
3. The parallel bars provide maximum stability and security for a patient during the beginning stages of ambulation or standing. The parallel bars are typically mounted to the floor and allow for all levels of weight bearing and gait patterns.
4. Axillary crutches can be used with all levels of weight bearing, however, require coordination for proper use. Axillary crutches can be used with two-point, three-point, four-point, swing-to, and swing-through gait patterns.

System Specific: Non-Systems
Content Outline: Equipment & Devices; Therapeutic Modalities

Exam Three: Question 135

A physical therapist observes that a number of aides appear to be unfamiliar with appropriate guarding techniques. The MOST appropriate remedial strategy to improve their performance is to:

1. offer assistance to the aides when the inappropriate behavior is observed
2. refer the aides to textbooks that explain proper guarding techniques
3. **develop a mandatory inservice on guarding techniques for the aides**
4. inform the director of rehabilitation that the aides are incompetent

> **Correct Answer: 3** (Nosse p. 217)

A mandatory inservice would allow the physical therapist to provide formal education for the aides to ensure consistent use of appropriate guarding techniques.

1. Aides must be competent with all guarding, transfers, and other duties within their job description. Offering assistance to an aide when they are guarding a patient incorrectly may assist with an isolated incident, however, does not fully address the issue of competency.
2. A textbook may be able to educate an aide on general guarding techniques, however, a textbook cannot take the place of an inservice or other forms of experiential training.
3. **An aide should receive mandatory inservicing for all expected job related duties. Each aide should be able to demonstrate proficiency during the inservice in order to ensure patient safety across the spectrum of activities.**
4. Informing the director that the aides are incompetent does not assist the department to improve the competency of the aides.

System Specific: Non-Systems
Content Outline: Safety & Professional Roles; Teaching/Learning; Research

Exam Three: Question 136

A physical therapist attends an inservice entitled "Principles of Exercise for the Obstetric Patient." During the session, the speaker identifies several conditions that are considered to result in high risk pregnancies. Which of the following conditions would NOT be considered high risk?

1. **diastasis recti**
2. incompetent cervix
3. pre-eclampsia
4. multiple gestation

> **Correct Answer: 1** (Kisner p. 804)

Diastasis recti refers to a separation of the two halves of the rectus abdominus muscle at the linea alba. This condition is often associated with pregnancy during the second and third trimesters, however, does not place a pregnancy at high risk.

1. **The etiology of diastasis recti is unknown with separation greater than two centimeters considered significant. This condition is not considered high risk for pregnancy, however, can produce low back pain due to a limited ability of the abdominal muscles to stabilize the pelvis and lumbar spine.**
2. The increase in pressure associated with pregnancy may cause the cervix to open prematurely. Incompetent cervix may lead to miscarriage or premature delivery and results in a high risk pregnancy. Causative factors include previous cervical surgeries, damage during a previous birth, malformed cervix or DES exposure.
3. Pre-eclampsia is a rapidly progressive condition characterized by high blood pressure and protein in the urine. Swelling, sudden weight gain, headaches, and changes in vision are common symptoms. The condition is considered a medical emergency with high risk to both the mother and baby.
4. Multiple gestation pregnancies are considered high risk since the fetal mortality rate for twins is four times that of single births. Twins have increased frequency of congenital anomalies, placenta previa, abruptio placenta, pre-eclampsia, cord accidents, and malpresentations.

System Specific: Other Systems
Content Outline: Foundations for Evaluation, Differential Diagnosis, & Prognosis

Exam Three: Question 137

A physical therapist reviews the medical record of a patient with a spinal cord injury. A note recently entered by the physician indicates that the patient contracted a respiratory infection. Which patient would be MOST susceptible to this condition?

1. **a patient with complete C4 tetraplegia**
2. a patient with a cauda equina lesion
3. a patient with Brown-Sequard's syndrome
4. a patient with posterior cord syndrome

Correct Answer: 1 (Umphred p. 626)

A patient with complete C4 tetraplegia will present with a loss of motor and sensory function secondary to damage to the spinal cord. Since the primary muscle of respiration, the diaphragm, is impaired the patient will be unable to voluntarily or effectively ventilate.

1. **A patient with complete C4 tetraplegia will have a reduced ventilatory capacity due to muscle paralysis. The patient will exhibit limited ability to clear secretions, impaired chest mobility, and alveolar hypoventilation.**
2. A cauda equina lesion is an injury that occurs below the L1 spinal level where the long nerve roots transcend. Cauda equina injuries are frequently incomplete due to the large number of nerve roots in the area and as a result are often considered to be peripheral nerve injuries. Characteristics include flaccidity, areflexia, and impairment of bowel and bladder function.
3. Brown-Sequard's syndrome is an incomplete lesion usually caused by a stab wound, which produces hemisection of the spinal cord. There is paralysis and loss of vibratory and position sense on the same side as the lesion due to the damage to the corticospinal tract and dorsal columns. There is a loss of pain and temperature sense on the opposite side of the lesion from damage to the lateral spinothalamic tract.
4. Posterior cord syndrome is an extremely rare condition that presents with a loss of proprioception, two-point discrimination, graphesthesia, and stereognosis below the level of the lesion. Patients typically present with a wide-based steppage gait.

System Specific: Other Systems
Content Outline: Foundations for Evaluation, Differential Diagnosis, & Prognosis

Exam Three: Question 138

A patient with a T3 spinal cord injury exercising on a treatment table in supine begins to exhibit signs and symptoms of autonomic dysreflexia including a dramatic increase in blood pressure. The MOST IMMEDIATE action to address the patient's blood pressure response is to:

1. elevate the patient's legs
2. call for assistance
3. **sit the patient upright**
4. check the urinary drainage system

Correct Answer: 3 (Pierson p. 344)

The physical therapist should immediately position the patient in sitting to address the autonomic nervous system response and reduce the patient's elevated blood pressure. After the patient has been positioned in sitting, the urinary drainage system should be checked since a blocked catheter is a common noxious stimulus that triggers the sympathetic response.

1. Elevation of the patient's legs would be contraindicated since the position would serve to increase the return of circulation and further increase blood pressure.
2. Calling for assistance is an acceptable option given the seriousness of autonomic dysreflexia, however, the action would not be the most immediate action to address the patient's blood pressure response.
3. **Autonomic dysreflexia is caused by a noxious stimulus below the level of the lesion that triggers the autonomic nervous system causing a sudden elevation in blood pressure. If untreated, this condition can lead to convulsions, hemorrhage, and death.**
4. The common causes of autonomic dysreflexia include distended or full bladder, kink or blockage in the catheter, bladder infections, pressure ulcers, extreme temperature changes, tight clothing or an ingrown toenail. A physical therapist should check the urinary drainage system immediately after moving the patient into a sitting position.

System Specific: Other Systems
Content Outline: Interventions

Exam Three: Question 139

A physical therapist treats a patient following a lower extremity amputation. The patient is currently one week post amputation and has a post-operative rigid dressing. Which of the following is NOT a benefit of the rigid dressing?

1. limits the development of post-operative edema in the residual limb
2. allows for earlier ambulation with the attachment of a pylon and foot
3. allows for earlier fitting of a definitive prosthesis
4. **allows for daily wound inspection and dressing changes**

Correct Answer: 4 (Seymour p. 126)

A rigid dressing, usually made from plaster of Paris or fiberglass, does not allow for wound inspection or dressing changes. The rigid dressing is applied in the operating room and remains on the residual limb approximately 7-14 days until the sutures are removed and proper shaping occurs.

1. The rigid dressing limits the development of post-operative edema by maintaining total contact with the surface of the residual limb.
2. The rigid dressing allows for earlier ambulation since the rigid construction of the cast allows for pylon attachment and weight bearing.
3. The rigid dressing allows for earlier fitting of a definitive prosthesis since healing occurs more rapidly. The limb also receives better protection and is less likely to develop a flexion contracture since the rigid dressing limits knee motion.
4. **A rigid dressing does not allow for wound inspection and dressing changes since the rigid dressing remains on the residual limb for an extended period of time. An elastic bandage or a shrinker would be examples of soft dressings that allow for frequent wound inspection and dressing changes.**

System Specific: Other Systems
Content Outline: Foundations for Evaluation, Differential Diagnosis, & Prognosis

Exam Three: Question 140

A patient rehabilitating from a traumatic head injury is lethargic since being placed on Phenobarbital. The PRIMARY purpose of the medication is to:

1. decrease agitation
2. **prevent seizures**
3. reduce spasticity
4. limit arrhythmias

Correct Answer: 2 (Ciccone p. 107)

Physical therapists must possess an awareness of commonly used pharmacological agents, their indications, and potential side effects. Failure to recognize anticipated side effects from a medication may significantly jeopardize patient safety.

1. The most common side effect of Phenobarbital is sedation. As a result, agitation is typically diminished, however, the primary purpose of the medication is to prevent seizures.
2. **Phenobarbital is classified as a barbiturate and is prescribed most often to prevent adult seizures. Side effects include sedation, vitamin deficiencies, nystagmus, and ataxia.**
3. There are many medications that treat spasticity, but the most common include Baclofen, Diazepam, and Dantrolene sodium.
4. Antiarrhythmic drugs are typically classified into four groups: sodium channel blockers, beta-blockers, drugs that prolong repolarization, and calcium channel blockers.

System Specific: Neuromuscular & Nervous Systems
Content Outline: Clinical Application of Foundational Sciences

Exam Three: Question 141

A patient with a transtibial amputation ambulates in the physical therapy gym. The patient exhibits an extended knee throughout early stance phase on the prosthetic side. The MOST appropriate action to resolve the patient's difficulty is:

1. plantar flex the foot
2. soften the heel wedge
3. move the foot anteriorly
4. **dorsiflex the foot**

Correct Answer: 4 (Rothstein p. 724)

The prosthesis requires slight ankle dorsiflexion to allow for subsequent knee flexion during early stance. A prosthesis with excessive plantar flexion will promote full knee extension during early stance.

1. A prosthetic foot that is plantar flexed will present with an increased extension moment and impede sufficient knee flexion during early stance. The prosthesis must be set into neutral or slight dorsiflexion to allow for knee flexion during stance phase.
2. Softening the heel wedge of a transtibial prosthesis will create an increased extension moment and impede sufficient knee flexion during stance phase.
3. Moving the foot of a transtibial prosthesis anteriorly will create an increased extension moment and impede sufficient knee flexion during stance phase.
4. **A prosthetic foot that is set in slight dorsiflexion will present with an increased flexion moment and assist with knee flexion during stance and when advancing the prosthesis.**

System Specific: Musculoskeletal System
Content Outline: Interventions

Exam Three: Question 142

A physical therapist examines a patient diagnosed with carpal tunnel syndrome. As part of the examination the therapist assesses end-feel. The therapist classifies the end-feel associated with wrist extension as firm. The MOST logical explanation is:

1. tension in the dorsal radiocarpal ligament and the dorsal joint capsule
2. contact between the ulna and the carpal bones
3. contact between the radius and the carpal bones
4. **tension in the palmar radiocarpal ligament and the palmar joint capsule**

Correct Answer: 4 (Norkin p. 122)

End-feel is the type of resistance that is felt when passively moving a joint through the end range of motion. Certain tissues and joints have a consistent end-feel and are described as firm, hard or soft. Pathology can be identified through noting the type of abnormal end-feel within a particular joint.

1. A firm end-feel with wrist flexion can result from tension in the dorsal radiocarpal ligament and the dorsal joint capsule.
2. The ulna articulates with the radius at the distal radioulnar joint, however, does not articulate with the carpal bones.
3. Contact between the radius and the carpal bones would result in a hard end-feel and not a firm end-feel.
4. **A firm end-feel with wrist extension can result from tension in the palmar radiocarpal ligament and the palmar joint capsule. Tension in the ulnocarpal ligament can also contribute to the firm end-feel.**

System Specific: Musculoskeletal System
Content Outline: Clinical Application of Foundational Sciences

Exam Three: Question 143

A physical therapist examines a patient diagnosed with patellofemoral syndrome. As part of the examination the therapist elects to measure the patient's Q angle. Which three bony landmarks are used to measure the Q angle?

1. anterior superior iliac spine, superior border of the patella, tibial tubercle
2. **anterior superior iliac spine, midpoint of the patella, tibial tubercle**
3. anterior superior iliac spine, inferior border of the patella, midpoint of the patella tendon
4. greater trochanter, midpoint of the patella, tibial tubercle

> **Correct Answer: 2** (Hertling p. 499)

The Q angle refers to the angle between the quadriceps muscles and the patella tendon. The angle represents the angle of quadriceps muscle force. Normal Q angle values are 13 degrees for males and 18 degrees for females. An increased Q angle above 18 degrees may be associated with patellar tracking dysfunction, subluxing patella, increased femoral anteversion or increased lateral tibial torsion.

1. The anterior superior iliac spine and tibial tubercle are landmarks used when measuring Q angle, however, the midpoint of the patella should be used as the axis instead of the superior border of the patella.
2. **The most accurate measure of quadriceps muscle force (i.e., Q angle) utilizes the origin and insertion of the quadriceps muscle and the midpoint of the patella.**
3. The inferior border of the patella is located too far distally to use as the axis when measuring Q angle. The midpoint of the patella tendon is relatively close to the axis and may be difficult to accurately locate compared to a bony landmark such as the tibial tubercle.
4. The greater trochanter is not associated with the origin of the quadriceps muscle and is located too far laterally to use as a landmark when measuring Q angle.

System Specific: Musculoskeletal System
Content Outline: Examination

Exam Three: Question 144

A patient in a rehabilitation hospital begins to verbalize about the uselessness of life and the possibility of committing suicide. The MOST appropriate physical therapist action is:

1. suggest the patient be placed on a locked unit
2. ask nursing to check on the patient every 15 minutes
3. **discuss the situation with the patient's case manager**
4. review the patient's past medical history for signs and symptoms of mental illness

> **Correct Answer: 3** (Bailey p. 317)

Any formal or informal indication that a patient may be suicidal should be taken seriously. The case manager communicates with all of the members of the rehabilitation team and is therefore an appropriate individual for the physical therapist to contact.

1. The physical therapist is not trained or qualified to determine a course of action for a patient that is potentially suicidal.
2. A nurse can frequently check on a patient, however, this action does not ensure the patient's safety given their tenuous mental state.
3. **The case manager would likely contact the attending physician or appropriate mental health provider for direct intervention.**
4. The patient's past medical history may or may not have any bearing on the patient's current status. In addition, the action does not address the patient's expressed suicidal intent.

System Specific: Other Systems
Content Outline: Foundations for Evaluation, Differential Diagnosis, & Prognosis

Exam Three: Question 145

A physical therapist positions a patient as shown prior to testing for clonus. The MOST appropriate action to complete the test is:

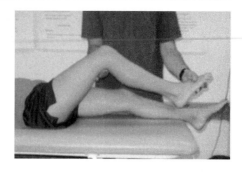

1. **provide a quick stretch to the plantar flexors**
2. provide a quick stretch to the dorsiflexors
3. provide a quick stretch to the plantar flexors while extending the knee
4. provide a quick stretch to the dorsiflexors while extending the knee

> **Correct Answer: 1** (DeMyer p. 311)

Clonus refers to rhythmic oscillation of a body part resulting from a quick stretch. The test is ideally performed by providing a stretch to the plantar flexors with the gastrocnemius in a relaxed position.

1. **Clonus is evaluated by supporting the knee in a partially flexed position, encouraging the patient to relax, and passively moving the foot. The therapist provides a quick stretch into dorsiflexion and observes any rhythmic oscillations between plantar flexion and dorsiflexion.**
2. When assessing clonus, the therapist provides a quick stretch to the plantar flexor muscle group, not the dorsiflexor muscle group.
3. When assessing clonus, the therapist provides a quick stretch to the plantar flexor muscle group, however, the knee should be partially flexed rather than extended in order to successfully place the gastrocnemius on slack and elicit the response.
4. When assessing clonus, the therapist should provide a quick stretch to the plantar flexor muscle group and maintain the knee in slight flexion. This option is completely opposite (i.e., quick stretch to the dorsiflexors while extending the knee).

System Specific: Neuromuscular & Nervous Systems
Content Outline: Examination

Exam Three: Question 146

A 29-year-old male diagnosed with ankylosing spondylitis reports progressive stiffening of the spine and associated pain for more than five years. The patient's MOST typical standing posture demonstrates:

1. posterior thoracic rib hump
2. **flattened lumbar curve, exaggerated thoracic curve**
3. excessive lumbar curve, flattened thoracic curve
4. lateral curvature of the spine with fixed rotation of the vertebrae

> **Correct Answer: 2** (Goodman – Differential Diagnosis p. 539)

Ankylosing spondylitis is a form of systemic rheumatic arthritis that is associated with an increase in thoracic kyphosis and loss of the lumbar curve. Ankylosing spondylitis occurs three times more often in males than females with a typical age of onset of 20-40 years.

1. A posterior thoracic rib hump is characteristic of scoliosis. The rotated vertebrae cause a rotation in the corresponding rib segments and result in posterior displacement of the rib cage.
2. **The clinical presentation of ankylosing spondylitis initially includes recurrent and insidious onset of back pain, morning stiffness, and impaired spinal extension. Chronic inflammation causes destruction of the ligamentous-osseous junction with subsequent fibrosis and ossification. The patient may exhibit flexion at the hips, spinal kyphosis, fatigue, weight loss, and peripheral joint involvement. If the costovertebral joints are affected there may be impaired chest mobility, compromised breathing, and decreased vital capacity.**
3. Excessive lumbar curve with a flattened thoracic curve is opposite from the typical clinical presentation of ankylosing spondylitis.
4. Lateral curvature of the spine with fixed rotation of the vertebrae is descriptive of scoliosis.

System Specific: Musculoskeletal System
Content Outline: Foundations for Evaluation, Differential Diagnosis, & Prognosis

Exam Three: Question 147

A physical therapist completes a developmental assessment on an infant. Which pediatric reflex would the therapist expect to be integrated at the youngest age?

1. plantar grasp reflex
2. Moro reflex
3. Landau reflex
4. **Galant reflex**

> **Correct Answer: 4** (Ratliffe p. 26)

Integration of a reflex refers to the period of time when a reflex is no longer present despite an appropriate stimulus.

1. The plantar grasp reflex is stimulated by placing pressure on the ball of the foot, generally in standing. The response is flexion and curling of the toes. The normal age of the response is from 28 weeks of gestation to nine months.

2. The Moro reflex is stimulated when an infant's head is suddenly allowed to fall into extension. The action causes a "startled look" followed by upper extremity abduction with the fingers open, then crossing the trunk into adduction. The normal age of the response is from 28 weeks of gestation to five months.

3. The Landau reflex is an equilibrium response that occurs when a child responds to prone suspension by aligning their head and extremities in line with the plane of the body. Although the response begins around three months of age, it is not fully integrated until the child's second year.

4. **The Galant reflex is stimulated by touching the skin along the spine from the shoulder to the hip. The response is lateral flexion of the trunk to the side of the stimulus. The normal age of the response is from 30 weeks of gestation to two months.**

System Specific: Neuromuscular & Nervous Systems
Content Outline: Examination

Exam Three: Question 148

A physical therapist examines a patient with a limited straight leg raise of 40 degrees due to inadequate hamstrings length. Which proprioceptive neuromuscular facilitation technique would be the MOST appropriate to increase the patient's hamstrings length?

1. **contract-relax**
2. rhythmic initiation
3. rhythmic stabilization
4. rhythmic rotation

> **Correct Answer: 1** (Sullivan p. 66)

Contract-relax is a proprioceptive neuromuscular facilitation (PNF) technique utilized to increase range of motion on one side of a joint. This technique utilizes isometric as well as isotonic contractions.

1. **Contract-relax is used to improve range of motion. As the extremity reaches the point of limitation, the patient performs a maximal contraction of the antagonistic muscle group. The therapist resists movement for eight to ten seconds followed by a period of relaxation. The technique is repeated until no further gains in range of motion are noted.**

2. Rhythmic initiation is used to initiate movement when hypertonia exists. Movement progresses from passive ("let me move you"), to active assistive ("help me move"), to slightly resistive ("move against resistance"). Movements are slow and rhythmical to reduce tone and allow for full range of motion.

3. Rhythmic stabilization is used to increase range of motion and coordinate isometric contractions. The technique requires isometric contractions of all muscles around a joint against progressive resistance. The patient should attempt to relax and move into the newly acquired range of motion.

4. Rhythmic rotation is a passive technique used to decrease hypertonia by slowly rotating an extremity around the longitudinal axis. Relaxation of the extremity promotes an increase in available range of motion.

System Specific: Neuromuscular & Nervous Systems
Content Outline: Interventions

Exam Three: Question 149

A physical therapist examines a patient following a transtibial amputation. The patient resides in a retirement community and describes herself as socially active. She is presently using a temporary prosthesis consisting of a plastic socket, a pylon, and a solid ankle cushion heel (SACH) foot. The patient expresses concern that the permanent prosthesis will look awful and will be obvious to everyone. Which type of prosthesis would be the MOST appropriate for the patient?

1.   endoskeletal shank and single-axis articulated foot-ankle assembly
2.   **endoskeletal shank and solid ankle cushion heel (SACH) foot**
3.   exoskeletal shank and single-axis articulated foot-ankle assembly
4.   exoskeletal shank and solid ankle cushion heel (SACH) foot

> ### Correct Answer: 2 (Tan p. 247)

An endoskeleton or modular shank is designed to incorporate a synthetic foam cover shaped like the opposite leg. As a result, the device is more cosmetically attractive and would likely make the patient more socially comfortable. A SACH foot is the most frequently prescribed foot-ankle assembly. It is considered to be a nonarticulated foot since it does not incorporate a mechanical joint at the ankle.

1.   An endoskeletal shank would be an appropriate choice given the patient's concerns, however, a single-axis articulated foot-ankle assembly would be heavier and requires more maintenance than the SACH foot. Since the patient is of retirement age and does not plan on heavy activity, this type of foot would not be appropriate.
2.   **Since the patient is of retirement age and expects low impact on the prosthesis, the endoskeletal shank and SACH foot will provide the patient with durability, low maintenance, and cosmesis.**
3.   An exoskeletal shank would not be appropriate for the patient since it less cosmetically desirable and heavier with the hard, thermoplastic resin shell. The single-axis articulated foot-ankle assembly would be heavier and require more maintenance than the SACH foot.
4.   An exoskeletal shank would not be as desirable for the patient as the endoskeletal shank. The SACH foot is appropriate for the patient.

System Specific: Non-Systems
Content Outline: Equipment & Devices; Therapeutic Modalities

Exam Three: Question 150

A physical therapist observes a patient during gait training. The patient has normal strength and equal leg length. As the patient passes midstance he slightly vaults and has early toe off. The MOST likely cause of this deviation is:

1.   weakness of the dorsiflexors
2.   weakness of the hip abductors
3.   limited plantar flexion
4.   **limited dorsiflexion**

> ### Correct Answer: 4 (Magee p. 964)

A patient with limited dorsiflexion may compensate with a vault or bounce through mid to late stance. Approximately ten degrees of dorsiflexion is required for late stance through toe off.

1.   Weakness of the dorsiflexors will typically create a "steppage gait pattern." The patient will present with foot slap at initial contact and compensate by lifting the knee higher than normal to clear the foot and avoid dragging the toe.
2.   Weakness of the hip abductors (gluteus medius and minimus) will typically create a contralateral dip of the pelvis during the stance phase of the weak side, also known as a Trendelenburg gait pattern. The observed contralateral dip of the pelvis results from the inability of the weak hip abductors to stabilize the pelvis during contralateral swing phase.
3.   Limited plantar flexion would not result in a vaulting gait pattern. The patient would require plantar flexion to vault (ascend onto the toes) during gait. Plantar flexion of 0-20 degrees is required for normal gait biomechanics with approximately 15 degrees during the loading response and 20 degrees during the pre-swing phase.
4.   **Limited dorsiflexion will typically result in premature elevation of the heel during midstance. The patient will appear to have a bounce during gait secondary to the gastroc-soleus tightness.**

System Specific: Musculoskeletal System
Content Outline: Foundations for Evaluation, Differential Diagnosis, & Prognosis

Exam Three: Question 151

A patient with an acute burn is referred to physical therapy less than 24 hours after being admitted to the hospital. The patient's burns range from superficial partial-thickness to deep partial-thickness and encompass approximately 35 percent of the patient's total body surface area. Which of the following findings would be MOST predictable based on the patient's injury?

1. **increased oxygen consumption**
2. hypernatremia
3. increased intravascular fluid
4. decreased core temperature

> **Correct Answer: 1** (Paz p. 266)

An acute burn produces hypermetabolism that results in increased oxygen consumption, increased minute ventilation, and an increased core temperature. Intravascular, interstitial, and intracellular fluids are all diminished.

1. **Pulmonary function is affected by the presence of a burn injury. In addition to increased oxygen consumption, the patient can also experience increased minute ventilation up to five times the normal value.**
2. Hyponatremia or low sodium concentration, initially occurs (within the first 36 hours) secondary to extracellular changes from the increased cellular permeability. In patients that sustain burns above 20% of the total body surface area, fluid and electrolyte replacement is a component of immediate medical management in order to control the hypermetabolic cycle that results from the burn.
3. Intravascular fluid will decrease due to the increased vascular permeability and overall hematologic changes. Cardiac output can decrease secondary to a combination of an increase in blood viscosity, decrease in intravascular fluid, and an overall increase in peripheral resistance.
4. A patient with a significant burn injury is at risk for an increased core temperature due to the increased metabolic and catabolic activity. The one to two degree increase occurs secondary to the "recalibrating" of the hypothalamic temperature centers in the brain. Patients that have sustained extensive burns require a warmer ambient temperature in order to reduce their metabolic rate. Average room temperature will create continued heat loss and perpetuate the hypermetabolic state.

System Specific: Integumentary System
Content Outline: Foundations for Evaluation, Differential Diagnosis, & Prognosis

Exam Three: Question 152

A patient sustains a deep partial-thickness burn to the anterior surface of the right upper extremity and a superficial partial-thickness burn to the anterior surface of the trunk. According to the rule of nines, the patient has burns over:

1. 13.5 percent of the body
2. **22.5 percent of the body**
3. 27 percent of the body
4. 36 percent of the body

> **Correct Answer: 2** (Rothstein p. 963)

The "rule of nines" is commonly utilized to assess the percentage of the body surface affected by a burn. Each area of the body has a specific percentage allotted to it in order to approximate the total percentage of the body surface affected. The values are as follows: head (9%), each upper extremity (9%), the trunk (36%), each lower extremity (18%), and the genital area (1%).

1. A value of 13.5% is less than the percentage of body surface affected. A candidate may have generated an answer of 13.5% by allocating only 9% for the anterior trunk instead of 18% and then adding 4.5% for the anterior surface of the upper extremity.
2. **The anterior surface of the right upper extremity equals 4.5% and the anterior surface of the trunk equals 18% (4.5%+18%=22.5%).**
3. A value of 27% is greater than the percentage of body surface affected in the described scenario. A candidate may have generated an answer of 27% by incorrectly allocating 9% for the anterior surface of the right upper extremity and then adding 18% for the anterior surface of the trunk.
4. The entire trunk is valued at 36% of the body using the "rule of nines."

System Specific: Integumentary System
Content Outline: Examination

Exam Three: Question 153

The treatment plan for a patient with hemiplegia is based on the theory of reinforcing normal movement through key points of control and avoiding all reflex movement patterns and associated reactions. This approach MOST closely resembles:

1. **Bobath**
2. Kabat
3. Rood
4. Brunnstrom

> **Correct Answer: 1** (Scott - Foundations p. 156)

The Bobath approach for neurological rehabilitation is often termed Neurodevelopmental Treatment (NDT). The patient learns to control movement through functional activities that promote normal movement patterns that integrate function.

1. **The Bobath approach recognizes that interference of normal brain function caused by central nervous system damage leads to a slowing down or cessation of motor development and the inhibition of righting reactions, equilibrium reactions, and automatic movements. Emphasis on normal movement and rotational patterns are key components of this therapeutic model.**

2. The Kabat, Knott, and Voss approach is based on the premise that stronger parts of the body are utilized to stimulate and strengthen weaker parts. Normal movement and posture is based on a balance between control of antagonist and agonist muscle groups. Movement patterns follow diagonals or spirals that each possess a flexion, extension, and rotatory component and are directed toward or away from midline.

3. The Rood approach is based on Sherrington and the reflex stimulus model. Rood believed that all motor output was the result of both past and present sensory input. Rood introduced the use of sensory stimulation to facilitate or inhibit responses, such as icing and brushing, in order to elicit desired reflex motor responses.

4. The Brunnstrom approach created and defined the term synergy and initially encouraged the use of synergy patterns during rehabilitation. The patient was encouraged to immediately practice synergy patterns and subsequently develop combinations of movement patterns outside of the synergy.

System Specific: Neuromuscular & Nervous Systems
Content Outline: Interventions

Exam Three: Question 154

A patient with several motor and sensory abnormalities exhibits signs of autonomic nervous system dysfunction. Which of the following is NOT an indicator of increased sympathetic involvement?

1. anxiety, distractibility
2. mottled, cold, shiny skin
3. **constriction of the pupils**
4. rapid, shallow breathing

> **Correct Answer: 3** (Sullivan p. 60)

The autonomic nervous system (sympathetic and parasympathetic divisions) function together to maintain homeostasis. The sympathetic division prepares the body for stressful situations using the "fight or flight" response. The parasympathetic division ("rest and digest") controls body processes during ordinary situations.

1. Anxiety and distractibility are characteristics seen with an increase in sympathetic activity. Increased sweating, abnormal circulation, a lowered pain threshold, and heightened reflex activity are additional characteristics of a sympathetic response.

2. Skin that appears mottled and shiny is indicative of an increase in sympathetic activity. Other characteristics include hypersensitivity to touch, a rapid heart rate, dilation of the lungs, and increased muscle tension and strength.

3. **Constriction of the pupils is characteristic of a parasympathetic response. The parasympathetic division will also decrease heart rate, stimulate digestion, constrict the lungs, and stimulate other internal organs.**

4. Rapid and shallow breathing is a characteristic of increased sympathetic activity. Treatment techniques to decrease sympathetic stimulation include maintained touch, massage, rocking, deep breathing, generalized warmth, and midline pressure.

System Specific: Other Systems
Content Outline: Foundations for Evaluation, Differential Diagnosis, & Prognosis

Exam Three: Question 155

A 55-year-old patient, six months status post CVA with right hemiparesis, attends physical therapy on an outpatient basis. As the patient lies supine on the mat, the physical therapist applies resistance to right elbow flexion. The therapist notes mass flexion of the right lower extremity as the resistance is applied. The therapist should document this as:

1. Raimiste's phenomenon
2. Souque's phenomenon
3. coordination synkinesis
4. **homolateral synkinesis**

Correct Answer: 4 (Sullivan p. 25)

Homolateral synkinesis is an associated reaction that can occur after neurological damage. Resistance to flexion of the involved upper extremity will cause flexion in the involved lower extremity.

1. Raimiste's phenomenon occurs when the involved lower extremity abducts or adducts with applied resistance to the uninvolved lower extremity in the same direction.
2. Souque's phenomenon is observed when a patient raises the involved upper extremity above 100 degrees with the elbow extended. This action produces extension and abduction of the involved fingers.
3. Coordination synkinesis refers to voluntary contraction of certain muscle groups on the involved side that, in turn, gives rise to involuntary contractions of synergistic muscles.
4. **Homolateral synkinesis is a condition often associated with hemiplegia where there is mutual dependency between the involved upper and lower extremities. Certain theories of neurological rehabilitation avoid utilizing associated reactions while other theories utilize them to increase movement.**

System Specific: Neuromuscular & Nervous Systems
Content Outline: Interventions

Exam Three: Question 156

A physical therapist orders a wheelchair for a patient with C4 tetraplegia. Which wheelchair would be the MOST appropriate for the patient?

1. manual wheelchair with friction surface handrims
2. manual wheelchair with handrim projections
3. **power wheelchair with sip and puff controls**
4. power wheelchair with joystick controls

Correct Answer: 3 (O'Sullivan p. 961)

A patient with C4 tetraplegia would require a power wheelchair with a sip and puff, head, mouth or chin controls. The wheelchair would also require a tilt-in-space frame to allow for pressure relief.

1. Friction surface handrims are used when patients do not have a functional grip or the strength necessary to adequately propel a wheelchair. Patients with C6-C7 tetraplegia commonly rely on this feature.
2. Handrim projections add depth to the wheel and allow the patient to more easily propel the wheelchair. This is indicated at C5 where the lowest innervation includes the biceps, brachialis, brachioradialis, deltoids, rhomboids, and supinator. Although a patient with C5 tetraplegia may utilize handrim projections, the necessary energy expenditure may necessitate the use of a power wheelchair for mobility.
3. **A patient with C4 tetraplegia will have innervation of the face and neck, diaphragm, and trapezius muscles. The patient should be able to verbally direct all aspects of wheelchair management and would be a candidate for a power wheelchair with head or mouth controls.**
4. A patient with C5 tetraplegia is appropriate for a power wheelchair with joystick control. Patients utilize a power wheelchair for community mobility secondary to the high energy expenditure of using a manual wheelchair with handrim projections.

System Specific: Non-Systems
Content Outline: Equipment & Devices; Therapeutic Modalities

Exam Three: Question 157

A child with a unilateral hip disarticulation works on advanced gait training activities. Which of the following activities would be the MOST difficult for the patient?

1. rising from a wheelchair
2. ascending stairs with a handrail
3. descending stairs with a handrail
4. **ascending a curb**

> **Correct Answer: 4** (Seymour p. 256)

Patients with amputations experience greater energy use when completing functional skills. The higher the level of amputation, the greater the metabolic demand will be for a given activity. A hip disarticulation refers to the surgical removal of the lower extremity from the pelvis.

1. Rising from a wheelchair is performed with double leg support allowing for use of the arm rests to provide assistance with upward movement during the transfer. This requires less energy expenditure than ascending a curb.
2. Ascending stairs with a handrail is a challenging activity for a patient with a hip disarticulation, however, the presence of a handrail likely provides the patient with the necessary balance and stability to complete the activity.
3. Descending stairs with a handrail is typically slightly less difficult for a patient with a hip disarticulation compared to ascending stairs since the patient does not need to overcome the force of gravity.
4. **A child with a hip disarticulation would have the greatest difficulty ascending a curb during prosthetic training since there are no external supports (handrails) to assist with the activity.**

System Specific: Musculoskeletal System
Content Outline: Foundations for Evaluation, Differential Diagnosis, & Prognosis

Exam Three: Question 158

A physical therapist examines the gait of a patient with a transtibial amputation. The patient exhibits delayed and limited knee flexion after heel strike on the prosthetic side. The MOST likely cause of the deviation is:

1. foot positioned in dorsiflexion
2. **heel wedge is too soft**
3. foot positioned too far posteriorly
4. socket is too large

> **Correct Answer: 2** (Seymour p. 203)

A physical therapist must be able to analyze the gait of a patient following amputation and identify any deviation from normal. Once identified, therapists should attempt to determine the likely cause of the deviation and if necessary make an adjustment or refer the patient to the prosthetist.

1. If the foot of the prosthesis is positioned in dorsiflexion the knee will move anteriorly in relation to the center of gravity and cause a greater flexion moment during heel strike and stance. The knee will subsequently exhibit excessive knee flexion during stance.
2. **If the heel wedge is too soft, it will create an extension moment at the knee. The prosthesis will not advance over the foot to allow for flexion that normally occurs after initial contact. The heel cushion should only compress approximately 3/8 inch.**
3. If the foot of the prosthesis is positioned too far posteriorly, it will cause a greater flexion moment and result in excessive flexion upon initial contact and stance. Conversely, a foot positioned too far anteriorly may delay and limit knee flexion due to the increased extension moment.
4. If the socket of the prosthesis is too large, it may cause a greater flexion moment due to diminished support between the socket and the residual limb. The residual limb will flex in an attempt to maintain the fit of the prosthesis causing premature knee flexion during initial contact and stance.

System Specific: Musculoskeletal System
Content Outline: Foundations for Evaluation, Differential Diagnosis, & Prognosis

Exam Three: Question 159

A physical therapist consults with an orthotist regarding the need for an ankle-foot orthosis for a patient status post CVA. The patient has difficulty moving from sitting to standing when wearing a prefabricated plastic ankle-foot orthosis (AFO). The therapist indicates the patient has poor strength at the ankle, intact sensation, and does not have any edema or tonal influence. The MOST appropriate type of AFO for the patient would incorporate:

1. **an articulation at the ankle joint**
2. tone reducing features
3. metal uprights
4. dorsiflexion assist

> **Correct Answer: 1** (Seymour p. 382)

A plastic AFO with an articulating ankle joint is more cosmetic and lighter than a metal upright AFO. The orthosis provides total contact and therefore should not be used on patients with fluctuating edema or significant sensory deficits.

1. **An articulation at the ankle joint would allow the tibia to advance forward over the fixed foot. This would assist the patient with weight shifting during the sit to stand transfer as well as during ambulation.**
2. This patient would not require an AFO with tone reducing features since they do not present with tonal influence. A total contact footplate can be used to normalize tonal abnormalities and improve function and gait in patients that present with increased tone.
3. A metal AFO consists of two metal uprights connected proximally to a calf band and distally to a mechanical ankle joint and shoe. The ankle joint can be locked or set to have limited anterior/posterior capability. Since this design does not provide total contact it does not pose a risk to patients with fluctuating edema or significant sensory deficits.
4. A posterior leaf spring (PLS) is a plastic AFO with a trim line posterior to the malleoli. The primary purpose of the orthosis is to provide a dorsiflexion assist to prevent foot drop. The patient's lack of strength at the ankle (i.e., poor) makes it unlikely that they would possess the necessary medial/lateral stability to use this orthotic.

System Specific: Non-Systems
Content Outline: Equipment & Devices; Therapeutic Modalities

Exam Three: Question 160

A physical therapist measures a patient for a straight cane prior to beginning ambulation activities. Which gross measurement method would provide the BEST estimate of cane length?

1. measuring from the head of the fibula straight to the floor and multiplying by two
2. measuring from the iliac crest straight to the floor
3. **measuring from the greater trochanter straight to the floor**
4. dividing the patient's height by two and adding three inches

> **Correct Answer: 3** (Pierson p. 221)

The straight cane can be used with a variety of gait patterns, but does not permit partial weight bearing. The patient should have 20-25 degrees of elbow flexion while grasping the handgrip. A straight cane provides minimal support and is used primarily for assisting with balance.

1. Measuring from the head of the fibula and multiplying by two would not be an accurate method to determine the appropriate length of a straight cane. The formula doesn't take into account the differences that may exist in sizing of a patient's long bones or overall body type.
2. Measuring from the iliac crest to the floor would be in excess of the required height for proper fit of a straight cane. If the straight cane is too long, the angle of elbow flexion will increase beyond 20-25 degrees and the cane will be less effective.
3. **The handgrip of a cane that is properly fit should be at the approximate level of the greater trochanter.**
4. Dividing the patient's height by two and adding three inches is not an accurate formula to fit a straight cane. The formula doesn't take into account where the greater trochanter lies in relation to height from the floor or the patient's body type.

System Specific: Non-Systems
Content Outline: Equipment & Devices; Therapeutic Modalities

Exam Three: Question 161

A physical therapist recommends a wheelchair for a patient rehabilitating from a CVA with the goal of independent mobility. The left upper and lower extremities are flaccid and present with edema. There is normal strength on the right, however, the patient's trunk is hypotonic. The patient is cognitively intact. The MOST appropriate wheelchair for the patient is:

1. solid seat, solid back, elevating legrests, and anti-tippers
2. sling seat, sling back, arm board, and elevating legrests
3. **light weight, solid seat, solid back, arm board, and elevating legrests**
4. light weight, solid seat, solid back, arm board, and standard footrests

> **Correct Answer: 3** (Pierson p. 140)

A physical therapist must carefully select a wheelchair for a patient that possesses the necessary adaptations to meet the patient's unique needs. Failure to select an adequately equipped wheelchair can significantly compromise the patient's progress in rehabilitation.

1. The flaccid upper extremity would need to be supported using an arm board. Anti-tippers would not typically be necessary for this patient.
2. A sling seat and sling back promote poor positioning and would not provide the necessary stability the patient requires.
3. **Independent propulsion is facilitated by the use of a lightweight wheelchair, while a solid seating system assists with posture and activities. An arm board allows the flaccid upper extremity to be supported and an elevating legrest will assist to decrease dependent edema.**
4. The wheelchair is appropriate for the patient, however, the presence of lower extremity edema makes it desirable to incorporate elevating legrests.

System Specific: Non-Systems
Content Outline: Equipment & Devices; Therapeutic Modalities

Exam Three: Question 162

A patient is scheduled to undergo a transtibial amputation secondary to gangrene of his left foot. In addition, the patient is one month status post right total knee arthroplasty due to osteoarthritis. Given the patient's past and current medical history, the physical therapist can expect which of the following tasks to be the MOST difficult for the patient following his amputation?

1. rolling from supine to sidelying
2. moving from sitting to supine
3. **moving from sitting to standing**
4. ambulating in the parallel bars

> **Correct Answer: 3** (O'Sullivan p. 1045)

All of the listed tasks are reasonable expectations for the patient, however, moving from sitting to standing would be the most difficult due to the required lower extremity strength and the necessary balance required to complete the activity.

1. Rolling from supine to sidelying should be a relatively easy task for the patient since they can utilize upper extremity strength to initiate the movement.
2. Transferring from sitting to supine should be a relatively easy task for the patient since it is a non-weight bearing activity. The patient's sitting balance should not be impaired and the patient should be able to transfer to sitting using upper extremity support.
3. **Transferring from sitting to standing would be the most difficult for the patient since the activity requires adequate strength and dynamic balance. The patient's strength will be decreased in the right lower extremity secondary to the recent total knee arthroplasty and balance will be altered due to the left transtibial amputation.**
4. Ambulating in the parallel bars requires greater strength and balance than performing bed mobility, however, the patient is able to use the parallel bars to provide a stable base of support. The patient can use upper extremity strength to decrease some of the demand on the right lower extremity and to maintain balance during the activity.

System Specific: Other Systems
Content Outline: Foundations for Evaluation, Differential Diagnosis, & Prognosis

Exam Three: Question 163

A patient diagnosed with T5 paraplegia is discharged from a rehabilitation hospital following 16 weeks of therapy. Assuming a normal recovery, which of the following MOST accurately describes the status of the patient's bathroom transfers?

1. independent with the presence of an attendant
2. independent with a sliding board
3. **independent with bathroom adaptations**
4. independent

Correct Answer: 3 (Umphred p. 619)

A patient with T5 paraplegia should be able to complete bathroom transfers with selected adaptations. The patient would possess full upper extremity innervation and limited trunk control.

1. An attendant would not be necessary based on the patient's upper extremity innervation and the availability of bathroom adaptations.
2. Use of a sliding board when transferring to or from a toilet or tub bench could create an unnecessary safety risk for the patient due to the inherent space limitations in the bathroom and the relative stability of the sliding board on different surfaces.
3. **A patient with T5 paraplegia should be independent for all transfers using bathroom adaptations such as a grab bar, tub bench or commode seat.**
4. A patient with any form of complete spinal cord lesion will require various adaptations in order to attain independence.

System Specific: Neuromuscular & Nervous Systems
Content Outline: Foundations for Evaluation, Differential Diagnosis, & Prognosis

Exam Three: Question 164

A physical therapist educates a patient status post transfemoral amputation on the importance of frequent skin checks. The MOST appropriate resource for the patient to utilize when inspecting the posterior aspect of the residual limb is:

1. **hand mirror**
2. video camera
3. nurse
4. prosthetist

Correct Answer: 1 (Seymour p. 138)

The use of a mirror during skin inspection of the residual limb will enable the patient to view the entire limb without being dependent on another person.

1. **A patient should regularly inspect all areas of the residual limb using a mirror in order to maintain healthy skin. Proper skin care is important for all patients following amputation.**
2. A video camera would not be the most appropriate resource to inspect the residual limb since it can be cumbersome to use and may not be readily available for all patients.
3. A nurse is capable of viewing areas of the residual limb that the patient cannot see, however, a mirror will enable the patient to inspect their skin independently.
4. A prosthetist, like the nurse, could inspect the skin, however, this option would result in the patient being dependent on another person.

System Specific: Integumentary System
Content Outline: Interventions

Exam Three: Question 165

A physical therapist examines a 26-year-old female whose subjective complaints include morning stiffness of her hands and visible swelling. The patient indicates that the stiffness seems to diminish with activity. This description BEST describes:

1. carpal tunnel syndrome
2. osteoporosis
3. **rheumatoid arthritis**
4. osteoarthritis

> **Correct Answer: 3** (Paz p. 375)

Rheumatoid arthritis is a chronic systemic autoimmune disorder of unknown etiology characterized by inflammatory changes in joints and related structures. The disease is two to three times more common in women than men.

1. Carpal tunnel syndrome is a medical condition caused by compression of the median nerve resulting in paresthesias, numbness, and muscle weakness in the hand. Symptoms include night pain, muscle atrophy, decreased grip strength, and decreased wrist mobility.

2. Osteoporosis is a metabolic condition that presents with a decrease in bone mass resulting in a greater risk of fracture. Symptoms include compression and other fractures, low thoracic or lumbar pain, loss of lumbar lordosis, kyphosis, decrease in height, Dowager's hump, and postural changes.

3. **Symptoms of rheumatoid arthritis include morning stiffness, limited range of motion, effusion, pain with movement, and low grade fever. Smaller peripheral joints are initially affected, however symptoms may progress to larger synovial joints.**

4. Osteoarthritis is a chronic disease that is characterized by degeneration of articular cartilage in weight bearing joints. Subsequent deformity and thickening of subchondral bone results in impaired functional status. The most commonly affected sites include the cervical spine (C5-C6), lumbar spine, hips, and knees.

System Specific: Other Systems
Content Outline: Foundations for Evaluation, Differential Diagnosis, & Prognosis

Exam Three: Question 166

A physical therapist provides pre-operative instructions to a patient scheduled for lower extremity amputation. Which of the following is the MOST common cause of lower extremity amputation?

1. tumor
2. trauma
3. **peripheral vascular disease**
4. cardiac disease

> **Correct Answer: 3** (Seymour p. 10)

Peripheral vascular disease refers to diseases of blood vessels outside the heart and brain. The condition is often caused by narrowing of vessels that carry blood to the legs, arms, stomach or kidneys.

1. Certain tumors will require extremity amputation, however, this is not the most common causative factor for lower extremity amputation. Sarcomas are the most common type of malignant tumor that require amputation.

2. Trauma may result in the need for amputation, however, this is not the most common causative factor for lower extremity amputation. Trauma remains the most common cause of upper extremity amputation.

3. **Peripheral vascular disease is caused by atherosclerotic or inflammatory processes causing lumen narrowing (stenosis), embolism, vasospasm, trauma or thrombus formation. Initially, symptoms may include intermittent claudication and in severe cases, the condition can progress to amputation. The relative risk of limb amputation is largely dependent on the number and severity of cardiovascular risk factors (i.e., smoking, hypertension, diabetes).**

4. Cardiac disease itself is not a common causative factor for lower extremity amputation.

System Specific: Other Systems
Content Outline: Foundations for Evaluation, Differential Diagnosis, & Prognosis

Exam Three: Question 167

A physical therapist instructs a patient diagnosed with C6 tetraplegia in functional activities. Which of the following activities would be LEAST appropriate?

1. independent raises for skin protection
2. manual wheelchair propulsion
3. assisted to independent transfers with a sliding board
4. **independent self-range of motion of the lower extremities**

Correct Answer: 4 (Umphred p. 617)

A patient with C6 tetraplegia does not have sufficient motor innervation to consistently perform independent self-range of motion of the lower extremities. The lowest motor innervation at the C6 level includes extensor carpi radialis, infraspinatus, latissimus dorsi, pectoralis major, teres minor, pronator teres, and serratus anterior.

1. A patient with C6 tetraplegia can provide pressure relief using a wheelchair with push handles or loops attached.
2. A patient with C6 tetraplegia can perform manual wheelchair propulsion with friction surface handrims or rim projections.
3. A patient with C6 tetraplegia can perform assisted to independent transfers using a sliding board. A patient with C7 tetraplegia is typically independent with transfers with or without a sliding board.
4. **A patient with C6 tetraplegia cannot typically perform self-range of motion of the lower extremities. The activity is more appropriate for a patient with C7 tetraplegia.**

System Specific: Neuromuscular & Nervous Systems
Content Outline: Interventions

Exam Three: Question 168

A physical therapist examines the residual limb of a patient following ambulation activities with a patellar tendon bearing prosthesis. The therapist identifies excessive redness over the patella. The MOST likely cause is:

1. **settling due to limb shrinkage**
2. socket not properly aligned
3. excessive withdrawal in sitting
4. excessive number of residual limb socks

Correct Answer: 1 (O'Sullivan p. 1048)

Redness over the patella most often occurs when a patient's residual limb sits too low in the prosthesis. This is most often caused by shrinking of the residual limb or an inadequate number of residual limb socks.

1. **A physical therapist may elect to add additional one-ply socks to the residual limb of a patient with excessive redness over the patella in order to more normally distribute weight bearing forces.**
2. If the socket was improperly aligned, it would be unlikely that the residual limb would only receive excess pressure directly over the patella.
3. If the patient's residual limb experienced excessive withdrawal during sitting, the patella would come further out of the socket as opposed to sitting lower within the socket. This would not cause excessive redness over the patella.
4. An excessive number of residual limb socks would elevate the patella tendon above the patella tendon bearing surface of the prosthesis. This would cause the patella to move further out of the socket and therefore would be unlikely to cause redness over the patella.

System Specific: Non-Systems
Content Outline: Equipment & Devices; Therapeutic Modalities

Exam Three: Question 169

A patient with increased sympathetic output is examined in physical therapy. Which treatment technique would NOT be beneficial in decreasing the level of sympathetic activity?

1. connective tissue massage
2. rotating the lower trunk in hooklying
3. **slow reversal hold of the quadriceps and hamstrings**
4. gentle manual pressure to the abdomen

Correct Answer: 3 (Sullivan p. 60)

The sympathetic division of the autonomic nervous system prepares the body for stressful situations using the "fight or flight" response. It increases heart rate, dilates the airways, and allows the body to release stored energy. This division also causes the palms to sweat, pupils to dilate, and hair to stand on end.

1. Connective tissue massage is a technique that can be used to decrease sympathetic activity. Massage can influence muscle tension via the circulatory and autonomic systems with noted changes in vital signs and muscle tone.
2. Passive rotation of the lower trunk while in a hooklying position is an example of rhythmical movement which produces reflexive autonomic changes and an overall calming effect.
3. **Slow reversal hold is a proprioceptive neuromuscular facilitation technique used primarily to improve stability surrounding a joint. The technique uses slow and resisted concentric contractions of agonists and antagonists around a joint with an isometric contraction that is performed at the end of each movement. Slow reversal hold would not decrease sympathetic activity.**
4. Maintained touch is used to promote a parasympathetic response and produce a generalized calming effect due to the stimulation of tonic sensory receptors. Gentle manual pressure to the abdomen is an example of maintained touch.

System Specific: Neuromuscular & Nervous Systems
Content Outline: Interventions

Exam Three: Question 170

A patient who sustained a CVA four weeks ago is beginning to show the ability to produce movement patterns outside of limb synergies. According to Brunnstrom, this patient is in which stage of recovery?

1. two
2. three
3. **four**
4. six

Correct Answer: 3 (Brunnstrom p. 45)

Brunnstrom separates neurological recovery into separate stages based on progression through abnormal tone and spasticity. The stages range from stage one "flaccidity" to stage seven "normal coordinated movement." The stages of recovery describe tone, reflex activity, and volitional movement.

1. Stage two is characterized by the appearance of basic limb synergies and the beginning of spasticity.
2. Stage three is characterized by voluntary movement within synergies and increased spasticity.
3. **Stage four is characterized by movement patterns beginning outside of synergy patterns with diminished spasticity.**
4. Stage six is characterized by isolated coordinated joint movements with the disappearance of spasticity.

System Specific: Neuromuscular & Nervous Systems
Content Outline: Examination

Exam Three: Question 171

A recent entry in the medical record indicates a patient exhibits dysdiadochokinesia. Based on the patient's documented deficit, which activity would be the MOST difficult for the patient?

1. **alternate supination and pronation of the forearms**
2. perform a standing squat
3. march in place
4. walk along a straight line

> **Correct Answer: 1** (Umphred p. 842)

Dysdiadochokinesia refers to the inability to perform rapid, alternating movements. This condition results in inappropriate timing of muscle firing and difficulty with cessation of ongoing movement.

1. **When the patient attempts pronation and supination of the forearms, the movement is slow and will lose range and rhythm quickly. The presence of dysdiadochokinesia is commonly associated with a cerebellar lesion.**
2. Performing a standing squat is not a velocity-based activity requiring alternating movement and therefore does not assess dysdiadochokinesia. The activity requires concentric and eccentric muscle control of the trunk and lower extremities.
3. Marching in place to a specific cadence is sometimes used to test for a cerebellar movement disorder. A positive test occurs when a patient is unable to follow the rhythm of the cadence.
4. Walking along a straight line is often used to identify signs of cerebellar pathology such as ataxia. Characteristics of an ataxic gait include uneven step length, increased base of support, inability to walk a straight line without lurching, impaired rhythm, and a high stepping pattern.

System Specific: Neuromuscular & Nervous Systems
Content Outline: Interventions

Exam Three: Question 172

A physical therapist recognizes that a child has significant difficulty flexing the neck while in a supine position. Failure to integrate which reflex could explain the child's difficulty?

1. **symmetrical tonic labyrinthine reflex**
2. Moro reflex
3. asymmetrical tonic neck reflex
4. symmetrical tonic neck reflex

> **Correct Answer: 1** (Ratliffe p. 26)

The symmetrical tonic labyrinthine reflex promotes a tendency for extension when a patient is in supine and reduced extensor influence when the patient is in prone. The persistence of a primitive reflex is generally seen with a neurological insult.

1. **The symmetrical tonic labyrinthine reflex serves to limit the child's ability to flex the neck when in a supine position. The child should lie in sidelying or in supine with hip flexion and/or knee flexion in order to decrease the influence of the reflex.**
2. The Moro reflex is elicited by a sudden change in the position of the head, usually having the head drop backwards. The typical response is crying along with extension and abduction of the upper extremities followed by flexion and adduction across the chest.
3. The asymmetrical tonic neck reflex is elicited through rotation of the neck. If the patient's head is turned, the upper and lower extremities on the face side extend and the upper and lower extremities on the skull side flex. The asymmetrical tonic neck reflex does not influence the child's ability to flex the neck while in a supine position.
4. The symmetrical tonic neck reflex is elicited by flexion or extension of the neck. When the head is flexed, upper extremities flex and lower extremities extend. When the head is extended, upper extremities extend and lower extremities flex. The symmetrical tonic neck reflex does not influence the child's ability to flex the neck while in a supine position.

System Specific: Neuromuscular & Nervous Systems
Content Outline: Interventions

Exam Three: Question 173

A physical therapist discusses the importance of a well-balanced diet with a patient diagnosed with type II diabetes mellitus. The MOST appropriate action to emphasize the importance of diet is:

1. provide a handout from the American Diabetes Association which outlines an appropriate diet
2. ask other patients that have made dietary changes to speak to the patient
3. **arrange for a consultation with a dietician**
4. provide copies of recent research articles which cite the benefit of a well-balanced diet

Correct Answer: 3 (Goodman - Pathology p. 490)

Type 2 diabetes mellitus is the most common form of diabetes. In type 2 DM, there is a combination of cellular resistance to insulin and an inadequate compensatory insulin secretory response. In most cases, this form of DM can be controlled with proper diet, exercise, weight control, and oral insulin supplementation.

1. A handout from the American Diabetes Association may serve as a helpful resource, however, type 2 diabetes mellitus is a condition where appropriate diet is critical to the management of the condition. As a result, a more proactive and formal action would be warranted.
2. Requesting that a patient with type 2 diabetes mellitus speak to other patients who have made dietary changes would qualify as a form of peer support, but would not provide the patient with enough information to make necessary dietary changes.
3. **Consultation with a dietician will provide the patient with education and a dietary program that typically includes a personal menu and recommendations for lifestyle modifications.**
4. Research articles on the benefits of a well-balanced diet may be of interest to some patients, however, the action would not be an appropriate substitute for a consultation with a dietician.

System Specific: Other Systems
Content Outline: Interventions

Exam Three: Question 174

A physical therapist instructs a patient in an exercise designed to increase pelvic floor awareness and strength. The exercise requires the patient to tighten the pelvic floor as if attempting to stop the flow of urine. The patient is instructed to hold the isometric contraction for five seconds and complete ten repetitions. The MOST appropriate INITIAL position for the exercise is:

1. **supine**
2. sitting
3. tall kneeling
4. standing

Correct Answer: 1 (Kisner p. 814)

The pelvic floor muscles follow the same general strengthening principles as other muscles of the body. As a result, the initial position for the pelvic floor exercise should remove or minimize the influence of gravity. As the patient demonstrates mastery of the initial position, the physical therapist can select positions that will provide the patient with a greater challenge.

1. **Kegel exercises or isometric contractions of the pelvic floor, are often utilized as part of a treatment program for incontinence. Supine and sidelying are the typical gravity-eliminated positions to initiate strengthening. A patient may also use a gravity-assisted position where the hips are above the level of the heart such as supported bridging or on elbows and knees in order to have gravity assist the contraction.**
2. A patient would progress to sitting once there is adequate strength and awareness of the pelvic floor muscles. Sitting requires exercise against gravity and therefore would not be the most appropriate initial position.
3. A patient would progress to tall kneeling once there is adequate strength and awareness of the pelvic floor in a sitting position. Tall kneeling requires proximal control and balance to maintain the position.
4. Standing is the highest level in the general progression of pelvic floor strengthening. The normal sequence is supine or sidelying followed by quadruped, sitting, tall kneeling, and standing.

System Specific: Other Systems
Content Outline: Interventions

Exam Three: Question 175

A physical therapist attempts to assess the dynamic balance of an elderly patient. Which screening tool would be the MOST helpful to test balance and gait?

1.   Functional Independence Measure
2.   **Tinetti Performance Oriented Mobility Assessment**
3.   Fugl-Meyer Assessment
4.   Barthel Index

> **Correct Answer: 2** (Physical Therapists Clinical Companion p. 123)

The Tinetti Performance Oriented Mobility Assessment is an outcome measurement tool used to identify if there is an increased risk for falling. The tool measures balance and gait using a two to three point ordinal scale and takes 5-15 minutes to administer. The risk of falling increases as the total score decreases.

1.   The FIM is a tool used in rehabilitation hospitals to determine a patient's level of disability and burden of care. A seven-point scale is utilized to examine 18 areas including self-care, sphincter control, transfers, locomotion, communication, and social cognitive activities. This tool is used as a predictor of disability.
2.   **The Tinetti Performance Oriented Mobility Assessment has two sections. The first section assesses balance through sit to stand and within the standing position. The second section assesses gait at normal and rapid speeds. There is a total maximum score of 28 with patients scoring less than 19 considered to be at high risk for falling.**
3.   The Fugl-Meyer Assessment is an ordinal scale used to measure recovery post CVA. The framework is based on Brunnstrom's sequence of recovery. The five areas of assessment are joint movement and pain, balance, upper extremity motor function, sensation, and lower extremity motor function. The maximum combined score for upper and lower extremity motor function is 100 and can be interpreted as a percentage of motor recovery. For example, a score of 63 indicates approximately 63% return of motor function.
4.   The Barthel Index is designed to measure the amount of assistance needed to perform ten different ADL and mobility activities with a total maximum score of 100. The index does not account for cognitive or safety issues and is not sensitive to higher level patients regarding their level of disability.

System Specific: Non-Systems
Content Outline: Safety & Professional Roles; Teaching/Learning; Research

Exam Three: Question 176

A physical therapist monitors the blood pressure of a 28-year-old male during increasing levels of physical exertion. Assuming a normal physiologic response, which of the following BEST describes the patient's blood pressure response to dynamic exercise?

1.   systolic pressure decreases, diastolic pressure increases
2.   systolic pressure remains the same, diastolic pressure increases
3.   systolic pressure and diastolic pressure remain the same
4.   **systolic pressure increases, diastolic pressure remains the same**

> **Correct Answer: 4** (Pierson p. 62)

The normal response to dynamic exercise is a progressive increase in systolic blood pressure, and no change or a slight decrease in diastolic pressure. The magnitude of increase in systolic blood pressure is approximately 5-10 mm Hg per metabolic equivalent.

1.   A decrease in systolic blood pressure and an increase in diastolic blood pressure are both abnormal responses.
2.   No change in systolic blood pressure and an increase in diastolic blood pressure are both abnormal responses. An increase in diastolic blood pressure of more than 10 mm Hg may be indicative of exertional ischemia.
3.   No change in either systolic or diastolic blood pressure is an abnormal response.
4.   **An increase in systolic blood pressure while diastolic blood pressure remains the same is a normal response to dynamic exercise.**

System Specific: Cardiac, Vascular, & Pulmonary Systems
Content Outline: Clinical Application of Foundational Sciences

Exam Three: Question 177

A physical therapist examines the reflex status of a patient. The therapist should use which technique to assess the patient's superficial reflexes?

1. brushing the skin with a light, feathery object
2. passive joint range of motion
3. **stroking the skin with a non-cutting, but pointed object**
4. tapping over a muscle tendon

Correct Answer: 3 (O'Sullivan p. 238)

Superficial cutaneous reflexes are elicited with a light stroke of the skin. The anticipated response is a small or brief contraction of the muscles innervated by a given spinal segment that received the light stroking.

1. Light touch sensation is assessed by brushing the skin with a light, feathery object.
2. Passive joint range of motion is performed to assess the influence of noncontractile structures on range of motion or tone (hypertonicity or hypotonicity).
3. **The plantar reflex (S1, S2) is an example of a superficial reflex. The reflex is elicited by stroking the lateral aspect of the foot from the heel to the ball of the foot with a blunt object. A normal response is indicated by flexion of the great toe, while an abnormal response is indicated by extension of the great toe with fanning of the four other toes (Babinski sign). The Babinski sign is often associated with upper motor neuron damage.**
4. Deep tendon reflexes are performed to test the integrity of the spinal reflex and are elicited by tapping over a muscle tendon. A physical therapist should strike the tendon with a reflex hammer after placing the tendon on slight stretch.

System Specific: Neuromuscular & Nervous Systems
Content Outline: Examination

Exam Three: Question 178

A patient returns to an outpatient physical therapy clinic two hours after a physical therapy session complaining of increased back pain. The patient has been in physical therapy for three previous visits and has had little difficulty with a program consisting of palliative modalities and pelvic stabilization exercises. The patient was referred to physical therapy after injuring his back two weeks ago. The MOST appropriate physical therapist action is:

1. contact the referring physician to discuss the patient's care plan
2. **instruct the patient to discontinue the pelvic stabilization exercises and re-examine the patient at his next visit**
3. refer the patient to the emergency room of a local hospital
4. instruct the patient to cancel existing physical therapy visits and schedule an appointment with the physician

Correct Answer: 2 (Criteria for Standards of Practice)

Physical therapists must carefully assess a patient's response to physical therapy interventions. The severity of the patient's signs and symptoms combined with the therapist's knowledge of their medical condition assists the therapist to make an informed decision regarding an appropriate course of action.

1. The patient's current complaints do not suggest the need for immediate consultation with the referring physician.
2. **The physical therapist should have the patient discontinue any activities that increase their pain. The therapist can re-examine the patient at the next scheduled visit and determine an appropriate course of action based on the findings.**
3. The patient's current complaints are not severe enough to warrant referral to an emergency room.
4. Physical therapists most often refer patients back to the referring physician due to a change in medical status or failure to make anticipated progress in physical therapy. The patient's recent increase in symptoms does not suggest that the patient is not a candidate for physical therapy.

System Specific: Musculoskeletal System
Content Outline: Interventions

Exam Three: Question 179

A physical therapist reviews the medical record of a patient rehabilitating from a stroke. The patient exhibits paralysis and numbness on the side of the body contralateral to the vascular accident. Which descending pathway is MOST likely damaged based on the patient's clinical presentation?

1. **corticospinal tract**
2. vestibulospinal tract
3. tectospinal tract
4. rubrospinal tract

Correct Answer: 1 (O'Sullivan p.195)

The corticospinal tract is the largest descending pathway where 80% of the fibers decussate and descend on the opposite side; 20% continue to descend ipsilaterally. The corticospinal tract carries information from the motor cortex directly to the spinal cord.

1. **The corticospinal tract is concerned with skilled fine motor control primarily of the distal limbs.**
2. The vestibulospinal tract is responsible for gross postural adjustments subsequent to head movements and acceleration.
3. The tectospinal tract is responsible for visual information related to spatial awareness. The tract ends at the cervical spine and controls the musculature of the neck as well as head position.
4. The rubrospinal tract communicates with the thalamus and cerebellum and plays an important role in the coordination of movement.

System Specific: Neuromuscular & Nervous Systems
Content Outline: Clinical Application of Foundational Sciences

Exam Three: Question 180

A patient exhibits pain and sensory loss in the posterior thigh, lateral calf, and dorsal foot. Extension of the hallux is poor, however, the Achilles reflex is normal. What spinal level would you expect to be involved?

1. L4
2. **L5**
3. S1
4. S2

Correct Answer: 2 (Magee p. 16)

Involvement of a specific spinal level often results in predictable impairments including diminished sensation, muscle weakness, impaired reflexes, and paresthesias.

1. L4 nerve root:
   Dermatome - medial buttock, lateral thigh, medial leg, dorsum of foot, great toe
   Myotome - tibialis anterior, extensor hallucis
   Reflexes - patellar

2. **L5 nerve root:**
   Dermatome - buttock, posterior and lateral thigh, lateral aspect of leg, dorsum of foot, medial half of sole, first, second, and third toes
   Myotome - extensor hallucis, peroneals, gluteus medius, dorsiflexors, hamstrings, plantar flexors
   Reflexes - medial hamstrings, posterior tibial

3. S1 nerve root:
   Dermatome - buttock, thigh, posterior leg
   Myotome - hamstrings, peroneals, plantar flexors
   Reflexes - Achilles

4. S2 nerve root:
   Dermatome - buttock, thigh, posterior leg
   Myotome - hamstrings, plantar flexors
   Reflexes - Achilles

System Specific: Neuromuscular & Nervous Systems
Content Outline: Clinical Application of Foundational Sciences

Exam Three: Question 181

A physical therapist performs goniometric measurements for elbow flexion with a patient in supine. In order to isolate elbow flexion the therapist should stabilize the:

1. **distal end of the humerus**
2. proximal end of the humerus
3. distal end of the ulna
4. proximal end of the radius

Correct Answer: 1 (Norkin p. 72)

When measuring elbow flexion the physical therapist should align the fulcrum of the goniometer over the lateral epicondyle of the humerus. The stationary arm should be aligned with the lateral midline of the humerus using the center of the acromial process as a reference. The moveable arm should be aligned with the lateral midline of the radius using the radial head and radial styloid process as references. Normal elbow flexion is 0-150 degrees.

1. **The distal end of the humerus should be stabilized when measuring elbow flexion to prevent flexion of the shoulder. The therapist should place a pad (i.e., folded towel) between the table and the distal humerus to prevent extension of the shoulder.**
2. Stabilization of the proximal end of the humerus is too far away from the elbow to adequately stabilize the joint during elbow flexion.
3. The distal end of the radius and ulna would be stabilized when measuring wrist flexion and extension or wrist radial and ulnar deviation.
4. Any attempt to stabilize the proximal end of the radius would interfere with elbow flexion range of motion.

System Specific: Musculoskeletal System
Content Outline: Examination

Exam Three: Question 182

A patient rehabilitating from a radial head fracture performs progressive resistive exercises designed to strengthen the forearm supinators. Which muscle would be of particular importance to achieve the desired outcome?

1. brachialis
2. brachioradialis
3. **biceps brachii**
4. anconeus

Correct Answer: 3 (Kendall p. 268)

A physical therapist should have a strong understanding of anatomy including primary and secondary actions of muscles and their innervations.

1. The brachialis muscle flexes the elbow joint. The muscle is innervated by the musculocutaneous nerve.
2. The brachioradialis muscle flexes the elbow joint and assists in supination and pronation when the movements are resisted. Although the muscle plays a role in supination of the forearm, the biceps brachii is a much more powerful supinator. The muscle is innervated by the radial nerve.
3. **The biceps brachii muscle flexes the elbow joint and supinates the forearm. The muscle is innervated by the musculocutaneous nerve.**
4. The anconeus muscle extends the elbow joint and assists to stabilize the ulna during supination and pronation. The muscle is innervated by the radial nerve.

System Specific: Musculoskeletal System
Content Outline: Clinical Application of Foundational Sciences

Exam Three: Question 183

A physical therapist examines a patient with a suspected injury to the thoracodorsal nerve. Which objective finding would be consistent with this injury?

1. shoulder medial rotation weakness
2. **shoulder extension weakness**
3. paralysis of the rhomboids
4. paralysis of the diaphragm

Correct Answer: 2 (Kendall p. 279)

The thoracodorsal nerve (C6, C7, C8) is a branch of the posterior cord of the brachial plexus. The nerve follows the course of the subscapular artery along the posterior wall of the axilla to the latissimus dorsi.

1. The medial rotators of the shoulder include the subscapularis, teres major, pectoralis major, latissimus dorsi, and anterior deltoid. The latissimus dorsi would be affected by an injury to the thoracodorsal nerve, however, the presence of a number of other muscles which act to medially rotate the humerus would be adequate to compensate for any impairment in the latissimus dorsi.

2. **The latissimus dorsi is innervated by the thoracodorsal nerve (C6, C7, C8). Weakness in this prime mover for shoulder extension would produce impaired strength during shoulder extension resistive testing despite the fact that several other muscles also function to extend the shoulder. These muscles include the posterior deltoid and teres major.**

3. The rhomboids are innervated by the dorsal scapular nerve (C4, C5).

4. The diaphragm is innervated by the phrenic nerve (C3, C4, C5).

System Specific: Neuromuscular & Nervous Systems
Content Outline: Clinical Application of Foundational Sciences

Exam Three: Question 184

A physical therapist works with a patient using a flotation device positioned vertically in the deep end of a pool. Which area of the patient's body would experience the GREATEST amount of hydrostatic pressure?

1. shoulders
2. torso
3. hips
4. **feet**

Correct Answer: 4 (Cameron p. 247)

Hydrostatic pressure refers to the pressure exerted by a fluid on a body immersed in the fluid. Hydrostatic pressure increases as the depth of immersion increases.

1. When positioned vertically, the shoulders would be only partially immersed since the patient is using a flotation device. The hydrostatic pressure on the shoulders would be negligible.

2. When positioned vertically, the torso will likely be partially or perhaps fully immersed. The hydrostatic pressure on the torso will be greater than the hydrostatic pressure on the shoulders, but less than the hydrostatic pressure on the hips or feet.

3. When positioned vertically, the hips will be fully immersed. The hydrostatic pressure on the hips will be less than the hydrostatic pressure on the feet since the feet are immersed to a greater depth.

4. **When positioned vertically, the feet would experience the greatest amount of hydrostatic pressure since they are the deepest immersed body part.**

System Specific: Other Systems
Content Outline: Clinical Application of Foundational Sciences

Exam Three: Question 185

A physical therapist elects to begin a trial of mechanical lumbar traction on a 165 pound male diagnosed with suspected nerve root impingement. The MOST appropriate amount of force to initiate the session is:

1. 15 lbs.
2. **30 lbs.**
3. 60 lbs.
4. 80 lbs.

Correct Answer: 2 (Cameron p. 302)

Mechanical traction refers to the application of forces to the body using a machine to separate joint surfaces and stretch periarticular structures. Traction is indicated for many diagnoses and allows for variation and adjustment of the established protocol based on individual patient needs. Traction affects many of the body's systems and requires ongoing monitoring and reassessment of treatment parameters.

1. 15 lbs. is an insufficient amount of force to use when initiating a trial of mechanical traction due to the relative weight of the patient's body.
2. **A traction force of 25-50 lbs. is recommended when initiating mechanical lumbar traction. The amount of force is low enough to reduce the risk of protective muscle guarding and spasm, but is sufficient to determine if traction is likely to aggravate the patient's symptoms.**
3. 60 lbs. is greater than the recommended range of 25-50 lbs. for initial treatment. This amount of force may cause muscle guarding secondary to patient fear, anxiety or pain.
4. 80 lbs. is almost 50% of the patient's body weight and corresponds to the approximate amount of force (i.e., 50%) necessary to cause mechanical separation in the lumbar spine. This amount of force may be appropriate depending on the established treatment objectives, however, would not be appropriate for the initial session.

System Specific: Non-Systems
Content Outline: Equipment & Devices; Therapeutic Modalities

Exam Three: Question 186

A physical therapist completes an examination on a patient diagnosed with Parkinson's disease. Results of the examination include 4/5 strength in the lower extremities, 10 degree flexion contracture at the hips, and exaggerated forward standing posture. The patient has difficulty initiating movement and requires manual assistance for gait on level surfaces. The MOST appropriate activity to incorporate into a home program is:

1. **prone lying**
2. progressive relaxation exercises
3. lower extremity resistive exercises with ankle weights
4. postural awareness exercises in standing

Correct Answer: 1 (Umphred p. 787)

Prone lying is a commonly employed positional technique designed to stretch the hip flexors in patients with Parkinson's disease. Increased flexibility of the hip muscles will improve standing posture and enable the body's center of gravity to remain within the base of support. Although some of the other options are appropriate, they would not provide the same degree of benefit for the patient based on the described clinical presentation.

1. **Prone lying is a static positioning activity designed to stretch the hip flexors. If the patient was unable to tolerate prone lying, the physical therapist could place one or more pillows under the patient's hips and gradually remove pillows over time as the patient improves their flexibility.**
2. Progressive relaxation exercises can be incorporated using gentle rocking or segmental trunk rotation, however, the patient needs to have adequate range of motion in the hip flexors to optimize their functional status.
3. Strengthening is a restorative intervention used with patients with Parkinson's disease, however, the patient's strength in the lower extremities is already good (i.e., 4/5) and therefore would not be an immediate treatment priority.
4. Postural awareness exercises in standing are an appropriate intervention, however, the relative benefit of the activity is limited without adequate muscle length. By improving the patient's hip flexibility, the patient would be able to exhibit improved standing posture.

System Specific: Other Systems
Content Outline: Interventions

Exam Three: Question 187

A patient four days status post right total hip arthroplasty loses his balance and falls to the ground during a physical therapy session. The patient is visibly shaken by the fall, but insists that he is uninjured. The physical therapist examines the right hip and although active motion elicits pain, all other findings are inconclusive. The therapist should:

1. continue with the current treatment so the patient does not focus on the incident
2. notify the supervisor about the incident
3. **document the incident and contact a physician to examine the patient before resuming treatment**
4. document the incident and gradually resume prior treatment

> **Correct Answer: 3** (Scott - Promoting Legal and Ethical Awareness p. 81)

If a patient has fallen or has been injured during physical therapy, the physical therapist must inform the patient's physician of the incident and request medical clearance prior to continuing with treatment. Failure to inform the physician would be considered a form of negligence.

1. A physical therapist must place the patient's well-being above any other present concern. An attempt to manipulate the patient for fear of personal liability is never an appropriate course of action.
2. A physical therapist may choose to notify their supervisor about the incident, however, the primary therapist action must be directed toward making sure the patient is unharmed and ensuring the integrity of the hip arthroplasty.
3. **The described incident combined with the patient's post-operative status provides adequate justification for physician involvement and documentation. In addition to traditional documentation, the physical therapist will need to complete an incident report.**
4. The incident must be documented, however, it would be inappropriate to resume treatment without first having the patient examined by a physician.

System Specific: Non-Systems
Content Outline: Safety & Professional Roles; Teaching/Learning; Research

Exam Three: Question 188

The medical record indicates a patient has been diagnosed with chronic respiratory alkalosis. The MOST consistent laboratory finding with this condition is:

1. **elevated arterial blood pH, low $PaCO_2$**
2. low arterial blood pH, elevated $PaCO_2$
3. elevated arterial blood pH, elevated $PaCO_2$
4. low arterial blood pH, low $PaCO_2$

> **Correct Answer: 1** (Rothstein p. 440)

Analysis of arterial blood gases provides information about acid-base balance, ventilation, and oxygenation.

1. **Elevated arterial blood pH and low $PaCO_2$ are consistent with respiratory alkalosis. This condition can be caused by alveolar hyperventilation due to dizziness or syncope.**
2. Low arterial blood pH and elevated $PaCO_2$ are consistent with respiratory acidosis. This condition can be caused by alveolar hypoventilation due to anxiety, confusion, and coma.
3. Elevated arterial blood pH and elevated $PaCO_2$ are consistent with a partially compensated metabolic alkalosis. Causes of metabolic alkalosis include bicarbonate ingestion, vomiting, diuretics, steroids, and adrenal disease.
4. Low arterial blood pH and low $PaCO_2$ are consistent with a partially compensated metabolic acidosis. Causes of metabolic acidosis include metabolic diseases or disturbances such as diabetes, lactic acid, uremic acidosis, and chronic diarrhea.

System Specific: Cardiac, Vascular, & Pulmonary Systems
Content Outline: Foundations for Evaluation, Differential Diagnosis, & Prognosis

Exam Three: Question 189

A patient with a transtibial amputation is observed ambulating with excessive knee flexion from heel strike through midstance on the prosthetic side. A possible cause for this deviation is:

1. the foot is set in neutral
2. the socket is set posterior in relation to the foot
3. the prosthesis is too short
4. **the socket is aligned in excessive flexion**

Correct Answer: 4 (Seymour p. 204)

If the socket of a transtibial prosthesis is aligned in excessive flexion, there will be excessive flexion during stance causing instability of the prosthetic limb. Anatomical contributing factors include a knee flexion contracture, knee extensor weakness or a hip flexion contracture.

1. A neutral foot setting would not cause excessive knee flexion from heel strike to midstance.
2. A transtibial socket that is set posteriorly to the foot will create an increased extension moment at the knee and result in insufficient knee flexion during early stance.
3. A prosthesis that is too short would typically create an increased extension moment at the knee and result in insufficient knee flexion during early stance. A prosthesis that is too long may cause excessive flexion during heel strike through midstance.
4. **A socket that is aligned in excessive flexion will create an increased flexion moment at the knee which will result in excessive flexion from heel strike through stance phase.**

System Specific: Musculoskeletal Systems
Content Outline: Examination

Exam Three: Question 190

A physical therapist monitors a patient's vital signs while completing 20 minutes of jogging at 5 mph on a treadmill. As the session approaches its conclusion, the therapist incorporates a cool down period. The anticipated response during the post-exercise period is:

1. a progressive increase in systolic blood pressure
2. **a progressive decrease in systolic blood pressure**
3. a progressive increase in diastolic blood pressure
4. a progressive increase in rate pressure product

Correct Answer: 2 (American College of Sports Medicine p. 55)

Incorporating a cool down period provides a gradual recovery and a return of the heart rate and blood pressure to near resting values. Additional benefits of cool down include enhanced venous return, increased dissipation of body heat, increased removal of lactic acid, and reduced likelihood of ventricular arrhythmias.

1. A progressive increase in systolic blood pressure is the normal response to an increase in workload and therefore would not be associated with the post-exercise period.
2. **A progressive decrease in systolic blood pressure is the normal post-exercise response.**
3. A progressive increase in diastolic blood pressure would be considered an abnormal response since it should not occur during an increase in work or during the post-exercise period.
4. Rate pressure product or double-product, is the product of heart rate and systolic blood pressure. Both heart rate and systolic blood pressure are expected to decrease during the post-exercise period. Rate pressure product is an indicator of myocardial oxygen consumption.

System Specific: Cardiac, Vascular, & Pulmonary Systems
Content Outline: Clinical Application of Foundational Sciences

Exam Three: Question 191

A patient status post stroke ambulates with a large base quad cane. The patient presents with left neglect and diminished proprioception. The MOST appropriate method to ensure patient safety is:

1. provide continuous verbal cues
2. utilize visual cues and demonstration
3. **offer manual assistance on the left side**
4. offer manual assistance on the right side

> **Correct Answer: 3** (O'Sullivan p. 1169)

A physical therapist must carefully consider a patient's current limitations and identify remedial strategies to assist the patient to achieve established goals. The presence of left neglect and diminished proprioception requires the therapist to take formal action to avoid jeopardizing patient safety.

1. Verbal cues may be beneficial for the patient, however, without concurrent manual assistance the patient would likely still have increased difficulty with ambulation and may be at increased risk for a fall.
2. Demonstration prior to practice is important, however, this type of educational strategy would not directly address the left neglect and diminished proprioception.
3. **The physical therapist should offer manual assistance on the patient's left side during ambulation activities. The manual assistance can facilitate motor activity and weight bearing, as well as proprioception on the affected side. Manual contact significantly reduces the risk for fall or injury.**
4. The patient presents with left neglect and as a result manual assistance would not typically be necessary on the right side of the body.

System Specific: Other Systems
Content Outline: Interventions

Exam Three: Question 192

A patient elevated on a tilt table to 60 degrees suddenly begins to demonstrate signs and symptoms of orthostatic hypotension. The MOST appropriate physical therapist action is to:

1. lower the tilt table 10 degrees and monitor the patient's vital signs
2. lower the tilt table 20 degrees and monitor the patient's vital signs
3. lower the tilt table 40 degrees and monitor the patient's vital signs
4. **lower the tilt table completely and monitor the patient's vital signs**

> **Correct Answer: 4** (Pierson p. 337)

Signs and symptoms of orthostatic hypotension include a 20 mm Hg or greater decrease in systolic blood pressure, dizziness, and nausea. The signs and symptoms are caused by reduced venous return from the lower extremities which is often precipitated by vertical positioning. The reduced venous return results in decreased filling of the left ventricle and diminished cardiac output and cerebral perfusion.

1. Lowering the tilt table 10 degrees would not likely be sufficient to adequately resolve the patient's current signs and symptoms of orthostatic hypotension.
2. Lowering the tilt table 20 degrees would serve as a relatively modest change in the degree of vertical positioning and would therefore be more appropriate if the patient had experienced only mild dizziness or another isolated sign or symptom of orthostatic hypotension.
3. Lowering the tilt table 40 degrees would be a viable option, however, the sudden onset of signs and symptoms of orthostatic hypotension make it more appropriate to lower the tilt table to a horizontal position.
4. **The magnitude of the positional change (i.e., 60 degrees to horizontal) would likely be adequate to reduce the patient's signs and symptoms of orthostatic hypotension. The patient's vital signs should be checked to ensure that the patient's blood pressure is within normal limits.**

System Specific: Cardiac, Vascular, & Pulmonary Systems
Content Outline: Interventions

Exam Three: Question 193

A physical therapist and a physical therapist assistant work as a team in an orthopedic private practice. Which activity would be inappropriate for the physical therapist assistant?

1. application of a superficial modality
2. **completing a discharge summary**
3. leading a group exercise program
4. performing an isokinetic test

Correct Answer: 2 (Guide to Physical Therapist Practice)

The physical therapist assistant is a technically educated health care provider who assists the physical therapist in the provision of physical therapy services. The physical therapist of record is directly responsible for the actions of the physical therapist assistant and should therefore possess a comprehensive understanding of the physical therapist assistant's scope of practice.

1. Physical therapist assistants routinely perform interventions such as the application of superficial modalities as part of an established plan of care.
2. **The physical therapist is solely responsible for the establishment of the discharge summary and the associated documentation.**
3. Physical therapist assistants often instruct individual patients and groups of patients in exercise programs. The activity would be within the physical therapist assistant's scope of practice.
4. An isokinetic test is a resistive test designed to collect data regarding a patient's strength. Physical therapist assistants perform tests and measures as part of their daily practice.

System Specific: Non-Systems
Content Outline: Safety & Professional Roles; Teaching/Learning; Research

Exam Three: Question 194

A physical therapist obtains a complete medical history prior to administering cryotherapy. Which condition would NOT be considered a contraindication to cryotherapy?

1. Raynaud's disease
2. cryoglobulinemia
3. **cancer**
4. cold urticaria

Correct Answer: 3 (Cameron p. 140)

Commonly used cryotherapeutic agents include cold whirlpool, ice packs, ice massage, cold sprays, and contrast baths. Physical therapists should be aware of indications and contraindications for all superficial agents.

1. Raynaud's disease is a condition that causes arteries supplying blood to the skin to narrow resulting in diminished circulation. Symptoms include pallor, rubor, cyanosis, and numbness and tingling in the digits and hand. Raynaud's disease is considered a contraindication for cryotherapy.
2. Cryoglobulinemia is a condition where abnormal blood protein transforms to gel when exposed to cold temperatures. The gel-like state can lead to ischemia and gangrene if prolonged exposure exists. Cryoglobulinemia is considered a contraindication for cryotherapy.
3. **Cryotherapy is not contraindicated for patient's with cancer, however, secondary impairments such as diminished sensation can make cryotherapy an unacceptable treatment option.**
4. Cold urticaria refers to an allergic-like response producing hives or large welts on the skin following exposure to cold. In more severe cases, the patient may experience a significant decrease in blood pressure, an increase in heart rate, and syncope. Cold urticaria is considered a contraindication for cryotherapy.

System Specific: Non-Systems
Content Outline: Equipment & Devices; Therapeutic Modalities

Exam Three: Question 195

A patient with T10 paraplegia is discharged from a rehabilitation hospital following 12 weeks of intense rehabilitation. Which of the following pieces of equipment would be the MOST essential to assist the patient with functional mobility?

1. ambulation with Lofstrand crutches
2. ambulation with Lofstrand crutches and ankle-foot orthoses
3. ambulation with Lofstrand crutches and knee-ankle-foot orthoses
4. **wheelchair**

> **Correct Answer: 4** (Rothstein p. 408)

A patient with a lesion above T12 would not be a functional ambulator due to the extreme energy demands and therefore would utilize a wheelchair as their primary mode of mobility.

1. A patient with an incomplete lesion may ambulate without an orthotic using Lofstrand crutches, however, this would not be an option for a complete spinal cord lesion.
2. A patient with a complete lesion at L4 or L5 would typically ambulate with crutches or canes and bilateral AFOs. The extensor digitorum, medial hamstrings, posterior tibialis, quadriceps, tibialis anterior, and low back muscles would be the lowest innervated muscles.
3. A patient with a complete lesion at L2 or L3 would typically ambulate with crutches and bilateral KAFOs. Patients at this level of injury may also use a manual wheelchair for energy conservation and convenience. The gracilis, iliopsoas, quadratus lumborum, rectus femoris, and sartorius would be the lowest innervated muscles.
4. **A patient with T10 paraplegia will require a wheelchair for community ambulation due to the increased energy expenditure associated with ambulation. The lower abdominals and intercostals would be the lowest innervated muscles.**

System Specific: Non-Systems
Content Outline: Equipment & Devices; Therapeutic Modalities

Exam Three: Question 196

A physical therapist instructs a patient's spouse to remove and reapply a bandage. Which of the following instructional methods would be the MOST appropriate to ensure the task is performed appropriately?

1. have the patient instruct the spouse how to remove and reapply the bandage
2. provide written instructions on how to remove and reapply the bandage
3. **instruct the spouse to remove and reapply the bandage and observe her performance**
4. instruct the spouse to contact the physical therapy department if she has specific questions on how to remove or reapply the bandage

> **Correct Answer: 3** (Hall p. 40)

The physical therapist should observe the removal and reapplication of the bandage in order to determine if the spouse is capable of performing the task. Although this will not ensure the task is done appropriately in the future, it will provide the patient with the opportunity for feedback based on their current performance.

1. If the patient instructs the spouse how to remove and reapply the bandage, the therapist can conclude that the patient can explain the task, but this does not ensure that the spouse can independently perform the task.
2. Written instructions are helpful for the patient and spouse as a resource, but will not ensure independence. Demonstration is the best instructional method to ensure proper technique and independence.
3. **Patient and family education is a critical component of a comprehensive plan of care following amputation. Direct observation of the spouse's performance is the best method to increase the probability that the activity will be performed correctly.**
4. The physical therapist would be exercising poor judgment if they requested the patient to call the department with questions on bandaging without providing additional instruction. The therapist must provide instruction and observe the family members' performance to ensure competence.

System Specific: Integumentary System
Content Outline: Interventions

Exam Three: Question 197

A physical therapist instructs a patient in an upper extremity proprioceptive neuromuscular facilitation pattern by telling the patient to begin by grasping an imaginary sword positioned in a scabbard on their left hip using their right hand. This type of command would be MOST appropriate to initiate:

1. D1 extension
2. D1 flexion
3. D2 extension
4. **D2 flexion**

> **Correct Answer: 4** (Kisner p. 196)

Proprioceptive neuromuscular facilitation (PNF) patterns are upper and lower extremity movement patterns that are designed to improve stability and strengthen the extremities, trunk, and neck. The patterns are performed unilaterally or bilaterally, symmetrically or asymmetrically. Resistance using tubing, weights or manual resistance can increase the level of difficulty.

1. The D1 extension pattern begins with the patient positioned in shoulder flexion, adduction, and lateral rotation. The patient follows the directive of "open your hand and push down and away from your body" to complete the diagonal pattern.
2. The D1 flexion pattern begins with the patient positioned in shoulder extension, abduction, and medial rotation. The patient follows the directive of "close your hand and pull up and across your body" to complete the diagonal pattern.
3. The D2 extension pattern begins with the patient positioned in shoulder flexion, abduction, and lateral rotation. The patient follows the directive of "close your hand and pull down and across your body" to complete the diagonal pattern.
4. **The D2 flexion pattern begins with the patient positioned in shoulder extension, adduction, and medial rotation. The patient follows the directive of "open your hand and pull up and away from your body" to complete the diagonal pattern.**

System Specific: Neuromuscular & Nervous Systems
Content Outline: Interventions

Exam Three: Question 198

A physical therapist develops a plan of care for a patient status post unilateral transtibial amputation that has been approved for inpatient rehabilitation. Assuming an uncomplicated recovery, what is the MOST appropriate amount of time for prosthetic training?

1. 1-2 days
2. **1-2 weeks**
3. 4-6 weeks
4. 6-8 weeks

> **Correct Answer: 2** (Lusardi p. 716)

A patient with a unilateral transtibial amputation would typically require one to two weeks for prosthetic training. Training includes donning and doffing, prosthetic management, transfers, ambulation, and stair training.

1. Prosthetic training requires careful observation of prosthetic fit and mastering all functional activities including gait, stairs, community training, transferring to and from the floor, and total care of the prosthesis. This cannot be accomplished in a one or two day period.
2. **A patient with a unilateral transtibial amputation would typically enter inpatient rehabilitation for one to two weeks for prosthetic training. This period permits sufficient time for the majority of patients to develop adequate proficiency in functional training activities.**
3. A patient with a unilateral transtibial amputation would not typically require four to six weeks of inpatient rehabilitation for prosthetic training. The patient should be able to master all aspects of prosthetic training within a one to two week time frame.
4. A patient with a unilateral transtibial amputation would not typically require six to eight weeks of inpatient rehabilitation for prosthetic training. A time frame of six to eight weeks would be more indicative of a patient with a complete spinal cord injury resulting in paraplegia.

System Specific: Musculoskeletal System
Content Outline: Foundations for Evaluation, Differential Diagnosis, & Prognosis

Exam Three: Question 199

After observing a patient during an exercise session, a physical therapist concludes that the patient commonly uses the Valsalva maneuver. Which activity would have the GREATEST probability of producing the Valsalva maneuver?

1. **lifting a 40 lb. package from the floor to a counter at waist level**
2. walking at 4 mph on a treadmill
3. stationary cycling at 80 revolutions per minute
4. using an upper extremity ergometer at 40 revolutions per minute

Correct Answer: 1 (Kisner p. 392)

The Valsalva maneuver refers to a contraction of the muscles of the abdomen, chest wall, and diaphragm in a forced expiratory effort against a closed glottis. This action produces an increase in intrathoracic and intra-abdominal pressures that lead to decreased venous blood flow to the heart.

1. **Patients commonly use the Valsalva maneuver during heavy resistance exercise. Forty pounds would be a sufficiently heavy load that would result in most patients straining and holding their breath while lifting the package from the floor.**
2. Walking at 4 mph on a treadmill is a rhythmical form of exercise that would not require the patient to hold their breath in a Valsalva maneuver. Patients typically establish a steady breathing pattern when walking at a constant speed on a treadmill.
3. Stationary cycling at 80 revolutions per minute is a rhythmical form of exercise. The continuous nature of the activity combined with the high revolutions per minute would not require the patient to hold their breath in a Valsalva maneuver.
4. Using an upper extremity ergometer at 40 revolutions per minute is a rhythmical form of exercise that requires continuous motion of the upper extremities. The Valsalva maneuver is more commonly observed in strenuous, shorter duration activities.

System Specific: Cardiac, Vascular, & Pulmonary Systems
Content Outline: Interventions

Exam Three: Question 200

A physical therapist receives a referral to instruct a patient in pelvic floor muscle strengthening exercises. Which of the following explanations would be the MOST effective to assist the patient to perform a pelvic floor contraction?

1. tighten your muscles like you were trying to expel a large amount of urine in a very short amount of time
2. **pull your muscles upward and inward as if attempting to stop the flow of urine**
3. tighten your abdominal muscles and anteriorly rotate your pelvis
4. gently push out as if you had to pass gas

Correct Answer: 2 (Hall p. 412)

The pelvic floor muscles support the pelvic organs against intra-abdominal pressure, provide closure of the urethra and rectum for continence, and support sexual function. Pelvic floor exercises, also known as Kegel exercises, assist to maintain the strength and function of the pelvic floor muscles.

1. Placing a downward pressure on the pelvic floor serves to increase intra-abdominal pressure and encourage protrusion or prolapse of the pelvic organs.
2. **The correct technique for pelvic floor exercises includes pulling the pelvic floor muscles up and in. Isometric contractions should be held for five to ten seconds with complete relaxation after each contraction. Five to ten contractions should be performed in a series and three to four series should be performed each day.**
3. Tightening the abdominal muscles will trigger reflexive contraction of the pelvic floor, however, anteriorly rotating the pelvis will lengthen the abdominal muscles. Performing both actions simultaneously will reduce the strength of any pelvic floor contraction.
4. The act of "pushing out as if you had to pass gas" places a downward pressure on the pelvic floor muscles. This action is opposite of the necessary action for pelvic floor strengthening.

System Specific: Other Systems
Content Outline: Interventions

Notes

Scoring Summary

Computer-Based Exams Scoring Summary

	Available Questions	Correct Questions	% Correct
Exam One	200		
Exam Two	200		
Exam Three	200		

Computer-Based Exams Index

Directions for Using the Computer-Based Exams Index

The Computer-Based Exams Index allows candidates to identify specific academic content in each of the three sample examinations. For example, consider the following entry: **Breathing exercises 2:** 146, 152; **3:** 8. The bold numbers represent the exam number and the non-bold numbers that follow represent the question number within the respective exam. Therefore, questions pertaining to breathing exercises are located in Exam Two: Question 146, 152 and in Exam Three: Question 8. The index provides candidates with an efficient and effective method to review selected academic content after completing each of the sample examinations.

Resource List

American Physical Therapy Association
1111 North Fairfax Street
Alexandria, Virginia 22314-1488
Phone: (800) 999-2782
Web site: **www.apta.org**

Federation of State Boards of Physical Therapy
124 West Street South, Third Floor
Alexandria, Virginia 22314
Phone: (703) 299-3100
Web site: **www.fsbpt.org**

Scorebuilders
P.O. Box 7242
Scarborough, Maine 04070-7242
Toll Free: (866) PTEXAMS
Phone: (207) 885-0304
Web site: **www.scorebuilders.com**
Fax: (207) 883-8377

State Licensing Agencies

Alabama

Alabama Board of Physical Therapy
100 N. Union Street
Suite 724
Montgomery, AL 36130-5040

(334) 242-4064
www.pt.alabama.gov/

Alaska

State PT & OT Board
333 Willoughby Avenue, 9th Floor
P.O. Box 11806
Juneau, AK 99811-0806

(907) 465-2580
www.commerce.state.ak.us/occ/pphy.htm

Arizona

Arizona State Board of Physical Therapy
4205 North 7th Avenue
Suite 208
Phoenix, AZ 85013

(602) 274-0236
www.ptboard.az.gov/public1/pages/home.asp

Arkansas

Arkansas State Board of Physical Therapy
9 Shackleford Plaza
Suite 3
Little Rock, AR 72211

(501) 228-7100
www.arptb.org/

California

Physical Therapy Board of California
2005 Evergreen Street
Suite 1350
Sacramento, CA 95815

(916) 561-8200
www.ptb.ca.gov/

Colorado

Colorado PT Licensure Division of Registrations
1560 Broadway
Suite 1350
Denver, CO 80202-5146

(303) 894-7851
www.dora.state.co.us/Physical-Therapy

Connecticut

Office of Practitioner Licensing & Certification
410 Capitol Avenue
MS #12APP
Hartford, CT 06134-0308

(860) 509-8377
www.ct.gov/dph/site/default.asp

Delaware

Division of Professional Regulation
861 Silver Lake Blvd.
Suite 203, Cannon Building
Dover, DE 19904-2467

(302) 744-4500
www.dpr.delaware.gov/boards/physicaltherapy

District of Columbia

District of Columbia Board of Physical Therapy
Health Professional Licensing Administration
717 14th Street, NW, Suite 600
Washington, DC 20005

(202) 724-8739
hpla.doh.dc.gov/

Florida

MQA/Board of Physical Therapy Practice
4052 Bald Cypress Way
Bin #C-05
Tallahassee, FL 32399-3255

(850) 245-4373
www.doh.state.fl.us/mqa/physical/

Georgia

Georgia Board of Physical Therapy
237 Coliseum Drive
Macon, GA 31217-3858

(478) 207-2440
www.sos.state.ga.us/plb/pt/

Hawaii

Hawaii Dept. of Commerce & Consumer Affairs
P.O. Box 3469
Honolulu, HI 96801

(808) 586-2694
www.hawaii.gov/dcca/areas/pvl/boards/

State Licensing Agencies

Idaho

Bureau of Occupational Licenses
1109 Main Street
Suite 220
Boise, ID 83702-5642

(208) 334-3233
www.ibol.idaho.gov/

Illinois

Illinois Dept. of Professional Regulation
Attn: Health Services Section
320 West Washington Street, 3rd Floor
Springfield, IL 62786

(217) 782-8556
www.idfpr.com/dpr/WHO/pt.asp

Indiana

Indiana Physical Therapy Committee
402 West Washington Street
Room W072
Indianapolis, IN 46204

(317) 234-2051
www.in.gov/pla/

Iowa

Iowa Department of Public Health
Lucas State Office Building
321 East 12th Street, 5th Floor
Des Moines, IA 50319-0075

(515) 281-4413
www.idph.state.ia.us/licensure/default.asp

Kansas

Kansas State Board of Healing Arts
Physical Therapy Examining Committee
235 South Topeka Blvd
Topeka, KS 66614

(785) 296-8563
www.ksbha.org/

Kentucky

Kentucky Board of Physical Therapy
312 Whittington Parkway
Suite 102
Louisville, KY 40222-5159

(502) 429-7140
www.pt.ky.gov/

Louisiana

Louisiana State Board of PT Examiners
104 Fairlane Drive
Lafayette, LA 70507

(337) 262-1043
www.laptboard.org/

Maine

Maine Dept. of Professional & Financial Reg.
Office of Licensing and Registration
35 State House Station
Augusta, ME 04333-0035

(207) 624-8603
www.maine.gov/pfr/

Maryland

Maryland Board of PT Examiners
4201 Patterson Avenue
#223
Baltimore, MD 21215-2299

(410) 764-4752
www.dhmh.state.md.us/bphte

Massachusetts

Massachusetts Board of Allied Health Prof.
Division of Registration
239 Causeway Street, Suite 500
Boston, MA 02114

(617) 727-3071
www.state.ma.us/reg/boards/ah/

Michigan

Physical Therapy State Boards
611 West Ottawa
1st Floor
Lansing, MI 48909-7518

(517) 335-0918
www.michigan.gov/mdch/

Minnesota

Minnesota Board of Physical Therapy
2829 University Avenue, SE
Suite 420
Minneapolis, MN 55414-3245

(612) 627-5406
www.physicaltherapy.state.mn.us/

State Licensing Agencies

Mississippi

Mississippi State Board of Physical Therapy
P.O. Box 55707
Jackson, MS 39296-5707

(601) 939-5124
www.msbpt.state.ms.us/

Missouri

Advisory Comm. for Prof. PTs & PTAs
P.O. Box 4
Jefferson City, MO 65102

(573) 751-0098
pr.mo.gov/physicaltherapists.asp

Montana

Montana Board of Physical Therapy
301 South Park, 4th Floor
P.O. Box 200513
Helena, MT 59620

(406) 841-2395
www.mt.gov/dli/ptp/

Nebraska

Nebraska Board of Physical Therapy DHHS,
Division of Public Health, Licensure Unit
301 Centennial Mall, P.O. Box 94986
Lincoln, NE 68509-4986

(402) 471-2299
www.dhhs.ne.gov/crl/rcs/pt/pt.htm

Nevada

Nevada Board of Physical Therapy Examiners
810 South Durango Drive
Suite 109
Las Vegas, NV 89145

(702) 876-5535
www.ptboard.nv.gov/

New Hampshire

PT Governing Board of New Hampshire
Office of Allied Health Professionals
2 Industrial Park Drive
Concord, NH 03301

(603) 271-8389
www.nh.gov/alliedhealth

New Jersey

New Jersey State Board of Physical Therapy
P.O. Box 45014
Newark, NJ 07101

(973) 504-6455
www.state.nj.us/lps/ca/medical/pt.htm

New Mexico

New Mexico Physical Therapy Board
P.O. Box 25101
Santa Fe, NM 87505

(505) 476-4880
www.rld.state.nm.us/PhysicalTherapy/index.html

New York

New York Physical Therapy Dispensing
Ofc. of the Professions, NYS Education Dept.
89 Washington Avenue
Albany, NY 12234

(518) 474-3817 x180
www.op.nysed.gov/pt.htm

North Carolina

North Carolina Board of Physical Therapy
18 West Colony Place
#140
Durham, NC 27705

(919) 490-6393
www.ncptboard2.org/

North Dakota

ND State Examining Committee for PT
Box 69
Grafton, ND 58237

(701) 352-0125
www.ndbpt.org/

Ohio

Ohio OT, PT, & Athletic Trainers Board
77 South High Street
16th Floor
Columbus, OH 43215-6108

(614) 466-3774
www.otptat.ohio.gov/

State Licensing Agencies

Oklahoma

Board of Medical Licensure & Supervision
Physical Therapy Advisory Committee
5104 North Francis, Suite C
Oklahoma City, OK 73118-0256

(405) 848-6845
www.okmedicalboard.org/

Oregon

Oregon Physical Therapy Licensing Board
800 NE Oregon Street
Suite 407
Portland, OR 97232-2187

(971) 673-0200
www.ptboard.state.or.us/

Pennsylvania

Pennsylvania State Board of PT
P.O. Box 2649
Harrisburg, PA 17105-2649

(717) 783-7134
www.dos.state.pa.us/physther

Puerto Rico

Office of Regulation and Certification
Call Box 10200
Santurce, PR 00908

(787) 725-8161 x209
www.salud.gov.pr/

Rhode Island

Rhode Island Department of Health
3 Capitol Hill
Room 104
Providence, RI 02908-5097

(401) 222-1750
www.health.ri.gov/

South Carolina

South Carolina Board of PT Examiners
110 Centerview Drive
P.O. Box 11329
Columbia, SC 29211

(803) 896-4655
www.llr.state.sc.us/

South Dakota

South Dakota State Board of Medical and Osteopathic
Examiners
125 South Main Avenue
Sioux Falls, SD 57104

(605) 367-7781
doh.sd.gov/boards/medicine/

Tennessee

Board of PT, PTA, Electrology & Reflexology
TN Health Licensure & Regulations
227 French Landing, Suite 300 Heritage Place, Metro Center
Nashville, TN 37243

(800) 778-4123 x25132
www.state.tn.us/health

Texas

Texas Board of PT Examiners
333 Guadalupe
Suite 2-510
Austin, TX 78701-3942

(512) 305-6900
www.ecptote.state.tx.us/

Utah

Div. of Occupational and Professional Licensing
160 East 300 South
Box 146741
Salt Lake City, UT 84114

(801) 530-6767
www.dopl.utah.gov/licensing/physical_therapist

Vermont

Physical Therapy Advisors
Office of Professional Regulation
National Life Building, North, FL 2
Montpelier, VT 05620-3402

(802) 828-2191
www.vtprofessionals.org

Virgin Islands

Virgin Islands Board of PT Examiners
DOH - Office of the Commissioner
48 Sugar Estate
St. Thomas, VI 00802

(340) 774-0117
www.fsbpt.org/Boards/VirginIslands/

State Licensing Agencies

Virginia

Virginia Board of Physical Therapy
Dept. of Health Professions
9960 Mayland Drive, Suite 300
Richmond, VA 23233-1463

(804) 367-4630
www.dhp.state.va.us/

Washington

Washington Board of Physical Therapy
P.O. Box 47867
Olympia, WA 98504-7867

(360) 236-4700
www.doh.wa.gov/hsqa/Professions/Physical_Therapy

West Virginia

West Virginia Board of Physical Therapy
642 Davisson Run Road
Clarksburg, WV 26301

(304) 627-2251
www.wvbopt.com/

Wisconsin

Wisconsin Dept. of Regulation & Licensing
1400 E. Washington Avenue/Room 178
P.O. Box 8935
Madison, WI 53708-8935

(608) 266-8098
drl.wi.gov/index.htm

Wyoming

Wyoming Board of Physical Therapy
1800 Carey Avenue
4th Floor
Cheyenne, WY 82002

(307) 777-3507
plboards.state.wy.us/ptherapy/index.asp

Prometric Testing Centers

Alabama
Birmingham
Dothan
Huntsville
Mobile
Montgomery

Alaska
Anchorage

Arizona
Casa Grande
Flagstaff
Goodyear
Phoenix
Tempe
Tucson

Arkansas
Arkadelphia
Fort Smith
Little Rock

California
Alameda
Anaheim
Camarillo
Culver City
Diamond Bar
Fair Oaks
Fremont
Fresno
Gardena
Glendale
Lake Forest
Rancho Cucamonga
Redlands
San Diego
San Francisco (2)
San Jose
Santa Rosa
South San Francisco
Van Nuys

Colorado
Colorado Springs
Grand Junction
Greenwood Village
Longmont

Connecticut
Glastonbury
Hamden
Norwalk

District of Columbia
Washington, D.C.

Delaware
New Castle

Florida
Boca Raton
Coral Springs
Davie
Fort Myers
Gainesville
Jacksonville
Maitland
Miami
Sarasota
Tallahassee
Tampa
Temple Terrace

Georgia
Athens
Atlanta (2)
Columbus
Macon
Marietta
Savannah
Valdosta

Hawaii
Honolulu

Idaho
Garden City
Pocatello

Illinois
Carterville
Champaign
Chicago
Deerfield
Homewood
Lombard
Peoria
Springfield
Sycamore

Indiana
Carmel
Evansville
Fort Wayne
Indianapolis (2)
Lafayette
Merrillville
Mishawaka
Terre Haute

Iowa
Ames
Bettendorf
Iowa City
Sioux City (2)
West Des Moines

Kansas
Hays
Overland Park
Pittsburg
Topeka
Wichita

Kentucky
Lexington
Louisville (2)

Prometric Testing Centers

Louisiana

Alexandria
Baton Rouge
Bossier City
Metairie

Maine

Bangor
Presque Isle
South Portland

Maryland

Baltimore (2)
Bethesda
Columbia
Salisbury
Towson

Massachusetts

Boston
Brookline
Burlington
Lowell
West Springfield
Worcester

Michigan

Ann Arbor
Grand Rapids
Lansing
Livonia
Sault Ste Marie
Troy

Minnesota

Duluth
Edina
Rochester
Woodbury

Mississippi

Jackson
Tupelo

Missouri

Jefferson City
Kansas City
Lees Summit
Springfield
St. Joseph
St. Louis

Montana

Billings
Helena

Nebraska

Columbus
Kearney
Lincoln
Omaha
Scottsbluff

Nevada

Las Vegas
Reno

New Hampshire

Concord
Portsmouth

New Jersey

Clark
Deptford
Fairlawn
Toms River
West Orange

New Mexico

Albuquerque (2)
Farmington
Las Cruces
Santa Fe

New York

Albany
Brooklyn
Buffalo
East Syracuse
Melville
New York City (3)
Poughkeepsie
Purchase
Queens
Rochester
Vestal
Westbury

North Carolina

Asheville
Charlotte
Greensboro
Greenville
Raleigh
Wilmington

North Dakota

Bismarck
Fargo

Ohio

Beavercreek
Cincinnati
Cleveland
Maumee
Mentor
Niles
Stow
Strongsville
Worthington

Oklahoma

Oklahoma City
Tulsa

Prometric Testing Centers

Oregon
Bend
Eugene
La Grande
Medford
Portland (2)

Pennsylvania
Allentown
Clarks Summit
Conshohocken
Erie
Harrisburg
Lancaster
Monroeville
Philadelphia
Pittsburgh
York

Texas
Abilene
Amarillo
Austin
Beaumont
Bedford
College Station
Corpus Christi
Dallas
El Paso
Houston (4)
Lubbock
McAllen
Odessa
San Antonio (3)
Tyler
Waco
Wichita Falls

West Virginia
Charleston
Morgantown

Wisconsin
Brookfield
Madison

Wyoming
Casper

Rhode Island
Warwick

South Carolina
Charleston
Columbia
Florence
Greenville (2)
N. Augusta
Rock Hill

South Dakota
Rapid City
Sioux Falls

Tennessee
Chattanooga
Clarksville
Cordova
Franklin
Knoxville
Madison
Memphis

Utah
Lindon
Saint George
Salt Lake City
Taylorsville

Vermont
Williston

Virginia
Bristol
Fairfax
Glen Allen
Lynchburg
Newport News
Roanoke

Washington
Mount Lake Terrace
Puyallup
Spokane

Bibliography

American Cancer Society, *www.cancer.org*, 2009

American College of Obstetricians and Gynecologists: *Exercise during Pregnancy and the Postpartum Period* (Technical Bulletin No 189), copyright ACOG, 1994

American College of Emergency Physicians: *First Aid, CPR, and AED*, Fifth Edition, Jones and Bartlett Publishers, Inc., 2007

American College of Sports Medicine: *ACSM's Resource Manual for Guidelines for Exercise Testing and Prescription*, Sixth Edition, Lippincott Williams & Wilkins, 2010

American Heart Association, *www.americanheart.org*, 2009

Anderson MK, Hall SJ, Martin M: *Fundamentals of Sports Injury Management,* Fourth Edition, Lippincott Williams & Wilkins, 2009

Anemaet W, Moffa-Trotter M: *Home Rehabilitation: Guide to Clinical Practice*, Mosby, 2000

Arends R: *Learning to Teach*, Third Edition, McGraw-Hill Inc., 2005

Bailey D, Robinson D: *Therapeutic Approaches in Mental Health/Psychiatric Nursing*, FA Davis Company, 1997

Belanger A: *Evidence-Based Guide to Therapeutic Physical Agents*, Lippincott Williams & Wilkins, 2003

Bennett S, Karnes J: *Neurological Disabilities: Assessment and Treatment*, Lippincott-Raven Publishers, 1998

Bickley L, Szilagyi P: *Bates' Guide to Physical Examination and History Taking*, Tenth Edition, Lippincott Williams & Wilkins, 2009

Bobath B: *Adult Hemiplegia: Evaluation and Treatment*, Third Edition Butterworth-Heinemann, 1990

Brannon F, Foley M, Starr J, Saul L: *Cardiopulmonary Rehabilitation: Basic Theory and Application*, FA Davis Company, 1998

Brotzman SB, Wilk KE: *Clinical Orthopedic Rehabilitation*, Mosby, 2003

Brunnstrom S: *Movement Therapy in Hemiplegia*, Harper and Row Publishers Inc., 1992

Cameron M: *Physical Agents in Rehabilitation: From Research to Practice*, Third Edition, WB Saunders Company, 2008

Campbell M: *Rehabilitation for Traumatic Brain Injury: Physical Therapy Practice in Context*, Churchill Livingstone, 2000

Campbell S: *Decision Making in Pediatric Neurologic Physical Therapy*, Churchill Livingstone, 1999

Campbell S: *Physical Therapy for Children*, Third Edition, WB Saunders Company, 2006

Carr J, Shepard R: *Neurological Rehabilitation: Optimizing Motor Performance*, Butterworth-Heinemann, 1998

Carr J, Shepard R: *Stroke Rehabilitation: Guidelines for Exercise and Training to Optimize Motor Skill*, Elsevier Science Limited, 2003

Centers for Disease Control and Prevention: *Guidelines for Isolation Precautions in Hospitals*, Atlanta, GA www.cdc.gov, 2009

Ciccone C: *Pharmacology in Rehabilitation*, Fourth Edition, FA Davis Company, 2007

Clark C, Bonfiglio M: *Orthopaedics: Essentials of Diagnosis and Treatment*, Churchill Livingstone, 1994

Clarkson HM: *Musculoskeletal Assessment*, Second Edition, Lippincott Williams & Wilkins, 2000

Code of Ethics, American Physical Therapy Association, HOD S06-00-12-23

Criteria for Standards of Practice for Physical Therapy, American Physical Therapy Association, BOD S03-06-16-38

Bibliography

Curtis K: **The Physical Therapist's Guide to Health Care**, Slack Inc., 1999

Davis C: **Patient Practitioner Interaction**, Fourth Edition, Slack Inc., 2006

De Domenico G, Wood E: **Beard's Massage**, Fifth Edition, WB Saunders Company, 2007

DeMyer W: **Technique of the Neurologic Examination**, McGraw-Hill Companies, 2004

Denegar C: **Therapeutic Modalities for Musculoskeletal Injuries**, Second Edition, Human Kinetics, 2005

Domholdt E: **Physical Therapy Research Principles and Application**, Second Edition, WB Saunders Company, 2000

Donatelli R, Wooden M: **Orthopedic Physical Therapy**, Third Edition, Churchill Livingstone, 2001

Drench M, Noonan A, Sharby N, Ventura S: **Psychosocial Aspects of Healthcare**, Second Edition, Prentice Hall, 2006

Dutton M: **Orthopaedic Examination, Evaluation, and Intervention**, Second Edition, McGraw-Hill Inc., 2008

Edelman C, Mandle C: **Health Promotion: Throughout the Lifespan**, Mosby, 2002

Falkenstein N, Weiss-Lessard S: **Hand Rehabilitation: A Quick Reference Guide and Review**, Second Edition, Mosby, 2004

Falvo DR: **Effective Patient Education**, Third Edition, Jones and Bartlett Publishers, 2004

Frownfelter D, Dean E: **Cardiovascular and Pulmonary Physical Therapy: Evidence and Practice**, Fourth Edition, Mosby-Year Book, Inc., 2006

Garrison S: **Physical Medicine and Rehabilitation Basics**, Second Edition, J.B. Lippincott Company, 2003

Giles S: **PTEXAM: The Complete Study Guide**, Scorebuilders, 2010

Goodman C, Boissonnault W, Fuller K: **Pathology: Implications for the Physical Therapist**, Third Edition, WB Saunders Company, 2008

Goodman C, Snyder T: **Differential Diagnosis in Physical Therapy**, Fourth Edition, WB Saunders Company, 2007

Guide for Conduct of the Physical Therapist Assistant, American Physical Therapy Association, 2004

Guide for Professional Conduct, American Physical Therapy Association, 2004

Guide to Physical Therapist Practice, Second Edition, American Physical Therapy Association, 2004

Haggard A: **Handbook of Patient Education**, Aspen Publishers, 1989

Hall C, Brody L: **Therapeutic Exercise: Moving Toward Function**, Second Edition, Lippincott Williams & Wilkins, 2004

Hamill J, Knutzen K: **Biomechanical Basis of Human Movement**, Third Edition, Lippincott Williams & Wilkins, 2008

Hertling D, Kessler R: **Management of Common Musculoskeletal Disorders**, Fourth Edition, Lippincott Williams & Wilkins, 2005

Hillegass E, Sadowsky H: **Cardiopulmonary Physical Therapy**, Second Edition, WB Saunders Company, 2001

Hislop HJ, Montgomery J: **Daniels and Worthingham's Muscle Testing: Techniques of Manual Examination**, Eighth Edition, WB Saunders Company, 2007

Hodgkin JE, Celli B, Connors G: **Pulmonary Rehabilitation: Guidelines to Success**, Fourth Edition, Lippincott Williams & Wilkins, 2008

Hoppenfeld S: **Physical Examination of the Spine and Extremities**, Appleton-Century-Crofts, 1982

Houglum P: **Therapeutic Exercise for Athletic Injuries**, Second Edition, Human Kinetics, 2005

Bibliography

Irwin S, Tecklin J: *Cardiopulmonary Physical Therapy: A Guide to Practice*, Fourth Edition, Mosby, 2004

Jacobs M, Austin N: *Splinting The Hand and the Upper Extremity: Principles and Process*, Lippincott Williams & Wilkins, 2003

Kendall F, McCreary E, Provance P: *Muscle Testing and Function*, Fifth Edition, Williams & Wilkins, 2005

Kisner C, Colby L: *Therapeutic Exercise Foundations and Techniques*, Fifth Edition, FA Davis Company, 2007

Kloth LC, McCulloch JM: *Wound Healing: Alternatives in Management*, Third Edition, FA Davis Company, 2002

Kongstvedt P: *Managed Care: What it is and How it Works*, Jones & Bartlett Publishers, Third Edition, 2008

Konin J, Wiksten D, Isear J, Brader H: *Special Tests for Orthopedic Examination*, Third Edition, Slack Inc., 2006

Kornblau B, Starling S: *Ethics in Rehabilitation: A Clinical Perspective*, Slack Inc., 2000

Levangie P, Norkin C: *Joint Structure and Function: A Comprehensive Analysis*, Fourth Edition, FA Davis Company, 2005

Long T, Toscano K: *Handbook of Pediatric Physical Therapy*, Second Edition, Lippincott Williams & Wilkins, 2002

Lundy-Ekman L: *Neuroscience Fundamentals for Rehabilitation*, Third Edition, WB Saunders Company, 2007

Lusardi M, Nielsen C: *Orthotics and Prosthetics in Rehabilitation*, Elsevier Inc., 2007

Magee D: *Orthopedic Physical Assessment*, Fifth Edition, WB Saunders Company, 2007

Malone T, McPoil T, Nitz A: *Orthopedic and Sports Physical Therapy*, Third Edition, Mosby-Year Book, Inc., 1997

Meyers B: *Wound Management: Principles and Practice*, Second Edition, Prentice Hall, 2007

Michlovitz S: *Thermal Agents in Rehabilitation*, Fourth Edition, FA Davis Company, 2005

Miller-Keane; *Encyclopedia and Dictionary of Medicine, Nursing, and Allied Health*, Seventh Edition, WB Saunders Company, 2003

Minor M, Minor S: *Patient Care Skills*, Fifth Edition, Appleton & Lange, 2006

Montgomery P, Connolly B: *Clinical Applications for Motor Control*, Slack Inc., 2003

National Physical Therapy Examinations Candidate Handbook, Federation of State Boards of Physical Therapy, 2009

Nelson R, Hayes K, Currier D: *Clinical Electrotherapy*, Third Edition, Appleton & Lange, 1999

Norkin C, White D: *Measurement of Joint Motion: A Guide to Goniometry*, Third Edition, FA Davis Company, 2003

Nosse L, Friberg D: *Managerial and Supervisory Principles for Physical Therapists*, Third Edition, Lippincott Williams & Wilkins, 2009

Nurse's 3-Minute Clinical Reference, Second Edition, Lippincott Williams & Wilkins, 2007

O'Sullivan S, Schmitz T: *Physical Rehabilitation: Assessment and Treatment*, Fifth Edition, FA Davis Company, 2007

Pagliarulo M: *Introduction to Physical Therapy*, Third Edition, Mosby, 2006

Paz J, West MP: *Acute Care Handbook for Physical Therapists*, Third Edition, Saunders, 2008

Physical Therapist's Clinical Companion, Springhouse Corporation, 2000

Pierson F: *Principles and Techniques of Patient Care*, Fourth Edition, WB Saunders Company, 2008

Placzek J, Boyce D: **Orthopaedic Physical Therapy Secrets**, Second Edition, Hanley and Belfus, Inc., 2006

Portney L, Watkins M: **Foundations of Clinical Research: Applications to Practice**, Third Edition, Prentice Hall, 2008

Prentice W: **Therapeutic Modalities for Physical Therapists**, Third Edition, McGraw-Hill Inc., 2005

Prentice W, Voight M: **Techniques in Musculoskeletal Rehabilitation**, McGraw-Hill Inc., 2001

Purtilo R, Haddad A: **Health Professional and Patient Interaction**, Seventh Edition, WB Saunders Company, 2007

Quinn L, Gordon J: **Functional Outcomes: Documentation for Rehabilitation**, Elsevier Science, 2003

Ratliffe K: **Clinical Pediatric Physical Therapy: A Guide for the Physical Therapy Team**, Mosby, 1998

Reese N, Bandy WD: **Joint Range of Motion and Muscle Length Testing**, Second Edition, WB Saunders Company, 2009

Richard R, Staley M: **Burn Care and Rehabilitation: Principles and Practice**, FA Davis Company, 1994

Robinson A, Snyder-Mackler L: **Clinical Electrophysiology**, Third Edition, Williams & Wilkins, 2007

Rothstein J, Roy S, Wolf S: **The Rehabilitation Specialist's Handbook**, Third Edition, FA Davis Company, 2005

Ruoti RG, Morris DM: **Aquatic Rehabilitation**, Lippincott Williams & Wilkins, 1997

Sahrman S: **Diagnosis and Treatment of Movement Impairment Syndromes**, Mosby, 2002

Saidoff DC, McDonough AL: **Critical Pathways in Therapeutic Intervention: Extremities and Spine**, Mosby, 2002

Sandstrom RW, Lohman H, Bramble JD: **Health Services: Policy and Systems for Therapists**, Second Edition, Prentice Hall, 2008

Saunders H: **Evaluation, Treatment, and Prevention of Musculoskeletal Disorders**, The Saunders Group, 1993

Scott R: **Foundations of Physical Therapy: A 21st Century-Focused View of the Profession**, McGraw-Hill Inc., 2002

Scott R: **Promoting Legal and Ethical Awareness**, Mosby, 2009

Seymour R: **Prosthetics and Orthotics: Lower Limb and Spinal**, Lippincott Williams & Wilkins, 2002

Shamus E, Shamus J: **Sports Injury: Prevention & Rehabilitation**, McGraw-Hill Inc., 2001

Shamus E, Stern D: **Effective Documentation for the Physical Therapy Professional**, McGraw-Hill Inc., 2004

Shepard K, Jensen G: **Handbook of Teaching for Physical Therapists**, Second Edition, Butterworth-Heinemann, 2002

Shumway-Cook A, Woollacott M: **Motor Control: Translating Research into Clinical Practice**, Third Edition, Lippincott Williams & Wilkins, 2007

Sine R, Liss S: **Basic Rehabilitation Techniques: A Self Instructional Guide**, Fourth Edition, Aspen Publishers, 2000

Standards of Ethical Conduct for the Physical Therapist Assistant, American Physical Therapy Association, HOD S06-00-13-24

Starkey C, Ryan J: **Evaluation of Orthopedic and Athletic Injuries**, FA Davis Company, 2002

Stephenson R, O'Connor L: **Obstetric and Gynecologic Care in Physical Therapy**, Second Edition, Slack Incorporated, 2000

Sullivan P, Markos P: *Clinical Decision Making in Therapeutic Exercise*, Appleton & Lange, 1995

Sultz H: *Health Care USA: Understanding Its Organization and Delivery*, Sixth Edition, Aspen Publishers, 2008

Sussman C, Bates-Jensen B: *Wound Care: A Collaborative Practice Manual for Physical Therapists and Nurses*, Third Edition, Aspen Publishers, 2007

Tan JC: *Practical Manual of Physical Medicine and Rehabilitation*, Second Edition, Mosby, 2005

Tecklin J: *Pediatric Physical Therapy*, Fourth Edition, Lippincott Williams & Wilkins, 2007

Tierney L: *Current Medical Diagnosis and Treatment*, 48th Edition, Appleton & Lange, 2008

Triola M: *Elementary Statistics*, 10th Edition, Pearson Addison Wesley Publishing Company Inc., 2007

Trofino R: *Nursing Care of the Burn Injured Patient*, FA Davis Company, 1991

Umphred D: *Neurological Rehabilitation*, Fifth Edition, Mosby, 2006

Van Deusen J: *Assessment in Occupational and Physical Therapy*, WB Saunders Company, 1997

Waxman S, deGroot J: *Correlative Neuroanatomy*, Appleton & Lange, 1995

PTEXAM: On-Campus Review Course

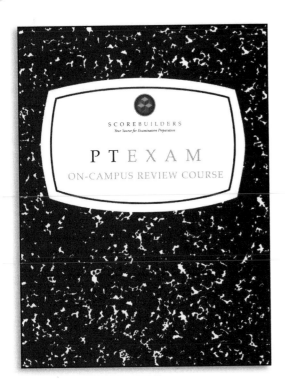

PTEXAM: Online Advantage

How Do You Measure Up Against the Competition?

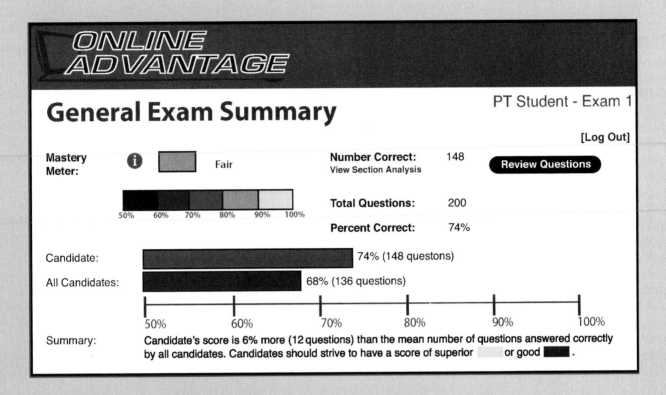

PT Student - Exam 1

General Exam Summary

[Log Out]

Mastery Meter: Fair

50% 60% 70% 80% 90% 100%

Number Correct: 148
View Section Analysis

Review Questions

Total Questions: 200

Percent Correct: 74%

Candidate: 74% (148 questons)

All Candidates: 68% (136 questions)

50% 60% 70% 80% 90% 100%

Summary: Candidate's score is 6% more (12 questions) than the mean number of questions answered correctly by all candidates. Candidates should strive to have a score of superior ▢ or good ▬ .

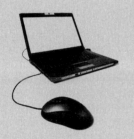

PTEXAM: Online Advantage

Price: $40.00 per examination or $60.00 for two exams each with 30 day access. Order directly online at **www.scorebuilders.com**

Visit our Online Advantage flash presentation at:
www.scorebuilders.com/oademo/

SCOREBUILDERS

P.O. Box 7242 • Scarborough, ME 04070-7242

Phone: 207-885-0304 • Toll Free: 866-PTEXAMS • Fax: 207-883-8377

WWW.SCOREBUILDERS.COM

TITLE

AN EVALUATION OF THE USEFULNESS OF A COMPREHENSIVE EXAMINATION AS A PREDICTOR OF SCORE ON THE NATIONAL PHYSICAL THERAPY EXAMINATION

AUTHORS

Giles, Scott M.[1]; Wetherbee, Ellen[2]

INSTITUTIONS

1. Department of Physical Therapy, University of New England, Portland, ME, USA.

2. Department of Physical Therapy, University of Hartford, West Hartford, CT, USA

ABSTRACT

Purpose/Hypothesis: Academic programs use a variety of methods to assist students with their preparation for the National Physical Therapy Examination (NPTE) including comprehensive examinations (CE). Previous research has suggested that CE scores can be used to predict NPTE scores, however, the studies have utilized data from only a single academic program and have used CEs developed by the program's academic faculty. The purpose of the study is to determine if there is a relationship between scores on a commercially available CE (PTEXAM: Online Advantage) and scores on the NPTE.

Number of Subjects: Academic programs using a CE product, PTEXAM: Online Advantage, in 2005-2006 were invited to participate in the research study.

Materials/Methods: Program chairs completed a survey describing how they administered the CE. Additionally, chairs provided data which anonymously compared students' CE scores and their associated scale scores on the NPTE. Descriptive statistics were used to analyze how the CE was administered. Regression analysis was used to identify a correlation coefficient between scores on the CE and scores on the NPTE; and to determine an individual's minimum CE score in order to obtain a NPTE scale score of 600 (i.e., minimum passing score) or greater with 95% confidence. The research study was approved by the University of New England Institutional Review Board.

Results: A geographically diverse sample of 12 physical therapist academic programs representing 332 students participated in the study. Ten (83.3%) of the academic programs offered the CE between 0-3 months before graduation and 11 (91.7%) administered the CE in a computer classroom. Nine (75%) of the academic programs encouraged students to prepare in advance and 8 (66.7%) established a minimum score for the CE. Minimum scores were established based on a variety of methods. A correlation coefficient of .674 was computed when comparing individual CE scores to individual NPTE scores. Linear regression was used to determine that a student who scores 144 (72.0%) on the CE has a 95% chance to score 600 or greater on the NPTE. There were no significant differences in the CE scores of students who were encouraged to prepare in advance or those whose academic programs required a minimum score.

Conclusions: Score on the CE using PTEXAM: Online Advantage was strongly correlated with score on the NPTE. The strength of the correlation suggests predictive validity of the CE and supports the use of CEs in physical therapist academic programs.

Clinical Relevance: A CE that is positively correlated with results on the NPTE may assist educators in identifying physical therapy students at risk for performing poorly on the NPTE. Early identification of "at risk" students has the potential to improve outcomes for academic programs and allow graduates to make more informed decisions on their readiness to take the actual examination.

Keywords: National Physical Therapist Examination, Comprehensive Examination.

*Abstract submitted and accepted for 2008 APTA Combined Sections Meeting in Nashville, Tennessee

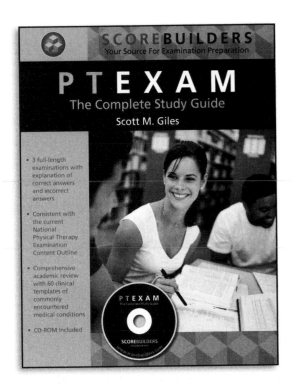
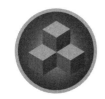

Using the PTEXAM CD-ROM

Please Read Before Installing PTEXAM: The Complete Study Guide CD-ROM

PTEXAM: The Complete Study Guide is optimized for the latest versions of Microsoft software. In order to take advantage of ***PTEXAM: The Complete Study Guide's*** enhanced performance, the Microsoft Setup Wizard may need to update some system files on your computer. If you are installing ***PTEXAM: The Complete Study Guide*** on a computer that requires updated system files, please follow installation step 3, which will quickly guide you through the update process. If your computer does not require updated system files, you will skip step 3.

Our software is compatible with the Windows operating system only (note: it is compatible with Intel-based Macs running Windows through Apple Boot Camp, Parallels Desktop, or VMware Fusion).

Installing PTEXAM: The Complete Study Guide CD-ROM

1. Close any applications you may be running.
2. Insert CD and the Windows auto-install program will automatically begin.
3. If the "Setup cannot continue because some system files are out of date on your system…" message appears, click the Yes button. If this message does not appear, continue to step 4. After clicking the Yes button you will be prompted to restart the computer. Repeat previous steps and then continue with step 4 once the computer restarts.
4. When the "**PTEXAM: The Complete Study Guide Setup**" dialog box appears, click the OK button.
5. When the next Setup dialog box appears, click the computer icon button.
6. When the Choose Program Group dialog box appears, click the Continue button.
7. If the "Version Conflict" message appears, click the Yes button. If this message does not appear, continue to step 8.
8. When the "setup completed successfully" dialog appears, click the OK button to end the installation process.

Starting PTEXAM: The Complete Study Guide CD-ROM

Click Start → All Programs → PTEXAM – The Complete Study Guide → Examination,

For any technical issues encountered while installing or using ***PTEXAM: The Complete Study Guide*** please visit us at **www.scorebuilders.com** and click on the "contact us" section for further assistance and problem solving.

SCOREBUILDERS

P.O. Box 7242 • Scarborough, ME 04070-7242
Phone: 207-885-0304 • Toll Free: 866-PTEXAMS • Fax: 207-883-8377
WWW.SCOREBUILDERS.COM